NCLEX-RN®
Questions & Answers

made
Incredibly
Easy!®

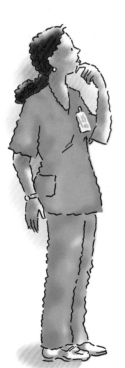

Seventh Edition

Clinical Editor
Susan Lisko, DNP, RN, CNE
Associate Professor of Nursing
Youngstown State University
Youngstown, Ohio

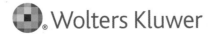
®. Wolters Kluwer

Philadelphia · Baltimore · New York · London
Buenos Aires · Hong Kong · Sydney · Tokyo

Senior Digital Product Manager, NCLEX: Renee A. Gagliardi
Associate Content Strategist: Dawn Lagrosa
Marketing Manager: Sarah Schuessler
Production Project Manager: Priscilla Crater
Design Coordinator: Elaine Kasmer
Manufacturing Coordinator: Kathleen Brown
Copyeditor: Dan Kraner
Prepress Vendor: SPi Global

Seventh Edition

Copyright © 2017 Wolters Kluwer

9 8 7 6 5 4 3 2 1

Printed in China

Library of Congress Cataloging-in-Publication Data
Names: Lisko, Susan, editor.
Title: NCLEX-RN questions & answers made incredibly easy! / clinical editor, Susan Lisko.
Other titles: NCLEX-RN questions and answers made incredibly easy!
Description: Seventh edition. | Philadelphia : Wolters Kluwer, [2017]
Identifiers: LCCN 2016008680 | ISBN 9781496325495
Subjects: | MESH: Nursing Care | Nursing | Examination Questions
Classification: LCC RT55 | NLM WY 18.2 | DDC 610.73076—dc23 LC record available at http://lccn.loc.gov/2016008680

LWW.com

Contents

About the Editor

Dr. Susan Lisko is an established nurse educator and NCLEX instructor with a passion for nursing. She earned a diploma in Nursing from St. Elizabeth Hospital Medical Center in Youngstown, Ohio, and then a BSN in Nursing from Youngstown State University, an MSN with a specialty in Nursing Education from Gannon University, and a Doctorate of Nursing Practice (DNP) from The Frances Payne Bolton School of Nursing, Case Western Reserve University. Most recently, she achieved certification as a Nurse Educator (CNE) from the National League for Nursing. The certification recognizes *excellence in the advanced specialty role of the academic nurse educator*. Dr. Lisko's awards for recognition 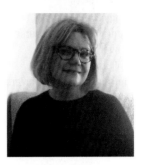 of expertise and contribution to nursing education include being named a 2011 Distinguished Professor of Teaching at Youngstown State University and Educator of the Year in Ohio. Throughout her career, she has published in refereed journals and in textbooks, and she has presented her scholarly research at nursing conferences throughout the country. She continues to teach at the undergraduate and graduate level, and she travels throughout the country teaching NCLEX-RN review courses. This is her second edition as Clinical Editor of this text.

Contributors

Peggy Baikie, DNP, RN, PNP-BC, NNP-BC
Program Manager/Nurse Practitioner
Denver Health
Affiliate Professor
Metropolitan State University of Denver
Denver, Colorado

Samantha H. Bishop, MN, RN, CPNP, CNE
Associate Professor of Nursing
Gordon State College School of Nursing and Health Sciences
Barnesville, Georgia

Linda Carman Copel, PhD, RN, PMHCNS, BC,CNE, ANEF, NCC, FAPA
Professor
College of Nursing
Villanova University
Villanova, Pennsylvania

Nancy Danou, MSN, RN
Instructor
Viterbo University
La Crosse, Wisconsin

Kelly L. Davis, MSN, RN, CNE
Instructor, Nursing Department
Delaware Technical and Community College—Owens
    Campus
Georgetown, Delaware

Jeff Dyck, BA, BSN, MSN
Faculty
British Columbia Institute of Technology School of
    Health Sciences
Burnaby, British Columbia, Canada

Don Laurino, MSN, CCRN, CMSRN, PHN, RN-BC
Instructor, VN (RN)
American Career College at St. Francis
Lynwood, California

Kathleen Lehmann, RN-BC, EdS, MEd, BSN, BA
Charge Nurse
Edith Nourse Rogers Memorial Veterans Hospital
Bedford, Massachusetts

J. Mari Beth Linder, PhD, RN, BC
Professor of Nursing
Department of Nursing
Missouri Southern State University
Joplin, Missouri

Karen Montalto, PhD, MSN, RN
Assistant Dean I, Director/Office of Nursing Student
    Success
Rutgers School of Nursing, Camden
Camden, New Jersey

Amanda C. Reichert, RN, MSN
Instructor of Nursing
Georgia Gwinnett College
Lawrenceville, Georgia

Nan Riedé, RN, MSN, CPN
Assistant Professor
Baptist College of Health Sciences
Memphis, Tennessee

Susan Rouse, PhD, RN
Assistant Professor
Indiana University Northwest
School of Nursing
Gary, Indiana

Mary L. Terwilliger, PhD, RN
Assistant Professor, Nursing
Clarion University of Pennsylvania
Clarion, Pennsylvania

Becky Ann Theil, DNP, RN, CNE
Acting Associate Provost
Shawnee State University
Portsmouth, Ohio

Susan K. Tucker, RN, MSN, DNP, CNE
Program Director, Nursing Education
Gadsden State Community College
Gadsden, Alabama

Linda Turchin, MSN
Assistant Professor of Nursing
Fairmont State University
Fairmont, West Virginia

Geri Tyrell, MSN, RN, CNE
Assistant Professor and Director
Department of Nursing
Bethel College
North Newton, Kansas

Lorna Walsh, BN, MEd, RN
Faculty
Year 1 and 2 Coordinator
BN (Collaborative) Program
Centre for Nursing Studies
St. John's, Newfoundland, Canada

Patricia Zrelak, RN, PhD, NEA-BC, CNRN
Nurse Researcher
University of California, Davis
Davis, California

Faculty

Janet Alexander, EdD, MSN, RN, CNE
Georgia Highlands College
Rome, Georgia

Lisa Alexander, MSN, RN, CS, NP
Georgia Perimeter College
Clarkston, Georgia

Danielle Artis, MSN, PNCB
Trinity Washington University
Washington, District of Columbia

Monique Bacher, RN, BScN, MSN(Ed)
George Brown College
Toronto, Ontario, Canada

Erin Bailey, DNP, RN, FNP-C
Stephen F. Austin State
   University
Nacogdoches, Texas

Lisette Barton, PhD, RN, FNP-BC, CNE
University of Houston
Sugar Land, Texas

Mary Beerman, MSN
Georgia Baptist School of Nursing
   at Mercer University
Atlanta, Georgia

Lyndele Bernard, BSN, MSN
Anne Arundel Community College
Arnold, Maryland

Samantha H. Bishop, MN, RN, CPNP,
   CNE
Gordon State College
Barnesville, Georgia

Mary Bjorklund, MSN, RN, CPN
Lone Star College at Kingwood
Houston, Texas

Wendy Blakely, PhD, RN
Capital University
Columbus, Ohio

Catherine Bock, RN, BSc, MAED
Kwantlen Polytechnic University
Surrey, British Columbia, Canada

Phil Bourget, RN, BA, BScN, MN
Georgian College
Barrie, Ontario, Canada

Cheryl Brady, RN, MSN, CNE
Kent State University
Salem, Ohio

Melissa Britt, RN, MSN
Robeson Community College
Lumberton, North Carolina

Daryle L. Brown, EdD, RN
Western Connecticut State
   University
Danbury, Connecticut

Robyn B. Caldwell, DNP, FNP-BC, CNE
Troy University—Montgomery
Montgomery, Alabama

Andrea Chute, RN, MN
MacEwan University
Edmonton, Alberta, Canada

Marcia Cook-Love, MSN, RN,
   PMHCNS-BC, FNP, CNE
Reading Hospital and Medical Center
West Reading, Pennsylvania

Cheryl Cummings, MSN
University of Saskatchewan
Saskatoon, Saskatchewan, Canada

Kelly Davis, MSN, RN, CNE
Delaware Technical Community
   College
Georgetown, Delaware

Fernande E. Deno, MSN, RN, CNE
Anoka-Ramsey Community College
Coon Rapids, Minnesota

Martie Dobbs, RN, BScN, MScN
University of Calgary
Calgary, Alberta, Canada

Andrea Doctor-Tyler, RN, MSN, CCRC,
   CCRC
University of the District of
   Columbia Community College
Washington, District of Columbia

Louise Dyjur, RN, BScN, MN, PhD
Red Deer College
Red Deer, Alberta, Canada

Jennifer Ellis, DNP, MSN, RN
University of Cincinnati Blue Ash
   College
Cincinnati, Ohio

Kathryn Ellis, RN, BScN, MA(Ed)
Centennial and George Brown
   Collaborative Nursing Degree
   Program
Toronto, Ontario, Canada

Sally Erdel, MS, RN, CNE
Bethel College
Mishawaka, Indiana

Michele Faxel, EdD, MS, RN
Samuel Merritt University
Oakland, California

Karen Ferguson, PhD, RNC, FNE
Martin Methodist College
Pulaski, Tennessee

Pasquale Fiore, MSc Health Adm,
   BScN, Cert. Ed, RN
British Columbia Institute of
   Technology School of Health
   Sciences
Vancouver, British Columbia,
   Canada

Nancy Fleming, RN, HBSCN, MAEd
Confederation College
Thunder Bay, Ontario, Canada

Jessica Flores, RN, BSN
Arizona State University
Tempe, Arizona

Sonya Franklin, RN, EdD/CI, MHA, MSN,
   BSN, AS, ADN
Cleveland State Community College
Cleveland, Tennessee

Louise S. Frantz, MHA, Ed, BSN, RN
Penn State University
Reading, Pennsylvania

Kathy Fukuyama, RN, BSN, MEd, EdD
Vancouver Community College
Vancouver, British Columbia, Canada

Karen E. Furlong, RN, MN, PhD
University of New Brunswick
Saint John, New Brunswick,
   Canada

Kimbra Gabhart, MSN
Elizabethtown Community and
   Technical College
Elizabethtown, Kentucky

Susan Golden, MSN, RN
Eastern New Mexico University—
  Roswell
Roswell, New Mexico

Lois Gotes, MSN, RN, APRN-CNP
Carl Albert State College
Poteau, Oklahoma

Sandy Gustafson, MA, RN, CNE
Hibbing Community College
Hibbing, Minnesota

Mona Haimour, RN, BScN, MSN, MPH(c)
MacEwan University
Edmonton, Alberta, Canada

Kathy Haley, MSN
Northwest Community College
Terrace, British Columbia, Canada

Carol Haus, RN, PhD, CNE
West Penn Hospital School of
  Nursing
Pittsburgh, Pennsylvania

Mindy Herrin, PhD(c), RN
Lakeview College of Nursing
Danville, Illinois

Barbara A. Hoglund, EdD, FNP-BC, CNE
Bethel University
St. Paul, Minnesota

Heidi Holmes, RN, MScN, GNC
Conestoga College
Kitchener, Ontario, Canada

Carole L. Hoveland, MS, RN
Sheridan College
Sheridan, Wyoming

Katherine Howard, MS, RN-BC, CNE
Middlesex County College—
  Raritan Bay Medical Center
Edison, New Jersey

Eleanor Hrabowych, RN, BN, MEd
University of Manitoba
Winnipeg, Manitoba, Canada

Roxanne Hurley, RN, MS
University of North Dakota
Grand Forks, North Dakota

Mohamed El Hussein, RN, BSN, MSN,
  PhD
Mount Royal University
Calgary, Alberta, Canada

Lenetra Jefferson, PhD, RN, CNE, LMT
Jefferson Parish Human Services
  Authority
New Orleans, Louisiana

Marian Yavorka Jobe, RN, MSN, MS
University of Pittsburgh Medical
  Center—Shadyside
Pittsburgh, Pennsylvania

Marlene Johnson, MSN/Ed, BSN, RN,
  HCRM
Concorde Career Institute
Miramar, Florida

Laly Joseph, DVM, DNP, MSN, ARNP,
  ANP, BC
University of Miami
Coral Gables, Florida

Eileen Kane, RN
UMass Memorial Medical Center
Anna Maria College
Paxton, Massachusetts

Angela Koller, DNP, MSN, RN
Ivy Tech Community College—
  Central Indiana
Indianapolis, Indiana

Christine L. Krause, MSN, CPNP
Aria School of Nursing
Penn State Abington
Trevose, Pennsylvania

Karen E. Kulhanek, RN, BSN, MEd,
  MSN
Kellogg Community College
Battle Creek, Michigan

Joanne Lavin, RN, EdD
City University of New York School
  of Professional Studies
New York, New York

Dana Law-Ham, PhD, RN, FNP, CNE
Central Maine Medical Center
  College of Nursing and Health
  Professions
Lewiston, Maine

Chrystal Lewis, MSN, PhD
University of Alabama
Tuscaloosa, Alabama

J. Mari Beth Linder, PhD, RN, BC
Missouri Southern State University
Joplin, Missouri

Christa Maclean, RN, BScN, MN
Saskatchewan Polytechnic
Regina, Saskatchewan, Canada

April Magoteaux, PhD, RN, CNS, NHA
Columbus State Community
  College
Columbus, Ohio

Tatayana Maltseva, MSN, ARNP,
  PMHNP-BC
Florida International University
North Miami, Florida

Andrea R. Mann, MSN, RN, CNE
Aria Health School of Nursing
Trevose, Pennsylvania

Maria A. Marconi, EdD, RN, CNE
University of Rochester
Rochester, New York

Kelly A. Martin, MS, RN, CNE
Colorado Northwestern
  Community College
Craig, Colorado

Cherie McCann, MSN, RN, BC, CPN
Armstrong State University
Savannah, Georgia

Melanie McClure, MSN, APRN, FNP-
  BC
University of St. Mary
Leavenworth, Kansas

Belle McGinty, MEd, RN, BSN
Brunswick Community College
Bolivia, North Carolina

Lisa Anne McKendrick, BScN, MN,
  RN
MacEwan University
Edmonton, Alberta, Canada

Janis McMillan, RN, MSN
Coconino Community College
Flagstaff, Arizona

Sybil Morgan, RN, BScN, MN
Saskatchewan Polytechnic
University of Regina
Saskatoon, Saskatchewan,
  Canada

Becky Murck, MSN, FNP-C
University of North Georgia
Dahlonega, Georgia

Michelle M. Murphy-Rozanski,
  PhD, MSN, RN, CRNP
Temple University Health System
Philadelphia, Pennsylvania

Catherine Myerholtz, MSN
The Medical College of Ohio
Chillicothe, Ohio

Audrey E. Nelson, PhD, RN
University of Nebraska Medical
  Center
Omaha, Nebraska

Mary Nifong, MSN, RN, CNE
Pikes Peak Community College
Colorado Springs, Colorado

Nancy Noble, MSN, RN, CNE
Marian University
Fond du Lac, Wisconsin

Tommie Norris, DNS, RN
University of Tennessee Health
   Science Center
Memphis, Tennessee

LaDonna Northington, DNS, RN, BC
University of Mississippi
Jackson, Mississippi

Sherry Obert, MSN, RN, NE-BC
Allegany College of Maryland at
   the Bedford County Campus
Everett, Pennsylvania

Sandra Olanitori, MS, RN
Norfolk State University
Norfolk, Virginia

Luella Orr, RN, BScN, MEd
Seneca College of Applied Arts
   and Technology
King City, Ontario, Canada

Rebecca Otten, EdD, RN
California State University—
   Fullerton
Fullerton, California

Diana Paladino, MSN, RN
Carlow University
Pittsburgh, Pennsylvania

Stephanie Palmersheim, MSN, RN
St. Luke's College
Sioux City, Iowa

Sudha C. Patel, BSN, MN, MA, DNS, RN
University of Louisiana at Lafayette
Lafayette, Louisiana

J. David (Dave) Patterson, RN, BN
University of Calgary
Calgary, Alberta, Canada

Lisa Peden, RN, MSN
Dalton State College
Dalton, Georgia

Sandra Pettit, RN, BScN, MVoc/Tech Ed
Saskatchewan Polytechnic
Regina, Saskatchewan, Canada

Judith T. Pfriemer, RN, MSN
Arkansas State University—
   Jonesboro
Jonesboro, Arkansas

Carswella Phillips, DNP, MSN, ARNP,
   AGPCNP-BC
Florida A&M University
Tallahassee, Florida

Tawna Pounders, BSN, MNSc
Baton Rouge Community
   College
Baton Rouge, Louisiana

Anne Purvis, RN, BSN, MEd, MSN, EdD,
   CNE
Gordon State College
Barnesville, Georgia

Nola Ragan, MSN
Sisseton Wahpeton Community
   College
Sisseton, South Dakota

Marisue Rayno, EdD, RN
Luzerne County Community
   College
Nanticoke, Pennsylvania

Janice Reilley, EdD, MSN, RN-BC
Immaculata University
Malvern, Pennsylvania

Montra Reinhardt, MSN, RN
Ivy Tech Community College
Bloomington, Indiana

Wendy J. Waldspurger Robb, PhD,
   RN, CNE
Cedar Crest College
Allentown, Pennsylvania

Carol Rodi, ASN, BSN, MSN
J. Sargeant Reynolds Community
   College
Richmond, Virginia

Julie Ross, MSN, RN
Wilkes-Barre Area Career &
   Technical Center
Wilkes-Barre, Pennsylvania

Beverly Rowe, RN, MSN, CNE
College of Coastal Georgia
Brunswick, Georgia

John E. Scarbrough, PhD, PT, RN, CNE
New Mexico State University
Las Cruces, New Mexico

Gwen Schmidt, BA
Bow Valley College
Calgary, Alberta, Canada

Charlotte Schober, MSN
Union College
Lincoln, Nebraska

Jean Schroeder, PhD, RN
The School of Nursing at Platt
   College
Aurora, Colorado

Camden Seal, MSN-Ed, RN
Hondros College
Columbus, Ohio

Susan Seiboldt, MSN, RN, CNE
Carl Sandburg College
Galesburg, Illinois

Carla Shapiro, RN, MN
University of Manitoba
Winnipeg, Manitoba, Canada

Vanessa Sheane, MN, RN
Grande Prairie Regional College
Grande Prairie, Alberta, Canada

Joy Shewchuk, RN, MSN
Humber College
Toronto, Ontario, Canada

Corey Sigurdson, MN, RN
Red River College
Winnipeg, Manitoba, Canada

Charla Smith, MSN, RN, CPN, CNE
Jackson State Community College
Jackson, Tennessee

Lisa B. Soontupe, EdD, RN, CNE
Nova Southeastern University
Fort Lauderdale, Florida

Laura Steadman, EdD, MSN, CRNP, RN
University of Alabama
Birmingham, Alabama

Margaret Swedish, BScN Nursing
MacEwan University
Edmonton, Alberta

Laurel R. Talabere, PhD, RN, AE-C
Capital University
Columbus, Ohio

Mary Tennies-Moseley, EdD, MN, BSN
Northern Virginia Community
   College
Annandale, Virginia

Landa Terblanche, PhD, RN
Trinity Western University
Langley, British Columbia,
   Canada

Nadia Torresan-Doodnaught, BScN,
   RNC, MN
Seneca College of Applied Arts
   and Technology
King City, Ontario, Canada

Bonny Townsend, RN, MSN
Grande Prairie Regional College
Grande Prairie, Alberta, Canada

Susan K. Tucker, DNP, RN, CNE
Gadsden State Community College
Gadsden, Alabama

Theresa Turick-Gibson, MSN
Hartwick College
Oneonta, New York

Bev Valkenier, MSN
University of British Columbia
Vancouver, British Columbia,
    Canada

Mary Anne Vanos, RN, BScN, MScN
Sheridan College
Brampton, Ontario, Canada

Stephen VanSlyke, RN, MN
University of New Brunswick
Fredericton, New Brunswick, Canada

Teresa Villaran, CNE, CCRN, APRN-BC
Berea College
Berea, Kentucky

Judy Voss, RN, MSN
The University of Texas Rio Grande
    Valley
Edinburg, Texas

Denacy Walker, MSN, ARNP, CNE
Miami Dade College
Miami, Florida

Gerry Walker, DHEd, MSN, RN
Park University
Parkville, Missouri

Judy Walloch, EdD, RN, CNE
Graham Hospital School of
    Nursing
Canton, Illinois

Lorna Walsh, BN, MEd, RN
Centre for Nursing Studies
St. John's, Newfoundland and
    Labrador

Michele A. Walters, DNP, APRN, FNP-
    BC, CNE
Morehead State University St.
    Claire Regional Medical Center
Morehead, Kentucky

Diane E. White, RN, PhD, CCRN
Georgia Gwinnett College
Lawrenceville, Georgia

Donna Wilsker, MSN, RN
Lamar University
Beaumont, Texas

Mary Williams, MS, RN
Gordon State College
Barnesville, Georgia

Karla Wolsky, PhD, RN
Lethbridge Community College
Lethbridge, Alberta, Canada

Jean Yockey, FNP-BC, CNE
University of South Dakota
Vermillion, South Dakota

Students

Jamie Everhart, RN
Saint Luke's Hospital
Kansas City, Missouri

Danielle Glover, RN-BSN
Pitman Manor, United Methodist
    Homes
Pitman, New Jersey

Chelsea Roberts, MSN, RN, CNL
The Christ Hospital Health
    Network
Cincinnati, Ohio

Emily Tang, BSN
Vanderbilt School of Nursing
Nashville, Tennessee

Erin L. Umberger, BSN, RN, ONS
Hefner VA Medical Center
Salisbury, North Carolina

Megan Vallance, BSN
University of Kentucky
Lexington, Kentucky

Julie Yoshioka, RN
University of Portland
Portland, Oregon

Preface

As a Nurse Educator for more than 30 years, my goal has been to encourage students to aspire to be the best nurse possible. To achieve that goal, many hours of instruction have been dedicated to providing students with a strong foundation of core concepts. Lectures, quizzes, theory examinations, case studies, clinical experiences, and simulations prepare them to complete the final phase of the educational process: passing the NCLEX® licensure exam.

If you, like so many students, reach the final phase and are in search of a resource to guide your preparation for success on the NCLEX, the seventh edition of *NCLEX–RN Questions & Answers Made Incredibly Easy!* has been developed to assist you in achieving that goal. This book provides you with more than 6,500 exemplary questions and answers designed to help you discover those areas in which you are strong and those areas in which some degree of review might be in order.

You will find questions written at the Apply and Analyze levels, reflecting the 2016 NCLEX-RN test plan, and including multiple-choice items and alternate-format items: multiple-response, multiple-choice (select all that apply); ordered response (drag and drop); hot spot; exhibit/chart; fill-in-the-blank with a calculation; graphic option; and audio (online). Each answer includes not only the rationale for the correct and incorrect responses but also information as to which aspects of nursing are being evaluated by that question. Thus, you will discover which parts of the nursing process are more problematic for you and which client needs categories are most challenging for you. Knowing this can help you focus on the further review needed for you to be successful.

Remember knowledge is power! To be successful on the NCLEX exam, plan your time, think positive, and practice, practice, practice! I wish you NCLEX SUCCESS.

—Susan Lisko, DNP, RN, CNE

NCLEX–RN Questions & Answers Made Incredibly Easy! will improve your knowledge while building your ability to apply that knowledge to real nursing scenarios. It also will strengthen your preparation for your licensure experience. Let's cut right to the chase! Here's how:

1. It will teach you all the important things you need to know about preparing for and passing the NCLEX. (And it will leave out all the fluff that wastes your time.)
2. It will direct your eye to the alternate-format questions.
3. It will help you remember what you've learned.
4. It will make you smile as it enhances your knowledge and skills.

Don't believe it? Try these features on for size:

- Reliable NCLEX preparation guidelines and hundreds of test-taking hints and strategies
- 3,500 NCLEX-style questions within the book itself to test your knowledge in all areas tested on the real examination
- Two-column format with questions on the left and answers and rationales on the right
- Book mark for you to hide the answers while reading the question
- Red font for alternate-format questions, and full color photographs and illustrations for graphic and hot spot questions
- Easy-to-use reference tables and charts for measurements, laboratory values, and heart and breath sounds
- Accompanying Web site with 3,000 additional questions in an interactive format—including graphic, ordered response, and audio questions

Plus, check out these updates:

- Alignment of all information with the 2016 NCLEX-RN test plan and NCSBN standards
- Full four-color design and art program integrated throughout
- Thorough content revision based on feedback from more than 100 nursing faculty and recent graduates across Canada and the United States to ensure the most up-to-date practices, highest quality questions, and appropriateness of content for review by students of both countries

- Revamping of all psychiatric nursing content for consistency with parameters of the *Diagnostic and Statistical Manual of Mental Disorders*, Fifth Edition (*DSM-5*)
- Appendices of commonly used metric abbreviations and English-to-metric conversions; normal adult and pediatric laboratory values; Erikson's stages of psychosocial development; sites for cardiac auscultation, posterior chest breath auscultation, and anterior chest breath palpation, percussion, and auscultation
- Free 7-day trial of *Lippincott NCLEX-RN PassPoint*

Plus, look for Joy, Jake, and friends in the margins throughout this book. As always, they will be there to explain key concepts, provide important hints, and offer reassurance. And, if you don't mind, we'll be spicing up the pages with a bit of humor along the way, to teach and entertain in a way that no other resource can.

Part I

Surviving the NCLEX®

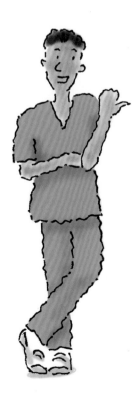

Chapter 1

Preparing for the NCLEX®

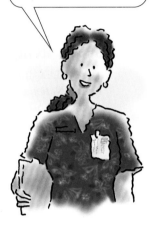

Understanding the NCLEX goals and structure is an important first step in proper preparation for the test. This chapter explains how best to prepare for this important examination.

Just the facts

In this chapter, you'll learn:
- ◆ about the NCLEX® and why you must take it
- ◆ what you need to know about taking the NCLEX by computer
- ◆ how to recognize and answer alternate-format questions
- ◆ strategies to use when answering NCLEX questions
- ◆ how to avoid common mistakes when taking the NCLEX.

Passing the National Council Licensure Examination (NCLEX®) is an important landmark in your career as a nurse. The first step on your way to passing the NCLEX is to understand what it is and how it's administered.

NCLEX® structure

The NCLEX is a test written by nurses who, like most of your nursing instructors, have an advanced degree and clinical expertise in a particular area. Only one small difference distinguishes nurses who write NCLEX questions: They're trained to write questions in the style you will see on the NCLEX.

If you've completed an accredited nursing program, you've already taken numerous tests written by nurses with backgrounds and experiences similar to those of the nurses who write for the NCLEX. The test-taking experience you've already gained will help you pass the NCLEX. So your NCLEX review should be just that—a review.

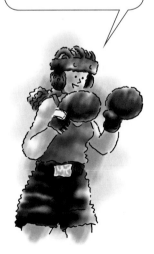

All your experience with testing means you're ready to do battle with this exam!

What's the point of it all?

The NCLEX is designed for one purpose: to determine whether it's appropriate for you to receive a license to practice as a nurse. By passing the NCLEX, you demonstrate that you possess the minimum level of knowledge necessary to practice nursing safely.

Studying abroad

If you completed your nursing education outside of the country in which you wish to practice, you must follow certain guidelines to be eligible to work as a registered nurse in the United States or Canada. To work in the United States you may need to obtain a certificate and credentials evaluation from the Commission on Graduates of Foreign Nursing Schools (CGFNS®, www.cgfns.org) and acquire a visa. To work in Canada, you may need to obtain registration/licensure to practice from the National Nursing Assessment Service (NNAS, www.nnas.ca).

Remember, the NCLEX is part of the nursing regulatory licensure/registration process. Site-specific policies are determined by the regulatory body or board of nursing in the jurisdiction in which you wish to practice.

Mix 'em up

In nursing school, you probably took courses that were separated into such subjects as pharmacology; nursing leadership; health assessment; adult health; and pediatric, maternal-neonatal, and psychiatric nursing. In contrast, the NCLEX is integrated, meaning that different subjects are mixed together.

As you answer NCLEX questions, you may encounter patients in any stage of life, from neonatal to geriatric. These patients—clients, in NCLEX terminology—may be of any background, and may be completely well or extremely ill, and may have any of a variety of disorders.

Client needs, front and center

The NCLEX draws questions from four categories of client needs that were developed by the *National Council of State Boards of Nursing* (NCSBN), the organization that sponsors and manages the NCLEX. *Client needs categories* ensure that a wide variety of topics appear on every NCLEX examination.

The NCSBN developed client needs categories after conducting a practice analysis of new nurses. All aspects of nursing care observed in the study were broken down into four main categories, some of which were broken down further into subcategories. (See *Client needs categories*, below.)

Remember, the NCLEX determines if you are able to give safe and effective care. By testing you across the client needs, the NCLEX will know you can practice safely in the setting of your choice.

What's the plan?

The categories and subcategories are used to develop the *NCLEX test plan*, the content guidelines for the distribution of test questions. Question writers and the people who put the NCLEX together use the test plan and client needs categories to make sure that a full spectrum of nursing activities is covered in the NCLEX. Client needs categories appear in most NCLEX review and question-and-answer books, including this one. As a test-taker, you don't have to concern yourself with client needs categories. You'll see those categories for each question and answer in this book, but they'll be invisible on the actual NCLEX.

Client needs categories

Each question on the NCLEX is assigned a category based on client needs. This chart lists client needs categories and subcategories and the percentages of each type of question that appears on an NCLEX examination.

Category	Subcategories	Percentage of NCLEX questions
Safe, effective care environment	• Management of care	17% to 23%
	• Safety and infection control	9% to 15%
Health promotion and maintenance		6% to 12%
Psychosocial integrity		6% to 12%
Physiological integrity	• Basic care and comfort	6% to 12%
	• Pharmacological and parenteral therapies	12% to 18%
	• Reduction of risk potential	9% to 15%
	• Physiological adaptation	11% to 17%

Testing by computer

Like most standardized tests today, the NCLEX is administered by computer. It is helpful to be familiar with taking tests on computers but, fortunately, the skills required to take the NCLEX on a computer are simple enough to allow you to focus on the questions, not the keyboard.

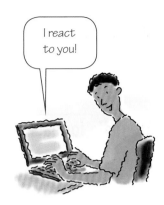

I react to you!

Feeling smart? Think hard!

The NCLEX is a *computer-adaptive test*, meaning that the computer reacts to the answers you give, supplying more difficult questions if you answer correctly and slightly easier questions if you answer incorrectly. Each test is thus uniquely adapted to the individual test-taker.

A matter of time

You have a great deal of flexibility with the amount of time you spend on individual questions. The examination lasts a maximum of 6 hours, however, so don't waste time. If you fail to answer a set number of questions within 6 hours, the computer will use the last 60 questions you answered to determine if you pass.

Most students have plenty of time to complete the test, so take as much time as you need to get the question right without wasting time. Keep moving at a decent pace to help maintain concentration.

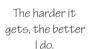

The harder it gets, the better I do.

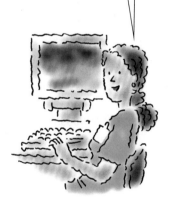

Difficult items = Good news

If you find as you progress through the test that the questions seem to be increasingly difficult, it's a good sign. The more questions you answer correctly, the more difficult the questions become.

Some students, though, knowing that questions get progressively harder, focus on the degree of difficulty of subsequent questions to try to figure out if they're answering questions correctly. Avoid the temptation to do this, as this may get you off track.

The finish line

The computer test finishes when one of these events occurs:
- You have demonstrated minimum competency, according to the computer program, which does so with 95% certainty that your ability exceeds the passing standard.
- You have demonstrated a lack of minimum competency, according to the computer program.
- You have answered the maximum number of questions (265 total questions).
- You have used the maximum time allowed (6 hours).

NCLEX® questions

During the exam, the candidate will be required to respond to a variety of formats. These items may include, but are not limited to, multiple-choice, multiple-response, fill-in-the-blank calculations, ordered response, and/or hot spots. All items may include multimedia, such as charts, tables, graphics, sound, or visuals. Certain strategies can help you understand and answer any type of NCLEX question.

Multiple choice

Many questions on the NCLEX are standard four-option, multiple-choice questions. This type of question will have only one correct answer.

Alternate formats

The first type of alternate-format item is the *multiple-response, multiple-choice question*. Unlike a traditional multiple-choice question, each multiple-response, multiple-choice question has more than one correct answer for every question, and it will contain more than four possible answer options. You'll recognize this type of question because it will ask you to select *all* answers that apply—not just the best answer (as may be requested in the more traditional multiple-choice questions).

Keep in mind that for each multiple-response, multiple-choice question, you must select at least one answer and you must select all correct answers for the item to be counted as correct. On the NCLEX, there's no partial credit in the scoring of these items.

Don't go blank!

The second type of alternate-format item is the *fill-in-the-blank*. These questions require you to provide the answer yourself, rather than select it from a list of options. You will perform a calculation, and then type your answer (a number without any words, units of measurement, commas, or spaces) in the blank space provided after the question. Rules for rounding are included in the question stem if appropriate. A calculator button is provided so you can easily do your calculations electronically.

Master that mouse!

The third type of alternate-format item is a question that asks you to identify an area on an illustration or graphic. For these so-called *"hot spot"* questions, the computerized exam will ask you to place your cursor and click over the correct area on an illustration. Try to be as precise as possible when marking the location. As with the fill-in-the-blanks, the identification questions on the computerized exam may require extremely precise answers to be considered correct.

Chart smarts

The fourth type of alternate-format item is the *exhibit/chart* format. Here you'll be given a problem, then a series of small screens containing additional information you'll need in order to answer the question. By clicking on the Tab button, you can access each screen in turn. Your answer can then be chosen from four multiple-choice answer options.

All in order

The fifth type of alternate-format item, *ordered response*, involves prioritizing or placing in correct order a series of statements, using a drag-and-drop technique. You'll decide which of the given options is first, click and hold it with the mouse, and then drag it into the first box given underneath and drop it into place. You'll repeat this process until you've placed all the available options in the lower boxes.

Now hear this!

The sixth alternate-format item type is the *audio item* format. You'll be given a set of headphones and you'll be asked to listen to an audio clip and select the correct answer from four options. You'll need to select the correct answer on the computer screen as you would with the traditional multiple-choice questions.

Picture perfect

The final alternate-format item type is the *graphic option* question. This varies from the exhibit format type because in the graphic option, your answer choices will be graphics, such as ECG strips. You'll have to select the appropriate graphic to answer the question presented.

The standard's still the standard

The NCSBN hasn't established a percentage of alternate-format items to be administered to each candidate. So relax; the standard, four-option, multiple-choice format questions compose the bulk of the test. (See *Sample NCLEX questions*, pages 7–9.)

(*text continues on page 9*)

Sample NCLEX® questions

Sometimes, getting used to the test format is as important as knowing the material covered. Try your hand at these sample questions and you'll have a leg up when you take the real test!

Sample four-option, multiple-choice question
A client's arterial blood gas (ABG) results are as follows: pH, 7.16; $Paco_2$, 80 mm Hg; Pao_2, 46 mm Hg; HCO_3^-, 24 mEq/L; Sao_2, 81%. This ABG result represents which condition?
1. Metabolic acidosis
2. Metabolic alkalosis
3. Respiratory acidosis
4. Respiratory alkalosis
Correct answer: 3

Sample multiple-response, multiple-choice question
The nurse is caring for a 45-year-old married client who has undergone hemicolectomy for colon cancer. The client has two children. Which concepts about families should the nurse keep in mind when providing care for this client? Select all that apply.
1. Illness in one family member can affect all members.
2. Family roles don't change because of illness.
3. A family member may have more than one role in the family.
4. Children typically aren't affected by adult illness.
5. The effects of an illness on a family depend on the stage of the family's life cycle.
6. Changes in sleeping and eating patterns may be signs of stress in a family.
Correct answer: 1, 3, 5, 6

Sample fill-in-the-blank calculation question
An infant who weighs 8 kg is to receive ampicillin 25 mg/kg I.V. every 6 hours. How many milligrams should the nurse administer per dose? Record your answer using a whole number.

_____ milligrams
Correct answer: 200

(continued)

Sample NCLEX® questions *(continued)*

Sample hot spot question
A client has a history of aortic stenosis. Identify the area where the nurse should place the stethoscope to best hear the murmur.

Correct answer:

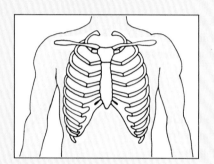

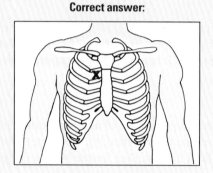

Sample exhibit/chart question
A 3-year-old client is being treated for severe status asthmaticus. After reviewing the progress notes (shown below), the nurse should determine that this client is being treated for which condition?

Progress notes	
4/5/16 0600	Pt. was acutely restless, diaphoretic, and with dyspnea at 0530. Dr. T. Smith notified and ordered ABG analysis. ABG drawn from ℝ radial artery. Stat results as follows: pH 7.28, Paco₂ 55 mm Hg, HCO₃- 26 mEg/L. Dr. Smith with pt. now. ———— J. Collins, R.N.

1. Metabolic acidosis
2. Respiratory alkalosis
3. Respiratory acidosis
4. Metabolic alkalosis

Correct answer: 3

Sample ordered response/drag-and-drop question
When teaching an antepartal client about the passage of the fetus through the birth canal during labor, the nurse describes the cardinal mechanisms of labor. Place these events in the sequence in which they occur. Use all the options.

Correct answer:

1. Flexion	3. Descent
2. External rotation	1. Flexion
3. Descent	5. Internal rotation
4. Expulsion	6. Extension
5. Internal rotation	2. External rotation
6. Extension	4. Expulsion

Sample NCLEX® questions *(continued)*

Sample audio question

Listen to the audio clip. What sound do you hear in the bases of this client with heart failure?

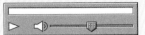

1. Crackles
2. Rhonchi
3. Wheezes
4. Pleural friction rub

Correct answer: 1

Sample graphic question

Which electrocardiogram strip should the nurse document as sinus tachycardia?

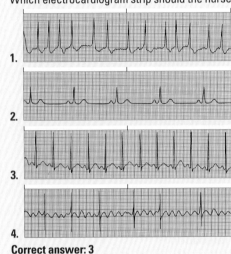

1.

2.

3.

4.

Correct answer: 3

Understanding the question

NCLEX questions are usually long. As a result, it's easy to feel overwhelmed with information. To focus on the question, apply proven strategies for answering NCLEX questions, including:
- determining what the question is asking
- determining relevant facts about the client
- rephrasing the question in your mind
- choosing the best option(s) before entering your answer.

Determine what the question is asking

Read the question twice. If the answer isn't apparent, rephrase the question in simpler, more personal terms. Breaking down the question into easier, less intimidating terms may help you to focus more accurately on the correct answer.

Give it a try

For example, a question might be, "A 74-year-old client with a history of heart failure is admitted to the coronary care unit with pulmonary edema. He's intubated and placed on a mechanical ventilator. Which parameter should the nurse monitor closely to assess the client's response to a bolus dose of furosemide I.V.?"

The options for this question—numbered from 1 to 4—may be:
1. Daily weight
2. 24-hour intake and output
3. Serum sodium levels
4. Hourly urine output

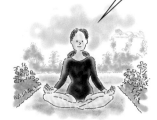

Focusing on what the question is really asking can help you choose the correct answer.

Hocus, focus on the question

Read the question again, ignoring all details except what's being asked. Focus on the last line of the question. It asks you to select the appropriate assessment for monitoring a client who received a bolus of I.V. furosemide.

Determine what facts about the client are relevant

Next, sort out the relevant client information. Start by asking whether any of the information provided about the client isn't relevant. For instance, do you need to know that the client has been admitted to the coronary care unit? Probably not; his reaction to I.V. furosemide won't be affected by his location in the hospital.

Determine what you do know about the client. In the example, you know that:
- he just received an I.V. bolus of furosemide, a crucial fact
- he has pulmonary edema, the most fundamental aspect of the client's underlying condition
- he's intubated and placed on a mechanical ventilator, suggesting that his pulmonary edema is serious
- he's 74 years old and has a history of heart failure, a fact that may or may not be relevant.

Rephrase the question

After you've determined relevant information about the client and the question being asked, consider rephrasing the question to make it more clear. Eliminate jargon and put the question in simpler, more personal terms. Here's how you might rephrase the question in the example: "My client has pulmonary edema. He requires intubation and mechanical ventilation. He's 74 years old and has a history of heart failure. He received an I.V. bolus of furosemide. What assessment parameter should I monitor?"

Choose the best option

Armed with all the information you now have, it's time to select an option. You know that the client received an I.V. bolus of furosemide, a diuretic. You know that monitoring fluid intake and output is a key nursing intervention for a client taking a diuretic, a fact that eliminates options 1 and 3 (daily weight and serum sodium levels), narrowing the answer down to option 2 or 4 (24-hour intake and output or hourly urine output).

You also know that the drug was administered by I.V. bolus, suggesting a rapid effect. (In fact, furosemide administered by I.V. bolus takes effect almost immediately.) Monitoring the client's 24-hour intake and output would be appropriate for assessing the effects of repeated doses of furosemide. Hourly urine output, however, is most appropriate in this situation because it monitors the immediate effect of this rapid-acting drug.

Key strategies

Regardless of the type of question, four key strategies will help you determine the correct answer for each question. These strategies are:
1. considering the nursing process
2. referring to Maslow's hierarchy of needs
3. reviewing patient safety
4. reflecting on principles of therapeutic communication.

Nursing process

One of the ways to answer a question is to apply the nursing process. Steps in the nursing process include:

- assessment
- diagnosis
- planning
- implementation
- evaluation.

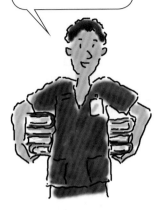

Say it 1,000 times: Studying for the NCLEX is fun... studying for the NCLEX is fun...

Process pointers

The nursing process may provide insights that help you analyze a question. According to the nursing process, assessment comes before analysis, which comes before planning, which comes before implementation, which comes before evaluation.

You're halfway to the correct answer when you encounter a four-option, multiple-choice question that asks you to assess the situation and then provides two assessment options and two implementation options. You can immediately eliminate the implementation options, which then gives you, at worst, a 50-50 chance of selecting the correct answer. Use the following sample question to apply the nursing process:

A client returns from an endoscopic procedure during which he was sedated. Before offering the client food, which action should the nurse take?

1. Assess the client's respiratory status.
2. Check the client's gag reflex.
3. Place the client in a side-lying position.
4. Have the client drink a few sips of water.

Assess before intervening

According to the nursing process, the nurse must assess a client before performing an intervention. Does the question indicate that the client has been properly assessed? No, it doesn't. Therefore, you can eliminate options 3 and 4 because they're both interventions.

That leaves options 1 and 2, both of which are assessments. Your nursing knowledge should tell you the correct answer—in this case, option 2. The sedation required for an endoscopic procedure may impair the client's gag reflex, so you would assess the gag reflex before giving food to the client to reduce the risk of aspiration and airway obstruction.

Watch phrasing

Why not select option 1, assessing the client's respiratory status? You might select this option, but the question is specifically asking about offering the client food, an action that wouldn't be taken if the client's respiratory status was at all compromised. In this case, you're making a judgment based on the phrase, "Before offering the client food." If the question was trying to test your knowledge of respiratory depression following an endoscopic procedure, it probably wouldn't mention a function—such as giving food to a client—that clearly occurs only after the client's respiratory status has been stabilized.

Maslow's hierarchy

Knowledge of Maslow's hierarchy of needs can be a vital tool for establishing priorities on the NCLEX. Maslow's theory states that physiological needs are the most basic human needs of all. Only after physiological needs have been met can safety concerns be addressed. Only after safety concerns are met can concerns involving love and belonging be addressed, and so forth. Apply the principles of Maslow's hierarchy of needs to the following sample question:

A client reports severe pain 2 days after surgery. Which action should the nurse perform **first**?
1. Offer reassurance to the client that he or she will feel less pain tomorrow.
2. Allow the client time to verbalize his or her feelings.
3. Check the client's vital signs.
4. Administer an analgesic.

Phys before psych

In this example, two of the options—3 and 4—address physiological needs. Options 1 and 2 address psychosocial concerns. According to Maslow, physiological needs must be met before psychosocial needs, so you can eliminate options 1 and 2.

Final elimination

Now, use your nursing knowledge to choose the best answer from the two remaining options. In this case, option 3 is correct because the client's vital signs should be checked before administering an analgesic (assessment before intervention). When prioritizing according to Maslow's hierarchy, remember your ABCs—airway, breathing, circulation—to help you further prioritize. Check for a patent airway before addressing breathing. Check breathing before checking the health of the cardiovascular system.

Tricky, tricky

Just because an option appears on the NCLEX doesn't mean it's a viable choice for the client referred to in the question. Always examine your choice in light of your knowledge and experience. Ask yourself, "Does this choice make sense for this client?" Allow yourself to eliminate choices—even ones that might normally take priority—if they don't make sense for a particular client's situation.

Patient safety

As you might expect, patient safety takes high priority on the NCLEX. You'll encounter many questions that can be answered by asking yourself, "Which answer will best ensure the safety of this client?" Use patient safety criteria for situations involving laboratory values, drug administration, activities of daily living, or nursing care procedures.

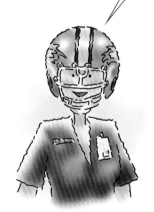

Patient safety takes high priority on the NCLEX.

Client first, equipment second

You may encounter a question in which some options address the client and others address the equipment. When in doubt, select an option relating to the client; never place equipment before a client.

For instance, suppose a question asks what the nurse should do first when entering a client's room where an infusion pump alarm is sounding. If two options deal with the infusion pump, one with the infusion tubing, and another with the client's catheter insertion site, select the one relating to the client's catheter insertion site. Always check the client first; the equipment can wait.

Therapeutic communication

Some NCLEX questions focus on the nurse's ability to communicate effectively with the client. Therapeutic communication incorporates verbal or nonverbal responses and involves:
- listening to the client
- understanding the client's needs
- promoting clarification and insight about the client's condition.

Room for improvement

Like other NCLEX questions, those dealing with therapeutic communication require choosing the best response. First, eliminate options that indicate the use of poor therapeutic communication techniques, such as those in which the nurse:

- tells the client what to do without regard to the client's feelings or desires (the "do this" response)
- asks a question that can be answered "yes" or "no," or with another one-syllable response
- seeks reasons for the client's behavior
- implies disapproval of the client's behavior
- offers false reassurances
- attempts to interpret the client's behavior rather than allowing the client to verbalize feelings
- offers a response that focuses on the nurse, not the client.

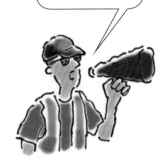

Listen up, some exam questions will focus on good therapeutic communication!

Ah, that's better!

When answering NCLEX questions, look for responses that:

- allow the client time to think and reflect
- encourage the client to talk
- encourage the client to describe a particular experience
- reflect that the nurse has listened to the client, such as through paraphrasing the client's response.

Avoiding pitfalls

Even the most knowledgeable students can get tripped up on certain NCLEX questions. (See *A tricky question,* page 14.) Students commonly cite three areas that can be difficult for unwary test-takers:

1. knowing the difference between the NCLEX and the "real world"
2. delegating care
3. knowing laboratory values.

NCLEX® versus the real world

Some students who take the NCLEX have extensive practical experience in health care. For example, many test-takers have worked as licensed practical nurses or unlicensed assistive personnel. In one of those capacities, test-takers might have been exposed to less than optimum clinical practice and may carry those experiences over to the NCLEX.

However, the NCLEX is a textbook examination—not a test of clinical skills. Take the NCLEX with the understanding that what happens in the real world may differ from what the NCLEX and your nursing school say should happen.

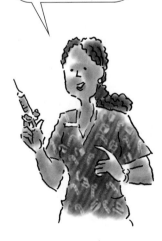

Remember, this is the real world. The NCLEX may not always reflect what happens in it.

Don't take shortcuts

If you've had practical experience in health care, you may know a quicker way to perform a procedure or tricks to get by when you don't have the right equipment. Situations such as staff shortages may force you to improvise. On the NCLEX, such scenarios can lead to trouble. Always check your practical experiences against textbook nursing care, selecting the response that follows the textbook.

A tricky question

The NCLEX occasionally asks a particular kind of question called the "further teaching" question, which involves patient-teaching situations. These questions can be tricky. You'll have to choose the response that suggests that the patient has *not* learned the correct information. Here's an example:

37. A client undergoes a total hip replacement. Which statement by the client indicates a need for further teaching?
1. "I'll need to keep several pillows between my legs at night."
2. "I'll need to remember not to cross my legs. It's such a bad habit."
3. "The occupational therapist is showing me how to use a 'sock puller' to help me get dressed."
4. "I don't know if I'll be able to get off that low toilet seat at home by myself."

The answer you should choose here is option 4 because it indicates that the client has a poor understanding of the precautions required after a total hip replacement and that he needs further teaching. *Remember:* If you see the phrase *further teaching* or *further instruction*, you're looking for a wrong answer by the patient.

Delegating care

On the NCLEX, you may encounter questions that assess your ability to delegate care. Delegating care involves coordinating the efforts of other health care workers to provide effective care for your client. On the NCLEX, you may be asked to assign duties to:
- licensed practical nurses or licensed vocational nurses
- direct care workers, such as unlicensed assistive personnel
- other support staff, such as nutrition assistants and housekeepers.

In addition, you'll be asked to decide when to notify a physician, a social worker, or another hospital staff member. In each case, you'll have to decide when, where, and how to delegate.

Shoulds and shouldn'ts

As a general rule, it's okay to delegate actions that involve stable clients or standard, unchanging procedures. Bathing, feeding, dressing, and transferring clients are examples of procedures that can be delegated.

Be careful not to delegate complicated or complex activities. In addition, don't delegate activities that involve assessment, evaluation, or your own nursing judgment. On the NCLEX and in the real world, these duties fall squarely on your shoulders. Make sure that you take primary responsibility for assessing and evaluating the client and for making decisions about the client's care. Never hand off those responsibilities to someone with less training.

Calling in reinforcements

Deciding when to notify a physician, a social worker, or another hospital staff member is an important element of nursing care. On the NCLEX, however, choices that involve notifying the physician are usually incorrect. Remember that the NCLEX wants to see you, the nurse, at work.

If you're sure the correct answer is to notify the physician, though, make sure the client's safety has been addressed before notifying a physician or another staff

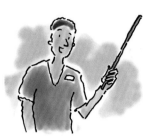

member. On the NCLEX, the client's safety has a higher priority than notifying other health care providers.

Knowing laboratory values

Some NCLEX questions supply laboratory results without indicating normal levels. As a result, answering questions involving laboratory values requires you to have the normal range of the most common laboratory values memorized to make an informed decision. The NCLEX uses units of measure that will be familiar to you. (See Appendix, page 919.)

Chapter 2

Passing the NCLEX®

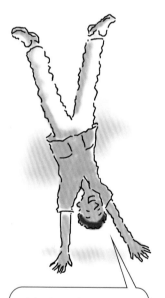

As you count down the weeks, days, and finally hours to the NCLEX, refer back to the information in this chapter. It's a recipe for NCLEX success!

Just the facts

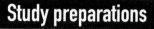

In this chapter, you'll learn:

◆ how to properly prepare for the NCLEX®

◆ how to concentrate during difficult study times

◆ ways to make more effective use of your time

◆ why creative studying strategies can enhance learning

◆ how to get the most out of NCLEX practice tests.

Study preparations

If you're like most people preparing to take the test, you're probably feeling nervous, anxious, or concerned. Keep in mind that most test-takers pass the NCLEX® the first time around.

Passing the test won't happen by accident, though; you'll need to prepare carefully and efficiently. To help jump-start your preparations:

• determine your strengths and weaknesses
• create a study schedule
• set realistic goals
• find an effective study space
• think positively
• start studying sooner rather than later.

Strengths and weaknesses

Most students recognize that, even at the end of their nursing studies, they know more about some topics than others. Because the NCLEX covers a broad range of material, you should make some decisions about how intensively you'll review each topic.

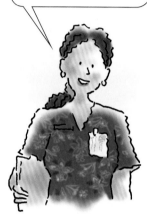

Most students pass the NCLEX on the first try. I know you can, too!

Make a list

Base those decisions on a list. Divide a sheet of paper in half vertically. On one side, list topics you think you know well. On the other side, list topics you need to review. Pay no attention if one side is longer than the other. When you're done studying, you'll feel strong in every area.

Where the list comes from

To make sure your list reflects a comprehensive view of all the areas you studied in school, look at the contents page in the front of this book. For each topic listed, place it in the "know well" column or "needs review" column. Separating content areas this way shows immediately which topics need less study time and which need more time.

You also may wish to integrate feedback you have received from your courses, instructors, and other products you have used to guide your understanding of strong and weak areas. For example, some products that use adaptive engines will assess your progress over time and give you feedback about areas that may pose challenges for you. Integrate this information into your plan.

Scheduling study time

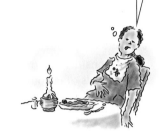

I'll cover difficult topics when I'm more alert.

Study when you're most alert. Most people can identify a period of the day when they feel most alert. If you feel most alert and energized in the morning, for example, set aside sections of time in the morning for topics that need a lot of review. Then you can use the evening, a time of lesser alertness, for topics that need some refreshing. The opposite is true as well; if you're more alert in the evening, study difficult topics at that time.

What and when

Set up a basic schedule for studying. Using a calendar or organizer, determine how much time remains before you'll take the NCLEX. (See *2 to 3 months before the NCLEX* below.) Fill in the remaining days with specific times and topics to be studied. Plan to start studying your weak areas early. Remember to schedule difficult topics during your most alert times.

Keep in mind that you shouldn't fill each day with studying. Be realistic and set aside time for normal activities. Try to create ample study time before the NCLEX and then stick to the schedule. Allow some extra time in the schedule in case you get behind or come across a topic that requires extra review.

Keep goals manageable

Part of creating a schedule means setting goals you can accomplish. You no doubt studied a great deal in nursing school, and by now you have a sense of your own capabilities. Ask yourself, "How much can I cover in a day?" Set that amount of time aside and then stay on task. You'll feel better about yourself—and your chances of passing the NCLEX—when you meet your goals regularly.

Study space

Find a space conducive to effective learning and then study there. Whatever you do, don't study with videos playing in the room or in an environment with multiple sources of distraction. Instead, find a quiet, inviting study space that:
- is located in a quiet, convenient place, away from normal traffic patterns
- contains a solid chair that encourages good posture (Avoid studying in bed; you'll be more likely to fall asleep and not accomplish your goals.)

To-do list

2 to 3 months before the NCLEX®

With 2 to 3 months remaining before you plan to take the examination, take these steps:
- Establish a study schedule. Set aside ample time to study but also leave time for social activities, exercise, family or personal responsibilities, and other matters.
- Become knowledgeable about the NCLEX-RN examination, its content, the types of questions it asks, and the testing format.
- Begin studying your notes, texts, and other study materials.
- Take some NCLEX practice questions to help you diagnose strengths and weaknesses as well as to become familiar with NCLEX-style questions.
- Focus on your areas of weakness. That way, you'll have time to review these areas again before the test date.

- uses comfortable, soft lighting with which you can see clearly without eye strain
- has a temperature between 65° and 70° F (18° and 21° C)
- contains flowers or green plants, familiar photos or paintings, and easy access to soft, instrumental background music.

Accentuate the positive

Consider hanging positive messages around your study space. Make signs with words of encouragement, such as, "You can do it!" "Keep studying!" and "Remember the goal!" These upbeat messages can help keep you going when your attention begins to waver.

Maintaining concentration

When you're faced with reviewing the amount of information covered by the NCLEX, it's easy to become distracted and lose your concentration. When you lose concentration, you make less effective use of valuable study time. To help stay focused, keep these tips in mind:

- Alternate the order of the subjects you study during the day to add variety to your study.
- Approach your studying with enthusiasm, sincerity, and determination.
- Once you've decided to study, begin immediately. Don't let anything interfere with your thought processes once you've begun.
- Concentrate on accomplishing one task at a time to the exclusion of everything else.
- Don't try to do two things at once, such as studying and watching videos or conversing with friends.
- Work continuously without interruption for a while but don't study for such a long period that the whole experience becomes grueling or boring.
- Allow time for periodic breaks to give yourself a change of pace. Use these breaks to ease your transition into studying a new topic.
- When studying in the evening, wind down from your studies slowly. Don't progress directly from studying to sleeping.

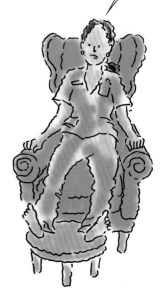

This chair invites slacking, not studying! You should find a chair that encourages good posture instead.

Taking care of yourself

Never neglect your physical and mental well-being in favor of longer study hours. Maintaining physical and mental health is critical for success in taking the NCLEX. (See *4 to 6 weeks before the NCLEX below.*)

To-do list

4 to 6 weeks before the NCLEX®

With 4 to 6 weeks remaining before you plan to take the examination, take these steps:
- Continue to focus on your areas of weakness.
- Find a study partner or form a study group.
- Take a practice test to gauge your skill level early.
- Take time to eat, sleep, exercise, and socialize to avoid burnout.

A few simple rules

You can increase your likelihood of passing the test by following these simple health rules:

- Get plenty of rest. You can't think deeply or concentrate for long periods when you're tired.
- Drink enough noncaffeinated beverages. Mild dehydration increases the effort required to concentrate and reason while distracting attention through feelings of fatigue and thirst.
- Eat nutritious meals. Maintaining your energy level is impossible when you're undernourished.
- Exercise regularly. Regular exercise, preferably 30 minutes daily, helps you work harder and think more clearly. As a result, you'll study more efficiently and increase the likelihood of success.

Memory power!

If you're having trouble concentrating but would rather push through than take a break, try making your studying more active by reading out loud. Active studying can renew your powers of concentration. By reading review material out loud to yourself, you're engaging your ears as well as your eyes—and making your studying a more active process. Hearing the material out loud also fosters memory and subsequent recall.

You can also rewrite in your own words a few of the more difficult concepts you're reviewing. Explaining these concepts in writing forces you to think through the material and can jump-start your memory.

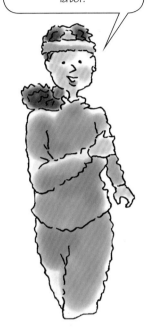

A short jog now will help us concentrate later.

Study schedule

When you were creating your schedule, you might have asked yourself, "How long should I study? One hour at a stretch? Two hours? Three?" To make the best use of your study time, you'll need to answer those questions.

Optimum study time

Consider studying in 20- to 30-minute intervals with a short break in between. You remember the material you study at the beginning and end of a session best and tend to remember less material studied in the middle of the session. The total length of time in each study session depends on you and the amount of material you need to cover.

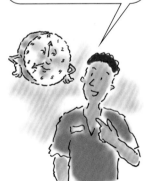

I've found that hour-and-a-half sessions work best for me.

To thine own self be true

So what's the answer? It doesn't matter as long as you determine what's best for *you*. At the beginning of your NCLEX study schedule, try study periods of varying lengths. Pay close attention to those that seem more successful.

Remember that you're an educated nurse who is competent at assessment. Think of yourself as a patient, and assess your own progress. Then implement the strategy that works best for you.

Finding time to study

So does that mean that short sections of time are useless? Not at all. We all have spaces in our day that might otherwise be dead time. (See *1 week before the NCLEX* on next page.) These are perfect times to review for the NCLEX but not to cover new material because by the time you get deep into new material, your time will be over.

Always keep some flash cards or a small notebook handy for situations when you have a few extra minutes. You may also want to use a mobile device to access NCLEX study tools available online.

You'll be amazed how many short sessions you can find in a day and how much reviewing you can do in 5 minutes. The following places offer short stretches of time you can use:
• eating breakfast
• waiting for, or riding on, a train or bus
• waiting in line at the grocery store, restaurant, or other places
• using exercise equipment, such as a treadmill.

Creative studying

Even when you study in a perfect study space and concentrate better than ever, studying for the NCLEX can get a little, well, dull. Even people with terrific study habits occasionally feel bored or sluggish. That is why it's important to have some creative tricks in your study bag to liven up your studying during those down times.

Creative studying doesn't have to be hard work. It involves making efforts to alter your study habits a bit. Some techniques that might help include studying with a partner or group and creating flash cards or other audiovisual study tools.

Study partners

Studying with a partner or group of students (3 or 4 students at most) can be an excellent way to energize your studying. Working with a partner allows you to test each other on the material you've reviewed. Your partner can give you encouragement and motivation. Perhaps most important, working with a partner can provide a welcome break from solitary studying.

Be choosy

Exercise some care when choosing a study partner or assembling a study group. A partner who doesn't fit your needs won't help you make the most of your study time. Look for a partner who:
• possesses similar goals to yours. For example, someone taking the NCLEX at approximately the same date who feels the same sense of urgency as you do might make an excellent partner.
• possesses about the same level of knowledge as you. Tutoring someone can sometimes help you learn, but partnering should be give-and-take so both partners can gain knowledge.
• can study without excess chatting or interruptions. Socializing is an important part of creative study, but remember, you've still got to pass the NCLEX—so stay serious!

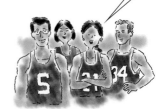

Find partners who can give you encouragement and motivation. But remember to stay focused!

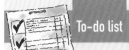

To-do list

The day before the NCLEX®

With 1 day before the NCLEX examination, take these steps:
- Drive to the test site, review traffic patterns, and find out where to park. If your route to the test site occurs during heavy traffic or if you're expecting bad weather, set aside extra time to ensure prompt arrival.
- Do something relaxing during the day.
- Avoid concentrating on the test.
- Eat and drink well and avoid dwelling on the NCLEX during nonstudy periods.
- Call a supportive friend or relative for some last-minute words of encouragement.
- Get plenty of rest the night before and allow for plenty of time in the morning.

Audiovisual tools

Flash cards and other audiovisual tools foster retention and make learning and reviewing fun.

Adobe flash? No, flash Cards!

Flash cards can provide you with an excellent study tool. The process of writing material on a flash card will help you remember it. In addition, flash cards are small and easily portable, perfect for those 5-minute slivers of time that show up during the day.

Creating a flash card should be fun. Use magic markers, highlighters, and other colorful tools to make them visually stimulating. The more effort you put into creating your flash cards, the better you'll remember the material contained on the cards.

Other visual tools

Flowcharts, drawings, diagrams, and other image-oriented study aids can also help you learn material more effectively. Substituting images for text can be a great way to give your eyes a break and recharge your brain. Remember to use vivid colors to make your creations visually engaging.

Hear's the thing

If you learn more effectively when you hear information rather than see it, consider recording key ideas using a phone app. Recording information helps promote memory because you say the information aloud when recording and then listen to it when playing it back. Like flash cards, these recordings are portable and perfect for those short study periods during the day. (See *The day before the NCLEX*, above.)

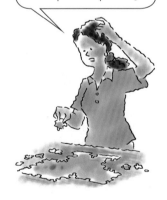

Charts, drawings, and diagrams make concepts less puzzling.

Practice tests

Practice questions should constitute an important part of your NCLEX study strategy. Practice questions can improve your studying by helping you review material and familiarizing yourself with the exact style of questions you'll encounter on the NCLEX.

Practice at the beginning

Consider working through some practice questions as soon as you begin studying for the NCLEX. For example, you might try a half-dozen questions from each chapter in this book.

If you score well, you probably know the material contained in that chapter fairly well and can spend less time reviewing that particular topic. If you have trouble with the questions, spend extra study time on that topic.

You're getting there

Practice questions can also provide an excellent means of marking your progress. Don't worry if you have trouble answering the first few practice questions you take; you'll need time to adjust to the way the questions are asked. Eventually, you'll become accustomed to the question format and begin to focus more on the questions themselves.

If you make practice questions a regular part of your study regimen, you'll be able to notice areas in which you're improving. You can then adjust your study time accordingly.

Practice makes perfect

As you near the examination date, continue to answer practice questions, but also set aside time to take an entire NCLEX practice test. (We've included three at the back of this book.) This will enable you to approximate the experience of taking the actual NCLEX. Using thePoint Web site that accompanies this resource (the code for which is found on this inside cover of this book), you can take practice tests with varying numbers of questions.

Because I've taken lots of practice tests, I understand how the questions work.

Additionally, a second code offers you a free 30-day trial of *Lippincott NCLEX-RN PassPoint*, which allows you to take adaptive quizzes across the curriculum as well as to take practice exams of varying lengths from 75 to 265 questions. These practice exams simulate the real NCLEX in every way. Note that 75 questions is the minimum number of questions you'll be asked on the actual NCLEX. By gradually tackling larger practice tests, you'll increase your confidence, build test-taking endurance, and strengthen the concentration skills that will enable you to succeed. (See *The day of the NCLEX* below.)

Online adaptive quizzing

Adaptive quizzing programs such as Lippincott NCLEX-RN PassPoint can help keep you engaged with learning because the quizzes and exams are individualized to your level of understanding. The more correct knowledge you demonstrate, the more challenging the learning experience becomes. PassPoint gives you ongoing feedback about your strengths and weaknesses so you know how to prioritize your study plan. It gives you an opportunity to take NCLEX-style exams of varying lengths to help you build your endurance and become more familiar with a simulated computer adaptive testing environment. By alternating your book review and quizzing with online learning, you can stay energized and prepare for NCLEX using the different media available to you.

To-do list

The day of the NCLEX®

On the day of the NCLEX examination, take these steps:

- Get up early.
- Wear comfortable clothes, preferably with layers you can adjust to fit the room temperature.
- Drink a glass of water and eat a small nutritious breakfast.
- Leave your house early.
- Arrive at the test site early with the required paperwork in hand.
- Avoid looking at your notes as you wait for your computer test.
- Listen carefully to the instructions given before entering the test room.
- Succeed, succeed, *succeed!*

Quick quiz

1. The best time to study is:
   A. in the morning.
   B. early in the evening.
   C. after eating a full meal.
   D. when you feel most alert.

Answer: 1. **D.** Study when you're most alert. If you feel most alert and energized in the morning, for example, set aside sections of time in the morning for topics that need a lot of review.

2. The temperature of the ideal study area should be between:
   A. 60° and 65° F (15° and 18° C).
   B. 65° and 70° F (18° and 21° C).
   C. 70° and 75° F (21° and 24° C).
   D. 75° and 80° F (24° and 27° C).

Answer: 2. **B.** The ideal study area has a temperature between 65° and 70° F (18° and 21° C).

3. To help you maintain concentration during long study periods, recommended study strategies include:
   A. Study the topics you find most interesting first, followed by the topics you find least interesting.
   B. Study the topics you find least interesting first, followed by the topics you find most interesting.
   C. Alternate the order of the subjects you study during the day.
   D. Study only the topics you find least interesting; you'll remember the others.

Answer: 3. **C.** Alternating the order of the subjects you study during the day adds variety to your study and helps you remain focused and make the most of your study time.

4. When selecting a study partner, choose one who:
   A. possesses similar goals as you.
   B. is highly social and will keep you entertained.
   C. isn't as knowledgeable as you so you can tutor him.
   D. likes to take a lot of breaks.

Answer: 4. **A.** A partner who doesn't fit your needs won't help you make the most of your study time. Look for a partner who has similar goals to yours, possesses about the same level of knowledge as you, and won't spend too much time socializing.

Scoring

⭐⭐⭐ If you answered all four questions correctly, wow! We hope the exam is ready for *you!*

⭐⭐ If you answered three questions correctly, terrific! You're cruising toward an exam day victory!

⭐ If you answered fewer than three questions correctly, fear not. By the time you're done practicing, you'll be an NCLEX success!

Part II

Care of the Adult

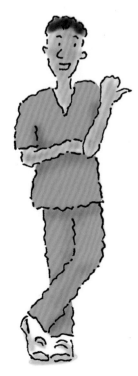

Chapter 3

Cardiovascular Disorders

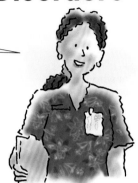

If you'd like to rummage through a Web site dedicated to cardiovascular disorders, check out the American Heart Association's at **www.heart.org**.

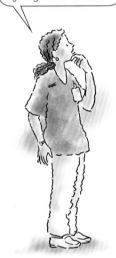

Hmm. Which artery is likely occluded? Can you give me a lead?

1. A client's electrocardiogram (ECG) is showing ST elevation in leads V2, V3, and V4. Which artery is **most** likely occluded?
   1. Circumflex artery
   2. Internal mammary artery
   3. Left anterior descending artery
   4. Right coronary artery

1. 3. The left anterior descending artery is the primary source of blood for the anterior wall of the heart. The circumflex artery supplies the lateral wall, the internal mammary artery supplies the anterior chest wall from clavicle to umbilicus, and the right coronary artery supplies the inferior wall of the heart. The ST elevation in leads V2, V3, and V4 suggests an anterior-wall myocardial infarction.
CN: Physiological integrity; CNS: Physiological adaptation; CL: Apply

2. A nurse, on a telemetry unit, teaches a client diagnosed with acute coronary syndrome about coronary blood flow. Which statement, made by the nurse, is correct?
   1. Most of the blood flow to coronary arteries is supplied during inspiration.
   2. Most of the blood flow to coronary arteries is supplied during diastole.
   3. Blood flow to coronary arteries is related to breathing patterns.
   4. Coronary arteries receive most of the blood flow during systole.

2. 2. Although the coronary arteries may receive a minute portion of blood during systole, most of the blood flow to coronary arteries is supplied during diastole. Breathing patterns are irrelevant to blood flow.
CN: Physiological integrity; CNS: Physiological adaptation; CL: Apply

Stop and think! Which of the markers rise because of cellular damage to the heart?

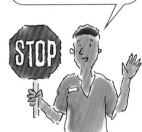

3. The nurse has just admitted a client to the telemetry floor with reports of acute chest pain radiating down the left arm. Which laboratory studies should the nurse order to evaluate myocardial damage? Select all that apply.
   1. Hemoglobin and hematocrit
   2. Serum glucose
   3. Creatinine phosphokinase (CK-MB)
   4. Troponin T and troponin I
   5. Myoglobin
   6. Blood urea nitrogen (BUN)

3. 3, 4, 5. Levels of CK-MB, troponin T, and troponin I rise because of cellular damage. Myoglobin elevation is an early indicator of myocardial damage. Neither hemoglobin, hematocrit, serum glucose, nor BUN levels provide information related to myocardial ischemia.
CN: Health promotion and maintenance; CNS: Prevention and early detection of disease; CL: Apply

CN: Client needs category   CNS: Client needs subcategory   CL: Cognitive level

4. A nurse has just completed teaching a client with atherosclerosis about the disease. The nurse determines that further teaching is necessary when the client states:
  1. "Plaques obstruct the coronary artery."
  2. "Plaques obstruct the coronary vein."
  3. "Hardened vessels can't dilate to allow blood to flow through."
  4. "Atherosclerosis can cause angina."

4. 2. Arteries, not veins, supply the myocardium with oxygen and other nutrients. Atherosclerosis is a direct result of plaque formation in the artery. Hardened vessels can't dilate properly and, therefore, constrict blood flow and oxygen, causing angina.
CN: Physiological integrity; CNS: Physiological adaptation; CL: Analyze

5. The nurse is assessing a client who is experiencing substernal chest pain. Which report of symptoms support a diagnosis of stable angina pectoris rather than a possible myocardial infarction? Select all that apply.
  1. "The pain began while I was watching television."
  2. "The pain goes up and down my left arm."
  3. "The pain lasts less than five minutes."
  4. "The pain started when I was eating breakfast and continued all morning."
  5. "One nitroglycerine tablet relieved the pain."

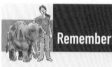

Remember

"Nitroglycerin nixes angina."

Nitroglycerin, a nitrate antianginal drug, helps prevent and treat acute attacks of angina.

5. 2, 3, 5. Stable angina pectoris is a temporary imbalance between the coronary artery's ability to supply oxygen, and the cardiac muscle's demand for oxygen. The substernal chest pain that occurs in this stable angina pectoris may radiate to an arm, is precipitated by exertion or stress, is relieved by rest or nitroglycerin, and lasts less than 15 minutes. Myocardial infarction occurs when myocardial tissue is abruptly and severely deprived of oxygen. The substernal chest pain that occurs in myocardial infarction radiates to the left arm, back, or jaw. It occurs without cause, usually in the morning, and is only relieved by opioids; and lasts 30 minutes or longer.
CN: Physiological integrity; CNS: Physiological adaptation; CL: Apply

6. The nurse is reviewing a client's lab work to determine if a risk for coronary artery disease is present. Which result would require an **immediate** intervention by the nurse?
  1. HDL = 100 mg/dl (5.5 mmol/l)
  2. LDL = 140 mg/dl (7.8 mmol/l)
  3. VLDL = 20%
  4. Total cholesterol = 240 mg/dl (13.3 mmol/l)

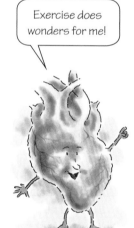

Exercise does wonders for me!

6. 4. Total cholesterol levels above 240 mg/dl (13.3 mmol/l) are considered excessive. They require dietary restriction and possibly medication. Exercise may also reduce cholesterol levels. The other levels listed are all nationally accepted levels for cholesterol and carry a lower risk of CAD.
CN: Physiological integrity; CNS: Reduction of risk potential; CL: Apply

7. A client is experiencing the classic signs and symptoms of acute coronary artery disease. What is the nurse's **priority** intervention?
  1. Remain with the client in order to decrease anxiety
  2. Apply supplemental oxygen
  3. Administer sublingual nitroglycerin
  4. Educate the client about the pathophysiology causing his symptoms

7. 2. Enhancing myocardial oxygenation is the priority when a client exhibits signs or symptoms of cardiac compromise. Without adequate oxygen, the myocardium suffers damage. Sublingual nitroglycerin is administered to treat acute angina, but its administration is not the first priority. Although educating the client and decreasing anxiety are important, neither are priorities when a client is compromised.
CN: Physiological integrity; CNS: Physiological adaptation; CL: Analyze

CN: Client needs category   CNS: Client needs subcategory   CL: Cognitive level

8. The nurse is preparing to educate a client about the long-term management of coronary artery disease. What information should the nurse include?
   1. The need to have cardiac catheterization done each year
   2. The use of coronary artery bypass surgery as preventative measure
   3. Daily oral administration of aspirin for prevention of blood clots
   4. The need to have percutaneous coronary intervention with routine cardiac catheterization

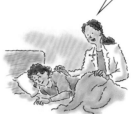

Conservative methods of treatment should always be your first course of action.

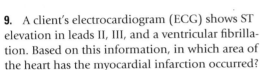

8. 3. Oral administration of aspirin is used to prevent the formation of blood clots in coronary arteries. Such a medication would be used initially and long term in the treatment of this disorder. Cardiac catheterization isn't a treatment but a diagnostic tool and is not done each year. Coronary artery bypass surgery and percutaneous transluminal coronary angioplasty are invasive, surgical treatments that are not necessarily initially used for treatment.
CN: Physiological integrity; CNS: Physiological adaptation; CL: Analyze

9. A client's electrocardiogram (ECG) shows ST elevation in leads II, III, and a ventricular fibrillation. Based on this information, in which area of the heart has the myocardial infarction occurred?
   1. Anterior left ventricle
   2. Apex
   3. Right inferior wall
   4. Lateral left atrium

9. 3. The right coronary artery supplies the right ventricle, or the inferior portion of the heart. An occlusion could produce an infarction in that area. The right coronary artery doesn't supply the anterior portion, lateral portion, or apical portion of the heart.
CN: Physiological integrity; CNS: Physiological adaptation; CL: Apply

10. A client with no history of cardiovascular disease comes to the ambulatory clinic with flu-like symptoms and a report of chest pain. What **priority** question should the nurse ask this client?
   1. "Can you describe the pain to me?"
   2. "Have you ever had this pain before?"
   3. "What makes the pain intensify?"
   4. "Can you rate the pain on a scale of 1 to 10, with 10 being the worst?"

10. 3. Chest pain is assessed by using the standard pain assessment parameters such as characteristics, location, duration, intensity, precipitating factors, and associated symptoms. Asking the client to describe the pain, if the pain has happened before, and to rate the pain are appropriate questions. These questions; however, do not help determine the cause of pain. Knowing what intensifies the pain will assist the nurse in determining a cause.
CN: Physiological integrity; CNS: Physiological adaptation; CL: Analyze

11. Where is the **best** site for the nurse to assess a client's pulse prior to administering digoxin?
   1. Inner aspect of right wrist at the base of the thumb
   2. At the left fifth intercostal space, midclavicular line
   3. The anterior aspect of the right arm at the antecubital fossa
   4. The left second intercostal space in the midclavicular line

11. 2. The administration of digoxin requires the assessment of the client's apical pulse. The correct landmark for obtaining an apical pulse is the left fifth intercostal space at the midclavicular line. This is the point of maximum impulse, and the location of the left ventricular apex. The left second intercostal space in the midclavicular line is where pulmonic sounds are auscultated.
CN: Physiological integrity; CNS: Basic care and comfort; CL: Apply

12. A client reports stabbing chest pain that increases in intensity with inspiration. The nurse understands that the **most** likely origin of this pain is:
1. cardiac.
2. gastrointestinal.
3. musculoskeletal.
4. pulmonary.

13. Where should the nurse auscultate to assess heart sounds associated with pulmonic stenosis?
1. The second intercostal space, to the right of the sternum
2. The fifth intercostal space in the midclavicular line
3. The second left intercostal space along the left sternal border
4. The third and fourth intercostal spaces along the left sternal border

14. The nurse is caring for a client receiving digoxin. Which symptoms would the nurse anticipate with a digoxin level of 2.3 ng/dl (0.08 nmol/l)? Select all that apply.
1. Nausea
2. Drowsiness
3. Photophobia
4. Increased appetite
5. Increased energy level
6. Seeing halos around bright objects

15. A client who had a myocardial infarction asks the nurse why he is receiving morphine. Which benefits of morphine should the nurse explain to this client? Select all that apply.
1. Sedation
2. Pain relief
3. Diminished anxiety
4. Decreased myocardial oxygen demand
5. Vasoconstriction of peripheral vessels
6. Increased urinary output

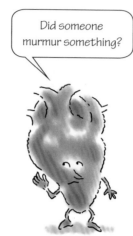

Did someone murmur something?

Remember

"Morphine pulverizes pain."

Morphine is the most potent opioid analgesic.

12. 4. Pulmonary pain is generally described by these symptoms. Musculoskeletal pain only increases with movement. Cardiac and gastrointestinal pains don't change with respiration.
CN: Physiological integrity; CNS: Physiological adaptation; CL: Understand

13. 3. Abnormalities of the pulmonic valve are auscultated at the second left intercostal space along the left sternal border. Aortic valve abnormalities are heard at the second intercostal space, to the right of the sternum. Mitral valve abnormalities are heard at the fifth intercostal space in the midclavicular line. Tricuspid valve abnormalities are heard at the third and fourth intercostal spaces along the left sternal border.
CN: Physiological integrity; CNS: Physiological adaptation; CL: Apply

14. 1, 2, 3, 6. Digoxin is a cardiac glycoside used to manage and treat heart failure, control ventricular rate in clients with atrial fibrillation, and treat and prevent recurrent paroxysmal atrial tachycardia. The therapeutic range of digoxin is 0.8 to 2.0 ng/dl (0.03 to 0.07 nmol/l). Signs of toxicity include gastrointestinal disturbances, neurological abnormalities, facial pain, personality changes, and ocular disturbances such as photophobia.
CN: Physiological integrity; CNS: Physiological adaptation; CL: Analyze

15. 1, 2, 3, 4. Morphine is administered because it decreases myocardial oxygen demand. Morphine will also decrease pain and anxiety while causing sedation. Vasodilation and urinary retention are associated with morphine administration.
CN: Physiological integrity; CNS: Pharmacological and parenteral therapies; CL: Apply

16. A client, with a history of cardiac problems, is concerned that he may incur a myocardial infarction (MI). What sign would alert the nurse that this client may be developing this acute condition?
1. Hoarseness
2. Pink, foamy sputum
3. Indigestion
4. Swelling of the feet and ankles

16. 3. A sensation, often described as heartburn, is commonly associated with an impending MI. Hoarseness is a classic sign of a thoracic aortic aneurysm which involves an outpouching of the vessel. Heart failure that can produce a pink foamy sputum. The swelling of the feet and ankles is associated with some cardiac conditions but is not is not directly associated with an MI.
CN: Physiological integrity; CNS: Physiological adaptation; CL: Analyze

17. A client is receiving furosemide for therapeutic diuresis. When administering furosemide, which level will require monitoring, and possible replacement, due to this diuresis?
1. Chloride
2. Magnesium
3. Potassium
4. Sodium

17. 3. Supplemental potassium may be administered with furosemide due to potassium loss that often occurs as a result of this diuretic. Neither chloride, magnesium nor sodium are lost during diuresis.
CN: Physiological integrity; CNS: Pharmacological and parenteral therapies; CL: Apply

18. A client is experiencing myocardial-infarction–induced heart failure. When assessing this client, the nurse should carefully auscultate for:
1. a third heart sound (S3).
2. a fourth heart sound (S4).
3. an aortic murmur.
4. aortic regurgitation.

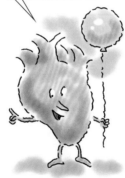

It's important to know what physiologic changes occur in your client after a heart attack.

18. 1. This client's condition can result in rapidly filling ventricles resulting in ventricular dilation. This can be auscultated as a third heart sound (S3). Systemic hypertension, or increased atrial contraction, can result in a fourth heart sound. Aortic valve malfunction is heard as a murmur while aortic regurgitation is the result of an incompetent aortic valve.
CN: Health promotion and maintenance; CNS: None; CL: Analyze

19. The nurse auscultates lung crackles in a client who has experienced an anterior-wall myocardial infarction (MI). Which diagnosis is supported by the presence of these sounds?
1. Left-sided heart failure
2. Pulmonic valve malfunction
3. Right-sided heart failure
4. Tricuspid valve malfunction

19. 1. The left ventricle is responsible for most of the cardiac output. An anterior-wall MI may result in a decrease in left ventricular function. Left ventricle malfunction results in left-sided heart failure, fluid accumulation in the interstitial and alveolar spaces and lungs crackles. Pulmonic and tricuspid valve malfunction will cause right-sided heart failure.
CN: Physiological integrity; CNS: Physiological; CL: Apply

20. The nurse has just admitted a client to the emergency department for evaluation of a possible myocardial infarction (MI). Which diagnostic intervention, by the nurse, would be **priority**?
1. Cardiac catheterization
2. Cardiac enzymes
3. Echocardiogram
4. Electrocardiogram (ECG)

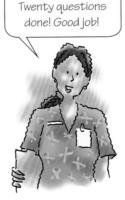

Twenty questions done! Good job!

20. 4. An ECG is the quickest, most accurate, and most widely used tool to determine the location of MI. Cardiac catheterization is an invasive study used to determine coronary artery disease. While it may also indicate the location of myocardial damage, the study may not be performed initially. Cardiac enzymes are used to diagnose MI but do not determine the location. An echocardiogram is used to view myocardial wall function after an MI has been diagnosed.
CN: Physiological integrity; CNS: Reduction of risk potential; CL: Apply

21. What is the **priority** nursing intervention for a client experiencing a myocardial infarction (MI)?
1. Administering morphine
2. Administering oxygen
3. Administering sublingual nitroglycerin
4. Obtaining an electrocardiogram (ECG)

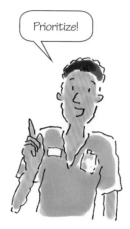

Prioritize!

21. 2. Administering supplemental oxygen to the client is the priority of care. The myocardium is deprived of oxygen during an infarction, so additional oxygen is administered to assist in oxygenation and prevent further damage. Morphine and sublingual nitroglycerin are also used to treat MI, but are commonly administered after oxygen. An ECG is the most common diagnostic tool used to evaluate MI.

CN: Safe, effective care environment; CNS: Management of care; CL: Analyze

22. A client who experienced a myocardial infarction (MI) tells the nurse that he is fearful of dying. Which statement, by the nurse, will help validate this client's feelings?
1. "Tell me more about your fear of dying."
2. "It must be very frightening to be told that you've had a MI."
3. "Facing death would certainly be a frightening experience for me."
4. "Please be assured that we're doing everything possible to prevent you from dying."

22. 2. The nurse should validate this client's feelings by acknowledging his fear. This provides the client with a sense of being understood, and demonstrates empathy. The nurse should explore this client's fear of dying after he is in more stable condition. Any response that focuses on the staff, rather than the client, is not appropriate and will not validate this client's feelings.

CN: Psychosocial integrity; CNS: None; CL: Analyze

23. The nurse understands that certain medications protect the ischemic myocardium by blocking catecholamines and sympathetic nerve stimulation. Which class of medications serve this function?
1. Beta-adrenergic blockers
2. Calcium channel blockers
3. Opioids
4. Nitrates

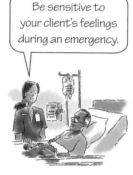

Be sensitive to your client's feelings during an emergency.

23. 1. Beta-adrenergic blockers work by blocking beta receptors in the myocardium, reducing the response to catecholamines and sympathetic nerve stimulation. They protect the myocardium, and help reduce the risk of another infarction by decreasing the workload of the heart and decreasing myocardial oxygen demand. Calcium channel blockers reduce the workload of the heart by reducing contractility and vasodilatation; thus, lowering afterload. Opioids reduce myocardial oxygen demand, promote vasodilation, and decrease anxiety. Nitrates reduce myocardial oxygen consumption by decreasing left ventricular end-diastolic pressure and systemic vascular resistance.

CN: Physiological integrity; CNS: Pharmacological and parenteral therapies; CL: Apply

24. A client who experienced a myocardial infarction (MI) 48 hours ago is **most** at risk for the developing:
1. cardiogenic shock.
2. heart failure.
3. arrhythmias.
4. pericarditis.

24. 3. Arrhythmias, caused by oxygen deprivation to the myocardium, are the most common complication of an MI. Cardiogenic shock, another complication of MI, is defined as the end stage of left ventricular dysfunction. The condition occurs in approximately 15% of clients with MI. Because the pumping function of the heart is compromised by an MI, heart failure is the second most common complication. Pericarditis most commonly results from a bacterial or viral infection but may occur one week after a MI.

CN: Physiological integrity; CNS: Physiological adaptation; CL: Apply

CN: Client needs category   CNS: Client needs subcategory   CL: Cognitive level

25. A client, diagnosed with heart failure, suddenly develops dyspnea at rest, disorientation, confusion, and crackles in the lung bases on auscultation. What are the important nursing interventions? Select all that apply.
1. Insert a Foley catheter
2. Monitor urinary output
3. Administer nasal oxygen
4. Administer a prescribed rapid-acting diuretic
5. Place the client in a modified Trendelenburg position
6. Administer the ordered 500-ml IV bolus of normal saline solution

25. 1, 2, 3, 4. Acute pulmonary edema is a life-threatening event in which the left ventricle of the heart fails to eject sufficient blood. Pressure in the lungs increases because of accumulated blood. The nurse should begin interventions to decrease this pressure. The client should be placed in high Fowler's position to facilitate respirations. The nurse should ensure that vascular access is available, but IV fluids are not administered because they will increase body fluid. Oxygen should be administered. The provider will often prescribe a rapid-acting diuretic to eliminate body fluid. A Foley catheter should be inserted to assess urinary output and to minimize exertion related to voiding.
CN: Physiological integrity; CNS: Physiologic adaptation; CL: Apply

26. The nurse is preparing to assess a client for jugular vein distention. How should the nurse position the head of this client's bed?
1. High Fowler's
2. Raised 10 degrees
3. Raised 30 degrees
4. Supine

26. 3. Jugular venous pressure is measured with a centimeter ruler to obtain the vertical distance between the sternal angle and the point of highest pulsation with the head of the bed inclined between 15 and 30 degrees. Increased pressure cannot be seen when the client is supine or when the head of the bed is raised 10 degrees because the point that marks the pressure level is above the jaw. The veins would be barely discernible above the clavicle if the client were in high Fowler's position.
CN: Physiological integrity; CNS: Health promotion and maintenance; CL: Analyze

Remember

"Digoxin rocks at treating heart failure."

Digoxin, a cardiac glycoside, treats heart failure by strengthening the contraction of the ventricles by increasing intracellular calcium at the cell membrane. It also slows the heart rate and can be used to treat certain cardiac arrhythmias.

27. The nurse is preparing to administer the initial dose of digoxin PO to a client. What is the nurse's **priority** assessment before administering this medication?
1. Apical heart rate
2. Blood pressure
3. Radial heart rate
4. Respiratory rate

27. 1. Assessing the client's apical heart rate is essential before administering digoxin. The apex of the heart is the most accurate pulse point in the body. Blood pressure is only affected if the heart rate is too low, in which case the nurse would withhold digoxin. The radial heart rate can be affected by cardiac and vascular disease and; therefore, will not accurately depict the heart rate. Digoxin has no effect on respiratory function.
CN: Physiological integrity; CNS: Pharmacological and parenteral therapies; CL: Apply

28. The nurse is performing a client's admission assessment. Which assessment finding would support the possibility that this client may have cardiovascular disease? Select all that apply.
1. Fatigue
2. Chest pain
3. Weight loss
4. Light-headedness
5. Dependent edema
6. Dyspnea when upright

28. 1, 2, 4, 5. Cardiovascular disease is any abnormal condition characterized by dysfunction of the heart and blood vessels. Common clinical manifestations of cardiovascular disease include chest pain, irregularities of the heart rhythm, cyanosis, fatigue, light-headedness, weight gain, dependent edema, and dyspnea. The client may report dyspnea when lying in a flat position, but not while upright.
CN: Physiological integrity; CNS: Physiological; CL: Apply

CN: Client needs category   CNS: Client needs subcategory   CL: Cognitive level

29. A nurse is monitoring a client for manifestations of cardiac tamponade. Which findings would support this diagnosis? Select all that apply.
1. Bradycardia
2. Hypertension
3. Restlessness
4. Muffled heart sounds
5. Widened pulse pressure
6. Distended neck veins

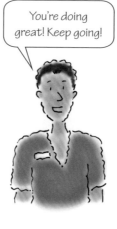

You're doing great! Keep going!

29. 3, 4, 6. Cardiac tamponade is a life-threatening condition caused by the accumulation of fluid in the pericardium. This fluid, which can be blood, pus, or air, compresses the heart and restricts blood flow to the ventricles. Symptoms of cardiac tamponade include elevated venous pressure, distended neck veins, Kussmaul's sign, hypotension and narrowed pulse pressure, tachycardia, dyspnea, restlessness, and anxiety, cyanosis of the lips and nails, diaphoresis, muffled heart sounds, pulsus paradoxus, decreased friction rub, decreased QRS voltage, and electrical alternans.
CN: Physiological integrity; CNS: Physiological adaptation; CL: Apply

30. While assessing a bedridden client, the nurse notes the presence of sacral edema. Which **most** likely has contributed to the edema?
1. Diabetes mellitus
2. Pulmonary emboli
3. Chronic kidney disease
4. Right-sided heart failure

30. 4. The sacral area is the most accurate area on the body to assess dependent edema in a bedridden client. Sacral, or dependent, edema is secondary to right-sided heart failure. Diabetes mellitus, pulmonary emboli, and chronic kidney disease aren't directly linked to sacral edema.
CN: Physiological integrity; CNS: Physiological adaptation; CL: Apply

31. A client experiencing right-sided heart failure is at greatest risk for developing:
1. hematuria.
2. polyuria.
3. oliguria.
4. polydipsia.

31. 3. Inadequate deactivation of aldosterone by the liver following right-sided heart failure will lead to fluid retention, which causes oliguria. Neither hematuria, polyuria, nor polydipsia are associated with right-sided heart failure.
CN: Physiological integrity; CNS: Physiological adaptation; CL: Apply

32. A client has been prescribed digoxin to increase the heart's ability to contract effectively. The nurse is teaching a client about common side effects of digoxin. Of which side effect should this client be aware?
1. Dizziness
2. Anxiety
3. Hyperactivity
4. Headache
5. Diarrhea
6. Weight loss

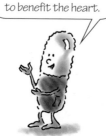

Make sure you understand how these different drugs work to benefit the heart.

32. 1, 2, 4, 5. Inotropic agents such as digoxin can trigger common side effects such as dizziness, anxiety, headache, and diarrhea. Changes in mood and alertness that include confusion and depression, rather than hyperactivity, may be observed. Weight loss is not associated with cardiac glycosides. The client should be instructed to notify their health care provider if any of these side effects become severe.
CN: Physiological integrity; CNS: Physiological adaptation; CL: Apply

33. What is the **priority** nursing intervention for a client experiencing a dysrhythmia that continues to deteriorate and requires converting?
1. Administer 1 mg of epinephrine IV
2. Defibrillate
3. Initiate CPR
4. Administer vasopressin 40 units IV

33. 2. To attempt to convert the rhythm, the nurse should first defibrillate the client. If this is unsuccessful, then CPR should be initiated. Epinephrine and vasopressin may be given, but only after two defibrillation attempts.
CN: Physiological integrity; CNS: Physiological adaptation; CL: Analyze

CN: Client needs category   CNS: Client needs subcategory   CL: Cognitive level

34. A nursing assessment confirms that a client, being evaluated for a cardiac-related diagnosis, is experiencing weight gain, nausea, and decreased urine output. The nurse suspects that this client may be experiencing:
  1. angina pectoris.
  2. cardiomyopathy.
  3. left-sided heart failure.
  4. right-sided heart failure.

34. 4. Weight gain, nausea, and decreased urine output are secondary effects of right-sided heart failure. Cardiomyopathy is usually identified as a symptom of left-sided heart failure. Left-sided heart failure primarily causes pulmonary symptoms rather than systemic ones. Angina pectoris doesn't cause weight gain, nausea, or a decrease in urine output.
CN: Physiological integrity; CNS: Physiological: CL: Apply

35. A client's cardiac rhythm strip shows a regular rhythm with atrial and ventricular rates of 70 beats per minute, a PR interval of 0.24 seconds, and a QRS duration of 0.08 seconds. The nurse interprets this rhythm as:
  1. Normal sinus rhythm (NSR)
  2. NSR with first-degree atrioventricular (AV) block
  3. Sinus arrhythmia
  4. Accelerated junctional rhythm.

35. 2. An increased PR interval is indicative of a first-degree AV block. NSR and sinus arrhythmia have normal PR intervals. The PR interval, if present, is less than 0.12 seconds in accelerated junctional rhythm.
CN: Physiological integrity; CNS: Physiologic adaptation; CL: Apply

36. While palpating a client's abdomen, the nurse notes a pulsating abdominal mass. How should the nurse interpret this assessment?
  1. Abdominal aortic aneurysm
  2. Enlarged spleen
  3. Gastric distention
  4. Gastritis

36. 1. The presence of a pulsating mass in the abdomen is an abnormal finding, and usually indicates an outpouching in a weakened vessel. The finding; however, can be normal on a very thin person. An enlarged spleen, gastric distention, and gastritis do not cause pulsation.
CN: Health promotion and maintenance; CNS: None; CL: Understand

37. The nurse understands that the **most** common symptom in a client with abdominal aortic aneurysm is:
  1. abdominal pain.
  2. diaphoresis.
  3. headache.
  4. upper back pain.

37. 1. Abdominal pain in a client with an abdominal aortic aneurysm results from the disruption of normal circulation in the abdominal region. Diaphoresis and headache are not associated with abdominal aortic aneurysm. Lower back pain usually signifies expansion and impending rupture of the aneurysm.
CN: Physiological integrity; CNS: Basic care and comfort; CL: Understand

38. A client with an abdominal aortic aneurysm is admitted to a step-down unit. The nurse should intervene **immediately** if this client experiences:
  1. a migraine-like headache.
  2. cramping in the legs.
  3. sudden, severe back pain.
  4. diaphoresis.

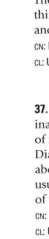

Looking good! Keep at it!

38. 3. If expansion and impending rupture of an abdominal aneurysm is suspected, the nurse should assess for acute and severe pain in the back or lower abdomen, which may radiate to the groin. None of the other options indicate a change in the status of the client's aneurysm.
CN: Physiological integrity; CNS: Physiological adaptation; CL: Apply

CN: Client needs category   CNS: Client needs subcategory   CL: Cognitive level

39. A client is scheduled for testing to diagnose an abdominal aortic aneurysm. What is the **most** definitive test for this condition?
1. Abdominal X-ray
2. Aortogram
3. Computed tomography (CT) scan
4. Ultrasound

39. 2. An aortogram accurately and directly depicts the vasculature, and clearly delineates the vessels and abnormalities. An abdominal aneurysm would only be visible on an X-ray if it were calcified. A CT scan or ultrasound don't give a direct view of the vessels, and don't yield as accurate a diagnosis as the aortogram.
CN: Health promotion and maintenance; CNS: None;
CL: Understand

40. The nurse is caring for a preoperative client with an abdominal aortic aneurysm. The nurse understands that this client is **most** at risk for:
1. hypertension.
2. aneurysm rupture.
3. cardiac arrhythmias.
4. diminished pedal pulses.

40. 2. Rupture of the aneurysm is a life-threatening emergency, and is the greatest concern for the nurse caring for this client. Hypertension should be avoided and controlled because it can cause the weakened vessel to rupture. Cardiac arrhythmias aren't directly linked to an aneurysm. Diminished pedal pulses, a sign of poor circulation to the lower extremities, are associated with an aneurysm, but aren't life threatening.
CN: Physiological integrity; CNS: Physiological adaptation;
CL: Understand

41. A client, who experienced a myocardial infarction, has received a thrombolytic agent. What is the **most** important nursing intervention during the next 24 hours?
1. Assessing for bleeding
2. Monitoring the client's potassium levels
3. Maintaining the client a supine position
4. Encouraging the client to ingest fluids

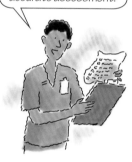

Knowing which symptom relates to which complication will help you to make a more accurate assessment.

41. 1. Thrombolytic agents are declotting agents that place the client at risk for hemorrhage from puncture wounds. All unnecessary needle sticks and invasive procedures should be avoided. The potassium level should be monitored in all cardiac clients, not just those receiving a thrombolytic agent. Although no specific position is required, most cardiac clients prefer semi-Fowler's position. The client's fluid balance must be carefully monitored. Encouraging fluids may be inappropriate at this time.
CN: Physiological integrity; CNS: Reduction of risk potential;
CL: Apply

42. The nurse is assessing the abdomen of a client admitted for a possible abdominal aneurysm. Where should the nurse palpate to determine this condition?
1. Right upper quadrant
2. Directly over the umbilicus
3. Middle lower abdomen to the left of the midline
4. Middle lower abdomen to the right of the midline

42. 3. The aorta lies directly left of the umbilicus; therefore, any other region is inappropriate for palpation.
CN: Physiological integrity; CNS: Basic care and comfort;
CL: Apply

43. The nurse is preforming an admission assessment on a client diagnosed with an abdominal aortic aneurysm. For which comorbidity should the nurse assess?
   1. Diabetes mellitus
   2. Hypertension
   3. Peripheral vascular disease
   4. Syphilis

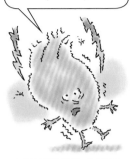

I'm suddenly feeling a little jittery, a little high-strung. (Get it?)

43. 2. Continuous pressure on the vessel walls from hypertension, can weaken the walls and cause an aneurysm. Diabetes mellitus doesn't have a direct link to aneurysm. Atherosclerotic changes can occur with peripheral vascular diseases, and are loosely linked to aneurysms. Only 1% of clients with syphilis experience an aneurysm.
CN: Health promotion and maintenance; CNS: None;
CL: Apply

44. When auscultating the abdominal region of a client with abdominal aortic aneurysm, the nurse hears a bruit. How should the nurse interpret this finding?
   1. Normal finding
   2. Reflects a partial arterial occlusion
   3. Indicates a collection of fluid in the lungs
   4. Shows an inflammation of the peritoneal surface

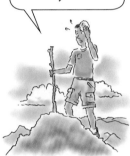

This is a real bruit of a question.

44. 2. A bruit is a vascular sound that reflects partial arterial occlusion. It is not a normal finding. Fluid in the lungs is called crackles. Inflammation of the peritoneal surface produces a friction rub.
CN: Physiological integrity; CNS: Basic care and comfort;
CL: Understand

45. The nurse assessing a client with an abdominal aortic aneurysm is **most** concerned when the client presents with:
   1. lower back pain, increased blood pressure, decreased red blood cell (RBC) count, and increased white blood cell (WBC) count.
   2. severe lower back pain, decreased blood pressure, decreased RBC count, increased WBC count.
   3. severe lower back pain, decreased blood pressure, decreased RBC count, decreased WBC count.
   4. intermittent lower back pain, decreased blood pressure, decreased RBC count, increased WBC count.

45. 2. Severe lower back pain indicates an aneurysm rupture, secondary to pressure being applied within the abdominal cavity. When rupture occurs, the pain is constant until the aneurysm is repaired. Blood pressure decreases due to the loss of blood after the aneurysm ruptures. The RBC count is decreased. The WBC count increases as cells migrate to the site of injury.
CN: Physiological integrity; CNS: Physiological adaptation;
CL: Apply

46. During the assessment of a client who had an abdominal aortic repair, the nurse notes a hematoma in the perineal area. The nurse interprets this as:
   1. a hernia.
   2. a stage-one pressure ulcer.
   3. a retroperitoneal rupture at the repair site.
   4. the rapid expansion of the aneurysm.

46. 3. Blood collects in the retroperitoneal space and is exhibited as a hematoma in the perineal area. This rupture is most commonly caused by leakage at the repair site. A hernia doesn't cause vascular disturbances, nor does a pressure ulcer. Because no bleeding occurs with rapid expansion of the aneurysm, a hematoma will not form.
CN: Physiological integrity; CNS: Physiological adaptation;
CL: Apply

47. A client, recently diagnosed with an aneurysm, asks the nurse if any genetic disease is closely linked to aneurysm formation. What is the nurse's **best** response?
1. Cystic fibrosis
2. Hemophilia
3. Marfan's syndrome
4. Sickle cell anemia

48. A client displays signs associated with a possible ruptured aortic aneurysm. What is the **priority** nursing intervention?
1. Administer prescribed antihypertensive medication
2. Prepare the client for an aortogram
3. Administer prescribed beta-adrenergic blocker medication
4. Prepare the client for surgical intervention

49. A nurse is teaching a group of nursing students about dilated cardiomyopathy (DCM). Which statements, made by the students, would indicate that teaching was effective? Select all that apply.
1. "Pregnancy may play a role in developing this form of cardiomyopathy."
2. "Initial symptoms of DCM are often increasing fatigue and dyspnea."
3. "Management of DCM focuses on decreasing cardiac workload."
4. "DCM is a rare form of cardiomyopathy."
5. "Obesity is a possible risk factor for DCM."
6. "DCM is curable with prompt, effective treatment."

50. Which type of cardiomyopathy is associated with childbirth?
1. Dilated
2. Hypertrophic obstructive
3. Myocarditis
4. Restrictive

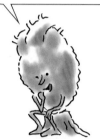

Think! This question is asking for a treatment, not a preventive measure.

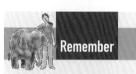

Remember

"-lol drugs make blood pressure fall."

Beta-adrenergic antagonists, which typically end in "-lol," are used for treating hypertension, along with arrhythmias and angina. Beta-adrenergic antagonists include the following:

- Atenolol
- Carvedilol
- Metoprolol
- Nadolol
- Propranolol

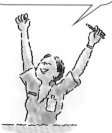

You've finished 50 questions! Good job!

47. 3. Marfan's syndrome results in the degeneration of the elastic fibers of the aortic media. Therefore, clients with this syndrome are more likely to develop an aneurysm. Although cystic fibrosis, hemophilia, and sickle cell anemia are all genetic diseases, they have not been linked to aneurysms.

CN: Health promotion and maintenance; CNS: None; CL: Apply

48. 4. When the vessel ruptures, prompt surgery is required for it's repair. Antihypertensive medications and beta-adrenergic blockers can help control hypertension, reducing the risk of rupture. An aortogram is a diagnostic tool used to detect an aneurysm.

CN: Physiological integrity; CNS: Basic care and comfort; CL: Apply

49. 1, 2, 3, 5. DCM, the most common form of cardiomyopathy, is associated with risk factors that include pregnancy and obesity. Initial symptoms include increasing fatigue, dyspnea and activity intolerance as well as the classic symptoms of heart failure. While DCM is a chronic, non-curable disease, management focuses on decreasing cardiac workload.

CN: Physiological integrity; CNS: Physiological; CL: Apply

50. 1. Dilated cardiomyopathy, defined as deterioration in cardiac function, typically presents between the last month of pregnancy and up to six months postpartum. The cause isn't entirely known. The condition may result from cardiomyopathy not apparent prior to pregnancy. Hypertrophic obstructive cardiomyopathy is an abnormal symmetry of the ventricles that has an unknown etiology but a strong familial tendency. Myocarditis isn't a form of cardiomyopathy. It is an inflammation of the cardiac muscle. Restrictive cardiomyopathy is rare and typically results in restricted ventricular filling.

CN: Physiological integrity; CNS: Physiological adaptation; CL: Apply

51. The nurse is reviewing an echocardiogram report of a client with hypertrophy of the ventricular septum. The nurse understands that this client should be further evaluated for:
  1. congestive cardiomyopathy.
  2. dilated cardiomyopathy.
  3. hypertrophic obstructive cardiomyopathy.
  4. restrictive cardiomyopathy.

51. **3.** In hypertrophic obstructive cardiomyopathy, hypertrophy of the ventricular septum is apparent. This abnormality isn't seen in other types of cardiomyopathy. Congestive cardiomyopathy does not exist.
CN: Physiological integrity; CNS: Physiological adaptation;
CL: Understand

52. A nurse, caring for a client with cardiomyopathy, is aware that this client is at high risk for developing:
  1. heart failure.
  2. diabetes mellitus.
  3. myocardial infarction (MI).
  4. pericardial effusion.

52. **1.** Because the structure and function of the heart muscle is affected, heart failure commonly occurs in clients with cardiomyopathy. Diabetes mellitus is unrelated to cardiomyopathy. Myocardial infarction results from prolonged myocardial ischemia due to reduced blood flow through one of the coronary arteries. Pericardial effusion is most predominant in clients with pericarditis.
CN: Physiological integrity; CNS: Physiological adaptation;
CL: Understand

53. While assessing a client with dilated cardiomyopathy, the nurse notices that the electrocardiogram (ECG) rhythm no longer has any P waves, only a fine wavy line. The ventricular rhythm is irregular with a QRS duration of 0.08 seconds. The heart rate is 110 bpm. The nurse interprets this rhythm as:
  1. atrial fibrillation.
  2. ventricular fibrillation.
  3. atrial flutter.
  4. sinus tachycardia.

53. **1.** Atrial fibrillation is defined as chaotic, asynchronous, electrical activity in the atrial tissue. On an ECG, uneven baseline fibrillating waves appear rather than distinguishable P waves. Ventricular fibrillation is a chaotic rhythm with no QRS complexes. In atrial flutter, there are flutter waves that are "sawtooth" in appearance. P waves are present in sinus tachycardia and represented as flutter waves.
CN: Physiological integrity; CNS: Physiological adaptation;
CL: Apply

54. The nurse performs an assessment on a newly-admitted client with a diagnosis of left-sided heart failure. What data should the nurse document to support this diagnosis? Select all that apply.
  1. Chronic cough
  2. Lower extremity edema
  3. Chest pain
  4. Rapid weight gain
  5. Flushed face
  6. Rapid pulse

These symptoms are classic, if you catch my drift.

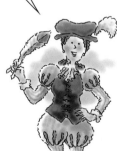

54. **1, 2, 4, 6.** Chronic cough, lower extremity edema, rapid weight gain, and rapid pulse are the classic symptoms of left-sided heart failure. A flushed face is usually associated with hypertension. Chest pain is usually associated with a myocardial infarction.
CN: Physiological integrity; CNS: Physiological adaptation;
CL: Apply

55. The nurse determines further teaching is necessary when a client with cardiomyopathy states:
  1. "Dilated cardiomyopathy decreases cardiac output."
  2. "Cardiac output increases in hypertrophic obstructive cardiomyopathy."
  3. "Cardiac output is not affected by hypertrophic obstructive cardiomyopathy."
  4. "Restrictive cardiomyopathy decreases cardiac output."

55. 2. Cardiac output isn't affected by hypertrophic obstructive cardiomyopathy, because the size of the ventricle remains relatively unchanged. Dilated cardiomyopathy and restrictive cardiomyopathy decrease cardiac output.
CN: Physiological integrity; CNS: Physiological adaptation; CL: Apply

56. The nurse, performing a cardiac assessment on a client, auscultates a fourth heart sound (S4). How should the nurse interpret this finding?
  1. Dilated aorta
  2. An older but normally functioning heart
  3. Decreased myocardial contractility
  4. Failure of the ventricle to eject all the blood during systole

It's important to know what the different sounds I make indicate.

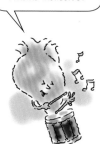

56. 4. An S4 occurs as a result of increased resistance to ventricular filling after atrial contraction. This increased resistance is related to decreased compliance of the ventricle. A dilated aorta doesn't cause an extra heart sound, though it does cause a murmur. Decreased myocardial contractility is heard as a third heart sound. An S4 isn't heard in a normally functioning heart.
CN: Physiological integrity; CNS: Physiological; CL: Understand

57. A client is being treated for dilated cardiomyopathy. Which medication would this client **most** likely receive?
  1. Anticoagulants
  2. Beta-adrenergic blockers
  3. Calcium channel blockers
  4. Nitrates

57. 2. By decreasing the heart rate and contractility, beta-adrenergic blockers improve myocardial filling and cardiac output, which are primary goals in the treatment of dilated cardiomyopathy. Anticoagulants are infrequently used to reduce the risk of emboli. Calcium channel blockers are sometimes used for the same reasons as beta-adrenergic blockers; however, they aren't as effective as beta-adrenergic blockers, and can cause increased hypotension. Nitrates aren't used because of their dilating effects, which would further compromise the myocardium.
CN: Physiological integrity; CNS: Pharmacological and parenteral therapies; CL: Apply

58. A client, diagnosed with cardiomyopathy, is demonstrating signs of left-sided heart failure with an ejection fracture is 50%. While providing this client with education regarding management of his condition, which interventions should the nurse include? Select all that apply.
  1. Implantable cardioverter defibrillator
  2. Low sodium diet
  3. Graduated exercise program
  4. Antidiuretic medication therapy
  5. Anticoagulant medication therapy
  6. ACE inhibitor medication therapy

58. 2, 3, 4, 6. The multi-faceted treatment will include a low sodium diet, gradual increase in activity and diuretic medication therapy to decrease fluid overload and cardiac workload. The use of ACE inhibitors, in conjunction with beta-adrenergic blockers will affect myocardial tissue remodeling. Anticoagulant therapy is not indicated in the management of these conditions at this time. An implantable cardioverter defibrillator becomes an option when the ejection fracture is below 35%.
CN: Physiological integrity; CNS: Physiological adaptation; CL: Analyze

59. A client, diagnosed with a form of angina, presents with a predictable level of pain that occurs during physical or emotional stress. What form of angina should the nurse focus on when preparing educational information?
1. Microvascular angina
2. Stable angina
3. Unstable angina
4. Variant angina

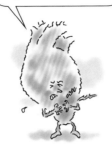

Stress can be a real pain in the heart.

60. After undergoing a cardiac catheterization, a client has a large puddle of blood under his buttocks. What is the nurse's **priority** action?
1. Call for help
2. Obtain vital signs
3. Ask the client to "lift up"
4. Assess the groin site

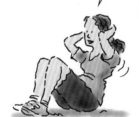

This is a tough one! Keep plugging along!

61. A client diagnosed with angina pectoris has a stat electrocardiogram (ECG) performed during an episode of chest pain. The nurse reviews the ECG and notes myocardial ischemia. How would myocardial ischemia be represented on an ECG?
1. Increased QRS duration
2. Shortened PR interval
3. Pathological Q-wave formation
4. T-wave inversion.

62. A client diagnosed with an impending myocardial infarction (MI) is experiencing angina. How should the nurse document this angina?
1. Variant angina
2. Chronic stable angina
3. Microvascular angina
4. Unstable angina

63. A client with a history of angina pectoris comes to the emergency room for treatment of the associated pain. For which medication would the nurse anticipate an order to relieve this pain?
1. Aspirin
2. Furosemide
3. Nitroglycerin
4. Nifedipine

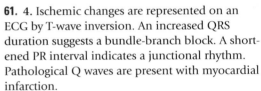

59. 2. The pain of stable angina is predictable in nature, builds gradually, and quickly reaches maximum intensity. Microvascular angina is characterized by pain lasting longer than 10 minutes. Unstable angina doesn't always need a trigger, is more intense, and lasts longer than stable angina. Variant angina usually occurs at rest, and not as a result of exertion or stress.
CN: Physiological integrity; CNS: Physiological adaptation; CL: Understand

60. 4. Assessment of the groin site is the priority. This establishes the source of the blood, and determines how much blood has been lost. The goal is to stop the bleeding. The nurse would call for help if needed after the assessment of the situation. After determining the extent of the bleeding, vital sign assessment is important. The nurse should never move the client, in case a clot has formed. Moving can disturb the clot and cause re-bleeding.
CN: Physiological Integrity; CNS: Physiologic Adaptation; CL: Apply

61. 4. Ischemic changes are represented on an ECG by T-wave inversion. An increased QRS duration suggests a bundle-branch block. A shortened PR interval indicates a junctional rhythm. Pathological Q waves are present with myocardial infarction.
CN: Physiological integrity; CNS: Physiological adaptation; CL: Analyze

62. 4. Unstable angina progressively increases in frequency, intensity, and duration and is related to an increased risk of MI within 3 to 18 months. Variant angina is related to coronary artery spasm, chronic stable angina is predictable and relieved by rest and nitrates. Microvascular angina is related to impairment of vasodilator reserve in normal coronary arteries.
CN: Physiological integrity; CNS: Physiological; CL: Apply

63. 3. Nitroglycerin is administered to reduce the myocardial demand, which decreases ischemia and relieves pain. In addition, nitroglycerin dilates the vasculature and reduces preload. Aspirin is administered to reduce the risk of myocardial infarction in clients with unstable angina. Furosemide is a loop diuretic that doesn't reduce pain or prevent angina. Nifedipine is a calcium channel blocker primarily used to decrease coronary artery spasm and hypertension.
CN: Physiological integrity; CNS: Pharmacological and parenteral therapies; CL: Analyze

CN: Client needs category   CNS: Client needs subcategory   CL: Cognitive level

64. While assessing a client diagnosed with angina, the client asks, "What causes this pain in my heart?" What is the nurse's **best** response?
1. Increased preload
2. Decreased afterload
3. Coronary artery spasm
4. Inadequate myocardial oxygenation

64. 4. Inadequate oxygen supply to the myocardium is responsible for the pain accompanying angina. Increased preload would be responsible for right-sided heart failure. Decreased afterload causes increased cardiac output. Coronary artery spasm is responsible for variant angina.
CN: Physiological integrity; CNS: Physiological adaptation;
CL: Apply

65. A nurse is preparing a client for cardiac catheterization. What is the nurse's **priority** assessment?
1. Weight and height
2. Known allergies
3. Apical heart rate
4. Cardiac rhythm

65. 2. Since cardiac catheterization involves the injection of a radiopaque dye. It is most important for the nurse to determine if this client has allergies to iodine or shellfish. The other three parameters are also part of the assessment, but are not the priority.
CN: Physiological integrity; CNS: Reduction of risk potential;
CL: Analyze

66. What is the nurse's **primary** treatment goal for a client diagnosed with angina?
1. Reversal of ischemia
2. Reversal of infarction
3. Reduction of stress and anxiety
4. Reduction of associated risk factors

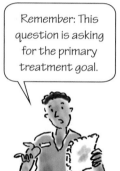

Remember: This question is asking for the primary treatment goal.

66. 1. Reversing the ischemia is the primary goal, achieved by reducing oxygen consumption and increasing oxygen supply. An infarction is permanent and can't be reversed. Reducing the associated risk factors, including stress and anxiety, will decrease the risk for angina attacks, but will not reverse the ischemia.
CN: Physiological integrity; CNS: Physiological adaptation;
CL: Apply

67. A client is experiencing chest pain at rest. The pain is unresponsive to nitroglycerine. The client is diagnosed with unstable angina, and the nurse immediately begins intervention. Which treatment is **most** appropriate for this client?
1. Cardiac catheterization
2. Echocardiogram
3. Heart transplantation
4. Percutaneous transluminal coronary angioplasty (PTCA)

67. 1. Cardiac catheterization is a diagnostic tool used to locate the blockage causing the angina. PTCA can alleviate the blockage and restore blood flow and oxygenation, but would not be done without the information provided by cardiac catheterization. An echocardiogram is a non-invasive diagnostic test used to identify various abnormalities in the heart muscle and valves. Heart transplantation involves replacing the client's heart with a donor heart, and is a treatment for end-stage cardiac disease.
CN: Physiological integrity; CNS: Physiological adaptation;
CL: Apply

68. The nurse is ambulating a client. The client experiences chest pain after ambulating 50 feet. What is the nurse's **priority** intervention?
1. Sit the client down
2. Get the client back to bed
3. Obtain an electrocardiogram (ECG)
4. Administer the ordered sublingual nitroglycerin

68. 1. The priority is to decrease oxygen consumption by sitting this client down. When the client's condition is stabilized, he can be returned to bed. An ECG can be obtained after the client is sitting down, and the ordered sublingual nitroglycerin could be administered.
CN: Physiological integrity; CNS: Basic care and comfort;
CL: Analyze

69. The nurse is assessing a client diagnosed with heart failure. Which nursing intervention would reduce the client's risk of developing cardiogenic shock?
1. Using aseptic technique
2. Administering supplemental oxygen
3. Applying elastic compression stockings
4. Assessing the client for known allergies

69. **2.** Cardiogenic shock is caused by reduced cardiac output and ineffective pumping of the heart. Supplemental oxygen would help manage these needs. Anaphylactic shock would result from an allergic reaction. An allergy assessment would be a focused intervention. The prevention of distributive shock involves supporting the client's cardiovascular and neurological function. Applying elastic compression stockings to help prevent blood from pooling in the legs would decrease the risk of distributive shock. Septic shock because is associated with systemic infection. The risk would be minimized by the strict implementation of aseptic technique for all invasive procedures.
CN: Physiological integrity; CNS: Physiological adaptation; CL: Analyze

70. Which condition would place a client at greatest risk for developing cardiogenic shock?
1. Acute myocardial infarction (MI)
2. Coronary artery disease
3. Decreased hemoglobin level
4. Hypotension

70. **1.** Fifteen percent of those who experience an acute MI will also experience cardiogenic shock secondary to the myocardial damage and decreased function. Coronary artery disease is a cause of MI. A decreased hemoglobin level is a result of bleeding. Hypotension is the result of a reduced cardiac output produced by the shock state.
CN: Physiological integrity; CNS: Reduction of risk potential; CL: Analyze

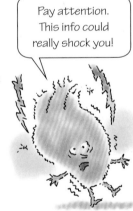

Pay attention. This info could really shock you!

71. Four clients have been admitted to the cardiac intensive care unit after experiencing acute myocardial infarctions. Each client has sustained a percentage of cardiac damage. Which client is **most** in need of interventions to prevent the development of cardiogenic shock?
1. The client with 10% damage
2. The client with 25% damage
3. The client with 40% damage
4. The client with 70% damage

71. **3.** At least 40% of the heart muscle must be involved for cardiogenic shock to develop. In most circumstances, the heart can compensate for up to 25% damage. An infarction involving 70% of the heart would have likely already caused cardiogenic shock.
CN: Physiological integrity; CNS: Physiological adaptation; CL: Understand

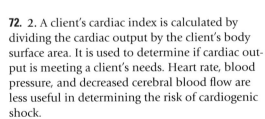

72. A client is at risk for developing cardiogenic shock. Which is a presenting symptom of this condition?
1. Decreased heart rate
2. Decreased cardiac index
3. Decreased blood pressure
4. Decreased cerebral blood flow

72. **2.** A client's cardiac index is calculated by dividing the cardiac output by the client's body surface area. It is used to determine if cardiac output is meeting a client's needs. Heart rate, blood pressure, and decreased cerebral blood flow are less useful in determining the risk of cardiogenic shock.
CN: Physiological integrity; CNS: Physiological adaptation; CL: Apply

73. The nurse is assessing a client who is display-ing the earliest sign of cardiogenic shock. The nurse would document this assessment finding as:
1. cyanosis.
2. decreased urine output.
3. presence of fourth heart sound (S4).
4. altered level of consciousness.

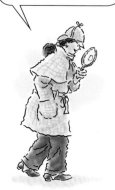

Pay attention. This question involves assessing the order of symptoms.

74. The nurse is monitoring the arterial blood gas (ABG) results of a client recovering from a myocar-dial infarction (MI). Which aspects of post-MI care are affected by ABG results? Select all that apply.
1. Fluid therapy
2. Physical activity
3. Oxygenation therapy
4. Ventilator support
5. Electrolyte therapy
6. Anticoagulation therapy

75. The nurse is planning care for a client in car-diogenic shock. What is the **priority** outcome for this client?
1. Correct hypoxia
2. Prevent infarction
3. Correct metabolic acidosis
4. Increase myocardial oxygen supply

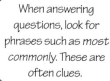

When answering questions, look for phrases such as *most commonly*. These are often clues.

76. Which class of drug is **most** commonly pre-scribed to increase cardiac output?
1. Beta-adrenergic agonist
2. Angiotensin-converting enzyme inhibitor
3. Loop diuretic
4. Beta blocker

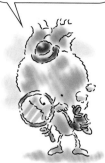

77. What is the nurse's **most** important tool for monitoring the severity of a shock state?
1. Arterial line
2. Indwelling urinary catheter
3. Electrocardiogram (ECG) monitor
4. Pulmonary artery catheter

73. 4. A decrease in cardiac output would initially result in decreased cerebral blood flow resulting in restlessness, agitation, or confusion. Cyanosis, decreased urine output, and the presence of an S4 are all later signs of shock.
CN: Physiological integrity; CNS: Physiological adaptation; CL: Apply

74. 1, 3, 4, 5. Arterial blood gas levels reflect cellular metabolism and oxygenation status. The nurse should evaluate the effectiveness of ther-apies, monitor the client's clinical status, and determine treatment needs based on ABG results. Arterial blood gas results are not a primary source of information used to formulate physical activity or anticoagulation therapy post MI.
CN: Reduction of Risk Potential; CNS: None; CL: Analyze

75. 4. A balance must be maintained between oxygen supply and demand. In a shock state, the myocardium requires more oxygen. If it can't get more oxygen, the effects of shock increase. Increasing oxygen will play a large role in correct-ing metabolic acidosis and hypoxia. Infarction typically causes the shock state, so prevention isn't an appropriate goal for this condition.
CN: Physiological integrity; CNS: Physiological adaptation; CL: Apply

76. 1. A Beta-adrenergic agonist, such as dobutamine is a direct-acting inotropic agent whose primary activity would result in an increase in cardiac output. An angiotensin-converting enzyme inhibitor directly lowers blood pressure. A loop diuretic doesn't have a direct effect on con-tractility or tissue perfusion. A beta blocker slows the heart rate and lowers blood pressure.
CN: Physiological integrity; CNS: Pharmacological and parenteral therapies; CL: Apply

77. 4. A pulmonary artery catheter will give accu-rate pressure measurements within the heart, that help determine the course of treatment. An arterial line, an indwelling urinary catheter, and an ECG monitor all provide valuable information related to the severity of a shock state but aren't the most important tools.
CN: Physiological integrity; CNS: Physiological adaptation; CL: Analyze

78. What would be heard during the first phase of Korotkoff's sounds?
1. Disappearance of sounds
2. Faint, clear tapping sounds
3. A murmur or swishing sounds
4. Soft, muffling sounds

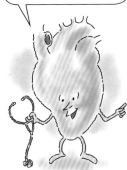

Did you hear that? Sounds like someone is dancing.

79. In what way do the kidneys attempt to normalize blood pressure when hypertension occurs?
1. The kidneys retain sodium and excrete water.
2. The kidneys excrete sodium and excrete water.
3. The kidneys retain sodium and retain water.
4. The kidneys excrete sodium and retain water.

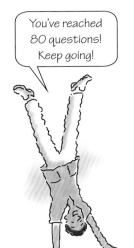

You've reached 80 questions! Keep going!

80. A nurse is teaching a client about the effects of angiotensin II on blood pressure. The nurse knows that teaching has been effective when the client states:
1. "It is a powerful vasodilator."
2. "It increases aldosterone secretion."
3. "It brings about a diuretic effect."
4. "It stimulates the parasympathetic nervous system."

81. How would the nurse **best** describe the characteristics of primary hypertension to a client?
1. It is uncontrollable, and has a rapid onset of complications.
2. It is a rapidly progressive increase in blood pressure.
3. It is a gradual and asymptomatic increase in blood pressure.
4. It can be corrected by treating the underlying conditions.

78. 2. Auscultation in phase I, would produce a faint, clear tapping sound that gradually increases in intensity. Phase II produces a murmur sound. Phase III produces a more intense murmur sound. A muffled sound that gives a soft blowing noise is heard in phase IV. Phase V, the final phase, is marked by the disappearance of sounds.
CN: Physiological integrity; CNS: Basic care and comfort;
CL: Remember

79. 2. The kidneys respond to a rise in blood pressure by excreting sodium and excess water. This response ultimately affects systolic blood pressure by regulating blood volume. Sodium or water retention would increase blood pressure. Sodium and water travel together across the membrane in the kidneys. One cannot travel without the other.
CN: Physiological integrity; CNS: Physiological adaptation;
CL: Understand

80. 2. Angiotensin II is a potent vasoconstrictor that increases aldosterone secretion and causes retention of sodium and water. Both of these affects result in an increase of blood pressure. Angiotensin II stimulates the sympathetic nervous system resulting in vasoconstriction.
CN: Physiological integrity; CNS: Physiological adaptation;
CL: Understand

81. 3. Primary hypertension is characterized by a progressive, gradual, usually asymptomatic increase in blood pressure. It is the most common type of hypertension. Malignant hypertension, also known as accelerated hypertension, is an uncontrollable, rapidly progressing form that causes a rapid onset of complications. Secondary hypertension occurs secondary to a known, correctable cause.
CN: Physiological integrity; CNS: Physiological adaptation;
CL: Understand

82. Prioritize the steps needed to perform an electrocardiogram (ECG).

| **1.** Wash hands |
| **2.** Clean the gel from the client's skin |
| **3.** Apply conductive gel to the client's skin |
| **4.** Disconnect the electrodes from the client |
| **5.** Attach electrodes to the client's skin and obtain a reading |
| **6.** Explain the importance of lying still, breathing normally, and refraining from talking during the test |

82. Ordered Response:

| **1.** Wash hands |
| **6.** Explain the importance of lying still, breathing normally, and refraining from talking during the test |
| **3.** Apply conductive gel to the client's skin |
| **5.** Attach electrodes to the client's skin and obtain a reading |
| **4.** Disconnect the electrodes from the client |
| **2.** Clean the gel from the client's skin |

CN: Physiological integrity; CNS: Physiological adaptation; CL: Apply

83. The nurse is evaluating the following telemetry strip. What information should the nurse document regarding this strip?

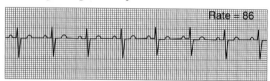

Rate = 86

1. Sinus tachycardia with a heart rate of 86 to 100
2. Normal sinus rhythm with heart rate of about 80
3. First-degree heart block with PR interval greater than 0.20 seconds
4. Pacemaker beat with a 1:1 capture

83. 2. Characteristics of normal sinus rhythm include the presence of uniform P waves preceding each QRS complex, a heart rate between 60 and 100/bpm, and regular rhythm. This is not sinus tachycardia because the heart rate is below 100. This is not first-degree heart block because the PR interval is 0.20 seconds, which is in the normal range. This is not pacemaker beat because it has uniform P waves, not spikes.
CN: Physiological integrity; CNS: Physiological adaptation; CL: Apply

84. Which statement **best** describes the action of furosemide for the treatment of hypertension?
1. It dilates peripheral blood vessels.
2. It decreases sympathetic cardioacceleration.
3. It inhibits the angiotensin-converting enzyme.
4. It inhibits reabsorption of sodium and water in the loop of Henle.

This question is asking for the mechanism of action of furosemide.

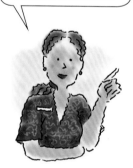

84. 4. Furosemide is a loop diuretic that inhibits sodium and water reabsorption in the loop of Henle, thereby causing a decrease in blood pressure. Vasodilators cause dilation of peripheral blood vessels, directly relaxing vascular smooth muscle and decreasing blood pressure. Adrenergic blockers decrease sympathetic cardioacceleration and decrease blood pressure. Angiotensin-converting enzyme inhibitors decrease blood pressure due to their action on angiotensin.
CN: Physiological integrity; CNS: Pharmacological and parenteral therapies; CL: Apply

85. A client with a history of hypertension has just had a total hip replacement. The provider orders hydrochlorothiazide 35 mg oral solution po/day. The label on the solution reads hydrochlorothiazide 50 mg/5 ml. How many milliliters should the nurse pour to administer the correct dose? Record your answer using one decimal place.

_____ ml

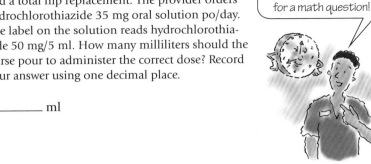

Yep. That's right. Time for a math question!

85. 3.5.

The correct formula to calculate a drug dosage is:

Dose on hand ÷ Quantity on hand = Dose desired ÷ X

In this example, the equation is:

$$50\ mg \div 5\ ml = 35\ mg \div X$$

$$X = 3.5\ ml$$

CN: Physiological integrity; CNS: Pharmacological and parenteral therapies; CL: Apply

86. Which statement, by a client with a history of hypertension, indicates that teaching regarding an annual eye exam has been effective?
1. "By examining your corneas, an ophthalmologist can visualize microvascular hemorrhages in your eyes."
2. "By examining the fovea in your eyes, an ophthalmologist can visualize microvascular venous occlusions in your eyes."
3. "By examining the retina in your eyes, an ophthalmologist can detect changes in the arteries in your eyes."
4. "By examining the sclera of your eyes, an ophthalmologist can detect changes in the arteries in your eyes."

86. 3. The retina is the only site in the body where arteries can be seen without invasive techniques. Changes in the retinal arteries signal similar damage to vessels elsewhere. The cornea is the nonvascular, transparent fibrous coat where the iris can be seen. The fovea is the point of central vision. The sclera is the fibrous tissue that forms the outer protective covering over the eyeball.

CN: Health promotion and maintenance; CNS: None; CL: Analyze

87. A nurse is assessing a client, with a history of varicose veins, for possible superficial thrombophlebitis. What would the nurse document? Select all that apply.
1. Redness
2. Induration
3. Warmth
4. Tenderness
5. Twisted appearance
6. Blue-color

87. 1, 2, 3, 4. Superficial thrombophlebitis is the inflammation of a superficial vein accompanied by the formation of a clot. Clinical manifestations of superficial thrombophlebitis include redness, induration, warmth, and tenderness along a vein. Discomfort may be relieved by applying heat. Activity is encouraged as prescribed, and a supportive wrap or stocking should be applied. Dilated blue-colored veins describe varicose veins.

CN: Physiological integrity; CNS: Physiological adaptation; CL: Apply

88. A nurse determines that a client understands the cause of primary varicose veins when the client states:
1. "Hypertension."
2. "Pregnancy."
3. "Thrombosis."
4. "Trauma."

88. 2. Primary varicose veins have a gradual onset and progressively worsen. In pregnancy, the expanding uterus and increased vascular volume impede blood return to the heart. The pressure places increased stress on the veins. Hypertension has no role in varicose vein formation. Thrombosis and trauma cause valvular incompetence and so are secondary causes of varicosities.

CN: Health promotion and maintenance; CNS: None; CL: Apply

89. Which manifestation of varicose veins would the nurse anticipate while assessing a woman in the third trimester of pregnancy? Select all that apply.
1. Leg fullness
2. Cool feet
3. Sharp calf pain
4. Leg ulcerations
5. Leg fatigue
6. Rest pain

89. 1, 5. Leg fatigue and fullness are classic signs of varicose veins, secondary to increased blood volume and edema. Sharp pain, leg ulcerations, rest pain and cool feet are symptoms of alteration in arterial blood flow.
CN: Physiological integrity; CNS: Physiological adaptation; CL: Understand

90. A nurse monitors a client, with a tumor of the esophagus, for signs of superior vena cava (SVC) syndrome. For which symptoms would the nurse assess this client? Select all that apply.
1. Epistaxis
2. Periorbital edema
3. Edema in the hands
4. Dyspnea
5. Mental status changes
6. Decrease in neck circumference

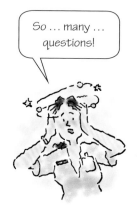

So ... many ... questions!

90. 1, 2, 3, 4, 5. SVC syndrome occurs when the SVC is compressed or obstructed by tumor growth. The manifestations result from the blockage of venous blood flow to the head, neck, and upper trunk. Early manifestations occur when the client arises after a night's sleep, and include edema of the face, especially around the eyes, and tightness of the shirt or blouse collar (Stokes' sign) due to edema. As the compression worsens, edema in the hands and arms, dyspnea, erythema of the upper body, and epistaxis occur. Late manifestations include hemorrhage, cyanosis, mental status changes, decreased cardiac output, and hypotension.
CN: Physiological integrity; CNS: Physiological adaptation; CL: Apply

91. Which condition is caused by increased hydrostatic pressure and chronic venous stasis?
1. Venous occlusion
2. Cool extremities
3. Nocturnal calf muscle cramps
4. Diminished blood supply to the feet

91. 3. Calf muscle cramps result from increased pressure and venous stasis secondary to varicose veins. An occlusion is a blockage of blood flow. Cool extremities and diminished blood supply to the feet are symptoms of arterial blood flow changes.
CN: Health promotion and maintenance; CNS: None; CL: Understand

92. The nurse is providing discharge instructions to a client with varicose veins. The nurse determines the need for further teaching when the client states:
1. "Exercise will make me feel better."
2. "I have to elevate my legs."
3. "Lying down can relieve my symptoms."
4. "Wearing tight clothing will not affect me."

92. 4. Tight clothing, especially below the waist, will increase vascular volume and impedes blood return to the heart. Exercise, leg elevations, and lying down usually relieve symptoms of varicose veins.
CN: Health promotion and maintenance; CNS: None; CL: Analyze

93. A client suspects that they have deep venous thrombosis (DVT). Which diagnostic studies should the nurse anticipate to verify this suspicion? Select all that apply.
1. Platelet count
2. D-dimer blood test
3. Electrocardiography
4. Venous duplex scanning
5. Magnetic resonance imaging (MRI)
6. International normalized ratio (INR)

93. 2, 4. Deep vein thrombosis is a disorder involving a thrombus in one of the deep veins of the body, most commonly the iliac or femoral veins. Venous duplex scanning is the primary diagnostic test for DVT because it allows visualization of the vein. The D-dimer blood test is also used in evaluation of DVT. The D-dimer is a product of fibrin degradation and is indicative of fibrinolysis, which occurs with thrombosis. A platelet count will not provide information related to the presence of DVT. An INR is a blood test used to evaluate the effectiveness of warfarin therapy. Electrocardiography evaluates the electrical activity of the heart. An MRI may be used for a variety of reasons, such as to detect the presence of a tumor. It will not diagnose DVT.

CN: Physiological integrity; CNS: Physiological adaptation; CL: Analyze

94. Which signs and symptoms associated with incompetent valves would the nurse anticipate in a client with secondary varicose veins?
1. Pallor and severe pain
2. Severe pain and edema
3. Edema and pigmentation
4. Absent hair growth and pigmentation

94. 3. Secondary varicose veins result from an obstruction of the deep veins. Incompetent valves lead to impaired blood flow, and edema and pigmentation result from venous stasis. Severe pain, pallor, and absent hair growth are symptoms of an altered arterial blood flow.

CN: Physiological integrity; CNS: Physiological adaptation; CL: Apply

95. Which intervention should the nurse include in teaching a client about post-venous ablation care for varicose veins?
1. Maintain bedrest for 24 to 36 hours
2. Keep the foot of the bed in a neutral position
3. Wear elastic compression stockings for two weeks
4. Apply moisturizing skin lotion to the extremities twice daily

95. 3. Nursing care, post venous ablation, includes the continuous application of elastic compression stockings for continuously for two weeks. Ambulation is encouraged as soon as anesthetic wears off, and progresses according to individual protocols. The foot of the bed should be elevated. Skin lotion should be avoided until incisions are completely healed.

CN: Physiological integrity; CNS: Reduction of risk potential; CL: Apply

96. Which client is **most** at risk for developing deep vein thrombosis (DVT)?
1. A 62-year-old female recovering from a total hip replacement
2. A 35-year-old female two days postpartum
3. A 33-year-old male runner with Achilles tendonitis
4. An ambulatory 70-year-old male who is recovering from pneumonia

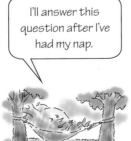

I'll answer this question after I've had my nap.

96. 1. DVT is most common in immobilized clients who have had surgical procedures such as total hip replacement. Pregnancy can cause varicose veins, which can lead to venous stasis, but it isn't a primary cause of DVT. Clients who are recovering from an injury or pneumonia may have decreased mobility, but these clients don't have the highest risk of developing DVT.

CN: Physiological integrity; CNS: Physiological adaptation; CL: Analyze

97. A client, admitted for lower extremity deep vein thrombosis (DVT), is experiencing dyspnea, chest pain, and diminished breath sounds. The nurse suspects that this client may be developing:
1. Hemothorax
2. Pneumothorax
3. Pulmonary embolism
4. Pulmonary hypertension

97. 3. A pulmonary embolism is a blood clot that forms in a vein, travels to the lungs, and lodges in the pulmonary vasculature. A hemothorax refers to blood in the pleural space. A pneumothorax is caused by an opening in the pleura. Pulmonary hypertension is an increase in pulmonary artery pressure, which increases the workload of the right ventricle.

CN: Physiological integrity; CNS: Physiological adaptation; CL: Apply

98. What term refers to the condition in which blood coagulates faster than normal, causing thrombin and other clotting factors to multiply?
1. Embolus
2. Hypercoagulability
3. Venous stasis
4. Venous wall injury

98. 2. Hypercoagulability is the condition of blood coagulating faster than normal, causing thrombin and other clotting factors to multiply. This condition, along with venous stasis and venous wall injury, accounts for the formation of deep vein thrombosis. An embolus is a blood clot or fatty globule that forms in one area and travels through the bloodstream to another area.

CN: Physiological integrity; CNS: Physiological adaptation; CL: Remember

99. A client is admitted with deep vein thrombosis (DVT). Which intervention would be **most** appropriate for pain relief?
1. Application of heat
2. Bed rest
3. Exercise
4. Leg elevation

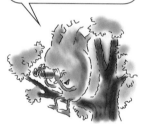

I see ... This question is asking you to characterize the type of pain experienced during deep vein thrombosis.

99. 4. Leg elevation alleviates the pressure caused by thrombosis and occlusion by easing venous return. The application of heat would dilate the vessels and cause blood to pool in the area of the thrombus, further increasing the risk of thrombus formation. Bed rest adds to venous stasis by increasing the risk of thrombosis formation. When DVT is diagnosed, exercise isn't recommended until the clot has dissolved.

CN: Physiological integrity; CNS: Basic care and comfort; CL: Apply

100. What assessment finding, by the nurse, would suggest that the client may have developed a deep vein thrombosis in the leg?
1. Coolness of the extremity
2. Calf tenderness
3. Appearance of a swollen vein
4. Decrease in calf size

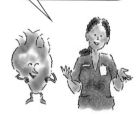

Congratulations! You've finished 100 questions! You're almost there!

100. 2. Clinical manifestations of obstruction of the deep veins include edema and swelling of the extremity because of the outflow of venous blood is inhibited. The extremity may feel warmer than the unaffected extremity and the superficial veins may appear more prominent. Tenderness is produced by inflammation of the vein wall and can be detected by gently palpating the extremity. A swollen vein is a sign of superficial thrombophlebitis

CN: Physiological integrity; CNS: Physiological adaptation; CL: Apply

101. The nurse is assessing a client with deep vein thrombosis (DVT). Which sign would be **most** supportive of this diagnosis?
1. Dyskinesia
2. Eversion
3. Positive Babinski's reflex
4. Pain on walking

102. A nurse is teaching a client about intermittent claudication. How would the nurse **best** describe this condition?
1. "It is caused by inadequate systemic blood supply."
2. "Leg position is the primary cause."
3. "A history of past leg trauma causes intermittent claudication."
4. "Inadequate muscle oxygenation is the cause of intermittent claudication."

103. The nurse anticipates that a client with intermittent claudication will receive:
1. analgesics.
2. warfarin.
3. heparin.
4. pentoxifylline.

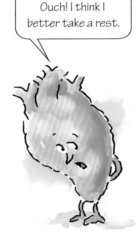

Ouch! I think I better take a rest.

104. Which oral medication would the nurse anticipate being prescribed to prevent further thrombus formation?
1. Warfarin
2. Heparin
3. Furosemide
4. Metoprolol

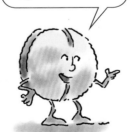

This question requires you to know how specific drugs are administered.

105. A client is experiencing acute pulmonary edema. How should the nurse position this client for maximum ventilation?
1. Lying flat in bed
2. Left side-lying
3. High-Fowler's position
4. Semi-Fowler's position

101. 4. Pain that occurs when walking is characteristic of DVT. Dyskinesia is the inability to perform voluntary movement. Eversion is the outward movement of the transverse tarsal joint. A positive Babinski's reflex is an extensor plantar response.
CN: Physiological adaptation; CNS: None; CL: Apply

102. 4. When a muscle is deprived of oxygen, it produces pain, much like that of angina. Inadequate systemic blood supply would cause necrosis, but the problem is actual oxygenation to the leg muscle. Leg position either alleviates or aggravates the condition. Leg trauma is not associated with this condition.
CN: Physiological integrity; CNS: Physiological adaptation; CL: Apply

103. 4. There are two main ways to treat claudication: medication and a surgical treatment, called revascularization. Pentoxifylline is one of the medications that are used. It decreases blood viscosity, increases red blood cell flexibility, and improves flow through small vessels. By improving the client's circulation, oxygenated blood flow is increased. When arterial pain becomes severe intermittent claudication progresses to rest pain. Analgesics would be prescribed rest pain relief. Warfarin and heparin are anticoagulants.
CN: Physiological integrity; CNS: Pharmacological and parenteral therapies; CL: Analyze

104. 1. Warfarin prevents vitamin K from synthesizing certain clotting factors. This oral anticoagulant can be given long term. Heparin is a parenteral anticoagulant that interferes with coagulation by readily combining with antithrombin. It cannot be administered orally. Neither furosemide nor metoprolol affects anticoagulation.
CN: Physiological integrity; CNS: Pharmacological and parenteral therapies; CL: Apply

105. 3. High-Fowler's position would maximize ventilation and facilitate breathing by reducing venous return. Lying flat and side-lying positions would worsen the breathing and increase the workload of the heart. Semi-Fowler's position will not reduce the workload of the heart as well as high-Fowler's position.
CN: Physiological adaptation; CNS: Basic care and comfort; CL: Apply

CN: Client needs category   CNS: Client needs subcategory   CL: Cognitive level

106. Which blood gas abnormality is **initially** suggestive of pulmonary edema?
1. Anoxia
2. Hypercapnia
3. Hyperoxygenation
4. Hypocapnia

106. 4. In an attempt to compensate for the increased work of breathing due to hyperventilation, CO_2 decreases, causing hypocapnia. If the condition persists, CO_2 retention occurs, and hypercapnia results. Although oxygenation is relatively low, the client isn't anoxic. Hyperoxygenation would result if the client was given oxygen in excess. This client would have a low oxygenation level secondary to fluid buildup.
CN: Physiological integrity; CNS: Physiological adaptation; CL: Apply

107. A nurse is caring for a client, with sick sinus syndrome, who is awaiting permanent pacemaker placement. Which assessment finding would indicate that this client is experiencing an acute drop in cardiac output and requires immediate pacemaker placement?
1. Decreased blood pressure
2. Alteration in level of consciousness (LOC)
3. Diuresis
4. Sustained tachycardia

107. 1. A decrease in blood pressure would indicate an acute decrease in cardiac output that requires immediate pacemaker placement. Alteration in LOC will only occur if the decreased cardiac output persists. This condition is characterized by alternating periods of bradycardia and tachycardia. Diuresis is not associated with a decrease in cardiac.
CN: Physiological integrity; CNS: Physiological adaptation; CL: Analyze

108. What action should the nurse take **first** when a client is coughing up pink, frothy sputum?
1. Place the client in high-Fowlers position
2. Plan to administer a diuretic
3. Start an IV line
4. Apply supplemental oxygen

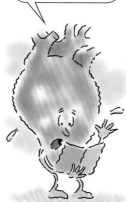

Don't panic! Just think about what to do first.

108. 1. Production of pink, frothy sputum is a classic sign of acute pulmonary edema Pulmonary edema requires immediate emergency treatment. The priority action is to place the client placed in high-Fowler's position to facilitate air exchange and improve oxygenation. After positioning the client, application of supplemental oxygen, IV access and drug therapy can be done. The goal of treatment is to reduce the amount of fluid in the lungs, improve gas exchange and heart function, and, if possible, correct the underlying disease. Because this client is at high risk for decompensation, the nurse should call for help without leaving the room.
CN: Physiological integrity; CNS: Physiological adaptation; CL: Analyze

109. The nurse is providing lifestyle teaching to a client who has experienced an acute episode of pulmonary edema. What instructions should the nurse provide? Select all that apply.
1. Limit caloric intake
2. Restrict carbohydrates
3. Measure the weight twice per day
4. Notify the provider of a daily weight gain greater than 3 lb (1.5 kg)
5. Follow a low-sodium diet
6. Engage in regular exercise

109. 4, 5, 6. Weight gain of 3 lb (1.5 kg) in one day is indicative of fluid retention that would increase the workload of the heart, and place the client at risk for acute pulmonary edema. Regular exercise and a low-sodium diet will help manage the workload of the heart. Limiting caloric intake doesn't influence fluid status. Restricting carbohydrates wouldn't affect fluid status. The client should be weighed each morning after the first urination. If the client is weighed later in the day, the finding will not be accurate because of fluid intake during the day.
CN: Physiological integrity; CNS: Reduction of risk potential; CL: Apply

110. A client with acute pulmonary edema has been taking an angiotensin-converting enzyme (ACE) inhibitor. The nurse explains that this medication has been ordered to:
1. promote diuresis.
2. increase cardiac output.
3. decrease contractility.
4. reduce blood pressure.

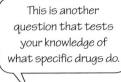

This is another question that tests your knowledge of what specific drugs do.

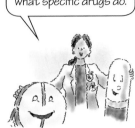

110. 4. ACE inhibitors are given to reduce blood pressure by inhibiting aldosterone production, which in turn decreases sodium and water reabsorption. ACE inhibitors also reduce production of angiotensin II, a potent vasoconstrictor. Diuretics are given to increase urine production. Vasodilators increase cardiac output. Negative inotropic agents decrease contractility.

CN: Physiological integrity; CNS: Pharmacological and parenteral therapies; CL: Apply

111. A client with acute pulmonary edema, caused by heart failure, asks the nurse which area of the heart has caused this condition. What is the nurse's **best** response?
1. Left atrium
2. Right atrium
3. Left ventricle
4. Right ventricle

111. 3. The left ventricle is responsible for the majority of force for cardiac output. If the left ventricle is damaged, the output decreases and fluid accumulates in the interstitial and alveolar spaces, causing pulmonary edema. Damage to the left atrium would contribute to heart failure, but wouldn't affect cardiac output or the onset of pulmonary edema. If the right atrium and right ventricle are damaged, right-sided heart failure would result.

CN: Physiological integrity; CNS: Physiological adaptation; CL: Apply

112. The nurse is assigned a client diagnosed with heart failure. Which statement **best** explains why the nurse should promptly report any changes in this client's respiratory rate?
1. Pulmonary edema, a life-threatening condition, can develop in minutes.
2. Severe acute respiratory syndrome (SARS) is a complication of heart failure.
3. Pneumonia is a consequence of inadequate ventilation with heart failure.
4. Pneumothorax, a life-threatening condition, can develop in minutes.

112. 1. Pulmonary edema can develop in minutes, secondary to a sudden fluid shift from the pulmonary vasculature to the lung interstitial alveoli. SARS and pneumonia are caused by infections. Pneumothorax is a collection of air or gas in the pleural space that causes a lung to collapse.

CN: Management of care; CNS: Reduction of risk potential; CL: Apply

113. The nurse evaluates previous teaching by asking the student nurse, "Which term is used to describe the amount of stretch on the myocardium at the end of diastole?" What is the student's **most** accurate response?
1. Afterload
2. Cardiac index
3. Cardiac output
4. Preload

113. 4. Preload is the amount of stretch of the cardiac muscle fibers at the end of diastole. The volume of blood in the ventricle at the end of diastole determines preload. Afterload is the force against which the ventricle must expel blood. Cardiac index is the individualized measurement of cardiac output, based on the client's body surface area. Cardiac output is the amount of blood the heart expels per minute.

CN: Physiological integrity; CNS: Physiological adaptation; CL: Understand

114. What is the **most** appropriate action for a nurse to take when administering a new blood pressure medication to a client?
1. Administer the medication to the client without explanation
2. Inform the client of the new drug only if he asks about it
3. Inform the client of the new medication, its name and use, and the reason for the medication
4. Administer the medication, and inform the client that the provider will later explain the medication

Which answer best promotes compliance?

114. 3. Informing the client of the medication, its use, and the reason for the medication change is important information for the client. Teaching the client about his treatment regimen promotes compliance. The other responses are inappropriate.
CN: Safe, effective care environment; CNS: Management of care; CL: Apply

115. The nurse is aware that antihypertensives should be used cautiously in clients already taking:
1. ibuprofen.
2. diphenhydramine.
3. thioridazine.
4. vitamins.

115. 3. Thioridazine affects the neurotransmitter norepinephrine, which causes hypotension and other cardiovascular effects. Administering an antihypertensive to a client who already has hypotension could have serious adverse effects. Ibuprofen is an anti-inflammatory that doesn't interfere with the cardiovascular system. Although diphenhydramine does have histaminic effects such as sedation, it isn't known to decrease blood pressure. Vitamins are not drugs and don't interfere with cardiovascular function.
CN: Physiological integrity; CNS: Pharmacological and parenteral therapies; CL: Apply

116. A client with a history of bronchial asthma is prescribed propranolol to control hypertension. Before administering propranolol, which **initial** action should the nurse take?
1. Monitor apical pulse rate
2. Instruct the client to take the medication with food
3. Question the provider about the order
4. Caution the client to rise slowly when standing

Note the word *initial* in question 116. It's the key to the right answer.

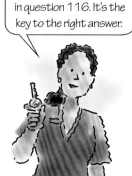

116. 3. Propranolol and other beta-adrenergic blockers are contraindicated in a client with bronchial asthma. The nurse should question the provider before giving the dose. The other responses are appropriate actions for a client receiving propranolol, but questioning the provider takes priority. The client's apical pulse should always be checked before giving propranolol. If the pulse rate is extremely low, the nurse should withhold the drug and notify the provider. Taking propranolol with food enhances its absorption. Because propranolol can cause light-headedness, the client should be told to rise slowly when standing.
CN: Physiological integrity; CNS: Pharmacological and parenteral therapies; CL: Apply

117. One hour after IV furosemide has been administered to a client with heart failure, a short burst of ventricular tachycardia appears on the cardiac monitor. Which electrolyte imbalance should the nurse suspect?
1. Hypocalcemia
2. Hypermagnesemia
3. Hypokalemia
4. Hypernatremia

117. 3. Furosemide is a potassium-depleting diuretic that can cause hypokalemia. In turn, hypokalemia increases myocardial excitability, leading to ventricular tachycardia. Hypocalcemia, which slows conduction through the atrioventricular junction, can cause such bradyarrhythmias as atrioventricular block. Hypermagnesemia may lead to bradycardia, not tachycardia. Hypernatremia may cause sinus tachycardia as a result of water loss.
CN: Physiological integrity; CNS: Physiological adaptation; CL: Apply

CN: Client needs category   CNS: Client needs subcategory   CL: Cognitive level

118. A client has a reduced serum high-density lipoprotein (HDL) level and an elevated low-density lipoprotein (LDL) level. Which dietary modification should the nurse recommend to this client?
1. Fiber intake of less than 10% of total calories daily
2. Less than 40% of calories from fat
3. Cholesterol intake of less than 300 mg daily
4. Less than 7% of calories from saturated fat

118. **4.** A client with low serum HDL and high serum LDL levels should get less than 7% of daily calories from saturated fat. Fiber intake should be at least 15% of total daily calories, total fat intake should be only 25% to 35% of daily calories, and cholesterol intake should be less than 200 mg daily.
CN: Physiological integrity; CNS: Reduction of risk potential;
CL: Apply

119. A paradoxical pulse occurs in a client who had coronary artery bypass graft (CABG) surgery two days ago. Which surgical complication would the nurse suspect?
1. Left-sided heart failure
2. Aortic regurgitation
3. Complete heart block
4. Pericardial tamponade

119. **4.** A paradoxical pulse can indicate pericardial tamponade, a complication of CABG surgery. Left-sided heart failure can cause pulsus alternans. Aortic regurgitation may cause bisferious pulse. Complete heart block may cause a bounding pulse.
CN: Physiological integrity; CNS: Physiological adaptation;
CL: Apply

120. A client was admitted to the coronary care unit (CCU) two days ago with an acute myocardial infarction. Which action would breach client confidentiality?
1. The CCU nurse gives a verbal report to the nurse on the telemetry unit before transferring the client to that unit.
2. The CCU nurse notifies the on-call provider about a change in the client's condition.
3. The emergency department (ED) nurse calls up the latest electrocardiogram results to check the client's progress.
4. At the client's request, the CCU nurse updates the client's wife on his condition.

120. **3.** The ED nurse is no longer directly involved with the client's care, and has no legal right to information about his present condition. Anyone directly involved in his care (such as the telemetry nurse and the on-call provider) has the right to information about his condition. Because this client asked the nurse to update his wife, doing so doesn't breach confidentiality.
CN: Safe, effective care environment; CNS: Management of care;
CL: Apply

121. A client is receiving CPR from paramedics as he arrives in the emergency department (ED). The paramedics are ventilating the client through an endotracheal tube placed prior to transport. During a pause in compressions, the cardiac monitor shows narrow QRS complexes and a heart rate of 55 bpm with a palpable pulse. Which action should the nurse take **first**?
1. Start an IV line and administer amiodarone
2. Check ET tube placement
3. Obtain an arterial blood gas (ABG) sample
4. Administer 1 mg atropine IV

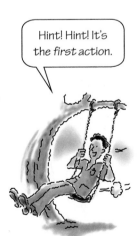

Hint! Hint! It's the first action.

121. **2.** Endotracheal tube placement should be confirmed as soon as the client arrives in the ED. Once the airway is verified, oxygenation and ventilation should be confirmed using an end-tidal carbon dioxide monitor and pulse oximetry. Next, the nurse should establish IV access. If the client experiences symptomatic bradycardia, atropine should be administered as ordered. The ABG sample would verify effectiveness of CPR ventilations. Amiodarone is indicated for ventricular tachycardia, ventricular fibrillation, and atrial flutter.
CN: Physiological integrity; CNS: Physiological adaptation;
CL: Apply

122. After unsuccessful CPR efforts, the nurse must prepare an Islamic client for the morgue. Which nursing action should the nurse take?
1. Asking the client's family if they want to perform the ritualistic washing
2. Doing nothing; the Burial Society will perform a ritual cleansing
3. Doing nothing; only the family and close friends may touch the body
4. Providing routine post-mortem care

122. 1. Physical care, at death, for a person of the Islamic faith consists of ritualistic washing by the family, with the client's body positioned toward Mecca. This action would be a family choice. The Burial Society may perform ritual cleansing for clients of the Jewish faith. Hindu clients believe that only family and close friends should touch the body. Routine post-mortem care is appropriate for Christian clients.
CN: Basic care and comfort; CNS: None; CL: Apply

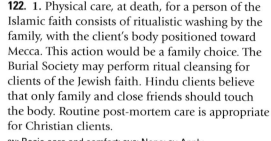

One of these medications will reduce the risk of coronary artery spasms.

123. A client has Prinzmetal's angina. Which type of medication should the nurse anticipate to reduce the risk of coronary artery spasms?
1. Beta-adrenergic blocker
2. Angiotensin-converting enzyme (ACE) inhibitor
3. Inotropic vasodilator
4. Calcium channel blocker

123. 4. A calcium channel blocker, such as diltiazem, is indicated for the management of Prinzmetal's angina. The class of medication would reduce the incidence of coronary artery spasm. A beta-adrenergic blocker, such as metoprolol, is used to treat angina by decreasing myocardial oxygen needs, and has no effect on coronary artery spasms. An ACE inhibitor, such as enalapril, is used to manage hypertension. An inotropic vasodilator, such as milrinone, is indicated for short-term IV therapy in heart failure.
CN: Physiological integrity; CNS: Pharmacological and parenteral therapies; CL: Apply

124. A client, with heart failure, is receiving furosemide, 40 mg IV. The provider orders 40 mEq of potassium chloride in 100 ml of dextrose 5% in water, to infuse over four hours. The client's most recent serum potassium level is 3.0 mEq/L. At which infusion rate should the nurse set the IV pump? Record your answer using a whole number.

_____ ml/hr

124. 25.
Use this formula to determine the infusion rate:

$$ml/hr = \frac{total\ volume\ (in\ ml)\ to\ be\ infused}{total\ time\ of\ infusion\ (in\ hr)}$$

$$ml/hr = \frac{100\ ml}{4\ hr}$$

$$ml/hr = 25$$

CN: Physiological integrity; CNS: Pharmacological and parenteral therapies; CL: Apply

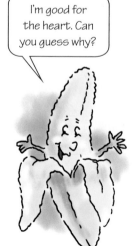

I'm good for the heart. Can you guess why?

125. A client diagnosed with electrolyte-imbalance induced ventricular tachycardia questions the need for more bananas in her diet. What is the **best** information the nurse can give this client?
1. Bananas are high in manganese.
2. Bananas are high in potassium.
3. Bananas are low in sodium.
4. Bananas are high in fiber.

125. 2. A low serum potassium level increases the risk of ventricular tachycardia. Therefore, the client should be instructed to eat potassium-rich foods such as bananas. None of the other options are associated with the prevention of ventricular tachycardia.
CN: Health promotion and maintenance; CNS: None; CL: Analyze

126. After cardiac surgery, a client's blood pressure measures 126/80 mmHg. How would the nurse interpret this client's mean arterial pressure (MAP), and organ perfusion status?
1. Organs are in danger of ischemia and perfusion pressure is critically low.
2. Organs are at risk for insufficient perfusion and perfusion pressure is borderline low.
3. Perfusion pressure is adequate to meet organs' perfusion needs.
4. Perfusion pressure minimally meets the organs' perfusion needs.

126. 3. Use this formula to calculate MAP:

$$MAP = \frac{systolic + 2\,(diastolic)}{3}$$

$$MAP = \frac{126\,mmHg + 2\,(80\,mmHg)}{3}$$

$$MAP = \frac{286\,mmHg}{3}$$

$$MAP = 95\,mmHg$$

This client's MAP is 95 mmHg. Normal MAP readings are 70 to 110. This client's organs are being adequately perfused.
CN: Physiological integrity; CNS: Reduction of risk potential; CL: Analyze

127. A client, who underwent femoral-popliteal (fem-pop) bypass surgery, is scheduled to return from the post-anesthesia care unit. Which staff member should receive this client?
1. Registered nurse with one year of experience
2. Licensed practical nurse (LPN) with five years of experience
3. Nursing assistant with 15 years of experience
4. Charge nurse with 10 years of experience

127. 1. Because this client requires frequent neurovascular assessments, a registered nurse should receive him. Although experienced and able to collect data, an LPN doesn't have the education to assess this client. The nursing assistant lacks the necessary assessment skills. The charge nurse needs to be available to direct the care of other clients.
CN: Safe, effective care environment; CNS: Management of care; CL: Analyze

128. A client, who recently had an upper respiratory infection, is admitted with suspected rheumatic fever. Which assessment findings confirm this diagnosis?
1. Erythema marginatum, subcutaneous nodules, and fever
2. Tachycardia, finger clubbing, and a loud second heart sound (S2)
3. Dyspnea, cough, and palpitations
4. Dyspnea, fatigue, and syncope

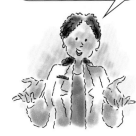

There are several findings here. Which answer confirms the diagnosis?

128. 1. A diagnosis of rheumatic fever requires that the client have either two major Jones criteria or one minor criterion, plus evidence of a previous streptococcal infection. Major criteria include carditis, polyarthritis, Sydenham's chorea, subcutaneous nodules, and erythema marginatum. Minor criteria include fever, arthralgia, elevated levels of acute phase reactants, and a prolonged PR interval on electrocardiography. Tachycardia, finger clubbing, and a loud S2 suggest transposition of the great arteries. Dyspnea, cough, and palpitations occur with mitral insufficiency. Dyspnea, fatigue, and syncope indicate aortic insufficiency.
CN: Physiological integrity; CNS: Physiological adaptation; CL: Apply

129. A client, with new onset of atrial fibrillation, is receiving warfarin to help prevent thromboemboli. The client will be discharged when the warfarin reaches therapeutic levels, and when the international normalized ratio (INR) ranges from:
1. 0.5 to 1 INR
2. 1.25 to 1.75 INR
3. 2 to 3 INR
4. 3.5 to 4 INR

129. 3. In a client with atrial fibrillation, the warfarin is at a therapeutic level when the INR ranges from 2 to 3. A range of 3.5 to 4 is too high, and increases the risk of hemorrhage. Discharge would be considered when the INR is within the therapeutic range.
CN: Physiological integrity; CNS: Reduction of risk potential; CL: Apply

130. A client comes to the emergency department stating, "My heart suddenly began to race." Cardiac monitoring identifies regular atrial and ventricular rhythm, a heart rate of 210 bpm, with the P wave hidden in the T wave. Which arrhythmia does the nurse identify from these characteristics?
1. Atrial flutter
2. Atrial fibrillation
3. Sinus tachycardia
4. Supraventricular tachycardia

130. 4. With supraventricular tachycardia, the rhythm is regular, the P wave is hidden in the preceding T wave, and the heart rate ranges from 140 to 250 bpm. A ventricular rate that varies with the degree of atrioventricular block, along with sawtooth P waves, characterizes atrial flutter. Irregular ventricular response, and absent P waves, characterize atrial fibrillation. Regular and equal atrial and ventricular rhythms and a rate of 100 to 160/bpm characterize sinus tachycardia.
CN: Physiological integrity; CNS: Physiological adaptation; CL: Apply

131. A client is receiving spironolactone to treat hypertension. Which instruction should the nurse provide?
1. Eat foods high in potassium
2. Take daily potassium supplements
3. Discontinue sodium restrictions
4. Avoid salt substitutes

131. 4. Because spironolactone is a potassium-sparing diuretic, the client should avoid salt substitutes because of their high potassium content. The client should also avoid potassium-rich foods and potassium supplements. To reduce fluid volume overload, sodium restrictions should continue.
CN: Physiological integrity; CNS: Pharmacological and parenteral therapies; CL: Apply

132. A client develops cardiac tamponade as a result of a motor vehicle collision. The provider performs a pericardiocentesis. Which assessment finding would indicate that this procedure has achieved the expected outcome?
1. Neck vein distention
2. Pulsus paradoxus
3. Increased blood pressure
4. Muffled heart sounds

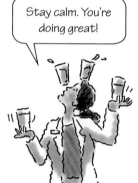

Stay calm. You're doing great!

132. 3. Cardiac tamponade is associated with decreased cardiac output, which in turn reduces blood pressure. By removing a small amount of blood from the pericardium, pericardiocentesis will increase blood pressure. Neck vein distention, pulsus paradoxus, and muffled heart sounds indicate persistent cardiac tamponade, and that pericardiocentesis hasn't been effective.
CN: Physiological integrity; CNS: Physiological adaptation; CL: Apply

133. A client, admitted with angina, reports severe chest pain and suddenly appears to lose consciousness and pulse. After calling for help and establishing unresponsiveness, which action should the nurse take **next**?
1. Deliver chest compressions
2. Open the client's airway
3. Check for breathing
4. Check for signs of circulation

133. 1. Compressions, airway, breathing guidelines state, immediately after calling out for help, and establishing unresponsiveness, the nurse should deliver chest compressions at a depth of at least two inches and at a rate of 100 compressions/min. After delivering 30 compressions, the nurse should open the airway by tilting the client's forehead back and lifting the chin. The nose should be pinched shut with forefinger and thumb, a normal-depth breath should be delivered over a one-second period of time, being sure the client's chest rises with each breath. After delivering two breaths, chest compressions should be continued. The nurse should deliver cycles of 30 compressions followed by two breaths until help arrives to supple the breaths and/or delivery an automatic external defibulator.
CN: Physiological integrity; CNS: Physiological adaptation; CL: Apply

134. A client is admitted with an acute inferior-wall myocardial infarction (MI). During the admission interview, the client states that he stopped taking his metoprolol five days ago because he was feeling better. For which complication should the nurse monitor this client?
1. Anxiety
2. Ineffective myocardial tissue perfusion
3. Sudden, acute pain
4. Hypertension

135. A client comes to the emergency department with acute shortness of breath and a cough that produces pink, frothy sputum. The client is restless and extremely anxious. Admission assessment reveals crackles and wheezes, a blood pressure of 82/45 mmHg, a heart rate of 120 bpm, and a respiratory rate of 38 breaths/min. The client's medical history includes hypertension, and heart failure. What is the nurse's **priority** intervention?
1. Providing supplemental oxygen
2. Elevating the head of the bed
3. Initiating intravenous access
4. Providing emotional support

136. The nurse is monitoring a client, who is six hours post embolectomy, for an acute arterial occlusion of the left leg. When a Doppler ultrasound fails to detect a pedal pulse, the nurse notifies the surgeon who requests that the client be prepared for immediate surgery. The client refuses to consider additional surgery. What is the nurse's **initial** intervention?
1. Reinforce the risks of not having the surgery
2. Notify the provider immediately
3. Notify the nursing supervisor
4. Record the client's refusal in the nurses' notes

137. The nurse is assigned to care for four clients. Which client should the nurse assess **first**?
1. A client admitted two days ago with heart failure, blood pressure of 126/76 mmHg, and a respiratory rate of 22 breaths/min
2. A client with end-stage, right-sided heart failure, with blood pressure of 78/50 mmHg, who is on hospice care
3. A client admitted one day ago with thrombophlebitis who is receiving IV heparin
4. A client admitted one hour ago with new-onset atrial fibrillation who is receiving IV diltiazem

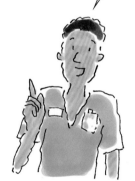

Here you're looking for the best initial response.

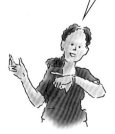

In answering this question, time is of the essence.

134. 2. Myocardial infarction results from prolonged myocardial ischemia caused by reduced blood flow through the coronary arteries. The priority for this client is to monitor for signs of ineffective myocardial tissue perfusion. While monitoring for anxiety, sudden and acute pain, as well as hypertension may be appropriate, such interventions are not the priority.
CN: Physiological integrity/adaptation; CNS: Management of care; CL: Analyze

135. 2. The most important intervention would be to facilitate air exchange. The priority action would be to elevate the head of the bed. Application of supplemental oxygen would be the next action. IV access and emotional support would follow.
CN: Physiological integrity; CNS: Reduction of risk potential; CL: Analyze

136. 2. The nurse should notify the health care provider. The health care provider is responsible for providing information regarding the procedure, risks, benefits and expected outcomes. After notifying the provider, the nurse should document the situation and client response in the client's record.
CN: Safe, effective care environment; CNS: Management of care; CL: Analyze

137. 4. The client with atrial fibrillation has the greatest potential to become unstable, and is on IV medication that requires close monitoring. After assessing this client, the nurse should assess the client with thrombophlebitis who is receiving a heparin infusion, and then the client admitted two days ago with heart failure. The client with end-stage right-sided heart failure, who is identified as a hospice client is of lowest priority.
CN: Safe, effective care environment; CNS: Management of care; CL: Analyze

138. A 23-year-old client admitted in hypovolemic shock. Which outcome suggests to the nurse that fluid resuscitation has been effective?
1. Urine output of 15 ml/hr
2. Urine output of 20 ml/hr
3. Urine output of 25 ml/hr
4. Urine output of 30 ml/hr

138. 4. In an adult, urine output below 30 ml/hr would indicate inadequate blood flow to the kidneys. Urine output of 30 ml/hr, or greater, reflects adequate fluid resuscitation.
CN: Physiological integrity; CNS: Physiological adaptation;
CL: Apply

139. A client is being monitored, via telemetry, using a three-lead system. Which illustration shows correct electrode placement to monitor modified chest lead one (MCL1)?

1.

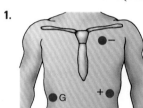

2.

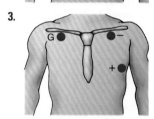

3.

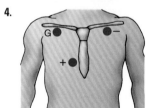

4.

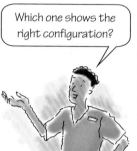

Which one shows the right configuration?

139. 4. Illustration four shows the correct electrode placement for MCL1. Illustration one shows the correct placement to monitor lead III. Illustration two shows the correct placement to monitor MCL6. Illustration three shows the correct placement to monitor lead II.
CN: Physiological integrity; CNS: Reduction of risk potential;
CL: Apply

140. An elderly client has a history of aortic stenosis. Where should the nurse should place the stethoscope to **best** hear the murmur?

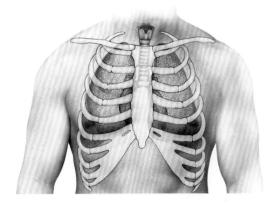

140. The murmur of aortic stenosis is low-pitched, rough, and rasping. It is heard loudest in second intercostal space to right of sternum.

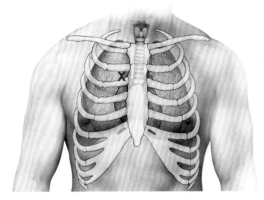

CN: Health promotion and maintenance; CNS: Physiological adaptation; CL: Apply

141. A client with deep vein thrombosis (DVT) has an IV infusion of heparin sodium infusing at 1,500 units/hr. The concentration in the bag is 25,000 units/500 ml. How many milliliters should the nurse document as intake from this infusion following an 8-hr shift? Record your answer using a whole number.

_____ ml

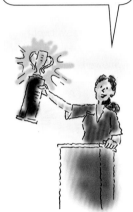

Congratulations! You finished the test!

141. 240.

First, calculate how many units are in each milliliter of the medication:

$$25,000 \ units/500 \ ml = 50 \ units/ml$$

Next, calculate how many milliliters the client receives each hr:

$$1 \ ml/50 \ units \times 1,500 \ units/hr = 30 \ ml/hr$$

Lastly, multiply by 8 hr:

$$30 \ ml/hr \times 8 \ hr = 240 \ ml$$

CN: Physiological integrity; CNS: Pharmacological and parenteral therapies; CL: Apply

Chapter 4

Hematologic & Immune Disorders

This challenging chapter covers HIV infection, AIDS, rheumatoid arthritis, ITP, and lots of other complex disorders. You can handle it, though, I know you can. Go for it!

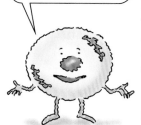

Remember to select all that apply—several answers will be right.

1. When reviewing the chart of a client recently diagnosed with AIDS, the nurse should expect to find which assessment data? Select all that apply.
   1. CD4+ count below 200 cells/μl
   2. Infection with HIV
   3. An alternative lifestyle
   4. Opportunistic infection
   5. T-cell count above 400 cells/μl

1. 1, 2, 4. According to the Centers for Disease Control and Prevention (CDC), three criteria must be met for an adult client to be diagnosed with AIDS. A person must be HIV-positive, have a CD4+ T-cell count below 200 cells/μl, and have an opportunistic infection such as tuberculosis, candidiasis, and cytomegalovirus. Because HIV attaches to the CD4+ receptor sites of the T cell, a T-cell value alone is incorrect.
CN: Physiological integrity; CNS: Physiological adaptation; CL: Apply

2. The nurse is gathering data on a client with pernicious anemia. Which data would support this diagnosis? Select all that apply.
   1. Angular cheilitis
   2. Smooth, bright-red tongue
   3. Hemoglobin of 14 g/dl (140 g/L)
   4. Sensitivity to cold
   5. Dyspnea on exertion

2. 1, 2, 4, 5. Pernicious anemia is a vitamin B_{12} deficiency due to lack of the intrinsic factor produced by gastric mucosa. Intrinsic factor is necessary for the absorption of vitamin B_{12}. Clinical manifestations include pallor, fatigue, dyspnea on exertion, angular chelitis (scaling of the surface of lips and fissures in the corner of the mouth), and sensitivity to cold. The client will also have a smooth, sore, bright red tongue because of the atrophy of the papillae of the tongue due to vitamin B_{12} deficiency. Hemoglobin of 14 g/dl (140 g/L) is normal.
CN: Physiological integrity; CNS: Physiological adaptation; CL: Apply

CN: Client needs category   CNS: Client needs subcategory   CL: Cognitive level

3. A nurse is assigned to care for a client who is a practicing Muslim. Which cultural considerations should the nurse include while caring for this client? Select all that apply.
  1. The administration of blood or blood products if necessary
  2. A preference for treatment by a health care worker of the same gender
  3. Meals that exclude pork but include other meat products from animals that have been ritually slaughtered
  4. The use of only the right hand when presenting items to the client
  5. Meals that do not combine meat and dairy products
  6. The refusal of organ donation or transplantation

3. 2, 3, 4. Muslims allow for the administration of blood and blood products. They prefer care from a health care worker of the same gender as themselves. Muslims do not eat pork, and only eat "halal" meat from ritually slaughtered animals. The nurse should always use the right hand in presenting items. The left hand is reserved for personal hygiene, and is considered unclean. Organ donation is allowed for the purpose of saving a life. Administration of blood and blood products is prohibited in Jehovah's Witness. Eating meat with milk is prohibited in Judaism.
CN: Psychosocial integrity; CNS: None; CL: Apply

4. A client is admitted to the hospital with pallor, fatigue, dry lips, and a smooth, bright-red tongue. A preliminary diagnosis of pernicious anemia has been made. Which diagnostic test would confirm this diagnosis?
  1. Bone marrow examination
  2. Ventilation-perfusion scan
  3. Schilling test
  4. Tensilon test

4. 3. Schilling test is performed to evaluate vitamin B_{12} absorption. It is used to diagnose pernicious anemia. Pernicious anemia is caused by lack of intrinsic factor produced by gastric mucosa, which is necessary for vitamin B_{12} absorption. In Schilling test, a radioactive vitamin B_{12} is given PO and then urine is collected over the next 24 hours to measure whether vitamin B_{12} is normally absorbed. Bone marrow examination is used for aplastic anemia. Ventilation-perfusion scan is used to help diagnose a client with pulmonary embolism. Tensilon test is a test for myasthenia gravis.
CN: Physiological integrity; CNS: Reduction of risk potential; CL: Apply

5. A client with HIV experiences frequent bouts of diarrhea. The nurse determines dietary teaching is effective when the client states the need to avoid which food?
  1. Milk
  2. Red licorice
  3. Chicken soup
  4. Broiled meat

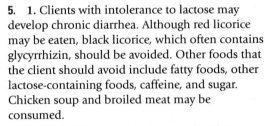

Spot on! A toast to your success.

5. 1. Clients with intolerance to lactose may develop chronic diarrhea. Although red licorice may be eaten, black licorice, which often contains glycyrrhizin, should be avoided. Other foods that the client should avoid include fatty foods, other lactose-containing foods, caffeine, and sugar. Chicken soup and broiled meat may be consumed.
CN: Physiological integrity; CNS: Basic care and comfort; CL: Apply

6. A nurse is preparing a dietary teaching plan for a client with rheumatoid arthritis. Which supplement will reduce inflammation for this client?
  1. Fish oil
  2. Vitamin D
  3. Iron-rich foods
  4. Calcium carbonate

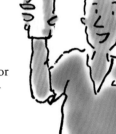

6. 1. Fish oil suppresses inflammatory mediator production (such as prostaglandins). Its mechanism of action is unknown. Iron-rich foods are recommended to decrease anemia associated with rheumatoid arthritis. Vitamin D and calcium supplements may help reduce bone resorption.
CN: Physiological integrity; CNS: Basic care and comfort; CL: Apply

7. A client diagnosed with uncomplicated rheumatoid arthritis is receiving naproxen. Which medication would require further intervention by the nurse prior to administration?
1. Cimetidine
2. Gabapentin
3. Dabigatran
4. Etanercept

8. The nurse is teaching a client about the transmission of HIV. Which statement demonstrates an understanding of the risks?
1. "I cannot have a routine teeth cleaning at the dentist's office."
2. "I may have intercourse with my spouse."
3. "I may engage in unprotected, non-insertive sexual contact."
4. "I should not engage in intercourse with a new partner without using a latex condom."

9. Which client is most likely to develop rheumatoid arthritis?
1. A 25-year-old woman
2. A 40-year-old man
3. A 65-year-old woman
4. A 70-year-old man

10. A nurse is caring for a client with AIDS. The client is receiving zidovudine. The client asked the nurse, "How does this drug work?" The nurse determines that teaching is effective when the client makes which statement?
1. "It kills HIV."
2. "It suppresses the replication of HIV virus."
3. "I won't infect anyone else when I take this drug."
4. "It's the only drug I need to take for HIV."

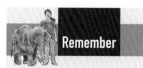

Remember

"Naproxen rocks at relieving rheumatoid arthritis."

Naproxen is a nonsteroidal anti-inflammatory drug (NSAID) used for clients with rheumatoid arthritis. Other NSAIDs are listed below.

NSAIDs
- Diclofenac
- Etodolac
- Fenoprofen
- Flurbiprofen
- Ibuprofen
- Indomethacin
- Ketoprofen
- Ketorolac
- Meloxicam
- Nabumetone
- Oxaprozin
- Piroxicam
- Sulindac

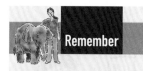

Remember

"Zidovudine zaps replication of the HIV virus."

Zidovudine is an antiviral drug that suppresses the replication of the HIV virus.

7. 3. Naproxen is a nonsteroidal anti-inflammatory drug (NSAID) used for clients with rheumatoid arthritis. NSAIDs are aspirin and aspirin-like medications that may increase the risk of bleeding when taken with an anticoagulant like dabigatran. Histamine H2 receptor antagonist drug used for peptic ulcer disease such as cimetidine, anticonvulsant drug gabapentin, and a tumor necrosis factor (TNF) blocker like etanercept will not cause serious drug interaction when taken with naproxen.
CN: Physiological integrity; CNS: Pharmacological and parenteral therapies; CL: Apply

8. 4. Intercourse with a new partner is risky because of the unknown intravenous drug use or sexual history of this partner. Using a latex condom may provide increased protection against HIV exposure. Absolute safe sex practices include autosexual activities, abstinence, and intercourse within a monogamous, uninfected partner. Very safe practices include non-insertive sexual contact. Having your teeth cleaned is not a risk factor if the dental office properly sterilizes the equipment.
CN: Health promotion and maintenance; CNS: None; CL: Analyze

9. 3. Rheumatoid arthritis affects women two to three times more often than men. The onset of rheumatoid arthritis in both men and women is highest among those in their 60s.
CN: Health promotion and maintenance; CNS: None; CL: Analyze

10. 2. Zidovudine is an antiviral drug that suppresses the replication of the HIV virus. It is most commonly used in conjunction with other anti-retroviral drugs. It also helps prevent the transmission of HIV from mother to fetus. Zidovudine is not a cure. It does not kill the HIV virus, and clients taking this medication remain infectious.
CN: Physiological integrity; CNS: Pharmacological and parenteral therapies; CL: Analyze

11. A nursing student is assigned to care for client with HIV. The student asks the staff nurse what precautions are necessary when measuring this client's blood pressure. What is the **best** information to give the student?
1. Wear gloves
2. Wear a gown
3. Use contact precautions
4. Wash hands

11. 4. Because measuring blood pressure doesn't involve contact with the client's blood or secretions, the nursing student should wash the hands before proceeding.
CN: Safe and effective care environment; CNS: Safety and infection control; CL: Apply

12. A nurse is caring for a client diagnosed with Kaposi's sarcoma. The client's lesions have scant serous drainage. What personal protective equipment should the nurse wear? Select all that apply.
1. Gloves
2. Gown
3. Surgical mask
4. Particulate mask
5. Shoe cover

12. 1, 2. Kaposi's sarcoma is a type of skin cancer seen in clients with AIDS. It presents as a brownish-red to blue skin lesion. The nurse should wear gloves and gown when in contact with this client. All the other options are not necessary.
CN: Safe and effective care environment; CNS: Safety and infection control; CL: Apply

13. The nurse determines that teaching was successful when the client with rheumatoid arthritis (RA) makes which statement?
1. "It will get better and worse again."
2. "Once it clears up, it will never come back."
3. "I will be cured."
4. "It will never get any better than it is right now."

13. 1. The client with RA needs to understand that it is an autoimmune disease characterized by periods of exacerbation and remission. There's no cure, but symptoms can be managed. Surgery may be indicated in some cases.
CN: Psychosocial integrity; CNS: None; CL: Apply

14. A client with joint pain, tenderness and swelling has been admitted to the hospital. A disease modifying anti-rheumatic drug (DMARD) is prescribed by the health care provider. Which medication should the nurse expect to administer?
1. Aspirin
2. Methotrexate
3. Ferrous sulfate
4. Prednisone

Remember

"DMARDs retard rheumatoid arthritis."

Disease-modifying anti-rheumatic drugs (DMARDs), such as methotrexate, treat rheumatoid arthritis.

14. 2. Methotrexate is considered a first-line DMARD for most clients with rheumatoid arthritis (RA). NSAIDs, such as aspirin, cannot be tolerated. Ferrous sulfate is not used to treat RA. Prednisone may be used to control inflammation when NSAIDs cannot be used.
CN: Physiological integrity; CNS: Pharmacological and parenteral therapies; CL: Apply

15. The nurse is reviewing a client's complete blood count (CBC) and notes an erythrocyte count of $2.7 \times 10^6/\mu l$ (2.70×10^{12}/L), leukocytes of $2,100/\mu l$ (2.10×10^9/L), and platelets of $90,000/\mu l$ (90×10^9/L). The nurse interprets this as indicative of what condition?
1. Pernicious anemia
2. Aplastic anemia
3. Sickle cell anemia
4. Polycythemia

15. 2. Aplastic anemia is a pathology of bone marrow dysfunction. Clients with aplastic anemia may have pancytopenia. Red blood cells, white blood cells, and platelets are all decreased. Bone marrow produces red blood cells, white blood cells, and platelets. The normal erythrocyte (red blood cells) count for an adult male is $4.6 \times 10^6/\mu l$ (4.60×10^{12}/L) to $6.2 \times 10^6/\mu l$ (6.20×10^{12}/L) and female is $4.2 \times 10^6/\mu l$ (4.20×10^{12}/L) to $5.4 \times 10^6/\mu l$ (5.40×10^{12}/L). The normal leukocyte (white blood cells) count is $4.500/\mu l$ (4.50×10^9/L) to $11,000/\mu l$ (11.00×10^9/L), and the normal thrombocytes (platelet) count is $150,000/\mu l$ (150×10^9/L) to $400,000/\mu l$ (400×10^9/L). Polycythemia is an abnormal increase in red blood cells, Sickle cell anemia results from defective hemoglobin with a sickle presence and pernicious anemia is the inability to absorb B_{12} from lack of intrinsic factor,
CN: Physiological integrity; CNS: Reduction of risk potential;
CL: Apply

16. A nurse is reviewing the laboratory results of a client with anemia. Which laboratory values are abnormal?
1. Erythrocyte count of $3.1 \times 10^6/\mu l$ (3.10×10^{12}/L)
2. Neutrophil count of $2,100/\mu l$ (2.10×10^9/L)
3. Leukocytes count of $2,300/\mu l$ (2.30×10^9/L)
4. Platelets count of $115,000/\mu l$ (115×10^9/L)

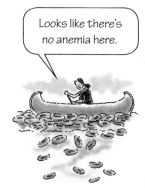

Looks like there's no anemia here.

16. 1. Anemia is defined as a decreased number of erythrocytes (red blood cells, RBC). The normal RBC count for an adult male is $4.6 \times 10^6/\mu l$ (4.60×10^{12}/L) to $6.2 \times 10^6/\mu l$ (6.20×10^{12}/L) and female is $4.2 \times 10^6/\mu l$ (4.20×10^{12}/L) to $5.4 \times 10^6/\mu l$ (5.40×10^{12}/L). The normal leukocyte (white blood cell, WBC) count is $4.500/\mu l$ (4.50×10^9/L) to $11,000/\mu l$ (11.00×10^9/L), and the normal thrombocyte (platelet) count is $150,000/\mu l$ (150×10^9/L) to $400,000/\mu l$ (400×10^9/L). Normal neutrophil count is 2,500 and 6,000. Leukopenia is a decreased number of WBC. Thrombocytopenia is a decreased number of thrombocytes (platelets). Lastly, neutropenia is a decreased number of neutrophils (a type of WBC).
CN: Physiological integrity; CNS: Reduction of risk potential;
CL: Apply

17. The nurse is assessing a client who has been experiencing black stools for the past month. The client suddenly reports chest and stomach pain. What is the **most** important action by the nurse?
1. Administer oxygen via nasal cannula
2. Assess the client's vital signs
3. Initiate cardiac monitoring
4. Draw blood for laboratory analysis

17. 2. Assessing vital signs would determine this client's hemodynamic stability. Monitoring the heart rhythm may be indicated based on assessment findings. Administering oxygen and drawing blood require a health care provider's order, and would not be part of a screening evaluation.
CN: Safe and effective care environment; CNS: Management of care; CL: Apply

18. A client arrives at the emergency department reporting chest and stomach pain and black, tarry stools for the past two months. Which orders should the nurse anticipate?
1. Cardiac monitoring, oxygen, creatine kinase, and lactate dehydrogenase (LD) levels
2. Prothrombin time (PT), partial thromboplastin time (PTT), fibrinogen, and fibrin split product levels
3. An electrocardiogram (ECG), complete blood count (CBC), occult blood screening, and comprehensive serum metabolic panel
4. An electroencephalogram (EEG), alkaline phosphatase (ALP) and aspartate aminotransferase levels (AST), and basic metabolic panel (BMP)

18. 3. An ECG is used to evaluate chest pain, a CBC detects anemia, and the test for occult blood detects blood in the stool. Cardiac monitoring, oxygen, creatine kinase, and LD levels are appropriate for a cardiac primary problem. A BMP (includes glucose, electrolytes, BUN, creatinine), and ALP and AST levels assess liver function. PT, PTT, fibrinogen, and fibrin split products are measured to verify bleeding dyscrasias. An EEG evaluates brain electrical activity.

CN: Physiological integrity; CNS: Reduction of risk potential; CL: Analyze

19. A client who received massive packed red blood cell (PRBC) blood transfusions due to trauma has a potassium level of 7.1 mEq/L (7.1 mmol/L). Which medication should the nurse expect to administer?
1. IV insulin
2. IV potassium chloride
3. Oral spironolactone
4. Oral lisinopril

19. 1. The client is experiencing transfusion-associated hyperkalemia. Storing packed red blood cell increases the potassium concentration. IV regular insulin pushes potassium from the blood into the cell decreasing the serum potassium level. Severe cases require hemodialysis. IV potassium chloride and spironolactone, a potassium-sparing diuretic, will further increase the potassium. Angiotensin-converting enzyme (ACE) inhibitor such as lisinopril causes hyperkalemia.

CN: Physiological integrity; CNS: Pharmacological and parenteral therapies; CL: Apply

20. A client diagnosed with anemia asks the nurse to explain the difference between anemia and thrombocytopenia. The nurse explains that anemia is caused by a decreased number of red blood cells and that thrombocytopenia results of:
1. an increase in red blood cells.
2. an increase in white blood cells.
3. a decrease in platelets.
4. a decrease in neutrophils.

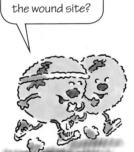

Wanna race to the wound site?

20. 3. Thrombocytopenia is caused by decreased number of platelets. An increase in red blood cells is called polycythemia vera. An increase in white blood cells is called leukocytosis. A decrease in neutrophils is called neutropenia.

CN: Physiological integrity; CNS: Physiological adaptation; CL: Analyze

21. Which factor increases a client's risk of developing anemia?
1. Colostomy following colon resection
2. Gastroesophageal reflux disease (GERD)
3. Gastrectomy
4. Bouts of dumping syndrome

21. 3. Lack of intrinsic factor following gastrectomy would cause pernicious anemia due to the client's inability to absorb vitamin B_{12}. The presence of a colostomy, GERD, or dumping syndrome would not directly affect the red blood cells.

CN: Physiological integrity; CNS: Reduction of risk potential; CL: Apply

22. The nurse is developing a dietary care plan for a client diagnosed with microcytic anemia. Which foods are most appropriate for this client?
1. Enriched breakfast cereal and hot tea
2. Eggs and yogurt
3. Chicken and brown rice
4. Split pea soup with ham

22. 4. Combining a nonheme iron source (split pea soup) with a heme iron source (ham) increases absorption of nonheme iron. Tea, calcium (in yogurt), and phytates (brown rice) block iron absorption.
CN: Physiological integrity; CNS: Basic care and comfort; CL: Apply

23. A client is admitted to the hospital with a preliminary diagnosis of rheumatoid arthritis (RA). Which screening test should the nurse anticipate for this client?
1. Antinuclear antibody (ANA) titer
2. Complete blood count (CBC)
3. Erythrocyte sedimentation rate (ESR)
4. Rheumatoid factor (RF)

23. 1. ANA is a commonly used screening tool for RA. Many people without RA can have an elevated titer for the disease. A positive ANA titer test may assist in the diagnosis of autoimmune diseases. ANA test results are just one factor considered when a diagnosis is being formulated. A client's clinical symptoms and other diagnostic tests must also be considered by the health care provider. The diagnosis of RA is based on multiple criteria, not simply a single test result. CBC, ESR, and RF are all used as diagnostic tools, and to monitor progress of the disease or response to therapy.
CN: Health promotion and maintenance; CNS: None; CL: Analyze

24. The nurse reviews the laboratory results of a postoperative female client two days following surgery, and notes a hemoglobin level of 11 g/dl (110 g/L). Which symptom would the nurse expect to see during assessment?
1. No abnormal symptoms
2. Pallor
3. Palpitations
4. Shortness of breath

24. 1. The normal hemoglobin for male is 14 to 18 g/dl (140 to 180 g/L) and female is 12 to 16 g/dl (120 to 160 g/L). Mild anemia usually has no clinical signs. Pallor, palpitations, and shortness of breath are associated with severe anemia.
CN: Physiological integrity; CNS: Reduction of risk potential; CL: Apply

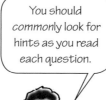

You should commonly look for hints as you read each question.

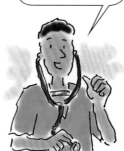

25. A client asks the nurse about a common cause of aplastic anemia. Which reply would be best?
1. Lack of intrinsic factor
2. Blood loss
3. Bone marrow suppression
4. Inadequate intake of iron

25. 3. Aplastic anemia is caused by bone marrow suppression. Lack of intrinsic factor is the cause of pernicious anemia. Blood loss will cause hypovolemic anemia. Iron deficiency anemia is due to inadequate intake of iron.
CN: Physiological integrity; CNS: Physiological adaptation; CL: Analyze

26. A nurse is reviewing the charts of four clients. Which client is at greatest risk for the development of anemia?
1. A client with Crohn's disease
2. A client with chronic renal failure (CRF)
3. A client with menorrhagia
4. A client with chronic obstructive pulmonary disease (COPD)

26. 2. Chronic renal failure will decrease the production of erythropoietin (EPO) which is needed for the production of red blood cells (RBC), thus resulting in anemia. A client with COPD will have polycythemia as hypoxia causes increased RBC production as a compensatory mechanism. Menorrhagia will cause hypovolemic anemia. As a result of blood loss, clients with Crohn's disease usually do not experience bleeding and, if they do, it is mild.
CN: Health promotion and maintenance; CNS: None; CL: Apply

27. A client has received an infusion of antibiotics and is now experiencing an anaphylactic reaction. What is the **priority** intervention by the nurse?
1. Administer a bolus of normal saline solution
2. Maintain a patent airway
3. Administer epinephrine
4. Monitor vital signs

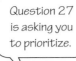

Question 27 is asking you to prioritize.

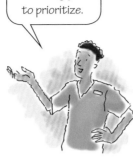

27. 2. The first priority is to maintain a patent airway. The client will then require an epinephrine injection. If hypotension develops, a saline bolus may be given. The client's vital signs should be monitored, but not as the first action.
CN: Safe, effective care environment; CNS: Management of care; CL: Apply

28. The nurse is assessing a postoperative client who is recovering from a partial gastrectomy. The nurse is aware that the client is at risk for developing:
1. anemia.
2. polycythemia.
3. purpura.
4. thrombocytopenia.

28. 1. Gastric surgery increases the risk of developing pernicious anemia. Polycythemia can occur from severe hypoxia due to congenital heart and pulmonary disease. Purpura and thrombocytopenia may result from decreased bone marrow production of platelets, and do not result from surgery.
CN: Physiological integrity; CNS: Reduction of risk potential; CL: Analyze

29. The nurse is reviewing the laboratory values of a 52-year-old client. The client's platelet count is 75,000/μl (75 × 10⁹/L). How would the nurse interpret this value?
1. Normal platelet count
2. Thrombocytopenia
3. Thrombocytopathy
4. Thrombocytosis

29. 2. Thrombocytopenia is a decreased number of platelets. A normal platelet count ranges from 150,000/μl (150 × 10⁹/L) to 400,000/μl (400 × 10⁹/L). Thrombocytopathy is platelet dysfunction, and thrombocytosis is an excess number of platelets.
CN: Physiological integrity; CNS: Reduction of risk potential; CL: Apply

30. What assessment findings should the nurse expect in a client with thrombocytopenia?
1. Weakness and fatigue
2. Dizziness and vomiting
3. Bruising and petechiae
4. Light-headedness and nausea

30. 3. Petechiae and bruising are classic signs of thrombocytopenia. Weakness and fatigue are signs of anemia. Light-headedness, nausea, dizziness, and vomiting are not classic signs of thrombocytopenia.
CN: Physiological integrity; CNS: Physiological adaptation; CL: Apply

Yahoo! I love it when you get the right answer.

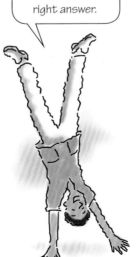

31. A nurse is teaching a client about the adverse reactions of kanamycin. What information should the nurse include? Select all that apply.
1. Decrease urine output
2. Bone damage
3. Hearing loss
4. Dry mouth
5. Increase blood glucose

31. 1, 3. Kanamycin is an aminoglycoside antibiotic. Adverse reactions to kanamycin include ototoxicity and nephrotoxicity. Bone damage, dry mouth, and hyperglycemia are not adverse effects of this medication.
CN: Physiological integrity; CNS: Pharmacological and parenteral therapies; CL: Apply

32. The nurse reviews the laboratory reports of a client who had coronary artery bypass graft (CABG) surgery three days ago. The nurse notes a decrease in the client's platelet count from 230,000/µl (230 × 10⁹/L) to 5,000/µl (5 × 10⁹/L). What complication may the client be developing?
1. Pancytopenia
2. Idiopathic thrombocytopenic purpura (ITP)
3. Disseminated intravascular coagulation (DIC)
4. Heparin-associated thrombosis and thrombocytopenia (HATT)

32. 4. HATT can occur after CABG surgery due to heparin use during surgery. Pancytopenia is a reduction in all blood cells. Although ITP and DIC cause platelet aggregation and bleeding, neither is common in a client after revascularization surgery.
CN: Physiological integrity; CNS: Physiological adaptation; CL: Apply

33. The nurse has instructed a client on self-administration of heparin injections. The nurse determines that teaching is effective when the client makes which statement?
1. "Heparin slows the time it takes for the blood to clot."
2. "Heparin stops the blood from clotting."
3. "Heparin thins the blood."
4. "Heparin dissolves clots in the arteries of the heart."

33. 1. Heparin prolongs the time needed for blood to clot. Heparin does not thin the blood. If given in large doses, heparin may stop the blood from clotting; however, this isn't why heparin is usually given. Heparin does not dissolve clots.
CN: Physiological integrity; CNS: Pharmacological and parenteral therapies; CL: Apply

34. A pregnant client arrives at the emergency department with abruptio placentae at 34 weeks gestation. The nurse is aware that the client is at risk for developing:
1. thrombocytopenia.
2. idiopathic thrombocytopenic purpura (ITP).
3. disseminated intravascular coagulation (DIC).
4. heparin-associated thrombosis and thrombocytopenia (HATT).

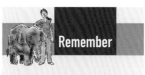

Remember

"Heparin helps halt blood clots."

Heparin, an antithrombolytic, prolongs the time needed for blood to clot.

34. 3. Abruptio placentae is a cause of DIC because of the activation of the clotting cascade after hemorrhage. Thrombocytopenia results from decreased bone marrow production. ITP can result in DIC but isn't associated with abruptio placentae. A client with abruptio placentae wouldn't receive heparin.
CN: Physiological integrity; CNS: Reduction of risk potential; CL: Apply

35. The nurse suspects that a client with disseminated intravascular coagulation (DIC) has now developed internal bleeding. For which condition should the nurse assess?
1. Hypertension
2. Jugular vein distension
3. Abdominal distension
4. Bradycardia

35. 3. As blood collects in the peritoneal cavity, dilation and distention of the abdomen occur. This is reflected by an increase in abdominal girth. The client with DIC would have hypotension and tachycardia. Jugular vein distension is a sign of fluid volume overload.
CN: Physiological integrity; CNS: Physiological adaptation; CL: Analyze

36. A 36-year-old client tells the nurse that he is experiencing fatigue, weight loss, low-grade fever, and also has pain in his fingers, elbows, and ankles. The nurse recognizes that these could be symptoms of which condition?
1. Anemia
2. Leukemia
3. Rheumatic arthritis
4. Systemic lupus erythematosus (SLE)

36. 3. Fatigue, weight loss, and a low-grade fever are all early signs of many immune system diseases, including anemia, leukemia, and SLE. However, only rheumatic arthritis is associated with pain in the fingers, elbows, wrists, ankles, and knees.
CN: Physiological integrity; CNS: Physiological adaptation; CL: Apply

CN: Client needs category   CNS: Client needs subcategory   CL: Cognitive level

37. The nurse is reviewing the platelet count of a client with possible essential thrombocytopenia. What test best confirms the diagnosis of this disorder?
1. Bleeding time
2. White blood cell (WBC) count
3. Immunoglobulin (Ig) G level
4. Prothrombin time (PT)

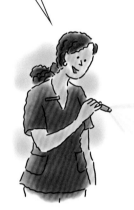

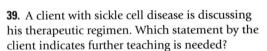

The word *first* should shed some light on the answer.

38. A nurse is assigned to four clients. Which client should the nurse see **first**?
1. A client who is being prepared for a major surgery receiving clopidogrel
2. A client who had open reduction internal fixation (ORIF) receiving fondaparinux
3. A client with a low white blood cell count receiving pegfilgrastim
4. A client with acquired immunodeficiency syndrome receiving emtricitabine

39. A client with sickle cell disease is discussing his therapeutic regimen. Which statement by the client indicates further teaching is needed?
1. "I should avoid vacationing or traveling in areas of high altitude."
2. "Cigarette smoking can cause a sickle cell crisis."
3. "I should drink 4 to 6 L of fluid each day."
4. "I should take one baby aspirin daily to help prevent sickle cell crisis."

40. A nurse is teaching a client who has HIV about the adverse effects of saquinavir. What information is important to include?
1. Hypoglycemia
2. Thrombocytopenia
3. Leukocytosis
4. Hypolipidemia

41. A client with thrombocytopenia, secondary to leukemia, develops epistaxis. The nurse would instruct the client to:
1. lie supine with his neck extended.
2. sit upright, leaning slightly forward.
3. tilt head backward while pinching the nose.
4. pinch nose while bending forward at the waist.

37. 1. After a platelet count, the test to determine thrombocytopenia is a bleeding time test. The platelet count is decreased, and bleeding time is prolonged. IgG assays are nonspecific but may help determine the diagnosis. A WBC count shows WBC values, and the PT monitor the effect of anticoagulation therapy with warfarin.
CN: Physiological integrity; CNS: Reduction of risk potential; CL: Analyze

38. 1. Clopidrogel is an anti-platelet drug that should be stopped seven days prior to surgery because it can increase the risk of bleeding. All the other options are correct. Fondaparinux can be given to a client who had ORIF to prevent blood clot formation. Pegfilgrastim is given to a client with low white blood cell (WBC). Emtricitabine is a nucleoside-nucleotide reverse transcriptase inhibitor (NNRTI) drug used for clients with HIV/AIDS.
CN: Physiological integrity; CNS: Pharmacological and parenteral therapies; CL: Apply

39. 4. Aspirin inhibits platelet aggregation and won't help prevent sickle cell crisis. Hydroxyurea is prescribed for some people to help prevent sickle cell crisis. High altitude increases oxygen demand and therefore can also precipitate a crisis. Tobacco, alcohol, and dehydration can precipitate a sickle cell crisis and should be avoided.
CN: Health promotion and maintenance; CNS: None; CL: Analyze

40. 2. Saquinavir is an antiretroviral-protease inhibitor used in combination with other antiretroviral medications to help manage HIV. Adverse effects include hyperglycemia, bone loss, hypersensitivity reaction, hyperlipidemia, thrombocytopenia, and leukopenia.
CN: Physiological integrity; CNS: Pharmacological and parenteral therapies; CL: Apply

41. 2. Sitting upright while leaning slightly forward avoids increasing the vascular pressure in the nose and helps the client avoid aspirating blood. Lying supine won't prevent aspiration of blood. Bending at the waist increases vascular pressure and promotes bleeding rather than stopping it.
CN: Physiological integrity; CNS: Physiological adaptation; CL: Apply

CN: Client needs category   CNS: Client needs subcategory   CL: Cognitive level

42. A client is receiving the drug oprelvekin? Which laboratory value shows the effectiveness of the drug?
1. Hemoglobin of 13 g/d (130 g/L)
2. Hematocrit of 44 percent (0.44)
3. White blood cell count of 7,000/µl (7.00 × 10⁹/L)
4. Platelet of 350,000/µl (350 × 10⁹/L)

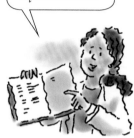

Which lab value equals success?

42. 4. Oprelvekin is given to a client with thrombocytopenia to stimulate the production of platelets. All the other options are not related to the drug's effectiveness.
CN: Physiological integrity; CNS: Pharmacological and parenteral therapies; CL: Analyze

43. The nurse is reviewing assessment data of clients who may be at risk for developing malignant lymphoma. Which client would be at highest risk?
1. A 22-year-old man with a history of mononucleosis
2. A 25-year-old man who smokes a pack of cigarettes a day
3. A 33-year-old man with a cousin with Hodgkin's lymphoma
4. A 40-year-old woman with HIV

43. 1. Malignant lymphoma has a peak incidence between ages 20 and 30, and after age 50. It's more common in men than women and is associated with a history of Epstein-Barr virus (which causes mononucleosis). There is also an increased incidence of the disease among siblings. There is no reported association between malignant lymphoma and smoking or HIV infection.
CN: Health promotion and maintenance; CNS: None; CL: Apply

44. A nurse is caring for client experiencing hypovolemic shock. Which findings should the nurse expect to assess?
1. Blood pressure of 132/85 mmHg, heart rate of 116, urine output of 45 ml/hr, and warm skin
2. Blood pressure of 149/92 mmHg, heart rate of 59, urine output of 57 ml/hr, and cold skin
3. Blood pressure of 87/58 mmHg, heart rate of 123, urine output of 20 ml/hr, and clammy skin
4. Blood pressure of 91/62 mmHg, heart rate of 99, urine output of 35 ml/hr, and pale skin

44. 3. Signs and symptoms of hypovolemic shock would include change in the level of consciousness, cool, clammy, and pale skin, hypotension, tachycardia, and tachypnea. The client will also have oliguria (decreased urine output) because of decreased circulation of fluid volume. Normal urine output is between 30 to 50 ml/hr.
CN: Physiological integrity; CNS: Physiological adaptation; CL: Apply

45. A nurse has been assigned to four clients. Which client should the nurse see **first**?
1. A client with systemic lupus erythematosus (SLE) with malar rash on the face
2. A client with rheumatoid arthritis who is receiving adalimumab for inflammation
3. A client with Hodgkin's lymphoma complaining of fatigue and night sweats
4. A client with hemophilia who is receiving acetylsalicylic acid (ASA) for joint pain

45. 4. A client with hemophilia should be seen first because ASA will increase bleeding. It should not be given to a client with hemophilia. Malar rash or "butterfly" rash is usually seen in clients with SLE. Adalimumab is a tumor necrosis factor (TNF) inhibiting anti-inflammatory drug given to clients with rheumatoid arthritis. A client with Hodgkin's lymphoma is expected to have fatigue and night sweats.
CN: Safe, effective care environment; CNS: Management of care; CL: Apply

46. The nurse determines that teaching was effective when the client with thrombocytopenia makes which statement?
1. "Platelets carry oxygen to the body cells."
2. "Platelets regulate the immune response."
3. "Platelets protect the body from inflammation and infection."
4. "Platelets stop the bleeding when arteries and veins are injured."

46. 4. Platelets clump together to plug small breaks in blood vessels. They also initiate the clotting cascade by releasing thromboplastin, which (in the presence of calcium) converts prothrombin into thrombin.
CN: Physiological integrity; CNS: Reduction of risk potential; CL: Apply

CN: Client needs category   CNS: Client needs subcategory   CL: Cognitive level

47. What manifestations are important for the nurse to assess in a 43-year-old client who has developed thrombocytopenia after undergoing colon cancer treatment? Select all that apply.
  1. Diarrhea
  2. Hematuria
  3. Ecchymosis
  4. Melena
  5. Epistaxis

47. 2, 3, 4, 5. Thrombocytopenia is an abnormal decrease in the number of blood platelets, which can result in bleeding. Hematuria, ecchymosis, melena, and epistaxis are all signs of bleeding. The client may have constipation but usually not diarrhea.
CN: Physiological integrity; CNS: Reduction of risk potential; CL: Apply

48. A client involved in a motor vehicle collision arrives in the emergency department unconscious, severely hypotensive, and with possible fractures of the pelvis and legs. Which parenteral fluid would the nurse expect to administer to this client?
  1. Fresh frozen plasma
  2. Normal saline solution
  3. Lactated Ringer's solution
  4. Packed red blood cells (RBCs)

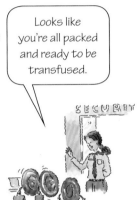

Looks like you're all packed and ready to be transfused.

48. 4. In a trauma situation, the first blood product given is unmatched (O negative) packed RBCs. Fresh frozen plasma is often used to replace clotting factors. Normal saline or lactated Ringer's solution is used to increase volume and blood pressure, but too much colloid will hemodilute the blood and won't improve the oxygen-carrying capacity that RBCs would.
CN: Physiological integrity; CNS: Physiological adaptation; CL: Apply

49. A client is receiving aspirin. Which statement made by the client needs follow-up?
  1. "I need to report if I have black stool."
  2. "I'll take the medication after a meal."
  3. "I can take Ginkgo biloba with aspirin."
  4. "I need to report loss of hearing in my ears."

49. 3. Aspirin, also known as acetylsalicylic acid, is used for mild to moderate pain, fever, inflammation, and atrial fibrillation stroke prevention. Aspirin may increase the bleeding when taken with herbal supplement Ginkgo biloba. The medication can cause gastrointestinal bleeding and ototoxicity. Nausea, vomiting, diaphoresis, and tinnitus are the earliest signs and symptoms of salicylate toxicity. Other early symptoms and signs are vertigo, hyperventilation, tachycardia, and hyperactivity. It should be taken with food especially if it causes stomach upset.
CN: Physiological integrity; CNS: Pharmacological and parenteral Therapies; CL: Apply

50. The nurse is making assignments for the next shift. Which client can be assigned to a licensed practical nurse/licensed vocational nurse (LPN/LVN)? Select all that apply.
  1. A client who just had coronary artery bypass graft (CABG)
  2. A client who needs initial admission assessment
  3. A client who needs assistance with colostomy irrigation
  4. A client who is receiving glargine subcutaneously
  5. A client who has C3 to C5 spine injury

50. 3, 4. An LPN/LVN can perform colostomy irrigation and administer subcutaneous injections. A client who just had CABG is unstable and needs to be monitored by an RN. The initial admission assessment should also be performed by an RN. C3 to C5 injury may cause respiratory compromise. Possible paralysis of diaphragm due to phrenic nerve involvement may occur. This client is unstable and should be assigned to an RN.
CN: Safe and effective care environment; CNS: management of care; CL: Apply

51. A nurse is caring for 70-year-old adult client and notes the laboratory results as listed in the chart below.

Progress notes		
2/10/17	Laboratory Results	
0800	Test	Result
	Hematocrit	61 percent (0.61)
	BUN	32 mg/dl (11.4 mmol/L)
	Sodium	159 mEg/L (159 mmol/L)

Based on the client's laboratory results, which interventions should the nurse include in the plan of care? Select all that apply.
1. Assess for neck vein distention
2. Test urine for specific gravity
3. Weigh the client daily
4. Record input and output
5. Limit fluid intake
6. Administer IV fluids

52. The nurse is assessing a client with an early diagnosis of stage I Hodgkin's disease. Which finding would the nurse likely observe?
1. Pericarditis
2. Night sweats
3. Splenomegaly
4. Persistent hypothermia

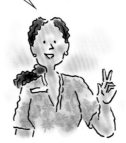

Don't break out in a sweat over this one. You'll figure it out.

53. A client has experienced an exacerbation of systemic lupus erythematosus (SLE). The nurse determines further teaching is necessary when the client makes which statement?
1. "I need to stay away from sunlight."
2. "I don't have to worry if I get strep throat."
3. "I need to work on managing the stress in my life."
4. "I don't have to worry about changing my diet."

54. The nurse is teaching a group of clients about some common physiologic changes of aging. What information should the nurse include in this teaching? Select all that apply.
1. Decreased cardiac output
2. Deceased residual urine
3. Decreased elasticity of skin
4. Decreased visual acuity
5. Decreased resistance to infection

51. 2, 3, 4, 6. The client is experiencing dehydration. Signs and symptoms include thirst, poor skin turgor, flat neck veins, weight loss, confusion, decreased urine output, increased heart rate, thready pulse, and postural hypotension. Fluid volume deficit will cause hemoconcentration. Hematocrit, BUN, and sodium will increase whenever the blood is concentrated. The normal hematocrit for males is 40 to 54 percent (0.40 to 0.54) and for female is 37 to 47 percent (0.37 to 0.47). The normal blood urea nitrogen (BUN) is from 8 to 23 mg/dl (2.9 to 8.2 mmol/L). Sodium level normal range is from 135 to 145 mEq/L (135 to 145 mmol/L). The kidneys will compensate by conserving the remaining fluid in the body leading to a decrease in urine output. Urine specific gravity will increase because the urine is concentrated. The nurse should replace the fluids through administration of intravenous solutions like lactated Ringer's solution or 0.9 percent sodium chloride per health care provider's order.
CN: Physiological integrity; CNS: Physiological adaptation; CL: Apply

52. 2. In stage I, signs and symptoms include a single enlarged lymph node (usually), unexplained fever, night sweats, malaise, and generalized pruritus. Although splenomegaly may be present in some clients, night sweats are generally more prevalent. Pericarditis isn't associated with Hodgkin's disease. Persistent hypothermia is associated with Hodgkin's but isn't an early sign of the disease.
CN: Health promotion and maintenance; CNS: None; CL: Analyze

53. 2. An infection, such as strep throat, may cause an exacerbation of SLE. Other factors that can precipitate an exacerbation are immunizations, sunlight exposure, and stress.
CN: Health promotion and maintenance; CNS: None; CL: Apply

54. 1, 3, 4, 5. Decreased cardiac output, decreased skin turgor, decreased visual acuity, and decreased resistance to infection are all common physiologic changes of aging. There will be an increase in residual volume of the urine due to the decrease in muscle tone of bladder.
CN: Health promotion and maintenance; CNS: None; CL: Apply

55. The nurse assesses a client with systemic lupus erythematosus (SLE) for signs of neurologic involvement. Which findings would the nurse document?
- **1.** Facial tic
- **2.** Psychosis
- **3.** Extremity weakness
- **4.** Cerebrovascular accidents

56. A nurse is reviewing the health care provider's orders for a client admitted with systemic lupus erythematosus (SLE). Which medication would the nurse expect to find in this client's plan of care?
- **1.** Morphine
- **2.** Ketoconazole
- **3.** Hydroxychloroquine
- **4.** Dimenhydrinate

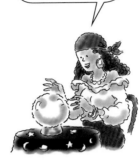

I see many correct answers in your future.

57. The nurse is reviewing the laboratory report of a client diagnosed with vitamin D deficiency.

Progress notes

2/10/17 1300	Test	Result
	Sodium	138 mEq/L (138 mmol/L)
	Potassium	4.1 mEq/L (4.1 mmol/L)
	Chloride	99 mEq/L (99 mmol/L)
	Calcium	5.2 mg/dL (1.3 mmol/L)
	Magnesium	1.5 mEq/L (0.75 mmol/L)
	Phosphorus	3.1 mg/dl (1 mmol/L)

Based on these laboratory results, which interventions should be included in the care plan? Select all that apply.
- **1.** Administer sodium polystyrene per health care provider's order.
- **2.** Encourage client to eat sardines, tofu, rhubarb, and collard greens.
- **3.** Administer magnesium sulfate per health care provider's order.
- **4.** Observe for muscle cramps and hyperactive deep tendon reflexes.
- **5.** Limit fluid intake and monitor for jugular vein distension (JVD).

55. 2. Neurologic involvement may be shown by psychosis, seizures, and headaches. Tics and cerebrovascular accidents aren't related to SLE. Weakness may be present, but it's usually related to muscle atrophy, not neurologic involvement.
CN: Physiological integrity; CNS: Physiological adaptation; CL: Apply

56. 3. Fatigue, photosensitivity and a "butterfly" rash on the face are all signs and symptoms of SLE. Hydroxychloroquine is used in the treatment of SLE to prevent inflammation. Pharmacological treatment of SLE also involves nonsteroidal anti-inflammatory drugs, corticosteroids, and immunosuppressive agents. Morphine is an opioid analgesic, ketoconazole is an antifungal agent, and dimenhydrinate is an antiemetic.
CN: Physiological integrity; CNS: Pharmacological and parenteral therapies; CL: Apply

57. 2, 4. The normal calcium level is 8.5 to 10.5 mg/dl (2.1 to 2.6 mmol/L). The client has hypocalcemia. Vitamin D is necessary for the absorption of calcium. The nurse should encourage client to eat foods high in calcium like sardines, tofu, rhubarb, and collard greens. The nurse should also monitor the client for signs and symptoms of hypocalcemia which includes muscle cramps, tetany, positive Chvostek's sign, positive Trousseau's sign, arrhythmias, and hyperactive deep tendon reflexes. The other laboratory results are within normal range. Sodium polystyrene sulfonate is used to lower potassium levels in clients with hyperkalemia. It is not necessary to administer magnesium sulfate since the magnesium level is normal. The client has no fluid volume overload so there's no need to limit fluids or monitor for jugular vein distension (JVD).
CN: Physiological integrity; CNS: Reduction of risk potential; CL: Apply

58. A client with a suspected diagnosis of systemic lupus erythematosus (SLE) is admitted to the hospital. Which laboratory results would support the diagnosis?
1. Leukopenia and an elevated serum complement level
2. Thrombocytosis and an elevated sedimentation rate
3. Pancytopenia and an elevated antinuclear antibody (ANA) titer
4. Leukocytosis and an elevated blood urea nitrogen (BUN) level

58. 3. Laboratory findings for clients with SLE usually show an elevated ANA titer, and decreased serum complement levels. Some clients also have anti-erythrocyte, anti-lymphocyte, anti-platelet antibodies which causes pancytopenia. Clients may have elevated BUN and creatinine levels from nephritis, but the increase does not indicate SLE.
CN: Physiological integrity; CNS: Reduction of risk potential; CL: Apply

59. The nurse is reviewing laboratory values of a client recently diagnosed with chronic lymphocytic leukemia. Which results should the nurse anticipate?
1. Sedimentation rate of 15 mm/hr
2. Aspartate aminotransferase of 30 units/L (0.50 μkat/L)
3. Platelet count of 95,000 /μl (95 × 10⁹/L)
4. Alanine aminotransferase of 10 units/L (0.17 μkat/L)

59. 3. Chronic lymphocytic leukemia shows a proliferation of small abnormal mature B lymphocytes and decreased antibody response. A low platelet count is often present. Uncontrolled proliferation of granulocytes occurs in myelogenous leukemia. Aspartate aminotransferase, alanine aminotransferase, and erythrocyte sedimentation rate values are not affected.
CN: Physiological integrity; CNS: Reduction of risk potential; CL: Apply

60. A client is scheduled for magnetic resonance imaging (MRI). Which client would require further assessment?
1. The client with a history of leukemia
2. The client who is allergic to barium
3. The client who is afraid being in a small room
4. The client who is sensitive to light

60. 3. During magnetic resonance imaging (MRI), the client will be confined in a small enclosed tube-shaped machine. The client who is afraid of being in a small room needs further assessment because that may indicate claustrophobia. All the other options are not associated with MRI.
CN: Physiological integrity; CNS: Reduction of risk potential; CL: Apply

61. The nurse determines that teaching about the adverse effects of pegfilgrastim was effective when the client makes which statement?
1. "I need to notify my health care provider when I experience bleeding."
2. "I need to notify my health care provider when I experience joint pain."
3. "I need to notify my health care provider when I experience nausea."
4. "I need to notify my health care provider if I experience hypotension."

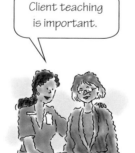

Client teaching is important.

61. 2. Pegfilgrastim is a leukocyte growth factor used to stimulate the production of white blood cells. It is used to decrease the incidence of infection in clients with neutropenia. Adverse effects include severe allergic reactions, acute respiratory distress syndrome, sickle cell crises, and spleen rupture. Joint pain is a sign of sickle cell crisis. The other options are not related to pegfilgrastim use.
CN: Physiological integrity; CNS: Pharmacological and parenteral therapies; CL: Apply

62. A client diagnosed with acute lymphocytic leukemia is about to begin chemotherapy. The nurse recognizes that further teaching is necessary when the client makes which statement?
1. "I'll have treatments only once a month."
2. "I'll be getting high doses of chemotherapy."
3. "I won't get sick at this stage of the treatment."
4. "The purpose of these treatments is to induce a remission."

62. 1. The initial phase of chemotherapy is called the induction phase and is designed to put the client into remission by giving high doses of the drugs. Treatments will occur more than once a month. Monthly treatments usually occur during the maintenance phase of chemotherapy. The other options indicate that the client understands chemotherapy.
CN: Physiological integrity; CNS: Basic care and comfort; CL: Apply

63. Which statement is correct, regarding the rate of cell growth activity during chemotherapy?
1. Rapidly-dividing cells are less susceptible to chemotherapy.
2. Slow-growing cells are more susceptible to chemotherapy.
3. Rapidly-dividing cells are more susceptible to chemotherapy.
4. Dividing cells are less susceptible to chemotherapy.

63. 3. The faster cells grow, the more susceptible they are to chemotherapy and radiation therapy. Slow-growing and non-dividing cells are less susceptible to chemotherapy. Repeated cycles of chemotherapy are used to destroy non-dividing cells as they begin active cell division.
CN: Physiological integrity; CNS: Physiological adaptation; CL: Apply

64. A client is receiving high-dose chemotherapy for a large, rapidly-dividing tumor. The nurse will monitor the client for 48 to 72 hours after the infusion, and assess which laboratory values?
1. Complete blood count, prothrombin time, and partial thromboplastin time
2. Myoglobin, troponin, and creatine kinase
3. Glucose, bilirubin, and alanine aminotransferase
4. Electrolytes, blood urea nitrogen (BUN), and creatinine

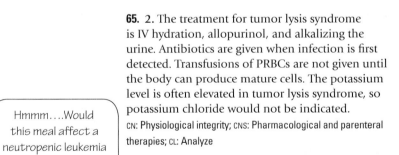

Look at all the progress you've made!

64. 4. The client is at high risk for developing lysis syndrome. Tumor lysis syndrome is an oncologic emergency that occurs as a result of rapid tumor cell breakdown in response to anti-cancer treatment. Because the client is at high risk for electrolyte imbalances and acute renal failure; electrolyte, BUN, and creatinine levels should be measured prior to treatment and for 48 to 72 hours after treatment. The other tests would not be indicated.
CN: Physiological integrity; CNS: Reduction of risk potential; CL: Apply

65. The nurse recognizes that the most appropriate treatment for clients with tumor lysis syndrome is:
1. antibiotics.
2. intravenous (IV) hydration.
3. packed red blood cells (PRBCs).
4. IV potassium chloride.

65. 2. The treatment for tumor lysis syndrome is IV hydration, allopurinol, and alkalizing the urine. Antibiotics are given when infection is first detected. Transfusions of PRBCs are not given until the body can produce mature cells. The potassium level is often elevated in tumor lysis syndrome, so potassium chloride would not be indicated.
CN: Physiological integrity; CNS: Pharmacological and parenteral therapies; CL: Analyze

Hmmm....Would this meal affect a neutropenic leukemia client in any way?

66. A client with leukemia has developed neutropenia. The nurse informs the client to avoid which food?
1. White bread
2. Carrot sticks
3. Stewed apples
4. Well-done steak

66. 2. Raw fruits and vegetables contain bacteria. A low-bacteria diet would be indicated.
CN: Safe and effective care environment; CNS: Safety and infection control; CL: Apply

CN: Client needs category   CNS: Client needs subcategory   CL: Cognitive level

67. A client diagnosed with leukemia is now experiencing neutropenia. Which assessment is a **priority** for the nurse?
1. Blood glucose
2. Bowel sounds
3. Heart sounds
4. Breath sounds

67. 4. Pneumonia, both viral and fungal, is a common cause of death in clients with neutropenia. Frequent assessment of respiratory rate and breath sounds is required. Although assessing blood pressure, bowel sounds, and heart sounds is important, it will not help detect pneumonia.
CN: Safe and effective care environment; CNS: Management of care; CL: Apply

68. The nurse is planning care for a client undergoing chemotherapy. What is the most appropriate instruction for the nurse to give this client?
1. Maintain bed rest
2. Perform activity as tolerated
3. Walk to the bathroom only
4. Get out of bed for brief periods

68. 2. It is important that the client be able to engage in activities that are of interest, and to maintain as much independence as possible. Bed rest is not necessary, nor is it necessary to limit the client's activity to only walking to the bathroom or to getting out of bed for brief periods.
CN: Health promotion and maintenance; CNS: None; CL: Apply

69. The nurse is examining charts to identify clients at risk for developing multiple myeloma. Which client is most at risk?
1. A 20-year-old Asian woman
2. A 30-year-old white man
3. A 50-year-old Hispanic woman
4. A 60-year-old black man

69. 4. Multiple myeloma is more common in middle-aged and older clients. The median age at diagnosis is 60 years. It is twice as common in blacks as it is in whites. It occurs most often in black men.
CN: Health promotion and maintenance; CNS: None; CL: Analyze

70. The nurse is monitoring the laboratory values of a client in the early stages of multiple myeloma. Which laboratory values would be abnormal?
1. Immunoglobulins
2. Platelets
3. Red blood cells (RBCs)
4. White blood cells (WBCs)

70. 1. Multiple myeloma is characterized by malignant plasma cells that produce an increased amount of immunoglobulin that isn't functional. As more malignant plasma cells are produced, there's less space in the bone marrow for RBC production. In late stages, platelets and WBCs are reduced as the bone marrow is infiltrated by malignant plasma cells.
CN: Physiological integrity; CNS: Reduction of risk potential; CL: Analyze

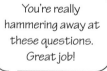

You're really hammering away at these questions. Great job!

71. A client has been diagnosed with multiple myeloma. The nurse should monitor this client for:
1. hypercalcemia.
2. hyperkalemia.
3. hypernatremia.
4. hypermagnesemia.

71. 1. Calcium is released when bone is destroyed. This causes an increase in serum calcium levels. Multiple myeloma doesn't affect potassium, sodium, or magnesium levels.
CN: Physiological integrity; CNS: Physiological adaptation; CL: Apply

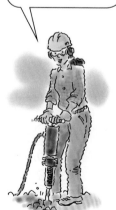

CN: Client needs category   CNS: Client needs subcategory   CL: Cognitive level

72. The nurse is making assignments for the unlicensed assistive personnel (UAP). Which tasks can be safely assigned to UAP? Select all that apply.
1. Assisting a client with a chest tube during ambulation
2. Feeding a client with swallowing difficulty
3. Teaching a client how to use a cane
4. Bathing a client with Alzheimer's disease
5. Turning a client who is poorly nourished

72. 4, 5. Unlicensed assistive personnel (UAP) can safely perform bathing and turning a client. Unstable clients cannot be delegated to UAP. Assisting a client with a chest tube, and feeding a client with swallowing difficulty cannot be assigned to UAP. The registered nurse should only delegate routine tasks, and tasks with lower priority. Teaching a client how to use a cane is not within their scope of practice.
CN: Safe and effective care environment; CNS: Management of care; CL: Apply

73. What assessment findings would the nurse anticipate in a client with a calcium level of 14.6 mg/dl (3.65 mmol/L)? Select all that apply.
1. Tetany
2. Renal calculi
3. Positive Chvostek's sign
4. Decreased bowel sounds
5. Hyperactive deep tendon reflexes (DTR)

73. 2, 4. A normal calcium level is 8.5 to 10.5 mg/dl (2.1 to 2.6 mmol/L). This client is experiencing hypercalcemia. Calcium has sedating effects. Too much calcium will cause lethargy, confusion, muscle weakness, decreased DTR, and decreased bowel sounds. Renal calculi form because most kidney stones are calcium stones, usually in the form of calcium oxalate. Tetany and Chvostek's sign are both signs of hypocalcemia where muscles are becoming tight due to decrease in calcium. Chvostek's sign is the twitching of the facial muscles in response to gentle tapping over the facial nerve in front of the ear.
CN: Physiological integrity; CNS: Physiological adaptation; CL: Apply

74. A client is schedule for bone marrow aspiration. Place these nursing actions in chronological order from most important to least important.

| 1. Apply direct pressure over the puncture site |
| 2. Explain procedure and obtain consent |
| 3. Monitor puncture site for bleeding |
| 4. Help the client maintain position |
| 5. Assess coagulation studies |
| 6. Position in lateral decubitus or prone |

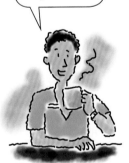

You're doing great! Don't quit now!

74. Ordered Response:

| 2. Explain procedure and obtain consent |
| 5. Assess coagulation studies |
| 6. Position in lateral decubitus or prone |
| 4. Help the client maintain position |
| 1. Apply direct pressure over the puncture site |
| 3. Monitor puncture site for bleeding |

CN: Physiological integrity; CNS: Reduction of risk potential; CL: Apply

75. The nurse is teaching the family of a client who has developed hypercalcemia and hyperurecemia as a result of multiple myeloma. What statement, by the family, indicates that teaching has been effective?
1. "We will keep the client on bed rest."
2. "We will be enforcing fluid restriction."
3. "We will make sure that the client drinks at least 3 quarts (3 liters) of fluid daily."
4. "We will always keep the lower extremities elevated."

75. 3. The client needs to drink 3 to 5 quarts (3 to 5 liters) of fluid each day to dilute calcium and uric acid, and to reduce the risk of renal dysfunction. Walking is encouraged to prevent further bone demineralization. The lower extremities do not need to be elevated.
CN: Physiological integrity; CNS: Basic care and comfort; CL: Apply

CN: Client needs category   CNS: Client needs subcategory   CL: Cognitive level

76. The nurse is aware that a client's physiologic response to a health crisis is important to the health outcome. Which nursing intervention should be addressed **first**?
1. Teaching the family how to care for the client
2. Helping the client effectively cope with the crisis
3. Maintaining intravenous access, medications, and diet
4. Teaching the client basic information about the illness

76. 2. Although all of the answers are important in the care of the client, if the individual isn't able to cope with the emotional, spiritual, and psychological aspects of his crisis, the other components of care may be ineffective as well.
CN: Psychosocial integrity; CNS: None; CL: Apply

77. What is the most appropriate nursing intervention to promote healing of a laceration?
1. Elevate the body part
2. Monitor blood pressure
3. Apply a pressure dressing and heat
4. Apply a pressure dressing and an ice pack

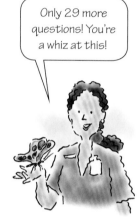

Only 29 more questions! You're a whiz at this!

77. 4. Pressure dressings help clotting by promoting the localization of microorganisms and the development of meshwork for repair and healing. Ice decreases blood flow to the site, slowing the bleeding. Elevating the body part helps reduce edema but doesn't directly promote healing. Monitoring blood pressure is important when the individual is bleeding but does nothing to promote clotting. Heat increases blood flow to the site, increasing the bleeding.
CN: Physiological integrity; CNS: Physiological adaptation; CL: Apply

78. A mother brings her 12-month-old child to the emergency department. The mother states the child's eyes are yellow. The nurse assesses the child and notes tachycardia and shortness of breath. Which diagnosis should the nurse anticipate?
1. Thalassemia
2. Hemophilia A
3. Sickle cell anemia
4. Leukemia

78. 3. Clinical signs do not appear in newborns. Signs and symptoms of sickle cell anemia often don't appear until an infant is at least 4 months old (fetal hemoglobin is replaced by adult hemoglobin) and may include swelling of hands and feet often in conjunction with a fever.
CN: Physiological integrity; CNS: Physiological adaptation; CL: Apply

79. Which therapeutic immune system response to an antigen is appropriate?
1. Widespread histamine release
2. Autoimmune reaction
3. Inflammatory response
4. Antibody production by T cells

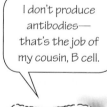

I don't produce antibodies— that's the job of my cousin, B cell.

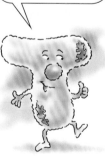

79. 3. Inflammation and increased body temperature are normal immune responses to detected antigens. Allergies are heightened responses to antigens. Widespread histamine release is an exaggerated response that can lead to anaphylaxis. Autoimmune response is one in which the immune system forms antibodies against the body's own tissues, resulting in disease. Antibodies are produced by B cells, not T cells.
CN: Physiological integrity; CNS: Reduction of risk potential; CL: Analyze

80. Which intervention has the most impact in delaying the development of AIDS once a client has been infected with HIV?
1. Monthly plasmapheresis
2. Eating a balanced diet
3. Compliance to treatment
4. Adequate rest and sleep

80. 3. Compliance with the complete therapeutic regimen is the most important intervention in delaying the onset of AIDS. This includes adhering to a healthy lifestyle, taking prescribed medications, and reducing risks from other infections. Eating a balanced diet and getting adequate rest and sleep are part of the overall therapeutic regimen. Plasmapheresis isn't a treatment for HIV/AIDS.
CN: Health promotion and maintenance; CNS: None; CL: Analyze

81. A child has developed chickenpox. Following recovery, the mother asks the nurse if her child has immunity against recurrence of the disease. Which response by the nurse is **best**?
1. "Your child has passive immunity."
2. "Your child has immunological immunity."
3. "Your child has active immunity."
4. "Your child has adaptive immunity."

81. 3. Active immunity results from the development of antibodies in response to the presence of antigens from a vaccination or an exposure to an infectious disease.
CN: Health promotion and maintenance; CNS: None; CL: Analyze

82. A client reports dyspnea, chills, headache, and flank pain while receiving a blood transfusion. Place the nurse's actions in order from highest to lowest priority?

1. Inform the primary care provider and blood bank
2. Monitor the client's vital signs
3. Stop the transfusion
4. Keep the IV line open with 0.9% sodium chloride
5. Return blood products to the blood bank
6. Document the transfusion-related occurrence

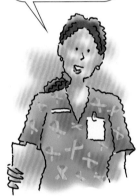

Ah—a question that asks you put steps in order. Time for some critical thinking!

82. Ordered Response:

3. Stop the transfusion
4. Keep the IV line open with 0.9% sodium chloride
1. Inform the primary care provider and blood bank
2. Monitor the client's vital signs
5. Return blood products to the blood bank
6. Document the transfusion-related occurrence

CN: Physiological integrity; CNS: Physiological adaptation; CL: Apply

83. Which assessment data would the nurse expect to see in the chart of a client admitted with *Pneumocystis jiroveci* pneumonia?
1. Blood pressure of 108/72 mmHg
2. Oxygen saturation 95 percent
3. Respiratory rate of 20
4. CD4 count below 200

83. 4. *Pneumocystis jiroveci* pneumonia (PJP) is a type of pneumonia caused by a *Pneumocystis jiroveci* fungus. It is an opportunistic infection seen in clients who are immunocompromised with a CD4 count below 200, particularly in clients with HIV/AIDS.
CN: Safe and effective care environment; CNS: Safety and infection control; CL: Analyze

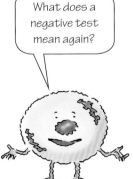

What does a negative test mean again?

84. The nurse determines that teaching was successful when a client with a negative HIV antibody test states:
1. "I'm not infected with HIV."
2. "I haven't produced antibodies to HIV."
3. "I'm immune to HIV."
4. "I have antibodies to HIV."

84. 2. A negative HIV antibody test means that HIV antibodies weren't in the client's blood at the time the test was performed. Antibodies may take three weeks to six months or longer to develop. A negative test result doesn't indicate immunity. If antibodies to HIV are present, the test result is positive.
CN: Physiological integrity; CNS: Reduction of risk potential; CL: Apply

CN: Client needs category   CNS: Client needs subcategory   CL: Cognitive level

85. A client is receiving 1 L of 0.9% sodium chloride IV to be infused for 12 hours. The IV infusion set has a drop factor of 15 gtts/ml. At how many drops per minute should the nurse set the IV to infuse? Record your answer using a whole number.

_____ gtts/min

85. 21.
Here are the calculations:

$$drops\ per\ minute = \frac{ml/hr}{60\ min/hr} \times drop\ factor$$

1,000 ml for 12 hours = 83 ml/hr

$$\frac{83\ ml/hr}{60\ min/hr} \times 15\ drop\ factor = 21\ gtts/min$$

CN: Physiological integrity; CNS: Pharmacological and parenteral therapies; CL: Apply

86. A client is admitted with hemophilia A. Which sports should the nurse recommend as safe for the client to participate? Select all that apply.
1. Basketball
2. Swimming
3. Baseball
4. Golf
5. Soccer

86. 2, 4. Hemophilia A or classic hemophilia is a bleeding disorder that results from a deficiency or abnormality of clotting factor VIII. A client with hemophilia should avoid contact sports like soccer, baseball, and basketball because of the risk of bleeding with injury. The client can safely participate in noncontact sports such as swimming and golf.

CN: Safe and effective care environment; CNS: Safety and infection control; CL: Apply

87. A client has been prescribed corticosteroids. The nurse would also anticipate an order for:
1. blood glucose checks every 6 hours.
2. fluid restriction to 1,000 ml in 24 hours.
3. lactulose 40 g in 4 oz (118 ml) of water daily.
4. serum platelet counts every 12 hours.

87. 1. Corticosteroids cause elevated blood glucose levels; insulin may be necessary to maintain normal blood glucose levels. Corticosteroids can cause edema, but fluid restrictions are generally unnecessary unless the client also has renal or cardiac disease. Lactulose is given for constipation and to treat hepatic encephalopathy. Platelet count every 12 hours is not necessary when monitoring clients undergoing corticosteroid therapy.

CN: Physiological integrity; CNS: Pharmacological and parenteral therapies; CL: Apply

88. A 32-year-old client is admitted with a tentative diagnosis of AIDS. The preliminary report of biopsies done on his facial lesions indicates Kaposi's sarcoma. What is the **most** appropriate action by the nurse?
1. Tell the client that Kaposi's sarcoma is common in people with AIDS
2. Pretend not to notice the lesions on the client's face
3. Inform the client of the biopsy results and support him emotionally
4. Explore the client's feelings about his facial disfigurement

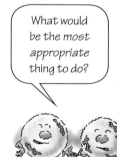

What would be the most appropriate thing to do?

88. 4. Facial lesions can contribute to decreased self-esteem and an altered body image. Discussing AIDS with a client whose diagnosis isn't final may be inappropriate and doesn't provide emotional support. Pretending not to notice visible lesions ignores the client's concerns. The health care provider—not the nurse—should inform the client of the biopsy results.

CN: Psychosocial integrity; CNS: None; CL: Apply

89. A client is receiving epoetin alfa. Which findings indicate the effectiveness of the drug?
1. Increase in white blood cells
2. Decrease in blood glucose
3. Increase in red blood cells
4. Decrease in blood coagulation

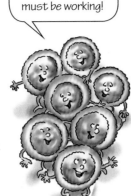

Hey! There are lots of us, now. The medicine must be working!

90. The nurse is performing mouth care on a client with AIDS. What is the **most** appropriate nursing intervention?
1. Use reverse isolation
2. Place the client in a private room
3. Put on a mask, gloves, and a gown
4. Wear gloves

91. The nurse is reviewing the laboratory values of a client with aplastic anemia. Which diagnostic findings would be consistent with this diagnosis?
1. A decreased production of T-helper cells
2. A decreased level of white blood cells, red blood cells, and platelets
3. An increased levels of white blood cells, red blood cells, and platelets
4. The presence of Reed-Sternberg cells and lymph node enlargement

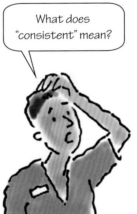

What does "consistent" mean?

92. The nurse is teaching a client with iron-deficiency anemia about ferrous gluconate therapy. Which statement, if made by the client, would indicate a correct understanding of the teaching?
1. "I will take the medication with an antacid."
2. "I will take the medication with a glass of milk."
3. "I will take the medication with whole-grain cereal."
4. "I will take the medication on an empty stomach with orange juice."

89. 3. Epoetin alfa is a man-made form of the protein human erythropoietin used to lessen the need for red blood cell transfusions. It stimulates the bone marrow to produce more red blood cells. The drug is used to treat anemia caused by chronic kidney disease, chemotherapy, and zidovudine, which is a drug used to treat HIV infection. The drug does not affect white blood cells or coagulation, nor does it cause blood glucose to decrease.
CN: Physiological integrity; CNS: Pharmacological and parenteral therapies; CL: Apply

90. 4. Standard precautions stipulate that a health care worker who anticipates coming into contact with a client's blood or body fluids must wear gloves. Reverse isolation is used to protect the client from the health care worker. A private room does not provide barrier protection, an essential step in standard precautions. A mask, gloves, and gown are needed only for anticipated contact with airborne droplets of blood or body fluids.
CN: Safe and effective care environment; CNS: Safety and infection control; CL: Apply

91. 2. The diagnostic findings for aplastic anemia include decreased levels of all the cellular elements of the blood (pancytopenia). T-helper cell production doesn't decrease in aplastic anemia. Reed-Sternberg cells and lymph node enlargement occur with Hodgkin's disease.
CN: Physiological integrity; CNS: Physiological adaptation; CL: Analyze

92. 4. Preferably, ferrous gluconate should be taken on an empty stomach with orange juice. Ferrous gluconate shouldn't be taken with antacids, milk, or whole-grain cereals because these foods reduce iron absorption.
CN: Physiological integrity; CNS: Pharmacological and parenteral therapies; CL: Apply

CN: Client needs category   CNS: Client needs subcategory   CL: Cognitive level

93. A nurse is working on a medical/surgical unit and notes that one of the assigned clients has a diagnosis of ankylosing spondylitis. The nurse would assess this client for:
1. red, painful, swollen joints.
2. fatigue and night sweats.
3. low back pain.
4. neck pain and stiffness.

93. 3. Typically, intermittent low back pain is the first indication of ankylosing spondylitis. Red, painful, swollen joints occur with rheumatoid arthritis. Although ankylosing spondylitis may cause fatigue, it rarely produces night sweats. Neck pain and stiffness from involvement of the cervical spine are relatively late manifestations.
CN: Physiological integrity; CNS: Physiological adaptation; CL: Analyze

94. A client is receiving oral prednisolone. Which side effects would the nurse expect to see from prolonged use of this medication? Select all that apply.
1. Weight loss
2. Hyperglycemia
3. Osteoporosis
4. Hirsutism
5. Cataract

94. 2, 3, 4, 5. Prednisolone is a corticosteroid used for inflammation. Prolonged use of this drug will cause hyperglycemia, osteoporosis, hirsutism, and cataract formation. Client will have weight gain not weight loss due to fluid retention.
CN: Physiological integrity; CNS: Pharmacological and parenteral therapies; CL: Apply

95. A young female client with a history of sickle cell disease reports abdominal pain. What is the **priority** intervention by the nurse?
1. Obtaining a history of the sequence of symptoms
2. Keeping the client nothing by mouth (NPO)
3. Administering IV fluids
4. Preparing the client for a computed tomography (CT) scan of the abdomen

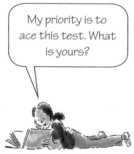

95. 1. Although the client may be in a sickle cell crisis and experiencing acute abdominal pain caused by sickling in the mesenteric circulation, it's important to remember that clients with sickle cell disease aren't spared from other intra-abdominal events. The history obtained from the client outlining the sequence of symptoms provides crucial assessment information. Other nursing interventions would include preparing the client for possible surgery by keeping her NPO and for diagnostic studies such as CT scanning. Administering IV fluids will help replenish fluid volume. Also, obtaining a history is a part of assessment. Nursing process always starts with assessment.
CN: Physiological integrity; CNS: Reduction of risk potential; CL: Apply

96. A nurse is developing a care plan for a neutropenic client with lymphoma. Which nursing intervention would be **most** appropriate?
1. Have the client use a soft toothbrush and electric razor, avoid using enemas, and watch for signs of bleeding
2. Wear a mask, gown, and gloves when entering the client's room
3. Provide a clear liquid, low-sodium diet
4. Have the client eliminate fresh fruits and vegetables from the diet, avoid using enemas, and practice frequent hand washing

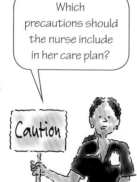

96. 4. Neutropenia occurs when the absolute neutrophil count falls below 1,000/µl (1 × 10⁹/L), and places the client at severe risk for infection. The nurse should eliminate fresh fruits and vegetables as part of a low-bacterial diet. Invasive procedures, such as enemas, should be avoided because the increase the risk of infection. Frequent hand washing lowers the risk of infection. The use of a soft toothbrush, avoidance of straight-edged razors and enemas, and monitoring for bleeding are precautions for thrombocytopenia. Wearing a mask, gown, and gloves when entering the client's room are reverse isolation measures. A neutropenic client doesn't require a clear liquid diet or sodium restrictions.
CN: Safe and effective care environment; CNS: Safety and infection control; CL: Apply

97. The nurse is reviewing a client's laboratory values and notes a deficiency of factor VIII. What diagnosis does the nurse suspect?
1. Sickle cell disease
2. Christmas disease
3. Hemophilia A
4. Thrombocytopenia

97. 3. Hemophilia A results from a deficiency of factor VIII. Sickle cell disease is caused by a defective hemoglobin molecule. Christmas disease, also called hemophilia B, results from a deficiency of factor IX. Thrombocytopenia is the deficiency of platelets in the blood.
CN: Physiological integrity; CNS: Physiological adaptation; CL: Analyze

98. A client admitted with heat stroke begins to show signs of disseminated intravascular coagulation (DIC). Which laboratory finding is **most** consistent with DIC?
1. Low platelet count
2. Elevated fibrinogen levels
3. Low levels of fibrin degradation products
4. Reduced prothrombin time (PT)

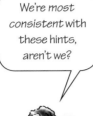

We're most consistent with these hints, aren't we?

98. 1. In DIC, platelets and clotting factors are consumed, resulting in microthrombi and excessive bleeding. As clots form, fibrinogen levels decrease and PT increases. Fibrin degradation products increase as fibrinolysis takes place.
CN: Physiological integrity; CNS: Physiological adaptation; CL: Analyze

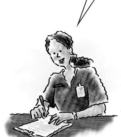

99. A client comes to the clinic reporting fever, drenching night sweats, and unexplained weight loss over the past three months. A physical examination reveals a single enlarged supraclavicular lymph node. The nurse suspects which probable diagnosis?
1. Influenza
2. Sickle cell anemia
3. Leukemia
4. Hodgkin's disease

99. 4. Hodgkin's disease typically causes fever, night sweats, weight loss, and lymph node enlargement. Influenza doesn't last for months. Clients with sickle cell anemia manifest symptoms of chronic anemia with pallor of the mucous membranes, fatigue, and decreased tolerance for exercise. Leukemia doesn't cause lymph node enlargement.
CN: Health promotion and maintenance; CNS: None; CL: Apply

100. A client has been informed by the health care provider that he has Hodgkin's disease. After the health care provider leaves the room, the client tells the nurse that he's afraid of dying. Which response by the nurse us **most** appropriate?
1. "Don't worry, many people survive this disease."
2. "Hodgkin's disease is very treatable."
3. "You're afraid of dying?"
4. "You should speak with your minister."

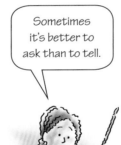

Sometimes it's better to ask than to tell.

100. 3. Repeating what the client has said encourages the client to elaborate on his thoughts and feelings. Telling him not to worry and saying that Hodgkin's disease is very treatable ignores his feelings, and offers false reassurance. Telling a client what to do, such as calling his minister, also ignores his feelings.
CN: Psychosocial integrity; CNS: None; CL: Apply

101. Before starting treatment for leukemia, a client receives IV fluids and allopurinol. These interventions reduce the risk for:
1. disseminated intravascular coagulation (DIC).
2. pancytopenia.
3. tumor lysis syndrome.
4. mucositis.

101. 3. During chemotherapy for leukemia, tumor lysis syndrome may occur as cell destruction releases intracellular components, resulting in hyperuricemia. Large fluid quantities and allopurinol therapy help reduce the amount of uric acid that result from tumor lysis syndrome but don't stop the cell lysis. Although DIC, pancytopenia, and mucositis are possible chemotherapy complications, they're not treated with IV fluids and allopurinol.
CN: Physiological integrity; CNS: Pharmacological and parenteral therapies; CL: Apply

102. A client with a gunshot wound requires an emergency blood transfusion. His blood type is AB negative. The nurse is aware that the **safest** blood type for this client to receive would be:
  1. AB Rh-positive.
  2. A Rh-positive.
  3. A Rh-negative.
  4. O Rh-positive.

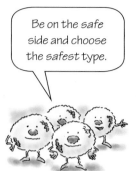

Be on the safe side and choose the safest type.

102. 3. It's important that a person with Rh-negative blood receives Rh-negative blood. If Rh-positive blood is administered to an Rh-negative person, the recipient develops anti-Rh agglutinins, and subsequent transfusions with Rh-positive blood may cause serious reactions with clumping and hemolysis of red blood cells.
CN: Physiological integrity; CNS: Pharmacological and parenteral therapies; CL: Apply

103. Which client is **most** at risk for developing acute lymphocytic leukemia?
  1. A 25-year-old black male
  2. A 4-year-old white female
  3. A 44-year-old white male
  4. A 51-year-old Asian female

103. 2. Acute lymphocytic leukemia is most common in young children and in adults age 65 and older. It's also more common in whites than in blacks or Asians.
CN: Health promotion and maintenance; CNS: None; CL: Analyze

104. A client with Hodgkin's disease who weighs 143 lb (65 kg) is to receive vincristine 25 mcg/kg IV. The nurse computes the correct dose in micrograms. How many micrograms should the client receive? Record your answer using a whole number.

_____ mcg

104. 1,625.
Multiply the weight in kilograms by the number of micrograms desired per kilogram:
65 kg × 25 = 1,625 mcg
CN: Physiological integrity; CNS: Pharmacological and parenteral therapies; CL: Apply

105. The nurse initiates the treatment for a delayed hypersensitivity reaction. What is the **most** appropriate treatment?
  1. Intravenous epinephrine
  2. Breathing treatment with albuterol
  3. Corticosteroids
  4. Benadryl

105. 3. Delayed hypersensitivity reactions are inflammatory reactions and require treatment with corticosteroids.
CN: Physiological integrity; CNS: Pharmacological and parenteral therapies; CL: Apply

106. Which non-pharmacologic interventions should be included in the plan of care for a client who has moderate rheumatoid arthritis? Select all that apply.
  1. Massaging inflamed joints
  2. Avoiding range-of-motion (ROM) exercises
  3. Applying splints to inflamed joints
  4. Using assistive devices at all times
  5. Selecting clothing that has Velcro fasteners
  6. Applying moist heat to joints

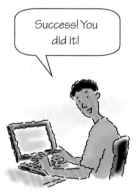

Success! You did it!

106. 3, 5, 6. Supportive, non-pharmacologic measures for the client with rheumatoid arthritis include applying splints to rest inflamed joints, using Velcro fasteners on clothes to aid dressing, and applying moist heat to joints to relax muscles and relieve pain. Inflamed joints should never be massaged because doing so can aggravate inflammation. A physical therapy program including ROM exercises and carefully individualized therapeutic exercises prevents loss of joint function. Assistive devices should be used only when marked loss of ROM occurs.
CN: Physiological integrity; CNS: Basic care and comfort; CL: Apply

Chapter 5

Respiratory Disorders

Looking for the latest information about respiratory disorders? Check out the American Association for Respiratory Care's Web site at **www.aarc. org**. It will respire—er, inspire—you.

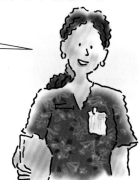

1. An immunosuppressed client is being treated for allergic bronchopulmonary aspergillosis. The client asked the nurse how he got this fungal infection. What is the nurse's **best** response?
  1. "You are more prone to react to this fungus because your immune system is weakened."
  2. "Fungal infections are more common at this time of year, so that is possibly what happened."
  3. "People who have allergy problems are more prone to getting viral, bacterial, and fungal infections."
  4. "There are many reasons a person gets a fungal infection, so let's look at the lab report to get the answer."

1. 1. Allergic bronchopulmonary aspergillosis is typically caused by being exposed to the fungus and having a compromised immune system. Exposure to the fungus can occur at any time of the year. Clients with heart disease and lung problems are more prone to respiratory infections than clients with allergies. The lab report will confirm the presence of an infection and identify the causative agent. It will not indicate how or why the person contracted the infection.
CN: Physiological integrity; CNS: Physiological adaptation;
CL: Analyze

2. Which client, diagnosed with pneumonia, is **most** likely to have community-acquired pneumonia?
  1. A client newly admitted to a long-term care facility
  2. A client who recently traveled on a cruise ship
  3. A client who has had multiple family visitors
  4. A client whose spouse recently died

In question 3, the terms *most likely causative* are a hint for finding the correct answer.

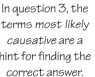

2. 1. The client who is a new resident in a long term care facility is at high risk for community-acquired infections. Traveling is not likely to cause community-acquired pneumonia. Legionnaires' disease is a risk if traveling on a confined cruise ship. Receiving family visits and the death of a spouse are not typically causative factors associated with developing community-acquired pneumonia.
CN: Physiological integrity; CNS: Reduction of risk potential;
CL: Apply

3. The nurse is reviewing the chart of a 58-year-old client with community-acquired pneumonia. Which bacteria are the **most** likely causative microorganisms?
  1. *Haemophilus influenzae*
  2. *Klebsiella pneumoniae*
  3. *Streptococcus pneumoniae*
  4. *Staphylococcus aureus*

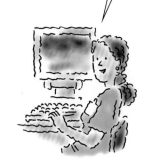

3. 3. Pneumococcal or streptococcal pneumonia is caused by *S. pneumonia*, and this bacterium is the most common cause of community-acquired pneumonia. *H. influenzae* is the most common cause of infection in children. *Klebsiella* species is the most common gram-negative organism found in the hospital setting. *S. aureus* is the most common cause of hospital-acquired pneumonia.
CN: Physiological integrity; CNS: Reduction of risk potential;
CL: Apply

CN: Client needs category CNS: Client needs subcategory CL: Cognitive level

4. An older adult client has developed pneumonia. What initial assessment finding would **most** concern the nurse?
 1. Confusion or delirium
 2. High grade fever and severe chills
 3. Hemoptysis and dyspnea
 4. Pleuritic chest pain and cough

4. **1.** The major sign of pneumonia in older adults may be a change in how clearly they think, or when an existing lung disease gets worse. Other common symptoms of pneumonia are fever, severe chills, hemoptysis, dyspnea, pleuritic chest pain and a productive cough. These symptoms tend to manifest later in elderly clients.
CN: Physiological integrity; CNS: Physiological adaptation; CL: Apply

5. A client has been diagnosed with pneumonia. What sound would the nurse anticipate while auscultating areas of consolidation?
 1. Bronchial
 2. Bronchovesicular
 3. Tubular
 4. Vesicular

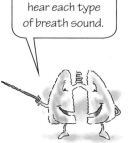

For question 5, think of where you normally hear each type of breath sound.

5. **1.** Chest auscultation would reveal bronchial breath sounds over areas of consolidation. Bronchovesicular breath sounds would be normal over mid-lobe lung regions. Tubular sounds are commonly heard over large airways. Vesicular breath sounds are commonly heard in the bases of the lung fields.
CN: Physiological integrity; CNS: Reduction of risk potential; CL: Apply

6. A client is exhibiting symptoms indicative of pneumonia. Which diagnostic test would the nurse anticipate to confirm this diagnosis?
 1. Arterial blood gas (ABG) analysis
 2. Chest X-ray
 3. Blood cultures
 4. Sputum culture and sensitivity

6. **4.** Sputum culture and sensitivity is the best way to identify the organism causing the pneumonia. ABG analysis will determine the extent of hypoxia present due to the pneumonia. A chest X-ray will show the area of lung consolidation. Blood cultures will help determine if the infection is systemic.
CN: Physiological integrity; CNS: Reduction of risk potential; CL: Apply

7. A 78-year-old client, admitted with a diagnosis of dehydration and a change in mental status, is being hydrated with IV fluids. On assessment, the nurse notes a temperature of 103.7° F (39.5° C), a cough producing yellow sputum, and pleuritic chest pain. How would the nurse interpret these symptoms?
 1. Acute respiratory distress syndrome (ARDS)
 2. Myocardial infarction (MI)
 3. Pneumonia
 4. Tuberculosis (TB)

The nurse can give oxygen without a health care provider's order to help her client breathe more easily.

7. **3.** Fever, productive cough, and pleuritic chest pain are common signs and symptoms of pneumonia. A client with ARDS would have dyspnea and hypoxia, with progressively worsening hypoxia if not aggressively treated. Pleuritic chest pain will vary with respiration, unlike the constant chest pain experienced with an MI. The client with TB will typically have a cough that produces blood-tinged sputum. A sputum culture would confirm the nurse's interpretation.
CN: Physiological integrity; CNS: Physiological adaptation; CL: Analyze

8. A client with pneumonia has developed dyspnea, has a respiratory rate of 32 breaths/min, and is having difficulty expelling secretions. The nurse auscultates the lung fields and hears bronchial sounds in the lower left lobe. Which action should the nurse take **first**?
 1. Administer antibiotics
 2. Encourage bed rest
 3. Apply oxygen
 4. Assess nutritional intake

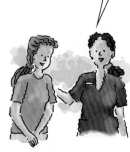

8. **3.** The client is having difficulty breathing, and is probably becoming hypoxic. As an emergency measure, the nurse should provide oxygen without waiting for a health care provider's order. Antibiotics may be warranted, but would require a provider's order. This client should be maintained on bed rest if he's dyspneic to minimize his oxygen demands, but providing additional oxygen will more immediately address his problem. The client will require nutritional support, but while dyspneic, the priority is oxygenation.
CN: Safe, effective care environment; CNS: Management of care; CL: Analyze

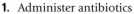

CN: Client needs category   CNS: Client needs subcategory   CL: Cognitive level

9. A client has just finished a 10-day course of antibiotic therapy for right lower lobe pneumonia. The client is scheduled to be discharged. Which assessment findings would indicate that this client is ready to be discharged?
1. Continued dyspnea
2. Fever of 102.7° F (38.97° C)
3. Respiratory rate of 32 breaths/min
4. Vesicular breath sounds in right base

9. **4.** If the client is to be discharged after receiving treatment for pneumonia, he should have stable vital signs, have clear breath sounds bilaterally, and have no evidence of shortness of breath.
CN: Physiological integrity; CNS: Physiological adaptation; CL: Analyze

10. A 20-year-old client is being treated for pneumonia. He has a persistent cough and reports severe pain when coughing. The nurse tells this client that the **most** effective way to reduce discomfort while coughing is to:
1. hold your cough in as much as possible.
2. place the head of your bed flat to help with coughing.
3. restrict fluids to help decrease the amount of sputum.
4. splint your chest wall with a pillow for comfort.

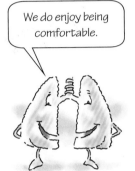

We do enjoy being comfortable.

10. **4.** Showing this client how to splint his chest wall will help decrease discomfort when coughing. Holding in coughs will only increase the amount of pain. Placing the head of the bed flat may increase the frequency of his cough and require more work. Increasing fluid intake will help thin his secretions, making then easier to clear. Promoting fluid intake is appropriate in this situation.
CN: Physiological integrity; CNS: Basic care and comfort; CL: Apply

11. A client in a long-term care facility has been receiving continuous tube feedings. The nurse notes that the client has a cough that produces tan sputum, and has a temperature of 102.7° F (38.9° C). The nurse auscultates the client's lung fields and hears bronchial breath sounds in the right middle lobe. The nurse suspects that the client may have developed:
1. bilateral atelectasis.
2. acute bronchitis.
3. aspiration pneumonia.
4. pulmonary embolism.

11. **3.** The client has likely aspirated the contents of his tube feedings and has developed aspiration pneumonia. This is the most common cause of pneumonia in clients with tube feedings. Atelectasis is not associated with a productive cough, and breath sounds would be decreased in the areas of atelectasis. A client with acute bronchitis would have a nonproductive or productive cough but secretions would usually be clear. A client with a pulmonary embolism wouldn't have a cough that produces tan sputum. Pulmonary embolisms aren't typically associated with high fever.
CN: Physiological integrity; CNS: Physiological adaptation; CL: Analyze

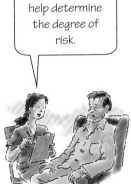

Asking a client questions will help determine the degree of risk.

12. A nurse, working in a rural county's public health department, has been alerted that there is an outbreak of tuberculosis (TB) in the area. Which client is at **highest** risk for developing TB?
1. A 16-year-old female high school student
2. A 35-year-old female day-care worker
3. A 43-year-old homeless man with a history of alcoholism
4. A 54-year-old businessman who travels worldwide

12. **3.** Clients who are economically disadvantaged, malnourished, and have reduced immunity, such as those with a history of alcoholism, are at extremely high risk for developing TB. A high school student, daycare worker, and a man traveling on business have a much lower risk of contracting TB.
CN: Physiological integrity; CNS: Physiological adaptation; CL: Apply

13. The nurse is conducting a class for the family members of clients diagnosed with tuberculosis (TB). The nurse determines that teaching has been effective when a family member states:
 1. "The disease is transmitted by sexual contact."
 2. "The disease is transmitted by contaminated needles."
 3. "The disease is transmitted through contaminated eating utensils."
 4. "The disease is transmitted by droplets exhaled from an infected person."

14. The nurse is performing a Mantoux skin test on an adult being screened for tuberculosis (TB). The client reports having negative tuberculin test results in the past. The nurse instructs the client to return and have the results interpreted:
 1. immediately after performing the test.
 2. 24 hours after performing the test.
 3. 48 hours after performing the test.
 4. one week after performing the test.

15. A client received a Mantoux skin test for tuberculosis (TB) on the right forearm. After 48 hours the site is reddened with an induration about 3 mm. The nurse interprets this result as:
 1. indeterminate.
 2. invalid, and must be repeated.
 3. negative.
 4. positive.

16. A client has recently been diagnosed with tuberculosis (TB). The nurse caring for the client anticipates that the client will develop:
 1. active TB within two weeks.
 2. active TB within one month.
 3. a fever that requires hospitalization.
 4. a positive skin test.

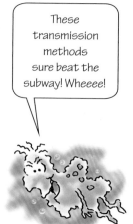

These transmission methods sure beat the subway! Wheeee!

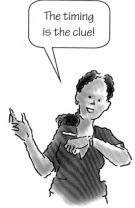

The timing is the clue!

13. 4. The TB bacillus is airborne and carried in droplets exhaled by an infected person. Sexual contact and contaminated needles don't spread TB bacillus, but may spread other communicable diseases. It's never advisable to use contaminated utensils, but, if cleaned thoroughly, these utensils may be reused.
CN: Safe, effective care environment; CNS: Safety and infection control; CL: Apply

14. 3. Mantoux skin tests should be read in 48 to 72 hours. If read too early or too late, the results won't be accurate.
CN: Physiological integrity; CNS: Reduction of risk potential; CL: Apply

15. 3. This test would be negative. An induration of 3 mm would be a positive result if the client had recent close contact with someone diagnosed with, or suspected of having, infectious TB. Follow-up should be done with this client, and a chest X-ray should be ordered. Indeterminate isn't a term used to describe results of a tuberculin test. The test can be repeated in six months to see if the client's test results change. If the tuberculin test is reddened, with an induration of 10 mm or more, it's considered positive according to the Centers for Disease Control and Prevention.
CN: Physiological integrity; CNS: Reduction of risk potential; CL: Analyze

16. 4. A primary TB infection occurs when the bacillus has successfully invaded the entire body after entering through the lungs. At this point, the bacilli are walled off and skin tests will read positive. The general population has a 10% risk of developing active TB over their lifetime, because of a break in the body's immune defenses, in many cases. Those with the active stage of the disease will show the classic symptoms of fever, hemoptysis, and night sweats.
CN: Physiological integrity; CNS: Physiological adaptation; CL: Analyze

17. A client was infected with the tuberculosis (TB) bacillus 10 years ago but never developed the disease. This client is now being treated for cancer, and begins to develop signs of TB. The nurse suspects that this client is exhibiting:
1. active infection.
2. latent infection.
3. superinfection.
4. tertiary infection.

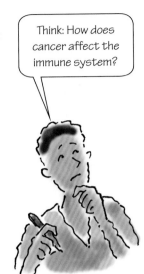

Think: How does cancer affect the immune system?

18. A client has been diagnosed with active tuberculosis (TB). The nurse should assess this client for:
1. chest and lower back pain.
2. chills, fever, night sweats, and hemoptysis.
3. fever of more than 104.7° F (40.7° C) and nausea.
4. headache and photophobia.

19. A client has received a preliminary diagnosis of tuberculosis (TB). In order to obtain a definitive diagnosis, the nurse anticipates that the health care provider will order which test?
1. Chest X-ray
2. Mantoux test
3. Sputum culture
4. Tuberculin test

20. A client has a positive Mantoux test, and a chest X-ray has been ordered. The client asks the nurse the reason for the X-ray. What is the nurse's **best** response?
1. To confirm the diagnosis of tuberculosis
2. To establish if a repeat skin test is needed
3. To determine the extent of lung involvement
4. To see if this is a primary or secondary infection

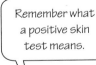

Remember what a positive skin test means.

21. A chest X-ray shows that a client's lungs are clear, following one Mantoux test that is positive with 10 mm of induration, and the previous Mantoux test was negative. The nurse explains to the client that these test results are possible because:
1. he had tuberculosis (TB) in the past and no longer has it.
2. he was successfully treated for TB, but skin tests always stay positive.
3. he's a "seroconverter," meaning the TB has entered his bloodstream.
4. he's a "tuberculin converter," which means he has been infected with TB since his last skin test.

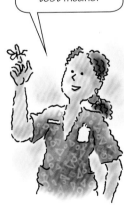

17. 1. Some people carry dormant TB infections that may develop into active disease. If there's no active disease, it's called a latent infection. The TB bacilli can remain latent for years and then become activate when the client's resistance is lowered. Superinfection doesn't apply in this case, and there's no such thing as tertiary infection.
CN: Physiological integrity; CNS: Physiological adaptation; CL: Apply

18. 2. Typical signs and symptoms are chills, fever, night sweats, and hemoptysis. Chest pain may be present from coughing but isn't usual. Clients with TB typically have low-grade fevers, not higher than 102.7° F (38.97° C). Nausea, headache, and photophobia aren't usual TB symptoms.
CN: Physiological integrity; CNS: Physiological adaptation; CL: Apply

19. 3. The sputum culture for Mycobacterium tuberculosis is the only method of confirming the diagnosis. Lesions in the lung may not be big enough to be seen on X-ray. Skin tests may be falsely positive or falsely negative.
CN: Physiological integrity; CNS: Reduction of risk potential; CL: Apply

20. 3. If the lesions are large enough, a chest X-ray will show their presence and the extent of lung involvement. A sputum culture will confirm the diagnosis. There can be false-positive and false-negative skin test results. A chest X-ray can't determine if this is a primary or secondary infection.
CN: Physiological integrity; CNS: Reduction of risk potential; CL: Apply

21. 4. A tuberculin converter's skin test will be positive, indicating that he has been exposed to, and infected with, TB and now has a cell-mediated immune response to the skin test. The client's blood and X-ray results may stay negative. This does not indicate that the infection has advanced to the active stage. Because the X-ray is negative, this client should be monitored every six months to detect changes in his chest X-ray or pulmonary examination. Being a seroconverter doesn't mean the TB has entered his bloodstream, it means that it can be detected by a blood test.
CN: Physiological integrity; CNS: Physiological adaptation; CL: Analyze

CN: Client needs category   CNS: Client needs subcategory   CL: Cognitive level

22. A client with a positive skin test for tuberculosis (TB) is not showing signs of active disease and is being treated with isoniazid, 300 mg daily. The nurse explains to the client that the medication should be taken for:
1. 10 to 14 days.
2. 2 to 4 weeks.
3. 3 to 6 months.
4. 9 to 12 months.

23. A hospitalized client, with a productive cough, chills, and night sweats is suspected of having active tuberculosis (TB). What is the nurse's **most** important intervention?
1. Maintain the client on respiratory isolation
2. Prepare the client to be discharged on bed rest
3. Administer the tuberculin test ordered by the health care provider
4. Administer the isoniazid ordered by the health care provider immediately before discharge

24. A 24-year old female client with active tuberculosis is receiving rifampin 600 mg daily. Which should this client avoid because of the significant interaction with rifampin?
1. Ginko biloba
2. Pancreatic enzymes
3. Oral contraceptives
4. Arthritis medications

25. What **priority** instruction should the nurse give a client taking medication for active tuberculosis (TB)?
1. "It's OK to miss a dose every day or two."
2. "If side effects occur, stop taking the medication."
3. "Only take the medication until you feel better."
4. "You must comply with the medication regimen to treat TB."

26. A client, diagnosed with active tuberculosis (TB), asks the nurse if he will be admitted to the hospital. The nurse responds that hospitalization would **most** likely occur to:
1. evaluate his condition.
2. determine his compliance.
3. prevent the spread of the disease.
4. determine the need for antibiotic therapy.

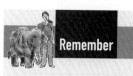

Remember

"Isoniazid tackles TB."

Isoniazid, a tuberculostatic agent, inhibits the growth of TB bacteria. It is commonly prescribed together with three other drugs to counteract drug-resistant TB strains:
- Rifampin
- Pyrazinamide
- Ethambutol or streptomycin

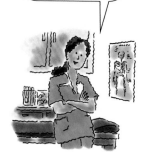

Keep in mind that TB is highly contagious.

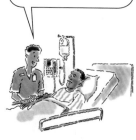

Noncompliance with your medication regimen could lead to the development of drug resistance.

22. 4. Because of the increasing incidence of resistant strains of TB, the disease must be treated from 9 to 12 months, or up to 24 months in some cases. Isoniazid is the most common medication used for the treatment of TB, but other antibiotics are often added to the regimen to obtain the best results.
CN: Physiological integrity; CNS: Pharmacological and parenteral therapies; CL: Apply

23. 1. This client is showing signs and symptoms of active TB and, because of the productive cough, is highly contagious. He should be admitted to the hospital and placed in respiratory isolation. Three sputum cultures should be obtained to confirm the diagnosis.
CN: Physiological integrity; CNS: Physiological adaptation; CL: Apply

24. 3. Oral contraceptives may have decreased effectiveness while taking rifampin, and may also cause breakthrough bleeding, spotting or pregnancy. Pancreatic enzymes and arthritis medications and supplements do not interfere with rifampin or cause adverse effects.
CN: Physiological integrity; CNS: Physiological adaptation; CL: Apply

25. 4. The regimen may last up to 24 months. It's essential that the client comply with therapy during that time or resistance will develop. At no time should the client stop taking the medications before his health care provider's authorization.
CN: Safe, effective care environment; CNS: Management of care; CL: Analyze

26. 3. A client with active TB is highly contagious until three consecutive sputum cultures are negative. This client should be put on respiratory isolation in a hospital setting.
CN: Safe, effective care environment; CNS: Safety and infection control; CL: Apply

27. A seven-year-old, who recently had a cold, is brought to the emergency department. The nurse assesses the child and finds that he is afebrile, has a respiratory rate of 36 breaths/min, and has a nonproductive cough. The nurse suspects that this child may be experiencing:
  1. acute asthma.
  2. bronchial pneumonia.
  3. chronic obstructive pulmonary disease (COPD).
  4. emphysema.

27. 1. Based on the child's history and symptoms, acute asthma is the most likely diagnosis. He's unlikely to have bronchial pneumonia without a productive cough and fever, and he's too young to have developed COPD and emphysema.
CN: Physiological integrity; CNS: Physiological adaptation; CL: Analyze

28. The nurse is performing an assessment on a client with a suspected diagnosis of asthma. Which assessment finding supports this diagnosis?
  1. Circumoral cyanosis
  2. Increased forced expiratory volume
  3. Inspiratory and expiratory wheezing
  4. Normal breath sounds

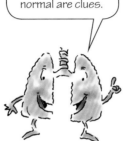

Listen to how we sound—any changes from normal are clues.

28. 3. Inspiratory and expiratory wheezes are typical findings in asthma. Circumoral cyanosis may be present in extreme cases of respiratory distress. The nurse would expect this client to have a decreased forced expiratory volume because asthma is an obstructive pulmonary disease. Breath sounds will be sound tight or markedly decreased.
CN: Physiological integrity; CNS: Physiological adaptation; CL: Analyze

29. A client recently experienced a common cold and a subsequent asthma attack. Based on the client's history, what type of asthma would the nurse suspect?
  1. Emotional
  2. Allergic
  3. Nonallergic
  4. Mediated

29. 3. Nonallergic asthma doesn't have an easily identifiable allergen, and can be triggered by the common cold. Extrinsic asthma is caused by emotional stressors. Allergic asthma is caused by dust, molds, and pet allergens. Mediated asthma doesn't exist.
CN: Physiological integrity; CNS: Physiological adaptation; CL: Analyze

30. A client with acute asthma is experiencing inspiratory and expiratory wheezing, and decreased forced expiratory volume. What is the nurse's **priority** intervention?
  1. Beta-adrenergic blockers
  2. Bronchodilators
  3. Inhaled steroids
  4. Oral steroids

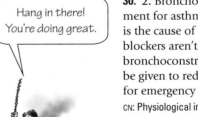

Hang in there! You're doing great.

30. 2. Bronchodilators are the first line of treatment for asthma because bronchoconstriction is the cause of reduced airflow. Beta-adrenergic blockers aren't used to treat asthma, and can cause bronchoconstriction. Inhaled or oral steroids may be given to reduce inflammation but aren't used for emergency relief.
CN: Physiological integrity; CNS: Pharmacological and parenteral therapies; CL: Apply

31. A 19-year-old client comes to the emergency department with acute asthma. His respiratory rate is 44 breaths/min, and he is in acute respiratory distress. What is the nurse's **priority** action?
  1. Take a full medical history
  2. Give a bronchodilator by nebulizer
  3. Apply a cardiac monitor to the client
  4. Provide emotional support to the client

31. 2. The client, having an acute asthma attack, needs to increase oxygen delivery to the lungs and body. Nebulized bronchodilators will open airways and increase the amount of oxygen delivered. The acute phase of the attack should be resolved, and then a full medical history should be obtained to determine the cause of the attack and how to prevent attacks in the future. It may not be necessary to place the client on a cardiac monitor unless he has a history of cardiac problems.
CN: Physiological integrity; CNS: Physiological adaptation; CL: Apply

32. A client tells the nurse that he was recently diagnosed with an allergy to the monosodium glutamate (MSG), found in some Chinese food, after he experienced an asthmatic attack. Which statement **best** describes this client's understanding of his diagnosis?

1. "I should only eat Chinese food once per month."
2. "I should use my inhalers before eating Chinese food."
3. "I should avoid Chinese food because it can trigger an asthma attack."
4. "I should investigate other causes of my asthma attacks, as Chinese food may not be a trigger."

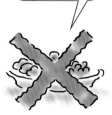

Sometimes the food you love doesn't love you back.

32. 3. If the trigger of an acute asthma attack is known, this trigger should be avoided at all times. Using an inhaler before eating will not prevent an attack. Food is commonly a trigger for an acute asthma attack.

CN: Physiological integrity; CNS: Physiological adaptation; CL: Apply

33. A 58-year-old client with a 40-year history of smoking one to two packs of cigarettes per day has a chronic cough that produces thick sputum, peripheral edema, and cyanotic nail beds. Based on this assessment, the nurse suspects the client may be experiencing:

1. acute respiratory distress syndrome (ARDS).
2. asthma.
3. chronic obstructive bronchitis.
4. emphysema.

33. 3. Because of his extensive history of smoking and symptoms, this client most likely has chronic obstructive bronchitis. Clients with ARDS will have acute symptoms of hypoxia and typically require large amounts of oxygen. Clients with asthma and emphysema tend not to have a chronic cough or peripheral edema.

CN: Physiological integrity; CNS: Physiological adaptation; CL: Apply

34. The nurse hears a health care provider refer to a client as a "blue bloater." The nurse is aware that this term refers to:

1. acute respiratory distress syndrome (ARDS).
2. asthma.
3. chronic obstructive bronchitis.
4. emphysema.

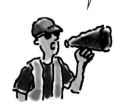

Looks like we've got another blue bloater. You know what to do.

34. 3. Clients with chronic obstructive bronchitis appear bloated. They have large barrel chests and peripheral edema, cyanotic nail beds, and, at times, circumoral cyanosis. Clients with ARDS are acutely short of breath and frequently need intubation for mechanical ventilation and large amounts of oxygen. Clients with asthma don't exhibit characteristics of chronic disease, and clients with emphysema appear pink and cachectic.

CN: Physiological integrity; CNS: Physiological adaptation; CL: Apply

35. The nurse views the term "pink puffer" on a client's chart. This assessment finding leads the nurse to suspect that the client may be experiencing:

1. acute respiratory distress syndrome (ARDS).
2. asthma.
3. chronic obstructive bronchitis.
4. emphysema.

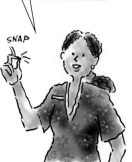

Terms like these make remembering symptoms a snap!

SNAP

35. 4. Because of the large amount of energy it takes to breathe, clients with emphysema are usually cachectic. They're pink and usually breathe through pursed lips, hence the term "puffer." Clients with ARDS are usually acutely short of breath. Clients with asthma don't have any particular characteristics, and clients with chronic obstructive bronchitis are bloated and cyanotic in appearance.

CN: Physiological integrity; CNS: Physiological adaptation; CL: Apply

36. A 66-year-old client has marked dyspnea at rest, is thin, and uses accessory muscles to breathe. The client is tachypneic, with a prolonged expiratory phase and has no cough. The client leans forward with the arms braced on the knees to support the chest and shoulders for breathing. Based on these assessment findings, the nurse suspects that the client is experiencing:

1. acute respiratory distress syndrome (ARDS).
2. asthma.
3. chronic obstructive bronchitis.
4. emphysema.

36. 4. These are classic signs and symptoms of emphysema. Clients with ARDS are acutely short of breath and require emergency care. Those with asthma are also acutely short of breath during an attack and appear very frightened. Clients with chronic obstructive bronchitis are bloated and cyanotic in appearance.

CN: Physiological integrity; CNS: Physiological adaptation; CL: Apply

37. A community health nurse is administering pneumococcal polysaccharide vaccinations and flu vaccinations to clients with asthma, chronic bronchitis, and emphysema. A client asks the nurse why these vaccines are recommended. What is the nurse's **best** response?

1. These vaccines are recommended for all clients.
2. These vaccines produce bronchodilation and improve oxygenation.
3. These vaccines help reduce the tachypnea these clients experience.
4. Respiratory infections can cause severe hypoxia and possibly death in these clients.

37. 4. It's highly recommended that clients with respiratory disorders receive vaccines to protect against respiratory infections. These clients may require intubation and mechanical ventilation if they become infected. The vaccines have no effect on bronchodilation or respiratory rate.

CN: Health promotion and maintenance; CNS: None; CL: Apply

38. A nurse is conducting a weekly support group for clients diagnosed with asthma, chronic bronchitis, and emphysema. The topic of today's class is exercise. The nurse determines teaching has been effective when a client states that exercise:

1. enhances cardiovascular fitness.
2. improves respiratory muscle strength.
3. reduces the number of acute attacks.
4. worsens respiratory function and is discouraged.

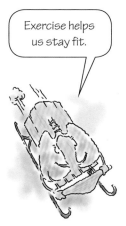

Exercise helps us stay fit.

38. 1. Exercise can improve cardiovascular fitness and help the client better tolerate periods of hypoxia, possibly reducing the risk of heart attack. Most exercise has little effect on respiratory muscle strength, and these clients can't tolerate the type of exercise necessary to do this. Exercise won't reduce the number of acute attacks. A client should check with his health care provider before starting any exercise program.

CN: Health promotion and maintenance; CNS: None; CL: Apply

39. A client with chronic obstructive bronchitis asks the nurse why he is receiving diuretic therapy. What is the nurse's **best** response?

1. To reduce fluid volume and reduce oxygen demand
2. To reduce fluid volume and improve your mobility
3. To reduce fluid volume and reduce sputum production
4. To reduce fluid volume and improve respiratory function

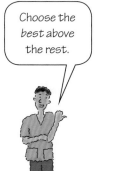

Choose the best above the rest.

39. 1. Reducing fluid volume will reduce the workload on the heart, which reduces oxygen demand and, in turn, reduces the respiratory rate. It may also reduce edema and slightly improve mobility. Sputum may become thicker, and make it more difficult to clear airways. Reducing fluid volume won't improve respiratory function but may improve oxygenation.

CN: Physiological integrity; CNS: Physiological adaptation; CL: Apply

40. The nurse is assessing a 69-year-old client who appears thin and cachectic. The client is short of breath at rest, dyspneic with the slightest exertion, and has diminished breath sounds with deep inspiration. The nurse interprets these assessment findings as indicative of:
1. acute respiratory distress syndrome (ARDS).
2. asthma.
3. chronic obstructive bronchitis.
4. emphysema.

40. 4. In emphysema, the wall integrity of the individual air sacs is damaged, reducing the surface area available for gas exchange. Very little air movement occurs in the lungs because of bronchiole collapse. In ARDS, the client's condition is more acute and typically requires mechanical ventilation. In asthma and bronchitis, wheezing is prevalent.
CN: Physiological integrity; CNS: Physiological adaptation; CL: Apply

41. A student nurse asks the staff nurse why a client with emphysema should receive only 1 to 3 L/min of oxygen, if needed. What is the **best** answer by the staff nurse?
1. This client doesn't notice when his body needs oxygen and he needs to breathe.
2. This client only breathes when his oxygen levels climb above a certain point.
3. This client only breathes when his oxygen levels dip below a certain point.
4. This client only breathes when his carbon dioxide level dips below a certain point.

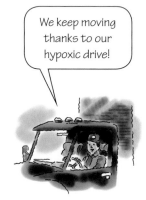

We keep moving thanks to our hypoxic drive!

41. 3. Clients with emphysema breathe when their oxygen levels drop to a certain level. This is known as the hypoxic drive. They don't take a breath when their levels of carbon dioxide are higher than normal, as do those with healthy respiratory physiology. If too much oxygen is given, this client will have little stimulus to take another breath, his carbon dioxide level will continue to climb, he will pass out, and respiratory arrest will occur.
CN: Physiological integrity; CNS: Physiological adaptation; CL: Analyze

42. What is the **most** important information for a nurse to teach a client with chronic obstructive pulmonary disease (COPD)?
1. How to assess his own pulse and respiratory rates
2. How to recognize when a change in his oxygen therapy is needed
3. How to treat respiratory infections without the use of antibiotics
4. How to recognize the signs of an impending respiratory infection

42. 4. Respiratory infection, in clients with a respiratory disorder, can be fatal. It's important that this client understands how to recognize the signs and symptoms of an impending respiratory infection. It isn't appropriate to teach this client how to listen to his own lungs or change his oxygen therapy regimen. If this client has signs and symptoms of an infection, he should contact his health care provider immediately.
CN: Health promotion and maintenance; CNS: None; CL: Apply

43. The nurse is caring for a client in the immediate postoperative period. The nurse's **priority** would be to prevent:
1. atelectasis.
2. bronchitis.
3. pneumonia.
4. pneumothorax.

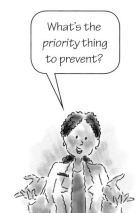

What's the priority thing to prevent?

43. 1. Atelectasis develops when there's interference with the normal negative pressure that promotes lung expansion. Clients in the postoperative phase often splint their breathing because of pain and positioning, which causes hypoxia. It's uncommon for any of the other respiratory disorders to develop.
CN: Physiological integrity; CNS: Reduction of risk potential; CL: Apply

44. A nurse is preparing a plan of care for a post-operative client. What is the **most** appropriate nursing intervention to prevent the development of atelectasis?
1. Chest physiotherapy
2. Mechanical ventilation
3. Reducing oxygen requirements
4. Use of an incentive spirometer

44. 4. Using an incentive spirometer will require the client to take deep breaths that promote lung expansion. Chest physiotherapy would help mobilize secretions but won't prevent atelectasis. Reducing oxygen requirements, or placing someone on mechanical ventilation won't affect the development of atelectasis.
CN: Physiological integrity; CNS: Reduction of risk potential; CL: Apply

45. A client is experiencing status asthmaticus. For which would the nurse anticipate an **immediate** order?
1. Inhaled Beta-2 adrenergic agonist
2. Inhaled corticosteroids
3. IV beta-adrenergic agents
4. Oral corticosteroids

45. 1. Inhaled beta-adrenergic agonists agents are the first line of therapy in status asthmaticus, as they help promote bronchodilation, which improves oxygenation. IV beta-adrenergic agents can be used, but must be carefully monitored because of their systemic effects. They are typically used when the inhaled beta-adrenergic agents do not work. Inhaled and oral corticosteroids are slow-acting, and their use won't reduce hypoxia in the acute phase.
CN: Physiological integrity; CNS: Physiological adaptation; CL: Apply

46. Which treatment goal is the nurse's **priority** for a client with status asthmaticus?
1. Avoiding intubation
2. Determining the cause of the attack
3. Improving exercise tolerance
4. Reducing secretions

For question 46, you need to choose the priority out of several possible goals.

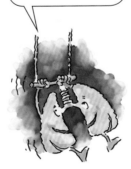

46. 1. Inhaled beta-adrenergic agents, IV corticosteroids, and supplemental oxygen are used to reduce bronchospasm, improve oxygenation, and avoid intubation. Determining the trigger for the client's attack and improving exercise tolerance are later goals. Typically, secretions aren't a problem in status asthmaticus.
CN: Physiological integrity; CNS: Physiological adaptation; CL: Apply

47. A client was given morphine for pain at 9 am. At 9:45 am, the nurse assesses the client and notes a respiratory rate of 4 breaths/min. The nurse recognizes that the client is at high risk:
1. an asthma attack.
2. respiratory arrest.
3. myoclonic seizures.
4. spontaneous arousal.

47. 2. Opioids, such as morphine, can cause respiratory arrest if given in large quantities. It's unlikely the client will have an asthma attack or myoclonic seizures or wake up on his own.
CN: Physiological integrity; CNS: Pharmacological and parenteral therapies; CL: Analyze

Looks like you're showing this test who's boss.

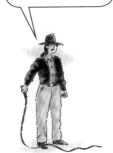

48. A client has a respiratory rate of 4 breaths/min. What are this nurse's **priority** assessments?
1. Arterial blood gas (ABG) and breath sounds
2. Level of consciousness and a pulse oximetry value
3. Breath sounds and reflexes
4. Pulse oximetry value and heart sounds

48. 2. This nurse should first attempt to rouse the client to increase the respiratory rate. Pulse oximetry and breath sounds should be assessed, and the provider informed of the findings. An ABG analysis may be ordered to determine specific carbon dioxide and oxygen levels, which would indicate the effectiveness of ventilation. An assessment of reflexes and heart sounds would be part of the more extensive examination done after the respiratory rate has stabilized.
CN: Physiological integrity; CNS: Physiological adaptation; CL: Apply

CN: Client needs category   CNS: Client needs subcategory   CL: Cognitive level

49. A nurse is assessing a client who has been given an opioid analgesic. Which arterial blood gas (ABG) value would indicate that this client is at risk for respiratory failure?
  1. $PaCO_2$ 15 mmHg
  2. $PaCO_2$ 30 mmHg
  3. $PaCO_2$ 40 mmHg
  4. $PaCO_2$ 80 mmHg

49. 4. A client with impending respiratory arrest will have inefficient ventilation, and will retain carbon dioxide. An ABG value of 80 mmHg would indicate retained CO_2. The other values are lower than expected.
CN: Physiological integrity; CNS: Physiological adaptation; CL: Analyze

50. A client's arterial blood gas (ABG) results are: pH: 7.16, $PaCO_2$: 80 mmHg, HCO_3: 24 mEq/L, SaO_2, 81%. Based on these values, this client is showing signs of:
  1. metabolic acidosis.
  2. metabolic alkalosis.
  3. respiratory acidosis.
  4. respiratory alkalosis.

50. 3. Because this client's $PaCO_2$ is high, and the HCO_3 is normal, this client has respiratory acidosis. This client's pH is less than 7.35, which eliminates metabolic and respiratory alkalosis as possibilities. If the HCO_3 was below 22 mEq/L, this client would have metabolic acidosis.
CN: Physiological integrity; CNS: Physiological adaptation; CL: Apply

51. Which client would be considered to be at the **highest** risk for respiratory failure?
  1. A client with breast cancer
  2. A client with cervical sprains
  3. A client with a fractured hip
  4. A client with Guillain-Barré syndrome

Examine each client's condition closely for the one placing the client at highest risk?

51. 4. Guillain-Barré syndrome is a progressive neuromuscular disorder that can affect the respiratory muscles and cause respiratory failure. The other conditions don't typically affect the respiratory system.
CN: Physiological integrity; CNS: Physiological adaptation; CL: Analyze

52. A client has started a new medication for hypertension. Thirty minutes after taking the medication, the client develops dyspnea, cardiac arrhythmias, and a decreased level of consciousness. How should the nurse interpret this reaction?
  1. Asthma attack
  2. Pulmonary embolism
  3. Anaphylactic shock
  4. Autoimmune response

52. 3. This client is having a reaction to the new medication and is exhibiting signs of impending anaphylactic shock, which could lead to respiratory and cardiac arrest. Although these signs could also indicate an asthma attack or a pulmonary embolism, the new medication should be the first suspect. An autoimmune response does not manifest these signs.
CN: Physiological integrity; CNS: Pharmacological and parenteral therapies; CL: Analyze

53. A client with chronic obstructive pulmonary disease (COPD) tells the home care nurse that he fell asleep in his car, while parked in the garage, with the engine running. A neighbor discovered the man an hour later. The client explained that he does this to keep warm in the winter months sometimes because his house is cold. What is the nurse's **priority** action?
  1. Contact the health department to ask for an inspection of the client's living conditions
  2. Notify the client's family members about what happened
  3. Refer the client for a psychiatric evaluation
  4. Collect more information about what happened from the neighbor

Set your priorities properly. What should be done first?

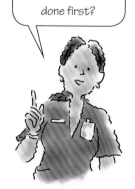

53. 3. A psychiatric evaluation is warranted since this client may have been attempting suicide or may be experiencing cognitive decline. The priority action must focus on the client's safety. The health department would be contacted when unintentional carbon monoxide poisoning occurs in a public or leased building. Contacting the extended family and the neighbor should be done with the client's permission.
CN: Physiological integrity; CNS: Physiological adaptation; CL: Analyze

54. A client, diagnosed with asthma, is experiencing an anaphylactic reaction to a medication. After administering initial emergency care, the nurse would:
1. administer beta-adrenergic blockers.
2. administer bronchodilators.
3. obtain serum electrolyte levels.
4. have the client lie flat in the bed.

55. A 19-year-old client is brought to the emergency after attending a party. A friend of the client reports that the client took some pills and was drinking alcohol. The nurse is unable to rouse the client. What would the nurse anticipate when assessing this client?
1. Hyperreflexive reflexes
2. Muscle spasms
3. Shallow respirations
4. Intermittent tachypnea

56. A nurse's initial client assessment indicates probable opioid overdose complicated by alcohol ingestion. What intervention should the nurse perform **first**?
1. Administer IV fluids
2. Administer IV naloxone
3. Continue monitoring of vital signs
4. Draw blood for a drug screen

57. A client has overdosed on an opioid while consuming alcohol. The client is now unconscious, and has been given naloxone. What is the nurse's **priority** action after the client rouses?
1. Determine dietary preferences and feed the client
2. Teach the client the effects of using pills and alcohol
3. Discharge the client from the hospital to home care
4. Seek admission, for the client, to a psychiatric facility

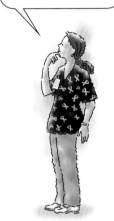

In a drug overdose, you'll want to do only one of these first. Which one?

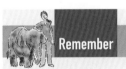

Remember

"Naloxone nullifies opioids."

Naloxone is an opioid antagonist, which means that it is administered to reverse the effects of opioids in cases such as respiratory depression or overdose.

54. 2. Bronchodilators will open the client's airway and improve oxygenation status. Beta-adrenergic blockers aren't indicated in the management of asthma because they may cause bronchospasm. Obtaining laboratory values wouldn't be done during an emergency, and having the client lie flat in bed could impede his ability to breathe.
CN: Physiological integrity; CNS: Physiological adaptation; CL: Analyze

55. 3. Most likely, this client can't be roused because of the combination of pills and alcohol he has ingested. This combination has caused shallow respirations, which, if not monitored, could lead to respiratory arrest. The nurse wouldn't expect to find intermittent tachypnea. Without additional information, the nurse wouldn't expect muscle spasms or hyperreflexia.
CN: Physiological integrity; CNS: Physiological adaptation; CL: Apply

56. 2. If a client has ingested opioids, naloxone would reverse the effects and rouse the client. Intravenous fluids would most likely be administered, and this client would be closely monitored over a period of several hours to several days. The client should be screened for drugs, but results may not come back for several hours.
CN: Physiological integrity; CNS: Physiological adaptation; CL: Analyze

57. 2. This client needs information about the dangers of taking pills and alcohol together. The client shouldn't be fed due to the risk of aspiration if the client's level of consciousness decreases. Discharge, at this point, is inappropriate and home care may not be necessary. Unless this client was trying to commit suicide, admission to a psychiatric facility isn't necessary.
CN: Physiological integrity; CNS: Physiological adaptation; CL: Analyze

58. A firefighter has been treated for smoke inhalation. The firefighter develops severe hypoxia 48 hours after the initial treatment, and requires intubation and mechanical ventilation. The nurse recognizes that this client is likely experiencing:
 1. acute respiratory distress syndrome (ARDS).
 2. pulmonary hypertension.
 3. bronchopulmonary dysplasia.
 4. hypersensitivity pneumonitis.

59. A client who experienced smoke inhalation has developed pulmonary edema. The nurse auscultates the client's breath sounds and anticipates hearing:
 1. crackles.
 2. decreased breath sounds.
 3. inspiratory and expiratory wheezing.
 4. upper airway rhonchi.

60. A client has vocal cord paralysis due to a complication experienced during thyroidectomy surgery. Which instructions should the nurse reinforce with the family caregiver prior to discharge?
 1. Inform the health care provider when the client experiences hoarseness
 2. Remind the client to take cough medication twice a day
 3. Have the client sit in an upright position when eating
 4. Prevent the client from drinking coffee on a daily basis

61. The nurse is explaining the process of acute respiratory distress syndrome (ARDS) to a client and her family. How should the nurse **best** describe this disease?
 1. Alveoli are over expanded.
 2. Alveoli increase perfusion.
 3. Alveolar spaces are filled with fluid.
 4. Alveoli improve gaseous exchange.

62. A 69-year-old client has developed acute shortness of breath and progressive hypoxia that requires mechanical ventilation following the repair of a fractured right femur. The nurse determines that the hypoxia was probably a result of:
 1. asthma attack.
 2. atelectasis.
 3. bronchitis.
 4. fat embolism.

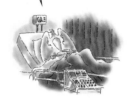

I feel so distressed. What about you?

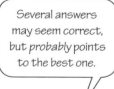

Several answers may seem correct, but probably points to the best one.

58. 1. Severe hypoxia, following smoke inhalation, is typically related to ARDS. The other conditions aren't typically associated with smoke inhalation and severe hypoxia.
CN: Physiological integrity; CNS: Physiological adaptation; CL: Apply

59. 1. In pulmonary edema, the most frequently heard sounds are crackles. Decreased breath sounds and inspiratory and expiratory wheezing are associated with asthma, and rhonchi is heard when there's sputum in the airways.
CN: Physiological integrity; CNS: Physiological adaptation; CL: Apply

60. 3. It is important that the caregiver keep client in an upright position while eating or drinking to prevent aspiration. Primary symptoms, that should be reported, include airway compromise and swallowing difficulties. Voice changes, such as hoarseness, croaky or breathy sounds should be monitored, but do not require immediate reporting. This client would not typically receive cough medication. There is no need to restrict coffee consumption. It is recommended that this client avoid alcohol and any form of tobacco.
CN: Physiological integrity; CNS: Physiological adaptation; CL: Apply

61. 3. ARDS leads to a buildup of fluid in the air sacs (alveoli). This fluid prevents enough oxygen from passing into the bloodstream. The fluid buildup also makes the lungs heavy and stiff, which decreases the lungs' ability to expand. The alveoli collapse, and gas exchange becomes impaired.
CN: Physiological integrity; CNS: Physiological adaptation; CL: Apply

62. 4. Long bone fractures are often correlated with fat emboli, which cause shortness of breath and hypoxia. It's unlikely that this client has developed asthma or bronchitis without a previous history of those conditions. This client could develop atelectasis, but that would not typically produce progressive hypoxia.
CN: Physiological integrity; CNS: Physiological adaptation; CL: Analyze

63. A client, who developed a fat embolism, is receiving 100% FiO$_2$ on a mechanical ventilator. The client continues to be hypoxic. What is the nurse's **most** important intervention?
1. Add positive end-expiratory pressure (PEEP)
2. Give beta-adrenergic blockers
3. Give diuretics
4. Increase the FiO$_2$ on the ventilator

64. A client, with a fat embolism, continues to be hypoxic following therapy with positive end-expiratory pressure (PEEP). What is the **priority** intervention to reduce oxygen demand?
1. Administer diuretics
2. Administer neuromuscular blockers
3. Put the head of the bed flat
4. Use bronchodilators

65. The client is receiving positive end-expiratory pressure (PEEP) therapy. The nurse anticipates that this client will exhibit:
1. bradycardia.
2. tachycardia.
3. increased blood pressure.
4. reduced cardiac output.

66. The nurse has placed a client diagnosed with acute respiratory distress syndrome (ARDS) in the prone position. The nurse determined that this position would:
1. improve cardiac output.
2. make the client more comfortable.
3. prevent reduce skin breakdown.
4. recruit more alveoli.

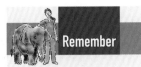

Remember

"-curium and -curonium drugs calm muscles."

Neuromuscular drugs, many of which end in either "-curium" or "-curonium," are used to relax skeletal muscles by disrupting the transmission of nerve impulses. These drugs include the following:
- Atracurium
- Cisatracurium
- Mivacurium
- Pancuronium
- Rocuronium
- Vecuronium

You're a natural! Keep going!

63. 1. PEEP can be added to open alveoli and keep them open. There's no reason to give this client beta-adrenergic blockers. The client may benefit from diuresis, but in the meantime, PEEP should be added to improve oxygenation. The highest amount of oxygen that can be delivered is 100% FiO$_2$.
CN: Physiological integrity; CNS: Physiological adaptation; CL: Apply

64. 2. Neuromuscular blockers will cause skeletal muscle paralysis, which reduces the amount of oxygen used by restless skeletal muscles. This action should improve oxygenation. Diuretics can be administered to reduce pulmonary congestion. The head of the bed should be partially elevated to facilitate diaphragm movement. Bronchodilators may be used, but they typically don't reduce the amount of hypoxia present. Diuretics, elevating the head of the bed, and bronchodilators would improve oxygen delivery, but would not reduce oxygen demand.
CN: Physiological integrity; CNS: Physiological adaptation; CL: Apply

65. 4. PEEP reduces cardiac output by increasing intrathoracic pressure and reducing the amount of blood delivered to the left side of the heart, thereby reducing cardiac output. It doesn't affect heart rate, but a decrease in cardiac output may reduce blood pressure, commonly causing compensatory tachycardia.
CN: Physiological integrity; CNS: Physiological adaptation; CL: Apply

66. 4. Turning the client to the prone position may recruit new alveoli in the posterior region of the lungs, and improve oxygenation status. A supine position may reduce the ability of the posterior alveoli to open and remain open. Cardiac output shouldn't be affected by the prone position. The prone position doesn't make a client more comfortable, and often requires sedation to be tolerable. Skin breakdown can still occur over the new pressure points.
CN: Physiological integrity; CNS: Physiological adaptation; CL: Apply

CN: Client needs category   CNS: Client needs subcategory   CL: Cognitive level

67. Which diagnosis is **most** likely to contribute to the development of acute respiratory distress syndrome (ARDS)?
  1. Acute appendicitis
  2. Massive trauma
  3. Receiving conscious sedation
  4. Right meniscus injury

67. 2. The client with massive trauma will require multiple transfusions. Blood products are preserved with citrate, which causes increased permeability in the lungs. Increased permeability allows ARDS to develop. Acute appendicitis, unless it causes overwhelming sepsis, won't lead to ARDS. Conscious sedation and injuries to the meniscus don't lead to ARDS.
CN: Physiological integrity; CNS: Physiological adaptation; CL: Analyze

Health care is a team sport. Don't forget to communicate with your teammates.

68. A nurse is reviewing the assessment of a client with acute respiratory distress syndrome (ARDS). Which clinical data **best** indicates improvement in this client?
  1. Arterial blood gas (ABG) values
  2. Bronchoscopy results
  3. Increased blood pressure
  4. Sputum culture and sensitivity results

68. 1. Improved ABG results would indicate that this client's oxygenation status has improved. Hypoxia occurs with ARDS, so bronchoscopy and sputum culture results may have no bearing on the improvement of ARDS. Increased blood pressure isn't relative to the client's respiratory condition.
CN: Physiological integrity; CNS: Physiological adaptation; CL: Analyze

69. A nurse is making a home visit and finds an older adult client who requires immediate treatment for exposure to carbon monoxide. What **priority** action would the nurse take prior to the arrival of the paramedics?
  1. Loosen all tight fitting clothing
  2. Expose the client to fresh air
  3. Monitor for breathing difficulties
  4. Provide warm clothing or a blanket

The doctor says we have "thoracic kyphoscoliosis." What does that mean? I don't know, but I feel so restricted.

69. 2. The priority action is to expose the client to fresh air. The client should be moved away from carbon monoxide area. If the person is unconscious, check for injuries before moving. Call 911 and begin CPR, if necessary.
CN: Physiological integrity; CNS: Physiological adaptation; CL: Apply

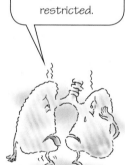

70. A client has been diagnosed with thoracic kyphoscoliosis. What effect will this diagnosis have on the client's lungs?
  1. Improve overall expansion
  2. Obstruct deflation
  3. Reduce alveolar compression during expiration
  4. Restrict expansion

70. 4. Thoracic kyphoscoliosis causes lung compression, restricts lung expansion, and results in more rapid and shallow respiration. It doesn't improve lung expansion because of the compression. It also doesn't cause obstruction or reduce alveolar compression during expiration.
CN: Physiological integrity; CNS: Physiological adaptation; CL: Apply

71. A 24-year-old client comes into the clinic reporting sudden-onset, right-sided chest pain and shortness of breath. While assessing the client, the nurse determines that the **most** important intervention is to:
  1. auscultate the breath sounds.
  2. order a chest X-ray.
  3. order an echocardiogram.
  4. order an electrocardiogram (ECG).

71. 1. Because this client is short of breath, listening to breath sounds will allow the nurse to obtain information to support care decisions and report information that will help identify the problem. Breath sounds may be decreased, abnormal or absent when a client is short of breath. The client may need a chest X-ray and an ECG, but a health care provider must order these tests. Unless a cardiac source for the client's pain is identified, an echocardiogram won't be necessary.
CN: Physiological integrity; CNS: Physiological adaptation; CL: Apply

72. A client with shortness of breath has decreased-to-absent breath sounds from the apex to the base of the lung on the right side. How would the nurse interpret this assessment finding?
1. Acute asthma
2. Chronic bronchitis
3. Pneumonia
4. Spontaneous pneumothorax

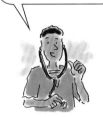

Listening to breath sounds sure helps diagnose a lot of conditions, doesn't it?

72. 4. A spontaneous pneumothorax occurs when the client's lung collapses, causing an acute decrease in lung function. A sudden collapse will cause chest pain and shortness of breath. Wheezes would be heard if asthma were present, and the client with bronchitis would have rhonchi. Pneumonia would have bronchial breath sounds over the area of consolidation.
CN: Physiological integrity; CNS: Physiological adaptation; CL: Analyze

73. The nurse anticipates that the **priority** treatment for a client with spontaneous pneumothorax is:
1. antibiotics.
2. bronchodilators.
3. chest tube placement.
4. hyperbaric chamber.

73. 3. The only way to re-expand a lung is to place a chest tube so air in the pleural space can be removed and the lung re-expanded. Antibiotics and bronchodilators would have no effect on lung re-expansion, nor would placing the client in a hyperbaric chamber.
CN: Physiological integrity; CNS: Physiological adaptation; CL: Apply

74. A 60-year-old client, involved in a motor vehicle accident, was brought to the emergency department by paramedics. During the assessment, the client reports difficulty breathing and chest pain. Auscultation of the lung fields reveals absent breath sounds in the left upper lobe. The nurse interprets this information as indicative of:
1. bronchitis.
2. pneumonia.
3. pneumothorax.
4. tuberculosis (TB).

74. 3. This client may have a left pneumothorax related to trauma. Auscultation would reveal rhonchi if this client had bronchitis, bronchial breath sounds if this client had pneumonia, and rhonchorous breath sounds with TB.
CN: Physiological integrity; CNS: Physiological adaptation; CL: Apply

75. A client is suspected of having a pneumothorax. The nurse anticipates that this diagnosis will be confirmed by:
1. auscultating breath sounds.
2. having the client use an incentive spirometer.
3. reviewing the chest X-ray report.
4. performing a thoracic puncture.

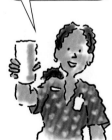

Cheers! You're doing a great job.

75. 3. A chest X-ray will reveal the area of collapsed lung, as well as the volume of air in the pleural space, if a pneumothorax is present. Listening to breath sounds won't confirm a diagnosis. An incentive spirometer is used to encourage deep breathing. A needle thoracostomy is performed by trained personnel, and only in an emergency situation.
CN: Physiological integrity; CNS: Physiological adaptation; CL: Apply

76. Following a motor vehicle collision, a client has a chest tube inserted in the left upper chest. The tube begins to drain dark red fluid. What does the nurse determine?
1. The chest tube was inserted improperly.
2. This is an expected result for this client.
3. An artery was nicked when the chest tube was placed.
4. The client is experiencing a hemothorax.

76. 4. This client has a hemothorax, in which blood collection causes a lung to collapse. The placement of a chest tube will drain blood from the space and re-expand the lung. An intercostal artery can be nicked during chest tube insertion, but the risk is minimal if the provider placing the tube is specifically trained. The initial chest X-ray would confirm the presence of blood, or air in the pleural space.
CN: Physiological integrity; CNS: Physiological adaptation; CL: Apply

CN: Client needs category   CNS: Client needs subcategory   CL: Cognitive level

77. A hospitalized client has a central IV catheter inserted in the subclavian vein. Shortly after placement, the client develops shortness of breath and appears restless. What is the nurse's **priority** action?
1. Administer a sedative
2. Advise the client to relax
3. Auscultate for breath sounds
4. Check for medication allergies

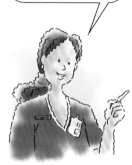

This question is checking you know the order of priority.

77. 3. The nurse should listen to the client's lungs to see if anything has changed. This client should not receive medication, especially sedatives, if dyspnea is present. This client should receive emotional support. The provider who placed the central venous access should be contacted. The nurse should check for medication allergies following the assessment.
CN: Physiological integrity; CNS: Physiological adaptation; CL: Analyze

78. A nurse is caring for a client who recently had a central venous catheter inserted. The client now appears short of breath and anxious. The nurse anticipates that the health care provider will order a:
1. chest X-ray.
2. electrocardiogram.
3. laboratory tests.
4. sedation.

78. 1. Inserting an IV catheter in the subclavian vein can result in pneumothorax. A chest X-ray should be done to confirm a pneumothorax. If the X-ray is negative, other tests should be done, but are not the first intervention. Sedation may further depress respirations.
CN: Physiological integrity; CNS: Reduction of risk potential; CL: Apply

79. A nurse is preparing a client for chest tube insertion in the upper right chest. What is the **priority** role of the nurse?
1. A nurse isn't required.
2. Preparing the chest tube drainage system
3. Bringing the chest X-ray to the client's room
4. Inserting the chest tube

79. 2. The nurse must anticipate that a drainage system will be required, and the system readied prior to chest tube for immediate connection following insertion. The chest X-ray need not be brought into the client's room. A trained provider will insert the chest tube.
CN: Physiological integrity; CNS: Physiological adaptation; CL: Apply

80. A nurse is auscultating the lungs of a client following chest tube insertion. What assessment finding would indicate correct chest tube placement?
1. Bronchial sounds heard at both bases
2. Vesicular sounds heard over the upper lung fields
3. Bronchovesicular sounds heard over both lung fields
4. Crackles heard on the affected side

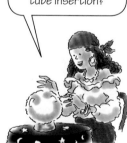

Which breath sounds do I predict hearing after chest tube insertion?

80. 3. If the chest tube is inserted correctly, normal bronchovesicular breath sounds should be heard and the client's oxygenation status should improve. A chest X-ray should be done to ensure re-expansion. All other sounds noted are abnormal.
CN: Physiological integrity; CNS: Reduction of risk potential; CL: Analyze

81. The nurse is caring for a client who has had a chest tube inserted for the treatment of a pneumothorax. Which assessment finding **best** indicates, to the nurse, that a chest tube is no longer needed?
1. There is minimal drainage from the chest tube.
2. Arterial blood gas (ABG) results are within normal range.
3. The client states he is not experiencing dyspnea.
4. No fluctuation in the water seal chamber occurs when no suction is applied.

81. 4. One indication of lung re-expansion is the cessation of fluctuation in the water seal chamber when suction isn't applied. Drainage should be minimal before the chest tube is removed. An ABG analysis may be done to ensure proper oxygenation, but isn't necessary if other clinical assessment criteria are met. A chest tube isn't removed until the client's lung has adequately re-expanded, and remains expanded.
CN: Physiological integrity; CNS: Physiological adaptation; CL: Analyze

CN: Client needs category   CNS: Client needs subcategory   CL: Cognitive level

82. A client is scheduled to have a chest tube removed. What is the **priority** nursing intervention prior to tube removal?
1. Disconnect the drainage system from the tube
2. Obtain a chest X-ray to document lung re-expansion
3. Obtain arterial blood gases (ABG) to document oxygen status
4. Sedate the client and have the health care provider remove the tube

82. 2. A chest X-ray should be done to ensure the lung is re-expanded and has remained expanded since suction was discontinued. The drainage system shouldn't be disconnected from the tube until it has been removed because a pneumothorax could reoccur. A pulse oximetry measurement, rather than ABG is sufficient to track oxygenation prior to tube removal. If the client can hold his breath while the chest tube is removed, there's less chance that air will be drawn back into the pleural space.
CN: Physiological integrity; CNS: Reduction of risk potential; CL: Apply

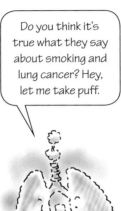

Do you think it's true what they say about smoking and lung cancer? Hey, let me take puff.

83. A nurse is teaching a client about lung cancer. The nurse determines that teaching was effective when the client states that which is the primary cause of lung cancer?
1. Genetics
2. Occupational exposures
3. Pipe smoking
4. Cigarette smoking

83. 4. As many as 90% of clients afflicted with lung cancer smoke cigarettes. Cigarette smoke contains several organ-specific carcinogens. There may be a genetic predisposition for the development of cancer. Occupational hazards, such as pollutants, can cause cancer. Pipe smokers inhale less often than cigarette smokers and tend to develop cancers of the lip and mouth.
CN: Health promotion and maintenance; CNS: None; CL: Apply

84. A nurse reinforces the teaching plan for a client who has recently been diagnosed with squamous cell carcinoma of the left lung. What is the **most** appropriate information for the nurse to give this client?
1. "You have a slow-growing cancer that rarely spreads."
2. "In terms of prognosis, you may have only a few months to live."
3. "Squamous cell cancer is a very rapid-growing cancer."
4. "The cancer has generally metastasized by the time diagnosis is made."

84. 1. Squamous cell carcinoma is a slow-growing, rarely metastasizing type of cancer. It has the most optimistic prognosis of all lung cancer types.
CN: Physiological integrity; CNS: Physiological adaptation; CL: Analyze

85. A nurse is obtaining assessment data from a client with possible lung cancer. The nurse is **most** concerned if the client exhibits which symptom?
1. Dizziness
2. Generalized weakness
3. Hypotension
4. Recurrent pleural effusions

85. 4. Recurring episodes of pleural effusions can be caused by a tumor, and should be investigated. Dizziness, generalized weakness, and hypotension aren't typically considered warning signs, but may occur in advanced stages of cancer.
CN: Physiological integrity; CNS: Physiological adaptation; CL: Apply

CN: Client needs category   CNS: Client needs subcategory   CL: Cognitive level

86. The nurse is admitting a client, diagnosed with a centrally located lung tumor, to the medical unit. On assessment, which symptom would the nurse anticipate from this client?
 1. Coughing
 2. Hemoptysis
 3. Pleuritic pain
 4. Shoulder pain

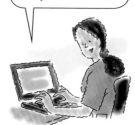

Centrally located. That's your clue for question 86.

86. 1. Centrally-located lung tumors are found in the upper airway, and usually produce such coughing, wheezing, and stridor. Small-cell tumors tend to be located in the lower airways and often cause hemoptysis. Tumors invading the pleural space may cause pleuritic pain. Pancoast tumors, which occur in the apices, may cause shoulder pain.
CN: Physiological integrity; CNS: Physiological adaptation; CL: Analyze

87. A client, with a suspected diagnosis of lung cancer, tells the nurse that the health care provider is scheduling tests to confirm the diagnosis. The nurse understands that the definitive diagnosis will be **best** determined by which test?
 1. Bronchoscopy
 2. Chest X-ray
 3. Computed tomography (CT) scan
 4. Surgical biopsy

87. 4. Only surgical biopsy with cytologic examination of the cells can give a definitive diagnosis of cancer and type. A biopsy taken during a bronchoscopy would not yield enough tissue to determine if a tumor is a carcinoid. Bronchoscopy gives positive results in only 30% of the cases. Chest X-ray and CT scan can identify location of abnormal tissue, but not confirm cancer.
CN: Physiological integrity; CNS: Physiological adaptation; CL: Apply

88. Which statements are true regarding lung cancer tumor staging? Select all that apply.
 1. Staging describes the severity of the cancer.
 2. Staging helps the health care provider plan appropriate treatment.
 3. Staging systems don't change over time.
 4. Surgical biopsy with cytologic cell examination is the only data collection method used to perform staging.
 5. Staging helps to determine whether the cancer has spread to distant areas of the body.

88. 1, 2, 5. Staging describes the extent and severity of the cancer, and helps the health care provider determine the most appropriate therapy. Staging systems continue to evolve as cancer is better understood. Multiple data collection methods, such as laboratory results, physical examinations, and imaging results, are used to determine the stage of a cancer.
CN: Physiological integrity; CNS: Physiological adaptation; CL: Analyze

89. The nurse understands that the **best** way to increase survival rates in those diagnosed with lung cancer is:
 1. routine bronchoscopy.
 2. early detection.
 3. high-dose chemotherapy.
 4. smoking cessation.

89. 2. Detecting cancer when the cells may be premalignant and potentially curable is most beneficial. A tumor must be one cm in diameter before it can be detected on a chest X-ray. A bronchoscopy can assist with early identification, but is often not ordered until an abnormal X-ray occurs. High-dose chemotherapy has minimal effect on long-term lung cancer survival. Smoking cessation won't reverse the process, but may prevent further decompensation.
CN: Health promotion and maintenance; CNS: None; CL: Apply

90. A client tells the nurse that his chest tube has been accidentally removed. What is the **most** appropriate action by the nurse?
1. Position the client on the left side
2. Position the client on the right side
3. Apply an occlusive dressing over the site
4. Reinsert the chest tube that fell out

90. 3. To prevent this client from sucking air into the pleural space and causing a pneumothorax, an occlusive dressing should be applied over the hole. The health care provider should be called, and the client checked for signs of respiratory distress. Positioning the client on either the left or right side won't make a difference. The old tube should not be reinserted because it's no longer sterile.
CN: Physiological integrity; CNS: Reduction of risk potential; CL: Apply

91. A client has been diagnosed with lung cancer and requires a wedge resection. The client asks the nurse to describe a wedge resection. The **most** appropriate response, by the nurse, is that the procedure involves resection of:
1. one entire lung.
2. a lobe of the lung.
3. a small, localized area near the surface of the lung.
4. a segment of the lung, including a bronchiole and its alveoli.

91. 3. A small area of tissue close to the surface of the lung is removed in a wedge resection. An entire lung is removed in a pneumonectomy. A lobe is removed in a lobectomy, and a segment of the lung is removed in a segmental resection.
CN: Physiological integrity; CNS: Physiological adaptation; CL: Apply

92. A nurse is caring for a client who has just returned to the unit following a lobectomy. During assessment, the nurse is aware that the lobectomy site:
1. remains empty.
2. is filled with a gel by the surgeon.
3. is filled with serous fluid.
4. is filled by overexpansion of the remaining lobes.

92. 4. The remaining lobe or lobes over expand slightly to fill the space previously occupied by the tissue that has been removed. The diaphragm is carried higher on the operative side to further reduce the empty space. The surgeon doesn't use gel to fill the space. Serous fluid overproduction would compress the remaining lobes, diminish their function, and, possibly, cause a mediastinal shift.
CN: Physiological integrity; CNS: Physiological adaptation; CL: Apply

93. A client, scheduled for a pneumonectomy, asks the nurse how the thoracic cavity will be filled. What is the nurse's **best** response?
1. The space remains filled with air only.
2. The surgeon fills the space with a gel.
3. Serous fluid fills the space and consolidates the region.
4. The lung tissue from the remaining lung grows in the space.

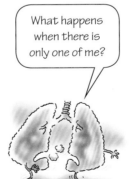

What happens when there is only one of me?

93. 3. In the immediately post-operative period air and serous fluid fills the space. Eventually the area consolidates, preventing extensive mediastinal shift of the heart and remaining lung. Air can't be left in the space. There's no gel that can be placed in the pleural space. The tissue from the other lung can't cross the mediastinum, although a temporary mediastinal shift exists until the space is filled.
CN: Physiological integrity; CNS: Physiological adaptation; CL: Apply

94. A client is scheduled to undergo a pneumonectomy. The nurse determines that the client understands the rationale for cutting the phrenic nerve and experiencing hemi-diaphragm paralysis when the client states the procedure will:
1. paralyze the diaphragm and reduce oxygen demand.
2. reduce the intensity of the postoperative pain.
3. increase the capacity of the remaining lung.
4. reduce the space left by the pneumonectomy.

94. 4. Because the hemi-diaphragm is a muscle that doesn't contract when paralyzed, it remains in an elevated position, reducing the space left by the pneumonectomy. Serous fluid has less space to fill, reducing the extent and duration of a mediastinal shift following surgery. Paralyzing the hemi-diaphragm doesn't decrease total-body oxygen demand or increase the capacity of the remaining lung. The client will experience postoperative pain. Although the client no longer needs the hemi-diaphragm on the operative side to breathe, this wouldn't be sufficient justification for cutting the phrenic nerve.
CN: Physiological integrity; CNS: Physiological adaptation; CL: Apply

95. A client with symptoms of acute asthma is ordered IV aminophylline 350 mg in 100 ml to be administered over 30 minutes. The nurse has vials of IV aminophylline labeled 250 mg/5 ml. How many milliliters of fluid contain the dose ordered? Record your answer using a whole number.

_____ ml

95. 7.

$$\frac{350\,mg}{X} = \frac{250\,mg}{5\,ml}$$

$$X = 7\,ml$$

CN: Physiological integrity; CNS: Physiological adaptation; CL: Apply

96. A client, with pre-existing pulmonary disease, has been diagnosed with lung cancer. The client is being evaluated for surgery. The nurse is aware that the impact of both conditions may:
1. have no effect on the surgery.
2. require the whole lung to be removed.
3. prevent the resection of the entire tumor.
4. prohibit the client from having the surgery done.

96. 4. If the client's pre-existing pulmonary disease is restrictive and advanced, it may be impossible to perform surgery, and the client may have to be treated with only chemotherapy and radiation.
CN: Physiological integrity; CNS: Physiological adaptation; CL: Apply

97. The nurse is performing preoperative teaching for a client scheduled for surgery. What should be the primary focus of this teaching?
1. Deciding if the client is an appropriate candidate for the surgery
2. Giving emotional support to the client and his family
3. Giving minute details of the surgery to the client and his family
4. Providing general information to reduce client and family anxiety

97. 4. The nurse's role is to provide general information about the surgery, explain expectations before and after surgery, and provide emotional support during this time. The nurse's role isn't to decide if the client should have surgery or to give minute details of the surgery unless the client or family requests them. The surgeon should answer most of the client's specific questions. Providing only emotional support, at this time, isn't sufficient.
CN: Physiological integrity; CNS: Reduction of risk potential; CL: Apply

CN: Client needs category   CNS: Client needs subcategory   CL: Cognitive level

98. A client, diagnosed with a large benign lung tumor, asks the nurse how it will be treated. What is the nurse's **best** response?
1. The tumor is treated with only radiation therapy.
2. The tumor is treated with only chemotherapy.
3. The tumor is left alone unless symptoms are present.
4. The tumor is removed with the least possible amount of tissue.

98. 4. The tumor is removed to prevent further compression of lung tissue as the benign tumor grows. If the tumor can't be removed, then radiation or chemotherapy may be used to reduce the size of the growth.
CN: Physiological integrity; CNS: Physiological adaptation; CL: Apply

99. The nurse is caring for a client with terminal lung cancer. What is the **priority** nursing intervention for this client?
1. Provide emotional support.
2. Provide nutritional support.
3. Provide pain control.
4. Prepare the client's will.

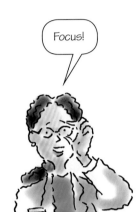

Focus!

99. 3. A client, with terminal lung cancer, may have extreme pleuritic pain and should be treated to reduce his discomfort. Preparing the client and their family for impending death and providing emotional support are also important, but shouldn't be the primary focus until the pain is under control. Nutritional support may be provided, but as the terminal phase advances, the client's nutritional needs greatly decrease. Nursing care doesn't focus on helping the client prepare a will.
CN: Physiological integrity; CNS: Basic care and comfort; CL: Analyze

100. A client, who weighs 165 lb (75 kg), with a pulmonary embolus, is ordered to receive heparin 20 units/kg/hr by IV infusion. How many units of heparin should the client receive each hour?
1. 1,000
2. 1,200
3. 1,500
4. 1,700

100. 3. Use the client's weight in kilograms.

$$20 \ units/kg/hr \times 75 \ kg = 1,500 \ units/hr$$

CN: Physiological integrity; CNS: Pharmacological and parenteral therapies; CL: Apply

101. A nurse is conducting a preoperative class for clients scheduled for gastric bypass surgery. One of the clients asks the nurse about the most common source of pulmonary embolism. What should be the nurse's response?
1. Amniotic fluid
2. Bone marrow
3. Septic thrombi
4. Venous thrombi

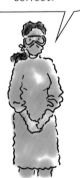

This clue asks you to select the most common, even when all answers are correct.

101. 4. Venous thrombi in the thigh and pelvis are the most common sources for pulmonary emboli. Clients who are immobile often form clots from these sites. When dislodged, the clots are carried through the bloodstream and lodge in the pulmonary vasculature. The other options are also sources but not the most common.
CN: Physiological integrity; CNS: Physiological adaptation; CL: Apply

102. Which client is at **highest** risk for developing a pulmonary embolism?
1. An ambulatory client who has inflammatory joint disease
2. An ambulatory client who has type 1 diabetes mellitus
3. A healthy client who is almost six months pregnant
4. A client who has fractures of the pelvis and right femur

102. 4. Thrombosis formation is caused by abnormalities in blood flow, vein wall integrity, and blood coagulation. The client with pelvic and femur fractures will be immobilized and probably have edema, which leads to venous stasis. This predisposes the client to the development of deep vein thrombosis. A pulmonary embolus commonly arises from clots in the deep veins of the leg that break off and travel to the pulmonary arteries. The risk of developing venous thrombosis isn't as high with the other conditions.
CN: Physiological integrity; CNS: Physiological adaptation; CL: Apply

103. The nurse is planning care for a client who has undergone a total knee replacement. What is the nurse's **priority** intervention to prevent the development of a pulmonary embolism?
1. Early ambulation
2. Chest X-ray detection
3. Lower extremity scans
4. Client intubation

Hint! Check out the words *priority intervention!*

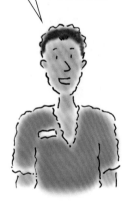

103. 1. Early ambulation will help reduce the pooling of blood, and decrease the tendency of blood to form a clot that could then dislodge. Frequent chest X-rays or lower extremity scans don't prevent pulmonary embolism. Intubation of the client won't prevent the occurrence of a pulmonary embolism.
CN: Physiological integrity; CNS: Reduction of risk potential; CL: Apply

104. Which physiologic effect of a pulmonary embolism would initially affect oxygenation?
1. A blood clot blocks ventilation without affecting perfusion.
2. A blood clot blocks ventilation, and produces hypoxia despite normal perfusion.
3. A blood clot blocks perfusion and ventilation, and produces profound hypoxia.
4. A blood clot blocks perfusion and produces hypoxia despite normal ventilation.

104. 4. A blood clot would block blood flow to a region of the lung tissue. The area would remain ventilated; however blood flow is blocked, and no gas exchange can occur in that region. A ventilation-perfusion mismatch occurs. Ventilation isn't initially affected by a blood clot because air can still move normally through the bronchial tree.
CN: Physiological integrity; CNS: Physiological adaptation; CL: Apply

105. A nurse is teaching the client about his pulmonary embolism. The client tells the nurse that he has a ventilation-perfusion mismatch. Which statement, by the client, **best** conveys an understanding of this diagnosis?
1. "The area of the lung being ventilated isn't being perfused."
2. "The area of the lung being perfused isn't being ventilated."
3. "The area of the lung being ventilated is also being perfused."
4. "The amount of ventilation occurring doesn't equal perfusion."

105. 1. A pulmonary embolism blocks the flow of blood past a region of lung tissue that is still being ventilated because no disorder of the bronchial tree exists. A pulmonary embolism blocks the pulmonary vasculature, not allowing blood to flow to the distal region of the lung and interferes with gas exchange. Blood must flow around each alveolus for the exchange of carbon dioxide and oxygen to occur. When an area of lung is ventilated but not perfused, there is a ventilation-perfusion mismatch specific to pulmonary embolism. A mismatch that shows impaired ventilation but normal perfusion would indicate a pathological state in the bronchial tree, such as pneumonia or atelectasis.
CN: Physiological integrity; CNS: Physiological adaptation; CL: Apply

106. A client has been exposed to radiation and is diagnosed with acute radiation syndrome. What symptoms would the nurse anticipate shortly after exposure?
1. Gastrointestinal system distress
2. Opportunistic infections occur
3. Decreased lymphocyte count
4. Increased intracranial pressure

106. 1. Gastrointestinal system distress. The classic symptoms for this stage are nausea, vomiting and diarrhea that occur from minutes to days following exposure, and may last up to several days.
CN: Physiological integrity; CNS: Physiological adaptation; CL: Apply

107. A client, diagnosed with a pulmonary embolism, tells the nurse that he feels a sense of extreme apprehension. The nurse recognizes that this manifestation is caused by:
1. an inflammation in the lung parenchyma.
2. loss of bilateral chest expansion.
3. loss of lung tissue area.
4. a sudden reduction in oxygenation.

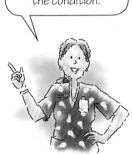

Here's a hint for question 107: Think about what causes the condition.

107. 4. The client with a pulmonary embolism has a portion of the lung that does not produce oxygenation, causing the client to feel extremely apprehensive. If the area involved is large, the apprehension can be great, giving the client the feeling of impending doom. The inflammatory reaction in the lung causes chest pain. There's no actual loss of lung tissue, and chest expansion isn't affected.
CN: Physiological integrity; CNS: Physiological adaptation; CL: Apply

108. 1A client with pulmonary embolism has developed hemoptysis. The nurse determines that this is **most** likely related to:
1. alveolar damage in the infarcted area.
2. blood vessel involvement where a clot was formed.
3. loss of lung parenchyma.
4. loss of lung tissue.

108. 1. The infarcted area produces alveolar damage that can lead to the production of bloody sputum, sometimes in massive amounts. Clot formation usually occurs in the legs. There's a loss of lung parenchyma and subsequent scar tissue formation, but these don't cause hemoptysis.
CN: Physiological integrity; CNS: Physiological adaptation; CL: Apply

109. A client with a massive pulmonary embolism is scheduled to have arterial blood gas analysis performed. The nurse expects the analysis will identify which condition?
1. Metabolic acidosis
2. Metabolic alkalosis
3. Respiratory acidosis
4. Respiratory alkalosis

109. 4. A client with a massive pulmonary embolism will have a large region of lung tissue that is unavailable for perfusion. This will cause the client to hyperventilate and blow off large amounts of carbon dioxide, which crosses the unaffected alveolar-capillary membrane more readily than does oxygen resulting in respiratory alkalosis.
CN: Physiological integrity; CNS: Physiological adaptation; CL: Analyze

110. A client, scheduled to have a ventilation-perfusion scan, asks the nurse to explain the tests. The nurse tells the client that the test will help diagnose a pulmonary embolism and provide information about:
1. amount of pleural surface and oxygenation present.
2. extent of the occlusion and amount of perfusion lost.
3. location and size of the pulmonary embolism.
4. presence of perfusion and atelectasis abnormalities.

110. 2. The ventilation-perfusion scan will provide information on the extent of occlusion caused by the pulmonary embolism and the amount of lung tissue involved in the area not perfused. It does not address the amount of pleural surface and oxygenation present, the size of a pulmonary emboli, or presence of perfusion and atelectasis abnormalities.
CN: Physiological integrity; CNS: Physiological adaptation; CL: Apply

CN: Client needs category   CNS: Client needs subcategory   CL: Cognitive level

111. A client, suspected of having a pulmonary embolism, asks the nurse how a definitive diagnosis is determined. Which test would definitively diagnosis a pulmonary embolism?
1. Arterial blood gas (ABG) analysis
2. Chest X-ray
3. Pulmonary angiogram
4. Ventilation-perfusion scan

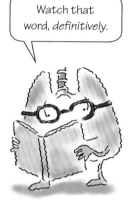

Watch that word, *definitively.*

111. 3. A pulmonary angiogram will definitively diagnose a pulmonary embolism. A catheter would be passed through the circulation to the region of the occlusion. The region would be outlined with an injection of contrast medium and viewed by fluoroscopy. This would show the location of the clot, as well as the extent of defective perfusion. ABG levels could define the amount of hypoxia present. A chest X-ray can't provide a definitive diagnosis of pulmonary embolism. The ventilation-perfusion scan can report whether there's a ventilation-perfusion mismatch present, and define the amount of tissue involved.
CN: Physiological integrity; CNS: Reduction of risk potential; CL: Apply

112. A definitive diagnosis of pulmonary embolism has been made for a client. Which medication would the nurse anticipate for this client?
1. Warfarin
2. Heparin
3. Streptokinase
4. Acyclovir

112. 2. Intravenous heparin is started once a pulmonary embolism is diagnosed to reduce clot formation. When a therapeutic level of heparin is established, warfarin is started. It can take up to three days before a therapeutic level of warfarin is achieved. Streptokinase is a fibrinolytic, usefulness in the management of pulmonary embolism. Acyclovir is an antiviral and is not prescribed after a pulmonary embolism.
CN: Physiological integrity; CNS: Pharmacological and parenteral therapies; CL: Apply

113. A nurse is teaching a client diagnosed with a pulmonary embolism about the prescribed heparin therapy. The nurse determines that teaching has been effective when the client states heparin is given to:
1. dissolve the clot.
2. break up the pulmonary embolism.
3. slow the development of other clots.
4. prevent clots from traveling to the lung.

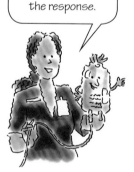

Knowing what a treatment should achieve will help you monitor the response.

113. 3. Heparin slows the development of other clots. It doesn't break up pulmonary embolisms or dissolve existing clots. Heparin doesn't stop clots from traveling to the lungs.
CN: Physiological integrity; CNS: Pharmacological and parenteral therapies; CL: Apply

114. A client, hospitalized for pulmonary embolism, is being discharged on warfarin therapy. The client asks the nurse to explain how warfarin works. What is the nurse's **best** response?
1. It inhibits the formation of blood clots.
2. It will reduce the size of the pulmonary embolism.
3. It will reduce blood pressure and prevent venous stasis.
4. It will dissolve an existing clot.

114. 1. Warfarin inhibits clot formation by interfering with clotting factors that are dependent on vitamin K. Warfarin doesn't dissolve clots, and won't reduce the size of a pulmonary embolus. It doesn't reduce blood pressure and won't prevent venous stasis. Coagulation studies will be performed every 2 to 4 weeks while the client is receiving warfarin.
CN: Physiological integrity; CNS: Pharmacological and parenteral therapies; CL: Apply

CN: Client needs category   CNS: Client needs subcategory   CL: Cognitive level

115. A client with a pulmonary embolism has been placed on oxygen therapy. The nurse is reviewing lab work and determines that the therapy is effective when the lab work shows which value?
1. $PaCO_2$ greater than 40 mmHg
2. $PaCO_2$ less than 40 mmHg
3. PaO_2 greater than 60 mmHg
4. PaO_2 less than 60 mmHg

115. 3. The goal of oxygen therapy for a client with a pulmonary embolism is to have a PaO_2 greater than 60 mmHg on FiO_2 of 40% or less. The normal range of the $PaCO_2$ is 35 to 45 mmHg. In the absence of other pathologic states, it should reach normal levels before the PaO_2 does on room air because carbon dioxide crosses the alveolar-capillary membrane with greater ease.
CN: Physiological integrity; CNS: Reduction of risk potential; CL: Analyze

116. A client, hospitalized with a pulmonary embolism, develops hypotension. The nurse determines that the hypotension was the result of:
1. pressure on the right side of the heart that caused a reduction in cardiac output.
2. reduced blood flow to the left lung that caused intermittent perfusion problems.
3. reduced blood return to the right side of the heart that lead to lower blood pressure.
4. increased pulmonary vascular resistance and reduced blood delivery to the left side of the heart.

116. 4. Blood meets resistance and can't perfuse the pulmonary vasculature because of the embolism. Pulmonary vascular resistance is increased, which reduces the amount of blood returned to the left side of the heart. This lowers cardiac output of the heart, and reduces blood pressure, sometimes significantly.
CN: Physiological integrity; CNS: Physiological adaptation; CL: Apply

117. A client with a pulmonary embolism is experiencing chest pain and apprehension. What is the nurse's **priority** intervention?
1. Administering ordered analgesic
2. Using visual guided imagery
3. Positioning the client on the left side
4. Providing emotional support

117. 1. Once a pulmonary embolism has been diagnosed and the amount of hypoxia determined, chest pain and the accompanying apprehension can be treated with analgesics as long as respiratory status isn't compromised. Guided imagery and emotional support can be used in conjunction with pain medication. Positioning the client on his left side when a pulmonary embolism is suspected may prevent a clot from breaking off and traveling through the heart into the arterial circulation.
CN: Physiological integrity; CNS: Physiological adaptation; CL: Apply

118. A client, with a pulmonary embolism, is scheduled to have an umbrella filter placed in the inferior vena cava. The nurse determines that teaching has been effective when the client states:
1. "The filter will prevent further blood clot formation."
2. "The filter will collect clots so they don't travel to the lungs."
3. "The filter will break the clots into small pieces."
4. "The filter contains anticoagulants that will dissolve any clots."

Always know the whys of a condition, especially the most common ones, like this one.

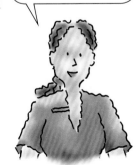

118. 2. The umbrella filter is placed in a client at high risk for the formation to collect clots so they don't travel to the lungs. The filter would trap large clot fragments and prevent them from traveling through the vena cava vein to the heart and lungs. It does not break clots into small pieces that would not significantly occlude the pulmonary vasculature. The filter doesn't prevent further clot formation and doesn't release anticoagulants.
CN: Physiological integrity; CNS: Physiological adaptation; CL: Apply

119. A nurse is providing preoperative teaching to a client scheduled for an embolectomy. The client is diagnosed with a pulmonary embolism. What **priority** information should the nurse provide to this client?
1. An embolectomy is done to remove an embolism in the lower extremity.
2. An embolectomy sucks an embolism out of the lung by bronchoscopy.
3. An embolectomy surgically removes the embolism source in the pelvis.
4. An embolectomy surgically removes the embolism in the pulmonary vasculature.

119. 4. If the pulmonary embolism is large and doesn't respond to treatment, an embolectomy may be necessary to restore perfusion to the lung. It's impossible to remove a pulmonary embolism through bronchoscopy because the defect isn't in the bronchial tree.
CN: Physiological integrity; CNS: Physiological adaptation; CL: Analyze

120. What is the nurse's **priority** intervention for a client diagnosed with a pulmonary embolism?
1. Assessing oxygenation status
2. Monitoring the oxygen delivery device
3. Monitoring for other sources of clots
4. Determining need for a ventilation-perfusion scan

120. 1. Nursing care should focus on assessing oxygenation status and ensuring that treatment is adequate. If the client's status begins to deteriorate, the nurse should contact the provider and attempt to improve oxygenation. Ensuring that the oxygen delivery device is working properly and monitoring for other clot sources aren't the primary focus of care. The provider would determine if the client required another ventilation-perfusion scan.
CN: Physiological integrity; CNS: Reduction of risk potential; CL: Apply

121. The nurse is obtaining a client's pulse oximetry reading. The nurse understands that pulse oximetry measures:
1. carbon dioxide in the blood.
2. oxygen in the blood.
3. the percentage of blood oxygen saturation.
4. the respiratory rate.

121. 3. Pulse oximetry indirectly monitors the oxygen saturation of a client's blood. This doesn't ensure that the oxygen being carried through the bloodstream is being perfused. Pulse oximetry doesn't provide information about the amount of carbon dioxide or oxygen in the blood or the client's respiratory rate.
CN: Physiological integrity; CNS: Physiological adaptation; CL: Apply

122. A nurse begins his shift by reading the following shift report. The nurse interprets these results as indicating which of the following?

Progress notes
Miscellaneous Reports
H.B. age 78
Hyperventilating, RR 36
Bpm. C/O dizziness, shortness of breath,
tingling in hands and feet, weakness. Anxious.
ABG: pH 7.48
Paco2: 33 mmHg

1. Metabolic acidosis
2. Acute respiratory failure
3. Respiratory alkalosis
4. Anxiety reaction

122. 3. Respiratory alkalosis is defined by a pH greater than 7.45 and $PaCO_2$ less than 35 mmHg, and generally is associated with deep, rapid breathing; light-headedness or dizziness; circumoral and peripheral paresthesia; and carpopedal spasms, twitching, and muscle weakness as it progresses. Metabolic acidosis is defined as a pH less than 7.3, $PaCO_2$ less than or equal to 34 mmHg depending on respiratory compensation, and HCO_3 less than 22 mEq/L and is caused by an underlying non-respiratory disorder. Acute respiratory failure is characterized by a pH less than 3, $PaCO_2$ greater than 50 mmHg, and markedly diminished oxygen saturation levels. Although the client may be anxious, the abnormal blood gas levels and corresponding symptoms indicate that treatment of respiratory alkalosis is the primary concern and may greatly reduce the client's anxiety level.
CN: Physiological integrity; CNS: Physiological adaptation; CL: Analyze

CN: Client needs category   CNS: Client needs subcategory   CL: Cognitive level

123. A client has been intubated and placed on a ventilator with positive end-expiratory pressure (PEEP). What is the primary purpose of PEEP?
1. Provide more oxygen and less carbon dioxide to the client
2. Open up bronchioles and allow more oxygen to the lungs
3. Open up the collapsed alveoli and help keep them open
4. Add pressure to the lung tissue and improve gas exchange

123. 3. PEEP delivers positive pressure to the lung at the end of expiration. This helps open collapsed alveoli and helps them stay open so gas exchange can occur in newly-opened alveoli, improving oxygenation. The bronchioles don't participate in gas exchange except to act as a conduit for inspired and expired air. The walls of the lungs are rigid enough that they generally don't collapse. PEEP doesn't add pressure directly to the lung tissue or provide more oxygen to the client.
CN: Physiological integrity; CNS: Physiological adaptation; CL: Apply

124. A nurse is reviewing a client's chest X-ray report. The report states that there are bilateral areas of collapsed alveoli in the bases. The nurse has initiated coughing and deep breathing exercises, reinforced the use of incentive spirometry, and encouraged the client to ambulate in the halls at least twice a day. Why did the nurse implement these interventions?
1. Alveoli need oxygen to live.
2. Alveoli have no effect on oxygenation.
3. Collapsed alveoli increase oxygen demand.
4. Gas exchange occurs in the alveolar membrane.

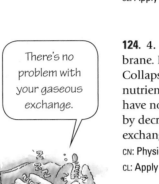

There's no problem with your gaseous exchange.

124. 4. Gas exchange occurs in the alveolar membrane. If alveoli collapse, no exchange occurs. Collapsed alveoli receive oxygen, as well as other nutrients from the bloodstream. Collapsed alveoli have no effect on oxygen demand, although by decreasing the surface area available for gas exchange, they decrease oxygenation of the blood.
CN: Physiological integrity; CNS: Physiological adaptation; CL: Apply

125. A hospitalized client is experiencing hypoxia. The health care provider orders continuous positive airway pressure (CPAP) per face mask. The family questions the nurse about the need for the mask. What is the **most** appropriate response by the nurse?
1. The mask provides 100% oxygen to the client.
2. The mask provides continuous air to the client.
3. The mask provides pressurized oxygen so the client can breathe more easily.
4. The mask provides pressurized oxygen at the end of expiration to open collapsed alveoli.

125. 3. The mask provides pressurized oxygen through inspiration and expiration. The mask can be set to deliver any amount of oxygen needed. By providing pressurized oxygen, the client has less resistance to overcome in taking in his next breath, making it easier to breathe. Pressurized oxygen, delivered at the end of expiration, is positive end-expiratory pressure, not CPAP.
CN: Physiological integrity; CNS: Physiological adaptation; CL: Apply

126. A client is being treated with bilevel positive airway pressure (BiPAP). The nurse anticipates that the use of BiPAP will provide:
1. 100% oxygen at both the inspiration and expiration periods.
2. pressurized oxygen so the client can breathe more easily.
3. pressurized oxygen at the end of expiration to open collapsed alveoli.
4. both continuous positive airway pressure (CPAP) and positive end-expiratory pressure (PEEP)

126. 4. BiPAP delivers both CPAP and PEEP. It provides differing pressures throughout the respiratory cycle to optimize oxygenation and ventilation. It's used in an effort to avoid intubation for mechanical ventilation. Inspiratory and expiratory pressures are set separately to optimize the client's ventilatory status, and the fraction of inspired oxygen is adjusted to optimize oxygenation. The second choice describes only the CPAP component of BiPAP, and the third choice describes the PEEP component.
CN: Physiological integrity; CNS: Physiological adaptation; CL: Apply

CN: Client needs category   CNS: Client needs subcategory   CL: Cognitive level

127. The nurse is caring for a client with a pleural effusion. The client asks, "What's a pleural effusion?" What is the nurse's **most** appropriate response?
1. Collapse of alveoli
2. Collapse of a bronchiole
3. Fluid in the alveolar space
4. Accumulation of fluid between the linings of the pleural space

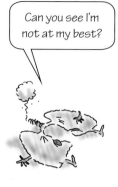

Can you see I'm not at my best?

127. 4. Pleural fluid normally seeps continually into the pleural space from the capillaries lining the parietal pleura. This fluid is reabsorbed by the visceral pleural capillaries and lymphatics. Any condition that interferes with either the secretion or drainage of this fluid will lead to a pleural effusion. The collapse of alveoli or a bronchiole has no particular name. Fluid within the alveolar space can be caused by heart failure or adult respiratory distress syndrome.

CN: Physiological integrity; CNS: Physiological adaptation; CL: Apply

128. A client, undergoing treatment for active pulmonary tuberculosis, is prescribed isoniazid tablets. The order is written for the client to receive 5 mg/kg of body weight up to a maximum of 300 mg daily. Based on the client's body weight of 143 lb (65 kg), how many 100-mg tablets should the nurse administer? Record your answer using a whole number.

_____ tablets

128. 3.

$$\frac{5\,mg}{1\,kg} = \frac{X\,mg}{65\,kg}$$

$$X = 325\,mg$$

The order reads not to exceed 300 mg; therefore, only three tablets are given.

CN: Physiological integrity; CNS: Physiological adaptation; CL: Apply

129. An 18-year-old client, who was involved in a motor vehicle accident, is admitted to the hospital with a diagnosis of pneumothorax. A chest tube is inserted and attached to a chest drainage system. The nurse notes almost constant bubbling in the water seal chamber. The nurse is aware that the bubbling is most likely the result of:
1. air leaks.
2. adequate suction.
3. inadequate suction.
4. kinked chest tubes.

129. 1. Bubbling in the water seal chamber of a chest drainage system stems from an air leak. In pneumothorax, an air leak can occur as air is pulled from the pleural space. Bubbling doesn't normally occur with either adequate or inadequate suction. A kinked chest tube can stop the suction and any pre-existing bubbling in the water seal chamber.

CN: Physiological integrity; CNS: Reduction of risk potential; CL: Apply

130. A comatose client requires nasopharyngeal airway suctioning. After the airway is inserted, the client gags and coughs. What is the **priority** nursing intervention?
1. Remove the airway and insert a shorter one
2. Reposition the airway
3. Leave the airway in place until the client gets used to it
4. Remove the airway and attempt suctioning without it

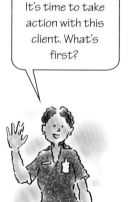

It's time to take action with this client. What's first?

130. 1. If a client gags or coughs during nasopharyngeal airway placement, it may indicate that the airway too long. The nurse should remove the airway and insert a shorter one. The client will not adjust to a catheter that is too long. Suctioning without a nasopharyngeal airway will cause trauma to the natural airway.

CN: Physiological integrity; CNS: Reduction of risk potential; CL: Apply

CN: Client needs category   CNS: Client needs subcategory   CL: Cognitive level

131. A nurse is teaching the family of an older adult client, who has a tracheostomy in place how to suction the client. The nurse determines that teaching was effective when the family uses:
1. intermittent suction while advancing the catheter.
2. continuous suction for no longer than 10 seconds while withdrawing the catheter.
3. continuous suction for no longer than 20 seconds while withdrawing the catheter.
4. continuous suction while advancing the catheter.

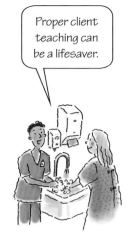

Proper client teaching can be a lifesaver.

131. 2. To prevent hypoxia, continuous suctioning shouldn't last more than 10 seconds with each pass during catheter withdrawal. Suction shouldn't be applied while the catheter is being advanced.
CN: Physiological integrity; CNS: Reduction of risk potential; CL: Apply

132. A client's arterial blood gas (ABG) analysis reveals a pH of 7.18, $PaCO_2$ of 73 mmHg, PaO_2 of 82 mmHg, and HCO_3 of 24 mEq/L. How would the nurse interpret these values?
1. Metabolic acidosis
2. Respiratory alkalosis
3. Metabolic alkalosis
4. Respiratory acidosis

132. 4. Normal ABG values include a pH of 7.35 to 7.45; $PaCO_2$ of 35 to 45 mmHg; PaO_2 of 80 to 100 mmHg; and HCO_3 of 22 to 26 mEq/L. This client's pH level is acidic, the $PaCO_2$ level is elevated, and the HCO_3 is normal, indicating respiratory acidosis. With metabolic acidosis, pH and HCO_3 are low and PaO_2 is normal. In respiratory alkalosis, the pH is elevated and $PaCO_2$ is low. In metabolic alkalosis, both pH and HCO_3 are elevated.
CN: Physiological integrity; CNS: Reduction of risk potential; CL: Analyze

133. A 67-year-old client is in respiratory distress after being admitted for an exacerbation of chronic obstructive pulmonary disease (COPD). How should the nurse position this client for optimal lung expansion?
1. Prone
2. Semi-Fowler's.
3. Reverse Trendelenburg's
4. Supine

What position will promote my expansion?

133. 2. Semi-Fowler's position promotes optimal lung expansion. A prone position would improve oxygenation in a client with acute respiratory distress syndrome, who's receiving mechanical ventilation, by recruiting new alveoli in the posterior region of the lungs. Reverse Trendelenburg's position may improve lung expansion but is less effective than semi-Fowler's position. Supine positioning aid lung expansion.
CN: Physiological integrity; CNS: Reduction of risk potential; CL: Apply

134. A client is admitted to the hospital with dehydration and pneumonia. On admission to the unit, the nurse notes that the IV has infiltrated. What is the **most** appropriate action by the nurse?
1. Stop the infusion and restart the infusion in another site
2. Remove the IV catheter and apply a cool compress to the site
3. Alternately apply moist heat and cold compresses to the site
4. Slow the infusion and gently massage the site

I've been infiltrated. What's the nurse's most appropriate action?

134. 1. After discovering an IV infiltration, the nurse should stop immediately the infusion, remove the IV catheter, and restart the infusion in another site. A warm compress should be applied to the infiltrated site. A cool compress doesn't promote fluid absorption. Moist heat shouldn't be applied until the infusion is stopped, the catheter is removed, and another catheter is inserted at a different site. Alternating moist heat and cold compresses to an infiltrated IV is contraindicated. Massaging the site is likely to cause pain and doesn't effectively treat an infiltration.
CN: Physiological integrity; CNS: Pharmacological and parenteral therapies; CL: Apply

CN: Client needs category   CNS: Client needs subcategory   CL: Cognitive level

135. Following a right lower lobectomy for lung cancer, a client returns to her room with a chest tube in place. The nurse formulates a care plan to promote air exchange in the postoperative period. The nurse determines the outcome has been met when the client:
1. sits upright, and leans slightly forward.
2. requests pain medication as needed.
3. maintains a pulse oximetry level above 93%.
4. takes deep breaths and is pain free.

135. 3. A pulse oximetry level above 93% and a normal respiratory rate demonstrates probable lung expansion and normal chest tube functioning. Sitting upright and leaning slightly forward would suggest that the client has impaired gas exchange because this position increases lung expansion. Taking deep breaths and requesting pain medication as needed, and remaining pain free are expected outcomes of nursing care for a post-operative client who underwent a lobectomy.
CN: Physiological integrity; CNS: Physiological adaptation; CL: Analyze

136. A client is involved in a motor vehicle accident. Upon admission to the emergency department, the client's heart rate was 130 bpm, with shallow respirations of 32 breaths/min, and a blood pressure of 90/60 mmHg. The breath sounds were diminished on the right side, and par-adoxical chest-wall movement appears on the right side. A chest X-ray reveals a right pneumothorax with multiple rib fractures. What diagnosis would the nurse anticipate for this client?
1. Tension pneumothorax
2. Flail chest
3. Ruptured diaphragm
4. Massive hemothorax

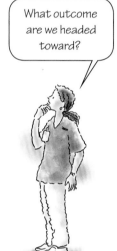

What outcome are we headed toward?

136. 2. Multiple rib fractures and paradoxical chest-wall movement would confirm a diagnosis of flail chest. Tension pneumothorax would cause severe respiratory distress, hypotension, diminished breath sounds over the affected area, hyperres-onance, distended neck veins, eventual tracheal shift, and, possibly, paradoxical chest-wall move-ment on the injured side. A ruptured diaphragm would lead to hyperresonance on percussion, hypotension, dyspnea, dysphagia, and shifting of heart and bowel sounds in the lower to middle chest. A massive hemothorax would produce signs of shock, dullness on percussion on the injured side, decreased breath sounds on the injured side, respiratory distress, and, possibly, mediastinal shift.
CN: Physiological integrity; CNS: Physiological adaptation; CL: Analyze

137. The emergency department health care pro-vider diagnoses a 35-year old client with a small peri-tonsillar abscess. The client's chart entry reads:

Discharge notes	
10/15/16 1400	The client is being discharged following a needle aspiration of the peri-tonsillar abscess. Clindamycin 600 mg/bid is order, and the client is to take ibuprofen 400 mg/ qid as needed for pain. Instructions were given to keep the follow-up appointment.

Based on this discharge note, what is the nurse's **priority** intervention?
1. Schedule an x-ray in the next 24 hours after the needle aspiration
2. Give the client a prescription for a follow-up lab test for mononucleosis
3. Tell the client there is a high risk for developing a second abscess
4. Instruct the client to report frequent swallowing or coughing up blood

137. 4. Hemorrhage and airway obstruction are the most common complications, and must be reported and treated immediately. X-rays are not frequently used in this situation. A culture would be performed on the exudate extracted from the abscess. If symptoms such as multiple swollen lymph nodes, fatigue or an enlarged spleen are present a test for mononucleosis would be performed. The risk of developing a second peri-tonsillar abscess is low.
CN: Physiological integrity; CNS: Physiological adaptation; CL: Apply

CN: Client needs category   CNS: Client needs subcategory   CL: Cognitive level

138. A 76-year-old client is admitted for elective knee surgery. Physical examination reveals shallow respirations but no signs of respiratory distress. What does this assessment finding indicate to the nurse?
1. Increased elastic recoil of the lungs
2. Increased number of functional capillaries in the alveoli
3. Decreased residual volume
4. Decreased vital capacity

I'm listening.

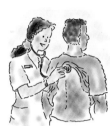

138. 4. A reduction in vital capacity is a normal physiological change in older adults. Other normal physiological changes include decreased elastic recoil of the lungs, fewer functioning capillaries in the alveoli, and an increase in residual volume.
CN: Health promotion and maintenance; CNS: None;
CL: Apply

139. An 89-year-old client is being discharged after spending five days in the hospital with a diagnosis of pneumonia. What information about the client's activities of daily living will the nurse give the caregiver prior to discharge?
1. Increase activities gradually
2. Exercise once a week
3. Walk daily until fatigued
4. Start to ride a stationary bike

139. 1. This client requires rest and a gradual increase in activities to avoid experiencing fatigue. An elderly client needs to build up exercise gradually by ambulating short distances. After an experience of pneumonia, the client should not walk until fatigued, as this may cause dyspnea. The nurse would not suggest a stationary bike unless the client used a stationary bike in his usual exercise routine.
CN: Physiological integrity; CNS: Physiological adaptation;
CL: Apply

140. An asthmatic client is being discharged with a prescription for cromolyn. The nurse determines that teaching is effective when the client states:
1. "I should use my inhaler no more than one hour before I exercise."
2. "I should use my inhaler whenever I feel an asthma attack coming on."
3. "I should stop taking steroids if I need a dose of my inhaler."
4. "I should avoid gargling and rinsing my mouth after using my inhaler."

140. 1. This inhaler should be used no more than one hour before exercise to prevent exercise-induced asthma. Cromolyn is not a rescue inhaler, and is contraindicated during an acute asthma attack. A client who is taking steroids should continue to take them if using cromolyn therapy. Gargling and rinsing the mouth after using cromolyn will reduce mouth dryness.
CN: Physiological integrity; CNS: Pharmacological and parenteral therapies; CL: Analyze

What's effective when it comes to exercise and asthma medication?

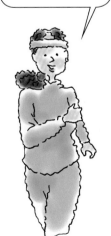

141. A nurse instructs the client on how to provide a sputum sample for analysis. The nurse determines teaching was effective when the client states:
1. "Fluids will be limited the day before the test, and restricted at midnight on the day before the test."
2. "I need to take several deep abdominal breaths, then take one more breath, and cough into the sterile container."
3. "If a bronchoscopy is required for specimen collection, I will have no oral intake for 12 hours before the procedure."
4. "After bronchoscopy, I will be reminded to start drinking water to prevent a sore throat."

141. 2. If a specimen will be collected by expectoration, the client should be instructed to take several deep abdominal breaths. When the client is ready to cough, he should take one more deep abdominal breath, bend forward, and cough into the provided sterile container. He should be instructed to drink plenty of fluids the day and night before the test. If the specimen will be collected during bronchoscopy, the client should fast for six hours before the procedure. After a bronchoscopy, the client will be observed for possible complications. Liquids can be consumed when the gag reflex returns.
CN: Physiological integrity; CNS: Reduction of risk potential;
CL: Apply

142. A 57-year-old client is admitted with acute bronchitis. During the admission interview, he tells the nurse he's allergic to bananas. To which may this client also be allergic?
1. Shellfish
2. Cephalosporins
3. Penicillins
4. Latex

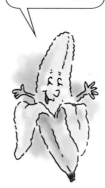

An allergy to bananas can cause which other allergy?

142. 4. Clients who are allergic to certain cross-reactive foods, including apricots, avocados, bananas, cherries, chestnuts, grapes, kiwis, passion fruit, peaches, and tomatoes, may also be allergic to latex. When exposed to latex, this client may have an allergic response similar to the one produced by these foods. Clients with allergies to shellfish are not usually allergic to bananas. Hypersensitivity reactions to cephalosporins are more common in clients with penicillin allergy. There's no link between food allergies and penicillin.
CN: Physiological integrity; CNS: Reduction of risk potential; CL: Apply

143. A client with pneumonia is ordered azithromycin 500 mg IV daily via a peripheral IV catheter. The medication is pre-mixed from the pharmacy in a 50 ml bag of solution to be infused over 30 minutes. The IV tubing delivers 15 gtts/ml. At what drip rate should the nurse set the infusion pump? Record your answer using a whole number.

_____ gtts/min

143. 25.

$$X = 50\,ml \times \frac{15\,gtt}{30\,min}$$

$$X = 25\,gtts/min$$

CN: Physiological integrity; CNS: Physiological adaptation; CL: Apply

144. A 20-year-old client with cystic fibrosis is being discharged with a high-frequency chest wall oscillating vest. Which statement, by the client, would indicate that the nurse's teaching, about the vest, has been effective?
1. "I'll wear the vest for five minutes each time a treatment is due."
2. "I'll lie down to use the vest."
3. "I'll require help in applying the vest."
4. "I can be in any position to use the vest."

144. 4. The vest system doesn't require special positioning or breathing to be effective. In most cases, treatments last 15 to 20 minutes and clients can manage therapy without any assistance.
CN: Safe, effective care environment; CNS: Safety and infection control; CL: Analyze

145. The chart entry, for a client being evaluated for cancer of the larynx, reads:

Progress notes	
10/15/16	A 70-year-old male is admitted for a
1130	diagnostic evaluation for possible cancer of
	the larynx. An intraoperative laryngoscopy is
	scheduled for the next day.

Based on this chart entry, what instruction should the nurse give this client?
1. Instruct the client not to drink irritating hot fluids prior to the test
2. Explain that medication will be given to decrease throat pain
3. Demonstrate mouth breathing so the client can perform it in the post-op period
4. Have the client do oral hygiene prior to the procedure to prevent pneumonia

145. 2. Prior to the laryngoscopy procedure, this client would be given medication for relaxation, for pain reduction and to decrease secretions. The client should be NPO prior to the test. There is no need to perform mouth breathing following a laryngoscopy. Although oral hygiene is appropriate nursing care, oral hygiene alone will not prevent hospital-acquired pneumonia.
CN: Physiological integrity; CNS: Reduction of risk potential; CL: Apply

CN: Client needs category   CNS: Client needs subcategory   CL: Cognitive level

146. A client tells the nurse that he has lost his appetite after receiving radiation treatment for lung cancer. What is the nurse's **most** appropriate response?

1. Drink plenty of fluids
2. Eat hot meats with spices to improve the taste
3. Limit activities immediately before and after meals
4. Consume food high in calories

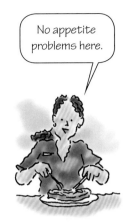

No appetite problems here.

146. 4. The client should consume high-calorie foods whenever he can, to help compensate for the times when he can't eat. Consuming large amounts of fluids will create a feeling of fullness, which can limit food intake. Hot meats tend to cause taste aversions during radiation therapy. Activity will increase the appetite.

CN: Physiological integrity; CNS: Physiological adaptation; CL: Apply

147. A client, with viral meningitis, tells the nurse that he is upset because his primary health care provider will not give him an antibiotic for his meningitis. How should the nurse respond to his statement?

1. "You will be better in 2 to 3 days, so no antibiotic treatment is necessary."
2. "You could talk to the provider again and I will be an advocate for you."
3. "You only need medication if you develop some meningitis complications."
4. "Antibiotics are only effective for bacterial infections."

147. 4. Clients with viral meningitis do not receive antibiotic treatment. Only clients with bacterial meningitis would receive antibiotic treatment. Clients with viral meningitis usually recover on their own in 7 to 10 days, and do not require antibiotic treatment.

CN: Physiological integrity; CNS: Physiological adaptation; CL: Apply

148. A nurse is teaching a group of police officers about the spread of tuberculosis (TB). Which statement, by an officer, would indicate that teaching has been effective?

1. " I could get TB by walking by someone who has the disease."
2. "I could get TB if I inhale droplets when an infected individual coughs."
3. "I could get TB if I search the home of someone infected with TB."
4. "I could get TB if I come in contact with blood from an infected person."

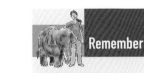

Here's a hint for you … cough, cough.

148. 2. Tuberculosis infection typically occurs from inhaling infected droplets after a person with TB coughs. Transmission usually requires close, frequent, prolonged contact. Human immunodeficiency virus is spread through contact with an infected person's blood or body fluids.

CN: Safe, effective care environment; CNS: Safety and infection control; CL: Analyze

149. A client receives midazolam, 2 mg IV, as sedation before bronchoscopy. Five minutes after he receives the drug, his respiratory rate drops to 4 breaths/min. What is the nurse's **most** appropriate action?

1. Administer naloxone
2. Administer protamine sulfate (Heparin antagonist)
3. Administer phentolamine
4. Administer flumazenil

Remember

"Flumazenil stills benzodiazepines."

Flumazenil reverses the effects of benzodiazepines such as midazolam.

149. 4. Flumazenil reverses the effects of benzodiazepines such as midazolam. Naloxone is used to reverse opioids, such as morphine. Protamine sulfate reverses the effects of heparin. Phentolamine is injected into the tissues to reverse the damaging effects of a dopamine infiltration.

CN: Physiological integrity; CNS: Pharmacological and parenteral therapies; CL: Apply

150. The nurse notes an order to change the client's chest drainage system from suction to gravity drainage. What is the **most** appropriate action by the nurse?
1. Detach tubing from the suction port to provide a vent
2. Clamp the client's drainage tube
3. Question the health care provider's order
4. Turn off the suction source and leave the tubing connected

151. A client with cancer develops pleural effusion. What sound would the nurse expect to hear during chest auscultation?
1. Crackles
2. Rhonchi
3. Diminished breath sounds
4. Wheezes

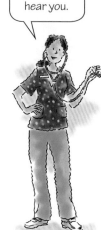

152. An IV of 1,000 ml 5% dextrose in water is ordered to infuse over eight hours for a client who is dehydrated after receiving chemotherapy. The IV drip rate is 10 gtts/ml. At what rate should the nurse set the infusion pump? Record your answer using a whole number.

_____ gtt/min

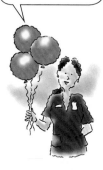

153. A 79-year-old client suddenly develops pulmonary edema. The health care provider prescribes furosemide 40 mg IV, and oxygen therapy using a non-rebreather mask. The nurse is aware that the mask will provide the client an oxygen concentration of:
1. 60% to 80%
2. 80% to 100%
3. 36%
4. 44%.

150. 1. When the suction source is turned off, the drainage system should be opened to the atmosphere so intrapleural air can escape from the system. Detaching the tubing from the suction port provides an exit vent for the air and, reduces the risk of tension pneumothorax. Clamping the tube may cause air to accumulate in the pleural space, leading to tension pneumothorax. There's no need to question the provider's order.
CN: Physiological integrity; CNS: Physiological adaptation; CL: Apply

151. 3. In pleural effusion, fluid accumulates in the pleural space, impairing transmission of normal breath sounds. Breath sounds will be diminished. Crackles commonly accompany atelectasis, interstitial fibrosis, and left-sided heart failure. Rhonchi suggest secretions in the large airways. Wheezes result from narrowed airways, as in asthma, chronic obstructive pulmonary disease, or bronchitis.
CN: Physiological integrity; CNS: Physiological adaptation; CL: Apply

152. 21.

$$8\,h \times 60\,min/h = 480\,min$$

$$X = \frac{1,000\,ml \times 10\,gtts/ml}{480\,min}$$

$$X = \frac{21\,gtts}{min}$$

CN: Physiological integrity; CNS: Physiological adaptation; CL: Apply

153. 2. The non-rebreather mask will deliver oxygen concentrations of 80% to 100%. It's reserved for emergency situations. A partial rebreather mask delivers concentrations of 60% to 80%. A nasal cannula delivers oxygen at flow rates of 1 to 6 l/min. A flow rate of 4 l/min delivers an oxygen concentration of 36%. A flow rate of 6 l/min delivers an oxygen concentration of 44%.
CN: Physiological integrity; CNS: Physiological adaptation; CL: Apply

154. A nurse, attending a neighborhood picnic, notices a motionless adult at the bottom of the swimming pool. She immediately calls for help and tries to rescue the person. When she pulls the adult out of the water, he's unresponsive and breathless, but has a pulse. What is the **most** appropriate action by the nurse?
1. Immediately start rescue breathing
2. Immobilize the cervical spine
3. Start chest compressions
4. Perform abdominal thrusts

154. 1. The nurse should immediately open the airway and begin rescue breathing. Immobilizing the cervical spine won't provide oxygenation. Chest compressions should only be delivered if a pulse is absent. Performing abdominal thrusts in an attempt to remove water from the lungs would delay the start of rescue breathing.

CN: Physiological integrity; CNS: Physiological adaptation; CL: Apply

155. A client, newly diagnosed with chronic obstructive pulmonary disease (COPD), presents to the clinic for a routine examination. The nurse teaches the client strategies to prevent airway irritation and infection. The nurse determines that teaching was successful when the client states:
1. "I should avoid crowded areas this summer."
2. "I only need to obtain the flu vaccine."
3. "I should use products with aerosol sprays."
4. "I should avoid being exposed to powders."

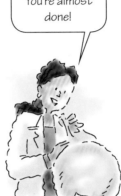

Keep going. You're almost done!

155. 4. A client with COPD should avoid powders, dusts, aerosol sprays, and smoke from cigarettes, pipes, and cigars. He should stay indoors when the humidity, temperature, and pollen counts are high, and avoid enclosed, crowded areas during cold and flu season. He should obtain immunizations against pneumococcal pneumonia as well as influenza.

CN: Health promotion and maintenance; CNS: None; CL: Analyze

156. A client, with a suspected pulmonary embolus, is brought to the emergency department reporting shortness of breath and pleuritic chest pain. Which assessment data would support this diagnosis? Select all that apply.
1. Low-grade fever
2. Thick green sputum
3. Bradycardia
4. Frothy sputum
5. Tachycardia
6. Blood-tinged sputum

156. 1, 5, 6. In addition to pleuritic chest pain and dyspnea, a client with a pulmonary embolus may also present with a low-grade fever, tachycardia, and blood-tinged sputum. Thick green sputum would indicate infection, and frothy sputum would indicate pulmonary edema. A client with a pulmonary embolus would be tachycardic.

CN: Physiological integrity; CNS: Physiological adaptation; CL: Apply

157. A health care provider prescribes an IV solution to infuse at a rate of 125 ml/hr. How many liters of solution will the client receive during an eight hour shift? Record your answer using a whole number.

_____ L

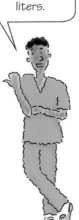

Don't forget to convert to liters.

157. 1.
The client should receive the solution at an infusion rate of 125 ml/hr.

$$125\,ml \times 8\,h = 1,000\,ml$$

Convert milliliters to liters by dividing by 1,000. The total volume in liters of normal saline solution that this client should receive in 8 hours is 1 liter.

CN: Physiological integrity; CNS: Pharmacological and parenteral therapies; CL: Apply

CN: Client needs category   CNS: Client needs subcategory   CL: Cognitive level

158. A client is admitted to the hospital with shortness of breath. The health care provider orders a stat hemoglobin and hematocrit level to be drawn. The client questions why blood is being drawn when he is having trouble breathing. What is the nurse's **best** response?
1. "We are just checking a baseline. However, hemoglobin has little to no effect on oxygenation."
2. "We want to see if you have more hemoglobin because it can decrease your respiratory rate."
3. "If we check your hemoglobin levels and they are low it tells us that you have reduced oxygen-carrying capacity."
4. "If we check your hemoglobin levels and they are low it tells us that you have increased oxygen-carrying capacity."

158. 3. Hemoglobin is the component of blood that carries oxygen. If the hemoglobin level is low, the amount of oxygen-carrying capacity is also low. More hemoglobin will increase the oxygen-carrying capacity and increase the total amount of oxygen available in the blood. If oxygen demand is higher than the available oxygen content, then an increase in hemoglobin may decrease the respiratory rate to normal levels.

CN: Physiological integrity; CNS: Reduction of risk potential; CL: Apply

159. The nurse is assessing a client's respiratory pattern. Which illustration represents Cheyne-Stokes respirations?

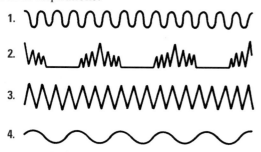

159. 2. In Cheyne-Stokes respirations, breaths gradually become faster and deeper than normal and then slower during a 30 to 170-second period with intermittent periods of apnea. Illustration one shows tachypnea, or shallow breathing with an increased respiratory rate. Illustration three shows Kussmaul's breathing, or rapid, deep breathing without pauses. Illustration four shows bradypnea, or regular breathing at a decreased rate.

CN: Physiological integrity; CNS: Reduction of risk potential; CL: Analyze

160. The chart entry for a client with chronic pharyngitis reads:

Progress notes	
10/15/16 0945	A 37-year-old female, who works in a textile factory, has returned to the clinic with symptoms of a persistent sore throat which makes swallowing uncomfortable and congestion that causes frequent episodes of coughing to expel mucous.

Based on this chart entry, how should the nurse teach this client how to manage these symptoms?
1. Recommend decreasing exposure to environmental irritants by wearing a mask
2. Instruct this client to ask the primary care provider for a complete cardiac evaluation
3. Suggest that the client increase the frequency of performing oral hygiene
4. Address the need to monitor for infection by taking a daily temperature reading

160. 1. Clients with chronic pharyngitis are often exposed to environmental irritants. Minimizing exposure, by wearing a disposable face mask, is a helpful intervention. A cardiac evaluation is not warranted for chronic pharyngitis. Good oral hygiene will decrease the symptoms, but will not address the underlying cause. Daily monitoring of this client's temperature is not warranted.

CN: Physiological integrity; CNS: Physiological adaptation; CL: Apply

161. A healthy client comes to the clinic for a routine examination. What type of breath sounds would the nurse anticipate while auscultating the lower lobes of the lungs?
1. Bronchial
2. Tracheal
3. Vesicular
4. Bronchovesicular

161. 3. Vesicular breath sounds are soft, low-pitched sounds normally heard over the lower lobes of the lung. They're prolonged on inhalation and shortened on exhalation. Bronchial breath sounds are loud, high-pitched sounds normally heard next to the trachea, and are loudest during exhalation. Tracheal breath sounds are harsh, discontinuous sounds heard over the trachea during inhalation or exhalation. Bronchovesicular breath sounds are medium-pitched, continuous sounds that occur during inhalation or exhalation and are best heard over the upper third of the sternum and between the scapulae.
CN: Health promotion and maintenance; CNS: None; CL: Apply

162. The nurse is preparing to obtain an arterial blood gas (ABG) sample on a client. Which action should the nurse take **first**?
1. Perform an Allen's test
2. Place a rolled towel under the client's wrist
3. Clean the puncture site with an alcohol or povidone-iodine pad
4. Palpate the artery with the index and middle fingers of one hand

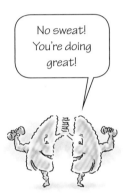

No sweat! You're doing great!

162. 1. An Allen's test to assess circulation should be performed first. Next, hands should be washed, gloves applied, and a rolled towel should be placed under the client's wrist for support. The artery should be located, and assessed for a strong pulse. The puncture site should be cleaned with an alcohol or povidone-iodine pad. The artery should be palpated with the index and middle fingers of one hand while holding the syringe over the puncture site with the other hand. Holding the needle bevel at a 30 to 45-degree angle, the skin and arterial wall should be punctured in one smooth motion. Blood should backflow into the syringe to the 5-ml mark. After collecting the sample, press a gauze pad over the puncture site for at least five minutes.
CN: Physiological integrity; CNS: Reduction of risk potential; CL: Apply

163. The chart entry for a client with a fungal infection in the maxillary sinus reads:

Progress notes	
10/15/16 1530	Client reports increased nasal discharge, a productive cough with green discharge, and increasing facial pain 60 minutes after pain medication was given. Recent vital signs: Temperature 98.2℉ F (37℃ C), Pulse 120, and Respirations 26.

What is the **priority** nursing action?
1. Assess for any type of vision changes
2. Limit the intake of oral fluids
3. Instruct the client to mouth breathe
4. Obtain a sputum sample

163. 4. The nurse should obtain a sputum sample and document the color and consistency of the discharge. The provider would indicate if the sputum needs to go to the lab for analysis. Vision changes are uncommon with fungal infections of the maxillary sinus. Oral fluids do not need to be limited. The nurse needs to monitor fluid intake and the client's state of hydration. The nurse would not encourage the client to mouth breath.
CN: Physiological integrity; CNS: Physiological adaptation; CL: Analyze

CN: Client needs category   CNS: Client needs subcategory   CL: Cognitive level

164. The nurse is assessing a client's chest tube and notes that it is not working properly. What is the nurse's **priority** action?
1. Check for disconnection of the tubing from the drainage unit
2. Clean the tips of the tubing and reconnect securely
3. Check patency of the chest tube
4. Submerge the end of the chest tube in one inch of sterile water

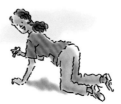

Don't let this one trip you up. Try reading it again.

164. 3. The most important action is to determine the patency of chest tube. Checking for a disconnection would be nurse's next action. Submerging the end of the chest tube in one inch of sterile water would only be necessary if the tube was disconnected and a chest drainage system was not available. Cleaning the tips of the tubing and reconnect securely would be necessary if the tube had become disconnected.
CN: Physiological integrity; CNS: Physiological adaptation; CL: Apply

165. A client with pneumonia is ordered ampicillin 200 mg/q4h. The vial is labeled 500 mg/10 ml. How many milliliters of the fluid contains the dose ordered? Record your answer using a whole number.

_____ ml

165. 4.
$$\frac{200\ mg}{X\ ml} = \frac{500\ mg}{10\ ml}$$
$$X = 4\ ml$$

CN: Physiological integrity; CNS: Physiological adaptation; CL: Apply

166. A client is scheduled for surgical resection after being diagnosed with lung cancer. The client correctly states that the procedure will remove:
1. the tumor and all the immediate surrounding tissue.
2. the tumor and as little surrounding tissue as possible.
3. all the tumor and any collapsed alveoli in the region.
4. as much tumor as possible, without removing any alveoli.

166. 2. The goal of surgical resection is to remove only tissue affected by the tumor while saving as much surrounding tissue as possible.
CN: Physiological integrity; CNS: Physiological adaptation; CL: Apply

167. A client has developed a pleural effusion. What intervention would the nurse anticipate the health care provider to perform?
1. Insert a chest tube
2. Perform a thoracentesis
3. Perform a paracentesis
4. Allow the pleural effusion to drain by itself

167. 2. Thoracentesis is used to remove excess pleural fluid and restore proper lung status. The fluid would be analyzed to determine if it's transudative or exudative. A chest tube is rarely necessary because the amount of fluid typically isn't large enough to warrant such a measure. Paracentesis is the removal of fluid from the abdomen. Pleural effusions can't drain by themselves.
CN: Physiological integrity; CNS: Physiological adaptation; CL: Apply

168. The care plan for a 42-year-old client with deep vein thrombosis (DVT) includes monitoring for complications. The nurse determines that this client is at highest risk of developing which complication?
1. Pulmonary embolism
2. Pneumothorax
3. Pulmonary edema
4. Pneumonia

168. 1. The most common etiology of pulmonary embolism is thromboembolism from a distant site, particularly from the deep veins of the legs and pelvis. Immobilization used to treat DVT is an additional clinical risk factor for pulmonary embolism. Pneumothorax and pulmonary edema aren't complications of DVT. Immobility also places this client at risk for pneumonia.
CN: Physiological integrity; CNS: Reduction of risk potential; CL: Apply

CN: Client needs category   CNS: Client needs subcategory   CL: Cognitive level

169. An employee-health nurse who performs annual purified protein derivative (PPD) testing instructs the staff about reading the PPD results. When should the results be read?
   1. 6 to 12 hours
   2. 12 to 24 hours
   3. 24 to 48 hours
   4. 48 to 72 hours

169. 4. To ensure accurate results, a PPD test must be read 48 to 72 hours after administration.
CN: Health promotion and maintenance; CNS: None;
CL: Apply

Chapter 6

Neurosensory Disorders

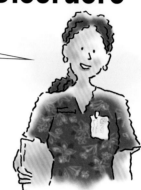

Stroke, subdural hematoma, laminectomy—they're all here in this comprehensive chapter on neurosensory disorders in adults. I've got a sixth sense, you're going to do great!

1. A nurse is caring for a client with the following visual field deficit.

What is the **most** important information for the nurse to teach this client?
1. Scan the environment on the affected side
2. Use memory aids such as pictures
3. Plan for adequate rest
4. Make simple, non-risky decisions

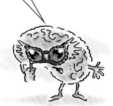

A stroke can make things look different.

1. 1. Scanning the environment can help a client with homonymous hemianopia overcome a loss in visual perception and prevent injury. Clients with other types of perceptual or memory loss may benefit from the interventions, nonspecific for a visual field loss, in the remaining answer choices.
CN: Physiological integrity; CNS: Physiological adaptation; CL: Apply

2. A client has recently experienced an embolic stroke, and is now stable. The client has been started on dabigatran. What information should the nurse provide to this client?
1. Dabigatran is the standard of care for preventing recurrent ischemic stroke.
2. Dabigatran is more effective than antiplatelet therapy in the presence of a thrombus.
3. Dabigatran is inexpensive and readily available, with few side effects.
4. Dabigatran helps prevent blood clots from forming in the presence of atrial fibrillation.

2. 4. Atrial fibrillation is the most common cause of embolic stroke. It is a newer anticoagulant medication approved for secondary stroke prevention in clients with atrial fibrillation of non heart valve origin. It helps prevent blood clots. Although anticoagulation is the standard of care for a client with stroke due to atrial fibrillation, antiplatelet medication remains the standard of care for non-cardiac thromboembolic stroke. Because of the increased risk of life-threatening bleeding, careful consideration is needed when ordering dabigatran.
CN: Physiological integrity; CNS: Pharmacological and parenteral therapies; CL: Apply

3. A 65-year-old client, who is experiencing a stroke, has been ordered alteplase. The order is for 0.9 mg/kg over one hour. The client weighs 110 lb (50 kg). What is the total dose in milligrams (mg) that the client will receive? Record your answer using a whole number.

_____ mg

3. 45.
Multiply 0.9 mg by 50 kg to obtain a dose of 45 mg. The total dose the client will receive is 45 mg.
CN: Physiological integrity; CNS: Pharmacological and parenteral therapies; CL: Apply

CN: Client needs category   CNS: Client needs subcategory   CL: Cognitive level

4. Which medication will the nurse administer to a client who experienced a thrombotic stroke two days ago?
1. Acetaminophen
2. Aspirin
3. Alteplase
4. Methylprednisolone

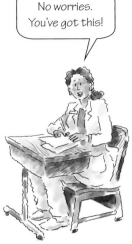

No worries. You've got this!

4. 2. Aspirin interferes with platelet aggregation to prevent blood clots from forming or growing larger and is used in the treatment, and secondary prevention, of ischemic stroke due to thrombosis. Antiplatelet medication, such as aspirin, should be given by day two in the absence of a bleeding complication. Alteplase is a potent medication that breaks down blood clots. It is approved by the U.S. Food and Drug Administration (FDA) for treatment within three hours of the onset of ischemic stroke. When alteplase is given, the client should have a brain scan 24-hours post infusion, and prior to the initiation of anti-platelet therapy. Methylprednisolone is a steroid with mild anticoagulant properties and is not indicated in acute stroke.
CN: Physiological integrity; CNS: Pharmacological and parenteral therapies; CL: Apply

5. A client is admitted to the emergency department with new onset of stroke-like symptoms. Prioritize the following nursing interventions.

| **1.** Assess airway, breathing, and circulation |
| **2.** STAT CT scan as ordered |
| **3.** Screen the client for ability to swallow |
| **4.** Administer atenolol to lower a BP of 181/106 mmHg |
| **5.** Administer alteplase per protocol. |

5. Ordered Response:

| **1.** Assess airway, breathing, and circulation. |
| **2.** STAT CT scan as ordered |
| **5.** Administer alteplase. |
| **4.** Administer atenolol to lower a BP of 181/106 mmHg |
| **3.** Screen the client for ability to swallow |

CN: Physiological integrity; CNS: Reduction of risk potential; CL: Apply

6. A client has had a moderate to large hemispheric stroke and has facial weakness. What would an assessment of this client reveal?
1. Complete upper and lower facial weakness on the affected side
2. Facial weakness with sparing of the forehead on the side of the paralysis
3. Client's smile is symmetric
4. Inability to open the client's closed eyes

6. 2. Hemispheric stroke is a result of damage to the upper motor neurons in the brain. This type of facial weakness is known as central facial paralysis. Because the muscles of the forehead receive input from both cerebral hemispheres, the forehead is spared on the side of the paralysis when the lesion is central. Full facial weakness is seen with direct injury to cranial nerve VII, such as in Bell's palsy. In both a central and peripheral palsy, the smile will be asymmetrical, and the nurse will be able open to the client's closed eyes.
CN: Physiological integrity; CNS: Physiological adaptation; CL: Apply

7. Why would the nurse need to conduct a swallow screen for a client following a stroke?
1. To assess the oral, pharyngeal, and esophageal phases of swallowing
2. To determine if it is safe for this client to take medications, fluids or food by mouth
3. To determine if a barium-swallow examination is required
4. To detects silent aspiration

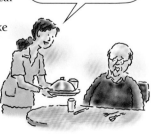

Careful what you serve to clients with stroke. They may have trouble swallowing it.

7. 2. A client with stroke must pass a swallow screen, or evaluation, prior to taking medications, fluids, or food by mouth. This screen is a minimally-invasive procedure that helps identify clients that might need further evaluation by a speech-language-pathologist or provider specialist. Based on the recommendations of these specialists, a barium swallow may be ordered. Screening will not detect aspiration that has occurred. Additional testing is required to determine the phase of swallowing affected.
CN: Physiological integrity; CNS: Reduction of risk potential; CL: Apply

CN: Client needs category   CNS: Client needs subcategory   CL: Cognitive level

8. What is the **priority** nursing intervention for client who has developed left arm swelling after a thromboembolic right hemispheric stroke?
1. Apply an arm split to prevent a contracture
2. Elevate the arm to improve venous return
3. Notify the provider of a potential brachial vein thrombosis
4. Obtain a physical therapy (PT) consult due to the client's decreased muscle strength

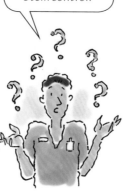

What functions does the brain stem control?

8. 2. In clients with hemiplegia or hemiparesis, loss of muscle contraction may decrease venous return resulting in swelling of the affected extremity. Elevating the extremity will help facilitate venous return and decrease swelling. Contractures may occur with a stroke, but don't typically present with swelling alone. Deep vein thrombosis may develop in clients with a stroke but are more likely to occur in the lower extremities. All clients with stroke should have a PT consult, especially in the presence of hemiparesis. CN: Physiological integrity; CNS: Physiological adaptation; CL: Apply

9. A client has experienced a cerebellar hemorrhage as indicated below. What is the nurse's **priority** assessment for this client?

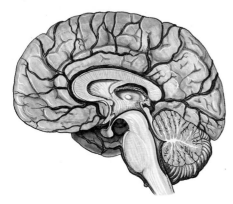

1. Aphasia
2. Bradypnea
3. Contralateral hemiplegia
4. Numbness and tingling of the face or arm

9. 2. A cerebellar hemorrhage is considered an emergency because of potential pressure on the brainstem. The brain stem contains the medulla, the vital cardiac, vasomotor, and respiratory center. The nurse should be most concerned with bradypnea. Symptoms of cerebellar stroke include ataxia, vertigo, dysarthria, and vertigo. Aphasia is associated with cortical stroke in the Brocha's or Wernicke areas. Sensory loss and hemiplegia are associated with strokes in areas other than the cerebellum. CN: Physiological integrity; CNS: Physiological adaptation; CL: Apply

10. What information should the nurse share with a client concerned about the risks for developing cataracts?
1. "Frequent streptococcal throat infections increase your risk."
2. "If your mother was exposed to rubella during pregnancy you have an increased risk."
3. "Increased intraocular pressure increases your risk."
4. "Prolonged use of steroidal anti-inflammatory agents increases your risk."

10. 4. Prolonged use of steroidal anti-inflammatory agents increase the risk for cataracts. The other risk factors don't contribute to the development of cataracts. CN: Health promotion and maintenance; CNS: None; CL: Apply

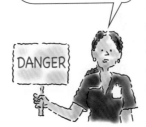

Which symptom is unexpected after surgery?

11. The nurse is caring for a client who has undergone cataract surgery. The nurse determines the need to notify the health care provider when the client reports:
1. blurred vision.
2. eye pain.
3. eye glare.
4. itching at the surgical site.

11. 2. Pain should not be present after cataract surgery. Pain may be an indication of hyphema, or clouding in the anterior chamber, and infection. The other symptoms may be present. CN: Physiological integrity; CNS: Physiological adaptation; CL: Apply

CN: Client needs category   CNS: Client needs subcategory   CL: Cognitive level

12. A client who experienced head trauma three hours ago now has clear fluid draining from her nose and mouth. What would the nurse suspect?
1. Basilar skull fracture
2. Cerebral concussion
3. Subdural hematoma
4. Sinus infection

13.

Progress notes	
2/10/17	19 year old male with mild concussion
1800	after slipping in school parking lot three
	hours prior. No loss of consciousness.
	No appreciable neurological deficits.
	CT scan normal. Client was preparing for
	discharge. Now reports a 5/s10 headache.
	Acetaminophen PO ordered.

When offered acetaminophen, the client's mother tells the nurse that she would like her son to have something stronger. What is the nurse's **best** response?
1. "Acetaminophen is strong enough for your son's mild concussion."
2. "We avoid giving aspirin to children and young adults because of the danger of Reye's syndrome."
3. "Opioids are avoided following a head injury because they may hide a deteriorating condition."
4. "Stronger medications may lead to vomiting, which increases the intracranial pressure (ICP)."

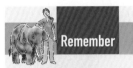

Remember

"Avoid opioids" when the client has a concussion.

They may mask changes in the level of consciousness that indicate increased intracranial pressure.

- Codeine
- Fentanyl citrate
- Hydrocodone
- Hydromorphone
- Levorphanol
- Meperidine
- Methadone
- Morphine
- Oxycodone
- Oxymorphone
- Propoxyphene
- Remifentanil
- Sufentanil

12. 1. Clear fluid draining from the ear or nose of a client may indicate a cerebrospinal fluid leak, which is common in basilar skull fractures. Concussion is associated with a brief loss of consciousness. Subdural hematoma occurs when there is bleeding between the dura and the arachnoid layers of the brain, and sinus infection is associated with facial pain and pressure with or without nasal drainage.

CN: Physiological integrity; CNS: Physiological adaptation; CL: Analyze

13. 3. Opioids may mask changes in the level of consciousness (LOC) that indicate increased ICP, and shouldn't be given as a first-line drug. Stating that acetaminophen is strong enough ignores the mother's question and isn't appropriate. Aspirin is contraindicated in conditions that include bleeding, and for children or young adults with viral illnesses due to the danger of Reye's syndrome. Stronger medications may not necessarily lead to vomiting, but will sedate the client, thereby masking changes in his LOC.

CN: Physiological integrity; CNS: Reduction of risk potential; CL: Apply

14. The nurse prepares the client for a lumbar puncture (LP) (see client chart below) to rule out a subarachnoid hemorrhage. Which assessment finding would require intervention before the procedure?

Progress notes	
2/10/17	56-year-old, right-handed female presents
1900	with severe onset of headache and
	projectile vomiting that started 45 minutes
	prior to admission. Physical examination
	findings include nuchal rigidity.

1. Severe vomiting
2. Suspected increased intracranial pressure (ICP)
3. Client requires mechanical ventilation
4. Blood in the cerebrospinal fluid (CSF)

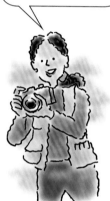

Stay focused. You'll spot the right answer.

14. 2. Sudden removal of CSF result in a lowered pressure in the lumbar area than in the brain which can cause brain herniation, especially in the presence of increased ICP. Therefore a LP is contraindicated when increased ICP is suspected. Vomiting may be caused by reasons other than increased ICP; therefore, LP isn't strictly contraindicated. A LP may be performed on clients requiring mechanical ventilation. Blood in the CSF is diagnostic for subarachnoid hemorrhage.
CN: Physiological integrity; CNS: Physiological adaptation; CL: Apply

15. The nurse is assessing a client with head trauma. The client has urine output of 300 ml/hr, dry skin, dry mucous membranes and high serum sodium. What is the nurse's **most** important intervention for this client?
1. Evaluate urine specific gravity
2. Anticipate treatment for renal failure
3. Provide emollients to the skin to prevent breakdown
4. Slow the IV fluids and notify the provider

15. 1. Urine output of 300 ml/hr in the presence of high serum sodium may indicate diabetes insipidus (DI). Sodium disturbances are common in clients with brain injury because of the major role that the central nervous system plays in the regulation of sodium and water homeostasis. Other related conditions include cerebral salt wasting and syndrome of inappropriate antidiuretic hormone (SIADH). DI may occur with increased intracranial pressure and head trauma. The nurse should evaluate for low urine specific gravity, increased serum osmolarity, and dehydration. There is no evidence that the client is experiencing renal failure. Providing emollients to prevent skin breakdown is important but not the priority. Slowing the rate of IV fluid would contribute to dehydration when polyuria is present.
CN: Physiological integrity; CNS: Physiological adaptation; CL: Analyze

16. The nurse anticipates that stool softeners will be given to a client prior to repair of a cerebral aneurysm. Why would stool softeners be given to this client?
1. To stimulate the bowel due to loss of nerve innervation
2. To prevent straining, which increases intracranial pressure (ICP)
3. To prevent the Valsalva maneuver that can result in a reflex bradycardia
4. To prevent constipation due to osmotic diuretics

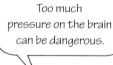

Too much pressure on the brain can be dangerous.

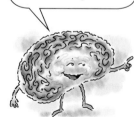

16. 2. Straining when having a bowel movement, sneezing, coughing, and suctioning may lead to increased ICP and should be avoided when the potential for increased ICP exists. Stool softeners don't stimulate the bowel and aren't used in combination with osmotic diuretics. Although the Valsalva maneuver may lead to an increase in ICP, it does not prevent reflex bradycardia.
CN: Physiological integrity; CNS: Reduction of risk potential; CL: Apply

CN: Client needs category   CNS: Client needs subcategory   CL: Cognitive level

17. A client with a subdural hematoma becomes restless and confused, with dilation of the ipsilateral pupil. What is the **most** important action by the nurse?

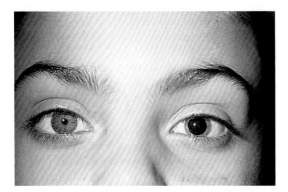

1. Elevate the head of the bed to reduce intraocular pressure
2. Preventing secondary acute tubular necrosis
3. Preparing to administer hypertonic saline or mannitol per provider order
4. Lower the head of the bed to improve cerebral perfusion

17. 3. Hypertonic saline and mannitol promote osmotic diuresis by increasing the pressure gradient, drawing fluid from intracellular to intravascular spaces. Therefore these agents are often used as first-line agents to decrease ICP while preparing the client for surgery. Elevating the head of the bed can also help facilitate venous return, targeting a decrease in ICP, not intraocular pressure. Although it is important to closely monitor fluid and electrolytes, preventing acute kidney injury is secondary.

CN: Physiological integrity; CNS: Pharmacological and parenteral therapies; CL: Apply

18. A client with a large cerebral intracranial hemorrhage was given mannitol to decrease intracranial pressure (ICP). What therapeutic effect should the nurse anticipate from mannitol?
1. Increased urine output
2. Pupils that are bilaterally 7 mm and nonreactive
3. Evidence of rebound cerebral hypertension
4. Normal blood urea nitrogen (BUN) and creatinine levels

18. 1. Mannitol promotes osmotic diuresis by increasing the pressure gradient in the renal tubules, thus increasing urine output. Fixed and dilated pupils are symptoms of increased ICP or cranial nerve damage, seen in herniation associated with a deteriorating cerebellar hemorrhage. No information is given about abnormal BUN and creatinine levels, or that mannitol is being given for renal dysfunction. Rebound cerebral hypertension is an adverse and undesired complication from ongoing mannitol use.

CN: Physiological integrity; CNS: Physiological adaptation; CL: Apply

19. The nurse is evaluating an arterial blood gas result from a client with a closed head injury and notes the $Paco_2$ is 30 mmHg. How should the nurse interpret this result?
1. Potentially appropriate, as modest lowering of carbon dioxide (CO_2) may reduce intracranial pressure (ICP)
2. This client is poorly oxygenated and requires emergent and aggressive hyperventilation
3. This is a normal $Paco_2$ value
4. This client has alveolar hypoventilation

19. 1. A normal $Paco_2$ value is 35 to 45 mmHg. CO_2 has vasodilating properties. Lowering $Paco_2$ through hyperventilation may lower ICP. Hyperventilation should only be used for short periods of time, when immediate control of ICP is necessary. Oxygenation is evaluated through PaO_2 and oxygen saturation. Alveolar hypoventilation would be reflected in an increased $Paco_2$.

CN: Physiological integrity; CNS: Physiological adaptation; CL: Analyze

20. The nurse notes that a client recovering from a brain injury may be developing foot drop and contractures. What is this nurse's **best** intervention?
1. High-topped sneakers, or other foot-up ankle support
2. Low-dose heparin therapy
3. Range of motion every shift
4. Sequential compression device

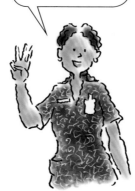

Remember these three things: relax, focus, and keep going.

20. 1. High-topped sneakers or other foot-up ankle support devices are used to prevent foot drop and contractures in neurological clients. Low-dose heparin therapy and sequential compression boots will prevent deep vein thrombosis. Although range of motion is important, it needs to be performed more frequently than once per shift to prevent foot drop.
CN: Physiological integrity; CNS: Basic care and comfort; CL: Apply

21. The nurse is observing a client who had a transsphenoidal hypophysectomy. Further intervention is required when the nurse observes:
1. bloody drainage from the ears.
2. frequent swallowing.
3. guaiac-positive stools.
4. hematuria.

21. 2. Frequent swallowing after brain surgery may indicate fluid or blood leaking from the sinuses into the oropharynx. Blood or fluid draining from the ear may indicate a basilar skull fracture, guaiac-positive stools indicate gastrointestinal bleeding, and hematuria may result from cystitis or other urological complications.
CN: Physiological integrity; CNS: Physiological adaptation; CL: Analyze

22. The nurse is preparing to administer vasopressin to a client who has undergone a hypophysectomy. What is the purpose of the medication?
1. To treat growth failure
2. To prevent syndrome of inappropriate antidiuretic hormone (SIADH)
3. To reduce cerebral edema and lower intracranial pressure
4. To replace antidiuretic hormone (ADH) normally secreted from the pituitary

22. 4. After hypophysectomy, or removal of the pituitary gland, the body can't synthesize ADH; therefore, vasopressin is administered. Somatropin or growth hormone is used to treat growth failure. SIADH results from excessive ADH secretion. Vasopressin is not used to treat cerebral edema.
CN: Physiological integrity; CNS: Pharmacological and parenteral therapies; CL: Apply

23. A client's intracranial pressure (ICP) is fluctuating between 20 and 25 mmHg. What is the nurse's best intervention?

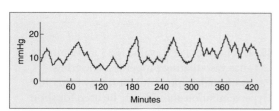

1. Ensuring that the mean arterial pressure (MAP) is less than 90 mmHg
2. Lowering the head of the bed to less than 15 degrees
3. Encouraging visitation
4. Reassessing the client's ABCs (airway, breathing, and circulation)

23. 4. The nurse should always reassess the client's ABCs when the ICP is elevated. Mean arterial pressure should be maintained at, or above, 90 mmHg to ensure adequate cerebral perfusion. The head of the bed should be elevated between 15 and 30 degrees to facilitate venous drainage. External stimulation, such as visitors, should be limited as it may increase ICP.
CN: Physiological integrity; CNS: Physiological adaptation; CL: Apply

CN: Client needs category   CNS: Client needs subcategory   CL: Cognitive level

24. A nurse is planning care for a client who has undergone a L4-L5 laminectomy. What is the **most** important intervention for the nurse to include on the first postoperative day?

Progress notes	
2/10/17	56-year-old client underwent a L4–L5
0900	lumbar laminectomy yesterday to alleviate
	pain caused by neural impingement from
	lumbar spinal stenosis. Client's progressing
	as expected.

1. Encourage the client to be out of bed
2. Apply maximum back bracing while in bed
3. Limit the client's movement in bed and reposition only when necessary
4. Provide a soft pressure mattress

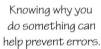

Knowing why you do something can help prevent errors.

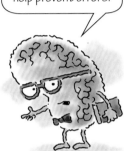

25. A client who has undergone a lumbar laminectomy is experiencing frequent voiding of small amounts of urine. What condition would the nurse associate with this symptom?
1. Diabetes insipidus
2. Diabetic ketoacidosis
3. Urine retention
4. Urinary tract infection (UTI)

26. What is the highest level of functioning a nurse would anticipate from a client with a spinal injury at the C6 level?
1. Significant loss of function at the biceps and shoulders
2. Potential loss of function at the shoulders and biceps and complete loss of function at the wrists and hands
3. Limited wrist control and complete loss of hand function
4. Lack of dexterity in the hands and fingers with limited use of arms

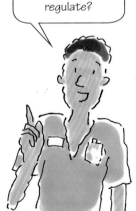

What functions do these areas regulate?

24. 1. In most cases, clients should be out of bed the first postoperative day to prevent the formation of blood clots and skin breakdown. Frequent repositioning, use of a chair-like brace for the lower back when out of bed, and a firm mattress will help minimize complications.
CN: Physiological integrity; CNS: Reduction of risk potential;
CL: Apply

25. 3. Swelling or pressure on the peripheral nerves controlling micturition, anesthesia, or use of an indwelling urinary catheter may lead to urine retention with frequent overflow of small amounts of urine. Diabetes insipidus and diabetic ketoacidosis cause polyuria. Symptoms of a UTI include dysuria and frequent voiding of small amounts of urine but would be less likely in this situation.
CN: Physiological integrity; CNS: Basic care and comfort;
CL: Analyze

26. 3. A lesion at C6 will result in limited wrist control and complete loss of hand function. Significant loss of function of the biceps and shoulder occurs with C4, with potential loss of function at the shoulder and biceps occurring at C5. An injury at C7 and T1 results in dexterity in the hands and finger but will limit the use of arms.
CN: Physiological integrity; CNS: Physiological adaptation;
CL: Apply

CN: Client needs category   CNS: Client needs subcategory   CL: Cognitive level

27. What is the nurse's **most** important action when preparing a client for magnetic resonance imaging (MRI)?
1. Question the client about allergy to contrast
2. Mark distal pulses on the foot in ink
3. Teach the client relaxation techniques
4. Tell the client he may be asked to cough or pant to clear the dye

27. 3. The MRI scanner is a narrow tube that contains a magnet. Although the MRI test is non-invasive, some clients may become claustrophobic during the test. Teaching relaxation techniques has been shown to help. Radiopaque contrast dye is used in MR angiogram, myelography, and cardiac catheterization, but not MRI. During cardiac catheterization, a client is asked to cough or pant to clear the dye. In procedures that include catheterization of the femoral artery, it is important to mark the pedal pulses.
CN: Physiological integrity; CNS: Reduction of risk potential; CL: Apply

28. A client is scheduled for chemonucleolysis with chymopapain to relieve the pain of a herniated disk. Which factor should be assessed **before** the procedure?
1. Allergy to meat tenderizers
2. Allergy to shellfish
3. Ability to lie flat during the procedure
4. Ability to perform full range of motion (ROM) on the affected side

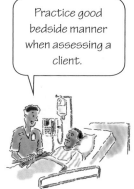

Practice good bedside manner when assessing a client.

28. 1. Chymopapain, derived from papaya, is an ingredient in meat tenderizers. Sensitivity to this substance may preclude the use of chymopapain. An allergy to shellfish is a dated contraindication to iodine-based contrast. There are unsubstantiated concerns of a cross reactivity between shellfish allergy and iodine/contrast allergy—some old medical forms still list this incorrectly as a contraindication. If you are allergic to shellfish, you do not need to avoid iodine or radiocontrast material. The client may be positioned in the side "C" position to allow access to the intervertebral area. Full ROM isn't needed for this procedure.
CN: Physiological integrity; CNS: Pharmacological and parenteral therapies; CL: Apply

29. A nurse is assigned four clients. Which client should the nurse see **first**?
1. A 17-year-old client 24 hours post appendectomy
2. A 33-year-old client with a recent diagnosis of Guillain-Barré syndrome
3. A 50-year-old client three days post myocardial infarction
4. A 50-year-old client with diverticulitis

29. 2. Guillain-Barré syndrome is characterized by ascending paralysis and potential respiratory failure. The order of client assessment should follow client priorities, with disorders of airway, breathing, and then circulation seen first. There is no information to suggest that the client with post myocardial infarction has an arrhythmia or other complication. There is no evidence to suggest hemorrhage or perforation for the remaining clients as a priority of care.
CN: Safe, effective care environment; CNS: Management of care; CL: Analyze

30. The nurse is teaching a client newly diagnosed with myasthenia gravis about the cause of this disease. The nurse determines that teaching has been effective when the client states:
1. "It is a post-viral illness, characterized by ascending paralysis."
2. "It causes loss of the myelin sheath surrounding peripheral nerves."
3. "It results from the inability of basal ganglia to produce sufficient dopamine."
4. "It is the destruction of acetylcholine receptors that causes muscle weakness."

30. 4. Myasthenia gravis, an autoimmune disorder, is caused by the destruction of acetylcholine receptors. Guillain-Barré syndrome is a post-viral illness characterized by ascending paralysis, multiple sclerosis is caused by loss of the myelin sheath, and Parkinson's disease is caused by the inability of basal ganglia to produce sufficient dopamine.
CN: Health promotion and maintenance; CNS: None; CL: Analyze

31. Which assessment finding would the nurse expect as an early sign of myasthenia gravis?
1. Dysphagia
2. Fatigue that improves by the end of the day
3. Ptosis
4. Respiratory distress

31. 3. Ptosis and diplopia are early signs of myasthenia gravis. Dysphagia and respiratory distress occur later. Symptoms are typically mild in the morning and may become exacerbated by stress or lack of rest.
CN: Health promotion and maintenance; CNS: None; CL: Apply

32. One hour after receiving pyridostigmine bromide for myasthenia gravis, a client reports difficulty swallowing and excessive respiratory secretions. What medication would the nurse anticipate to reverse the effects of pyridostigmine bromide?
1. Additional pyridostigmine bromide
2. Atropine
3. Edrophonium
4. Acyclovir

Remember

"Atropine is mean to acetylcholine."

Anticholinergics, such as atropine, block cholinergic agonists, such as acetylcholine, from activating cholinergic receptors.

- Atropine
- Belladonna
- Hyoscyamine
- Methscopolamine
- Scopolamine
- Glycopyrrolate
- Propantheline
- Dicyclomine
- Oxybutynin
- Tolterodine

32. 2. These symptoms suggest cholinergic crisis or excessive acetylcholinesterase medication, typically appearing 45 to 60 minutes after the last dose of acetylcholinesterase inhibitor. Atropine, an anticholinergic drug, is used to antagonize acetylcholinesterase inhibitors. The other drugs are acetylcholinesterase inhibitors. Edrophonium is used for diagnosis, and pyridostigmine bromide is used to treat myasthenia gravis and would worsen these symptoms. Acyclovir is an antiviral and would not be used to treat these symptoms.
CN: Physiological integrity; CNS: Pharmacological and parenteral therapies; CL: Analyze

33. A client with suspected myasthenia gravis is to undergo a test with edrophonium. The client asks if edrophonium can be used to treat myasthenia gravis. What is the nurse's **best** response?
1. It isn't available in an oral form
2. With repeated edrophonium use, immunosuppression may occur
3. Dry mouth and abdominal cramps may be intolerable adverse effects
4. The short half-life of edrophonium makes it impractical for long-term use

33. 4. Edrophonium is not available in an oral form and the duration of action is 1 to 2 minutes, making it impractical for the long-term management of myasthenia gravis. Immunosuppression with repeated use is an adverse effect of steroid administration. Dry mouth and abdominal cramps are adverse effects of increased acetylcholine in the parasympathetic nervous system.
CN: Physiological integrity; CNS: Pharmacological and parenteral therapies; CL: Apply

34. What explanation, by the nurse, **best** describes the effect of plasmapheresis therapy for clients with myasthenia gravis?
1. It prevents exacerbation of myasthenia gravis when the client is pregnant or under stress.
2. It removes T and B lymphocytes that attack acetylcholine receptors.
3. It delivers acetylcholinesterase inhibitor directly into the bloodstream.
4. It separates and removes acetylcholine receptor antibodies from the blood.

Talk your way through the question and the answer will come to you.

34. 4. The purpose of plasmapheresis in myasthenia gravis is to separate and remove circulating acetylcholine receptor antibodies from the blood of clients who do not respond to the usual therapies or who are in crisis. Although stress or pregnancy, may precipitate crisis, this is not the purpose of this procedure. Plasmapheresis does not remove T and B lymphocytes, nor does it deliver acetylcholinesterase inhibitor directly into the bloodstream.
CN: Physiological integrity; CNS: Pharmacological and parenteral therapies; CL: Apply

CN: Client needs category   CNS: Client needs subcategory   CL: Cognitive level

35. What would the nurse expect when assessing a client with glaucoma?
1. Reports of double vision
2. Reports of halos around lights
3. Intraocular pressure of 15 mmHg
4. Soft globe on palpation

35. 2. Reports of halos around lights are common in clients with glaucoma. Symptoms of glaucoma don't include double vision, but can include loss of peripheral vision or blind spots, reddened sclera, firm globe, decreased accommodation, halos around lights, and occasional eye pain. Some clients may be asymptomatic. Normal intraocular pressure is 10 to 21 mmHg.

CN: Physiological integrity; CNS: Physiological adaptation; CL: Apply

36. What statement, by a client with glaucoma, demonstrates an understanding of the need for medication compliance?
1. "I will experience diplopia if I don't take my medication as ordered."
2. "If I don't take my medication as ordered I will experience permanent vision loss."
3. "It is important to take my medication as ordered to avoid progressive loss of peripheral vision."
4. "I will experience pupillary constriction if I don't take my medication as ordered."

36. 2. Without treatment, glaucoma may progress to irreversible blindness. Treatment won't restore visual damage, but will halt disease progression. Blurred or foggy vision, not diplopia, is typical in glaucoma. The loss of central vision is typical with glaucoma. Miotics, which constrict the pupil, are used to treat glaucoma, and to permit outflow of the aqueous humor.

CN: Physiological integrity; CNS: Pharmacological and parenteral therapies; CL: Understand

37.

Progress notes	
2/10/17 2100	18-year-old college student presents to the emergency department with a severe headache and onset of bizarre behavior that started approximately five hours ago. Client is oriented to person, but not place or time. Physical assessment includes petechiae. Oral temperature is 104° F (40° C). HR: 128/bpm. RR: 24/min, O₂: 95% on room air. Lumbar puncture ordered. Client is being evaluated for bacterial meningitis.

37. 4. This client's rapid course, and petechiae suggest that she is at risk for a fulminant presentation of meningitis, which can include circulatory collapse. Intravenous access may be needed, not only for immediate antibiotics to address the infection, but also for fluids and vasopressors. The client does not currently require intubation. Immunization will not prevent disease in persons who have already been exposed. An analgesic may be given, but IV access is the top priority.

CN: Physiological integrity; CNS: Physiological adaptation; CL: Apply

What is the **most** important action by the nurse?
1. Prepare this client for endotracheal intubation
2. Administer the meningitis vaccination per order
3. Administer an analgesic per order
4. Obtaining IV access in preparation of antibiotic administration

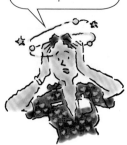

This question is making my head spin.

38. A nurse is evaluating a client to determine the extent of Parkinson's disease. Which symptoms would the nurse expect to see? Select all that apply.
1. Bulging eyeballs
2. Diminished distal sensation
3. Shuffling gait
4. Muscle rigidity
5. Changes in speech

38. 3, 4, 5. Parkinson's disease is characterized by the slowing of voluntary muscle movement, muscular rigidity, and resting tremors. Clients with Parkinson's disease often have a distinctive shuffling gait. Clients may speak in a softened voice, often in monotone manner, and may slur or hesitate before speaking. Exophthalmos occurs in Graves' disease. Diminished distal sensation does not occur in Parkinson's disease.
CN: Physiological integrity; CNS: Physiological adaptation; CL: Apply

39. The nurse is assessing a client with Parkinson's disease and documents the following: "The client's face is expressionless, and the client's speech is monotone." How should the nurse interpret this?
1. The client is most likely depressed
2. These are common symptoms that produce an undesired façade of an alert and responsive individual.
3. The client's antipsychotic medication may need to be adjusted.
4. The client probably has dementia.

39. 2. The nurse should recognize that these are common symptoms of Parkinson's disease. The symptoms do not indicate depression or dementia, although these are common in Parkinson's disease. Antipsychotic medication will often mimic Parkinson's disease extrapyramidal symptoms and is not indicated. Parkinson's disease is caused by degeneration of the substantia nigra in the basal ganglia of the brain, where dopamine is produced and stored. This degeneration results in motor dysfunction, resulting in symptoms such as an expressionless face and monotone speech.
CN: Physiological integrity; CNS: Physiological adaptation; CL: Apply

40. Which client would be **most** at risk for secondary Parkinson's disease caused by pharmacotherapy?
1. A 30-year-old client with schizophrenia who is taking chlorpromazine
2. A 50-year-old client taking nitroglycerin tablets for angina
3. A 60-year-old client who is taking prednisone for chronic obstructive pulmonary disease
4. A 75-year-old client using naproxen for rheumatoid arthritis

40. 1. Phenothiazines such as chlorpromazine deplete dopamine, which may lead to extrapyramidal effects. The other drugs don't place the client at a greater risk for developing Parkinson's disease.
CN: Physiological integrity; CNS: Pharmacological and parenteral therapies; CL: Apply

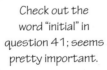

Check out the word "initial" in question 41; seems pretty important.

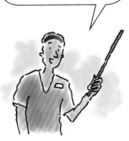

41. What are the **initial** symptoms of Parkinson's disease?
1. Akinesia
2. Aspiration of food
3. Dementia
4. Pill rolling movements of the hand

41. 4. Early symptoms of Parkinson's disease include coarse resting tremors of the fingers and thumb. Akinesia and aspiration are late signs of Parkinson's disease. Dementia occurs in only 20% of clients with Parkinson's disease.
CN: Health promotion and maintenance; CNS: None; CL: Apply

42. Which assessment findings demonstrate an effective outcome of levodopa-carbidopa medication therapy for a client with Parkinson's disease? Select all that apply.
1. Improved visual acuity
2. Decreased dyskinesia
3. Reduction in short-term memory
4. Reduced rigidity and tremor
5. Less frequent "freezing"

43. A client reports a dry mouth two days after starting therapy with trihexyphenidyl for Parkinson's disease. What is the **best** action by the nurse?
1. Offer the client ice chips and frequent sips of water
2. Withhold the medication and notify the provider
3. Change the client's diet to clear liquid until the symptoms subside
4. Encourage the use of supplemental puddings and shakes to maintain weight

44. Which antiparkinsonian drug can cause drug tolerance or toxicity if taken for too long?
1. Amantadine
2. Levodopa-carbidopa
3. Pergolide
4. Selegiline

45. A young client was recently diagnosed with multiple sclerosis (MS) and wants more information on the disease. Which statement is **most** accurate for the nurse to give?
1. MS is an autoimmune disease.
2. MS is more common in men than women.
3. MS is characterized by remyelination.
4. MS is an acute and curable disease.

46. A client with multiple sclerosis (MS) is started on 20 mg of glatiramer subcutaneously daily. Immediately after the injection, the client experiences flushing and chest pain. What is the **most** appropriate nursing intervention?
1. Call a code
2. Call the provider to inform him of the client's adverse reaction
3. Administer oxygen
4. Monitor the client to see if the symptoms quickly dissipate

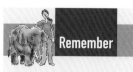

Remember

"Dopa- drugs increase dopa-mine"—that's the straight dope on dopaminergic drugs!

Dopaminergics are one group of drugs that treat Parkinson's disease, which is characterized by dopamine deficiency.

- Levodopa
- Carbidopa-levodopa
- Amantadine
- Bromocriptine
- Ropinirole
- Pramipexole
- Pergolide
- Selegiline

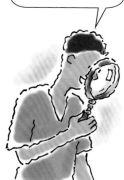

Aha! I spy some clues in these questions. Do you?

42. 2, 4. Levodopa-carbidopa will increase the amount of dopamine in the central nervous system, allowing for more smooth and purposeful movements. The drug doesn't affect visual acuity, and should improve dyskinesia and short-term memory. It does not affect "freezing" or problems with autonomic functions, such as constipation, urinary problems, impotence, or pain.
CN: Physiological integrity; CNS: Pharmacological and parenteral therapies; CL: Apply

43. 1. Trihexyphenidyl is an anticholinergic agent that causes blurred vision, dry mouth, constipation, and urinary retention. There is no need to withhold the drug unless hypotension or tachyarrhythmia occurs. A clear liquid diet isn't indicated at this time. I doesn't provide adequate nutrition, and may be more difficult to swallow than thickened liquids if dysphagia is present. Although weight loss may occur with Parkinson's disease, it is not a side effect of trihexyphenidyl.
CN: Physiological integrity; CNS: Pharmacological and parenteral therapies; CL: Analyze

44. 2. Long-term therapy with levodopa-carbidopa can result in drug tolerance or toxicity manifested by confusion, hallucinations, or decreased drug effectiveness. The other drugs listed don't require the client to take a drug holiday.
CN: Physiological integrity; CNS: Pharmacological and parenteral therapies; CL: Understand

45. 1. MS is a chronic autoimmune disease that is more common in women than in men. It is characterized by multiple areas of demyelination and sclerosis of the underlying nerve fibers. There are no known cures for MS, although treatment can help promote remissions and prevent exacerbations.
CN: Physiological integrity; CNS: Physiological adaptation; CL: Apply

46. 4. Glatiramer helps to decrease the number of relapses in the MS client. Flushing, chest pain, palpitations, anxiety, shortness of breath, and itching occur in some clients following administration of the medication. They typically are transient and self-limiting and don't need specific treatment.
CN: Physiological integrity; CNS: Pharmacological and parenteral therapies; CL: Analyze

CN: Client needs category   CNS: Client needs subcategory   CL: Cognitive level

47. What would the nurse expect to assess in a client experiencing early symptoms of multiple sclerosis (MS)?
1. Diplopia
2. Grief
3. Paralysis
4. Dementia

48. What information is important for the nurse to include when teaching a client with multiple sclerosis (MS) about ways to avoid exacerbation of the disease?
1. Patching the affected eye
2. Sleeping eight hours each night
3. Taking hot baths for relaxation
4. Drinking 1,500 to 2,000 ml of fluid daily

49. The nurse is caring for a 19-year-old client recently diagnosed with multiple sclerosis (MS). What interventions would be important for the nurse to include when teaching this client ways to prevent the exacerbation of symptoms? Select all that apply.
1. Suggesting a support group or meditation to decrease stress
2. Providing a hot bath or shower to promote relaxation
3. Decreasing fluid intake
4. Planning activities to avoid fatigue
5. Promoting daily exercise

50. A client with suspected multiple sclerosis (MS) undergoes a lumbar puncture. The nurse understands that the results of the cerebrospinal fluid (CSF) may show:
1. blood or increased red blood cells.
2. elevated white blood cells (WBCs) or purulent drainage.
3. increased glucose concentrations.
4. increased protein levels.

51. A nurse observes a client experiencing repetitive and involuntary horizontal, rhythmic movements of the eyes. The nurse interprets these movements as:
1. diplopia.
2. exophthalmos.
3. nystagmus.
4. oculogyric crisis.

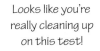

Looks like you're really cleaning up on this test!

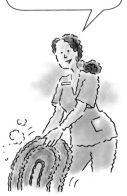

47. **1.** Early symptoms of MS include slurred speech and diplopia. Grief isn't a clinical manifestation. Paralysis is a late symptom of MS. Although depression and a short attention span may occur, dementia is rarely associated with MS.
CN: Physiological integrity; CNS: Physiological adaptation;
CL: Apply

48. **2.** MS is exacerbated by exposure to stress, fatigue, and heat. Clients should balance activity with rest. Patching the affected eye may result in improved vision and balance, but won't prevent exacerbation of the disease. Adequate hydration will help prevent urinary tract infections. Hot baths will have negligible impact on the disease process.
CN: Physiological integrity; CNS: Reduction of risk potential;
CL: Apply

49. **1, 4, 5.** Heat, stress, and fatigue may exacerbate MS. Support groups and meditation can help decrease stress. A cool shower may help reduce heat symptoms. Daily exercise is important, but not to the point of fatigue. Decreasing fluids may predispose the client to dehydration, stress and infection and can increase symptoms.
CN: Physiological integrity; CNS: Reduction of risk potential;
CL: Apply

50. **4.** Elevated gamma globulin fraction in CSF occurs in MS without an elevated level in the blood. Elevated WBCs or purulent drainage indicate infection. Blood may be found with trauma or subarachnoid hemorrhage. Increased glucose concentration is a non-specific finding indicating infection or subarachnoid hemorrhage.
CN: Physiological integrity; CNS: Physiological adaptation;
CL: Analyze

51. **3.** Nystagmus is characterized by repetitive and uncontrolled movements of the eyes. Eye movements can occur from side to side, up and down, or in a circular pattern. Diplopia means double vision. Exophthalmos refers to bulging eyeballs, as seen in Graves' disease. Oculogyric crisis is defined as a rotating movement of the eyes, but often presents as a prolonged involuntary upward deviation of the eyes.
CN: Health promotion and maintenance; CNS: None;
CL: Understand

52. What is the nurse's **most** important intervention for a client having a tonic-clonic seizure?
1. Protect the client from further injury
2. Time the duration of the seizure
3. Note the origin of seizure activity
4. Insert a padded tongue blade to prevent the client from biting his tongue

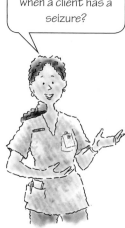

What's the first thing you should do when a client has a seizure?

52. 1. The priority during and after a seizure is to protect the person from injury by keeping them from falling to the floor. Furniture or other objects that be a source of injury during the seizure should be moved out of the client's way. Timing the seizure, and noting the origin of the seizure are important, but are not the priority. Nothing should be placed in the client's mouth during a seizure because teeth may be dislodged or the tongue pushed back, further obstructing the airway.
CN: Safe, effective care environment; CNS: Management of care; CL: Apply

53. A client recalls smelling an unpleasant odor before a seizure. How would the nurse interpret this information?
1. Atonic seizure
2. Seizure with aura
3. Icterus
4. Postictal experience

53. 2. An aura occurs in some clients as a warning before a seizure. The client may experience a certain smell, a vision such as flashing lights, or a sensation. Atonic seizure or drop attack refers to an abrupt loss of muscle tone. Icterus refers to jaundice. Postictal experience occurs after a seizure, during which the client may be confused, somnolent, and fatigued.
CN: Physiological integrity; CNS: Physiological adaptation; CL: Understand

54. A client with new-onset seizures of unknown cause is started on phenytoin. The health care provider has ordered a loading dose of 15 mg/kg IV to be given at a rate of 40 mg/min. What is the loading dose in milligrams if the client weighs 176 lb (80 kg)? Record your answer using a whole number.

_____ mg

54. 1,200.

$$15 \frac{mg}{kg} \times 80 \, kg = 1,200 \, mg$$

CN: Physiological integrity; CNS: Pharmacological and parenteral therapies; CL: Apply

55. A client, weighing 132 lb (60 kg), is to receive phenobarbital 2 mg/kg/day to be given in a divided into three equal doses. How many milligrams of phenobarbital will the client receive in each dose? Record your answer using a whole number.

_____ mg

55. 40.

$$2 \, mg/kg/day \, (total \, dose) \times 60 \, kg$$
$$(client's \, weight) = 120 \, mg/day$$

The total dose per day is 120 mg. Dividing 120 mg by 3 equal doses provides the final answer of 40 mg per dose.
CN: Physiological integrity; CNS: Pharmacological and parenteral therapies; CL: Apply

56. A client, who has just started taking phenytoin, asks the nurse if there are any adverse effects of this medication. What is the nurse's **best** response?
1. Dry mouth
2. Furry tongue
3. Somnolence
4. Tachycardia

56. 3. Adverse effects of phenytoin include sedation, somnolence, gingival hyperplasia, blood dyscrasia, and toxicity. The other symptoms aren't adverse effects of phenytoin.
CN: Physiological integrity; CNS: Pharmacological and parenteral therapies; CL: Apply

57. The laboratory has just notified the nurse that a client on the unit has a phenytoin level of 32 mg/dl. Which symptoms should the nurse anticipate from this client?
1. Ataxia and confusion
2. Sodium depletion
3. Tonic-clonic seizure
4. Urinary incontinence

58. What **priority** intervention should the nurse implement when administering phenytoin to a client who has a nasogastric (NG) tube for feeding?
1. Check the phenytoin level after giving the drug to check for toxicity
2. Elevate the head of the bed before giving phenytoin through the NG tube
3. Give phenytoin one hour before or two hours after NG tube feedings to ensure absorption
4. Verify proper placement of the NG tube by placing the end of the tube in a glass of water and observing for bubbles

59.

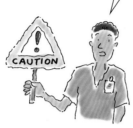

Progress notes

2/10/17	56-year-old client presents with sudden
1100	onset of stroke-like symptoms that started
	45 minutes prior to admission. Presenting
	National Institute of Health Stroke Scale
	(NIHSS) Score = 20. Head CT negative
	for blood. Past medical history includes
	hypertension treated with an ACE inhibitor.
	Alteplase 68 mg IV, given over one hour.

At the end of the alteplase infusion, the nurse notes that the client's tongue was swollen. What is the nurse's **priority** action?
1. Document this is a normal finding for the client
2. Draw arterial blood gases and prepare for immediate intubation
3. Have the client chew ice chips every 15 minutes
4. Administer antihistamines, intravenous corticosteroids, and or epinephrine

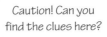

Caution! Can you find the clues here?

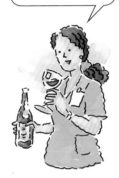

So, why doesn't alcohol get along with phenytoin?

57. 1. A level of 32 mg/dl indicates phenytoin toxicity. Symptoms of toxicity include confusion and ataxia. Phenytoin doesn't cause hyponatremia, seizure, or urinary incontinence. Incontinence may occur during or after a seizure.
CN: Physiological integrity; CNS: Pharmacological and parenteral therapies; CL: Analyze

58. 3. Phenytoin is protein bound. It is important to allow time for adequate absorption before resuming feedings. Nutritional supplements and milk interfere with the absorption of phenytoin, decreasing its effectiveness. Phenytoin levels are checked before giving the drug, and the drug is withheld for elevated levels to avoid compounding toxicity. The head of the bed is elevated when giving all drugs or solutions and isn't specific to phenytoin administration. The nurse verifies NG tube placement by checking for stomach contents before giving drugs and feedings. If placed in water to check, the client could aspirate.
CN: Physiological integrity; CNS: Pharmacological and parenteral therapies; CL: Apply

59. 4. The client has orolingual angioedema, a rare allergic reaction to alteplase that is more common in those taking ACE inhibitors. The nurse should prepare to administer antihistamines, intravenous corticosteroids, or epinephrine per provider orders. When caught early, intubation can often be prevented. If the client is in respiratory distress, and swelling is significant, the nurse should prepare for immediate intubation to protect the airway. Arterial blood gases are not needed pre-intubation, as airway obstruction is the immediate concern. Ice chips are contraindicated. A swollen tongue is not a symptom of stroke.
CN: Physiological integrity; CNS: Pharmacological and parenteral therapies; CL: Apply

60. When assessing vital signs in a client with new onset of seizures, which assessment is **most** important?
1. Checking for a pulse deficit
2. Checking for pulsus paradoxus
3. Obtaining an accurate temperature
4. Checking the blood pressure for an auscultatory gap

61. What nursing interventions are appropriate for a client is experiencing status epilepticus? Select all that apply.
1. Protect the client from harm
2. Insert a padded tongue blade in the mouth
3. Assess for hypoglycemia
4. Administer lorazepam per health care providers order
5. Place in prone position
6. Remain with client and give verbal reassurance

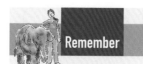

Remember

The "-one" drugs (corticosteroids) "own" inflammation— that is, they help reduce it.

- Beclomethasone
- Cortisone
- Dexamethasone
- Hydrocortisone
- Methylprednisolone
- Prednisolone
- Prednisone
- Triamcinolone

60. 3. High temperatures can induce seizures. It is important to obtain an accurate temperature in a safe manner. Pulse deficit occurs in an arrhythmia. Pulsus paradoxus may occur with cardiac tamponade. An auscultatory gap occurs in hypertension.
CN: Physiological integrity; CNS: Reduction of risk potential; CL: Apply

61. 1, 3, 4, 6. Status epilepticus is a medical emergency. Stay with the client, protecting them from harm, and call for help. Ensure that the airway is open and provide supplemental oxygen. Do not force an airway with a tongue blade. It is important to assess cardiac and respiratory function. Blood glucose should be checked to rule out hypoglycemia. Secure an IV and prepare to give lorazepam or a similar first-line agent. When the seizure ceases, turn the client on their side to protect the airway. Stay with the client during the postictal stage, and give verbal reassurance as the client may be confused and scarred.
CN: Safe, effective care environment; CNS: Management of care; CL: Apply

62. An alert and oriented client comes to the emergency department after hitting his head in a motor vehicle accident. What should the nurse do **first**?
1. Assess range of motion (ROM) to determine the extent of injuries
2. Call for an immediate chest X-ray
3. Immobilize the client's head and neck
4. Open the airway with the head-tilt, chin-lift maneuver

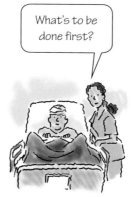

What's to be done first?

62. 3. All clients with a head injury are treated as if a cervical spine injury is present until an X-ray confirms otherwise. ROM would be contraindicated at this time. There is no indication that the client needs an immediate chest X-ray, although one may be done after stabilizing the spine. The airway doesn't need to be opened since the client appears alert and not in respiratory distress. The head-tilt, chin-lift maneuver wouldn't be used until cervical spine injury is ruled out.
CN: Safe, effective care environment; CNS: Management of care; CL: Apply

63. What information is important for the nurse to consider when planning care for a client admitted with a complete C6 spinal injury?
1. Causes aphasia
2. Causes hemiparesis
3. Causes paraplegia
4. Causes quadriplegia

63. 4. Quadriplegia occurs as a result of complete cervical spine injuries, and results in paralysis of arms and legs. Nursing care will need to be adapted to meet this client's needs. Aphasia refers to difficulty expressing or understanding spoken words and is caused by injury to the Broca and or Wernicke areas of the brain. Hemiparesis describes weakness of one side of the body. Paraplegia occurs as a result of injury to the thoracic cord and below.
CN: Physiological integrity; CNS: Physiological adaptation; CL: Understand

CN: Client needs category   CNS: Client needs subcategory   CL: Cognitive level

64. The nurse is caring for a client with damage to the hippocampus, amygdala, and fornix. How should the nurse plan care for this client?
1. Monitor vital signs frequently
2. Assess coordination during activity
3. Evaluate memory and emotion during interaction with family
4. Monitor interventions for pain control

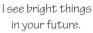

I see bright things in your future.

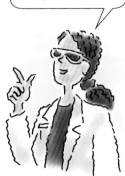

64. 3. The hippocampus, amygdala, and fornix make up the limbic system, which regulates emotions. The hippocampus and associated structures are also important for short-term memory. Coordination is a function of the cerebellum. The midbrain, pons, medulla oblongata, and reticular formation regulate vital functions.
CN: Safe, effective care environment; CNS: Management of care; CL: Apply

65. A 30-year-old client is admitted to the progressive care unit with a C5 fracture from a motorcycle accident. What would be the nurse's **priority** assessment?
1. Bladder distention
2. Neurological deficit
3. Pulse oximetry readings
4. Client feelings about the injury

65. 3. After a spinal cord injury, ascending cord edema may cause a higher level of injury. The diaphragm is innervated at the C4 level, so assessment of adequate oxygenation and ventilation is necessary. Although the other options are important, observation for respiratory failure is the priority.
CN: Safe, effective care environment; CNS: Management of care; CL: Apply

66. While in the emergency department, a client with C8 quadriplegia develops a blood pressure of 80/44 mmHg, pulse of 48 beats per minute, and respiratory rate of 18 breaths per minute. Which condition would the nurse suspect?
1. Autonomic dysreflexia
2. Hemorrhagic shock
3. Neurogenic shock
4. Pulmonary embolism

What condition fits these symptoms?

66. 3. Symptoms of neurogenic shock include hypotension, bradycardia, and warm, dry skin due to loss of adrenergic stimulation below the level of the lesion. Hypertension, bradycardia, flushing, and sweating are seen with autonomic dysreflexia. Hemorrhagic shock presents with anxiety, tachycardia, and hypotension. This would not be suspected without an injury. Pulmonary embolism presents with chest pain, hypotension, hypoxemia, tachycardia, and hemoptysis. This may be a later complication of spinal cord injury due to immobility.
CN: Physiological integrity; CNS: Physiological adaptation; CL: Analyze

67. A client is experiencing hearing loss, buzzing, and ringing in the ears. Which type of brain tumor would the nurse suspect for a client with these symptoms?
1. Acoustic neuroma
2. Astrocytoma
3. Craniopharyngioma
4. Ependymoma

67. 1. An acoustic neuroma is a benign tumor affecting the eighth cranial nerve. Symptoms include loss of hearing in one ear, buzzing or ringing in the ear, and occasionally some dizziness. The other tumors listed do not usually affect hearing.
CN: Physiological integrity; CNS: Physiological adaptation; CL: Remember

68. What is the **best** nursing intervention for a client who has just been diagnosed with a glioblastoma?
1. Providing honest, accurate information while maintaining hope
2. Discussing a referral to palliative care
3. Reviewing medication required to treat potential complications
4. Educating the client on the importance of receiving the influenza vaccine prior to initiating chemotherapy

68. 1. It is most important for the nurse to provide honest and accurate information while maintaining hope. Glioblastoma are highly malignant tumors with a 50% mortality rate at one year. The other options are premature.
CN: Physiological integrity; CNS: Physiological adaptation; CL: Apply

CN: Client needs category   CNS: Client needs subcategory   CL: Cognitive level

69. A 22-year-old client with quadriplegia in supine position is apprehensive and flushed, with a blood pressure of 210/100 mmHg and heart rate of 50 bpm. Which nursing intervention should be done **first**?
1. Place the client flat in bed
2. Assess patency of the indwelling urinary catheter
3. Give one sublingual nitroglycerin tablet
4. Raise the head of the bed immediately to 90 degrees

69. 4. Anxiety, flushing above the level of the lesion, piloerection, hypertension, and bradycardia are symptoms of autonomic dysreflexia, typically caused by such noxious stimuli as a full bladder, fecal impaction, or pressure ulcer. Putting the client flat will cause the blood pressure to increase more. The indwelling urinary catheter should be assessed immediately after the head of the bed is raised. Nitroglycerin is given to relieve chest pain and reduce preload. It isn't used for hypertension or dysreflexia.
CN: Safe, effective care environment; CNS: Management of care; CL: Analyze

70. A client with paraplegia from a T10 injury is getting ready to transfer to a rehabilitation hospital. When the nurse offers to assist him, the client throws his suitcase on the floor and says, "You don't want to help me." What is the nurse's **most** appropriate response?
1. "I just offered to help you."
2. "I'll pick these things up for you and come back later."
3. "You seem angry today. Going to rehab can be scary."
4. "When you get to rehab, they won't let you behave like this."

70. 3. The nurse should always focus on the feelings underlying a particular action. Answers one and four are confrontational. Offering to pick up the client's belongings doesn't deal with the situation, and assumes that he can't do it alone.
CN: Psychosocial integrity; CNS: None; CL: Apply

71. A client with a cervical spine injury is placed in a Minerva body vest. The client is uncomfortable and would like to try a different device. What is the **best** response by the nurse?
1. The vest protects the neck against excessive motion.
2. The vest will provide for immobilization of the midcervical segments.
3. The vest will provide significant immobilization including lateral flexion.
4. There are other soft-type collars that can be used.

71. 3. The Minerva vest will provide significant immobilization including lateral flexion. Most soft collars do not limit cervical motion but act as a reminder against excessive motion. More rigid devices such as the Philadelphia collar provide reasonable immobilization of the midcervical segments for flexion and extension but not for lateral flexion.
CN: Physiological integrity; CNS: Physiological adaptation; CL: Apply

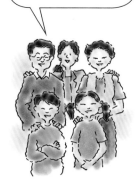

Include the whole family when teaching; it will help the client remember better.

72. A client with a halo vest is being discharged from the hospital. What is the **most** important information for the nurse to give the client and family?
1. "Don't use the wheelchair while the halo vest is in place."
2. "Clean the pin sites with peroxide."
3. "Keep the wrench that opens the vest attached at all times."
4. "Perform range-of-motion (ROM) exercises to the neck and shoulders four times daily."

72. 3. The wrench to remove the vest must be attached at all times in case the client needs cardiopulmonary resuscitation. The vest is designed to improve mobility. This client may use a wheelchair. Peroxide, especially full strength, can disrupt the healing process and normal flora. The purpose of the vest is to immobilize the neck. Range-of-motion exercises to the neck are prohibited, but should be performed to other areas.
CN: Physiological integrity; CNS: Reduction of risk potential; CL: Apply

73. A client is admitted with intervertebral disk prolapse, and shows new symptoms of urinary incontinence and paralysis of both legs. What is the **priority** action by the nurse?
1. Obtain an order for a urinary drainage device
2. Notify the provider immediately
3. Increase the frequency of vital signs
4. Administer medication to decrease inflammation

73. 2. Cauda equina syndrome occurs when there is compression on the nerve roots. It affects areas below the level of these nerve roots. It is an emergency that requires surgical intervention. If not treated, it may lead to permanent loss of bladder and bowel control and paralysis of the legs. Inserting a urinary drainage device, increasing the frequency of vital signs, and administering anti-inflammatory medication may be interventions that are needed; however, they are not the priority.
CN: Safe, effective care environment; CNS: Management of care; CL: Analyze

74. Which intervention describes an appropriate bladder program for a client in rehabilitation for a recent spinal cord injury?
1. Insert an indwelling urinary catheter.
2. Schedule intermittent catheterization every two to four hours.
3. Perform a straight catheterization every eight hours while the client is awake
4. Perform the Crede maneuver to the lower abdomen before the client voids

74. 2. Intermittent catheterization should begin every two to four hours early in treatment. When residual volume is less than 400 ml, the schedule may advance to every four to six hours. Indwelling catheters may predispose the client to infection and are removed as soon as possible. The Crede maneuver is applied after voiding to enhance bladder emptying.
CN: Physiological integrity; CNS: Basic care and comfort; CL: Apply

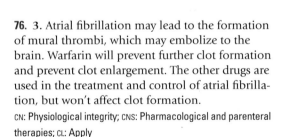

Methinks you are halfway through the test—bravo!

75. A 46-year-old client with breast cancer reports back pain and difficulty moving her legs. Which nursing intervention is the **most** appropriate?
1. Notify the provider
2. Position the client on her side, and prop her with a foam wedge
3. Ask the provider for a physical therapy consultation
4. Give acetaminophen, and reassure the client that the pain will disappear soon

75. 1. Back pain and neurological deficits may be symptoms of metastasis. The provider should be notified. Repositioning the client, physical therapy, or giving acetaminophen may help the pain but can delay evaluation and treatment.
CN: Health promotion and maintenance; CNS: None; CL: Analyze

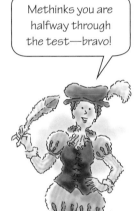

76. A client was admitted to the hospital because of a transient ischemic attack (TIA) secondary to atrial fibrillation. The nurse anticipates that the provider will prescribe:
1. digoxin.
2. diltiazem.
3. warfarin.
4. quinidine gluconate.

76. 3. Atrial fibrillation may lead to the formation of mural thrombi, which may embolize to the brain. Warfarin will prevent further clot formation and prevent clot enlargement. The other drugs are used in the treatment and control of atrial fibrillation, but won't affect clot formation.
CN: Physiological integrity; CNS: Pharmacological and parenteral therapies; CL: Apply

77. A client has been newly diagnosed with Ménière's disease. What is the nurse's **priority** of care for this client?
1. Controlling the client's symptoms
2. Encouraging the client to increase their dietary salt intake
3. Reassuring the client that hearing loss is temporary
4. Preparing the client for surgery

77. 1. Ménière's disease is a chronic disease without a definitive curative treatment. It is most important for the nurse to focus on symptom relief and non-interventional treatment, especially for a newly-diagnosed client. Non-interventional treatment would include lifestyle adjustments, medical therapies, and rehabilitation. Interventional therapy is limited to clients who have intractable vertigo symptoms that significantly impair quality of life despite aggressive medical management. Hearing loss fluctuates and is progressive. Dietary interventions include avoiding foods with high salt or sugar content.
CN: Safe, effective care environment; CNS: Management of care; CL: Analyze

78. How should the nurse position a client who has just undergone a stapedectomy?
1. On the affected side
2. On the unaffected side
3. Prone
4. In Sims' position

79. The nurse is planning care for a client with classic Ménière's disease. Which assessment finding would require intervention?
1. Epistaxis
2. Facial pain
3. Ptosis
4. Tinnitus

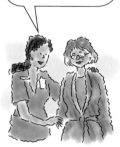

Offer extra help to clients who are unsteady on their feet.

80. A client presents with a foreign body protruding from his eye. What is the nurse's **most** important intervention?
1. Irrigate the eye with sterile saline
2. Assess visual acuity with a Snellen chart
3. Remove the foreign body with sterile forceps
4. Patch both eyes until seen by the ophthalmologist

81. A client with severe eye pain requests a prescription for the topical anesthetic that the ophthalmologist instilled. What is the nurse's **best** response to this request?
1. Topical anesthetic provides a way for pathogens to enter.
2. Topical anesthetic can cause dependence and rebound pain.
3. Damage could occur to the cornea due to lack of sensation caused by topical anesthetic.
4. Topical anesthetic causes mydriasis and blurred vision making activity hazardous.

82. The nurse is assessing an 86-year-old client who is hearing impaired. Which intervention should the nurse implement?
1. Obtain an ear wick
2. Shout into the better ear
3. Lower your voice pitch while facing the client
4. Ask the family to go home and get the client's hearing aid

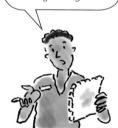

Be clear and precise when giving instructions about drug dosages.

78. 2. The client should be positioned on the unaffected side with the operative ear up. Although Sims' position is a side-lying position, it doesn't consider which side is best for after ear surgery.
CN: Physiological integrity; CNS: Physiological adaptation; CL: Apply

79. 4. Tinnitus, dizziness, and vertigo occur in Ménière's disease. Intervention is necessary as the client is at risk to fall and develop injury. Epistaxis may occur with a variety of blood dyscrasias or local lesions. Facial pain may occur with trigeminal neuralgia. Ptosis occurs with a variety of conditions, including myasthenia gravis.
CN: Physiological integrity; CNS: Physiological adaptation; CL: Apply

80. 4. One or both eyes should be patched to prevent pain with extraocular movement or accommodation. Chemicals or small foreign bodies may be irrigated. Assessment of visual acuity isn't a priority, although it may be done after treatment. Protruding objects aren't removed by the nurse because the vitreous body may rupture.
CN: Safe, effective care environment; CNS: Management of care; CL: Apply

81. 3. Corneal damage may occur with the prolonged use of topical anesthetics. If the bottle isn't touched to the eye or lashes, the entry of pathogens should be limited. Dependence and rebound don't occur from topical anesthetics. Anesthetics don't cause mydriasis.
CN: Physiological integrity; CNS: Reduction of risk potential; CL: Apply

82. 3. Hearing loss in an elderly client typically involves the upper ranges. Lowering the pitch of your voice and facing the client will provide other means of understanding, such as lip reading. An ear wick is used to allow medications to enter the ear canal. Shouting is typically in the upper ranges and could cause anxiety to an already anxious client. Alternative means of communication such as writing may also be used to assess chest pain while waiting for the family to bring the hearing aid from home.
CN: Physiological integrity; CNS: Basic care and comfort; CL: Apply

CN: Client needs category   CNS: Client needs subcategory   CL: Cognitive level

83. A client is scheduled for magnetic resonance imaging (MRI) of the head. What is the nurse's **priority** prior to the MRI?
1. Allow the client no food for eight hours prior to the MRI
2. Assess the client for a prostheses or pacemaker
3. Assess for the presence of carotid artery disease
4. Be sure that the client has voided prior to the MRI

83. 2. Strong magnetic waves may dislodge metal in the client's body, causing tissue injury. Although the client may be told to restrict food for eight hours, particularly if contrast is used, metal is an absolute contraindication for this procedure. Voiding beforehand would make the client more comfortable and better able to remain still during the procedure, but isn't essential for the scan. Having carotid artery disease isn't a contraindication to having an MRI.
CN: Safe, effective care environment; CNS: Safety and infection control; CL: Apply

84. Which nursing intervention is important while caring for a client who has expressive aphasia?
1. Place the client in busy room
2. Include detailed instructions about all procedures
3. Avoid yes or no questions
4. Encourage the client to use hand gestures, or other alternate methods to communicate

84. 4. A client with aphasia should be encouraged to use alternate ways to communicate, such as pointing, picture boards, hand gestures, and drawing. Clients with aphasia should be placed in a quiet room without a lot or noise or distractions. Ask questions in a way that the client can answer with a "yes" or "no." Don't burden this client with excessive information.
CN: Physiological integrity; CNS: Management of Care; CL: Apply

85. A nurse is preparing to instill ear drops in a 28-year-old client with otitis externa. What is the correct procedure for instillation?
1. Pull the pinna down and back
2. Pull the pinna up and back
3. Pull the tragus up and back
4. Separate the palpebral fissures with a clean gauze pad

85. 2. To straighten the ear canal of an adult, the pinna is pulled up and back. Options 1 and 3 aren't appropriate methods for preparing the ear to receive eardrops. The palpebral fissures are in the eye.
CN: Physiological integrity; CNS: Pharmacological and parenteral therapies; CL: Understand

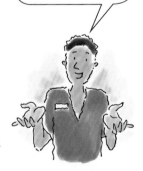

Make sure the client understands your teaching before moving on.

86. The nurse has just completed discharge teaching for a client who has undergone cataract surgery. What statement, by the client, alerts the nurse that further teaching is needed?
1. "I need to avoid bending and straining."
2. "I need to avoid high-sodium foods to reduce intraocular pressure."
3. "I need to avoid driving and sleeping on the affected side."
4. "I need to avoid using makeup on the affected eye."

86. 2. After cataract surgery, there is no need to restrict sodium. Using makeup, bending, straining, lifting, vomiting, and sleeping on the affected side may increase intraocular pressure and put strain on the sutures.
CN: Physiological integrity; CNS: Reduction of risk potential; CL: Apply

87. Which sign of increased intracranial pressure (ICP), after head trauma, would appear **first**?
1. Bradycardia
2. Large amounts of very dilute urine
3. Restlessness and confusion
4. Widened pulse pressure

87. 3. The earliest symptom of increased ICP is a change in mental status. Bradycardia, widened pulse pressure, and bradypnea occur later. The client may void large amounts of very dilute urine if there's damage to the posterior pituitary.
CN: Physiological integrity; CNS: Physiological adaptation; CL: Analyze

CN: Client needs category   CNS: Client needs subcategory   CL: Cognitive level

88. A client admitted to the emergency department for head trauma is diagnosed with an epidural hematoma. What would **most** likely cause this condition?
   1. Laceration of the middle meningeal artery
   2. Rupture of the carotid artery
   3. Trauma to the middle cerebral artery
   4. Venous bleeding from the arachnoid space

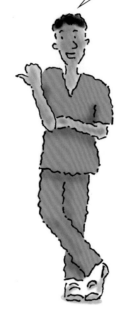

Did you catch the words "most likely"? Good! You're starting to catch on.

89. A 23-year-old client has been hit on the head with a baseball bat. The nurse notes clear fluid draining from his ears and nose. What is the nurse's **priority** intervention?
   1. Position the client flat in bed
   2. Notify the provider of a potential cerebrospinal fluid leak
   3. Suction the nose to maintain airway patency
   4. Pack the nose and ears with sterile gauze

90. The nurse is teaching the parents of a child who is in the lucid period following head trauma. Which statement **best** describes the lucid period?
   1. An interval when the child's speech is garbled
   2. An interval when the child is alert but can't recall recent events
   3. An interval when the child is oriented, but then becomes somnolent
   4. An interval when the client has a warning symptom, such as an odor or visual disturbance

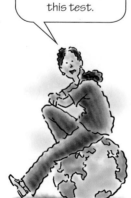

Oh yeah. You are so dominating this test.

91. The nurse is teaching the family how to suction the tracheostomy of a client with C4 quadriplegia. What information should the nurse include in these instructions?
   1. Limit suction to 10 seconds at a time
   2. Regulate the suction machine to minus 300 cm of suction
   3. Apply suction only while inserting the catheter
   4. Pass the suction catheter 2 to 3 cm into the opening of the tracheostomy tube

88. 1. Epidural hematoma or extradural hematoma are usually caused by laceration of the middle meningeal artery. Trauma to the middle cerebral artery would be associated with intracerebral hemorrhage or stroke. Venous bleeding from the arachnoid space is usually observed with subdural hematoma.
CN: Physiological integrity; CNS: Physiological adaptation;
CL: Remember

89. 2. Clear or light pink tinged liquid from the nose or ear in the presence of a head injury may be leakage of cerebral spinal fluid due to a basilar skull fracture. The provider should be notified, and precautions to prevent infection should be taken. Placing the client flat in bed may increase intracranial pressure and promote pulmonary aspiration. The nose shouldn't be suctioned because of the risk of inadvertently suctioning brain tissue through the sinuses. Nothing should be inserted into the ears or nose of a client with a skull fracture because of the risk of infection.
CN: Physiological integrity; CNS: Management of Care ;
CL: Analyze

90. 3. A lucid interval is described as a brief period of unconsciousness followed by alertness, and then unconsciousness. This is most common with an epidural hematoma. Clients should be closely monitored and swift action taken if the client deteriorates. Garbled speech is known as dysarthria. An interval in which the client is alert but can't recall recent events is known as amnesia. Warning symptoms, or auras, typically occur before seizures.
CN: Physiological integrity; CNS: Reduction of risk potential;
CL: Apply

91. 1. Suction should be applied for no longer than 10 seconds at a time to prevent hypoxia. Suction pressure of up to 120 mmHg for open-system suctioning and up to 160 mmHg for closed-system suctioning can be used. Suction should be regulated to −80 to −120 cm. Higher suction may cause tissue damage. Suction should only be applied while withdrawing the catheter. When suctioning the trachea, the catheter is inserted 10 to 15 cm, or until resistance is felt.
CN: Physiological integrity; CNS: Reduction of risk potential;
CL: Apply

92. What information should the nurse include when providing discharge teaching for a client with a hemorrhagic stroke?

1. Share the facts about the occurrence of coronary artery disease
2. Emphasize the importance of follow-up with their regular provider for new, or worsening stroke symptoms
3. Explain the relationship between hypertension and their stroke
4. Explain the need to take a daily aspirin or other anti-platelet medication

92. 3. Clients need to be educated about how to decrease their specific risk factor for recurrent stroke, such as better blood pressure management, and the need to contact emergency medical services promptly for new stroke symptoms. Unlike uncontrolled hypertension, coronary artery disease is not a major risk factor for hemorrhagic stroke. Daily aspirin and anti-platelet medication are routine medications in clients with ischemic, not hemorrhagic strokes.

CN: Physiological integrity; CNS: Reduction of risk potential; CL: Understand

93. Which nifedipine-related side effect should the nurse be **most** concerned with when caring for a new stroke admission?

1. Dehydration
2. Hypocarbia
3. Hypotension
4. Weakness

93. 3. Nifedipine is a calcium channel blocker used to lower blood pressure. It is avoided in acute stroke due to the potential of hypotension. Hypotension in acute ischemic stroke reduces brain perfusion and is associated with poor stroke outcomes. Treatment for an acute stroke includes permissive hypertension. Hypocarbia, dehydration, and weakness are not common side effects of nifedipine.

CN: Physiological integrity; CNS: Physiological adaptation; CL: Apply

94. Which client on the rehabilitation unit is at greatest risk for the development of autonomic dysreflexia?

1. A client with brain injury
2. A client with herniated nucleus pulposus
3. A client with a high cervical spine injury
4. A client with a stroke

94. 3. Autonomic dysreflexia refers to uninhibited sympathetic outflow in clients with spinal cord injuries most commonly above the level of T6. Autonomic dysreflexia is characterized by severe paroxysmal hypertension associated with throbbing headaches, profuse sweating, nasal stuffiness, flushing of the skin above the level of the lesion, bradycardia, apprehension, and anxiety. It is sometimes accompanied by cognitive impairment. The other clients aren't prone to dysreflexia.

CN: Safe, effective care environment; CNS: Management of care; CL: Apply

95. Which condition indicates that spinal shock is resolving in a client with C7 quadriplegia?

1. Absence of pain sensation in the chest
2. Return of reflexes below the injury
3. Spontaneous respirations
4. Urinary continence

95. 2. The return of reflexes and spasticity are signs of resolving shock. Spinal or neurogenic shock are characterized by hypotension, bradycardia, dry skin, flaccid paralysis, or the absence of reflexes below the level of injury. The absence of pain sensation in the chest doesn't apply to spinal shock. Spinal shock descends from the injury, and respiratory difficulties occur at C4 and above. Slight muscle contraction at the bulbocavernosus reflex occurs but not enough for urinary continence.

CN: Physiological integrity; CNS: Physiological adaptation; CL: Analyze

CN: Client needs category CNS: Client needs subcategory CL: Cognitive level

96. A client is being discharged from the hospital following a laminectomy. The nurse recognizes that the client needs further teaching when he states:

1. "I'll sleep on a firm mattress."
2. "I won't drive for 2 to 4 weeks."
3. "When I pick things up, I'll bend my knees."
4. "I can't wait to pick up my one-year-old granddaughter."

97. When assessing a client with herniated nucleus pulposus of L4-L5, the nurse suspects spinal cord compression. Which finding supports the nurse's assessment?

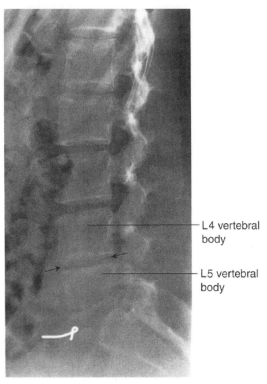

L4 vertebral body

L5 vertebral body

1. Lower back pain
2. Pain radiating across the buttocks
3. Positive Kernig's sign
4. Urinary incontinence

98. What actions should the nurse include in the plan of care to prevent autonomic dysreflexia in a client with a T6 injury?

1. Treating headache
2. Avoiding excessive position changes
3. Preventing fecal impaction
4. Avoiding urinary catheterization

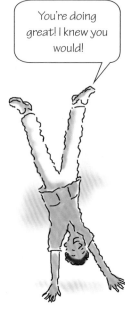
You're doing great! I knew you would!

96. 4. Lifting more than 10 lb (4.5 kg) for several weeks after surgery is contraindicated. The other responses are appropriate.

CN: Physiological integrity; CNS: Reduction of risk potential; CL: Analyze

97. 4. Progressive neurological deficits at L4-L5, including worsening muscle weakness, paresthesia, and loss of bowel and bladder control, are symptoms of spinal cord compression. The other symptoms usually occur in clients with herniated nucleus pulposus without spinal cord compression. Kernig's sign is a symptom of meningitis and is characterized by severe stiffness of the hamstrings causing an inability to straighten the leg when the hip is flexed to 90 degrees.

CN: Physiological integrity; CNS: Physiological adaptation; CL: Apply

98. 3. The avoidance of fecal impaction and the prevention of bladder distention are the mainstays in preventing episodes of autonomic dysreflexia. An indwelling or intermittent urinary catheter may be required. Skin breakdown can also be a source of noxious stimuli. This client should be repositioned frequently to prevent skin breakdown. Headache is a symptom but not a cause of autonomic dysreflexia.

CN: Physiological integrity; CNS: Physiological adaptation; CL: Apply

CN: Client needs category   CNS: Client needs subcategory   CL: Cognitive level

99. A client experiencing an episode of autonomic dysreflexia becomes hypertensive. What is the **most** important intervention by the nurse?
  1. Elevate the client's legs
  2. Place the client flat in bed
  3. Place the client in Trendelenburg's position
  4. Place the client in high Fowler's position

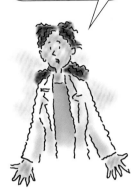

Don't freak out! Take a deep breath and re-read the question.

99. 4. Putting the client in high Fowler's position can help reduce blood pressure below dangerous levels until other treatment can be started. Elevating the client's legs, putting the client flat in bed, or putting the bed in Trendelenburg's position would place this client in positions that could increase blood pressure.
CN: Physiological integrity; CNS: Reduction of risk potential; CL: Apply

100. A client, recovering from a spinal cord injury, has a great deal of spasticity. Which medication would the nurse anticipate to relieve spasticity?
  1. Hydralazine
  2. Baclofen
  3. Lidocaine
  4. Methylprednisolone

100. 2. Baclofen is a skeletal muscle relaxant used to decrease spasms. It may be given orally or intrathecally. Hydralazine is an antihypertensive and afterload-reducing agent. Lidocaine is an antiarrhythmic and a local anesthetic agent. Methylprednisolone is an anti-inflammatory drug used to decrease spinal cord edema in the acute phase.
CN: Physiological integrity; CNS: Pharmacological and parenteral therapies; CL: Apply

101. As part of cervical traction, a client has just had Gardner-Wells tongs inserted into his scalp. What should the nurse be **most** concerned about?
  1. Preventing anxiety and promoting cooperation by offering emotional support, evaluation and education
  2. Meticulous pin and site care to prevent infection
  3. Prophylaxis prevention for deep vein thrombosis (DVT)
  4. A complete physical assessment including breath sounds q4h to detect spinal shock

101. 4. While all of these interventions are important, the most important is a complete physical assessment including breath sounds every q4h to detect changes in condition such as spinal shock. Spinal shock results in severe bradycardia, profound hypotension, warm dry skin, and absent reflexes below the level of the lesion. These symptoms are potentially life threatening and require immediate intervention.
CN: Physiological integrity; CNS: Reduction of risk potential; CL: Apply

102. A client with a T1 spinal cord injury arrives at the emergency department with a blood pressure of 82/40 mmHg, pulse of 34 bpm, dry skin, and flaccid paralysis of the lower extremities. Which condition would the nurse suspect?
  1. Autonomic dysreflexia
  2. Hypervolemia
  3. Neurogenic shock
  4. Sepsis

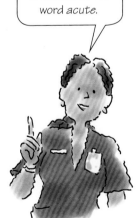

Pay close attention to the word acute.

102. 3. Loss of sympathetic control and unopposed vagal stimulation below the level of injury typically cause hypotension, bradycardia, pallor, flaccid paralysis, and warm, dry skin during neurogenic shock. Hypervolemia is indicated by a rapid and bounding pulse and edema. Autonomic dysreflexia occurs after neurogenic shock abates. Signs of sepsis would include elevated temperature, increased heart rate, and increased respiratory rate.
CN: Physiological integrity; CNS: Physiological adaptation; CL: Analyze

103. A client has a cervical spine injury at the level of C5. Which condition would the nurse anticipate during the acute phase?
  1. Absent corneal reflex
  2. Decerebrate posturing
  3. Movement of only the right or left half of the body
  4. The need for mechanical ventilation

103. 4. The diaphragm is stimulated by nerves at the level of C4. Initially, this client may need mechanical ventilation due to cord edema. This may resolve in time. Absent corneal reflexes, decerebrate posturing, and hemiplegia occur with brain injuries, not spinal cord injuries.
CN: Physiological integrity; CNS: Physiological adaptation; CL: Apply

CN: **Client needs category**   CNS: **Client needs subcategory**   CL: **Cognitive level**

104. When caring for a client with quadriplegia, which nursing intervention is the **priority**?
 1. Forcing fluids to prevent renal calculi
 2. Maintaining skin integrity
 3. Obtaining adaptive devices for more independence
 4. Preventing atelectasis

104. 4. Clients with quadriplegia have paralysis or weakness of the diaphragm, abdominal, or intercostal muscles. Maintenance of airway and breathing take top priority. Although forcing fluids, maintaining skin integrity, and obtaining adaptive devices for more independence are all important interventions, preventing atelectasis is the priority.
CN: Physiological integrity; CNS: Reduction of risk potential; CL: Apply

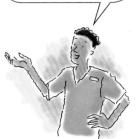

Speak slowly and use words the client can understand.

105. A client with C7 quadriplegia is flushed, anxious and reports a pounding headache. Which symptoms would the nurse anticipate?
 1. Decreased urine output or oliguria
 2. Hypertension and bradycardia
 3. Respiratory depression
 4. Symptoms of shock

105. 2. Hypertension, bradycardia, anxiety, blurred vision, and flushing above the lesion occur with autonomic dysreflexia due to uninhibited sympathetic nervous system discharge. The other options are incorrect. The most common cause of autonomic dysreflexia is bowel impaction or bladder distension.
CN: Physiological integrity; CNS: Physiological adaptation; CL: Analyze

106. A nurse is explaining the difference between stroke and transient ischemic attack (TIA). How would the nurse **best** describe the difference?
 1. A TIA resolves in less than 24 hours, usually within 30-minutes
 2. A TIA may be hemorrhagic in origin
 3. A TIA may cause permanent motor or sensory deficit
 4. A TIAs is a small strokes

106. 1. A transient ischemic attack is a ischemic processes that presents like stroke, but resolves prior to any permanent brain damage. Symptoms usually resolve within 30-minutes, but by definition, within 24 hours. Although TIA is a risk factor for stroke, they are not small strokes, as there is no permanent brain damage or sustained symptoms.
CN: Physiological integrity; CNS: Physiological adaptation; CL: Analyze

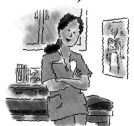

You're on your way to becoming a professional!

107. A client has had a right stroke and now has a flaccid left side. Which nursing intervention would **best** prevent shoulder subluxation for this client?
 1. Splint the wrist
 2. Use an air splint
 3. Put the affected arm in a sling
 4. Perform range-of-motion exercises on the affected side

107. 3. Due to the weight of the flaccid extremity, the shoulder may disarticulate. A sling will support the extremity. The other options won't support the shoulder. Air splints are used to support fractured or broken bones.
CN: Physiological integrity; CNS: Basic care and comfort; CL: Apply

108. A 40-year-old paraplegic client must perform intermittent catheterization of the bladder at home. How should the nurse instruct this client to perform this task?
 1. Clean the meatus from back to front
 2. Measure the quantity of urine
 3. Gently rotate the catheter during removal
 4. Clean the meatus with soap and water

108. 4. Intermittent catheterization may be performed at home using clean technique, with soap and water to clean the urinary meatus. A woman should always clean the meatus from front to back, and a man should use an expanding circles technique working outward from the meatus. It isn't necessary to measure the urine. The catheter doesn't need to be rotated during removal.
CN: Physiological integrity; CNS: Basic care and comfort; CL: Apply

109. Which method should the nurse use when assessing a client's pupil accommodation?
1. Assess peripheral vision of the client
2. Touch the cornea lightly with a wisp of cotton
3. Have the client follow an object upward, downward, obliquely, and horizontally
4. Observe for pupil constriction and convergence while focusing on an object coming toward the client

109. 4. Accommodation refers to convergence and constriction of the pupil while following a focusing on a near object, then looking at distant object. A pen light should be used to determine pupil constriction. Assessing for peripheral vision refers to visual fields. Touching the cornea lightly with a wisp of cotton describes assessment of the corneal reflex. Having the client follow an object upward, downward, obliquely, and horizontally refers to cardinal fields of gaze.
CN: Physiological integrity; CNS: Reduction of risk potential; CL: Apply

Breathe in. Breathe out.

110. A client at the eye clinic reports difficulty seeing at night. Which nutritional deficiency could contribute to this difficulty?
1. Vitamin A
2. Vitamin B$_6$
3. Vitamin C
4. Vitamin K

110. 1. Nyctalopia may be caused by a vitamin A deficiency or dysfunctional rod receptors. None of the other deficiencies listed lead to nyctalopia.
CN: Health promotion and maintenance; CNS: None; CL: Apply

111. A client with a spinal cord injury has a neurogenic bladder. When planning for discharge, the nurse should anticipate that this client will require:
1. intermittent catheterization program.
2. a Kock pouch.
3. transurethral prostatectomy.
4. ureterostomy.

111. 1. Intermittent catheterization, should start at two-hour intervals and increase to 4 to 6-hour intervals, to manage neurogenic bladder. A Kock pouch is a type of urinary diversion. Transurethral prostatectomy is indicated for an obstruction to urinary outflow by benign prostatic hyperplasia or for the treatment of cancer. An ileostomy or ureterostomy is not necessary.
CN: Physiological integrity; CNS: Basic care and comfort; CL: Apply

112. When using a Snellen alphabet chart, a nurse records a client's vision as 20/40. Which statement **best** describes 20/40 vision?
1. The client has alterations in near vision and is legally blind.
2. The client can see at 20 feet what the person with normal vision sees at 40 feet.
3. The client can see at 40 feet what the person with normal vision sees at 20 feet.
4. The client has a 20% decrease in acuity in one eye, and 40% decrease in the other eye.

112. 2. The numerator refers to the client's vision compared to the denominator, which refers to normal vision. Legal blindness refers to 20/150 or less. Alterations in near vision may be due to loss of accommodation caused by the aging process presbyopia or farsightedness.
CN: Physiological integrity; CNS: Reduction of risk potential; CL: Analyze

113. Which illustrations represent an intact vestibuloocular reflex response?

1.

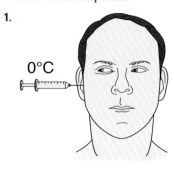

0°C

3.

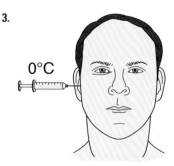

0°C

2.

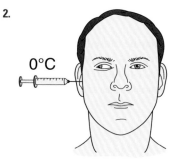

0°C

4.

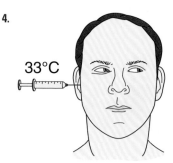

33°C

113. 1. An intact vestibuloocular reflex to cold water results in eye deviation of both eyes toward the ear being stimulated. Eyes deviate to the opposite direction when warm water is used. No eye deviation is an ominous sign.

CN: Physiological integrity; CNS: Physiological adaptation; CL: Remember

114. The nurse instills atropine drops into both eyes for a client undergoing an ophthalmic examination. Which instruction should this client follow until the medication wears off?
1. "Use caution because your blink reflex is paralyzed."
2. "Avoid wearing your regular glasses when driving."
3. "Be aware that the pupils may be unusually small."
4. "Wear dark glasses in bright light because the pupils are dilated."

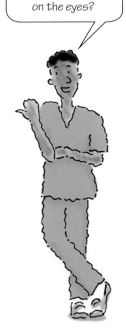

What effects does atropine have on the eyes?

114. 4. Atropine, an anticholinergic drug, has mydriatic effects such as pupil dilation. This allows more light onto the retina, and may cause photophobia and blurred vision. Atropine doesn't paralyze the blink reflex or cause miosis. Driving may be contraindicated due to blurred vision.

CN: Physiological integrity; CNS: Pharmacological and parenteral therapies; CL: Apply

115. A client with a history of a beer-laden diet is admitted with severe hyponatremia due to low serum sodium. Which statement is true regarding low serum sodium?
1. It is important to correct the hyponatremia as quickly as possible.
2. Rapid correction of the sodium may result in infarction of the pons.
3. The client should be placed on a low-protein, low-salt diet.
4. This condition will reverse itself when the client sobers up, and no treatment is necessary.

115. 2. Care must be taken not to correct the hyponatremia too quickly. Beer diets are low in sodium and protein. The body utilizes the calories in beer prior to breaking down endogenous energy sources. This leads to low solute levels in the blood and kidneys. Although healthy, the kidneys are unable to pull water from the serum to make urine. When solutes are given, rapid diuresis occurs and the serum sodium quickly corrects. When this happens to fast, osmolar demylination syndrome can occur resulting in an infarct of the pons or other vulnerable areas in the brain. A low-protein, low-salt diet is not indicated.

CN: Physiological integrity; CNS: Physiological adaptation; CL: Understand

116.

Progress notes	
2/10/17	46-year-old male admitted for intracranial
0800	hemorrhage four days ago. Morning
	laboratory results demonstrate a low
	serum sodium of 121 meEq/L, a low serum
	osmolality of 256 mOsm/kg, a high urine
	osmolality of 588 mOsm/kg, and a high
	urine sodium of 89 mmol/L. Vital signs
	are stable. Urine output is high, averaging
	greater than 100 cc/hr.

Which nursing interventions should the nurse include when planning care for a client with cerebral salt wasting (CSW) syndrome?
1. Fluid restriction
2. Sodium and fluid replacement
3. Sodium restriction
4. Synthetic vasopressin replacement

116. 2. Cerebral salt wasting syndrome is a volume-depleted and sodium-wasting state, requiring fluid replacement with isotonic solutions to prevent further deterioration. Its presentation is similarly to the syndrome of inappropriate antidiuretic hormone secretion (SIADH), which is treated with free water restriction. Synthetic vasopressin replacement is used to treat central diabetes insipidus.
CN: Physiological integrity; CNS: Pharmacological and parenteral therapies; CL: Apply

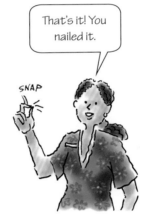

That's it! You nailed it.

SNAP

117. Which statement indicates that a client requires additional teaching following cataract surgery?
1. "I'll avoid eating until the nausea subsides."
2. "I can't wait to get back to the gym."
3. "I'll avoid bending over to tie my shoelaces."
4. "I'll avoid touching the dropper to my eye when using my eye drops."

117. 2. Lifting, which can involve the Valsalva maneuver, increases intraocular pressure (IOP), and can strain the surgical site. Preventing nausea and subsequent vomiting, avoiding bending, or placing the head in a dependent position will also prevent increased IOP. Touching the eye dropper to the eye will contaminate the dropper and the entire bottle of medication.
CN: Physiological integrity; CNS: Reduction of risk potential; CL: Analyze

118. A client has had cataract surgery resulting in aphakia. How would the nurse **best** describe this condition?
1. Absence of the crystalline lens
2. A "keyhole" pupil
3. Loss of accommodation
4. Retinal detachment

118. 1. Aphakia means without lens due to surgical removal. In cataract surgery, the diseased lens is removed and replaced with an intraocular lens. A keyhole pupil results from iridectomy. Loss of accommodation is a normal response to aging. Retinal detachment is usually associated with retinal holes created by vitreous traction.
CN: Physiological integrity; CNS: Physiological adaptation; CL: Understand

119. The nurse is developing a, educational program about glaucoma for the community. What information should the nurse include in this program?
1. Glaucoma is easily corrected with eyeglasses.
2. White and Asian individuals are at the highest risk for glaucoma.
3. Yearly screening is recommended for people between the ages of 20 to 40.
4. Glaucoma can be painless and vision may be lost before the person is aware of a problem.

119. 4. Open-angle glaucoma causes a painless increase in intraocular pressure (IOP) with loss of peripheral vision. A variety of miotics and agents to decrease IOP, and occasionally surgery, are used to treat glaucoma. African-Americans have a three-fold-greater chance of developing glaucoma, and blindness than other groups. Individuals over age 40 years should be screened.
CN: Health promotion and maintenance; CNS: None; CL: Apply

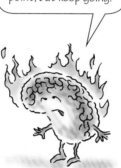

I know you're feeling fried at this point, but keep going!

120. Which medication would the nurse anticipate for a client having an episode of acute angle-closure glaucoma?
1. Acetazolamide
2. Atropine
3. Furosemide
4. Urokinase

120. 1. Acetazolamide, a carbonic anhydrase inhibitor, decreases intraocular pressure (IOP) by decreasing the secretion of aqueous humor. Atropine dilates the pupil and decreases outflow of aqueous humor, causing an increase in IOP. Furosemide is a loop diuretic, and urokinase is a thrombolytic agent. They aren't used in the treatment of glaucoma.
CN: Physiological integrity; CNS: Pharmacological and parenteral therapies; CL: Apply

121. A client presents with a detached retina. Which symptoms would the nurse anticipate with this condition?
1. Flashing lights and floaters
2. Homonymous hemianopia
3. Loss of central vision
4. Ptosis

121. 1. Signs and symptoms of retinal detachment include abrupt flashing lights, floaters, loss of peripheral vision, or a sudden shadow or curtain in the vision. Occasionally, vision loss is gradual.
CN: Physiological integrity; CNS: Physiological adaptation; CL: Apply

122. A client has undergone an enucleation of the right eye for a malignancy. A prosthesis has been placed in the socket. Which intervention should the nurse perform?
1. Instill miotics as ordered to the affected eye
2. Teach the client to clean the prosthesis in soap and water
3. Assess reactivity of the pupils to light and accommodation
4. Teach the client to prevent straining which can lead to increased intraocular pressure

122. 2. Enucleation of the eye refers to the surgical removal of the entire eye. This client needs instructions about the prosthesis. There are no activity restrictions, and there is no need for miotic eyedrops. Prophylactic antibiotics may be used in the immediate postoperative period. Miotic eyedrops are used in acute glaucoma to inhibit visual field loss and slow optic nerve damage.
CN: Physiological integrity; CNS: Physiological adaptation; CL: Apply

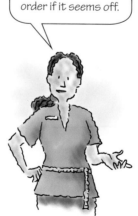

Don't be afraid to question an order if it seems off.

123. Which circumstance would cause the nurse to question an order to irrigate the ear canal?
1. Ear pain
2. Hearing loss
3. Otitis externa
4. Perforated tympanic membrane

123. 4. Irrigation of the ear canal is contraindicated when there is a perforation of the tympanic membrane because solution, entering the inner ear, may cause dizziness, nausea, vomiting, and infection. The other conditions aren't contraindications to irrigation of the ear canal.
CN: Physiological integrity; CNS: Reduction of risk potential; CL: Apply

CN: Client needs category   CNS: Client needs subcategory   CL: Cognitive level

124. How should the nurse proceed when instilling neomycin and polymyxin B sulfates and hydrocortisone optic suspension, two drops in the right ear?
1. Verify the proper client and route
2. Warm the solution to prevent dizziness
3. Hold an emesis basin under the client's ear
4. Position the client in the semi-Fowler's position

124. 1. When giving medications, a nurse should follow the five "Rs" of medication administration: right client, right drug, right dose, right route, and right time. The drops may be warmed to prevent pain or dizziness, but this action isn't essential. An emesis basin would be used for irrigation of the ear. The client should be placed in the lateral position for five minutes, not semi-Fowler's position, to prevent the drops from draining.
CN: Physiological integrity; CNS: Pharmacological and parenteral therapies; CL: Apply

125. When teaching a client with Ménière's disease, which instruction should the nurse give regarding vertigo?
1. Report dizziness at once
2. Drive in daylight hours only
3. Get up slowly, turning the entire body
4. Change your position using the logroll technique

125. 3. Turning the entire body, not the head, will prevent vertigo. Dizziness is expected, and can often be prevented or lessened through self-care interventions. The client shouldn't drive because she may reflexively turn the wheel to correct for vertigo. Turning the client slowly and smoothly while in bed will be helpful. Logrolling is not necessary.
CN: Physiological integrity; CNS: Reduction of risk potential; CL: Apply

126. What is the nurse's **priority** action when administering phenytoin to a client intravenously?
1. Administer rapidly
2. Withhold other anticonvulsants
3. Mix phenytoin with saline solution only
4. Use only dextrose solution when flushing the IV catheter

126. 3. Phenytoin is only compatible with saline solutions. Dextrose will cause an insoluble precipitate to form. Phenytoin should be administered at a rate of less than 50 mg/min. There is no need to withhold additional anticonvulsants.
CN: Physiological integrity; CNS: Pharmacological and parenteral therapies; CL: Apply

127. An 18-year-old client was hit in the head with a baseball during practice. What instruction would the nurse give when discharging this client to the care of his mother?
1. Watch him for keyhole pupil for the next 24 hours
2. Expect profuse vomiting for 24 hours after the injury
3. Wake him every hour and assess his orientation to person, time, and place
4. Notify the provider immediately if he has a headache

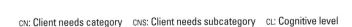

Communicate with the client's mother in a quiet, calm place.

127. 3. Changes in level of consciousness (LOC) may indicate expanding lesions such as subdural hematoma. Orientation and LOC are assessed frequently for the first 24 hours. A keyhole pupil is found after iridectomy. Profuse or projectile vomiting is a symptom of increased intracranial pressure, and should be reported immediately. A slight headache may last for several days after concussion. Severe or worsening headaches should be reported.
CN: Physiological integrity; CNS: Physiological adaptation; CL: Apply

128. A client has been prescribed carbamazepine. Which complication should the nurse be alert to?
1. Acute respiratory distress syndrome
2. Diplopia
3. Elevated levels of phenytoin
4. Leukocytosis

128. 2. Complications of carbamazepine include diplopia, dizziness, ataxia, and rash. Acute respiratory distress syndrome isn't a complication of carbamazepine. Carbamazepine decreases blood levels of phenytoin and hormonal contraceptives. It also causes agranulocytosis because of the reduction in leukocytes.
CN: Physiological integrity; CNS: Pharmacological and parenteral therapies; CL: Apply

129. For a client has sustained damage to the caudate nucleus, putamen, and globus pallidus. This client should be monitored for:
1. eye movement.
2. modulation of sounds.
3. motor movement.
4. muscle coordination.

129. **3.** Motor movement is regulated by the basal ganglia, which consists of the caudate nucleus, putamen, and globus pallidus. Eye movement is too vague because there are several cranial nerves responsible for various forms of eye movement. Modulation of sounds occur from the occipital lobe. The cerebellum regulates muscle coordination.

CN: Safe, effective care environment; CNS: Management of care; CL: Apply

130. Which assessment findings might the nurse observe in a client with injury to the thalamus?
1. Burning or aching sensation over one half of the body
2. Seizures
3. Problems initiating movement
4. Memory lapses

130. **1.** Damage to the thalamus may result in thalamic syndrome, which is characterized by pain, burning, or an aching sensation over the contralateral side of the body. It is often accompanied by mood swings. Problems initiating movement are associated with the basal ganglia and memory problems with the hippocampus. Seizures are not specific to thalamic injury.

CN: Physiological integrity; CNS: Physiological adaptation; CL: Apply

131. What is the best technique for the nurse to use when communicating with a client experiencing second-stage Alzheimer's disease?
1. Listen carefully and decipher word substitutions
2. Avoid repeating messages, as this may agitate the client
3. Avoid "yes" or "no" questions
4. Avoid using subject-verb-object sentence structure

The key to this one is remembering the functions of the different parts of the brain.

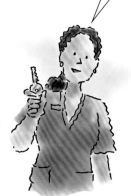

131. **1.** Listening and deciphering word substitutions is most helpful, as the client may have difficulty expressing thoughts. Sentences should be repeated as often as needed. It is helpful to use "yes" or "no" questions or multiple-choice questions with this client to facilitate ease of communication. Sentences should be short and literal, following the subject-verb-object format.

CN: Psychosocial integrity; CNS: None; CL: Apply

132. A client was admitted to the hospital with a first-degree burn from touching a hot oven. The family tells the nurse that this client could not feel the how hot the oven was. Which area of the brain would the nurse suspect as cause of this dysfunction?
1. Frontal lobe
2. Occipital lobe
3. Parietal lobe
4. Temporal lobe

132. **3.** The parietal lobe regulates sensory function, which would include the ability to detect hot or cold. The frontal lobe regulates thinking, planning, and judgment, and the occipital lobe is primarily responsible for vision function. The temporal lobe regulates memory.

CN: Physiological integrity; CNS: Physiological adaptation; CL: Apply

133. Which cranial nerve (CN) controls a client's pupillary reaction?
1. II
2. III
3. IV
4. V

133. **2.** CN III, the oculomotor nerve, controls pupil constriction. CN II is the optic nerve, which controls vision. CN IV is the trochlear nerve, which coordinates eye movement. CN V is the trigeminal nerve, which innervates the muscles used for chewing.

CN: Physiological integrity; CNS: Physiological adaptation; CL: Apply

134. A client has experienced a massive cerebral hemorrhage with loss of consciousness and requires an electroencephalogram (EEG). The client's family asks why this test is necessary. The nurse explains that an EEG is used to measure:
1. the extent of intracranial bleeding.
2. the precise location of the brain injury.
3. activity of the brain.
4. the percentage of functional brain tissue.

134. **3.** An EEG measures the electrical activity of the brain. The extent of intracranial bleeding and location of the injury site would be determined by computerized tomography or magnetic resonance imaging. The percentage of functional brain tissue would be determined by a series of tests.
CN: Physiological integrity; CNS: Reduction of risk potential; CL: Apply

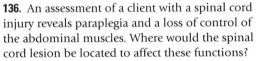

You're almost done. Then you can have cake.

135. A nurse is teaching a client, who has Parkinson's disease, and his family about dietary practices. Which signs and symptoms are **most** important for the nurse to address? Select all that apply.
1. Fluid overload
2. Drooling
3. Aspiration
4. Choking
5. Dysphagia
6. Diarrhea

135. **2, 3, 4, 5.** Eating problems associated with Parkinson's disease include dysphagia, risk of choking, drooling, aspiration, and constipation. Fluid overload and diarrhea aren't problems specifically related to Parkinson's disease.
CN: Physiological integrity; CNS: Reduction of risk potential; CL: Analyze

136. An assessment of a client with a spinal cord injury reveals paraplegia and a loss of control of the abdominal muscles. Where would the spinal cord lesion be located to affect these functions?
1. Cervical
2. Lumbar
3. Sacral
4. Thoracic

136. **4.** Complete injuries at or below the thoracic spinal levels result in paraplegia and the inability to control the abdominal muscles. Trunk stability is also affected. Functions of the hands, arms, neck, and breathing are associated with cervical injuries. The effects of injuries to the lumbar or sacral regions of the spinal cord include decreased control of the legs and hips, urinary system, and anus.
CN: Physiological integrity; CNS: Physiological adaptation; CL: Apply

137. A nurse performs a neurological assessment on a client who reports headache and dizziness. Which assessment technique would help assess the motor function of cranial nerve VII?
1. Ask the client to clench his jaw
2. Test the gag reflex by placing an applicator against the pharynx
3. Ask the client to frown, smile, and raise his eyebrows
4. Ask the client to swallow

137. **3.** To assess the motor function of cranial nerve VII, the nurse should ask the client to frown, smile, and raise his eyebrows. If these facial expressions are symmetrical, motor function is intact. Jaw clenching tests the function of cranial nerve V. Testing the gag reflex by placing an applicator against the pharynx, and assessing swallowing ability are ways to evaluate cranial nerve IX function. Testing the gag reflex would assess the function of cranial nerve X.
CN: Health promotion and maintenance; CNS: None; CL: Apply

138. An 18-year-old client is admitted with a closed head injury sustained in a motor vehicle accident. His intracranial pressure (ICP) shows an upward trend. Which intervention should the nurse perform **first**?
1. Reposition the client to avoid neck flexion
2. Administer 1 g of mannitol IV as ordered
3. Increase the ventilator's respiratory rate to 20 breaths/min
4. Administer 100 mg of pentobarbital IV as ordered

138. **1.** The nurse should first reposition the client to avoid neck flexion, which will increase venous return and lower ICP. If nursing measures prove ineffective, notify the provider.
CN: Safe, effective care environment; CNS: Management of care; CL: Apply

CN: Client needs category   CNS: Client needs subcategory   CL: Cognitive level

139. A client arrives at the emergency department after slipping on a patch of ice and hitting his head. A computed tomography (CT) scan of the head reveals a collection of blood between the skull and dura mater. Which type of head injury does this finding suggest?
1. Subdural hematoma
2. Subarachnoid hemorrhage
3. Epidural hematoma
4. Contusion

139. 3. An epidural hematoma occurs when blood collects between the skull and dura mater. In a subdural hematoma, venous blood collects between the dura mater and arachnoid mater. In a subarachnoid hemorrhage, blood collects between the pia mater and arachnoid membrane. A contusion is a bruise on the brain's surface.
CN: Physiological integrity; CNS: Physiological adaptation; CL: Apply

140. After falling 208 feet (63.4 m), a 36-year-old construction worker sustains a C6 fracture with spinal cord transection. Which additional findings should the nurse anticipate?
1. Quadriplegia with gross arm movement and diaphragmatic breathing
2. Quadriplegia and loss of respiratory function
3. Paraplegia with intercostal muscle loss
4. Loss of bowel and bladder control

140. 1. A client with a spinal cord injury at levels C5-C6 has quadriplegia with gross arm movement and diaphragmatic breathing. Injuries at levels C1-C4 lead to quadriplegia with total loss of respiratory function. Paraplegia with intercostal muscle loss occurs with injuries at T1-L2. Injuries below L2 cause paraplegia and loss of bowel and bladder control.
CN: Physiological integrity; CNS: Physiological adaptation; CL: Apply

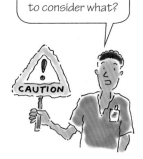

Hint! Hint! It's most important to consider what?

141. A client with a subarachnoid hemorrhage is prescribed a 1,000 mg loading dose of IV phenytoin. What information is **most** important when administering this dose?
1. Therapeutic drug levels should be maintained between 20 and 30 mg/ml.
2. Rapid phenytoin administration can cause cardiac arrhythmias.
3. Phenytoin should be mixed in dextrose in water before administration.
4. Phenytoin should be administered through an IV catheter in the client's hand.

141. 2. Intravenous phenytoin should not exceed 50 mg/min, as rapid administration can depress the myocardium, causing lethal dysrhythmias. Therapeutic drug levels range from 10 to 20 mg/ml. Phenytoin is only compatible with normal saline, not dextrose in water. Phenytoin is very irritating to the blood vessels, and may cause purple glove syndrome when administered IV into a hand.
CN: Physiological integrity; CNS: Pharmacological and parenteral therapies; CL: Apply

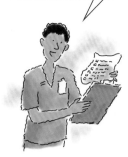

Which instruction shall I include in the teaching plan?

142. What instruction should the nurse include when developing a discharge teaching plan for a client who has been prescribed phenytoin?
1. "Take the drug on an empty stomach."
2. "You can consume alcoholic beverages in moderation."
3. "You can take any phenytoin brand because all brands are the same."
4. "Don't stop taking the drug except with medical supervision."

142. 4. Abrupt cessation of phenytoin may trigger status epilepticus, so the client should be warned not to stop the drug unless approved by the provider. Taking phenytoin with food minimizes GI distress. Alcoholic beverages can decrease the drug's effectiveness. Changing phenytoin brands may alter the therapeutic effect.
CN: Physiological integrity; CNS: Pharmacological and parenteral therapies; CL: Apply

143. A 20-year-old client, who fell approximately 31 feet (9.45 m), is unresponsive and breathless. A cervical spine injury is suspected. What is the **priority** action by the nurse?
1. Inserting a nasopharyngeal airway
2. Inserting an oropharyngeal airway
3. Performing the jaw-thrust maneuver
4. Performing the head-tilt, chin-lift maneuver

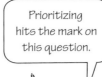

Prioritizing hits the mark on this question.

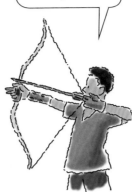

143. 3. If the client has a suspected cervical spine injury, the jaw-thrust maneuver should be used to open the airway. If the tongue or relaxed throat muscles are obstructing the airway, a nasopharyngeal or oropharyngeal airway can be inserted; however, the client must have spontaneous respirations when the airway is open. The head-tilt, chin-lift maneuver requires neck hyperextension, which can worsen a cervical spine injury.
CN: Physiological integrity; CNS: Physiological adaptation; CL: Analyze

144. An 87-year-old client is admitted following a stroke. During the admission interview and assessment the client's speech is slow, non-fluent, and labored. How should the nurse document this finding?
1. Receptive aphasia
2. Wernicke's aphasia
3. Expressive aphasia
4. Global aphasia

144. 3. Expressive aphasia results from damage to Broca's area, located in the frontal lobe of the brain's dominant hemisphere. Typically, the client with expressive aphasia has difficulty expressing himself and his speech is slow, non-fluent, and labored; however, comprehension of written and verbal communication is intact. With receptive aphasia the client can't comprehend written or verbal communication. His speech is normal, but he conveys information poorly. With global aphasia, a combination of receptive and expressive aphasia, most of the brain's communication system is damaged. Global aphasia results from extensive damage to Broca's and Wernicke's areas.
CN: Physiological integrity; CNS: Physiological adaptation; CL: Apply

145. What information should the nurse include when developing a teaching plan for a client who will undergo a stapedectomy for treatment of otosclerosis?
1. Tinnitus is common after surgery.
2. Vertigo and dizziness are common after surgery.
3. Hearing should return immediately after surgery.
4. Excessive drainage is common after surgery.

145. 2. Vertigo is the most frequent complication of stapedectomy. The client should move slowly to avoid triggering or worsening vertigo, and should ask for assistance with ambulation. Tinnitus rarely follows this surgery and should be reported to the provider. Hearing typically decreases after surgery because of ear packing and tissue swelling, but commonly returns over the next two to six weeks. Usually, postoperative drainage and pain are minimal. Excessive drainage should be reported.
CN: Physiological integrity; CNS: Reduction of risk potential; CL: Apply

146. What is the nurse's **priority** while caring for a client recently diagnosed with primary open-angle glaucoma?
1. Preventing the risk for injury related to peripheral vision loss
2. Treating chronic pain related to increased intraocular pressure
3. Addressing the adverse effects of medication
4. Teaching related to the new diagnosis of glaucoma

146. 1. Risk for injury related to peripheral vision loss takes priority because open-angle glaucoma limits peripheral vision. The client risks injury from stumbling over objects that he cannot see. Angle-closure glaucoma commonly causes acute pain. Primary open-angle glaucoma is an incurable disease that requires lifelong treatment. Adverse effects of medications are common. Although ineffective health maintenance and is an appropriate diagnosis for this client, safety is the priority. Client teaching is also important for any client with a new diagnosis, but the top priority is client safety.
CN: Physiological integrity; CNS: Reduction of risk potential; CL: Analyze

147. What information should the nurse give the client about mydriatic agents?
1. "Your pupils will be small and your night vision will be diminished."
2. "Blurred vision is an adverse effect, and you should report it to the provider immediately."
3. "Eye pain is common after administration."
4. "Compress the lacrimal sac for one minute after instillation."

147. 4. To prevent systemic absorption, the client should compress the lacrimal sac for one minute after instilling a mydriatic agent. The drug dilates the pupils and causes light sensitivity. Blurred vision is an expected effect of mydriatics, and do not need not be reported immediately. The client should discontinue the drug if eye pain occurs.
CN: Physiological integrity; CNS: Pharmacological and parenteral therapies; CL: Apply

148. A nurse is performing a neurological assessment on a client during a routine physical examination. Where should the nurse place the tongue blade to begin an assessment of Babinski's reflex?

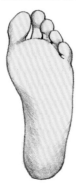

148. To test for the Babinski reflex, use a tongue blade to slowly stroke the lateral side of the foot's sole. Start at the heel and move toward the great toe. The normal response in an adult is plantar flexion of the toes. Upward movement of the great toe and fanning of the little toes, called the Babinski reflex, is abnormal.
CN: Health promotion and maintenance; CNS: None; CL: Apply

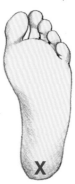

149. The nurse is assessing a client's deep tendon reflexes. Which photo shows an assessment of the bicep reflex?

1.

2.
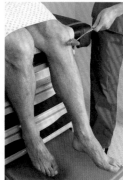

3.
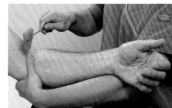

4.
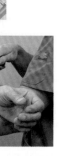
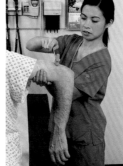

149. 3. To test the biceps reflex, the client's elbow is flexed at a 45-degree angle. The nurse places her thumb or index finger over the bicep tendon and strikes the tendon with the pointed end of the reflex hammer, assessing the contraction of the bicep muscle and flexion of the forearm. Photo one shows an assessment of the patellar reflex. Photo two shows an assessment of the brachioradialis reflex. Photo four shows an assessment of the tricep reflex.
CN: Physiological integrity; CNS: Reduction of risk potential; CL: Analyze

Chapter 7

Musculoskeletal Disorders

Here's a test that covers nursing care for clients with a disorder of the musculoskeletal system. So get moving! (Get it? Moving? Hmmm, I must be losing my touch.)

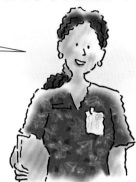

1. A 70-year-old female client who reports back pain is diagnosed with osteoporosis. The nurse is aware that this client is **most** at risk for:
  1. acute pain.
  2. fracture.
  3. compartment syndrome.
  4. paralysis.

2. A 76-year-old woman, with a history of osteoporosis is 24-hours postoperative for a total right hip replacement. What is the **priority** nursing action for this client?
  1. Managing pain
  2. Ambulating 50 feet
  3. Caring for the surgical wound
  4. Promoting nutrition

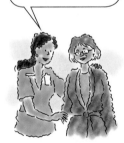

A client may have different postoperative risk factors.

3. The nurse is teaching a client about the risk factors for developing osteoporosis. What is the **most** important information for the nurse to include? Select all that apply.
  1. Inadequate dietary intake of calcium
  2. Blood pressure medications
  3. Family history
  4. Smoking
  5. Oral hypoglycemics

4. The nurse is teaching the client about the cause of primary osteoporosis. What is the **most** accurate answer for the nurse to provide?
  1. Alcoholism
  2. Malnutrition
  3. Hormonal imbalance
  4. Osteogenesis imperfecta

1. 2. Bones weaken with osteoporosis, and there's a decrease in bone matrix and remineralization resulting in fracture. Pain may occur, but a fracture can be life threatening.
CN: Physiological integrity; CNS: Physiological adaptation; CL: Apply

2. 1. Adequate pain relief will enable this client to engage in initial mobility exercises and prevent potential complications. Ambulating 50 feet is a longer-term goal. Wound care and nutrition are important post-surgical priorities to ensure wound healing, but are not the priority.
CN: Physiological and safety integrity; CNS: Physiological adaptation; CL: Analyze

3. 1, 3, 4. Inadequate dietary intake of calcium, family history, and smoking are risk factors of osteoporosis. There is no evidence that blood pressure medications or oral hypoglycemics are risk factors.
CN: Physiological integrity; CNS: Physiological adaptation; CL: Apply

4. 3. Primary osteoporosis, is the result of a normal physiological process, such as menopause/hormonal imbalance or aging. Alcoholism, malnutrition, osteogenesis imperfecta, rheumatoid arthritis, liver disease, scurvy, lactose intolerance, hyperthyroidism, and trauma cause secondary osteoporosis.
CN: Physiological integrity; CNS: Physiological adaptation; CL: Apply

CN: Client needs category   CNS: Client needs subcategory   CL: Cognitive level

5. A 42-year-old client recently had a total hysterectomy and bilateral oophorectomy. Which of response, by the client, would indicate an understanding about osteoporosis?
   1. "Osteoporosis only affects women over 65 year of age."
   2. "My risk for osteoporosis is low because I still have my thyroid gland."
   3. "I'm still producing hormones, so I don't have to worry about osteoporosis."
   4. "I need to take precautions to prevent osteoporosis because I have had surgically induced menopause."

5. 4. Menopause, at any age, puts a woman at risk for osteoporosis because of the associated hormonal imbalance. This client's thyroid gland won't protect her from osteoporosis. With her ovaries removed, she's no longer producing progesterone or estrogen.
CN: Physiological integrity; CNS: Physiological adaptation;
CL: Analyze

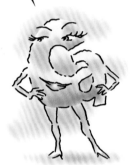

I'm a primary means of prevention.

6. The nurse is teaching a class on primary prevention of osteoporosis. What is the **most** important information for the nurse to provide?
   1. Maintain optimal calcium intake
   2. Place necessary items within reach of the client
   3. Install safety rails in the bathroom to prevent falls
   4. Use a professional alert system in the home in case a fall occurs when the client is alone

6. 1. Primary prevention of osteoporosis includes maintaining optimal calcium intake. Placing items within reach of the client, using a professional alert system in the home, and installing bars in bathrooms are all secondary and tertiary methods of preventing falls.
CN: Health promotion and maintenance; CNS: None;
CL: Apply

7. The nurse is providing discharge teaching for a client who was hospitalized with gout. The nurse determines that teaching was effective when the client states the need to reduce intake of which food?
   1. Tofu
   2. Liver
   3. Tomatoes
   4. Blackberries

7. 2. A client with gout should reduce their intake of purine-rich food, such as liver. Blackberries, tofu, and tomatoes are not rich in purine.
CN: Physiological integrity; CNS: Basic care and comfort;
CL: Apply

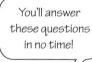

You'll answer these questions in no time!

8. The nurse is planning interventions for a client who is having an acute gout attack. What is the **priority** nursing intervention for this client?
   1. Instruct the client to change their dietary intake
   2. Instruct the client about relaxation techniques
   3. Administer prescribed analgesics
   4. Encourage increased fluid intake

8. 3. Administering prescribed analgesics to relieve pain would be the priority. The other actions are appropriate measures, but aren't the priority.
CN: Physiological integrity; CNS: Physiological adaptation;
CL: Analyze

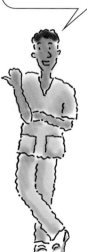

9. A nurse is interviewing a client who has a pattern of non-chronic gout. Which statement, by the client, **best** describes the pattern of non-chronic gout?
   1. "I have a continuous low pain level."
   2. "I have a continuous high pain level."
   3. "I have occasional painful attacks with pain-free periods between attacks."
   4. "I have occasional painful attacks with continuous low pain between attacks."

9. 3. The usual pattern of gout involves painful attacks with pain-free periods between attacks. Chronic gout may lead to frequent attacks with persistently painful joints.
CN: Physiological integrity; CNS: Physiological adaptation;
CL: Apply

10. The health care provider has prescribed a diet that limits purine-rich foods. Which foods should this client avoid? Select all that apply.
1. Bananas, wine, and cheese
2. Milk, ice cream, vegetables, and yogurt
3. Anchovies, sardines, and kidneys
4. Sweetbreads, red meats, and alcohol
5. Chicken, fish, and dried fruits

11. The nurse has provided teaching to a client newly diagnosed with gout. The nurse determines that teaching has been effective when the client states:
1. "Weight loss will decrease purine levels."
2. "Weight loss will decrease inflammation."
3. "Weight loss will increase uric acid levels and decrease stress on joints."
4. "Weight loss will decrease uric acid levels and decrease stress on joints."

12. The nurse informs a client diagnosed with gout that his X-rays are normal. Which statement, by the nurse, is **most** appropriate when the client asks if he still has gout?
1. "No, you're cured."
2. "Yes, X-rays are unreliable."
3. "Yes, X-rays remain normal in the early stages of gout."
4. "Yes, X-ray changes are only seen with acute attacks."

13. The nurse is evaluating the effectiveness of colchicine, prescribed for a client recently been diagnosed with gout. What outcomes would indicate that this medication has been effective? Select all that apply.
1. Decreased inflammation
2. Decreased infections
3. Fewer gout attacks
4. Effective pain management
5. The client is able to perform daily living activities

14. Which statement, by a client diagnosed with gout, would indicate an understanding of the discharge instructions?
1. "I'll increase my fluids so that the inflammation will be reduced."
2. "Increasing fluid intake will increase the calcium my body absorbs."
3. "Increasing fluid intake will cause my body to excrete more uric acid."
4. "Increasing fluids will help provide a cushion for my bones."

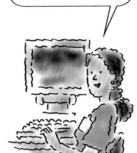

Question 12 asks you to choose the *most appropriate* answer. That means more than one may be suitable.

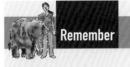

Remember

"Colchicine flouts gout."

Colchicine alleviates inflammation associated with acute gouty arthritis attacks.

10. 3, 4. Anchovies, sardines, kidneys, sweetbreads, and lentils are very high in purines. Bananas and dried fruits are high in potassium. Milk, ice cream, and yogurt are rich in calcium. Wine, cheese, preserved fruits, meats, and vegetables contain tyramines.
CN: Physiological integrity; CNS: Basic care and comfort; CL: Apply

11. 4. Weight loss will decrease uric acid levels and decrease stress on joints. Weight loss will not decrease purine levels, increase uric acid levels, or decrease inflammation.
CN: Health promotion and maintenance; CNS: None; CL: Apply

12. 3. X-rays can be very valuable in the diagnosis of gout, and are normal in the early stages of the condition. Telling the client that he's cured is incorrect, because he may be in the early stages of gout when X-rays appear normal. With chronic gout, X-rays will show damage to cartilage and bone. When X-ray changes occur, the changes will be present during both attacks and remissions.
CN: Physiological integrity; CNS: Physiological adaptation; CL: Apply

13. 1, 3, 4, 5. The action of colchicine is to decrease inflammation by reducing the migration of leukocytes to synovial fluid, which will decrease pain and the frequency of gout attacks. Colchicine doesn't decrease infection.
CN: Physiological integrity; CNS: Pharmacological and parenteral therapies; CL: Apply

14. 3. Increasing fluid intake will promote the excretion of uric acid. Fluids do not decrease inflammation, increase calcium absorption, or provide a cushion for weakened bones.
CN: Physiological integrity; CNS: Physiological adaptation; CL: Apply

CN: Client needs category   CNS: Client needs subcategory   CL: Cognitive level

15. The nurse is performing an admission assessment on a client with osteoarthritis. Which clinical manifestations would the nurse anticipate in this client?
1. Joint pain following exercise that is relieved by rest
2. Symmetrical swelling of the joints in both hands
3. Morning stiffness that lasts longer than 30 minutes
4. Elevated body temperature

15. 1. The most common symptom of osteoarthritis is joint pain following exercise or weight-bearing, that is usually relieved by rest. The other options are all symptoms of rheumatoid arthritis.
CN: Physiological integrity; CNS: Physiological adaptation; CL: Apply

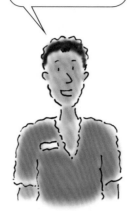

Your client depends on you for information.

16. The health care provider has prescribed indomethacin for a client with gout. What is the **most** important information for the nurse to give the client about this medication?
1. Bleeding is not a problem with NSAIDs.
2. Take NSAIDs with food to avoid an upset stomach.
3. Take NSAIDs on an empty stomach to increase absorption.
4. Don't take NSAIDs at bedtime because they may cause wakefulness.

16. 2. Indomethacin, like other NSAIDs, should be taken with food because it can be irritating to the gastrointestinal (GI) mucosa and lead to GI bleeding. Indomethacin can cause drowsiness, not excitement, and potential bleeding complications.
CN: Physiological integrity; CNS: Pharmacological and parenteral therapies; CL: Apply

17. The nurse is obtaining a health history from a client who has been taking ibuprofen. What **priority** questions should the nurse ask this client? Select all that apply.
1. "How often do you take this medication?"
2. "Have you had any difficulty breathing?"
3. "Do you monitor your blood pressure regularly?"
4. "Have you ever had tarry, black stools?"
5. "Have you ever vomited blood?"

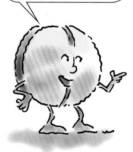

I'm just a little guy, but I'm ready to take action.

17. 1, 2, 4, 5. Questions four and five are appropriate for a client who is taking ibuprofen because the medication can lead to irritation of the gastrointestinal (GI) mucosa, which can increase the risk of a GI bleed and vomiting. Knowing how often the client takes the medication is important because the client should not exceed 3,600 mg/day. Over medication can lead to renal failure, which will cause the blood pressure to increase. If the client has a history of respiratory problems, ibuprofen can increase the risk for developing hypersensitivity reactions.
CN: Physiological integrity; CNS: Pharmacological therapies; CL: Apply

18. A client asks the nurse for information about osteoarthritis. What is the **most** appropriate information for the nurse to include?
1. Osteoarthritis is rarely debilitating.
2. Osteoarthritis is a rare form of arthritis.
3. Osteoarthritis afflicts people over age 60.
4. Osteoarthritis is the most common form of arthritis.

18. 4. Osteoarthritis is the most common form of arthritis, and can be extremely debilitating. It can affect people of any age, although most are elderly.
CN: Physiological integrity; CNS: Physiological adaptation; CL: Apply

19. The health care provider orders 2 g of ampicillin in 50 ml of D5W, to infuse IV piggyback (IVPB) over 30 minutes, for a client who had a right total knee replacement secondary to osteoarthritis. At what rate would the nurse set the IV infusion pump in milliliters per hour? Record your answer using a whole number.

_____ ml/h

19. 100.

$$60 \div 30 \times 50 \, ml/hr = 100 \, ml/hr$$

CN: Physiological integrity; CNS: Pharmacological and parenteral therapies; CL: Apply

CN: Client needs category   CNS: Client needs subcategory   CL: Cognitive level

20. The health care provider orders heparin, 7,500 units subcutaneous, for a client who had a left total hip replacement secondary to osteoarthritis. The pharmacy sent heparin 5,000 units/0.5 ml to the unit. How many milliliters should the nurse administer to this client? Record your answer using two decimal places.

_____ ml

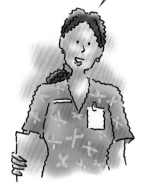

Don't be fooled. What does primary mean in this question?

20. 0.75.

$$\frac{5{,}000 \; units}{7{,}500 \; units} = \frac{0.5 \; ml}{X \; ml}$$

$$X = 0.5 \; ml \times \frac{7{,}500}{5} = 0.75 \; ml$$

CN: Physiological integrity; CNS: Pharmacological and parenteral therapies; CL: Apply

21. What are the causes of primary osteoarthritis?
1. Overuse of joints, aging, and obesity
2. Obesity, aging, and diabetes mellitus
3. Congenital abnormality, aging, overuse of joints
4. Diabetes mellitus, congenital abnormality, aging

21. 1. Primary osteoarthritis may be caused by the overuse of joints, aging, or obesity. Congenital abnormalities and diabetes mellitus can cause secondary osteoarthritis.

CN: Physiological integrity; CNS: Physiological adaptation; CL: Apply

22. A nurse is caring for a client with osteoarthritis of the knee. The nurse determines that discharge teaching has been effective when the client states:
1. "I'll take my ibuprofen on an empty stomach."
2. "I'll try taking a warm shower in the morning."
3. "I'll wear my knee splint every night."
4. "I'll jog at least a mile every morning."

22. 2. A client with osteoarthritis has joint stiffness that may be partially relieved by a warm shower in the morning. Ibuprofen should be taken with food, as should all nonsteroidal anti-inflammatory medications. Splints are usually used by clients with rheumatoid arthritis. Because the problem is continued stress on the joint, the client should attempt exercise that puts less strain on the joint, such as swimming.

CN: Physiological integrity; CNS: Basic care and comfort; CL: Apply

23. The health care provider has prescribed salicylates for a client with osteoarthritis. The nurse assesses the client and determines that intervention is necessary when the client exhibits:
1. hearing loss.
2. increased pain in joints.
3. decreased calcium absorption.
4. increased bone demineralization.

23. 1. Many elderly people already have diminished hearing, and salicylate use can lead to further or total hearing loss. Salicylates do not increase pain in joints, decrease calcium absorption, or increase bone demineralization.

CN: Physiological integrity; CNS: Pharmacological and parenteral therapies; CL: Apply

24. A debilitated 69-year-old client has been admitted to the medical-surgical unit from a nursing home with a diagnosis of osteoarthritis. During the health history, the nurse learns that the client has been on prolonged bed rest. What is the **most** appropriate nursing intervention for this client?
1. Encourage and educate coughing and deep breathing and limit fluid intake
2. Turn the client every two hours and encourage coughing and deep breathing
3. Provide only passive range of motion (ROM) and decrease stimulation
4. Have the client lie as still as possible and give adequate pain medicine

24. 2. A bedridden client should be turned every two hours, have adequate nutrition, and cough and deep breathe. Hydration, active and passive ROM, and adequate pain medication are also appropriate nursing measures. To prevent contractures, the client shouldn't limit fluid intake or lie as still as possible.

CN: Physiological integrity; CNS: Basic care and comfort; CL: Apply

CN: Client needs category   CNS: Client needs subcategory   CL: Cognitive level

25. A client asks the nurse, "What is the difference between rheumatoid arthritis (RA) and osteoarthritis (OA)?" What is the nurse's **most** appropriate response?
1. OA is gender specific; RA is not.
2. OA is a systemic disease; RA is localized.
3. OA is a localized disease; RA is systemic.
4. OA has dislocations and subluxations; RA does not.

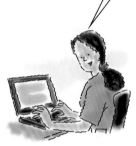

It's important to know the difference between these two common diseases.

25. 3. OA is a degenerative disease caused primarily from wear and tear on the joints, whereas RA is an autoimmune disease. Both types of arthritis are more common in women than men. OA and RA are more prevalent in older adults, but RA can develop at any age. Clients have dislocations and subluxations in both disorders.
CN: Physiological integrity; CNS: Physiological adaptation;
CL: Apply

26. A nurse is performing an assessment on a client diagnosed with osteoarthritis. Which clinical manifestations would the nurse anticipate in this client?
1. Elevated sedimentation rate
2. Multiple subcutaneous nodules
3. Asymmetrical joint involvement
4. Localized warmth, fever, and malaise

26. 3. Asymmetrical joint involvement is present in osteoarthritis. Elevated sedimentation rate, multiple subcutaneous nodules, inflammation, fever, and malaise are all present with rheumatoid arthritis.
CN: Physiological integrity; CNS: Physiological adaptation;
CL: Analyze

27. A nurse is teaching about primary prevention of injury to a client diagnosed with osteoarthritis. Examples of primary prevention include: Select all that apply.
1. Avoiding repetitive tasks
2. Avoiding physical activity
3. Warming up before exercising
4. Performing only repetitive tasks
5. Using isometric exercises

27. 1, 3. Examples of primary prevention of injury from osteoarthritis include warming up before exercise, and avoiding repetitive tasks. Bed rest would contribute to many other systemic complications. Physical activity is a key component of remaining fit and healthy, and maintaining joint function. Isometric exercises are a type of strength training in which the joint angle and muscle length do not change during contraction. Isometric exercises are done in static positions, rather than being dynamic through a range of motion.
CN: Health promotion and maintenance; CNS: None;
CL: Apply

28. The client asks the nurse for information about osteoarthritis. What is the **most** appropriate information for the nurse to include about the disease?
1. It is a systemic inflammatory joint disease.
2. It is a disease involving fusion of the joints in the hands.
3. It is an inflammatory joint disease, with degeneration and loss of articular cartilage in synovial joints.
4. It is a non-inflammatory joint disease, with degeneration and loss of articular cartilage in synovial joints.

28. 4. Osteoarthritis is a non-inflammatory joint disease, with degeneration and loss of articular cartilage in synovial joints. Rheumatoid arthritis is a systemic inflammatory joint disease. Arthrodesis is fusion of the joints.
CN: Physiological integrity; CNS: Physiological adaptation;
CL: Apply

CN: Client needs category   CNS: Client needs subcategory   CL: Cognitive level

29. The **most** appropriate clothing for a client with osteoarthritis would include:
1. zippered clothing.
2. shoes that firmly tie to promote stability.
3. velcroed clothing, slip-on shoes, and rubber grippers.
4. buttoned clothing, slip-on shoes, and rubber grippers.

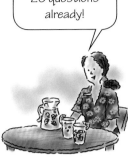

You've finished 29 questions already!

29. 3. Velcroed clothing, slip-on shoes, and rubber grippers will make it easier for the client with osteoarthritis to dress and grip objects. Zippers, ties, and buttons may be difficult for this client to use.
CN: Physiological integrity; CNS: Basic care and comfort; CL: Apply

30. A nurse is caring for a client, diagnosed with osteoarthritis, who refuses to perform independent care. What is the **most** important nursing intervention for this client?
1. Perform all care activities for this client
2. Explain the purpose of maintaining complete independence
3. Encourage and support the client to perform as much self-care as possible
4. Explain that once the care task has been completed independently, pain medication will be administered

30. 3. A client, with osteoarthritis, should be encouraged to perform as much self-care as possible. The nurse's goal is to allow the client to maintain as many self-care abilities as possible with minimal help as needed. It is never appropriate to use pain medication as a bargaining tool.
CN: Psychosocial integrity; CNS: None; CL: Analyze

31. The nurse asks a client, in the late stages of osteoarthritis, to describe the pain. The nurse anticipates that this client will describe the pain how?
1. Grating
2. Dull ache
3. Dull and deep aching pain
4. Deep aching pain that is only relieved by rest

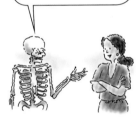

What your client says about pain can help you know the stage of osteoarthritis.

31. 1. In the late stages of osteoarthritis, the client often describes the joint pain as grating. As the disease progresses, the cartilage covering the ends of bones is destroyed and bones rub against each other. Osteophytes, or bone spurs, may form on the ends of bones. A dull ache or deep aching pain, with or without relief with rest, is often seen in the early stages of osteoarthritis.
CN: Physiological integrity; CNS: Physiological adaptation; CL: Apply

32. A client is admitted to the medical-surgical unit for osteoarthritis and weakness in the left lower extremity. The client uses a walker at home. The health care provider orders a cane and physical therapy for the client. The client asks the nurse about the difference between the cane and walker. What is the nurse's **best** response?
1. A walker is a better choice than a cane.
2. The cane should be used on the affected side.
3. The cane should be used on the unaffected side.
4. A client with osteoarthritis should be encouraged to ambulate without the cane.

32. 3. A cane should be used on the unaffected side. A client with osteoarthritis should be encouraged and educated to ambulate with a cane, walker, or other assistive device as needed. The assistive device takes the weight and stress off of joints.
CN: Physiological integrity; CNS: Basic care and comfort; CL: Apply

33. The nurse is providing discharge teaching to a client with osteoarthritis. What is the **most** important information for the nurse to include?
1. Walk and increase distance gradually
2. Remain as sedentary as possible
3. Return to a normal level of activity
4. Include vigorous exercise in your daily routine

33. 1. A client with osteoarthritis should pace their activities and avoid over exertion. Over exertion can increase joint degeneration and cause pain. Becoming sedentary will increase the risk of developing pneumonia and contractures.
CN: Physiological integrity; CNS: Basic care and comfort; CL: Apply

CN: Client needs category   CNS: Client needs subcategory   CL: Cognitive level

34. A 79-year-old client has been admitted to the unit. The client is diagnosed with a left hip fracture secondary to a fall, and is scheduled for a left total hip replacement (LTHR). The client's comorbidities are hypertension and diabetes. The client is a full code with no known allergies (NKA). What is the nurse's **priority** action for this client?
1. Promote sleep and rest
2. Encourage therapeutic communications
3. Maintain standard precautions
4. Pain management

34. 4. Addressing acute pain is the priority for this client. Maintaining an acceptable level of pain will allow this client to participate in the plan of care. The other nursing interventions would be lower priorities.
CN: Physiological integrity; CNS: Physiological adaptation; CL: Apply

35. A client asks the nurse what factors affect how long it will take for a hip to heal following hip replacement surgery. What are the **best** responses by the nurse? Select all that apply.
1. The age of the client
2. The height of the client
3. The gender of the client
4. The client's comorbidities
5. The client's marital status

35. 1, 4. The age and comorbidities of the client are important because they can affect the blood supply to the fracture, which can affect the healing process. An older client, or one with comorbidities such as hypertension and diabetes, will have slower bone healing due to a decrease in blood supply. The height of the client does not directly delay bone healing. The client's gender and marital status have no effect on healing.
CN: Physiological integrity; CNS: Physiological adaptation; CL: Apply

36. A nurse is providing pin site care for a client in skeletal traction. Prioritize the nurse's steps for performing proper pin care.

| 1. Apply clean gloves |
| 2. Inspect sites for color, erythema, drainage |
| 3. Perform hand hygiene |
| 4. Clean each pin site with prescribed solution |
| 5. Prepare supplies |

36. Ordered Response:

| 3. Perform hand hygiene |
| 5. Prepare supplies |
| 1. Apply clean gloves |
| 2. Inspect sites for color, erythema, drainage. |
| 4. Clean each pin site with prescribed solution. |

Hand washing will decrease the risk of contamination. Supplies should be gathered and organized, then clean gloves should be applied. The sites should be inspected for erythema or drainage and then each pins site should be clean per provider's order.
CN: Physiological Integrity; CNS: Reduction of Risk potential; CL: Apply.

37. A client was prescribed an anti-inflammatory drug for osteoarthritis five days ago. The client says the pain has decreased a little but not completely. Which nursing intervention would be the **most** appropriate?
1. Notify the health care provider and suggest increasing the dose
2. Notify the health care provider and suggest stopping the medication
3. Notify the health care provider and suggest adding another medication
4. Continue the present dose and offer other pain relief measures

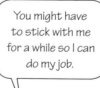

You might have to stick with me for a while so I can do my job.

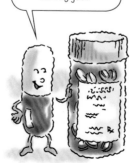

37. 4. Anti-inflammatory medications may take 2 to 3 weeks to provide full benefits. If the client can tolerate the pain, the prescribed pain medication should be continued, and other pain measures, such as rest, massage, heat, or cold should be offered. Increasing, stopping, or adding another medication is not appropriate because the medication hasn't been taken long enough to provide full benefit.
CN: Physiological integrity; CNS: Pharmacological and parenteral therapies; CL: Apply

CN: Client needs category   CNS: Client needs subcategory   CL: Cognitive level

38. A client has been diagnosed with a herniated nucleus pulposus. Which statement, by the nurse, **best** describes this condition?
 1. The disk slips out of alignment.
 2. The disk shatters, and fragments place pressure on nerve roots.
 3. The disk remains intact, and the surrounding tissue is displaced.
 4. The disk causes pressure on the nerve root

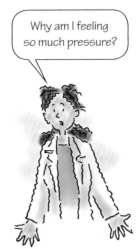

Why am I feeling so much pressure?

38. 4. With a herniated nucleus pulposus, or herniated disk, the nucleus of the disk puts pressure on the annulus, causing pressure on the nerve root. The disk itself does not slip, rupture, or shatter. The nucleus tissue usually moves from the center of the disk.
CN: Physiological integrity; CNS: Physiological adaptation; CL: Apply

39. The nurse is caring for a client admitted for a herniated nucleus pulposus. The client reports a pain level of 7 out of 10 and is currently using the ordered morphine sulfate patient-controlled analgesia pump for pain management. What is the **priority** nursing assessment for this client?
 1. Neurological system
 2. Respiratory system
 3. Gastrointestinal system
 4. Cardiovascular system

39. 2. The respiratory system is the highest priority nursing assessment because morphine sulfate can lead to respiratory depression, which can cause death for the client. The other systems should be monitored, but are not the priority.
CN: Physiological integrity; CNS: Physiological adaptation; CL: Analyze

40. A client reports low back pain that radiates down the right leg, with numbness and weakness in the same leg. Based on subjective data, the nurse would suspect that these symptoms are related to:
 1. herniated nucleus pulposus.
 2. muscular dystrophy.
 3. Parkinson's disease.
 4. osteoarthritis.

40. 1. Compression of nerves by the herniated nucleus pulposus can cause back pain that radiates into the leg, with numbness and weakness of the leg. Muscular dystrophy causes wasting of skeletal muscles. Parkinson's disease is characterized by progressive muscle rigidity and tremors. Osteoarthritis causes deep, aching joint pain.
CN: Physiological integrity; CNS: Physiological adaptation; CL: Analyze

41. The nurse is examining the hands of a client with osteoarthritis and notes Heberden's nodes on the second finger. Where, on the finger, would the nurse observe the node?

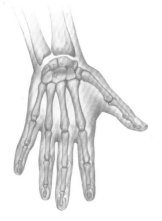

41. Heberden's nodes appear on the distal interphalangeal joints. These bony and cartilaginous enlargements are usually hard and painless, and typically occur in middle-aged and elderly clients with osteoarthritis.

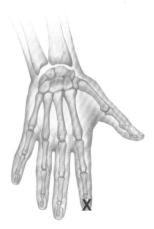

CN: Health Promotion and Maintenance; CNS: Physiological adaptation; CL: Apply

CN: Client needs category   CNS: Client needs subcategory   CL: Cognitive level

42. Which preoperative instructions should the nurse include while teaching a client scheduled for spine surgery? Select all that apply.
1. An incentive spirometer will be used following surgery.
2. Intense physical therapy is needed after the procedure.
3. There is a greater risk associated with spine surgery compared to other surgeries.
4. Recovery time is twice as long following spine surgery compared to other surgeries.
5. The client should be turned every two hours after surgery using a logroll technique.
6. The client will be using a pain rating scale to rate pain.

42. 1, 5, 6. An incentive spirometer is used to prevent atelectasis. Physical therapy may not be necessary. There is no greater risk, and no longer recovery time with spine surgery compared to any other surgery. The client should be logrolled following surgery. The client will be asked to rate their pain using a pain rating scale.
CN: Physiological integrity; CNS: Reduction of risk potential; CL: Apply

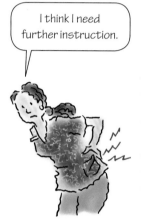

I think I need further instruction.

43. A nurse has provided teaching to a client with a herniated lumbar disk. The nurse determines that further teaching is necessary when the client states:
1. "I can strengthen my back muscles by doing pelvic tilt exercises."
2. "I need to maintain a healthy weight to limit back strain."
3. "I should bend at the waist when picking up objects."
4. "I should increase my fiber and fluid intake."

43. 3. The client should bend at the knees, not the waist, to maintain proper body mechanics. Pelvic tilt exercises are recommended to strengthen back muscles. Increasing fiber and fluid intake will help soften stool and prevent straining that could increase intraspinal pressure. Any extra weight carried by the client increases back strain.
CN: Physiological integrity; CNS: Physiological adaptation; CL: Apply

44. A nurse is caring for a client with low back pain. Which action could the nurse delegate to the unlicensed assistive personnel (UAP)?
1. Assess pain level
2. Palpate the abdomen for distension
3. Reposition the client from side-lying to back
4. Assess the client's skin for skin breakdown

44. 3. The nursing assistant is able to perform routine tasks. The registered is responsible for assessment, teaching, and evaluation of clients.
CN: Safe, effective care environment; CNS: Management of care; CL: Apply

45. A client asks the nurse why a cold pack should be applied to a sprained ankle. What is the nurse's **best** response?
1. It decreases pain and increases circulation.
2. It numbs the nerves and dilates the blood vessels.
3. It promotes circulation and reduces muscle spasm.
4. It constricts local blood vessels and decreases swelling.

Nice moves! Looks like you've found your groove.

45. 4. Application of a cold pack will cause blood vessels to constrict, which reduces the leakage of fluid into the tissues and prevents swelling. It may also have an effect on muscle spasms. Cold therapy may reduce pain by numbing the nerves and tissues. Cold therapy doesn't promote circulation or dilate the blood vessels.
CN: Physiological integrity; CNS: Basic care and comfort; CL: Apply

46. The nurse is teaching a community class about back injuries. Which site is common for vertebral herniation?
1. L1-L2, L4-L5 vertebrae
2. L1-L2, L5-S1 vertebrae
3. L4-L5, L5-S1 vertebrae
4. L5-S1, S2-S3 vertebrae

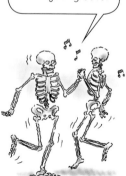

46. 3. The most common areas of herniation are lumbar four and five vertebrae, and sacral one vertebra.
CN: Health promotion and maintenance; CNS: None; CL: Apply

CN: Client needs category   CNS: Client needs subcategory   CL: Cognitive level

47. A 50-year-old client is admitted to the emergency department with severe lower back pain, weakness, and atrophy of the right leg muscles. Based on the clinical manifestations, which diagnostic tests would the nurse anticipate for this client?
1. Chest X-ray, magnetic resonance imaging (MRI), and computed tomography (CT) scan
2. Lumbar puncture, chest X-ray, MRI, and CT scan
3. Lumbar puncture, chest X-ray, and myelography
4. Myelography, MRI, and CT scan

47. 4. Tests used to diagnose a herniated nucleus pulposus include myelography, MRI, and CT scan. Chest X-ray and lumbar puncture are not conclusive for a herniated disk.
CN: Physiological integrity; CNS: Physiological adaptation; CL: Apply

48. A nurse is preparing a client, with a history of back pain, for discharge. Which discharge instructions should the nurse include when teaching this client how to prevent back injury?
1. Sleep on your side and carry objects at arm's length
2. Sleep on your back and carry objects at arm's length
3. Sleep on your side and carry objects close to your body
4. Sleep on your back and carry objects close to your body

48. 3. Sleeping in a lateral position, and carrying objects close to the body will put less strain on the back. Sleeping in a prone position, and carrying objects at arm's length will add pressure to the back.
CN: Health promotion and maintenance; CNS: None; CL: Apply

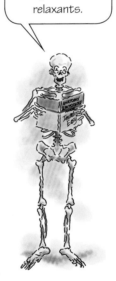

Now I know why they call them relaxants.

49. A client is being discharged with a prescription for skeletal muscle relaxants. What **priority** information should the nurse share with this client?
1. Change your position quickly to avoid dizziness
2. Double a missed dose to ensure proper muscle relaxation
3. Cough and cold medications are appropriate to take, if needed
4. Muscle relaxants can decrease alertness and may cause drowsiness

49. 4. This client should avoid activities that require alertness because muscle relaxants can cause drowsiness. This client should change position slowly to avoid dizziness. A missed dose should not be doubled, and taking cold medication can increase the risk of adverse effects.
CN: Physiological integrity; CNS: Pharmacological and parenteral therapies; CL: Apply

50. The nurse suspects that a client, with a recent fracture, has developed compartment syndrome. Which assessment finding would be **most** concerning to the nurse? Select all that apply.
1. An overall decrease in bone mass
2. A palpable growth in and around the bone tissue
3. The inability to perform active movement
4. The inability to perform passive movement
5. Intense, throbbing pain unresponsive to analgesics
6. Absent pulses distal to the fracture site

50. 3, 5, 6. When compartment syndrome is present, the client will not be able to perform active movement, and pain will occur with passive movement. Osteoporosis brings an overall decrease in bone mass. A bone tumor will show growth in and around the bone tissue. Symptoms of compartment syndrome include pain, decreased movement and absent pulses distal to the fracture site.
CN: Physiological integrity; CNS: Physiological adaptation; CL: Apply

51. The nurse is caring for a client who has returned to the unit following the application of a cast for a fracture of the right ulna. The client is now reports severe pain, numbness, and tingling of the right arm. What is the nurse's **most** important action?
1. Administer acetaminophen as prescribed
2. Lower the arm below the level of the heart
3. Immediately report the client's symptoms
4. Apply a heating pad

51. 3. Severe pain, numbness, and tingling are symptoms of impaired circulation due to compartment syndrome, which is a medical emergency. Don't give analgesics until the client has been assessed and treated. Lowering the arm below the level of the heart and applying heat will decrease venous outflow and further impair circulation.
CN: Physiological integrity; CNS: Physiological adaptation; CL: Apply

52. The nurse is assessing a client with a hematoma and compartment syndrome in the same extremity. Which symptoms would the nurse anticipate? Select all that apply.
1. Edema
2. Increased venous pressure
3. Decreased venous circulation
4. Increased arterial circulation
5. Decreased pain on movement

52. 1, 2, 3. The hemorrhage in compartment syndrome would cause edema, increased venous pressure, and decreased venous and arterial circulation. Compartment syndrome would cause increased pain.
CN: Physiological integrity; CNS: Physiological adaptation; CL: Apply

53. A client has developed compartment syndrome following the application of a cast for a fractured tibia. What is the **priority** goal of care for this client?
1. Prevent tissue death, which can occur within 2 to 4 hours
2. Decrease the swelling in the extremity
3. Prevent nonunion of the fracture
4. Decrease the client's level of pain

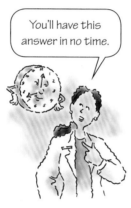

You'll have this answer in no time.

53. 1. Following the development of compartment syndrome, there is an increase in pressure within the affected compartment that compromises circulation to the muscle tissue and nerves. This may lead to tissue necrosis within two to four hours. Decreasing pain levels, preventing nonunion of the fracture, and decreasing the swelling in the affected extremity are important goals of treatment, but they are not the priority.
CN: Physiological integrity; CNS: Physiological adaptation; CL: Apply

54. The nurse is caring for a client with compartment syndrome. Which intervention would the nurse anticipate for this client?
1. Casting
2. Amputation
3. Fasciotomy
4. Observation

54. 3. Treatment of compartment syndrome includes fasciotomy, which involves cutting the fascia over the affected area to permit muscle expansion. Amputation and casting are not treatments for compartment syndrome.
CN: Physiological integrity; CNS: Physiological adaptation; CL: Apply

55. The nurse prepares to give penicillin to a client with osteomyelitis. The health care provider has ordered 700 mg IM. The vial is a mix-o-vial containing drug powder and sterile water for injection. When mixed together the vial contains 1 g/3.4 ml. How much should the nurse draw up to give this client? Record your answer using one decimal place.

_____ ml

55. 2.4.

$$X = \frac{\text{Dose Desired}}{\text{Dose on Hand or Dose Available}} \times \frac{\text{milliliters}}{\text{grams}}$$

$$X = \frac{700\text{ mg}}{1,000} \times \frac{3.4\text{ ml}}{1\text{ g}} = 2.4\ ml$$

CN: Physiological integrity; CNS: Pharmacological and parenteral therapies; CL: Apply

56. A nurse is admitting a client who is experiencing new signs and symptoms of paresthesia. What is the **most** appropriate question for the nurse to ask the client?
  1. "Have you had any changes in range of motion (ROM)?"
  2. "Do you have any numbness and tingling?"
  3. "Do you have any pain and blanching?"
  4. "How long have you had fever and chills?"

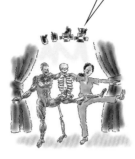

You're doing great! I'm beside myself with joy.

56. **2.** Paresthesia is described as numbness and tingling. It is not associated with fever and chills or changes in ROM, nor is it described as pain or blanching.

CN: Physiological integrity; CNS: Physiological adaptation; CL: Analyze

57. A client has undergone a fasciotomy for the treatment of compartment syndrome. What is the **priority** nursing intervention for this client?
  1. Demonstrating the use of incentive spirometer
  2. Assessing the dressing at the surgical site
  3. Performing a bladder scan
  4. Measuring pulse oximetry

57. **2.** The assessment of the wound dressing is a priority following a fasciotomy. A fasciotomy involves the excision of the fascia that leaves the wound unsutured. The wound is covered with dressings that are moistened with sterile saline. The client may develop infection in this open wound. Gas exchange and cardiac output should not be affected by a fasciotomy.

CN: Physiological integrity; CNS: Physiological adaptation; CL: Analyze

58. The community health nurse found an elderly female client lying in the snow. The client was unable to move her right leg because of a fracture. Which action should the nurse take **first**?
  1. Immobilize the fracture in its present position
  2. Elevate the leg on whatever is available
  3. Realign the fracture ends
  4. Reduce the fracture

58. **1.** Initial treatment of obvious and suspected fractures includes immobilizing and splinting the limb. Any attempt to realign or reset the fracture at the stem may cause further injury and complications. The leg may be elevated only after immobilization.

CN: Safe, effective care environment; CNS: Management of care; CL: Analyze

59. A nurse is caring for a client experiencing difficulty swallowing following a spinal cord injury and the placement of a halo traction device. Which nursing interventions are most appropriate for this client? Select all that apply.
  1. Place client in an upright position to eat
  2. Verify that a cough reflex is present
  3. Verify that a gag reflex is present
  4. Instruct the client to tilt their chin upward when swallowing
  5. Assist the client to select foods from a mechanical soft diet

59. **1, 2, 3, 5.** These are appropriate interventions for a client with dysphagia. The risk of aspiration is life threatening. Sitting upright will allow for easier swallowing. Verifying reflexes is important to prevent possible aspiration. Swallowing is easier with the chin down, rather than up.

CN: Physiological integrity; CNS: Reduction of risk potential; CL: Apply

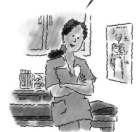

Knowing normal signs will alert you to what is wrong.

60. Which symptoms are indicative of a fracture?
  1. Tingling, coolness, and loss of pulses
  2. Loss of sensation, redness, and coolness
  3. Coolness, redness, and pain at the site of injury
  4. Redness, warmth, and pain at the site of injury

60. **4.** Signs of a fracture may include redness, warmth, numbness or loss of sensation, pain at the site of injury Coolness, tingling, and loss of pulses are signs of a vascular problem.

CN: Physiological integrity; CNS: Physiological adaptation; CL: Apply

---

CN: Client needs category   CNS: Client needs subcategory   CL: Cognitive level

61. A nurse is performing a neurovascular assessment. What should the nurse include in this assessment?
  1. Orientation, movement, pulses, and warmth
  2. Capillary refill, movement, pulses, and warmth
  3. Orientation, pupillary response, temperature, and pulses
  4. Respiratory pattern, orientation, pulses, and temperature

61. 2. A correct neurovascular assessment should include capillary refill, movement, pulses, and warmth. Neurovascular assessment involves nerve and blood supply to an area. Respiratory pattern, orientation, temperature, and pupillary response aren't part of a neurovascular examination.
CN: Physiological integrity; CNS: Reduction of risk potential; CL: Apply

62. A nurse has instructed a client to accurately measure the circumference of both calves each morning and to report any increase in size. The nurse determines that these instructions were understood when the client states:
  1. "I'll use a measuring tape to check circumference."
  2. "I'll use the standardized chart for limb circumference."
  3. "I only have to call if one leg is significantly larger than the other."
  4. "I can measure my calves either near the knee or closer to the ankle."

62. 1. The correct method for measuring calf circumference is to use a measuring tape. The calf should always be measured where the circumference is largest. The client should report any increase in circumference. An increase in calf circumference could be unilateral or bilateral. There's no standardized chart for limb circumference.
CN: Health promotion and maintenance; CNS: None; CL: Apply

63. A nurse is performing a neurovascular assessment on a client admitted with a fractured right femur. The nurse notices that the pulses are not palpable. What is the nurse's **most** important action?
  1. Alert the charge nurse immediately
  2. Reassesses the pulses again in one hour
  3. Notify the health care provider immediately
  4. Verify the clinical findings with Doppler ultrasonography

63. 4. If pulses are not palpable, they should be reassessed using Doppler ultrasonography. If pulses cannot be found with Doppler ultrasonography, immediately notify the provider.
CN: Safe, effective care environment; CNS: Management of care; CL: Apply

64. A client with a left arm cast reports a foul odor emanating from the cast. What is the appropriate action by the nurse?
  1. Assess further because this may be a sign of an infection
  2. Teach the client proper cast care, including hygiene measures
  3. This is normal, especially when a cast is in place for a few weeks
  4. Assess further because this may be a sign of neurovascular compromise

64. 1. A foul odor emanating from a cast may be a sign of an infection. The nurse should assess for fever, malaise, and, possibly, an elevation in white blood cells. Odor is not a sign of neurovascular compromise, which would include decreased pulses, coolness, and paresthesia.
CN: Physiological integrity; CNS: Reduction of risk potential; CL: Analyze

65. The nurse is collaborating with the orthopedic technician regarding interventions to reduce the roughness of a cast. What is the nurse's **best** intervention?
  1. Petal the edges
  2. Elevate the limb
  3. Break off the rough area
  4. Distribute pressure evenly

65. 1. Petaling the edges will reduce the roughness of the cast. Elevating the limb will prevent swelling. Never break a rough area off the cast. Distributing pressure evenly will prevent pressure ulcers.
CN: Physiological integrity; CNS: Basic care and comfort; CL: Apply

CN: Client needs category   CNS: Client needs subcategory   CL: Cognitive level

66. The nurse is aware that elevating a casted limb will prevent swelling. How should the nurse elevate a casted limb?
1. Place the limb with the cast close to the body
2. Place the limb with the cast at the level of the heart
3. Place the limb with the cast below the level of the heart
4. Place the limb with the cast above the level of the heart

67. A client asks the nurse to explain why a plaster cast cannot get wet. What is the nurse's **best** response?
1. A wet cast can cause a foul odor.
2. A wet cast will weaken or could be destroyed.
3. A wet cast is heavy and difficult to maneuver.
4. It is okay to get the cast wet, just use a hair dryer to dry it off.

68. A client visits the emergency department with a report of dull, deep bone pain unrelated to movement. The client asks the nurse if this could be a fracture. What is the nurse's **best** response?
1. These are classic symptoms of a fracture.
2. Fracture pain is sharp and related to movement.
3. Fracture pain is sharp and unrelated to movement.
4. Fracture pain is dull and deep and related to movement.

69. A nurse is caring for a client with skeletal traction to the right leg. The client reports severe right leg pain. Which action should the nurse perform **first**?
1. Perform pin care
2. Notify the health care provider
3. Check the client's alignment in bed
4. Remove the weights from the traction

70. A 70-year-old male client is admitted to the medical-surgical unit with a fractured femur. The client is placed in Russell's traction. The client asks the nurse to help him with back care. What is the nurse's **most** appropriate intervention?
1. Tell the client that he will not have back care while in traction
2. Tell the client to use the trapeze to lift his back off the bed
3. Support the weight to give the client more freedom of movement
4. Remove the weight to give the client more freedom of movement

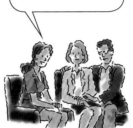

Your client depends on you to know the answers.

66. 4. To reduce swelling, the casted limb should be placed above the level of the heart, and extended away from the body. Placing it below or at the level of the heart will not reduce swelling.
CN: Physiological integrity; CNS: Basic care and comfort;
CL: Apply

67. 2. A wet cast will weaken or could be destroyed. A foul odor is a sign of infection.
CN: Physiological integrity; CNS: Reduction of risk potential;
CL: Apply

68. 2. Fracture pain is sharp and related to movement. Pain that is dull and deep and unrelated to movement is not typical of a fracture.
CN: Health promotion and maintenance; CNS: None; CL: Analyze

69. 3. A client who reports severe leg pain may need realignment to ease some pressure on the fracture site. If this is ineffective, then the provider should be notified. The weights ordered may be too heavy, but the nurse can't remove them without a provider's order. Performing pin care isn't appropriate at this time.
CN: Safe, effective care environment; CNS: Management of care;
CL: Apply

70. 2. The traction must not be disturbed to maintain correct alignment, and the trapeze should be used lift his back off the bed. The client can have back care as long as he uses the trapeze and does not disturb the alignment. The weight should not be moved without a health care provider's order. It should hang freely without touching anything.
CN: Physiological integrity; CNS: Basic care and comfort;
CL: Apply

CN: Client needs category   CNS: Client needs subcategory   CL: Cognitive level

71. The trauma nurse is caring for a client who was involved in an automobile accident. The client was wearing a seat belt at the time of the accident. Which area would the trauma nurse assess for fracture?
1. Brachial and clavicle
2. Brachial and humerus
3. Humerus and clavicle
4. Occipital and humerus

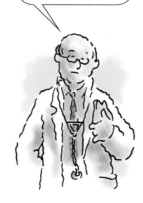

It's important to understand the different types of fractures.

71. 3. Classic fractures that occur with trauma from an automobile accident are those of the humerus and clavicle. There are no brachial bones, and occipital bones are not involved in a traumatic injury.
CN: Physiological integrity; CNS: Physiological adaptation;
CL: Analyze

72. The nurse is caring for a client who has been placed in traction prior to surgery. The client asks the nurse why he has been placed in traction. What is the nurse's **best** response?
1. Traction allows for more activity.
2. Traction will help prevent skin breakdown.
3. Traction helps with repositioning while in bed.
4. Traction helps to prevent trauma and overcome muscle spasms.

72. 4. The purpose of traction is to guide the body part back into place and hold it steady. Traction may be used to stabilize and realign bone fractures to decrease trauma to an area, help reduce the pain of a fracture before surgery, treat bone deformities caused by certain conditions, correct stiff and constricted muscles, joints, tendons, or skin and prevent painful muscle spasm.
Traction doesn't help in preventing skin breakdown, repositioning the client, or allowing the client to become active.
CN: Physiological integrity; CNS: Basic care and comfort;
CL: Apply

73. A 75-year-old client with Paget's disease is undergoing diagnostic exams for a suspected fracture. What type of fracture would the nurse anticipate for this client?
1. Linear
2. Oblique
3. Transverse
4. Longitudinal

73. 3. A transverse fracture commonly occurs with such bone diseases as osteomalacia and Paget's disease. Linear, longitudinal, and oblique fractures generally occur with trauma.
CN: Physiological integrity; CNS: Physiological adaptation;
CL: Apply

74. A nurse is caring for a client admitted to the hospital with a diagnosis of Paget's disease and hypertension. Which assessment data are **most** important in planning care for this client?
1. The client lives alone and experiences social isolation.
2. The client reports frequent crying spells.
3. The client reports having stiff legs and pain when walking.
4. The client does not have a primary care provider.

74. 3. Paget's disease presents with mobility issues caused by loss of bone structure. Chronic Paget's disease can lead to isolation and ineffective coping, but physical needs are the priority. Not having a primary care provider is not related to the disease process.
CN: Physiological integrity; CNS: Physiological adaptation;
CL: Apply

75. The emergency room nurse is caring for a 20-year-old female client who reports severe pain in her upper right arm. The nurse suspects domestic abuse. Which X-ray finding would indicate the need for additional investigation?
1. Longitudinal fracture
2. Transverse fracture
3. Oblique fracture
4. Spiral fracture

75. 4. Spiral fractures seen in the upper extremities are commonly related to physical abuse. Longitudinal and oblique fractures generally occur with trauma. A transverse fracture commonly occurs bone diseases such as osteomalacia and Paget's disease.
CN: Physiological integrity; CNS: Physiological adaptation;
CL: Apply

CN: Client needs category   CNS: Client needs subcategory   CL: Cognitive level

76. A 25-year-old male client has just had a plaster cast applied to his right forearm following the reduction of a closed radius fracture due to an inline skating accident. What is the **priority** nursing assessment for this client?
1. Sensation and movement of the fingers
2. Whether the client is having any pain
3. Whether the cast is completely dry
4. Whether the cast needs petaling

76. 1. Neurovascular checks are most important because they are used to determine if any impairment exists after cast application. Checking to see if the cast is completely dry isn't the nurse's highest priority. Petaling to smooth the cast's edge is done when the cast is completely dry.
CN: Physiological integrity; CNS: Reduction of risk potential; CL: Apply

77. A nurse is caring for a client with a femoral shaft fracture. Which assessment finding would warrants an **immediate** intervention by nurse?
1. Decreased urine output
2. Constipation
3. Hemorrhage
4. Pain

77. 3. Femoral shaft fractures may cause hemorrhage, with as much as 1,000 to 1,500 ml of blood loss. Constipation and decreased urine output aren't direct complications of a fracture. Pain may occur, but it can be controlled with analgesia.
CN: Physiological integrity; CNS: Physiological adaptation; CL: Analyze

78. The nurse is assessing a client admitted for a long bone fracture. Which complication, from this type of fracture, would be life threatening?
1. Fat emboli
2. Bone emboli
3. Serous emboli
4. Platelet emboli

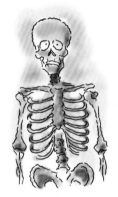

Wow! This is a serious complication.

78. 1. A life-threatening complication of long bone fractures is the development of fat emboli. Bone or platelet emboli are rare occurrences, and are infrequently associated with long bone fractures. There are no emboli known as serous emboli.
CN: Physiological integrity; CNS: Physiological adaptation; CL: Analyze

79. The nurse is obtaining a specimen of wound drainage from a client with osteomyelitis. Prioritize the nurse's steps necessary to collect this specimen.

1.	Return swab to culture tube
2.	Insert tip of swab into the wound in the area of the drainage and rotate
3.	Open sterile culture tube
4.	Apply clean gloves
5.	Complete hand hygiene
6.	Identify client using two identifiers

79. Ordered Response:

6.	Identify client using two identifiers
5.	Complete hand hygiene
4.	Apply clean gloves
3.	Open sterile culture tube
2.	Insert tip of swab into the wound in the area of the drainage and rotate
1.	Return swab to culture tube

CN: Physiological integrity; CNS: Reduction of risk potential; CL: Apply

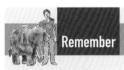

Remember

"Xanthines zap bronchospasm."

Methylxanthines, such as theophylline, relieve or prevent bronchospasm and treat asthma by relaxing the smooth muscles of the bronchi.

80. A client has developed a fat emboli. Which treatments would the nurse anticipate?
1. Antibiotics, IV fluids, steroids, and oxygen
2. Theophylline, morphine, oxygen, and IV fluids
3. Morphine, oxygen, IV fluids, and antibiotics
4. Albuterol, oxygen, IV fluids, and steroids

80. 1. Treatment of fat emboli may include oxygen, IV fluids, steroids to counteract inflammation in the lungs and correct cerebral edema, and antibiotics to prevent infection. Albuterol, morphine, and theophylline aren't commonly used to treat fat emboli.
CN: Physiological integrity; CNS: Physiological adaptation; CL: Analyze

CN: Client needs category   CNS: Client needs subcategory   CL: Cognitive level

81. A nurse is caring for a client diagnosed with a fracture. The health care provider has ordered a high-protein diet for the client. The nurse explains to the client that a high-protein diet is ordered because protein:
1. promotes gluconeogenesis.
2. has anti-inflammatory properties.
3. promotes cell growth and bone union.
4. decreases pain medication requirements.

81. 3. High protein intake promotes cell growth and bone union. Protein does not promote gluconeogenesis, exert anti-inflammatory properties, or decrease pain medication requirements.
CN: Physiological integrity; CNS: Basic care and comfort; CL: Apply

82. A nurse is instructing an unlicensed assistive personnel (UAP) on the proper care of a client in Buck's extension traction following a fracture of the left fibula. Which observation would indicate that teaching has been effective?
1. The leg in traction is kept externally rotated.
2. The weights are allowed to hang freely over the end of the bed.
3. The UAP instructs the client to perform ankle rotation exercises.
4. The UAP lifts the weights while assisting the client as he moves up in bed.

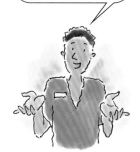

Observation is a key skill for nurses in every field.

82. 2. In Buck's traction, the weights should hang freely without touching the bed or floor. Lifting the weights would break the traction. The client should be moved up in bed, allowing the weight to move freely along with the client. The leg should be kept in straight alignment. Performing ankle rotation exercises could cause the leg to go out of alignment.
CN: Physiological integrity; CNS: Basic care and comfort; CL: Apply

83. A client has been diagnosed with gout. Which foods should the nurse instruct the client to eat in moderation? Select all that apply.
1. Green, leafy vegetables
2. Chocolate
3. Sardines
4. Liver
5. Shrimp
6. Eggs

83. 3, 4, 5. Clients with gout should avoid foods that are high in purines, such as liver, cod, shrimp, and sardines. They should also avoid anchovies, sweetbreads, lentils, and alcoholic beverages, especially beer and wine. Green, leafy vegetables, chocolate, and eggs are not high in purines.
CN: Physiological integrity; CNS: Basic care and comfort; CL: Apply

84. A client is receiving nutritional counseling following the application of a plaster cast for a fracture. The client asks the nurse why vitamin D intake is important. What is the nurse's **best** response?
1. It increases the absorption and use of potassium and phosphorus.
2. It increases the absorption and use of calcium and phosphorus.
3. It aids in the excretion of calcium and phosphorus.
4. It aids in the excretion of potassium and calcium.

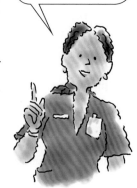

Placing the client in the correct position after hip surgery is critical.

84. 2. Vitamin D increases the absorption and use of calcium and phosphorus. Vitamin D does not affect potassium, nor does it reduce the absorption or affect the excretion of calcium and phosphorus.
CN: Physiological integrity; CNS: Pharmacological and parenteral therapies; CL: Apply

85. Which position would be **best** for a client following surgical repair of the hip?
1. Prone
2. Adduction
3. Abduction
4. Subluxated

85. 3. After surgical repair of the hip, the desired position of the legs and hips is abduction. Adduction, prone, or subluxated positions do not keep the prosthesis within the acetabulum.
CN: Physiological integrity; CNS: Reduction of risk potential; CL: Apply

CN: Client needs category   CNS: Client needs subcategory   CL: Cognitive level

86. A nurse is providing discharge teaching to a client following a left hip replacement. The nurse determines that discharge teaching has been effective when the client states:
1. "I must remain on bed rest."
2. "I have no activity restrictions."
3. "I am allowed limited weight bearing."
4. "I cannot bear any weight for two months."

86. 3. After a hip replacement, the client will have limited weight bearing restrictions. The client will be allowed to move with restrictions for approximately two to three months. The hip should not be flexed more than 90 degrees. Abduction past the midline of the body is prohibited. Progressive weight bearing reduces the complications of immobility.

CN: Physiological integrity; CNS: Basic care and comfort; CL: Apply

87. A client has undergone hip surgery. Which intervention, by the nurse, would help prevent postoperative deep vein thrombosis?
1. Complete bed rest with gradual re-introduction of minimal activity
2. Elevate head of bed, turn the client every two hours
3. Vigorous pulmonary hygiene using an incentive spirometer
4. Administer the ordered subcutaneous enoxaparin and pneumatic compression boots

87. 4. Enoxoparin is a low molecular weight heparin injection that inhibits clot formation. Pneumatic boots will prevent stasis of fluid in the lower extremities that could precipitate clot formation. Complete bed rest would promote stasis of blood flow, which could precipitate clot formation. Pulmonary care or elevated head positioning will not prevent clot formation.

CN: Physiological integrity; CNS: Reduction of risk potential; CL: Apply

88. A client with a spinal cord injury has dexamethasone 16 mg ordered IV. The drug vial contains 24 mg/ml. The nurse plans to use a tuberculin syringe to measure the dose. How much should the nurse draw up to give to this client? Record your answer using two decimal places.

_____ ml

88. 0.67.

$$X = \frac{\text{Dose Desired}}{\text{Dose on Hand or Dose Available}}$$

$$X = \frac{16\ mg}{24\ \dfrac{mg}{ml}} = 0.67\ ml$$

CN: Physiological integrity; CNS: Pharmacological and parenteral therapies; CL: Apply

89. A nurse has witnessed an automobile accident. Which nursing interventions are **best** for a client with a suspected fracture at the scene of this accident? Select all that apply.
1. Do not move the client
2. Immobilize the extremity
3. Move the client to safety immediately
4. Sit the client up to facilitate the airway
5. Begin chest compressions

Make sure your initial intervention is the correct one.

89. 2, 3. At the scene of an accident, a client with a suspected fracture should have the extremity immobilized and then be moved to safety. If the client is in a safe place, do not try to move him. Do not sit the client up, as this could make the fracture worse. Chest compressions would only be done if the nurse determines that the client is unresponsive.

CN: Safe, effective care environment; CNS: Safety and infection control; CL: Apply

90. The nurse is evaluating a client on crutches who is using a three-point gait. Which assessment, made by the nurse, would indicate that the client is using the crutches correctly?
1. The client is placing weight on the feet.
2. The client is placing weight on the axillary areas.
3. The client is placing weight on the palms of the hands.
4. The client is placing weight on the palms and axillary areas.

90. 3. To avoid damage to the brachial plexus nerves in the axilla, the palms of the hands should bear the client's weight. Minimal weight should be placed on the affected leg.
CN: Physiological integrity; CNS: Basic care and comfort; CL: Apply

91. A client, with a right hip fracture, reports left-sided leg pain and left lower leg edema. Based on the client's report, which complication would the nurse anticipate?
1. Deep vein thrombosis (DVT)
2. Pulmonary embolism
3. Fat emboli
4. Infection

91. 1. Unilateral leg pain and edema might be symptoms of DVT. Symptoms of fat emboli include restlessness, tachypnea, and tachycardia and are more common in long bone injuries. An infection is unlikely, and would occur on the opposite side of the fracture. Tachycardia, chest pain, and shortness of breath may be symptoms of a pulmonary embolism.
CN: Physiological integrity; CNS: Reduction of risk potential; CL: Apply

92. Which nursing intervention would be appropriate for a client in traction?
1. Add and remove weights as the client wants
2. Assess the pin sites every shift and as needed
3. Make sure the knots in the rope catch on the pulley
4. Give range of motion to all joints, including those immediately proximal and distal to the fracture, every shift

92. 2. Nursing care for a client in traction may include assessing pin sites every shift, and making sure the knots in the rope do not catch on the pulley. Weights should be added and removed per health care provider orders. Range of motion exercise should be provided to all joints, except those immediately proximal and distal to the fracture, every shift.
CN: Physiological integrity; CNS: Basic care and comfort; CL: Apply

93. A nurse is assisting the health care provider with the application of a cast. Which nursing interventions would be included in the immediate cast care?
1. Rest the cast on the bedside table
2. Dispose of the plaster water in the sink
3. Support the cast with the palms of the hands
4. Wait until the cast dries before cleaning the surrounding skin

93. 3. After assisting the health care provider with the cast application, the cast should be supported with the palms of the hands. The cast should not be rested on a hard or sharp surface. The plaster water should be disposed of in a sink with a plaster trap or in a garbage bag. The skin surrounding the cast should be cleaned before the cast dries.
CN: Safe, effective care environment; CNS: Management of care; CL: Apply

94. The health care provider has just removed a cast from a 20-year-old client's lower leg. During the removal, a small superficial abrasion occurred over the ankle. Which statement, by the client, would indicate a need for additional instruction?
1. "The dry, peeling skin will go away by itself."
2. "I must use a moisturizing lotion on the dry areas."
3. "I can wash the abrasion on my ankle with soap and water."
4. "I will wait until the abrasion is healed before I go swimming."

94. 2. The dry, peeling skin will heal in a few days with normal cleaning, and without lotion. Vigorous scrubbing isn't necessary. Washing the abrasion, and delaying swimming until healing are correct procedures following cast removal.
CN: Physiological integrity; CNS: Reduction of risk potential; CL: Apply

CN: Client needs category   CNS: Client needs subcategory   CL: Cognitive level

95. A nurse is providing teaching to a client who has recently had a plaster cast applied. Which statement would indicate that the nurse's teaching has been effective?
1. "Heat is a normal sensation as the cast dries."
2. "I'll call my health care provider if I feel any heat."
3. "The cast will need to be removed if I feel any heat."
4. "The heat I feel is most likely caused by an infection."

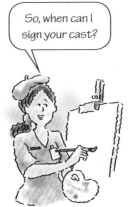

So, when can I sign your cast?

95. 1. It is normal for a client to report heat from the cast as it dries. The cast will not need to be removed if this occurs, and the heath care provider should not be notified. Heat from the cast is not a sign of infection.
CN: Physiological integrity; CNS: Reduction of risk potential; CL: Apply

96. A nurse is providing care for a client with a leg cast. Which action, by the nurse would, be the **most** appropriate to help prevent foot drop?
1. Encouraging bed rest
2. Supporting the foot with 45 degrees of flexion
3. Supporting the foot with 90 degrees of flexion
4. Placing a stocking on the foot to provide warmth

96. 3. To prevent foot drop in a leg with a cast, the foot should be supported with 90 degrees of flexion. Bed rest can cause foot drop. Keeping the extremity warm will not prevent foot drop.
CN: Health promotion and maintenance; CNS: None; CL: Apply

97. The nurse is teaching the caregivers of a client with a hip-spica cast about the need to avoid gas-forming foods. Which statement would indicate that teaching has been effective?
1. "Gas-forming foods should be avoided to prevent flatus."
2. "Gas-forming foods should be avoided to prevent diarrhea."
3. "Gas-forming foods should be avoided to prevent constipation."
4. "Gas-forming foods should be avoided to prevent abdominal distension."

97. 4. A client with a hip-spica cast should avoid gas-forming foods to prevent abdominal distension that could cause pressure on the cast. Gas-forming foods may cause flatus, but that is not a reason to avoid them. Gas-forming foods generally do not cause diarrhea or constipation.
CN: Physiological integrity; CNS: Reduction of risk potential; CL: Apply

98. The nurse instructs a client with a femur fracture to walk with crutches using a four-point gait, beginning with the left foot. Prioritize the steps of this nurse's instructions.

| 1. Move the right foot forward to the level of right crutch |
| 2. Move the left crutch forward 4 to 6 inches (10 to 15 cm) |
| 3. Move the left foot forward to the level of left crutch |
| 4. Move the right crutch forward 4 to 6 inches (10 to 15 cm) |
| 5. Assume tripod position baring weight on the handgrips |

98. Ordered Response:

| 5. Assume tripod position baring weight on the handgrips |
| 4. Move the right crutch forward 4 to 6 inches (10 to 15 cm) |
| 3. Move the left foot forward to the level of left crutch |
| 2. Move the left crutch forward 4 to 6 inches (10 to 15 cm) |
| 1. Move the right foot forward to the level of right crutch |

CN: Physiological integrity; CNS: Reduction of risk potential; CL: Apply

CN: Client needs category   CNS: Client needs subcategory   CL: Cognitive level

99. A client has attended a sports medicine clinic to learn how to reduce the risk of experiencing a sports-related injury. Which activity would indicate that this client understands how to prevent a sports-related injury?
1. Warming up
2. Building strength
3. Pacing the activity
4. Working with moderate intensity

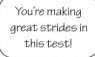

You're making great strides in this test!

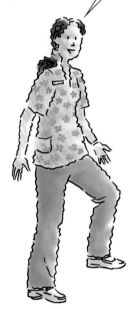

99. **1.** The best way to prevent a sports-related injury is to warm up. Pacing the activity, building strength, and using moderate intensity are also prevention measures, but warming up is the most effective.
CN: Physiological integrity; CNS: Reduction of risk potential; CL: Apply

100. A client has just returned from the post-anesthesia care unit following internal fixation of a left femoral neck fracture. In which way should the nurse position this client?
1. On his back with two pillows between his legs
2. On his left side with his right knee bent
3. On his right side with his left knee bent
4. Seated at a 90-degree angle

100. **1.** The operative leg must be kept abducted to prevent dislocation of the hip. Placing the client on the left or right side with knee bent does not promote abduction. Acute flexion of the affected hip may cause dislocation. The head of the bed may be raised 35 to 49 degrees.
CN: Physiological integrity; CNS: Reduction of risk potential; CL: Apply

101. Which clinical manifestations would lead the nurse to suspect a fat embolus in a client who has a left femur fracture?
1. Dyspnea
2. Sudden headache
3. Numbness in the left leg
4. Muscle spasm in the left thigh

101. **1.** A fat embolism usually presents as acute respiratory distress. Symptoms include chest pain, cyanosis, dyspnea, tachypnea, and apprehension. A sudden headache is not a symptom of a fat embolism. Muscle spasms in the left thigh are a neuromuscular response of the local muscle around the femoral fracture. Numbness would be a neurovascular response.
CN: Physiological integrity; CNS: Physiological adaptation; CL: Apply

102. Which statement **best** explains an open reduction of a fractured femur?
1. Traction will be used.
2. A cast will be applied.
3. Crutches will be used after surgery.
4. Some form of screw, plate, nail, or wire is usually used to maintain alignment.

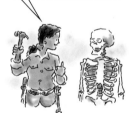

Screws, nails, wires—who knew nursing was so much like home repair?

102. **4.** Open reduction means that the tissue must be surgically opened and the fractured bones realigned. To maintain proper alignment, a screw, plate, nail, or wire is inserted into the bone to prevent the bones from separating. Although traction may have been used before surgery, it won't be needed once the fracture is reduced. A cast or crutches may be used after surgery, but this question refers to a surgical procedure.
CN: Physiological integrity; CNS: Physiological adaptation; CL: Apply

103. Which clinical manifestations would lead the nurse to suspect that the client has a dislocation of the left hip?
1. Pain relieved with pressure
2. Pain in the inguinal area, and an abnormal gait
3. Internal rotation of the knee, abduction of the leg
4. Pain in the hip, the thigh appears longer than the unaffected leg

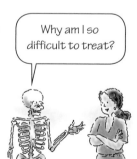

Why am I so difficult to treat?

103. **2.** A dislocated hip will create problems with walking. Pain is often due to a pinched nerve in the joint. Pressure should not be applied to a painful joint or fracture unless there's hemorrhage. The leg is usually adducted and shortened.
CN: Physiological integrity; CNS: Physiological adaptation; CL: Analyze

104. A 20-year-old client has developed osteomyelitis two weeks after a fishhook was removed from his foot. Which rationale **best** explains the need for long term antibiotic therapy?
1. Bone has poor circulation.
2. Tissue trauma requires antibiotics.
3. Feet are normally more difficult to treat.
4. Fishhook injuries are highly contaminated.

104. 1. An infection of the bone is difficult to treat because bone has very poor blood circulation. This infection would require the use of long-term IV antibiotics to make sure the infection is cleared. Tissue trauma does not always require antibiotics. Feet are not more difficult to treat than other parts of the body unless the client has a circulatory problem or diabetes mellitus. Fishhooks may not be more contaminated than another instrument that caused an injury.
CN: Physiological integrity; CNS: Pharmacological and parenteral therapies; CL: Apply

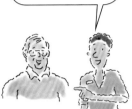

After providing teaching, always check in with your client to make sure he has understood it.

105. The nurse is teaching a client, diagnosed with degenerative joint disease, about the condition. The nurse recognizes that teaching has been effective when the client states:
1. "It is a non-inflammatory joint disease."
2. "It is an immune-mediated joint disease."
3. "It is a joint inflammation after a viral infection."
4. "It is a joint inflammation related to systemic infections."

105. 1. Degenerative joint disease is joint disease due to non-inflammatory wear and tear on joints, and is often seen in athletes. It is not immune-mediated, inflammatory, or caused by systemic infections.
CN: Physiological integrity; CNS: Physiological adaptation; CL: Apply

106. What information should the nurse include in client education about gout?
1. Good foot care will reduce complications.
2. Increased dietary intake of purine is needed.
3. Production of uric acid in the kidneys affects joints.
4. Uric acid crystals cause inflammatory destruction of the joint.

106. 4. The client should understand that uric acid crystals collect in the joint of the great toe and cause inflammation. The kidneys excrete uric acid, an end product of metabolism. A diet low in purines would be indicated for a client with gout. Good foot care does not affect the development of gout, but increasing water intake may help prevent urinary stone formation.
CN: Physiological integrity; CNS: Reduction of risk potential; CL: Apply

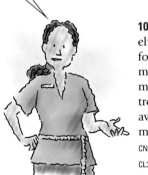

The words most appropriate in question 107 are a clue to the answer.

107. A client has been treated with IV antibiotics for osteomyelitis. The treatment has not been effective. Which intervention would be the **most** appropriate for this client?
1. Bone grafts
2. Hyperbaric oxygen therapy
3. Amputation of the extremity
4. Debridement of necrotic tissue

107. 4. The tissues may need to be debrided to eliminate necrotic tissue and allow new tissue to form. A bone graft would be done after debridement. Hyperbaric oxygen therapy is a new treatment modality that has been used in the successful treatment of osteomyelitis, but it is not universally available. Amputation is not indicated in the treatment of acute osteomyelitis.
CN: Physiological integrity; CNS: Physiological adaptation; CL: Apply

108. A client asks why a high-protein diet has been ordered while he recovers from a fracture. What is the nurse's **best** explanation?
1. Protein promotes gluconeogenesis.
2. Protein has anti-inflammatory properties.
3. Protein promotes cell growth and bone union.
4. Protein decreases pain medication requirements.

108. 3. High-protein intake will promote cell growth and bone union. Protein does not decrease pain medication requirements, have anti-inflammatory properties, or promote gluconeogenesis.
CN: Physiological integrity; CNS: Basic care and comfort; CL: Apply

109. A nurse is caring for a client who has been admitted to the hospital with a musculoskeletal injury. Why has cold therapy been ordered for this client?
1. It promotes analgesia and circulation.
2. It numbs the nerves and dilates the vessels.
3. It promotes circulation and reduces muscle spasms.
4. It causes local vasoconstriction and prevents edema or muscle spasm.

109. 4. Cold causes the blood vessels to constrict, which reduces the leakage of fluid into the tissues and prevents swelling and muscle spasms. Cold therapy may reduce pain by numbing the nerves and tissues. Heat therapy promotes circulation, enhances flexibility, reduces muscle spasms, and also provides analgesia.
CN: Physiological integrity; CNS: Basic care and comfort; CL: Apply

110. What discharge information should the nurse provide to a client with a cast?
1. Use powder under the cast as needed
2. Itching under the cast indicates infection
3. Keep the extremity in a dependent position
4. Report fever and foul odors around the cast

110. 4. Fever, foul odor, and warmth over a specific area of the cast after it is dry may be signs of infection. Itchy skin results from dry skin, and powder should not be used. The extremity should be elevated for 24 to 48 hours.
CN: Health promotion and maintenance; CNS: None; CL: Apply

111. The nurse is assessing a client in traction and determines. Which condition places the client at risk for traction-related complications?
1. Coronary artery disease
2. Diabetes mellitus
3. Hypertension
4. Hip fracture

111. 2. Because people with diabetes commonly have microvascular compromise and delayed wound healing, they require careful monitoring for early signs of skin breakdown. The other conditions do not increase the risk of traction-related complications.
CN: Physiological integrity; CNS: Reduction of risk potential; CL: Analyze

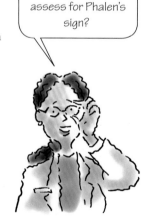

Which action will help the nurse assess for Phalen's sign?

112. A client tells the nurse that she experiences pain and numbness in her fingers when typing on a computer keyboard. Which action will help the nurse assess for Phalen's sign?
1. Having the client hold both wrists in acute flexion with the dorsal surfaces touching for 60 seconds
2. Having the client hold both hands above her head with her arms straight for 30 seconds
3. Having the client extend her wrists while the nurse provides resistance
4. Tapping gently over the median nerve in the wrist

112. 1. Acute wrist flexion places pressure on the inflamed median nerve, causing the pain and numbness of Phalen's sign. Holding the hands above the head with arms straight for 30 seconds is not an assessment technique. Tapping gently over the median nerve tests for Tinel's sign, which is another sign of carpal tunnel syndrome. Placing the wrists in extension against resistance tests the strength.
CN: Physiological integrity; CNS: Physiological adaptation; CL: Apply

113. A client has had a knee-high cast removed six weeks after suffering an ankle fracture. Palpation reveals a hard, non-tender lump at the fracture site. How should the nurse interpret this finding?
1. The bone may have healed in misalignment, possibly from the short leg cast.
2. Remodeling should have occurred by now, so this finding would suggest malunion.
3. Callus formation normally occurs at this stage and may feel like a lump on the bone.
4. Swelling and bruising may persist after a traumatic fracture.

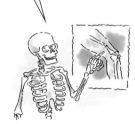

How would you interpret this finding?

113. 3. Callus formation is a normal stage of bone repair. It is characterized by an overgrowth of bone that is reabsorbed gradually during the remodeling stage. This deformity is painless, whereas misalignment and malunion typically cause pain. Swelling and bruising should have disappeared by this time.
CN: Physiological integrity; CNS: Physiological adaptation; CL: Analyze

CN: Client needs category   CNS: Client needs subcategory   CL: Cognitive level

114. A client visits the emergency department with a suspected fracture of the right hip. Which assessment finding would the nurse anticipate? Select all that apply.
   1. The right leg is longer than the left leg.
   2. The right leg is shorter than the left leg.
   3. The right leg is externally rotated.
   4. The right leg is internally rotated.
   5. The right leg is abducted.
   6. The right leg is adducted.

114. 2, 3, 6. With a hip fracture, the affected leg will be shorter, adducted, and externally rotated.
CN: Physiological integrity; CNS: Physiological adaptation; CL: Apply

115. A client who is receiving acetaminophen for osteoarthritis reports continuing pain. The health care provider prescribes celecoxib. What important information regarding this medication, should the nurse share with this client?
   1. Report black and tarry stools to the health care provider
   2. Use a stool softener or fiber laxative daily to prevent constipation
   3. If you miss a dose, take a double dose the next day
   4. Don't take the medication with dairy products

115. 1. Black and tarry stools are a sign of gastrointestinal (GI) bleeding, and may necessitate a medication change. Dairy products can help reduce GI irritation. The celecoxib dose should never be doubled. Constipation isn't an adverse effect of this medication.
CN: Physiological integrity; CNS: Pharmacological and parenteral therapies; CL: Apply

116. A client has had an above-the-knee amputation four days after a traumatic injury. The postoperative dressing has loosened and fallen off the stump. What is the **most** appropriate nursing intervention?
   1. Ask the provider to assess the client immediately
   2. Apply a cool, moist compress to the operative site
   3. Wrap the stump with an elastic compression bandage
   4. Instruct the client to lie quietly in bed without movement

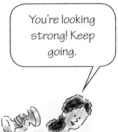

You're looking strong! Keep going.

116. 3. Rewrapping the stump should be completed first. The surgeon may want to see the unwrapped surgical site, but does not need to be notified immediately. Incisions should be kept dry and clean. A moist, cool compress would not be appropriate. The client does not need to lie still or avoid movement.
CN: Psychosocial integrity; CNS: None; CL: Analyze

117. A nurse is assigned to care for a 70-year-old client with acute rheumatoid arthritis. Which finding would the nurse anticipate during assessment of this client?
   1. Radial deviation of the distal phalanges
   2. Tender, painful, and stiff joints
   3. Heberden's nodes
   4. Bouchard's nodes

117. 2. Tender, painful, and stiff joints characterize acute rheumatoid arthritis. The other assessment findings characterize osteoarthritis, including Heberden's nodules and Bouchard's nodes.
CN: Physiological integrity; CNS: Physiological adaptation; CL: Apply

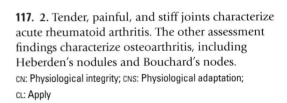

118. A client with lactose intolerance requires dietary teaching. Which foods should the nurse advise the client to eat to ensure adequate calcium intake?
1. Cheese and yogurt
2. Beef liver and broccoli
3. Bananas and avocados
4. Collard greens and spinach

118. **4.** Dark green, leafy vegetables are the best non-dairy sources of calcium. Bananas and avocados are good sources of vitamin K. Beef liver and broccoli supply iron. Cheese and yogurt should be avoided because of the lactose intolerance.

CN: Physiological integrity; CNS: Basic care and comfort;
CL: Apply

119. The nurse is teaching a 57-year-old female client about post-menopausal bone loss. Which factors are **most** likely to cause bone loss in this client? Select all that apply.
1. Chronic use of stool softeners
2. Calcium channel blocker use
3. Lack of sunlight exposure
4. Increased estrogen level
5. Decreased estrogen level
6. Increased progesterone level

119. **3, 5.** Lack of sunlight exposure decreases absorption of vitamin D, which must be present for calcium to be absorbed from the small intestine. Calcium channel blockers do not affect serum calcium levels. Stool softeners do not increase peristalsis, so they do not impair calcium absorption. Decreased estrogen levels lead to bone loss. Increased estrogen and progesterone levels occur in the pregnant client, not the postmenopausal client.

CN: Health promotion and maintenance; CNS: None;
CL: Analyze

120. A client with a torn meniscus, caused by a football injury, arrives at the outpatient surgery clinic for an arthroscopic meniscectomy. What is the **most** important information for the nurse to give the client?
1. Exactly how the procedure will be performed
2. Avoidance of weight bearing for two weeks following surgery
3. Postoperative exercises, such as straight-leg raising and quadriceps sitting
4. The possibility of severe postoperative pain for 24 to 48 hours after surgery

120. **3.** The best time to teach about postoperative care is preoperatively. Straight-leg raising and quadriceps sitting exercises help maintain the strength of the affected extremity. The health care provider, not the nurse, should explain the surgical procedure. Weight bearing may begin as soon as the day of surgery. Usually, pain is mild to moderate after arthroscopic surgery.

CN: Physiological integrity; CNS: Basic care and comfort;
CL: Apply

121. A client is ready to be discharged following arthroscopic knee surgery. Which instruction would the nurse anticipate from the health care provider?
1. Ice and elevate the extremity for 12 hours after discharge
2. Infection isn't a potential problem because of the small incision size
3. Swelling and coolness of the joint and limb are normal right after surgery
4. Take acetaminophen with codeine every four hours as necessary for pain relief

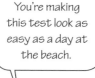

You're making this test look as easy as a day at the beach.

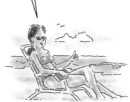

121. **4.** Mild to moderate pain is normal after this type of surgery and can be relieved by oral narcotic analgesics. To minimize swelling, the client should ice and elevate the extremity for at least 24 hours following surgery. Infection is a potential problem after any invasive procedure. Swelling and coolness of the joint and limb may indicate complications from tourniquet use during surgery.

CN: Physiological integrity; CNS: Basic care and comfort;
CL: Apply

122. A perimenopausal client is at high risk for osteoporosis because of family history, lactose intolerance, and small body frame. This client asks the nurse how she can prevent osteoporosis. What is the nurse's **best** response?
1. Increase the amount of calcium and vitamin D in your diet
2. Hormone replacement therapy (HRT) is recommended
3. Have a bone density test yearly
4. It is not necessary to stop smoking

122. 1. Adequate calcium and vitamin D intake are an important part of an overall prevention program. Bone density tests can evaluate the risk for osteoporosis but do not need to be done yearly. Smoking is a risk factor for developing osteoporosis. Studies show that estrogen in HRT may influence the development of breast and uterine cancers.
CN: Physiological integrity; CNS: Pharmacological and parenteral therapies; CL: Analyze

123. The nurse is reviewing the tests ordered for a client diagnosed with Ewing's sarcoma. What test would determine the extent of metastasis?
1. Bone scan
2. Computed tomography (CT) scan
3. Magnetic resonance imaging (MRI)
4. Positron emission tomography (PET)

123. 1. A bone scan views the entire skeletal structure, indicating areas of possible metastases. CT scan, MRI, and PET scan visualize only one body area at a time.
CN: Physiological integrity; CNS: Reduction of risk potential; CL: Apply

124. An 80-year-old client with pneumonia has been admitted to the hospital. The client's medical history includes chronic rheumatoid arthritis. Which assessment finding would the nurse anticipate for this client?
1. Thickened plaque overlying the flexor tendon of the ring finger
2. Cystic swelling on the dorsum of the wrist
3. Flattened thenar eminence
4. Swan-neck deformity

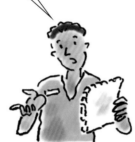

Pay close attention to the word *chronic* and what it implies.

124. 4. In chronic rheumatoid arthritis, the fingers may show hyperextension of the proximal interphalangeal joints with fixed flexion of the distal interphalangeal joints, referred to as swan-neck deformities. Flattened thenar eminence characterizes thenar atrophy, a condition that suggests an ulnar nerve disorder. The first sign of a Dupuytren's contracture is a thickened plaque overlying the flexor tendon of the ring finger and possibly the little finger at the level of the distal palmar crease. Ganglia are cystic, round, usually non-tender swellings located along tendon sheaths or joint capsules. Ganglia frequently involve the dorsum of the wrist.
CN: Physiological integrity; CNS: Physiological adaptation; CL: Apply

125. The nurse provides crutch walking instructions to a client following arthroscopic knee surgery. Which statement, by the client, would indicate a need for further teaching?
1. "When I sit down, I can hold both crutches in my right hand."
2. "When I go up the stairs, I should advance the affected leg first."
3. "I should not put my body weight on my underarms when I use my crutches."
4. "I will move both crutches forward together, and move my affected leg forward with the crutches."

125. 2. The client should assume the tripod position and transfer weight to crutches. When going up stairs, the unaffected leg should go up first while the crutches and the operative leg stay on the lower step. The affected leg should advance after the crutches and the unaffected leg.
CN: Physiological integrity; CNS: Physiological adaptation; CL: Apply

126. An elderly client, with rheumatoid arthritis, is being treated with prednisone. Which complications can occur with long-term steroid therapy?
1. Breast and uterine cancer
2. Osteoporosis and diabetes mellitus
3. Weight loss and lactose intolerance
4. Deep vein thrombosis (DVT), pulmonary embolus, and stroke

126. 2. Long-term prednisone therapy can increase the loss of calcium from bones, slow down the formation of new bone tissue, resulting in osteoporosis, and alter glucose metabolism. Breast and uterine cancer, DVT, pulmonary embolus, stroke, weight loss, and lactose intolerance are not common adverse effects of prednisone.

CN: Physiological integrity; CNS: Pharmacological and parenteral therapies; CL: Analyze

127. A nurse is caring for a client with a history of spinal cord injury. Which nursing actions can reduce the risk for autonomic dysreflexia? Select all that apply.
1. Instruct the client to wear a medical alert bracelet at all times
2. Observe the client for a pattern of temperament changes
3. Monitor the patency of the indwelling urinary catheter
4. Promote a high fiber diet, and the use of a stool softener
5. Perform a digital rectal exam to remove fecal impaction if evacuation doesn't occur within 24 hours

127. 3, 4. Bowel and bladder distention are common causes of autonomic dysreflexia (AD). A digital rectal exam is contraindicated for fecal impaction, as it could cause an episode of AD. No bowel movement within 24 hours does not necessarily indicate fecal impaction.

CN: Physiological integrity; CNS: Reduction of risk potential; CL: Apply

128. The nurse is assessing a client's response to skeletal traction that has been applied to a lower extremity. Which finding would be considered to be normal?
1. Coolness and pallor below the fracture level
2. Moderate to severe muscle spasms around the fracture area
3. Serous drainage and crust formation at the pin insertion site
4. Erythema and swelling immediately around the pin insertion site

128. 3. Serous drainage around the pin insertion site is a normal finding. Some facilities do not recommend crust removal because of its protective nature. A pale extremity may indicate arterial compromise. Erythema and swelling signal infection. Severe muscle spasms may indicate improper alignment of the body or traction.

CN: Physiological integrity; CNS: Reduction of risk potential; CL: Analyze

129. A client with type 2 diabetes mellitus has been placed in skeletal traction following a motor vehicle collision. The provider is concerned because the client demonstrates symptoms of developing osteomyelitis. The provider orders IV antibiotics, blood culture, recreation therapy, and pin site care. What is the **priority** nursing intervention for this client?
1. Ask the recreation therapist to see the client for diversional activities
2. Administer the antibiotic
3. Obtain a blood specimen for culture
4. Perform pin site care

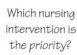

Which nursing intervention is the priority?

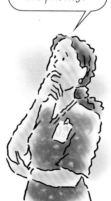

129. 3. The client is demonstrating symptoms of osteomyelitis. The first priority would be to obtain the blood culture prior to starting the first dose of antibiotic. The antibiotic can then be administered. The other options are included in care of the client. However, the priority is to obtain the culture. Osteomyelitis is a dangerous bone infection that's hard to eradicate it.

CN: Physiological integrity; CNS: Reduction of risk potential; CL: Analyze

130. A client in skeletal traction reports pain and has received an analgesic one hour ago. In addition, the nurse offers this client an alternative pain management measure. What actions may be implemented based on the nurse's scope of practice?
1. Acupressure and shiatsu
2. Relaxation and imagery
3. Hypnosis and therapeutic touch
4. Swedish massage and the Feldenkrais method

131. A client has decided on conservative treatment for a herniated nucleus pulposus. The nurse anticipates that this treatment will include:
1. surgery.
2. bone fusion.
3. bed rest, pain medication, physiotherapy.
4. strenuous exercise, pain medication, physiotherapy.

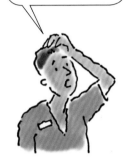

I wonder what the word conservative means in this question?

132. The nurse is caring for a 70-year-old client who has undergone a right total hip replacement. How should the nurse plan to reposition the client?
1. Every 1 to 2 hours, from the unaffected side to the back
2. Every 4 to 6 hours, from the unaffected side to the back
3. Every 1 to 2 hours, from the affected side to the back
4. Every 4 to 6 hours, from the affected side to the back

133. A client is being discharged from the emergency department after cast application for a fracture of the tibia. Based on this diagnosis, what is the **most** important information for the nurse to teach this client?
1. Cough and deep breathe at least every two hours
2. Restrict your fluid intake to one liter per day
3. Keep the leg elevated and apply ice for the first 24 to 48 hours
4. Call the provider immediately if you experience apprehensiveness, shortness of breath, fever, or palpitations.

130. 2. Relaxation and imagery are effective adjuncts to pharmacological pain management that the nurse can implement without a provider's order. Although the other therapies may promote pain management, they require special training or certification.
CN: Physiological integrity; CNS: Basic care and comfort; CL: Apply

131. 3. Conservative treatment of a herniated nucleus pulposus may include bed rest, pain medication, and physiotherapy. Aggressive treatment may include surgery such as a bone fusion.
CN: Physiological integrity; CNS: Reduction of risk potential; CL: Apply

132. 1. The client should be turned at least every two hours, and always from the unaffected side to the back. The client should never be placed on the affected side. Turning the client every 4 to 6 hours presents a greater risk for skin breakdown.
CN: Physiological integrity; CNS: Reduction of risk potential; CL: Apply

133. 4. Fat embolism is a complication of a long bone fracture. Signs and symptoms include apprehension, altered mental status, respiratory distress, tachycardia, tachypnea, fever, and petechiae over the neck, upper arms, and chest. Coughing and deep-breathing exercises as well as leg elevations with ice applications can help prevent other complications of a long bone fracture but have no effect on fat emboli. The client should also be instructed that drinking plenty of fluids to stay well hydrated will help him avoid embolic complications.
CN: Physiological integrity; CNS: Reduction of risk potential; CL: Apply

134. The nurse is examining an older adult client with a fracture. What is the **most** common site of fractures in older adults?

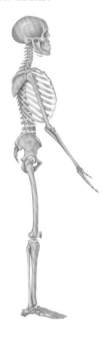

134. Hip fracture is the most common injury in the elderly population, and has a high rate of mortality due to complications of surgery, and prolonged immobility.

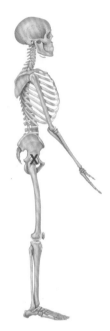

CN: Physiological integrity; CNS: Reduction of risk potential; CL: Apply

135. A client reports a flare-up of acute gout. What is the **most** common site of acute gout?

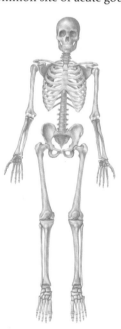

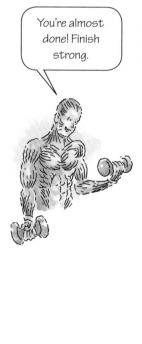

You're almost done! Finish strong.

135. Pain and inflammation of gout usually occurs in one or more small joints of the great toe. The metatarsophalangeal joint of the great toe is most common.

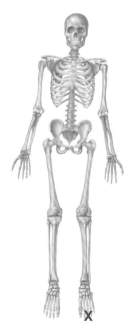

CN: Physiological integrity; CNS: Reduction of risk potential; CL: Apply

CN: Client needs category   CNS: Client needs subcategory   CL: Cognitive level

136. A nurse is caring for a postsurgical client. Identify the **most** common site for deep vein thrombosis (DVT) for this client.

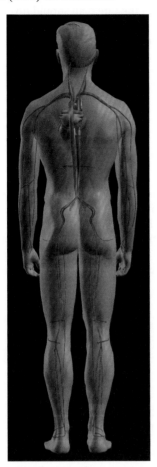

136. DVT is a blood clot that forms in a vein deep in the body. Most deep vein blood clots occur in the client's lower leg.

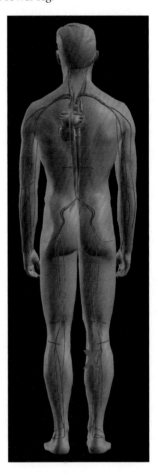

CN: Physiological integrity; CNS: Reduction of risk potential; CL: Apply

137. A nurse is caring for a client who is two days postoperative from open reduction and internal fixation of a fractured left tibia/fibula. The client reports severe pain in the left leg. The nurse administers the prescribed morphine sulfate, 2 mg IV. The client continues to report severe pain. The client's right leg appears normal. The nurse assesses the left leg and finds that it's cool, pale, and has absent pulses and a capillary refill greater than three seconds. What is the nurse's **priority** action?

1. Notify the health care provider
2. Document the clinical findings
3. Administer another dose of the prescribed morphine sulfate
4. Reassess the left lower extremities within one hour

137. 1. Skin that is cool to touch, has no pulse, and with capillary refill greater than three seconds would indicate that the client has impaired circulation. Several complications such as compartment syndrome or deep vein thrombosis, can impede circulation and would require immediately action to prevent damage to the nerves and tissues and necrosis. The nurse should collaborate with the health care provider for additional plans of care. Pain that is caused by tissue ischemia will not be relieved by morphine sulfate. Reassessing the left leg in one hour would delay care and cause additional complications.

CN: Physiological integrity; CNS: Physiological adaptation; CL: Apply

138. A client, with a femoral fracture, is in skeletal traction. During the initial shift assessment, the nurse finds that the weight used in traction is heavier than specified by the nursing care plan. What action should the nurse take **first**?
1. Ask the health care provider, during rounds, if the order was changed
2. Check the health care provider's orders to see if the orders included a weight change
3. Assume that the health care provider ordered the weight change
4. Remove the weight and replace it with the weight specified in the plan

138. 2. The nurse should check the provider's orders to see if a weight change was ordered first. If it was, the nurse responsible for ensuring implementation of the care plan should investigate why the change was not incorporated in the plan.
CN: Safe, effective care environment; CNS: Management of care; CL: Analyze

139. A client is receiving discharge teaching regarding the early signs and symptoms of compartment syndrome. The nurse recognizes that teaching has been effective when the client states:
1. "I will contact my health care provider if I notice redness."
2. "I will contact my health care provider if I notice swelling."
3. "I will contact my health care provider if I notice numbness and tingling."
4. "I will contact my health care provider if I notice a change in my skin color."

139. 3. Numbness and tingling are known as paresthesia, which is the earliest sign of compartment syndrome. Pain, heat, and swelling are later signs and symptoms of compartment syndrome. Skin pallor isn't a sign of compartment syndrome.
CN: Physiological integrity; CNS: Physiological adaptation; CL: Analyze

140. A nurse explains the process of cane usage to a hospitalized client with left-sided weakness. Prioritize the steps of proper cane usage.

1. Place the cane in the right hand
2. Hold the cane on the right side and advance the left leg
3. Advance the cane 6 to 10 inches (15 to 25 cm) with each step
4. Perform hand hygiene
5. Secure a gait belt around client's waist

140. Ordered Response:

4. Perform hand hygiene
5. Secure a gait belt around client's waist
1. Place the cane in the right hand
2. Hold the cane on the right side and advance the left leg
3. Advance the cane 6 to 10 inches (15 to 25 cm) with each step

CN: Physiological integrity; CNS: Reduction of risk potential; CL: Apply

141. Which signs and symptoms would the nurse anticipate while assessing a client diagnosed with fat emboli?
1. Tachypnea, tachycardia, shortness of breath, and paresthesia
2. Paresthesia, bradypnea, bradycardia, and petechial rash on chest and neck
3. Bradypnea, bradycardia, shortness of breath, and petechial rash on chest and neck
4. Tachypnea, tachycardia, shortness of breath, and petechial rash on chest and neck

141. 4. Signs and symptoms of fat emboli include tachypnea, tachycardia, shortness of breath, and a petechial rash on the chest and neck. The fat molecules enter the venous circulation and travel to a lung, obstructing pulmonary circulation. Bradycardia, bradypnea, and paresthesia are not usual symptoms.

CN: Health promotion and maintenance; CNS: None; CL: Analyze

142. A client is demonstrating his understanding of touchdown weight bearing prior to being discharged. Which outcome would demonstrate this understanding?
1. The ability to bear full weight on the affected extremity
2. The ability to bear 30% to 50% of weight on the affected extremity
3. The ability to touch the floor with the extremity with no weight bearing
4. Keeping the extremity elevated at all time with no weight bearing

142. 3. Touchdown weight bearing allows the client to touch the floor with the extremity with no weight bearing. Full weight bearing allows for full weight to be put on the affected extremity. Partial weight bearing allows for 30% to 50% weight bearing on the affected extremity. Non–weight bearing is no weight on the extremity.

CN: Physiological integrity; CNS: Basic care and comfort; CL: Apply

143. A nurse is providing teaching to a client with a brace for a fractured foot. The nurse determines that teaching has been effective when the client states:
1. "The brace will act as a splint."
2. "The brace will allow for movement."
3. "The brace will help to prevent infection."
4. "The brace will encourage direct contact."

143. 1. The purpose of the brace is to act as a splint, maintain immobility, and prevent direct contact. A brace does not prevent infection.

CN: Physiological integrity; CNS: Reduction of risk potential; CL: Apply

No bones about it. You did it!

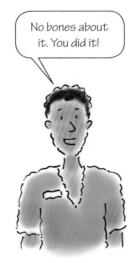

144. What instructions are **most** important for the nurse to provide a client who has been discharged following hip surgery?
1. Do not flex your hip more than 30 degrees; do not cross your legs, and get help putting on your shoes
2. Do not flex your hip more than 60 degrees; do not cross your legs, and get help putting on your shoes
3. Do not flex your hip more than 90 degrees; do not cross your legs, and get help putting on your shoes
4. Do not flex your hip more than 120 degrees; do not cross your legs, and get help putting on your shoes

144. 3. Discharge instructions should include not flexing the hip more than 90 degrees, not crossing the legs, and to ask for help to put on shoes. These restrictions prevent dislocation of the new prosthesis.

CN: Physiological integrity; CNS: Reduction of risk potential; CL: Apply

CN: Client needs category   CNS: Client needs subcategory   CL: Cognitive level

Chapter 8

Gastrointestinal Disorders

From hiatal hernias to diverticulitis to pancreatitis, this chapter covers all the GI disorders you could ask for, in one handy package. Gotta love it!

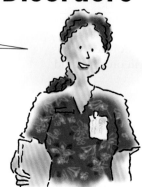

1. A client asks the nurse what caused the development of a hiatal hernia? What is the nurse's **best** response?
   1. "It is a genetic condition."
   2. "It is caused by a weak esophageal muscle."
   3. "It is caused by increased pressure in your gastrointestinal tract."
   4. "It is caused by weakness of the diaphragmatic muscle."

A healthy diet and a healthy weight can prevent many health problems.

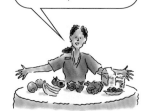

2. Which client is at highest risk of developing a hiatal hernia?
   1. The client with a BMI of 35
   2. The client with chronic constipation
   3. The client with irritable bowel syndrome
   4. The client with decreased peristalsis

3. A client is admitted with a hiatal hernia. Which symptoms would the nurse expect to find on assessment? Select all that apply.
   1. Heartburn
   2. Dysphagia
   3. Esophageal reflux
   4. Abdominal cramping
   5. Diarrhea

4. The nurse will be assisting with the diagnostic tests for a client who may have a hiatal hernia. For which test should the nurse prepare to assist?
   1. Colonoscopy
   2. Magnetic resonance imaging (MRI)
   3. Barium swallow with fluoroscopy
   4. Barium enema

CN: Client needs category   CNS: Client needs subcategory   CL: Cognitive level

1. 4. A hiatal hernia is caused by weakness of the diaphragmatic muscle, and increased intra-abdominal pressure. This weakness allows the stomach to slide into the esophagus. The esophageal supports weaken; however, the esophageal muscle weakness or increased esophageal muscle pressure is not a factor in hiatal hernia. The hernia is not the result of a genetic condition.
CN: Physiological integrity; CNS: Physiological adaptation; CL: Apply

2. 1. Obesity may cause increased abdominal pressure that pushes the lower portion of the stomach into the thorax. Clients with a BMI over 30 are considered obese. Constipation, irritable bowel and decreased peristalsis do not have an effect on the development of a hiatal hernia.
CN: Physiological integrity; CNS: Physiological adaptation; CL: Analyze

3. 1, 2, 3. Heartburn, dysphagia and esophageal reflux can be associated with hiatal hernia. Abdominal cramping and diarrhea are not associated with this disorder. Abdominal cramping and diarrhea can be caused by many other abdominal conditions such as irritable bowel and infections.
CN: Physiological integrity; CNS: Physiological adaptation; CL: Apply

4. 3. A barium swallow with fluoroscopy shows the position of the stomach in relation to the diaphragm. A colonoscopy and a lower GI series show disorders of the intestine. An abdominal X-ray series will show structural defects, but not necessarily a hiatal hernia, unless it's sliding or rolling at the time of the X-ray.
CN: Health promotion and maintenance; CNS: None; CL: Apply

5. What symptoms would the nurse expect to find for a client with appendicitis? Select all that apply.
1. Right lower quadrant pain
2. Anorexia
3. Nausea
4. Hypothermia
5. Projectile vomiting

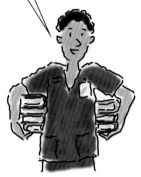

Hmm. I remember reading about that somewhere.

5. 1, 2, 3. The client experiencing appendicitis would most likely present with right lower quadrant pain, anorexia, and nausea. A low grade fever is often present, but not hypothermia. Projectile vomiting is not seen with this condition.
CN: Physiological integrity; CNS: Physiological adaptation; CL: Analyze

6. How would the nurse expect a client with appendicitis to describe the pain?
1. "I have aching in my lower abdomen."
2. "The pain comes on very quickly and goes away just as quickly."
3. "The pain occurs every hour for just a few minutes."
4. "The pain is steady and is a 7 on a scale of 1 to 10."

6. 4. The pain begins in the epigastrium or periumbilical region and then shifts to the lower right quadrant then becomes steady. The pain may be moderate to severe. Clients do not describe the pain as intermittent, fleeting or aching.
CN: Physiological integrity; CNS: Physiological adaptation; CL: Apply

7. A client diagnosed with an appendicitis states that his pain is an 8 on a scale of 1 to 10. What is the nurse's **best** intervention to assist this client?
1. Position the client prone
2. Sit the client on the side of the bed, leaning on the bedside table
3. Ambulate the client with assistance
4. Position the client on his back with legs drawn up towards the abdomen

7. 4. Lying still with the legs drawn up toward the chest helps relieve tension on the abdominal muscles, which helps to reduce the pain. Lying flat, sitting and ambulating may increase the amount of pain experienced.
CN: Physiological integrity; CNS: Physiological adaptation; CL: Apply

8. What is the **priority** nursing intervention for a client with acute appendicitis?
1. Teaching the client about surgery
2. Encouraging oral intake of clear fluids
3. Maintaining the client on bed rest
4. Assessing for symptoms of peritonitis

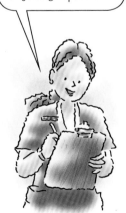

Be thorough when you assess a client so you don't miss anything important.

8. 4. The focus of care is to assess for peritonitis, or inflammation of the peritoneal cavity. Peritonitis is most commonly caused by appendix rupture and invasion of bacteria, which could be lethal. The nurse should discourage oral intake in preparation for surgery. Keeping the client on bed rest is important; however, in the acute phase, management should focus on minimizing preoperative complications and recognizing when complications may occur.
CN: Safe, effective care environment; CNS: Management of care; CL: Apply

CN: Client needs category   CNS: Client needs subcategory   CL: Cognitive level

9. The nurse is teaching a client about gastritis. The nurse determines that teaching was effective when the client states?
  1. "Gastritis is caused by erosion of the gastric mucosa."
  2. "Gastritis is an inflammation of a diverticulum."
  3. "Gastritis is an inflammation of the gastric mucosa."
  4. "Gastritis is caused by a reflux of stomach acid into the esophagus."

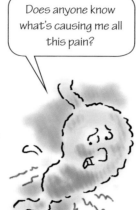

Does anyone know what's causing me all this pain?

9. 3. Gastritis is an inflammation of the gastric mucosa that may be acute or chronic. Erosion of the mucosa results in ulceration. Inflammation of a diverticulum is called diverticulitis. Reflux of stomach acid is known as gastroesophageal reflux disease.
CN: Physiological integrity; CNS: Physiological adaptation; CL: Analyze

10. A client reports that heartburn and belching occurs one to two 2 hours after eating, and when lying down. For which should the nurse assess?
  1. Cardiac enzymes
  2. Lumbar strain
  3. Potential hiatal hernia
  4. Intestinal infection

10. 3. Symptoms of hiatal hernia may include heartburn, belching, difficulty swallowing and abdominal pain or chest pain. A client's position after eating can intensify the symptoms. This condition seems to be associated with chronic exposure of the lower esophageal sphincter to the lower pressure of the thorax, making it less effective. Lumbar strain produces back pain. Infection of the intestinal tract may present with diarrhea, nausea, abdominal pain, and loss of appetite. Cardiac enzymes would be assessed to determine the presence of an early myocardial infarction.
CN: Physiological integrity; CNS: physiological adaptation; CL: Analyze

11. Which nursing intervention should be included in the immediate postoperative management of a client who has undergone gastric resection?
  1. Monitoring gastric pH
  2. Assessing for bowel sounds
  3. Teaching about dumping syndrome
  4. Monitoring for symptoms of hemorrhage

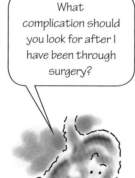

What complication should you look for after I have been through surgery?

11. 4. This client should be monitored closely for signs and symptoms of hemorrhage, such as bright red blood in the nasogastric tube suction, tachycardia, or a drop in blood pressure. Gastric pH may be monitored to evaluate the need for H2 receptor antagonists. Bowel sounds may not return for up to 72 hours postoperatively. Dumping syndrome is a complication of surgery; however, it does not occur in the immediate postoperative period.
CN: Physiological integrity; CNS: Reduction of risk potential; CL: Apply

12. A client has been diagnosed with acute gastritis. What is the **most** important information for the nurse to provide to the client?
  1. "You need to decrease stress."
  2. "You will need surgery."
  3. "We need to assess for the underlying cause."
  4. "You will need to have enteral tube feedings."

12. 3. Discovering and treating the cause of gastritis is the appropriate approach. Treatment of gastritis depends on the cause, and can include dietary management, but not enteral feedings, medications such as antacids or H2 blockers, antibiotics for *Helicobacter pylori*, lifestyle changes such as smoking cessation, surgery, or stress management.
CN: Physiologic integrity; CNS: Physiological adaptation; CL: Apply

13. Which client is **most** at risk for developing chronic gastritis?
1. A client who is 25 years old
2. A client who has had frequent upper respiratory infections
3. A client who had a cholecystectomy
4. A client who has *Helicobacter pylori* infection

13. 4. Chronic gastritis typical occurs in an older adult, but can occur at any age. There are many causes, *H. pylori* infection, autoimmune factors, exposure to toxic substances in the workplace, radiation therapy, smoking, and alcohol. Frequent upper respiratory infections and gall bladder surgery do not produce chronic gastritis.

CN: Physiological integrity; CNS: reduction of risk potential; CL: Analyze

14. A client with chronic gastritis asks why vitamin B$_{12}$ injections are needed. What is the nurse's **best** response?
1. "Your white blood cell count is low."
2. "This will decrease your pain."
3. "Your stomach cannot absorb vitamin B$_{12}$."
4. "This will cure your disorder."

14. 3. With gastritis, the stomach lining becomes thin and atrophic, which impairs the production of gastric intrinsic factor. Decreased production of intrinsic factor leads to reduced absorption of vitamin B$_{12}$, and pernicious anemia. The client cannot absorb vitamin B$_{12}$. Vitamin B$_{12}$ does not decrease pain. The treatment of vitamin B$_{12}$ injections will not cure the disorder.

CN: Physiological integrity; CNS: Physiological adaptation; CL: Analyze

15. What is the **most** important information for the nurse to teach a client who is diagnosed with gastroesophageal reflux disease (GERD)?
1. Decrease smoking to one or two cigarettes a day
2. Take non-steroidal anti-inflammatory drugs (NSAIDs) for pain
3. Decrease alcoholic consumption to one to two drinks daily
4. Sleep in the right-side lying position

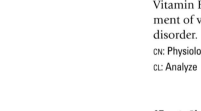

Remember

With NSAIDs, remember the three "A's":
- Analgesic
- Antipyretic
- Anti-inflammatory

15. 4. Sleeping in the right-side lying position decreases the incidence of reflux. The client should refrain from smoking and drinking alcohol, as both habits can aggravate GERD. NSAIDs reduce esophageal sphincter pressure which allows reflux to occur. The condition does not typically cause pain.

CN: Health promotion and maintenance; CNS: None; CL: Apply

16. What should the nurse include in the discharge teaching plan for a client who has diverticulitis? Select all that apply.
1. Decrease daily fluid intake
2. Adhere to a high fiber diet
3. Avoid strawberries and tomatoes
4. Decrease carbohydrates
5. Avoid nuts and corn

16. 2, 3, 5. Twenty-five to 35 grams of fiber daily are recommended to prevent the recurrence of diverticulitis in diverticular disease. Strawberries, tomatoes, nuts, and corn should all be avoided, as well as any foods with seeds. These seeds can become lodged in the diverticula causing inflammation and infection. Decreasing fluid intake can result in constipation and exacerbate the condition. Decreasing carbohydrates is not recommended.

CN: Physiological integrity; CNS: Basic care and comfort; CL: Apply

17. The nurse is preparing a teaching plan for a client diagnosed with diverticulosis. What is the **most** important information for the nurse to provide to this client? Select all that apply.
1. "You should not experience any pain."
2. "Peritonitis may be a complication of this condition."
3. "Antibiotics may be prescribed."
4. "Constipation may lead to the development of the disease."
5. "Laxative use is a common cause of the disease."

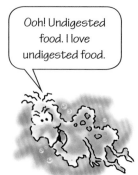

Ooh! Undigested food. I love undigested food.

17. 2, 3, 4. Constipation is linked to the development of diverticula, which develops as a result of increased pressure. The condition often progresses to diverticulitis. Peritonitis can result from ruptured diverticula. Undigested food can block the diverticulum, decreasing blood supply to the area, and potentiating an invasion of bacteria. Antibiotics may be prescribed. Clients may have cramping or lower abdominal pain. Laxative use does not cause diverticulitis.
CN: Physiological integrity; CNS: Physiological adaptation; CL: Analyze

18. A client diagnosed with diverticulosis states, "I never knew I had this!" What is the nurse's **best** response?
1. "Many clients don't know they have diverticulosis, as there are often no symptoms."
2. "You probably have not had this for long."
3. "Have you ever had constipation?"
4. "Symptoms are very similar to many other conditions."

18. 1. Diverticulosis is often an asymptomatic condition. Clients can have the disease for a while and not realize they have it. A history of constipation does not mean the client has diverticulosis. Symptoms generally occur when the condition progresses to diverticulitis, with inflammation and infection.
CN: Physiological integrity; CNS: Physiological adaptation; CL: Analyze

19. Which test should the nurse expect to be ordered for a client suspected of having diverticulosis?
1. Abdominal ultrasound
2. Barium enema
3. Barium swallow
4. Gastroscopy

19. 2. A barium enema will cause diverticula to fill with barium and become easily visible on an X-ray. An abdominal ultrasound can tell more about structures, such as the gallbladder, liver, and spleen, rather than the intestine. A barium swallow and gastroscopy view upper gastrointestinal structures.
CN: Health promotion and maintenance; CNS: None; CL: Apply

20. The nurse has provided discharge teaching for a client who was hospitalized and treated for acute diverticulitis. Which statement by the client indicates an understanding of the discharge instructions?
1. "I'll reduce my fluid intake."
2. "I'll decrease the fiber in my diet."
3. "I'll take all of my antibiotics."
4. "I'll exercise to increase my intra-abdominal pressure."

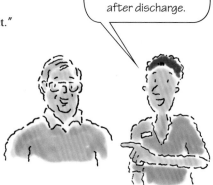

Listen to your client. Make sure he understands what he's supposed to do after discharge.

20. 3. Antibiotics are used to reduce the inflammation and potential infectious process. The client typically is not allowed anything orally until the acute episode subsides. Parenteral fluids are given until the client feels better. It is recommended that the client drink 64 oz (2 L) of water per day, and gradually increase fiber in the diet to improve intestinal motility. During the acute phase, activities that increase intra-abdominal pressure should be avoided to decrease pain and reduce the possibility of an intestinal obstruction.
CN: Physiological integrity; CNS: Physiological adaptation; CL: Analyze

21. Crohn's disease can be described as a chronic relapsing disease. Which area of the gastrointestinal system may be involved with this disease?
1. The entire length of the large colon
2. Only the sigmoid area
3. The layers of mucosa and submucosa
4. The small intestine and colon, affecting the entire thickness of the bowel

21. 4. Crohn's disease more commonly involves any segment of the small intestine, the colon, or both, affecting the entire thickness of the bowel. However, it can also affect the digestive system anywhere from the mouth to the anus. Ulcerative colitis affects the entire length of the large colon and the layers of mucosa and submucosa. Only the sigmoid area is very specific and, therefore, not likely.
CN: Physiological integrity; CNS: Physiological adaptation; CL: Apply

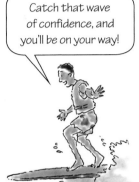

Catch that wave of confidence, and you'll be on your way!

22. A client presents with a recurrence of Crohn's disease. Which area of the alimentary canal does the nurse suspect is involved?
1. Ascending colon
2. Descending colon
3. Sigmoid colon
4. Terminal ileum

22. 4. Studies have shown that the terminal ileum is the most common site for recurrence in clients with Crohn's disease. The other areas may be involved but aren't as common.
CN: Physiological integrity; CNS: Physiological adaptation; CL: Apply

23. A nurse is preparing the teaching plan for a client with Crohn's disease. Which factor should the nurse include as a possible link to the development of this disease?
1. Constipation
2. Diet
3. Heredity
4. Lack of exercise

23. 3. Although the definitive cause of Crohn's disease is unknown, it's thought to be associated with infectious, immune, or psychological factors. Because it has a higher incidence in siblings, it may have a genetic cause.
CN: Health promotion and maintenance; CNS: None; CL: Analyze

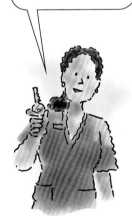

A key to answering a question is reading it carefully and eliminating answer choices.

24. A nurse is teaching a client, recently diagnosed with ulcerative colitis, about iron supplements. What information should the nurse include in the teaching plan?
1. "Iron is necessary to treat the ulcer."
2. "Iron supplements treat anemia."
3. "Iron prevents constipation."
4. "Iron potentiates immunosuppression."

24. 2. Clients with ulcerative colitis often have chronic blood loss through the intestines. Iron supplements help with iron deficiency anemia. Iron does not treat the ulcers. Often iron supplements cause constipation. Iron does not cause or potentiate immunosuppression.
CN: Health promotion and maintenance; CNS: None; CL: Analyze

25. What condition is a client with an anorectal fistula at risk for developing?
1. Crohn's disease
2. Diverticulitis
3. Diverticulosis
4. Ulcerative colitis

25. 1. In advanced cases, the lesions of Crohn's disease become transmural, and involve all thicknesses of the bowel. These lesions may perforate the bowel wall, forming fistulas with adjacent structures. Fistulas don't develop in diverticulitis or diverticulosis. The ulcers that occur in the submucosal and mucosal layers of the intestine in ulcerative colitis usually don't progress to fistula formation as in Crohn's disease.
CN: Physiological integrity; CNS: Physiological adaptation; CL: Analyze

26. A client with Crohn's disease has been experiencing 20 watery stools per day. What is the nurse's **priority** assessment?
1. Heart rate
2. Urinary output
3. Blood pressure
4. Electrolytes

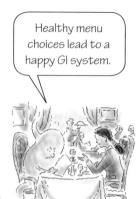

Healthy menu choices lead to a happy GI system.

26. 4. The client who has 20 watery stools per day is at high risk for fluid and electrolyte imbalance. Electrolyte imbalance leads to dysrhythmias and acid base alteration. The highest priority is to assess electrolytes, then assess heart rate, blood pressure and finally urinary output. Electrolyte and fluid replacement is a priority for this client.
CN: Physiological integrity; CNS: Physiological adaptation; CL: Analyze

27. What precautions should the nurse take while caring for a client infected with *Clostridium difficile*? Select all that apply.
1. Wash hands with antimicrobial soap before leaving the room
2. Wear gloves when entering the room
3. Provide client with disposal dishes
4. Provide mask for client when going to X-ray
5. Place patient in room away from the nurses' station

27. 1, 2. The nurse should wear gloves when entering this client's room, and wash his hands with antimicrobial soap before leaving. Clients can leave their room if precautions are taken. Disposable dishes are not necessary for contact precautions. A mask is not necessary when leaving the room. Room location does not matter; however, clients are kept in isolation and should not share a room with clients with other infections.
CN: Safety and effective care environment; CNS: Safety and infection control; CL: Apply

28. What information should the nurse give to a client with *Clostridium difficile* infection?
1. Antibiotic use can cause *C. difficile* to proliferate in the bowel
2. Steroid therapy often causes *C. difficile* diarrhea
3. Malabsorption causes *C. difficile* to grow in the bowel
4. Genetic abnormalities are the most common cause of *C. difficile* diarrhea

28. 1. Antibiotic use can cause *C. difficile* to proliferate in the bowel and result in diarrhea. The condition is not caused by steroid therapy, malabsorption or genetic abnormalities.
CN: Physiological integrity; CNS: Physiological adaptation; CL: Analyze

29. What information, about transmission and recovery, is essential for the client diagnosed with hepatitis B?
1. Most clients with hepatitis B recover and clear the virus from their system.
2. Hepatitis B has a short incubation period
3. Alcohol consumption will not affect recovery in the acute phase of illness
4. Hepatitis B is not a risk factor for cirrhosis and liver cancer

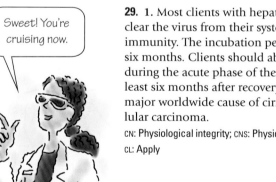

Sweet! You're cruising now.

29. 1. Most clients with hepatitis B recover and clear the virus from their system and then develop immunity. The incubation period is from one to six months. Clients should abstain from alcohol during the acute phase of the illness and for at least six months after recovery. Hepatitis B is a major worldwide cause of cirrhosis and hepatocellular carcinoma.
CN: Physiological integrity; CNS: Physiological adaptation; CL: Apply

30. A client diagnosed with hepatitis B states, "How did I develop this condition?" How should the nurse respond?
1. "Common risks include unprotected sex with an infected partner."
2. "Blood transfusions are the most common risk."
3. "Contaminated food is the most common cause."
4. "Swimming in contaminated water is a primary risk."

30. 1. Clients who have unprotected sex with an infected partner risk transmission. Accidental needle sticks, sharing needles, and hemodialysis are also potential causes of hepatitis B. Blood transfusions are not currently a risk. It is not spread through food or water.
CN: Safe, effective care environment; CNS: Safety and infection control; CL: Understand.

CN: Client needs category   CNS: Client needs subcategory   CL: Cognitive level

31. The nurse is caring for a client on total parenteral nutrition (TPN). What is the nurse's **priority** intervention for the client?
1. Monitoring electrolytes
2. Monitoring urinary output
3. Assessing ability to swallow
4. Assessing consistency of stool

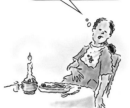

Ugh! I think I need to give my stomach a break.

31. **1.** The high glucose content of TPN can contribute to excess urine output and fluid and electrolytes imbalance. Serum electrolytes and glucose should be monitored daily, or per facility protocol. There is no need to assess the client's ability to swallow, as the TPN is administered intravenously. Monitoring urinary output and the consistency of stool is not as high a priority as monitoring electrolytes but should be completed.
CN: Physiological integrity; CNS: Physiological adaptation; CL: Apply

32. A client is receiving total parenteral nutrition (TPN) and has less than 50 ml of solution left in their TPN bag. There is a delay, and the next bag is not available from the pharmacy. What is the **best** action for the nurse to take?
1. Hang 500 ml normal saline at 100 ml/hr
2. Infuse 10% dextrose at the ordered rate of the TPN
3. Flush the intravenous line and convert it to a heparin lock
4. Assess blood glucose continuously

32. **2.** This client should continue to receive IV fluid because of the potential for fluid and electrolyte shifts and an alteration in blood glucose levels. Normal saline will not stabilize the client's blood glucose. Continuous blood glucose monitoring is not necessary; however, the nurse should continuously evaluate the client's fluid and electrolyte balance.
CN: Physiological integrity; CNS: Reduction of Risk potential; CL: Apply

33. A client presents to the emergency department with chest pain, achalasia, and unintentional weight loss. What additional assessment findings will the nurse expect to find in a client with achalasia?
1. Difficulty swallowing
2. Positive cardiac enzymes
3. Elevated serum potassium
4. Diarrhea

33. **1.** Difficulty swallowing is another symptom of achalasia. The esophageal sphincter usually relaxes when a client swallows. In achalasia, it does not relax, and peristalsis is reduced. Cardiac enzymes are not elevated in this condition. Serum potassium is not elevated in achalasia. Diarrhea is not a symptom associated with this disorder.
CN: Physiological Integrity; CNS: Physiological Adaptation; CL: Analyze

34. Which condition increases the risk for surgery in a client with ulcerative colitis?
1. Bowel intussusception
2. Bowel herniation
3. Bowel outpouching
4. Bowel perforation

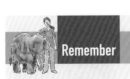

Remember

With acetaminophen, remember the two "A's":
- Analgesic
- Antipyretic

34. **4.** Bowel perforation, obstruction, hemorrhage, and toxic megacolon are common complications of ulcerative colitis that may require surgery. Gastritis and herniation are not associated with irritable bowel disease, and outpouching of the bowel wall is diverticulosis.
CN: Physiological integrity; CNS: Physiological adaptation; CL: Apply

35. The nurse is preparing to administer pain medication to a client diagnosed with irritable bowel disease (IBD). Which medication would the nurse anticipate for this client?
1. Acetaminophen
2. Fentanyl
3. Prednisone
4. Docusate

35. **3.** The pain of IBD is caused by inflammation, which steroids can reduce. Acetaminophen has little effect on pain, and opiates won't treat its underlying cause. Stool softeners do not treat the pain of irritable bowel disease
CN: Physiological integrity; CNS: Pharmacological and parenteral therapies; CL: Analyze

CN: Client needs category   CNS: Client needs subcategory   CL: Cognitive level

36. The nurse is caring for a client two days post abdominal surgery. The surgery resulted in the creation of a stoma. What is the nurse's **priority** while caring for this client?
1. Assessing the client's body image
2. Teaching the client how to care for the stoma
3. Addressing the client's sexual concerns
4. Explaining dietary changes

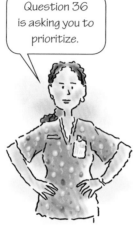

Question 36 is asking you to prioritize.

36. 2. Although these are all concerns that the nurse should address, caring for the stoma is crucial before discharge. Dietary changes would be the next highest priority. Assessing for needs related to body image and sexual concerns would follow.
CN: Physiological integrity; CNS: Physiological adaptation; CL: Apply

37. Which condition might the nurse find in the medical history of a client with colon cancer?
1. Appendicitis
2. Hemorrhoids
3. Hiatal hernia
4. Ulcerative colitis

37. 4. Chronic ulcerative colitis, granulomas, and familial polyposis seem to increase a person's chance of developing colon cancer. The other conditions listed have no known effect on colon cancer risk.
CN: Health promotion and maintenance; CNS: None; CL: Apply

38. A nurse is providing nutritional teaching for a client with a family history of colon cancer. Which choice demonstrates an understanding of the appropriate diet for the client?
1. Vegetarian chili
2. Hot dogs and sauerkraut
3. Egg salad on rye bread
4. Spaghetti and meat sauce

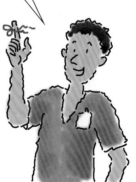

Don't forget. Screening for colon cancer should be on the "to do" list of anyone over 50 years old.

38. 1. A high-fiber, low-fat food, such as vegetarian chili, increases motility, decreases the chance of constipation, and is recommended to help avoid colon cancer. The other choices are not high-fiber and low-fat choices.
CN: Physiological integrity; CNS: Basic care and comfort; CL: Apply

39. The nurse teaches a client, who is over 50 years of age and at risk for colon cancer, about health promotion interventions. What is the **most** important information for the nurse to provide?
1. Abdominal computed tomography (CT) scan
2. Abdominal X-ray
3. Colonoscopy
4. Fecal occult blood test

39. 4. Surface blood vessels of polyps and cancers are fragile and often bleed with the passage of stools. A fecal occult blood test should be performed annually. Abdominal X-ray and CT scan can help establish tumor size and metastasis. A colonoscopy can help to locate a tumor as well as polyps, but is only recommended every 10 years.
CN: Health promotion and maintenance; CNS: None; CL: Apply

40. A client with colon cancer is scheduled to receive radiation therapy prior to surgery. What should the nurse include in the teaching plan about the use of radiation therapy?
1. It helps reduce the size of the tumor.
2. It eliminates the malignant cells.
3. It may cure the cancer.
4. It helps heal the bowel after surgery.

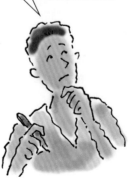

Hmm. If radiation therapy is used before surgery, what is its purpose?

40. 1. Radiation therapy is used before surgery to reduce the size of the tumor, making it easier to be resected. Radiation therapy isn't curative, can't eliminate malignant cells, and could slow postoperative healing.
CN: Physiological integrity; CNS: Physiological adaptation; CL: Apply

CN: Client needs category   CNS: Client needs subcategory   CL: Cognitive level

41. Which symptoms would the nurse anticipate in a client newly diagnosed with colon cancer?
1. A change in appetite
2. A change in bowel habits
3. An increase in body weight
4. An increase in body temperature

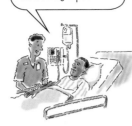

It's important to ask the client about symptoms.

41. 2. The most common report of the client with colon cancer is a change in bowel habits. The client may have anorexia, secondary abdominal distention, or weight loss. Fever isn't related to colon cancer.
CN: Physiological integrity; CNS: Physiological adaptation; CL: Apply

42. A client is in the immediate postoperative stage following a bowel resection. What assessments are important for the nurse to make? Select all that apply.
1. Breath sounds
2. Temperature
3. Wound infection
4. Swallowing reflex
5. Reflux assessment

42. 1, 2, 3. After bowel surgery, the client is at risk for infection and respiratory compromise. The first line of defense has been breached for the surgical incision. The nurse should assess breath sounds to determine adequate gas exchange and the possible development of hypostatic pneumonia. Monitoring temperature will determine if the client is normothermic, or experiencing potential complications of malignant hyperthermia. Wound infection does not occur immediately after surgery. It is generally occurs four to five days postoperative. Swallowing reflex and assessment for reflux are not priority assessments, and are not related to colon surgery.
CN: Physiological integrity; CNS: Physiological adaptation; CL: Apply

43. Which symptom, if reported by a client, would lead the nurse to suspect gastric cancer?
1. Abdominal cramping
2. Constant hunger
3. Feeling of fullness
4. Weight gain

43. 3. The client with gastric cancer may report a feeling of fullness in the stomach but not enough to cause him to seek medical care. Abdominal cramping isn't associated with gastric cancer. Anorexia and weight loss are common symptoms of gastric cancer.
CN: Physiological integrity; CNS: Physiological adaptation; CL: Apply

44. A client is seen in the outpatient surgical clinic for a suspected diagnosis of gastric cancer. Which diagnostic test should the nurse anticipate for this client?
1. Barium enema
2. Colonoscopy
3. Endoscopy
4. Serum chemistry levels

44. 3. An endoscopy will allow direct visualization of the tumor. A colonoscopy or a barium enema will help diagnose colon cancer, not gastric cancer. Serum chemistry levels don't contribute useful data to the assessment of gastric cancer.
CN: Health promotion and maintenance; CNS: None; CL: Apply

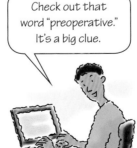

Check out that word "preoperative." It's a big clue.

45. A client with gastric cancer anticipates having surgery for a gastric resection. What is the **most** important nursing intervention during the preoperative period?
1. Discharge planning
2. Correction of nutritional deficits
3. Prevention of deep vein thrombosis
4. Instruction regarding radiation treatment

45. 2. Clients with gastric cancer commonly have nutritional deficits and may be cachectic. Discharge planning before surgery is important, but correcting the nutritional deficit is a higher priority. Prevention of deep-vein thrombosis is not a high priority prior to surgery. Radiation therapy has not been proven effective for gastric cancer, and teaching about it preoperatively would not be appropriate.
CN: Safe, effective care environment; CNS: Management of care; CL: Apply

46. Which is the **priority** care need of a client following gastric resection surgery?
1. Body image
2. Nutritional needs
3. Skin care
4. Spiritual needs

46. 2. After gastric resection, a client may require total parenteral nutrition, or have jejunostomy tube feedings to maintain adequate nutritional status to promote healing. Body image is not a priority at this time because clothing can cover the incision site. Incisional care is necessary to prevent infection; otherwise, the skin should not be affected. Spiritual needs may be a concern, and should be addressed as the client demonstrates readiness.
CN: Safe, effective care environment; CNS: Management of care; CL: Analyze

47. What is the **most** important information for the nurse to teach a client who has been diagnosed with hepatitis C? Select all that apply.
1. "This disease is spread by airborne transmission."
2. "Hepatitis C can cause liver failure."
3. "You should not drink alcohol if you have this diagnosis."
4. "Constipation is a common manifestation of this disorder."
5. "Rest, vitamins and diet will prompt remission."

47. 2, 3. Hepatitis C is a leading cause of cirrhosis and liver failure. It is an infectious blood borne illness that becomes chronic. Inflammation, caused by infection, leads to scarring of the liver. Alcohol consumption contributes to disease progression, and increases the severity of the liver damage. Rest, vitamins and diet are beneficial, but will not prompt remission. Constipation is not a common manifestation, and the hepatitis C is not airborne.
CN: Physiological integrity; CNS: Reduction of risk potential; CL: Apply

48. A client reports having several episodes of rectal bleeding, ribbon-shaped stools, and abdominal cramping. What is the nurse's **priority** action?
1. Assess for hemorrhoids and constipation
2. Auscultate bowel sounds and percuss the abdomen
3. Assist the client with preparation for colonoscopy
4. Palpate the liver and assess for jugular vein distention

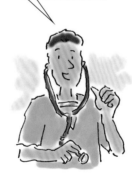

Take a listen to what your client's stomach is trying to tell you.

48. 3. Rectal bleeding, ribbon-shaped stool, and abdominal cramping are all associated with colorectal cancer. Further assessment will be made by having a colonoscopy. The nurse should teach the client about this diagnostic test. Hemorrhoids do not cause ribbon-shaped stools and cramping. Auscultation of bowel sounds and percussion will help determine the client's condition. The symptoms are not associated with liver failure or jugular vein distention.
CN: Physiological integrity; CNS: Physiological adaptation; CL: Analyze

49. A nurse cares for multiple clients with obesity. Which client does the nurse consider the **best** candidate for bariatric surgery?
1. The client with a BMI of 29
2. The client with truncal obesity
3. The client with arthritis
4. The client with peptic ulcer disease

49. 3. Bariatric surgery is an intervention for clients who have not responded to other interventions, and who have medical risks affected by obesity, such as arthritis. A BMI of 29 is not high enough for consideration for this intervention. Truncal obesity might be a sign of an endocrine disorder, and other assessments should be made prior to considering surgery. A peptic ulcer is a contraindication for this type of surgery.
CN: Health promotion and maintenance; CNS: None; CL: Analyze

CN: Client needs category   CNS: Client needs subcategory   CL: Cognitive level

50. A client is considering gastric bypass versus minimally invasive gastric surgery. What fact is appropriate to tell this client?
1. Gastric bypass surgery is rarely performed
2. Dumping syndrome is associated with minimally invasive surgery
3. Recovery time is quicker for minimally invasive surgery
4. There is less scarring with gastric bypass surgery.

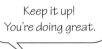
Keep it up! You're doing great.

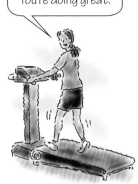

50. 3. Recovery is quicker for minimally invasive surgery, and there are relatively few side effects. Gastric bypass surgery is a common surgery. There is less scarring with minimally invasive surgery. Dumping syndrome is not associated with minimally invasive surgery.
CN: Safe, Physiological integrity; CNS: Reduction of Risk Potential; CL: Apply

51. Which condition may lead to hemorrhoids?
1. Diarrhea
2. Diverticulosis
3. Portal hypertension
4. Rectal bleeding

51. 3. Portal hypertension and other conditions associated with persistently high intra-abdominal pressure, such as pregnancy, can lead to hemorrhoids. The passing of hard stool, not diarrhea, can aggravate hemorrhoids. Diverticulosis has no relationship to hemorrhoids. Rectal bleeding can be a symptom of hemorrhoids.
CN: Physiological integrity; CNS: Physiological adaptation; CL: Analyze

52. Which assessment is **most** relevant with the diagnosis of hemorrhoids?
1. Abdominal assessment
2. Diet history
3. Digital rectal examination
4. Sexual history

52. 3. A digital rectal examination is important to assess for internal hemorrhoids, and to determine if other causes of the pain and bleeding are present. Abdominal assessment is not necessary for hemorrhoids. Dietary history is relevant because constipation can worsen hemorrhoids, but it isn't as important to diagnosis as a digital rectal examination. Sexual history may also be relevant, but isn't as important as a digital rectal examination.
CN: Physiological integrity; CNS: Physiological adaptation; CL: Analyze

53. A client has been diagnosed with Barrett's esophagus. What should the nurse teach this client regarding his diagnosis?
1. "This condition increases the risk of esophageal cancer."
2. "This condition can cause vomiting."
3. "Diarrhea often results from this condition."
4. "A yearly colonoscopy is necessary for screening."

53. 1. Barrett's esophagus is a complication of gastroesophageal reflux disease. Normal tissue lining the esophagus changes to tissue resembling the lining of the intestine. While there are no specific symptoms, it increases the risk of developing esophageal adenocarcinoma. Routine screening is recommended; however, yearly colonoscopies are not necessary for this upper gastrointestinal problem.
CN: Physiological integrity; CNS: Physiological adaptation; CL: Apply

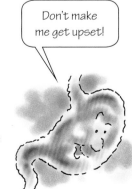
Don't make me get upset!

54. A client asks why he is having a vagotomy to treat his peptic ulcer. What is the nurse's **best** response?
1. "To repair a hole in the stomach."
2. "To reduce the ability of the stomach to produce acid."
3. "To prevent the stomach from sliding into the chest."
4. "To remove a potentially malignant lesion in the stomach."

54. 2. A vagotomy is performed to eliminate the acid-secreting stimulus to gastric cells. A perforation would be repaired with a gastric resection. Repair of a hiatal hernia prevents the stomach from sliding through the diaphragm. Removal of a potentially malignant tumor would not reduce the entire acid-producing mechanism.
CN: Physiological integrity; CNS: Reduction of risk potential; CL: Apply

CN: Client needs category   CNS: Client needs subcategory   CL: Cognitive level

55. A client is admitted with peritonitis. Which condition, found in the client's history, is **most** likely to have contributed to this inflammation?
1. Cholelithiasis
2. Gastritis
3. Perforated ulcer
4. Incarcerated hernia

55. 3. The most common cause of peritonitis is a perforated ulcer, which can pour contaminants into the peritoneal cavity, causing inflammation and infection within the cavity. The other conditions are not direct causes of peritonitis. If cholelithiasis leads to rupture of the gallbladder, gastritis leads to erosion of the stomach wall, or an incarcerated hernia leads to rupture of the intestines, peritonitis may also develop.
CN: Physiological integrity; CNS: Physiological adaptation; CL: Analyze

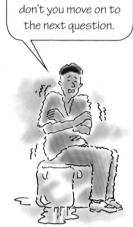

Brain freeze? Why don't you move on to the next question.

56. A client is admitted in the early stages of peritonitis. What is the nurse's **priority** assessment?
1. Abdominal distention
2. Abdominal pain and rigidity
3. Hyperactive bowel sounds
4. Right upper quadrant pain

56. 2. Abdominal pain, causing rigidity of the abdominal muscles, is characteristic of peritonitis. Abdominal distention may occur as a late sign. Bowel sounds may be normal or decreased. Right upper quadrant pain is characteristic of cholecystitis or hepatitis.
CN: Health promotion and maintenance; CNS: None; CL: Apply

57. Which laboratory result would the nurse anticipate in a client with peritonitis?
1. Partial thromboplastin time above 100 seconds
2. Hemoglobin level below 10 mg/dl
3. Potassium level above 5.5 mEq/L
4. White blood cell (WBC) count above 15,000/µl

57. 4. Because of infection, the client's WBC count will be elevated. A partial thromboplastin time longer than 100 seconds may suggest disseminated intravascular coagulation (DIC), a serious complication of septic shock. A hemoglobin level below 10 mg/dl may occur from hemorrhage. A potassium level above 5.5 mEq/L may suggest renal failure.
CN: Physiological integrity; CNS: Reduction of risk potential; CL: Apply

58. A recently admitted client is suspected of having peritonitis. He's requesting a glass of water to drink. Which would be the nurse's **best** response to the client?
1. "I can give you small amounts of water frequently."
2. "I will get you some sugar free candy."
3. "I'll check with the health care provider."
4. "Until your diagnosis is confirmed and bowel function returns, it would not be safe to give you anything to drink."

58. 4. The client with peritonitis is not commonly allowed anything orally until the source of the peritonitis is confirmed and treated. Intravenous fluids are given to maintain hydration, hemodynamic stability and to replace electrolytes. Sugar free candy does not provide fluid and may result in abdominal pain and diarrhea. Checking with the health care provider isn't necessary.
CN: Physiological integrity; CNS: Physiological adaptation; CL: Apply

59. What is the nurse's **priority** while caring for a client with peritonitis?
1. Fluid and electrolyte balance
2. Gastric irrigation
3. Pain management
4. Psychosocial issues

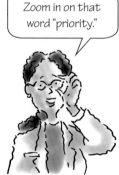

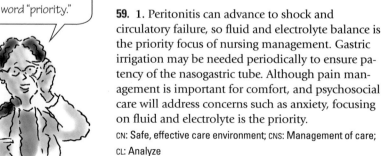

Zoom in on that word "priority."

59. 1. Peritonitis can advance to shock and circulatory failure, so fluid and electrolyte balance is the priority focus of nursing management. Gastric irrigation may be needed periodically to ensure patency of the nasogastric tube. Although pain management is important for comfort, and psychosocial care will address concerns such as anxiety, focusing on fluid and electrolyte is the priority.
CN: Safe, effective care environment; CNS: Management of care; CL: Analyze

60. What is the **most** important information for the nurse to teach the client about the development of pancreatitis?
1. Alcohol abuse
2. Hypercalcemia
3. Hyperlipidemia
4. Pancreatic duct obstruction

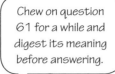

Chew on question 61 for a while and digest its meaning before answering.

60. 1. Alcohol abuse is the major cause of acute pancreatitis in males, although gallbladder disease is more commonly implicated in women. Hypercalcemia, hyperlipidemia, and pancreatic duct obstruction are also less common causes of pancreatitis.
CN: Physiological integrity; CNS: Reduction of risk potential; CL: Apply

61. Which intervention is a **priority** within the first 24 hours following bariatric surgery?
1. Activity
2. Pain control
3. Diet teaching
4. Exercise

61. 2. Pain control is the priority in the first 24 hours following any type of bariatric surgery. Dietary teaching should be completed prior to discharge, but is not a higher priority than pain control. Information about exercise for weight loss can be included in the discharge plan.
CN: Physiological integrity; CNS: Physiological adaptation; CL: Apply

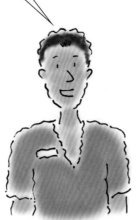

62. Which laboratory test would the nurse anticipate to help diagnose pancreatitis?
1. Amylase level
2. Hemoglobin level
3. Blood glucose level
4. White blood cell count

62. 1. Amylase is an enzyme secreted by the pancreas. When elevated, it's useful in diagnosing pancreatitis. Hemoglobin level can be low in pancreatitis, but there can be other causes for this. The blood glucose level may be elevated with pancreatitis, but this factor is not diagnostic. The white blood cell count may be elevated in pancreatitis, but this symptom can be due to infection.
CN: Health promotion and maintenance; CNS: None; CL: Analyze

63. A client with pancreatitis may exhibit Cullen's sign on physical examination. Which assessment finding best describes Cullen's sign?
1. Jaundiced sclera
2. Pain that occurs with movement
3. Spasms of the arm when a blood pressure cuff is applied
4. Bluish discoloration of the periumbilical area

63. 4. Cullen's sign is bluish discoloration of the periumbilical area from subcutaneous intraperitoneal hemorrhagic pancreatitis. Jaundiced sclera occurs with hepatitis. Pain with movement is a common finding with peritonitis. One Trousseau sign seen in hypocalcemia is spasms of the arm when a blood pressure cuff is applied.
CN: Health promotion and maintenance; CNS: None; CL: Analyze

64. Which factor should be the **initial** focus of nursing management in a client with acute pancreatitis?
1. Dietary management
2. Prevention of skin breakdown
3. Management of hypoglycemia
4. Pain control

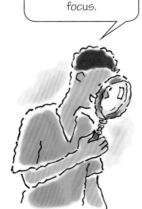

Look for the initial focus.

64. 4. The priority is to provide adequate pain control. This is essential to minimize discomfort and restlessness, which may stimulate pancreatic secretion further. Initially, the client with acute pancreatitis isn't permitted food and oral intake. Although prevention of skin breakdown is important, it isn't the initial focus. Clients are at risk for hyperglycemia, not hypoglycemia.
CN: Physiological integrity; CNS: Physiological adaptation; CL: Analyze

CN: Client needs category   CNS: Client needs subcategory   CL: Cognitive level

65. What should the nurse assess for while admitting a client to the hospital with suspected acute pancreatitis?
1. Hypoglycemia
2. Hypernatremia
3. Hypocalcemia
4. Hyperkalemia

65. **3.** The client with acute pancreatitis may exhibit hypocalcemia due to the deposit of calcium in areas of fat necrosis. Hyperglycemia, not hypoglycemia, may occur due to reduced insulin production caused by the islet of Langerhans involvement. Hypokalemia and hyponatremia may occur because potassium is lost in emesis, but hypernatremia is unlikely.
CN: Physiological integrity; CNS: Physiological adaptation; CL: Analyze

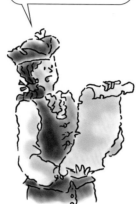

Hear ye, hear ye! Local nursing student aces NCLEX exam!

66. If a client's gastric ulcer perforates, which action should the nurse include in the management of care?
1. Removal of the nasogastric (NG) tube
2. Antacid administration
3. H2-receptor antagonist administration
4. Fluid and electrolyte replacement

66. **4.** The client should be treated with antibiotics as well as fluid, electrolyte, and blood replacement per provider's order. NG tube suction should also be performed to prevent further spillage of stomach contents into the perineal cavity. Antacids and H2-receptor antagonists are not helpful in this situation.
CN: Physiological integrity; CNS: Physiological adaptation; CL: Apply

67. A client presents to the emergency department with abdominal pain, weight loss, steatorrhea, and a random glucose of 417 mg/dl. Which diagnostic test should the nurse anticipate?
1. Abdominal computed tomography scan
2. Lower gastrointestinal series
3. Ultrasound of the abdomen
4. Colonoscopy

67. **3.** The symptoms correlate with chronic pancreatitis. An abdominal ultrasound could reveal pancreatic changes. The other tests are of no value in evaluating the pancreas.
CN: Physiological integrity; CNS: Physiological adaptation; CL: Analyze

Remember

With aspirin (acetylsalicylic acid), remember the four "A's":
- Analgesic
- Antipyretic
- Anti-inflammatory
- Anticoagulant

68. Which intervention is **most** appropriate to reduce the exacerbation of pain for a client with pancreatitis?
1. Lying in a supine position
2. Taking aspirin
3. Eating a low-fat diet
4. Abstaining from alcohol

68. **4.** Abstaining from alcohol is imperative to reducing pancreatic injury, and may completely control pain. Lying in a supine position usually aggravates the pain because it stretches the abdominal muscles. Taking aspirin can cause bleeding in hemorrhagic pancreatitis. During an attack of acute pancreatitis, the client is not allowed to ingest anything orally.
CN: Physiological integrity; CNS: Reduction of risk potential; CL: Apply

69. A client with cirrhosis reports that his skin always feels itchy. Which abnormality, associated with cirrhosis, results in itching?
1. Prolonged prothrombin time
2. Decreased protein level
3. Increased bilirubin level
4. Increased aspartate aminotransferase level

69. **3.** High bilirubin levels irritate peripheral nerves, causing an intense itching sensation. Itching is not a symptom of prolonged prothrombin time, decreased protein levels, or increased aspartate aminotransferase levels.
CN: Physiological integrity; CNS: Physiological adaptation; CL: Analyze

CN: Client needs category   CNS: Client needs subcategory   CL: Cognitive level

70. A client presents with dark urine, fatigue, and generalized pruritus. Lab results reveal elevated serum bilirubin and increased bile salts. The diagnosis of biliary cirrhosis is made. The client asks what is happening in his body. What is the nurse's **best** response?
1. "There is an obstruction of the bile ducts causing biliary inflammation."
2. "Your liver is releasing toxins, which are poisonous to your circulation."
3. "The alcohol you have consumed has caused small nodules to form in your liver."
4. "The weakened heart muscle has limited blood flow to the liver."

71. The nurse is assessing a client admitted to rule out cirrhosis. Which assessment finding would support this diagnosis?
1. Dry skin
2. Hepatomegaly
3. Peripheral edema
4. Pruritus

72. Which diagnostic test will confirm a client's diagnosis of cirrhosis?
1. Albumin level
2. Bromsulphthalein dye excretion
3. Liver biopsy
4. Liver enzyme levels

73. Which assessment finding does the nurse expect to find in a client with a diagnosis of cirrhosis?
1. Increased carbon dioxide level
2. Increased pH level
3. Increased prothrombin time
4. Increased white blood cell (WBC) count

74. Which is the **priority** nursing action while caring for a client with esophageal varices?
1. Assessing for hemorrhage
2. Controlling blood pressure
3. Encouraging nutritional intake
4. Teaching the client about varices

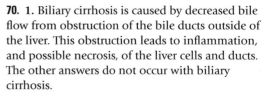

Remember to feed your brain well to stay sharp.

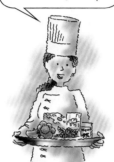

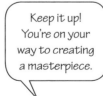

Keep it up! You're on your way to creating a masterpiece.

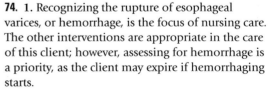

70. 1. Biliary cirrhosis is caused by decreased bile flow from obstruction of the bile ducts outside of the liver. This obstruction leads to inflammation, and possible necrosis, of the liver cells and ducts. The other answers do not occur with biliary cirrhosis.
CN: Physiological integrity; CNS: Physiological adaptation; CL: Analyze

71. 2. The client with cirrhosis has a liver that is enlarged, fibrotic, and nodular, which makes it palpable. The client may develop dry skin, pruritus, and peripheral edema, but these symptoms may have other causes.
CN: Physiological integrity; CNS: Physiological adaptation; CL: Analyze

72. 3. A liver biopsy can reveal the exact cause of hepatomegaly. The albumin level will be low, but that can be caused by poor nutritional states. Bromsulphthalein dye excretion may be reduced, but could be caused by other hepatocirculatory disorders. Liver enzymes may be elevated, but other liver conditions may cause these elevations.
CN: Physiological integrity; CNS: Physiological adaptation; CL: Apply

73. 3. Clotting factors may not be produced normally when a client has cirrhosis, increasing the potential for bleeding. There is no associated change in carbon dioxide level or pH unless the client is developing other comorbidities, such as metabolic alkalosis. The WBC count can be elevated in acute cirrhosis but it is not always altered.
CN: Physiological integrity; CNS: Physiological adaptation; CL: Apply

74. 1. Recognizing the rupture of esophageal varices, or hemorrhage, is the focus of nursing care. The other interventions are appropriate in the care of this client; however, assessing for hemorrhage is a priority, as the client may expire if hemorrhaging starts.
CN: Physiological integrity; CNS: Reduction of Risk Potential; CL: Apply

CN: Client needs category   CNS: Client needs subcategory   CL: Cognitive level

75. Several children at a day care center have been infected with hepatitis A virus. What is the **most** important information the nurse can provide to the parents and day care workers to reduce the risk of hepatitis A transmission?
1. Hand washing after diaper changes
2. Isolation of the sick children
3. Use of masks during contact with the children
4. Sterilization of all eating utensils

75. 1. Children in day care centers are at risk of hepatitis A infection, which is transmitted via fecal-oral route due to poor hand hygiene practices and poor sanitation. Isolation of sick children, use of mask during contact, and sterilization of all eating utensils would not be useful in breaking the chain of infection.
CN: Safe, effective care environment; CNS: Safety and infection control; CL: Apply

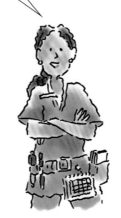

Remember all the tools you have in your tool belt when you answer a question.

76. A client is being evaluated for hepatitis A. Which activity places the client at greatest risk for the development of hepatitis A?
1. Helping his roommate with an epistaxis episode
2. Receiving an elective blood transfusion after surgery
3. Eating a shrimp platter at a local restaurant
4. Having sexual intercourse with his fiancée

76. 3. Hepatitis A can be caused by contact with contaminated feces, and may be transmitted through infected water, milk, or food, especially shellfish from contaminated waters. Hepatitis B is caused by blood contact and sexual contact. Hepatitis C is usually caused by contact with infected blood, including blood transfusions.
CN: Health promotion and maintenance; CNS: None; CL: Apply

77. The nurse is providing discharge teaching to a client diagnosed with a peptic ulcer. The client asks the nurse which type of pain medication he can take. Which response, by the nurse, would be the **best**?
1. Aspirin
2. Acetaminophen
3. Naproxen
4. Ibuprofen

77. 2. Acetaminophen is recommended for pain relief because it does not promote irritation of the mucosa. Aspirin and nonsteroidal anti-inflammatory drugs such as naproxen and ibuprofen may cause irritation of the mucosa and subsequent bleeding.
CN: Physiological integrity; CNS: Pharmacological and parenteral therapies; CL: Apply

78. The nurse is performing an assessment on a client being evaluated for viral hepatitis. Which symptom will the nurse most likely assess on this client?
1. Arthralgia
2. Irritability
3. Headache
4. Polyphagia

78. 1. Arthralgia is common in clients with viral hepatitis. Other symptoms of viral hepatitis include lethargy, flulike symptoms, anorexia, nausea and vomiting, abdominal pain, diarrhea, constipation, and fever. Excitability, headache, and polyphagia are not symptoms of viral hepatitis.
CN: Physiological integrity; CNS: Physiological adaptation; CL: Apply

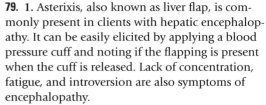

You're making this look easy!

79. A client is admitted with a diagnosis of hepatic encephalopathy. What would the nurse's assessment documentation include?
1. Asterixis
2. Migraines
3. Nuchal rigidity
4. Abdominal distention

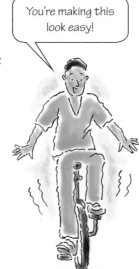

79. 1. Asterixis, also known as liver flap, is commonly present in clients with hepatic encephalopathy. It can be easily elicited by applying a blood pressure cuff and noting if the flapping is present when the cuff is released. Lack of concentration, fatigue, and introversion are also symptoms of encephalopathy.
CN: Physiological integrity; CNS: Physiological adaptation; CL: Apply

80. Which dietary instructions should the nurse provide to a client with toxic hepatitis?
1. Increase fiber in the diet
2. Decrease carbohydrates in the diet
3. Decrease protein in the diet
4. Eat high-calorie foods

80. 4. Instructions to a client with toxic hepatitis should include consuming a high-calorie diet. The client is allowed to eat and drink, and does not need to consume low-calorie or low-residue foods.
CN: Physiological integrity; CNS: Basic care and comfort;
CL: Apply

81. A client with suspected liver cancer is admitted to the hospital. Which diagnostic test does the nurse anticipate the healthcare provider to order as confirmation of this diagnosis?
1. Abdominal ultrasound
2. Abdominal X-ray
3. Cholangiogram
4. Computed tomography (CT) scan

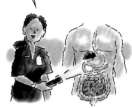

Which test sheds the most light on liver cancer?

81. 4. A client with suspected liver cancer will likely undergo CT imaging to identify tumors. The results of a CT scan are much more definitive than the findings of an ultrasound or X-ray. A cholangiogram evaluates the gallbladder, not the liver.
CN: Health promotion and maintenance; CNS: None;
CL: Apply

82. The nurse is caring for a client following a liver biopsy. What is a **priority** assessment for this client?
1. Abdominal cramping
2. Hemorrhage
3. Nausea and vomiting
4. Temperature

82. 2. The liver is very vascular, and a biopsy could cause the client to hemorrhage. The client may experience some discomfort but, typically, not cramping. Nausea and vomiting may be present, and infection may occur but not immediately after the procedure, therefore, increases in temperature are unlikely.
CN: Physiological integrity; CNS: Reduction of risk potential;
CL: Apply

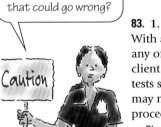

What's the worst that could go wrong?

83. A client with a liver disorder is scheduled to have an invasive procedure. Which test result should the nurse monitor to ensure client safety?
1. Coagulation studies
2. Liver enzymes
3. Serum chemistry
4. White blood cell count

83. 1. The liver produces six blood clotting factors. With any liver disease or trauma, production of any of these factors may be altered, placing the client at risk for hemorrhage. The other laboratory tests should also be monitored, but the results may not necessarily relate to the safety of the procedure.
CN: Physiological integrity; CNS: Reduction of risk potential;
CL: Analyze

84. A nurse is providing instructions to a client who will undergo a liver biopsy the next morning. The client asks the nurse about potential problems. Information about what potential complication should the nurse plan to include in his teaching plan?
1. Paralytic ileus
2. Hemorrhage
3. Renal shutdown
4. Constipation

84. 2. Because the most common adverse effect of a liver biopsy is bleeding, the nurse should provide relevant information regarding the potential for hemorrhage. There is no reason to provide the client with information about paralytic ileus. Renal shutdown is not an expected complication after a liver biopsy. The nurse would have no reason to suspect that the client will have a problem with constipation after a liver biopsy.
CN: Physiological integrity; CNS: Reduction of risk potential;
CL: Apply

CN: Client needs category   CNS: Client needs subcategory   CL: Cognitive level

85. A client is diagnosed with a tumor in the liver, and radiation therapy is started. What information should the nurse include in the teaching plan?
1. Radiation may cause skin irritation.
2. Therapy is usually scheduled once a month.
3. This therapy has no systemic effects.
4. Radiation is often used in isolation.

85. 1. Radiation therapy usually causes skin irritation which can range from redness to blistering. Therapy is given five days a week. Radiation does cause some systemic effects, such as fatigue. This therapy is often used in combination with other therapies for liver cancer.
CN: Physiological integrity; CNS: Physiological adaptation;
CL: Apply

86. Which risk factors would place a client at risk for the development of cholelithiasis? Select all that apply.
1. Use of oral contraceptives
2. History of diabetes mellitus
3. Increased daily exercise
4. Obesity
5. Age less than 25 years

86. 1, 2, 4. Stone formation is frequent in people who use oral contraceptives, estrogen or clofibrate. The incidence of stone formation increases with age, and is greater in those who have diabetes. Daily exercise will not contribute to stone formation.
CN: Health promotion and maintenance; CNS: None;
CL: Apply

87. A client is admitted with the diagnosis of gall stones. Which assessment finding does the nurse expect with this client?
1. Pain on urination
2. Black stools
3. A positive Murphy's sign
4. A positive Trousseau's sign

87. 3. Murphy's sign is elicited when the client reacts to pain, and stops inhaling when the examiner's fingers are on the location of the gallbladder. It's a common finding in clients with cholecystitis. The nurse should teach the client about possible interventions for gallstones. In addition, the nurse should evaluate the client's risk factors for gallstones to determine the cause and prevent future occurrences.
CN: Physiological integrity; CNS: Physiological adaptation;
CL: Apply

88. A 30-year-old female client is suspected of having cholecystitis. What questions should the nurse ask this client? Select all that apply.
1. "Has anyone in your family ever been diagnosed with cholecystitis?"
2. "What is your daily activity routine?"
3. "Do you take birth control pills?"
4. "Are you on hormone replacement therapy?"
5. "Are you a vegetarian?"

88. 1, 2, 3, 4. Risk factors for cholecystitis include a family history, a sedentary lifestyle, and the use of birth control pills. This client is 30 years old, and may have undergone gynecological surgery that would require hormone replacement therapy. A vegetarian diet does not place a client at risk for the development of this disorder.
CN: Health promotion and maintenance; CNS: None;
CL: Apply

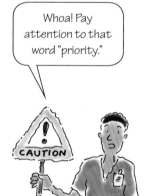

Whoa! Pay attention to that word "priority."

89. The nurse is caring for a client with acute cholecystitis. What is a **priority** intervention for this client?
1. Administration of antibiotics
2. Assessment of vital signs
3. Assessment of white blood cell count
4. Preparation for surgery

89. 2. Assessing vital signs would be a priority to determine any hemodynamic changes such as bleeding or perforation. After the baseline, determination of status labs and antibiotics can be reviewed and treated. Surgery is generally preformed after the acute episode has subsided.
CN: Safe, effective care environment; CNS: Management of care;
CL: Apply

CN: Client needs category   CNS: Client needs subcategory   CL: Cognitive level

90. A nurse has given discharge instructions to a client with chronic cholecystitis. The nurse understands that teaching has been effective when the client states:
  1. "I need to rest more."
  2. "I should avoid taking antacids."
  3. "I should increase the fat in my diet."
  4. "I will take my anticholinergic medications as prescribed."

90. **4.** Conservative therapy for chronic cholecystitis includes weight reduction by increasing physical activity, a low-fat diet, antacid use to treat dyspepsia, and anticholinergic use to relax smooth muscles and reduce ductal tone and spasm.
CN: Physiological integrity; CNS: Reduction of risk potential; CL: Apply

91. Which sign would a nurse's assessment most likely reveal in a client diagnosed with a duodenal ulcer?
  1. Hematemesis
  2. Malnourishment
  3. Melena
  4. Pain with eating

91. **3.** The client with a duodenal ulcer may have bleeding at the ulcer site, which shows up as melena. The other findings are consistent with a gastric ulcer.
CN: Physiological integrity; CNS: Physiological adaptation; CL: Apply

92. What should the nurse instruct a client to do to reduce occurrences of dumping syndrome?
  1. Sip fluids with meals
  2. Eat three meals daily
  3. Lie down after meals for 30 minutes
  4. Eat a high-carbohydrate, low-fat, and low-protein diet

92. **3.** To reduce occurrences of dumping syndrome, clients should be lie down for 30 minutes after eating. They should eat small, frequent low-carbohydrate, high-protein, moderate-fat meals, and avoid sweets. Eating in a semi-recumbent position is also helpful.
CN: Physiological integrity; CNS: Reduction of risk potential; CL: Apply

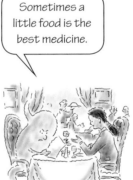

Sometimes a little food is the best medicine.

93. The nurse assesses a client diagnosed with a duodenal ulcer. Which finding would the nurse anticipate?
  1. Early satiety
  2. Pain on eating
  3. Dull upper epigastric pain
  4. Pain when the stomach is empty

93. **4.** Pain of a duodenal ulcer occurs on an empty stomach, and is relieved by eating food or antacids. The other symptoms are those of a gastric ulcer.
CN: Physiological integrity; CNS: Physiological adaptation; CL: Apply

94. The nurse has just admitted a client to "rule out" peptic ulcer. Which diagnostic study would the nurse anticipate?
  1. Abdominal X-ray
  2. Barium swallow
  3. Computed tomography (CT) scan of the abdomen
  4. Esophagogastroduodenoscopy (EGD)

94. **4.** The EGD can visualize the entire upper gastrointestinal tract as well as allow for tissue specimens and electrocautery as needed. The barium swallow could locate a gastric ulcer and may be an initial test performed. A CT scan and an abdominal X-ray aren't useful in the diagnosis of an ulcer.
CN: Health promotion and maintenance; CNS: None; CL: Apply

95. The nurse is preparing to administer ranitidine to a client diagnosed with peptic ulcer disease. What assessment finding indicates the client has had a therapeutic response to the medication?
  1. The client is hungry.
  2. The client has less gastric pain.
  3. The client has less belching.
  4. The client has no diarrhea.

95. **2.** Ranitidine is an H2-receptor antagonist that reduces acid secretion by inhibiting gastrin secretion. It will decrease gastric pain and irritation. The medication will not stimulate hunger, decrease belching or decrease diarrhea in clients who have peptic ulcer disease.
CN: Physiological integrity; CNS: Pharmacological and parenteral therapies; CL: Apply

CN: Client needs category   CNS: Client needs subcategory   CL: Cognitive level

96. The nurse is caring for a client admitted with acute pancreatitis. Which intervention is the **highest** priority for this client's care?
1. Assessment of pancreatic enzymes results
2. Assessment of skin color
3. Assessment of lung sounds
4. Assessment of urinary output

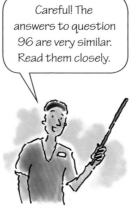

Careful! The answers to question 96 are very similar. Read them closely.

96. 3. Airway and breathing is the priority for this client. Respiratory complications can occur, such as pleural effusion, atelectasis, and pneumonia. An assessment of lung sounds is a priority, and is crucial to the assessment of these conditions. Assessment of skin color for jaundice is important; however, signs such as Cullen and Grey-Turner would indicate development of a necrotizing form of pancreatitis, which would be significant. Urinary output is also important as the client is usually on IV fluids, and it may reflect kidney function.
CN: Physiological integrity; CNS: Physiological adaptation; CL: Analyze

97. Which dietary discharge instruction should the nurse include to prevent a recurrence of the client's pancreatitis?
1. Decrease carbohydrate intake in diet
2. Decrease calories consumed daily
3. Decrease alcohol consumption to one or two drinks per day
4. Avoid beverages that contain caffeine

97. 4. A client with pancreatitis must avoid foods or beverages that can cause a relapse of the disease. Caffeine must be avoided because it's a stimulant that may irritate the pancreas. The client with pancreatitis must avoid all alcohol because it is one of the causes of pancreatitis. The diet should be low in fats and high in calories, especially carbohydrates.
CN: Physiological integrity; CNS: Reduction of risk potential; CL: Apply

98. In which position should the nurse place the client, following a liver biopsy?
1. Left side-lying position, with the bed flat
2. Right side-lying position, with the bed flat
3. Trendelenburg position.
4. High fowlers position.

98. 2. Lying the client on his right side, with the bed flat will splint the biopsy site and minimize bleeding. The other positions will not put pressure on the biopsy site and may allow the client to bleed after the procedure.
CN: Physiological integrity; CNS: Reduction of risk potential; CL: Apply

99. Which breakfast food choices are appropriate for the client diagnosed with irritable bowel syndrome (IBS)?
1. Coffee, scrambled eggs, bacon and toast with butter
2. Skim milk, shredded wheat, toast and jelly
3. Tea with skim milk, pancakes with syrup, sausage
4. Orange juice, vegetable omelet, toast with margarine

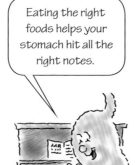

Eating the right foods helps your stomach hit all the right notes.

99. 2. The client with irritable bowel syndrome needs to be on a diet that contains at least 25 g of fiber per day. Fatty foods should be avoided because they may precipitate symptoms. Skim milk, shredded wheat, toast and jelly is the choice that is lowest in fat and highest in fiber for this client.
CN: Physiological integrity; CNS: Basic care and comfort; CL: Apply

100. A client presents to the emergency department, reporting that he has been vomiting every 30 to 40 minutes for the past eight hours. Which intervention is a **priority** for this client?
1. Assess pain and administer opioids
2. Assess hydration and administer fluids
3. Assess nutrition and insert a nasogastric tube
4. Assess blood gasses and replace electrolytes

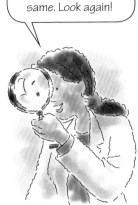

Tricky, tricky. The answers to question 100 all look the same. Look again!

100. 4. The highest risk is that constant vomiting has decreased this clients' acid content, and caused an electrolyte imbalance. Excessive loss of upper gastric fluid causes the client to develop metabolic alkalosis. Electrolytes and bicarbonate needs to be replaced to prevent cardiovascular problems. The second priority is to assess hydration and begin to replace fluids. In this client, pain and nutrition are a lower priority. Once vomiting is controlled a decision may be reached about ways to support nutrition.
CN: Physiological integrity; CNS: Reduction of risk potential; CL: Analyze

101. Five days after undergoing abdominal surgery, a client develops a small-bowel obstruction. Which is the **priority** assessment for this client?
1. Nutritional status
2. Pain
3. Fluid status
4. Bowel sounds

101. 3. Fluid shifts to the site of the bowel obstruction, causing a fluid deficit in the intravascular spaces. If the obstruction isn't resolved immediately, the client may experience imbalanced nutrition and other problems. Because this client can develop more severe problems, and even cardiovascular collapse, if fluid status is not addressed, pain relief should be addressed after fluid status.
CN: Physiological Integrity; CNS: Reduction of Risk Potential; CL: Analyze

102. A client diagnosed with gastroesophageal reflux disease (GERD) presents to the clinic for a follow-up appointment. Which dietary instruction is appropriate for the nurse to provide?
1. "Eat a small snack before bedtime."
2. "Avoid alcohol and caffeine."
3. "Drink 16 oz (0.5 L) of water with each meal."
4. "Eat three well-balanced meals every day."

102. 2. A client with GERD should avoid alcohol, caffeine, and foods that increase acidity, all of which can cause epigastric pain. To further prevent reflux, the client should remain upright for two to three hours after eating, avoid eating before bedtime, avoid bending and wearing tight clothing, avoid drinking large volumes of fluid with meals, and eat small, frequent meals to help reduce gastric acid secretion.
CN: Physiological integrity; CNS: Reduction of risk potential; CL: Apply

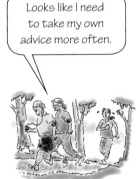

Looks like I need to take my own advice more often.

103. Which instruction should the nurse include when teaching an elderly client how to prevent constipation?
1. "Drink 48 oz (1.5 L) of fluid each day."
2. "Avoid grain products and nuts."
3. "Your diet should include no more than 15 g of fiber per day."
4. "Be sure to get regular exercise."

103. 4. Exercise helps prevent constipation. Fluids and dietary fiber promote normal bowel function. The client should drink 48 oz (1.5 L) of fluid per day. Daily dietary intake of 25 to 30 g/day of fiber is recommended, especially for treatment of constipation in the older adult.
CN: Health promotion and maintenance; CNS: None; CL: Apply

104. The nurse is assessing a client with diarrhea. Which outcome would indicate that fluid resuscitation has been successful?
1. The client passes formed stools at regular intervals.
2. The client reports a decrease in stool frequency and liquidity.
3. The client exhibits firm skin turgor.
4. The client no longer experiences perianal burning.

104. 3. Firm skin turgor would be one indication of successful fluid resuscitation. Other indications would include moist mucous membranes and urine output of at least 30 ml/hr. Passage of formed stools at regular intervals, and a decrease in stool frequency and liquidity indicate successful resolution of diarrhea. The absence of perianal burning indicates that the irritation from the diarrhea is gone.
CN: Physiological integrity; CNS: Basic care and comfort; CL: Analyze

105. Which information does the nurse include in a community education class about the prevention of colon cancer?
1. Limit fat intake to 20 to 25 percent of your total daily calories
2. Include 15 to 20 g of fiber in your daily diet
3. Schedule an annual rectal examination after age 35
4. Undergo sigmoidoscopy annually after age 50

105. 1. To help prevent colon cancer, fats should account for no more than 20 to 25 percent of total daily calories, and the diet should include 25 to 30 g of fiber per day. A digital rectal examination is not recommended as a stand-alone test for colorectal cancer. A colorectal cancer screening is advised for clients over age 50, including a flexible sigmoidoscopy every five years, yearly fecal occult blood tests, a double-contrast barium enema every five years, or a colonoscopy every 10 years.
CN: Health promotion and maintenance; CNS: None; CL: Apply

106. A 30-year-old client has gluten-induced enteropathy. The nurse instructs the client on foods that need to be eliminated from her diet. The nurse determines that teaching was successful when the client chooses to eliminate:
1. milk and dairy products.
2. protein-containing foods.
3. wheat products.
4. fresh fruits and vegetables.

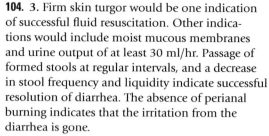

Pick your food carefully.

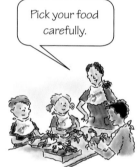

106. 3. To manage gluten-induced enteropathy, the client must eliminate gluten, including all cereal grains except rice and corn. During initial disease management, clients will eat a high-calorie, high-protein diet with mineral and vitamin supplements to help normalize the nutritional status. Lactose intolerance is sometimes an associated problem, so milk and dairy products are limited until improvement occurs.
CN: Physiological integrity; CNS: Basic care and comfort; CL: Apply

107. After a right hemicolectomy for the treatment of colon cancer, a 57-year-old client is reluctant to turn while on bed rest. What is the **most** appropriate intervention by the nurse?
1. Asking a coworker to help turn the client
2. Explaining to the client why turning is important
3. Allowing the client to turn when he's ready to do so
4. Telling the client that the health care provider's order states he must turn every two hours

107. 2. The appropriate action is to explain the importance of turning to avoid postoperative complications. Asking a coworker to help turn the client against his will would infringe on his rights. Allowing the client to turn when he's ready would increase his risk for postoperative complications. Telling the client that he must turn because of the health care provider's orders would put him on the defensive, and exclude him from participating in care decisions.
CN: Physiological integrity; CNS: Reduction of risk potential; CL: Apply

CN: Client needs category   CNS: Client needs subcategory   CL: Cognitive level

108. A nurse assists a health care provider during paracentesis. When documenting the procedure, which information should the nurse include?
1. The nurse's role during the procedure
2. The reason for the procedure
3. The health care provider's name and the client's response to the procedure
4. Diagnostic tests performed before obtaining the specimen

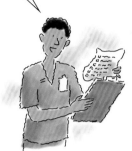

Good record keeping is a key factor in client care.

109. A client has a percutaneous endoscopic gastrostomy (PEG) tube inserted for continuous tube feedings. The nurse should place the client in which position before starting the feeding?
1. Semi-Fowler's
2. Supine
3. Reverse Trendelenburg
4. Prone

110. An enema is prescribed for a client with suspected appendicitis. What is the **most** appropriate action by the nurse?
1. Prepare 750 ml of irrigating solution warmed to 100° F (37.8° C).
2. Question the health care provider about the order
3. Provide privacy and explain the procedure to the client
4. Assist the client to left lateral Sim's position

111. A 75-year-old client is admitted to the hospital with lower gastrointestinal bleeding. The client's hemoglobin on admission to the emergency department is 7.3 g/dl. The health care provider prescribes two units of packed red blood cells (RBCs) to infuse over one hour each. Each unit of packed RBCs contains 250 ml. The blood administration set has a drip factor of 10 gtt/ml. What is the flow rate in drops per minute? Record your answer using a whole number.

_____ gtt/min

108. 3. The nurse should document the date and time of the procedure, the health care provider's name, pertinent information about the procedure (including tests done on the specimen obtained), the client's response, and client teaching. Documentation should include the client's response to interventions during the procedure. The reason for the procedure does not need to be documented.

CN: Physiological integrity; CNS: Reduction of risk potential; CL: Analyze

109. 1. To prevent aspiration of stomach contents, the nurse should place the client in semi-Fowler's position. The supine and reverse Trendelenburg positions may cause aspiration.

CN: Physiological integrity; CNS: Reduction of risk potential; CL: Apply

110. 2. Enemas are contraindicated in an acute abdominal condition of unknown origin, as well as after recent colon or rectal surgery or myocardial infarction. Questioning the health care provider about the order would be the correct thing to do. The other answers are correct if enema administration is appropriate.

CN: Safe, effective care environment; CNS: Safety and infection control; CL: Apply

111. 42.
Each unit of packed RBCs contains 250 ml. Each unit is to infuse over one hr. Use the following equation:

$$\frac{250\, ml}{60\, minutes} = 4.16 \frac{ml}{minute}$$

Multiply by the drip factor:

$$4.16 \frac{ml}{minute} \times 10 \frac{gtt}{ml} = 41.6 \frac{gtt}{minute}$$

Round to 42 gtt/minute.

CN: Physiological integrity; CNS: Pharmacological and parenteral therapies; CL: Analyze

112. A nurse is assessing a client's abdomen. Identify the area where the nurse's hand should be placed to palpate the liver.

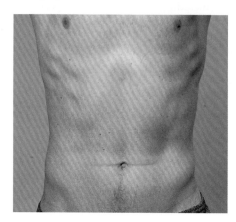

112. The nurse can palpate the liver by standing at the client's right side and placing her right hand on the client's abdomen to the right of midline. The nurse should point the fingers of her right hand toward the client's head, just under the right rib margin.

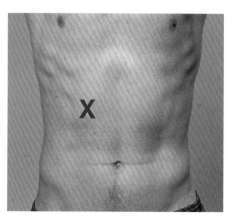

CN: Health promotion and maintenance; CNS: None; CL: Apply

113. A nurse is caring for a client who has had extensive abdominal surgery and is in critical condition. Dextrose 5% in half-normal saline solution is infusing through a triple-lumen central catheter at 125 ml/hr. The health care provider's orders include gentamicin 80 mg IV piggyback in 50 ml D5W over 30 minutes; ranitidine 50 mg IV in 50 ml D5W over 30 minutes; one unit of 250 ml of packed red blood cells (RBCs) over three hours; and a nasogastric tube flush with 30 ml normal saline solution every two hours. How many milliliters should the nurse document as the intake for the 8-hour shift? Record your answer using a whole number.

_____ ml

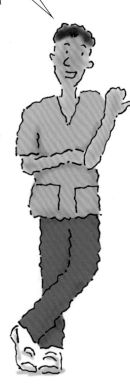

113. 1,470.
The regular IV at 125 ml × 8 hrs = 1,000 ml; gentamicin piggyback = 50 ml; ranitidine piggyback = 50 ml; packed RBCs = 250 ml; and nasogastric flushes of 30 ml × 4 = 120 ml.

$$(1,000 + 50 + 50 + 250 + 120) \; ml = 1,470 \; ml$$

CN: Physiological integrity; CNS: Pharmacological and parenteral therapies; CL: Apply

Chapter 9

Endocrine Disorders

This chapter covers diabetes mellitus and other endocrine disorders, typically a difficult area for nursing students. Don't worry, though, I'll help you through all the tough spots.

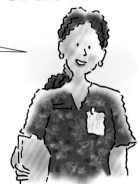

1. The nurse admits a client diagnosed with a new onset of type 1 diabetes mellitus. Which symptoms should the nurse expect to find during his initial physical assessment?
  1. Polydipsia, polyuria, and weight loss
  2. Weight gain, tiredness, and bradycardia
  3. Irritability, diaphoresis, and tachycardia
  4. Diarrhea, abdominal pain, and weight loss

"Poly" means "much"—much thirst, much urination ... you get the idea.

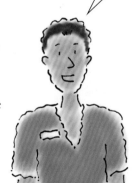

1. 1. Symptoms of uncontrolled type 1 diabetes mellitus include polydipsia, polyuria, and weight loss. Weight gain, tiredness, and bradycardia are symptoms of hypothyroidism. Irritability, diaphoresis, and tachycardia are symptoms of hypoglycemia. Symptoms of Crohn's disease include diarrhea, abdominal pain, and weight loss.
CN: Physiological integrity; CNS: Reduction of risk potential;
CL: Analyze

2. A client presents with diaphoresis, palpitations and tachycardia approximately two hours after receiving 20 units of insulin regular. What is the nurse's **most** appropriate intervention?
  1. Administer 15 grams of a simple carbohydrate
  2. Administer additional insulin based on a sliding scale
  3. Administer lorazepam per PRN order
  4. Draw blood for a glucose level

2. 1. These symptoms suggest hypoglycemia. The priority action would be to administer a simple carbohydrate to rapidly increase the blood glucose level. Drawing blood to assess blood glucose would require additional time, and the client could experience severe hypoglycemia. Additional insulin should not be administered as symptoms indicate hypoglycemia. Lorazepam is for anxiety, and would not treat hypoglycemia.
CN: Physiological integrity; CNS: Physiological adaptation;
CL: Apply

3. The nurse is caring for a preoperative client who has type 1 diabetes mellitus. Which action should the nurse take on the morning of the surgery?
  1. Clarify the insulin dose with the healthcare provider
  2. Hold all insulin for the day
  3. Administer oral anti-diabetic agents only
  4. Administer the full daily insulin dose

3. 1. The nurse should clarify this client's insulin dose with the healthcare provider on the day of surgery. A client who takes daily insulin may be given a reduced dose of intermediate or long acting insulin, or may be given rapid acting insulin based on their blood glucose levels. An IV infusion of 5% dextrose in water may be given with the insulin to prevent low blood glucose during surgery. The client's blood glucose will continue to rise even if the client is not eating, so insulin will not be held for the day. The full daily dose will most likely not be given, as the client will need to adjust their dose based on the blood glucose level. Clients with type 1 diabetes don't take oral anti-diabetic agents.
CN: Physiological integrity; CNS: Physiological adaptation;
CL: Apply

CN: Client needs category   CNS: Client needs subcategory   CL: Cognitive level

4. The nurse is teaching health promotion to a group of adults in the community. Which action would the nurse advise to decrease the risk factors for type 2 diabetes mellitus?
  1. Following a fat-free diet and non-impact exercise three times a week
  2. Maintaining an ideal weight and participation in daily exercise
  3. Following a very low carbohydrate diet that includes moderate amounts of fat
  4. Smoking cessation and a diet high in protein and fat

5. The nurse is caring for a client with type 2 diabetes mellitus. One hour after taking an oral diabetic medication, the client becomes nauseous and vomits. The nurse should:
  1. administer another dose of the drug.
  2. administer subcutaneous insulin.
  3. monitor blood glucose closely, and assess for signs of hypoglycemia.
  4. monitor blood glucose closely, and assess for signs of hyperglycemia.

6. What priority information regarding diet and exercise should the nurse teach a client newly diagnosed with type 1 diabetes mellitus?
  1. Exercise will increase blood glucose
  2. Fluid, protein, and electrolytes should be managed
  3. Calorie intake should be reduced prior to exercise
  4. Dietary goals, dietary composition, and physical activity are key

7. A nurse is teaching a client recently diagnosed with type 1 diabetes mellitus about the chronic complications associated with the disease. Which information should the nurse include?
  1. Buy shoes that are a half size larger
  2. Schedule yearly eye examinations
  3. Exercise will increase insulin resistance
  4. Podiatry visits are necessary every five years

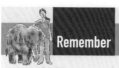

Remember

"Insulin" is derived from the Latin word insula, which means island.

This makes sense, as this hormone is produced by the beta cells of the "islets" of Langerhans in the pancreas.

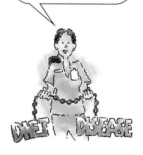

Diabetes mellitus is a disease with many links—one change leads to another.

DIET DISEASE

4. 2. Achieving and maintaining ideal body weight and participating in daily exercise are key to preventing type 2 diabetes. A low-fat diet can be encouraged, but some fat is required in all diets. Carbohydrates should make up the majority of a healthy diet. Diets high in fat are never encouraged.
CN: Health promotion and maintenance; CNS: None; CL: Apply

5. 3. When a client who has taken an oral antidiabetic agent vomits, the nurse should monitor blood glucose, and frequently assess for signs of hypoglycemia. After one hour, most of the medication would have been absorbed. Any food ingested may be lost, and repeating the dose would further lower glucose levels. Giving subcutaneous insulin would also lower glucose levels, causing hypoglycemia. Since most of the medication would have been absorbed, this client wouldn't have hyperglycemia.
CN: Physiological integrity; CNS: Pharmacological and parenteral therapies; CL: Analyze

6. 4. Clients with diabetes must understand the relationship between dietary goals, dietary composition, and regular physical activity. Exercise will usually decrease blood glucose. Management of fluids, proteins, and electrolytes is important for a client with acute renal failure. The client with diabetes may require additional calories prior to exercise.
CN: Health promotion and maintenance; CNS: None; CL: Apply

7. 2. Retinopathy is a chronic complication of diabetes mellitus. Yearly eye examinations are recommended. Shoes should fit properly and be the correct size because of the risk of serious foot injury. Exercise decreases insulin resistance. A podiatrist should be seen at least once a year.
CN: Physiological integrity; CNS: Reduction of risk potential; CL: Apply

8. The nurse is teaching a client newly diagnosed with type 1 diabetes mellitus about the rotation of insulin injection sites. The nurse determines that teaching was effective when the client states:
1. "Rotate injection sites within one anatomical region."
2. "Rotate injection sites from one anatomic region to another."
3. "Rotation of injection sites does not affect speed of absorption."
4. "Rotation of injection sites does not prevent lipohypertrophy."

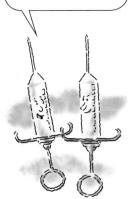

Remember to pick a different injection site this time—but stay in the same basic area.

8. 1. Rotation of insulin injections within one anatomic site is preferred to prevent day-to-day changes in absorption. Speed of absorption is affected by choice of site. Lipohypertrophy can be prevented by rotation of sites.
CN: Physiological integrity; CNS: Pharmacological and parenteral therapies; CL: Apply

9. The nurse is providing education to a group of clients newly diagnosed with type 1 diabetes mellitus. One client asks why the glycosylated hemoglobin blood test (HbA1c) is done. What is the nurse's **best** response?
1. HbA1c measures hemoglobin level in addition to blood glucose level.
2. HbA1c is used to assess long-term glycemic control.
3. HbA1c provides information about conditions that effect a red blood cell's life span.
4. HbA1c provides information about serum protein and albumin.

9. 2. The HbA1c results gives your average blood glucose (blood sugar) control for the past two to three months. It is a good indicator of the average blood glucose level during the 120-day life span of red blood cells. It is used to assess long-term glycemic control. It does not provide the current hemoglobin or serum blood glucose level. It does not provide information about serum protein or albumin.
CN: Physiological integrity; CNS: Reduction of risk potential; CL: Apply

10. The nurse is providing diabetes education to a group of clients previously diagnosed with type 1 diabetes mellitus. One of the clients asks about the advantage of using a continuous subcutaneous insulin infusion (CSII) pump. What nurse's best response would be:
1. "CSII is easy to use, and requires very little education."
2. "CSII eliminates the potential for ketoacidosis."
3. "CSII is cheaper to use than traditional insulin injections."
4. "CSII allows for flexibility in meal timing."

10. 4. CSII provides a basal dose of insulin which at mealtimes, and controls blood glucose levels better than a multiple-injection schedule. CSII allows for flexibility in meal timing because the mealtime dose of insulin is not given if a meal is skipped or eaten later than planned. The use of this pump requires intensive education for the client. The potential for more frequent and severe ketoacidosis may increase because of inexperience in pump use, infection, or accidental cessation, or obstruction of the infusion. CSII is more costly than traditional insulin injections, and not all costs may be covered by insurance.
CN: Physiological integrity; CNS: Pharmacological and parenteral therapies; CL: Apply

11. The nurse is admitting a client with a diagnosis of myxedema. During the initial assessment, which findings would the nurse be **most** concerned about?
1. Hypertension and weight loss
2. Heat intolerance and emotional lability
3. Corneal ulcerations and increased appetite
4. Bradycardia and decreased intellectual function

11. 4. Myxedema is caused by hypothyroidism. The symptoms of hypothyroidism include bradycardia and decreased intellectual functions, such as slurred speech, impaired memory, and inattentiveness. Hypertension, weight loss, heat intolerance, emotional lability, and increased appetite are all symptoms of hyperthyroidism. Corneal ulcerations may be seen in hyperthyroidism due to exophthalmos which may prevent eyelids from closing completely.
CN: Physiological integrity; CNS: Physiological adaptation; CL: Analyze

12. The nurse is caring for a client who is one day postoperative from a total thyroidectomy. Which symptom would prompt the nurse to immediately call the rapid response team (RRT) for intervention?
   1. Blood pressure of 150/92 mmHg
   2. Harsh, high-pitched respiratory sounds
   3. Weak voice or hoarseness
   4. Decreased deep tendon reflexes

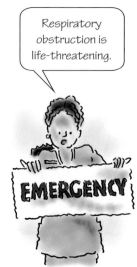

Respiratory obstruction is life-threatening.

EMERGENCY

12. 2. Stridor, or harsh, high-pitched respiratory sounds, indicate respiratory obstruction, which may be caused by laryngeal spasms or swelling. A blood pressure of 150/92 mmHg is high, but does not warrant a call to the RRT. A weak voice or hoarseness can be expected if the laryngeal nerve has been affected. Decreased deep tendon reflexes are not a concern. Hyperactive deep tendon reflexes would indicate a low calcium level, which may occur with damage to the parathyroid glands.
CN: Physiological integrity; CNS: Reduction of risk potential; CL: Apply

13. The nurse is educating a client newly diagnosis of papillary thyroid cancer that has metastasized. What is the **most** important information for the nurse to share about brachytherapy?
   1. Brachytherapy includes a short surgical procedure.
   2. Brachytherapy is rarely used for this type of cancer.
   3. Brachytherapy uses radioactive isotopes to destroy the cancer.
   4. Brachytherapy involves an external radiation source.

13. 3. Brachytherapy means "short" or "close" therapy. Brachytherapy uses radioactive isotopes to destroy the cancer. Radioactive iodine (RAI), also known as I-131 is ingested or injected, and the iodine concentrates in the thyroid gland to destroy the cancer. There is no surgical procedure involved in this therapy. The radiation source is internal. Radioactive iodine therapy improves the survival rate of patients with papillary or follicular thyroid cancer (differentiated thyroid cancer) that has spread to the neck or other body parts, and this treatment is now standard practice in such cases.
CN: Physiological integrity; CNS: Reduction of risk potential; CL: Analyze

14. The nurse is preparing a teaching plan for a client diagnosed with papillary thyroid carcinoma who is scheduled for surgery. Which information is a **priority** for the nurse to share?
   1. Information on oral chemotherapy
   2. The possibility of disease recurrence
   3. Risk factors for development of cancer
   4. Preoperative instructions for the scheduled surgery

14. 4. A partial or total thyroidectomy is often utilized for treatment, and the client needs to be informed about and pre-, and postoperative care. The health care provider is responsible for providing information regarding the surgical procedure, expectations, side effects and potential complications of treatment. Papillary carcinoma is the most common type of thyroid cancer. It can be present for years without obvious symptoms. Early diagnosis increases the chance of cure, because the cancer is confined to the thyroid gland at that stage. Metastasis is more likely with other types of thyroid cancers, although early diagnosis is key.
CN: Physiological integrity; CNS: Pharmacological and parenteral therapies; CL: Apply

15. The nurse is assessing a client who is being treated for hypothyroidism. Which symptom would indicate a potentially serious complication?
   1. Chills, fever, and hypotension
   2. Palpitations and chest pain
   3. Decreased visual acuity
   4. Low platelet count

15. 2. Palpitations and chest pain are cardiac symptoms, which can be precipitated by thyroid replacement therapy in clients with pre-existing heart disease. Chills, fever, and hypotension could indicate several complications, such as sepsis related to infection, or a transfusion reactions unrelated to hypothyroid therapy. Decreased visual acuity and a low platelet count are not related to hypothyroidism.
CN: Physiological integrity; CNS: Physiological adaptation; CL: Apply

CN: Client needs category   CNS: Client needs subcategory   CL: Cognitive level

16. Which test should the nurse anticipate for a client experiencing weight gain, intolerance to cold, constipation, and lethargy?
1. Liver function tests
2. Hemoglobin A1c (HbA1c)
3. T4 and thyroid-stimulating hormone
4. 24-hour urine free cortisol measurement

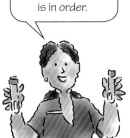

Looks like some blood collection is in order.

17. A nurse is admitting a client with hypothyroidism. What is the **priority** assessment?
1. Polyuria, polydipsia, and weight loss
2. Heat intolerance, nervousness, weight loss, and hair loss
3. Coarsening of facial features and extremity enlargement
4. Tiredness, cold intolerance, weight gain, and constipation

18. A client is started on steroid therapy after an adrenalectomy. Which information is **most** important to share with this client? Select all that apply.
1. Take the prescribed dose daily, and do not miss a dose
2. Notify your healthcare provider if you experience increased urination
3. Discontinue steroid therapy after two weeks
4. Take this medication for the rest of your life
5. Take two doses if you miss a dose

19. A client is receiving supplemental steroid therapy for a respiratory illness and reports waking up five times a night to urinate. What is the nurse's **priority** action?
1. Assist the client in obtaining a bedside commode
2. Make certain the client has a clear path to the toilet
3. Tell the client to take naps during the day
4. Assess the client's blood glucose level

16. 3. The client's symptoms suggest hypothyroidism. Levels of thyroid-stimulating hormone and T4 should be measured if hypothyroidism is suspected. Liver function tests are used to determine liver disease. HbA1C measurement is used to assess long-term blood glucose levels. As part of the screening process for Cushing's syndrome, a 24-hour urine free cortisol measurement is completed.
CN: Physiological integrity; CNS: Physiological adaptation; CL: Apply

17. 4. Tiredness, cold intolerance, weight gain, and constipation are symptoms of hypothyroidism, secondary to a decrease in cellular metabolism. Polyuria, polydipsia, and weight loss are symptoms of type 1 diabetes mellitus. The symptoms of hyperthyroidism include heat intolerance, nervousness, weight loss, and hair loss. Coarsening of facial features and extremity enlargement are symptoms of acromegaly.
CN: Physiological integrity; CNS: Physiological adaptation; CL: Apply

18. 1, 2, 4. Steroid therapy following an adrenalectomy will continue for the rest of the client's life. It is important to take the dose daily, and not miss a dose. The client should be instructed about potential side effects such as hyperglycemia, which could manifest as symptoms such as increased urination. Clients should take the medication as soon as they remember the missed dose, but should not double the dose the next day.
CN: Physiological integrity; CNS: Physiological adaptation; CL: Analyze

19. 4. Steroid therapy can increase blood glucose levels. As hyperglycemia leads to increased urination, the nurse should assess the client's blood glucose level, and notify the health care provider if it is elevated. Assessment is required prior to intervention. The remaining choices are interventions that could be completed after an assessment.
CN: Physiological integrity; CNS: Reduction of risk potential; CL: Apply

20. The nurse is caring for a client who has experienced a cerebral vascular accident (CVA). The client's urinary output has decreased to 10 ml/hr. What is the nurse's **priority** assessment?
1. Thyroid hormones
2. Cardiac status
3. Adrenocorticotrophic hormone (ACTH) level
4. Serum sodium level

20. 4. Urine output of 10 ml/hr is defined as oliguria. Oliguria is often linked to electrolyte imbalance and the syndrome of inappropriate antidiuretic hormone (SIADH). The client with SIADH retains fluid causing dilutional hyponatremia. Assessment of serum sodium can confirm the diagnosis of SIADH. Assessment of thyroid hormone is not indicated with this symptom. Assessment of cardiac status or ACTH level would not be indicated in this situation. Hyponatremia is a common electrolyte disorder encountered with clients who have neurological disorders.
CN: Physiological integrity; CNS: Reduction of risk potential; CL: Apply

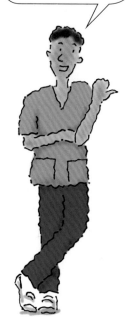

The answers to question 21 all look similar, don't they? Read them carefully.

21. The nurse admits a client with a diagnosis of chronic adrenal insufficiency. Which assessment findings confirm this diagnosis? Select all that apply.
1. Hyponatremia
2. Hyperkalemia
3. Hyperglycemia
4. Hypercalcemia
5. Hypocalcemia

21. 1, 2, 4. Adrenal insufficiency is manifested by hyponatremia, hyperkalemia, hypoglycemia, and hypercalcemia. BUN is generally increased.
CN: Physiological integrity; CNS: Reduction of risk potential; CL: Apply

22. A nurse is caring for a client diagnosed with diabetes insipidus. Which laboratory value is **most** important for the nurse to monitor?
1. Glucose
2. Hemoglobin
3. Creatinine
4. Sodium

22. 4. Diabetes insipidus occurs as a result of decreased release of antidiuretic hormone, which disturbs fluid and electrolyte balance, especially sodium. Clients need to be closely monitored for hypernatremia.
CN: Physiological integrity; CNS: Reduction of risk potential; CL: Analyze

23. A client diagnosed with Addison's disease is concerned about dark areas of skin around his knees and elbows. The nurse's best response would be:
1. "This finding is not related to Addison's disease. I will refer you to a dermatologist."
2. "This skin change is related to your medication therapy, and should subside in a few weeks."
3. "This is related to hormonal changes caused by Addison's disease."
4. "This change is related to sun exposure and should not be a concern."

23. 3. Addison's disease causes melanin stimulating hormone (MSH) levels to elevate as the pituitary gland is stimulated. MSH secretion results in areas of increased pigmentation. The changes in skin pigmentation is not related to sun exposure or medication therapy. The changes do not damage the skin, and there is no reason to refer this client to a dermatologist.
CN: Physiological integrity; CNS: Physiological adaptation; CL: Apply

CN: Client needs category   CNS: Client needs subcategory   CL: Cognitive level

24. The nurse is caring for a postoperative client who has undergone a transsphenoidal hypophysectomy. Which assessments would be **most** important for this client? Select all that apply.
1. Urinary output
2. Psychological status
3. Fluid and electrolyte balance
4. Gastrointestinal status
5. Visual assessment

24. 1, 3, 5. A common complication of neurologic disorders, trauma or surgery is diabetes insipidus (DI). DI results from a lack of antidiuretic hormone (ADH). This causes the kidneys to excrete very dilute urine with a low specific gravity. Urinary output must be monitored. In addition, fluid and electrolyte imbalances results from fluid and hormonal changes. Due to the location of the pituitary gland, inflammation and trauma in this area can cause visual changes. Psychosocial status and gastrointestinal status are not priority assessments for the client.
CN: Physiological integrity; CNS: Physiological adaptation; CL: Apply

25. The nurse is caring for a postoperative client who has undergone surgical removal of the pituitary gland (hypophysectomy), and has now developed diabetes insipidus (DI). The nurse should assess for:
1. hypertension and bradycardia.
2. glucosuria and weight gain.
3. fluid overload and hyponatremia.
4. severe dehydration and hypernatremia.

25. 4. A client with DI excretes high volumes of urine, even without fluid replacement. Limiting fluid intake will cause severe dehydration and hypernatremia. A client undergoing a fluid deprivation test may experience tachycardia and hypotension. Weight loss, and normal urine glucose levels are common in a client with DI. Fluid overload and hypernatremia are signs of syndrome of inappropriate antidiuretic hormone (SIADH).
CN: Physiological integrity; CNS: Physiological adaptation; CL: Analyze

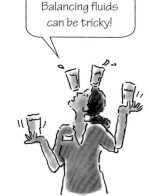

Balancing fluids can be tricky!

26. The nurse is caring for a client with diabetes insipidus (DI). What is the nurse's **priority** intervention?
1. Watching for signs and symptoms of septic shock
2. Maintaining adequate hydration
3. Checking weight every three days
4. Monitoring urine for specific gravity >1.030

26. 2. Maintaining fluid intake is essential in a client with DI. The client is at risk for developing hypovolemic shock because of increased urine output. Weight should be measured daily to monitor fluid balance. Urine specific gravity should be monitored for low osmolality, generally <1.005, due to the body's inability to concentrate urine.
CN: Safe, effective care environment; CNS: Management of care; CL: Apply

27. The nurse has just completed an assessment of a client who has suffered a head injury. Which assessment finding requires intervention?
1. The client states she is not thirsty.
2. The client's urine has a specific gravity <1.005.
3. The client has a mild headache.
4. The client's potassium level is 3.5 mEq/L.

27. 2. Increased urinary output with a specific gravity of 1.001 to 1.005 could indicate the development of diabetes insipidus (DI). DI often occurs in clients with head trauma or surgery, and results from a lack of antidiuretic hormone (ADH). Lack of thirst is not of concern, and a mild headache is expected. The potassium level noted is within normal limits.
CN: Physiological integrity; CNS: Physiological adaptation; CL: Analyze

28. A client diagnosed with diabetes insipidus (DI) is receiving desmopressin. Which symptom would require **immediate** intervention?
1. Rash and difficulty breathing
2. Abdominal cramping
3. Burning at the injection site
4. Headache

28. 1. Rash and difficulty breathing may indicate an allergic reaction to the medication, which requires immediate intervention. The other symptoms may occur, but are not life threatening.
CN: Physiological integrity; CNS: Pharmacological and parenteral therapies; CL: Apply

CN: Client needs category CNS: Client needs subcategory CL: Cognitive level

29. The nurse is caring for a client who is diagnosed with diabetes insipidus (DI). The nurse should carefully assess this client to prevent:
1. decreased hemoglobin and hyponatremia.
2. hypertension and bradycardia.
3. hypotension and increased urine output.
4. high urine specific gravity and hypertension.

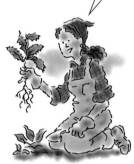

Weed out the wrong answers and the right one will be obvious.

29. 3. A lack of antidiuretic hormone (ADH) causes diabetes insipidus (DI). This causes the kidneys to excrete large amounts of very dilute urine with a low specific gravity. The loss of large amounts of urine can cause hypovolemic hypotension and tachycardia. It also causes hemodilution, which results in increased hemoglobin and hypernatremia.
CN: Physiological integrity; CNS: Physiological adaptation; CL: Apply

30. The nurse is caring for a client admitted with a suspected diagnosis of hypopituitarism. Which assessment finding requires a **priority** intervention?
1. Global headache
2. Decreased thyroid stimulating hormone (TSH)
3. Fatigue
4. Deficiency of gonadotropic hormones

30. 2. A deficiency of TSH is the most life threatening finding. This will result in an overall decrease in functioning that can affect all systems of the body. Headaches, fatigue and a deficiency of gonadotropic hormones can result from hypopituitarism, however, these are not priority findings. Hypothyroidism, resulting from hypopituitarism can affect cardiac and respiratory functions.
CN: Physiological integrity; CNS: Reduction of risk potential; CL: Analyze

31. The nurse is admitting a client suspected of having Addison's disease. An initial serum chemistry test is done. Which findings should the nurse expect?
1. Hyponatremia and hyperkalemia
2. Hypernatremia and hypokalemia
3. Hyperglycemia and hypernatremia
4. Hypercalcemia and hyperglycemia

31. 1. Addison's disease is characterized by hyponatremia, and hyperkalemia. Serum glucose is low due to decreased glyconeogenesis and depletion of muscle and liver glycogen. Serum calcium is not usually affected to a significant degree.
CN: Physiological integrity; CNS: Physiological adaptation; CL: Apply

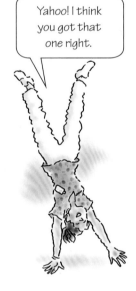

Yahoo! I think you got that one right.

32. Which assessment findings should the nurse expect in a patient with Addison's disease?
1. Weight gain and loss of skin pigment
2. Fatigue and muscle weakness
3. Hypertension and hypernatremia
4. Increased appetite and hypokalemia

32. 2. Manifestations of adrenal insufficiency or Addison's disease include fatigue, muscle weakness, weight loss, hyperpigmentation, hypotension, hyponatremia, decreased appetite, and hyperkalemia.
CN: Physiological integrity; CNS: Physiological adaptation; CL: Apply

33. The nurse is caring for a client with Addison's disease. Which laboratory value would indicate that treatment has been effective?
1. Sodium of 147 mEq/L
2. Potassium of 2.9 mEq/L
3. Sodium of 142 mEq/L
4. Potassium of 6.0 mEq/L

33. 3. Adrenal insufficiency causes a low sodium level, and a high potassium level. A sodium value of 142 mEq/L is within the normal range, and indicates that therapy has been effective. All of the other values are outside the normal range.
CN: Physiological integrity; CNS: Physiological adaptation; CL: Apply

34. The nurse is caring for a client admitted with Addisonian crisis. Which outcome is the **priority**?
1. Preventing irreversible shock
2. Preventing infection
3. Relieving anxiety
4. Lowering blood pressure

34. 1. A client in Addisonian crisis has an uncontrolled loss of sodium in the urine, and impaired mineralocorticoid function, which results in a loss of extracellular fluid, low blood volume, and possible irreversible shock. Preventing infection isn't an appropriate goal in this life-threatening situation. Relieving anxiety is appropriate after the client is stabilized. The client in Addisonian crisis is hypotensive, and blood pressure should be raised not lowered.
CN: Safe, effective care environment; CNS: Management of care; CL: Analyze

35. The nurse is caring for a client preliminarily diagnosed with hypothyroidism. Which laboratory serum values should the nurse expect?
1. High T3 and T4, and low thyroid-stimulating hormone (TSH)
2. High T3 and T4, and normal TSH
3. Low T3 and T4, and low TSH
4. Low T3 and T4, and high TSH

35. 4. Thyroid cells may fail to produce sufficient levels of thyroid hormones. This causes low serum levels, and the client has a decreased metabolic rate. As a result, the hypothalamus and anterior pituitary gland produce more TSH in an attempt to trigger the production of more T3 and T4 from the thyroid gland.
CN: Physiological integrity; CNS: Physiological adaptation; CL: Apply

36. What assessment finding is expected for a client diagnosed with Addison's disease?
1. Fatigue
2. Edema
3. Heat intolerance
4. Respiratory acidosis

36. 1. Clients with Addison's disease experience fatigue related to decreased metabolic energy production and altered body chemistry. Clients with Addison's disease experience decreased fluid loss, secondary to decreased mineralocorticoid secretion. Heat intolerance is a symptom of hyperthyroidism. The respiratory system isn't directly affected, and gas exchange shouldn't be affected.
CN: Health promotion and maintenance; CNS: None; CL: Analyze

37. The nurse is planning care for a client with Addison's disease. What is an appropriate outcome for this client?
1. Fluid intact of less than 1,000 ml a day
2. Participating in daily relaxation techniques
3. Ambulating in the hall five to six times per day
4. Choosing low sodium foods

What is the most important thing to teach a client with Addison's disease?

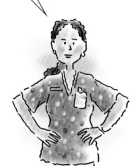

37. 2. Stress can precipitate a hypotensive crisis in clients with Addison's disease. Clients need to learn ways to identify and cope with stressors. Fluids should not be restricted. Intake should be 3 qt (3 L) or more per day. Activity should be monitored closely to avoid fatigue and weakness. Sodium should not be restricted.
CN: Physiological integrity; CNS: Physiological adaptation; CL: Analyze

38. The nurse is providing education about disease management to a client with Addison's disease. The nurse's teaching should include:
1. eating a low-sodium diet.
2. decreasing fluids to 1,000 ml/day.
3. wearing a Medic-Alert bracelet.
4. taking daily cortisone on an empty stomach.

38. 3. Clients with Addison's disease should wear a Medic-Alert bracelet to inform health care providers of the possibility of Addisonian crisis. Clients with Addison's disease are commonly hyponatremic and should not restrict their sodium or fluid intake. Steroid replacement therapy should be taken with food or milk to prevent gastric distress.
CN: Physiological integrity; CNS: Physiological adaptation; CL: Apply

CN: Client needs category   CNS: Client needs subcategory   CL: Cognitive level

39. The nurse is admitting a client to the unit with Cushing's syndrome. The nurse is likely to find which signs or symptoms during his initial assessment?
  1. "Moon face" and truncal obesity
  2. Weight loss and heat intolerance
  3. Changes in skin texture and low body temperature
  4. Polyuria and dehydration

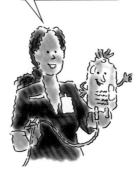

This question calls for a concentrated effort.

39. 1. Overproduction of adrenocortical hormone results in redistribution of fat, which manifests as a "moon face," truncal obesity, and a "buffalo hump." Weight loss and heat intolerance indicate thyroid hormone overproduction. Changes in skin texture and low body temperature indicate underproduction of thyroid hormone. Polyuria and dehydration indicate diabetic ketoacidosis.
CN: Physiological integrity; CNS: Physiological adaptation; CL: Apply

40. The nurse is planning care for a client diagnosed with Cushing's syndrome. Which potential complication should the nurse instruct this client about?
  1. Dehydration
  2. Infections
  3. Breathing difficulty
  4. Acute pain

40. 2. High levels of corticosteroids cause reduced inflammatory and immune responses, putting the client with Cushing's syndrome at increased risk for infection. Sodium and water are retained in clients with Cushing's syndrome, causing fluid overload. Breathing difficulty and acute pain are not generally associated with this condition.
CN: Physiological integrity; CNS: Physiological adaptation; CL: Apply

41. The nurse is aware that the client with Cushing's syndrome is at risk for:
  1. hypoglycemia and dehydration.
  2. hypotension and hyperkalemia hyperglycemia.
  3. hyponatremia and dehydration.
  4. hypertension and heart failure.

41. 4. An increase in mineralocorticoid activity in a client with Cushing's syndrome results in sodium and water retention, which commonly contributes to hypertension and heart failure. Hypoglycemia and dehydration are uncommon in a client with Cushing's syndrome. Clients with Cushings syndrome may have a decrease in potassium or hypokalemia. Diabetes mellitus and hyperglycemia may develop, but hypotension is not part of the disease process. Dehydration also is not a complication of Cushing's syndrome.
CN: Physiological integrity; CNS: Physiological adaptation; CL: Analyze

42. The nurse is admitting a client with newly diagnosed Cushing's syndrome. Which laboratory values should the nurse expect to find?
  1. Decreased sodium and decreased glucose
  2. Decreased cortisol and decreased glucose
  3. Increased cortisol and decreased sodium
  4. Increased cortisol and increased sodium

42. 4. Increased cortisol, glucose, and sodium are found in clients with Cushing's syndrome.
CN: Physiological integrity; CNS: Physiological adaptation; CL: Apply

43. The nurse is caring for a client who is diagnosed with Cushing's syndrome. What is the **priority** assessment?
  1. Serum glucose
  2. Daily weight
  3. Urinary output
  4. Abdominal girth

43. 1. Cushing's syndrome results in the increased secretion of cortisol from the adrenal cortex. It is caused by either an abnormality in the adrenal cortex itself, the anterior pituitary gland, or the hypothalamus. The presence of excess glucocorticoids affects the metabolism, and all body systems. An increase in total body fat results from slow turnover of plasma fatty acids. This fat is redistributed, producing truncal obesity, "buffalo hump," and "moon face." An increase in the breakdown of tissue protein, and an increase in urine nitrogen excretion also occur, resulting in decreased muscle mass and strength, thin skin, and fragile capillaries. The effect on minerals leads to bone density loss. Glucose metabolism is profoundly affected by hypercortisolism. The liver is stimulated to convert more glycogen into glucose, and insulin receptors are less sensitive causing decreased blood glucose movement into the cells.
CN: Physiological integrity; CNS: Physiological adaptation; CL: Apply

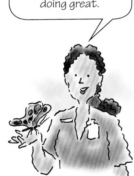

Butterflies in your stomach? Don't worry—you're doing great.

44. The nurse is caring for a client in the post anesthesia care unit (PACU) following an adrenalectomy. What is the nurse's **priority** action?
  1. Assessing serum potassium
  2. Assessing blood pressure
  3. Administering dextrose in water
  4. Administering opioids

44. 2. Removing a major source of adrenal hormones may cause a state of temporary adrenal insufficiency. After an adrenalectomy, the patient is usually sent to a critical care unit. Immediately after surgery, the patient should be assessed every 15 minutes for shock due to possible insufficient glucocorticoid replacement. Assessment is a priority over interventions. Assess the blood pressure, then electrolytes, and finally assess the client for fluid replacement and pain management needs.
CN: Physiological integrity; CNS: Physiological adaptation; CL: Analyze

45. The nurse is caring for a client recently diagnosed with Cushing's syndrome. Which assessment finding should the nurse expect to find?
  1. Bruising and hypotension
  2. Truncal obesity and abdominal striae
  3. Hypertension and emaciation
  4. Weight loss and "moon face"

45. 2. Cushing's syndrome causes truncal obesity and striae due to fat redistribution. Other manifestations include hypertension and weight gain in the abdominal area with muscle wasting in the extremities.
CN: Physiolongogical integrity; CNS: Physiological adaptation; CL: Apply

46. The nurse is providing education for a client with Cushing's syndrome. Which information should the nurse include in the teaching plan?
  1. Dietary sodium should be increased
  2. Physical changes are disease related
  3. High fluid intake is important
  4. Dietary protein should be restricted

46. 2. The client may have a disturbed body image related to fat redistribution, "moon face," "buffalo hump," striae, acne, and hirsutism. Explaining that these changes are disease related will help the client address these feelings. Clients with Cushing's should reduce sodium intake. Fluids are often restricted, and a high-protein diet is encouraged.
CN: Physiological integrity; CNS: Physiological adaptation; CL: Apply

CN: Client needs category   CNS: Client needs subcategory   CL: Cognitive level

47. The nurse is providing community education to a group of clients about the prevention of type 2 diabetes mellitus. Which client would be at **highest** risk for the development of diabetes mellitus?
1. A young adult who plays basketball regularly
2. An elderly woman who is sedentary
3. A middle-age woman who delivers mail
4. A middle-age man with a basal metabolic rate within normal limits

47. 2. The risk for developing type 2 diabetes mellitus is increased in clients over 65 years of age. Maintaining a normal weight and basal metabolic rate, along with exercise decrease the risk. The risk is increased with a lack of exercise.
CN: Physiological integrity; CNS: Reduction of risk potential; CL: Apply

48. A client with type 1 diabetes mellitus often skips his ordered dose of insulin. What **priority** information should the nurse give to this client regarding the omission of insulin doses?
1. May lead to ketoacidosis
2. May cause hypoglycemic coma
3. May lead to pancreatitis
4. May cause diabetes insipidus

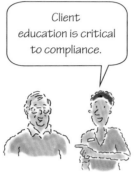

Client education is critical to compliance.

48. 1. A client who fails to regularly take insulin is at risk for hyperglycemia, which could lead to diabetic ketoacidosis. Hypoglycemia would not occur because the lack of insulin would lead to increased levels of sugar in the blood. A client with chronic pancreatitis may develop diabetes, but insulin-dependent diabetes mellitus does not lead to pancreatitis. Diabetes insipidus isn't caused by alteration in insulin levels.
CN: Physiological integrity; CNS: Physiological adaptation; CL: Apply

49. A client with type 1 diabetes mellitus presents with polyphagia, polydipsia, and polyuria. Further assessment shows signs of dehydration. The nurse determines that this client may be experiencing:
1. Diabetes insipidus
2. Diabetic ketoacidosis
3. Hypoglycemia
4. Syndrome of inappropriate antidiuretic hormone (SIADH)

49. 2. Early manifestations of diabetic ketoacidosis include polydipsia, polyphagia, and polyuria. Diabetes insipidus may result in dehydration but not polyphagia and polydipsia. Symptoms of hypoglycemia include diaphoresis, tachycardia, and nervousness. A client with SIADH is unable to excrete dilute urine, causing hyponatremia.
CN: Physiological integrity; CNS: Physiological adaptation; CL: Apply

50. The nurse is admitting a client diagnosed with primary hyperthyroidism. Which laboratory results should the nurse expect? Select all that apply.
1. Elevated thyroid stimulating hormone
2. Decreased thyroid stimulating hormone
3. Elevated T3 levels
4. Elevated T4 levels
5. Decreased T3 levels
6. Decreased T4 levels

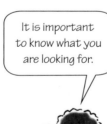

It is important to know what you are looking for.

50. 2, 3, 4. The best indicator of primary hyperthyroidism is the suppression of TSH below 0.1 µg/ml. This occurs when circulating levels of thyroid hormones are elevated. High levels of thyroid hormones signal the pituitary gland to cease production of TSH. This is a crucial differentiation between thyroid and pituitary dysfunction.
CN: Physiological integrity; CNS: Reduction of risk potential; CL: Analyze

51. A client exhibiting exophthalmos, weight loss, and tachycardia would be evaluated by checking which levels?
1. Amylase, lipase, and trypsin
2. Triiodothyronine (T3), thyroxine (T4), and thyroid-stimulating hormone (TSH)
3. Glucocorticoids, mineralocorticoids, and androgens
4. Vasopressin and oxytocin

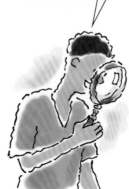

51. 2. The symptoms reflect a potential dysfunction of the thyroid gland. T3, T4, and TSH are all secreted by the thyroid gland. Amylase, lipase, and trypsin are enzymes produced by the pancreas that aid in digestion. Glucocorticoids, mineralocorticoids, and androgens are produced by the adrenal gland. The pituitary gland secretes vasopressin and oxytocin.
CN: Health promotion and maintenance; CNS: None; CL: Analyze

CN: Client needs category   CNS: Client needs subcategory   CL: Cognitive level

52. The nurse is teaching a client diagnosed with hypothyroidism. Which statement should the nurse include in the teaching?
1. "Your adrenal glands will need to be assessed."
2. "We will need to measure your parathyroid hormone."
3. "You will need to take hormones daily for life."
4. "A CT scan is necessary to determine the cause of your problem."

52. 3. Hypothyroidism is a life threatening condition, and clients need to take replacement hormones for life. The adrenal gland should not be affected by hypothyroidism. Parathyroid hormone is not routinely assessed. A CT scan is not usually necessary to determine the cause of hypothyroidism. Hormone assessment will assist in the diagnosis.
CN: Physiological integrity; CNS: Physiological adaptation; CL: Apply

53. The nurse is admitting a client diagnosed with hyperthyroidism. The client asks what can be done for this disorder. Which is the nurse's **best** reply?
1. "You will need to take thyroid hormones."
2. "A Lithotripsy will be scheduled."
3. "You will most likely have radioactive iodine therapy."
4. "A Laryngectomy will be scheduled."

53. 3. This client will most likely receive radioactive iodine (RAI) in the form of oral I-131. The thyroid gland absorbs the RAI, and some of the thyroid-producing cells will be destroyed by the local radiation. Lithotripsy is a procedure to break up stones, such as found in the renal system. Oral thyroid hormones are contraindicated because the client currently produces too much. A laryngectomy involves removal of the larynx.
CN: Physiological integrity; CNS: Reduction of risk potential; CL: Apply

54. A nurse is teaching a group of nursing students about the thyroid gland and aging. Which information should the nurse plan to teach?
1. The thyroid gland increases in size with increasing age.
2. Older adults require higher doses of replacement therapy.
3. Thyroid hormone secretion increases with age.
4. The basal metabolic rate decreases with age.

54. 4. The basal metabolic rate decreases with age, because the thyroid gland decreases in size and hormone output as the client ages. Older adults require lower doses of replacement thyroid hormone. A large dose of thyroid hormone can adversely affect the heart muscle.
CN: Physiological integrity; CNS: Reduction of risk potential; CL: Apply

I hate getting caught in a storm.

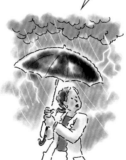

55. A client with hyperthyroidism develops a high fever, tachycardia, and systolic hypertension. The nurse suspects:
1. hepatic coma.
2. thyroid storm.
3. myxedema.
4. laryngeal spasm.

55. 2. Thyroid storm is a form of severe hyperthyroidism that can be precipitated by stress, injury, or infection. Hepatic coma occurs in clients with profound liver failure. Myxedema is related to hypothyroidism. Laryngeal spasms are a possible complication following thyroid surgery, and do not involve fever or hypertension.
CN: Physiological integrity; CNS: Physiological adaptation; CL: Analyze

56. The nurse is caring for a client diagnosed with Graves' disease. What is the nurse's **priority** intervention for this client?
1. Insertion of eye drops
2. Assessment of temperature
3. Decreasing stress
4. Promoting comfort

56. 2. The highest priority intervention is the assessment of the client's body temperature. An increase in temperature can indicate a rapid decline in the patient's condition, and the onset of thyroid storm.
CN: Physiological integrity; CNS: Reduction of risk potential; CL: Apply

57. A client is admitted with a diagnosis of hyperparathyroidism. Which symptoms should the nurse anticipate?
1. Exophthalmos
2. Renal calculi
3. Weight gain
4. Weight loss

57. 2. Hyperparathyroidism is over production of parathyroid hormone, characterized by elevated serum calcium, bone calcification, or renal calculi. Exophthalmos and weight loss are signs of hyperthyroidism, and weight gain is a sign of hypothyroidism.
CN: Physiological integrity; CNS: Physiological adaptation;
CL: Apply

58. A client presents with flushed skin, exophthalmos, irritability, and palpitations. What is the nurse's **priority** intervention?
1. Assessing thyroid hormone levels
2. Assessing parathyroid hormones
3. Providing the client with hypothermia blanket
4. Sitting with client

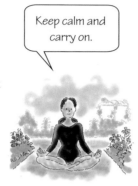

Keep calm and carry on.

58. 1. Signs and symptoms of hyperthyroidism include nervousness, palpitations, irritability, exophthalmos, heat intolerance, weight loss, and weakness. The nurse should first assess thyroid hormone levels. Hyperparathyroidism is characterized by weakness and anorexia. A hypothermia blanket is not a priority intervention for a client who is flushed. Sitting with a client who is irritable due to elevated thyroid hormones may not assist in calming.
CN: Physiological integrity; CNS: Physiological adaptation;
CL: Analyze

59. What should the nurse assess in a female client with anterior pituitary hypofunction?
1. Date of least menstrual period
2. Weight gain
3. Changes in urinary output
4. Chest pain

59. 1. Amenorrhea is a sign of decreased follicle-stimulating hormone, which is one of the anterior pituitary hormones. Weight gain is associated with Cushing's syndrome. Urinary output is related to posterior pituitary function, and chest pain is not related to hormone levels.
CN: Health promotion and maintenance; CNS: None;
CL: Apply

60. Two days after admission for a brain stem contusion, a client begins urinating two to three liters a day, and has a serum sodium level of 155 mEq/dl (155 mmol/L). For which condition should the plan to assess?
1. Myxedema coma
2. Diabetes insipidus
3. Type 1 diabetes mellitus
4. Syndrome of inappropriate antidiuretic hormone (SIADH)

60. 2. Two leading causes of diabetes insipidus are hypothalamic or pituitary tumors, and closed head injuries. Myxedema coma is a form of hypothyroidism. Type 1 diabetes mellitus isn't caused by a brain injury. A client with SIADH would have hyponatremia and oliguria.
CN: Physiological integrity; CNS: Reduction of risk potential;
CL: Apply

61. A client with type 1 diabetes mellitus is exhibiting Kussmaul's respirations, abdominal discomfort, and lethargy. What intervention should the nurse perform?
1. Assess complete blood count (CBC)
2. Administer insulin as ordered
3. Start an intravenous infusion of dextrose
4. Assess neurological status

61. 2. Clients with Kussmaul's respirations, abdominal discomfort, and lethargy, are symptomatic of diabetic ketoacidosis (DKA). The nurse should administer insulin to decrease blood glucose levels. A CBC and neurological status assessment will not aid in the diagnosis of this condition. An intravenous infusion of dextrose would elevate the client's glucose level.
CN: Physiological integrity; CNS: Reduction of risk potential;
CL: Apply

CN: Client needs category   CNS: Client needs subcategory   CL: Cognitive level

62. The nurse is admitting a client diagnosed with diabetic ketoacidosis (DKA). What is the nurse's **priority** intervention?
   1. Subcutaneous glucagon administration
   2. Transfusion of whole blood
   3. Glucocorticoid administration
   4. Intravenous insulin

63. The nurse is caring for a client diagnosed with diabetic ketoacidosis (DKA). The client is receiving insulin and IV fluids. Which laboratory test would be a **priority** for the nurse to monitor?
   1. Serum potassium
   2. Hemoglobin A1C (HbA1c)
   3. Serum calcium
   4. Serum nitrogen

64. The home health nurse is visiting a client newly diagnosed with type 1 diabetes mellitus. The client reports nausea and abdominal pain. The nurse observes dehydration and dry skin. What question should the nurse ask the client?
   1. "What did you drink today?"
   2. "Are you taking your insulin daily?"
   3. "When is the last time you had a checkup?"
   4. "Did you weigh yourself today?"

65. The nurse is preparing to administer IV insulin to a client diagnosed with diabetic ketoacidosis (DKA). What will the nurse monitor while the client is receiving this intervention?
   1. Hypokalemia and hypoglycemia
   2. Hypocalcemia and hyperkalemia
   3. Hyperkalemia and hyperglycemia
   4. Hypernatremia and hypercalcemia

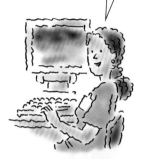

Make sure you know which disorder the question is asking you to treat.

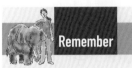

Remember

"Gluc-agon increases gluc-ose."

Insulin decreases it.

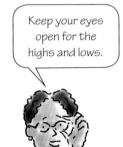

Keep your eyes open for the highs and lows.

62. **4.** A client with DKA should receive IV insulin to lower glucose and IV fluids to correct hypotension. Glucagon is given to treat hypoglycemia and is not appropriate for DKA. Blood products aren't needed to correct DKA. Glucocorticoids are not used to treat DKA, and may aggravate the hyperglycemia.
CN: Physiological integrity; CNS: Pharmacological and parenteral therapies; CL: Apply

63. **1.** Insulin therapy reduces serum potassium levels as insulin allows potassium to enter cells. Hypokalemia will cause cardiac complications and is a common cause of death in the treatment of DKA. HbA1c values indicate overall glucose control over a three to four month span. Serum calcium and nitrogen are not priorities in managing DKA.
CN: Physiological integrity; CNS: Reduction of risk potential; CL: Apply

64. **2.** The nurse should ask if the client is taking their insulin, as a common cause of DKA is missed insulin. Classic symptoms of diabetic ketoacidosis (DKA) include polyuria, weight loss, nausea and vomiting, altered mental status, abdominal pain, and Kussmaul's respirations. The nurse should also check a blood glucose level. Asking the client what he drank, if he weighed himself, and when he had a check-up will not help identify the cause of the current symptoms.
CN: Physiological integrity; CNS: Reduction of risk potential; CL: Apply

65. **1.** The nurse should monitor for decreased potassium and decreased glucose. Hypoglycemia might occur if too much insulin is administered, or insulin is administered too quickly. Intravenous insulin forces potassium into cells, thereby lowering plasma levels of potassium. The client may have hyperkalemia prior to starting the insulin therapy, but hypokalemia will occur with insulin administration. Calcium and sodium levels should not be affected.
CN: Physiological integrity; CNS: Pharmacological and parenteral therapies; CL: Apply

66. A client diagnosed with hyperosmolar hyperglycemic nonketotic syndrome (HHNS) is **most** at risk for the development of:
1. infection.
2. confusion.
3. dehydration.
4. skin breakdown.

66. 3. A client with HHNS has severe dehydration, which requires immediate intervention. The other potential problems are a lower priority.
CN: Physiological integrity; CNS: Physiological adaptation;
CL: Analyze

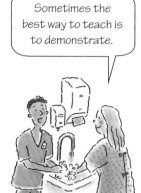

Sometimes the best way to teach is to demonstrate.

67. The nurse teaches a client diagnosed with hyperglycemic hyperosmolar state (HHS) how to monitor his condition. What is a potential warning sign of this condition?
1. Symptoms of hyperglycemia
2. Symptoms of hypoglycemia
3. Ketones in the urine
4. Rapid and deep respirations

67. 1. Both HHS and ketoacidosis (DKA) are caused by hyperglycemia and dehydration. It is important to teach the client the signs and symptoms of increased blood glucose, dehydration and how to assess for ketones in the urine. HHS differs from DKA in that ketone levels are low, or absent and blood glucose levels are much higher. In HHS as well as DKA, the serum potassium level may drop quickly when insulin therapy allows potassium to enter cells.
CN: Physiological integrity; CNS: Reduction of risk potential;
CL: Apply

68. The nurse is administering an insulin infusion for a client diagnosed with diabetic ketoacidosis (DKA). Which outcome indicates that treatment has been effective?
1. Lowered blood glucose level to normal limits within one hour
2. The replacement of fluids during the first 24 hours
3. An increase in anion gap within 24 hours
4. An increase in blood glucose levels within the first three hours

68. 2. The goal of treatment for DKA is to lower the blood glucose level gradually while replacing fluids during the first 24 hours of treatment. Lowering blood glucose levels too quickly will result in complications, and is not a desirable outcome. The anion gap should be decreased with treatment.
CN: Physiological integrity; CNS: Pharmacological and parenteral therapies; CL: Apply

69. A client with type 2 diabetes mellitus comes to the emergency department with weakness, thirst, and an inability to concentrate. What should the nurse assess?
1. Thyroid hormones
2. Weight
3. Apical pulse
4. Blood glucose

69. 4. This client's symptoms suggest HHS. The nurse should assess blood glucose levels to determine if the client is hyperglycemic. The other assessments will not help rule out this disorder.
CN: Physiological integrity; CNS: Physiological adaptation;
CL: Apply

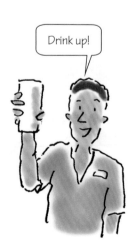

Drink up!

70. The nurse is providing education about sick-day rules to a group of clients with type 1 diabetes mellitus. Which information is appropriate to include?
1. Monitor blood glucose at least once a day
2. Do not take insulin until you feel well
3. Drink 8 to 12 oz of fluid each waking hour
4. If nauseous, do not eat or drink

70. 3. To prevent dehydration, sick clients should drink 8 to 12 oz of sugar-free liquids every waking hour. Clients who are ill should monitor their blood glucose at least every four hours and continue to take insulin or oral agents. If nauseated, clients should consume more easily tolerated foods or liquids equal to the carbohydrate content of usual meals.
CN: Physiological integrity; CNS: Pharmacological and parenteral therapies; CL: Analyze

71. The nurse is caring for a client with type 1 diabetes mellitus. At 3:00 AM, the nurse finds the client disoriented to time and place, diaphoretic, and complaining of palpitations. What is the nurse's **priority** intervention?
1. Give 10 to 15 g of carbohydrate orally
2. Call the healthcare provider for additional insulin order
3. Administer 1 mg of glucagon subcutaneously
4. Check blood glucose level

71. 4. Check the blood glucose level first when symptoms arise, then proceed with treatment according to the results. If the client is hypoglycemic, administration of a simple carbohydrate is appropriate. If the client is conscious, the carbohydrate may be given orally. If consciousness is altered, subcutaneous or intramuscular glucagon is appropriate. This client is showing symptoms of hypoglycemia, additional insulin would further lower the blood glucose.
CN: Physiological integrity; CNS: Reduction of risk potential; CL: Apply

72. A client presents to the health clinic with a toxic multinodular goiter. What is the **priority** concern for this client?
1. Heat intolerance
2. Exophthalmos
3. Dysrhythmias
4. Extreme mood swings

72. 3. Cardiovascular concerns are the priority concern for clients who have a goiter. Goiters are seen with hyperthyroidism. Hyperthyroidism can result in all of these symptoms.
CN: Physiological integrity; CNS: Reduction of risk potential; CL: Apply

73. The nurse is caring for an athletic client with hyperparathyroidism. The client is currently showing signs of apathy and depression, and despite the client's athleticism, the nurse's assessment finds flabby musculature. The nurse should assess for:
1. hypercalcemia.
2. hypocalcemia.
3. hypernatremia.
4. hyponatremia.

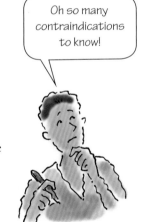

Oh so many contraindications to know!

73. 1. The client is demonstrating signs of hypercalcemia. An overactive parathyroid gland produces an increased amount of parathyroid hormone. This increase promotes the release of calcium from the bone and increases serum calcium. Hypocalcemia would cause muscle cramps and possible tetany. Hyperparathyroidism does not directly affect sodium levels.
CN: Physiological integrity; CNS: Reduction of risk potential; CL: Analyze

74. The nurse is providing education to a client diagnosed with hyperparathyroidism. The nurse determines further teaching is necessary when the client states that they will continue to take:
1. acetaminophen.
2. aspirin.
3. potassium-wasting diuretics.
4. thiazide diuretics.

74. 4. Thiazide diuretics shouldn't be taken by a client with hyperparathyroidism as they decrease renal excretion of calcium, and increase serum calcium levels. There are no contraindications to acetaminophen or aspirin for clients with hyperparathyroidism. Potassium loss is not a concern for clients with hyperparathyroidism.
CN: Physiological integrity; CNS: Pharmacological and parenteral therapies; CL: Apply

Remember

"Diuretic" is derived from the Greek word diourein, which means "to urinate," which is exactly what diuretic drugs make you do.

They promote excretion of water and electrolytes by the kidneys, which results in greater urine output. One class of diuretics is the thiazides:

- Bendroflumethiazide
- Chlorothiazide
- Hydrochlorothiazide
- Methyclothiazide

CN: Client needs category   CNS: Client needs subcategory   CL: Cognitive level

75. The serum calcium level of a client with hyperparathyroidism is 14.6 mg/dl (0.81 mmol/L). Which intervention is **most** appropriate?
1. Withholding fluids
2. Starting oral calcium supplements
3. Administering vitamin D supplements
4. Administering intravenous fluids at 200 ml/hr

75. 4. Normal calcium levels range from 8.5 to 10.5 mg/dl (0.47 to 0.58 mmol/L). A level of 14.6 mg/dl (0.81 mmol/L) is dangerously high. To decrease the calcium level, intake of calcium should be reduced, and calcium excretion should be promoted by administering IV, and oral fluids as well as diuretics. Vitamin D increases the calcium level.
CN: Physiological integrity; CNS: Physiological adaptation; CL: Analyze

76. Which assessment would be a **priority** for a nurse caring for a client with hypoparathyroidism?
1. Decreased calcium
2. Increased thyroid hormone
3. Decreased phosphate
4. Increased potassium

76. 1. The parathyroid gland works to balance calcium by decreasing bone calcium and increasing serum calcium. Decreased calcium can result in bone fractures for the client. Calcium and phosphorus levels are inversely related. Therefore, a low-functioning parathyroid gland would manifest as hyperphosphatemia and hypocalcemia. Thyroid hormone and potassium are not directly affected.
CN: Physiological integrity; CNS: Physiological adaptation; CL: Analyze

77. What is the **priority** nursing intervention for the client with hyperthyroidism?
1. Keeping warm
2. Increasing activity
3. Providing a calm, restful environment
4. Placing the client in high Fowler's position

77. 3. Clients with hyperthyroidism are typically anxious, diaphoretic, nervous, and fatigued. They need a calm, restful environment in which to relax and get adequate rest. Clients with hyperthyroidism are usually warm and need a cool environment. Activity should not be increased. A high Fowler's position would benefit a client who is dyspneic, but not usually necessary for the client with hyperthyroidism.
CN: Safe, effective care environment; CNS: Management of care; CL: Apply

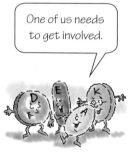

One of us needs to get involved.

78. What should the nurse teach a client receiving vitamin D therapy for hypoparathyroidism?
1. Vitamin D is taken to increase absorption of calcium.
2. Vitamin D will cure hypoparathyroidism.
3. Vitamin A and C will increase absorption of calcium.
4. Vitamin D therapy will stabilize potassium levels.

78. 1. A client with hypoparathyroidism has a decreased serum calcium level. Variable doses of vitamin D preparations enhance the absorption of calcium from the gastrointestinal tract. This does not cure the client's hypoparathyroidism. Vitamins A, C, and E are not involved with this process. Vitamin D therapy will not assist in stabilizing potassium.
CN: Physiological integrity; CNS: Pharmacological and parenteral therapies; CL: Analyze

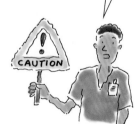

Read series answers carefully to be certain all are correct.

79. The nurse is caring for a client admitted with joint pain and weakness. The client describes a gradual coarsening of facial features and enlargement of hands and feet over the past year. What assessment is appropriate for this client?
1. Growth hormone levels
2. Cortisol levels
3. Thyroid hormones
4. Insulin levels

79. 1. Acromegaly is marked by coarsening of facial features and soft tissue, and swelling of the hands and feet. The cause is overproduction of growth hormone. Cortisol levels are increased in Cushing's syndrome, which causes thin extremities, truncal obesity, and a "moon face." Thyroid hormones are not related to these symptoms. Graves' disease causes exophthalmos, weight loss, and heat intolerance. Changes in insulin levels do not cause this client's symptoms.
CN: Physiological integrity; CNS: Physiological adaptation; CL: Apply

80. A nurse is teaching a client about mixing insulin. The healthcare provider has ordered, regular insulin 6 units mixed with long-acting insulin 10 units. Place the following steps in the correct order.

1. Withdraw 6 units of regular insulin

2. Inject 10 units of air into the long-acting insulin vial

3. Inject 6 units of air into the regular insulin

4. Withdraw 10 units of long-acting insulin

5. Roll bottle of long-acting insulin gently to mix

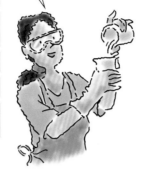

Make sure you get the steps right for mixing insulin. It's important!

80. Ordered Response:

5. Roll bottle of long-acting insulin gently to mix

2. Inject 10 units of air into the long-acting insulin vial

3. Inject 6 units of air into the regular insulin

1. Withdraw 6 units of regular insulin

4. Withdraw 10 units of long-acting insulin

CN: Physiological integrity; CNS: Pharmacological and parenteral therapies; CL: Analyze

81. What should the nurse teach a client with a diagnosis of a pituitary tumor?
1. This type of tumor can have effects on many hormones.
2. Pituitary tumors cannot be removed.
3. Surgical removal is not necessary.
4. Radioactive iodine is the treatment of choice.

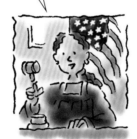

Here's a case for knowing your hormones cold.

81. 1. Tumors that affect the pituitary gland can cause many hormonal changes. The symptoms depend on the area of the gland affected, and if the tumor is secreting or causing the pituitary to secrete added hormones. Surgery through a transsphenoidal hypophysectomy is usually the preferred treatment. Radioactive iodine is used for thyroid gland problems.
CN: Physiological integrity; CNS: Physiological adaptation; CL: Apply

82. The nurse is reviewing a client's chart and notes a low serum calcium level. What is the nurse's **priority** assessment for the client?
1. Chvostek's sign
2. Phosphorous levels
3. Trousseau's sign
4. Airway

82. 4. Hypocalcemia can cause muscle spasms. The priority intervention is the protection of the airway and replacement of serum calcium. Assessing Chvostek's and Trousseau sign will help determine if the client has hypocalcemia, however, this is not as high a priority as protecting the client's airway. Assessment of phosphorous levels is also not a high a priority
CN: Physiological integrity; CNS: Reduction of risk potential; CL: Apply

83. After undergoing a thyroidectomy, a client develops tetany. What statement by the nurse is **most** accurate?
1. "This is a temporary condition and will resolve on its own."
2. "This condition can be life threatening and needs immediate treatment."
3. "This condition is related to hypothyroidism."
4. "This condition is very rare."

83. 2. Immediate treatment is necessary for a client who develops hypocalcemia and tetany following a thyroidectomy. The condition will not resolve until treated with supplemental calcium gluconate. The condition is related to damage of the parathyroid glands, not hypothyroidism.
CN: Physiological integrity; CNS: Pharmacological and parenteral therapies; CL: Analyze

84. After a thyroidectomy, the cline develops a positive Trousseau's sign. What is the nurse's **priority** action?

1. Administer levothyroxine therapy
2. Administer liothyronine therapy
3. Administer potassium chloride
4. Administer calcium gluconate

84. 4. Damage to the parathyroid glands can inadvertently occur during a thyroidectomy. This may cause a decrease in serum calcium, which causes muscle hyperexcitability and tetany. The treatment for a client who develops hypocalcemia and tetany following a thyroidectomy is calcium gluconate. Hypokalemia does not cause a positive Trousseau's sign. Decreased thyroid hormones will not cause tetany, however, the client will have to take thyroid replacement therapy following a thyroidectomy.
CN: Physiological integrity; CNS: Reduction of risk potential;
CL: Analyze

85. Which test should a nurse expect for a client with severe abdominal pain in the midepigastric region, back tenderness, nausea, and vomiting?

1. Amylase
2. C-peptide
3. Stool culture
4. Colonoscopy

85. 1. Severe abdominal pain in the midepigastric region, back tenderness, nausea, and vomiting may be due to irritation of the pancreas. An amylase level test should be ordered. C-peptide, a stool culture, and a colonoscopy would not be ordered for the presenting symptoms.
CN: Physiological integrity; CNS: Physiological adaptation;
CL: Analyze

86. A client has been admitted with acute abdominal pain in the midepigastric region. The diagnosis of "rule out acute pancreatitis" is made. What assessments would the nurse conduct for this client? Select all that apply.

1. Back pain and tenderness
2. Nausea and vomiting
3. Lower extremity edema
4. Rebound abdominal tenderness
5. Hemoglobin and hematocrit

86. 1, 2. The signs and symptoms of acute pancreatitis include midepigastric abdominal pain, back pain, nausea, and vomiting. There should be no reason for changes in hemoglobin and hematocrit or pedal edema. Rebound tenderness is generally assessed with acute appendicitis.
CN: Physiological integrity; CNS: Physiological adaptation;
CL: Apply

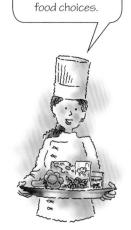

Teach your client the importance of making healthy food choices.

87. The nurse is updating the plan of care for a client recovering from acute pancreatitis. Which interventions should be included in the care plan?

1. Eat small, frequent meals that are bland, high carbohydrate, high protein, and low fat
2. Consume no more than one alcoholic drink per day and limit coffee to three cups per day
3. Include fruits and vegetables that are high in vitamin C and K and increase fiber
4. Maintain a diet that is low residue, low protein, and high in calcium

87. 1. In order to restore energy and nutrients, small, frequent meals that are high carbohydrate, high protein, and low fat are advised. Spicy foods, caffeine, and alcohol should be avoided. The other instructions do not relate to pancreatitis.
CN: Physiological integrity; CNS: Basic care and comfort;
CL: Apply

88. A client is diagnosed with an attack of acute pancreatitis secondary to gallstones and gallbladder disease. Which type of diet will this client require?

1. High-calorie, high-protein diet
2. High-fiber diet, with high fluid intake
3. Low-fat diet, avoiding heavy meals
4. A diet high in protein, calcium, and vitamin D

88. 3. A client who survives an acute pancreatitis attack caused by gallstones or gallbladder disease should maintain a low-fat diet and avoid heavy meals. A high-calorie, high-protein diet is appropriate for clients with hyperthyroidism. A diet high in fiber, with high fluid intake, is recommended for constipation. A client with Cushing's syndrome should follow a diet high in protein, calcium, and vitamin D.
CN: Physiological integrity; CNS: Reduction of risk potential;
CL: Apply

89. A client who has been treated for type 1 diabetes mellitus for five years reports numbness and tingling in the lower extremities. What should the nurse teach this client?
1. Inspect your feet daily
2. Soak your feet daily
3. Keep your feet elevated whenever possible
4. Massage your lower extremities daily

89. 1. Clients with type 1 diabetes mellitus are at increased risk for peripheral vascular disease as well as peripheral neuropathy. When this client experiences numbness, they may not be aware of a break in their skin or infection. Visually inspecting the feet daily will allow them to see any potential signs of infection. The client should not soak their feet, as this leads to maceration and open areas that can become infected. Keeping feet elevated is recommended if there is edema with vascular disease, however, this is not an intervention for numbness and tingling. Massaging the lower limbs can lead to clots being dislodged from the venous or arterial vasculature.
CN: Physiological integrity; CNS: Reduction of risk potential; CL: Apply

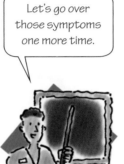

Let's go over those symptoms one more time.

90. A client has developed diabetic ketoacidosis (DKA), secondary to infection. The nurse should assess for which potential problems?
1. Kussmaul's respirations and a fruity odor to the breath
2. Shallow respirations and severe abdominal pain
3. Decreased respirations and increased urine output
4. Cheyne-Stokes respirations and foul-smelling urine

90. 1. Severe acidosis leads to Kussmaul's respirations and a fruity odor to the breath. Shallow respirations and severe abdominal pain may be symptoms of pancreatitis. Decreased respirations and increased urine output are not symptoms related to DKA. Cheyne-Stokes respirations and foul-smelling urine do not result from DKA.
CN: Physiological integrity; CNS: Physiological adaptation; CL: Apply

91. A client diagnosed with a toxic nodular goiter questions the nurse about the cause of the disorder. What is the nurse's **best** response?
1. "It is an autoimmune disorder."
2. "It is a directly inherited genetic disorder."
3. "It is a type of cancer."
4. "It is a condition resulting from environmental toxins."

91. 1. Toxic nodular goiter or Hyperthyroidism has many causes, the most common of which is Graves' disease. Graves' disease is an autoimmune disorder. While research is being performed that suggests a genetic link, there is currently no proof of direct inheritance. This is not a cancerous condition and links to environmental toxins have not been proven.
CN: Physiological integrity; CNS: Pharmacological and parenteral therapies; CL: Apply

92. A client with type 1 diabetes mellitus has developed influenza. What is the **most** important information for the nurse to teach the client?
1. "Do not administer insulin if you are nauseous."
2. "Monitor your glucose every four hours when you are sick."
3. "Hold insulin when vomiting."
4. "Decrease fluid intake to decrease vomiting."

92. 2. It is important for the client to test blood glucose every four hours and administer insulin based on a sliding scale. During periods of infection or illness, insulin-dependent clients may require additional insulin to compensate for increased blood glucose levels. Insulin should not be held when vomiting or nauseous. Fluids should be increased to prevent dehydration.
CN: Physiological integrity; CNS: Pharmacological and parenteral therapies; CL: Apply

93. A client was diagnosed with type 2 diabetes mellitus five years ago, and has now started insulin therapy. What is the **most** important information to teach the client?
1. "Your diabetes was not controlled with several drugs, so insulin therapy is the next step."
2. "This therapy is not usually warranted."
3. "All clients with type 2 diabetes mellitus need insulin therapy."
4. "This therapy is only temporary."

93. 1. For treatment of type 2 diabetes mellitus, oral agents are started at the lowest effective dose and increased every one to two weeks until the client reaches the desired blood glucose control or the maximum dosage. If the maximum dosage of one agent does not control blood glucose levels, a second agent with a different mechanism of action may be added. Insulin therapy is indicated for the patient with type 2 diabetes mellitus when blood glucose cannot be controlled with the use of two or three different antidiabetic agents. This is the standard therapy, and the therapy would be lifelong.
CN: Health promotion and maintenance; CNS: None; CL: Apply

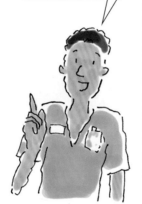

Make sure you know the standard guidelines of common disorders.

94. A client is being screened for diabetes mellitus and has two recent fasting blood glucose results of 132 mg/dl (7.33 mmol/L) and 146 mg/dl (8.10 mmol/L). How should these results be interpreted?
1. These are normal results. No further action is needed.
2. These results indicate diabetes mellitus. Follow-up is required.
3. The fasting blood glucose tests should be repeated two more times.
4. The client should be scheduled for a hemoglobin A1c (HbA1c) test.

94. 2. These are not normal results. Criteria for the diagnosis of diabetes mellitus include A1C ≥6.5%, FPG ≥126 mg/dl (7.0 mmol/L), Fasting defined as no caloric intake for ≥8 hrs. 2-hr PG ≥200 mg/dl (11.1 mmol/L) during OGTT (75-g). Performed as described by the WHO, using glucose load containing the equivalent of 75 g anhydrous glucose dissolved in water. Random PG ≥200 mg/dl (11.1 mmol/L). In the absence of unequivocal hyperglycemia results should be confirmed using repeat testing.
CN: Physiological integrity; CNS: Reduction of risk potential; CL: Analyze

95. A client diagnosed with a unilateral pheochromocytoma is scheduled for surgery to remove the left adrenal gland. What condition is the client **most** at risk for developing during surgery?
1. Hypertension
2. Renal failure
3. Hyponatremia
4. Thyroid storm

95. 1. A pheochromocytoma is a benign tumor of the adrenal medulla that secretes epinephrine and norepinephrine, resulting in hypertension and paroxysmal tachycardia. During surgical manipulation, the tumor can secrete epinephrine and norepinephrine, resulting in rapid fluctuations of blood pressure and heart rate. This client requires close monitoring during surgery. Renal failure, thyroid storm and sodium fluctuation are not commonly associated with this surgery.
CN: Physiological integrity; CNS: Reduction of risk potential; CL: Analyze

96. A client is newly diagnosed with a tumor of the adrenal medulla. What is the **priority** nursing assessment?
1. Tetany
2. Glucose
3. Blood pressure
4. Cortisol levels

96. 3. Tumors of the adrenal medulla usually produce hypertension because they release epinephrine and norepinephrine. Tetany is not a consequence of this type of tumor. Glucose and cortisol levels are not necessarily affected, however, assessing for changes in these levels would be a lower priority than assessment of blood pressure.
CN: Physiological integrity; CNS: Physiological adaptation; CL: Apply

CN: Client needs category   CNS: Client needs subcategory   CL: Cognitive level

97. What is a nurse's **priority** assessment for a client who has just began corticosteroid therapy?
1. Serum sodium levels
2. Serum glucose levels
3. Basal metabolic rate
4. Adrenocorticotropic hormone (ACTH) levels

97. 2. A major adverse effect of corticosteroid therapy is an elevation in glucose levels. Slowing of the metabolism is also expected, but not the priority. Sodium can be affected. ACTH levels might change, however, this should not affect therapy or the client's status.
CN: Physiological integrity; CNS: Pharmacological and parenteral therapies; CL: Analyze

98. What is the **priority** assessment for a client diagnosed with hyperparathyroidism?
1. Urinary output
2. Thyroid hormones
3. Calcium levels
4. Tetany

98. 4. Check for tetany by assessing for Trousseau's or Chvostek's sign at the bedside prior to other assessments. Tetany is the hyper-excitability of nerves and muscles that can cause the airway to spasm and close. Urinary output, thyroid hormones and calcium levels should all be assessed, but are not the priority.
CN: Physiological integrity; CNS: Physiological adaptation; CL: Analyze

99. A client with type 2 diabetes mellitus is prescribed capsaicin cream 0.075% What should the nurse include in a teaching plan for this medication?
1. "This cream should be applied daily to prevent dry skin."
2. "This cream should be applied to open sores to prevent infection."
3. "This cream should be applied to necrotic areas of ulcers to aid in debridement."
4. "Apply capsaicin cream four times daily to decrease neuropathic pain sensations."

99. 4. This drug reduces amounts of substance P, which is involved in pain transmission. The nurse should teach the client to apply the cream four times daily for several weeks. The cream does not prevent dry skin, debride or treat infections.
CN: Physiological integrity; CNS: Physiological adaptation; CL: Analyze

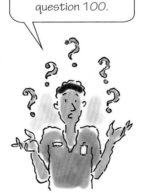

The words most important are a clue to how to answer question 100.

100. The nurse is providing education for a client newly diagnosed with Addison's disease. The client is receiving a maintenance dose of steroids. What **priority** information should the nurse include?
1. Fluid maintenance
2. Symptoms of hypo and hyperglycemia
3. Taking steroids exactly as prescribed
4. Exercise schedule

100. 3. A client with Addison's disease requires more steroids than the body produces. It is most important to teach a client to take steroids exactly as they are prescribed to prevent complications. Taking a lower dose may trigger an Addisonian crisis. Taking a higher dose increases the effects of potassium depletion, hyperglycemia, and fluid retention which can lead to a life-threatening situation. Information regarding fluid maintenance, the symptoms of hypo- and hyperglycemia and exercise are important, but not the priority.
CN: Physiological integrity; CNS: Pharmacological and parenteral therapies; CL: Apply

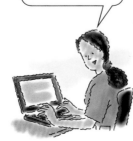

Be careful! Combo answers can be tricky!

101. A client is being treated for Addisonian crisis. Which laboratory values are **most** important for the nurse to monitor?
1. Serum bicarbonate and sodium
2. Serum glucose and ketones
3. Serum sodium and potassium
4. Serum calcium and magnesium

101. 3. If steroid replacement therapy is inadequate, sodium loss and potassium retention persist. If the steroid dose is too high, sodium and water are retained, and large amounts of potassium are excreted. Steroid replacement can affect glucose, but the replacement doesn't have as great an impact on ketones, bicarbonate, calcium, or magnesium as it does on sodium and potassium.
CN: Physiological integrity; CNS: Reduction of risk potential; CL: Analyze

CN: Client needs category   CNS: Client needs subcategory   CL: Cognitive level

102. A client diagnosed with diabetic ketoacidosis (DKA) had a serum glucose level of 485 mg/dl (26.92 mmol/L). After treatment, the serum glucose level dropped to 185 mg/dl (10.27 mmol/L). The client developed an irregular heart rate. Which assessment finding **most** likely caused this irregularity?
1. Decreased serum chloride level
2. Decreased serum potassium level
3. Elevated serum glucose level
4. Elevated serum sodium level

102. 2. Correction of an elevated serum glucose level may alter the serum potassium level, predisposing the client to dysrhythmias. Serum chloride and sodium changes are more likely to contribute to an altered level of consciousness, whereas elevated serum glucose contributes to the long-term effects of diabetes mellitus, such as coronary artery disease, hypertension, and peripheral vascular disease.
CN: Physiological integrity; CNS: Physiological adaptation; CL: Analyze

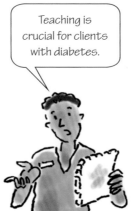

Teaching is crucial for clients with diabetes.

103. When teaching a client with diabetes about nutritional planning, which food choice would be considered one serving of a healthy carbohydrate?
1. One small orange
2. 1/2 cup of vanilla ice cream
3. Two slices of white bread
4. Two cups of whole-grain rice

103. 1. One small orange is considered one serving of a healthy carbohydrate. The orange provides vitamins, fiber and water content. Vanilla ice cream contains both carbohydrate and saturated fat. Two slices of white bread are two servings of carbohydrate. Two cups of whole-grain rice are approximately three to four servings of a carbohydrate.
CN: Physiological integrity; CNS: Basic care and comfort; CL: Apply

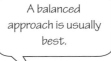

A balanced approach is usually best.

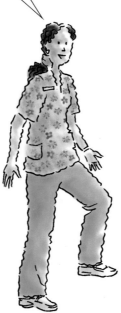

104. An unemployed client without health insurance has not filled his prescription. Which assessment finding indicates that this client is not taking her levothyroxine as prescribed?
1. Diarrhea
2. Rapid heart rate
3. Warm, dry, flushed skin
4. Temperature of 94° F (34.4° C)

104. 4. Levothyroxine is prescribed for hypothyroidism, which causes a hypodynamic state. Failure to maintain levothyroxine therapy can lead to a low body temperature as well as slowing all metabolic processes. The other assessments indicate a hypermetabolic state, which could be symptomatic of an increase in thyroid hormones
CN: Physiological integrity; CNS: Physiological adaptation; CL: Apply

105. A client newly diagnosed with type 1 diabetes mellitus is ready for discharge. What **priority** information should the nurse include?
1. Foot care
2. How to balance diet, exercise, and medication
3. Regular healthcare provider visits
4. How to maintain the self-blood glucose monitor

105. 2. With type 1, type 2, or gestational diabetes mellitus, balancing diet, exercise, and medication is essential to disease control, and is priority information. Foot care, regular healthcare visits and maintenance of the self-blood glucose monitor are all important things to teach the client about managing diabetes mellitus, but not the priority.
CN: Physiological integrity; CNS: Physiological adaptation; CL: Apply

106. Which statement indicates to the nurse that a client with type 1 diabetes mellitus understands proper foot care?
1. "I'll call for a healthcare provider's appointment if my feet start to ache."
2. "I will soak my feet daily."
3. "I'll go barefoot around the house to avoid pressure areas on my feet."
4. "I'll wear cotton socks with well-fitting shoes."

106. 4. Cotton socks wick moisture away from the skin, and help prevent fungal infections and maceration. Proper shoe fit helps avoid pressure areas. Aching isn't a common sign of foot problems, however, a tingling sensation in the feet indicates neurovascular changes. Soaking feet can cause maceration and possible infection and is not recommended. Going barefoot can cause injury.
CN: Physiological integrity; CNS: Reduction of risk potential; CL: Analyze

CN: Client needs category   CNS: Client needs subcategory   CL: Cognitive level

107. An adolescent client who has type 1 diabetes mellitus has a decreased level of consciousness and a serum glucose level of 45. Which is the **priority** nursing intervention?
1. Placing a Salem sump tube and providing tube feedings
2. Administering a 500-ml bolus of normal saline solution
3. Administering 1 mg of glucagon intramuscularly or subcutaneously
4. Calling the healthcare provider for orders

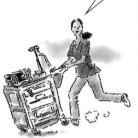

Blood glucose that low constitutes an emergency. What's the right response?

107. 3. Administering 1 mg of glucagon intramuscularly or subcutaneously helps restore the client's physiological integrity. Providing a feeding tube is time consuming, and appropriate only in a less urgent situation. A bolus of normal saline solution would only correct the client's fluid status, not her glucose level. Calling the healthcare provider would delay treatment at a time when rapid intervention is crucial.
CN: Physiological integrity; CNS: Physiological adaptation; CL: Apply

108. A client is admitted to the medical floor with a diagnosis of pancreatitis. What is the **priority** nursing intervention?
1. Maintain oral intake and avoid analgesics
2. Control pain and maintain NPO status
3. Allow the client to dictate food and alcohol servings
4. Support surgical management interventions

108. 2. The priority for client care is to provide pain control and decrease gastrointestinal activity. Alcohol and caffeine are contraindicated in pancreatitis because they exacerbations symptoms. Surgery is not a primary intervention for treatment of pancreatitis.
CN: Physiological integrity; CNS: Physiological adaptation; CL: Apply

109. The nurse is providing education for a client diagnosed with Cushing's syndrome. Which statement indicates an understanding of the disease?
1. "My blood sugar is low, so I don't need to watch my diet."
2. "I should increase my fluid intake to three liters a day."
3. "I will weigh myself daily and report any gain."
4. "With this disease process, it is okay to increase my sodium intake."

109. 3. Excess fluid volume can be a complication of Cushing's syndrome due to sodium and water retention. This can quickly lead to fluid overload, heart failure, and pulmonary edema. Weight gain is an indicator of fluid retention and should be reported. Sodium intake should be kept to a minimum, and fluid restriction may be needed to maintain balance. Hyperglycemia occurs instead of hypoglycemia.
CN: Health promotion and maintenance; CNS: None; CL: Apply

110. The nurse is admitting a client diagnosed with untreated hypothyroidism. What manifestations can the nurse expect to find during the initial assessment? Select all that apply.
1. Cold intolerance
2. Tachycardia
3. Hypotension
4. Weight gain
5. Mental sluggishness

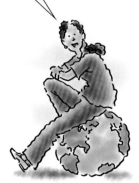

You should feel on top of the world! You're almost finished.

110. 1, 3, 4, 5. Cardiac functions are decreased resulting in bradycardia and hypotension. Weight gain is common due to decreased metabolism. Intolerance to cold often occurs due to lowered body temperature and slowed metabolism. Neurological manifestations include slurred or slowed speech, impaired memory, and inattentiveness, all of which result is mental sluggishness.
CN: Physiological integrity; CNS: Physiological adaptation; CL: Analyze

CN: Client needs category   CNS: Client needs subcategory   CL: Cognitive level

111. A client is admitted with a diagnosis of diabetic ketoacidosis. An insulin drip is initiated with 50 units of insulin in 100 ml of normal saline solution. The IV is being infused via an infusion pump, and the pump is currently set at 10 ml/hr. How many units of insulin each hour is this client receiving? Record your answer using whole number.

_____units

112. A client with Addison's disease is scheduled for discharge after being hospitalized for an adrenal crisis. Which statements would indicate that the nurse's teaching has been effective? Select all that apply.
1. "I have to take my steroids for 10 days."
2. "I need to weigh myself daily to be sure I don't eat too many calories."
3. "I need to call my healthcare provider to discuss my steroid needs before I have dental work."
4. "I will call the healthcare provider if I start to feel fatigued, weak, or dizzy."
5. "If I feel like I have the flu, I'll carry on as usual because this is an expected response."
6. "I need to obtain and wear a medical alert bracelet."

113. A client who suffered a brain injury after falling off a ladder has recently developed syndrome of inappropriate antidiuretic hormone (SIADH). What findings indicate that the treatment being received for SIADH is effective? Select all that apply.
1. Decrease in body weight
2. Rise in blood pressure; drop in heart rate
3. Absence of wheezes in the lungs
4. Increase in urine output
5. Decrease in urine osmolarity

111. 5.
To determine the number of insulin units the client is receiving per hour, the nurse must first calculate the number of units in each milliliter of fluid:

$$\frac{50\ units}{100\ mL} = 0.5\ units/mL$$

Next, multiply the units/ml by the rate of mL/hour:

$$0.5\ units \times 10\ \frac{mL}{hour} = 5\ \frac{units}{hour}$$

CN: Physiological integrity; CNS: Pharmacological and parenteral therapies; CL: Apply

112. 3, 4, 6. Dental work can be a cause of physical stress, therefore, the client's healthcare provider should be informed, and may need to adjust the steroid dosage. Fatigue, weakness, and dizziness are symptoms of inadequate dosing. The healthcare provider should be notified if these symptoms occur. A medical alert bracelet allows health care providers to access the client's history of Addison's disease if it can't be communicated by the client. For this client, routine administration of steroids is a lifetime treatment. Daily weight is monitored for changes in fluid balance, not caloric intake. Influenza is an added physical stressor. The client's healthcare provider should be informed, and steroid dosage may need adjusted.
CN: Physiological integrity; CNS: Reduction of risk potential; CL: Analyze

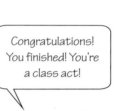

Congratulations! You finished! You're a class act!

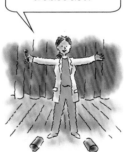

113. 1, 4, 5. SIADH is an abnormality involving an excessive release of antidiuretic hormone. The predominant feature is water retention with oliguria, edema, and weight gain. Successful treatment should result in a reduction of weight, increased urine output, and a decrease in urine concentration osmolarity.
CN: Physiological integrity; CNS: Physiological adaptation; CL: Analyze

Chapter 10

Genitourinary Disorders

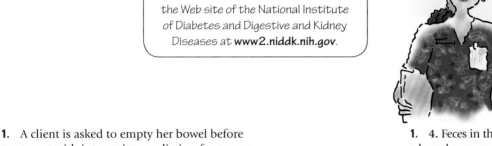

For more information about genitourinary system disorders, visit the Web site of the National Institute of Diabetes and Digestive and Kidney Diseases at **www2.niddk.nih.gov**.

1. A client is asked to empty her bowel before treatment with intracavitary radiation for cancer of the cervix. Which statement by the nurse **best** explains why this is important?
  1. Feces in the bowel increase the risk for ileus.
  2. An empty bowel allows the applicator to be positioned with little or no discomfort.
  3. Bowel movements increase the risk of inadvertent contamination of the vagina and urethra.
  4. Pressure changes in the pelvis associated with bowel movements can alter the position of the applicator and the radiation source.

1. 4. Feces in the bowel increase the likelihood of a bowel movement, which can change the position of the applicator and radiation source. Pressure changes that occur during a bowel movement may cause a position change of the radioactive implant resulting in the delivery of radiation and injury to healthy tissue and less to the malignant lesion Feces in the bowel do not increase the risk of ileus or inadvertent contamination of the vagina and urethra from a bowel movement. Applicators are usually inserted under anesthesia in the operating room.
CN: Physiological integrity; CNS: Reduction of risk potential;
CL: Analyze

2. A health care provider tells a client diagnosed with a sexually transmitted infection to return one week after antibiotic treatment to have a repeat culture done to verify the cure. This order would be appropriate for a client who has:
  1. genital warts.
  2. genital herpes.
  3. gonorrhea.
  4. syphilis.

2. 3. Gonococcal infections can be completely eliminated by drug therapy. This is documented by a negative culture four to seven days after therapy is complete. Genital warts are not curable, and are identified by appearance, not culture. Genital herpes is not curable, and is identified by the appearance of the lesions, or by cytologic studies. The diagnosis of syphilis is by Darkfield microscopy or serological tests.
CN: Physiological integrity; CNS: Physiological adaptation;
CL: Apply

3. What is the **best** question a nurse can ask a client when determining the type of incontinence the client has developed?
  1. "Do you drink alcohol daily?
  2. "Do you have a busy job?"
  3. "Are you incontinent when you cough or laugh?
  4. "How old are you?"

3. 3. Stress incontinence is the most common type of incontinence. The primary symptom is the loss of small amounts of urine when the client coughs, sneezes, jogs, or lifts. The person with stress incontinence cannot tighten their urethra enough to prevent leakage. The nurse should ask this question to determine if the incontinence occurs at these times. Alcohol, busy jobs and age are not significant risk factors. Stress incontinence can also occur after childbirth.
CN: Physiological integrity; CNS: Physiological adaptation;
CL: Analyze

CN: Client needs category   CNS: Client needs subcategory   CL: Cognitive level

4. A client has been diagnosed with a chlamydial infection. Which statement indicates that this client understands the potential complications of this infection?
1. "I'm glad that I'm not pregnant. This disease can cause birth defects."
2. "I hope this medicine works before this disease destroys my kidneys."
3. "I should have used birth control pills to decrease my risk of this disease."
4. "This infection can lead to infertility, and I need to have it treated."

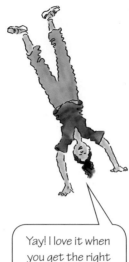

Yay! I love it when you get the right answer.

5. A client with genital herpes asks the nurse to recommend comfort measures for the virus. What is the nurse's **best** response?
1. "Wear loose cotton underwear."
2. "Apply a water-based lubricant to the lesions."
3. "Rub rather than scratch in response to an itch."
4. "Pour hydrogen peroxide and water over the lesions."

6. It is **most** important for the nurse to provide teaching of breast self-examinations to clients who have:
1. cervical dysplasia.
2. a dermoid cyst.
3. endometrial polyps.
4. ovarian cancer.

7. A 38-year-old client attends a follow-up visit after having a vaginal hysterectomy. She has an elevated temperature and decreased hematocrit. The nurse understands that these symptoms could indicate:
1. hematoma.
2. hypovolemia.
3. infection.
4. thromboembolism.

4. 4. Chlamydia is a common cause of pelvic inflammatory disease and infertility. It does not cause birth defects or affect the kidneys. It can cause conjunctivitis and respiratory infection in neonates exposed to infected cervicovaginal secretions during delivery. Using birth control pills does not decrease the risk of infection.
CN: Physiological integrity; CNS: Reduction of risk potential; CL: Apply

5. 1. Wearing loose cotton underwear promotes drying, and decreases irritation of the lesions. Other types of underwear, such as silk and synthetic, tends to trap moisture. The use of lubricants is contraindicated because they can prolong healing time, and increase the risk of secondary infection. Lesions should not be rubbed or scratched because of the risk of tissue damage and additional infection. Cool, wet compresses can be used to soothe the itch. The use of hydrogen peroxide and water on lesions is not recommended.
CN: Physiological integrity; CNS: Basic care and comfort; CL: Apply

6. 4. Clients with ovarian cancer have an increased risk for breast cancer. Breast self-examination are crucial to early detection and treatment. There is no known relationship between breast cancer and cervical dysplasia, endometrial polyps, or dermoid cysts.
CN: Health promotion and maintenance; CNS: None; CL: Apply

7. 1. An elevated temperature and decreased hematocrit are symptoms of hematoma. Symptoms of hypovolemia include increased hematocrit and hemoglobin values. Elevated temperature is a classic sign of infection, but a decreased hematocrit is not. Abrupt onset of fever is a symptom of thromboembolism, but other symptoms include dyspnea, chest pain, cough, hemoptysis, restlessness, and signs of shock.
CN: Physiological integrity; CNS: Reduction of risk potential; CL: Apply

---

CN: Client needs category   CNS: Client needs subcategory   CL: Cognitive level

8. Which client is at greatest risk for dehydration?
1. A 48-year-old having intracavitary radiation for cancer of the cervix
2. A 59-year-old one week after a radical vulvectomy
3. A 67-year-old receiving adjuvant tamoxifen therapy for breast cancer
4. A 72-year-old with a vesicovaginal fistula

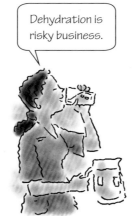

Dehydration is risky business.

8. 1. Dehydration can occur from fluid loss secondary to tissue destruction at the site of irradiation at any age. After radical vulvectomy, wound drains are generally removed by postoperative day four or five, and don't create a significant risk of dehydration. Tamoxifen therapy is unrelated to dehydration. Although urine may escape through the vagina as a result of a vesicovaginal fistula, it does not cause the loss of an unusual amount of urine or other fluid.
CN: Physiological integrity; CNS: Physiological adaptation; CL: Analyze

9. Which client would benefit most from information explaining the importance of receiving an annual Papanicolaou (PAP) test?
1. A client with a history of recurrent candidiasis
2. A client who had her first pregnancy before the age of 20
3. A client infected with the human papillomavirus (HPV)
4. A client who has used oral contraceptives for 27 years

9. 3. HPV causes genital warts, which are associated with an increased incidence of cervical cancer. Recurrent candidiasis, pregnancy before age 20, and the use of oral contraceptives have not been shown to increase the risk of cervical cancer.
CN: Health promotion and maintenance; CNS: None; CL: Analyze

10. A client develops candidiasis. Which is the **most** likely contributor?
1. Nulliparity
2. Menopause
3. Use of corticosteroids
4. Use of spermicidal jelly

10. 3. Small numbers of the fungus *Candida albicans* are commonly found in the vagina. Because corticosteroids suppress the immune system, they increase the risk of candidiasis. Pregnancy, not nulliparity, increases the risk of candidiasis. It is thought that higher estrogen levels and higher glycogen content in vaginal secretions during pregnancy increase a woman's risk of developing Candidiasis. Candidiasis is rare before menarche or after menopause. The use of oral contraceptives, not spermicidal jelly, increases the risk of candidiasis. Oral contraceptives contain an excess in the amount of estrogen, resulting an increase of blood sugar levels, which yeast feeds on. As a result, an overgrowth of yeast occurs.
CN: Health promotion and maintenance; CNS: None; CL: Apply

11. A client visits the clinic with a primary concern of a "frothy, greenish, vaginal discharge." Which diagnosis does the nurse anticipate?
1. Candidiasis
2. Gardnerella vaginalis vaginitis
3. Gonorrhea
4. Trichomoniasis

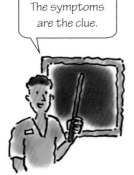

The symptoms are the clue.

11. 4. The discharge associated with infection caused by Trichomonas organisms is homogenous, greenish-gray, watery, and frothy or purulent. The discharge associated with candidiasis is thick and white in appearance. An infection due to *Gardnerella vaginalis* would present with a discharge that is thin and grayish white, with a fishy odor. Gonorrhea is asymptomatic in many women, but can present with a purulent vaginal discharge.
CN: Physiological integrity; CNS: Physiological adaptation; CL: Apply

CN: Client needs category   CNS: Client needs subcategory   CL: Cognitive level

12. A woman reports an intermittent, milky, vaginal discharge. She is not sexually active and denies an itching or burning sensation. What is the nurse's **best** intervention?
   1. Teach the client how to clean the perineal area more completely
   2. Evaluate the client for an allergy to a feminine hygiene product
   3. Teach the client that this is normal
   4. Ask the client if she wears tight clothing

12. 3. The nurse should teach the client that this is a normal discharge. Vaginal fluid is clear, milky, or cloudy, depending on the fluctuating levels of estrogen and progesterone. A milky-appearing vaginal discharge is normal and is not associated with inadequate cleaning, sensitivity, or a reaction to heat or moisture.
CN: Health promotion and maintenance; CNS: None;
CL: Apply

13. What is the **priority** nursing intervention for a client in the immediate post-operative stage following breast reconstructive surgery?
   1. Prevent hypothermia
   2. Maintain even pressure on the wound
   3. Position the client on the operative side
   4. Raise the client's arms over her head four times daily

13. 1. Hypothermia causes a decrease in surface circulation. This can lead to ischemia of the skin or muscle graft, and ultimately to tissue necrosis in clients who had breast reconstruction surgery. Maintaining good circulation is crucial, and pressure on the breast wound must be avoided. The client should be positioned on her back or on her non-operative side. Arms should not be lifted above shoulder level for four to six weeks.
CN: Physiological integrity; CNS: Reduction of risk potential;
CL: Apply

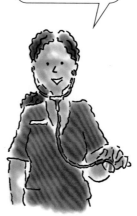

Which answer is most likely to be correct?

14. A client who had intracavitary radiation treatment for cancer of the cervix one month ago reports small amounts of vaginal bleeding. This client is most likely experiencing:
   1. recurrence of the carcinoma.
   2. development of a rectovaginal fistula.
   3. expected effect of the radiation therapy.
   4. infection secondary to a change in vaginal flora.

14. 3. After intracavitary radiation, some vaginal bleeding occurs for one to three months following treatment. Intermittent, painless, vaginal bleeding is a classic symptom of cervical cancer, but given this client's history, the bleeding is more likely a result of the radiation than recurrent cancer. The passage of feces through the vagina, is a sign of rectovaginal fistula. Vaginal infections show various types of vaginal discharge, but not vaginal bleeding.
CN: Physiological integrity; CNS: Physiological adaptation;
CL: Apply

15. A nurse enters the room of a client who had a left modified mastectomy eight hours ago. Which assessment finding requires further intervention?
   1. The client is squeezing a ball in her left hand.
   2. The client is wearing a robe with tight elastic cuffs.
   3. The client's affected arm is elevated on a pillow.
   4. A blood pressure cuff is on the client's right arm.

15. 2. Elastic cuffs can contribute to the development of lymphedema, and should be avoided. Simple exercises, such as squeezing a ball, help promote circulation and should be started as soon as possible after surgery. Elevation of the affected arm promotes venous and lymphatic return from the extremity. Blood pressure measurements in the affected arm should also be avoided.
CN: Safe, effective care environment; CNS: Management of care;
CL: Analyze

16. The client has a wound dehiscence and is at risk for evisceration. For which should the nurse assess this client?
1. Tachycardia accompanied by a weak, thready pulse
2. Hypotension with a decreased level of consciousness (LOC)
3. Shallow, rapid respirations and increasing vaginal drainage
4. Low-grade fever with increasing serosanguineous incisional drainage

16. 4. Evisceration, the protrusion of wound contents may occur as a result of dehiscence and is a serious complication. Signs of impending evisceration are a low-grade fever, and increasing serosanguineous drainage. Tachycardia, a weak, thready pulse, hypotension, decreased LOC, shallow respirations, and vaginal drainage are all unrelated to impending evisceration, but may be associated with other serious problems such as shock.
CN: Physiological integrity; CNS: Reduction of risk potential; CL: Apply

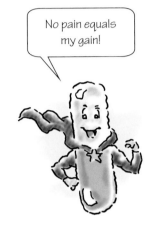

No pain equals my gain!

17. Oxycodone is being administered to a client with metastatic breast cancer. Which assessment finding indicates that this medication is having a therapeutic effect?
1. Bone density is increased
2. Pain is 0 to 2 on a 10-point scale
3. Alpha-fetoprotein level is decreased
4. Serum calcium level is within normal range

17. 2. Oxycodone is an opioid analgesic used for alleviating severe pain, especially in terminal illness. If a client's pain has decreased to 0 to 2 on a 10-point scale, the medication is having a therapeutic effect. This medication does not directly affect bone density, alpha-fetoprotein level, or serum calcium level.
CN: Physiological integrity; CNS: Pharmacological and parenteral therapies; CL: Analyze

18. Which instruction should the nurse give to a client with prostatitis who is receiving double strength co-trimoxazole?
1. Don't expect improvement of symptoms for 7 to 10 days
2. Drink six to eight glasses of fluid daily while taking this medication
3. If a sore mouth or throat develops, take the medication with milk or an antacid
4. Use a sunscreen of at least SPF-15 with para-aminobenzoic acid (PABA)

18. 2. Six to eight glasses of fluid daily are needed to prevent renal problems, such as crystalluria and stone formation. The symptoms should improve in a few days if the drug is effective. Sore throat and sore mouth are adverse effects that should be reported right away. The drug causes photosensitivity, but a PABA-free sunscreen should be used because PABA can interfere with the drug's action.
CN: Physiological integrity; CNS: Pharmacological and parenteral therapies; CL: Apply

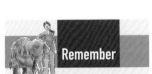

Remember

Alpha-adrenergic blockers get "RID" of hypertension by:
- **R**elaxing smooth muscle in blood vessels
- **I**ncreasing dilation of blood vessels
- **D**ecreasing blood pressure

Alpha-adrenergic blockers include the following drugs:
- Phentolamine
- Prazosin
- Doxazosin
- Terazosin

19. What is the most important assessment for the nurse to make when administering tamsulosin to a client with benign prostatic hyperplasia (BPH)?
1. Voiding pattern
2. Size of the prostate
3. Creatinine clearance
4. Serum testosterone level

19. 1. The alpha-adrenergic blocker tamsulosin relaxes the smooth muscle of the bladder neck and prostate, so the urinary voiding symptoms of BPH are reduced in many clients. These drugs do not affect the size of the prostate, renal function, or the production or metabolism of testosterone.
CN: Physiological integrity; CNS: Pharmacological and parenteral therapies; CL: Apply

20. The nurse is assigned four clients. Which client is at **highest** risk for impaired skin integrity?
1. A client with endometriosis
2. A client taking oral contraceptives
3. A client with a vaginal packing in place
4. A client having reconstructive breast surgery

20. 4. Reconstructive breast surgery places the client at risk for insufficient blood supply to the muscle graft and skin, which can lead to tissue necrosis. Endometriosis and oral contraceptives aren't generally associated with altered tissue perfusion. Pressure from vaginal packing can sometimes put pressure on the bladder neck and interfere with voiding.
CN: Physiological integrity; CNS: Reduction of risk potential; CL: Analyze

CN: Client needs category   CNS: Client needs subcategory   CL: Cognitive level

21. A client is diagnosed with priapism. What condition is the client at risk for developing?
1. Disseminated intravascular coagulation (DIC)
2. Hydronephrosis
3. Penile gangrene
4. Testicular atrophy

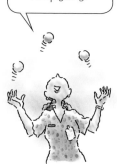

You've got it all under control. Keep going!

22. The nurse is teaching a client how to decrease their risk for toxic shock syndrome. What is the **best** information for a nurse to share?
1. Avoid douching
2. Wear loose cotton underwear
3. Use pads, not tampons
4. Avoid sexual intercourse during menses

23. The nurse is reviewing discharge instructions for a client who had a dilation and curettage procedure. Which statement should the nurse include in the discharge instructions?
1. Tampons may be used during exercise.
2. Avoid strenuous work and sexual intercourse for at least two weeks.
3. Stay on bed rest for three days, then gradually resume normal activity.
4. Take a soaking tub bath each day to promote relaxation.

24. Which assessment finding is expected in a client receiving bicalutamide and leuprolide for advanced prostate cancer?
1. Abdominal distention
2. Acromegaly
3. Colicky pain
4. Hot flashes

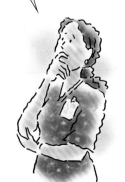

What is *abnormal* about this client's findings?

25. Which assessment finding is abnormal in a 72-year-old male client?
1. Increased sperm count
2. Small, firm testes on palpation
3. History of slowed sexual response
4. Decreased plasma testosterone level

21. 3. Priapism is a condition in which the penis is persistently erect and painful. It's a urological emergency because gangrene, secondary to ischemia, can result if venous drainage of the corpora cavernosa does not occur. Priapism does not cause DIC, hydronephrosis, or testicular atrophy.
CN: Physiological integrity; CNS: Reduction of risk potential; CL: Apply

22. 3. The cause of toxic shock syndrome is a toxin produced by *Staphylococcus aureus* bacteria. It most commonly occurs in menstruating women who use tampons. Tampons, particularly when left in place for more than eight hours, are believed to provide an ideal environment for bacterial growth. The bacteria then enters the bloodstream through breaks in the vaginal mucosa. Douching, use of loose cotton underwear, and sexual intercourse during menstruation have no direct association with toxic shock syndrome.
CN: Health promotion and maintenance; CNS: None; CL: Analyze

23. 2. Strenuous work, which can result in increased bleeding, should be avoided for two weeks to allow time for healing. Sexual intercourse should also be avoided for two weeks to allow healing and decrease the risk of infection. Tampons and tub baths should be avoided for one week. Overall activity should be gradually resumed, reaching preoperative levels within two-weeks. Bed rest and other restrictions aren't usually necessary.
CN: Physiological integrity; CNS: Reduction of risk potential; CL: Apply

24. 4. Bicalutamide, a nonsteroidal antiandrogen, and leuprolide, a gonadotropin-releasing hormone agonist, decrease the production of testosterone. This helps decrease the production of cancer cells involved in prostate cancer. Because androgens are responsible for the development of male genitalia and secondary male sex characteristics, low androgen levels can cause genital atrophy, breast enlargement, and hot flashes. Abdominal distention, acromegaly, and colicky pain aren't caused by bicalutamide and leuprolide therapy.
CN: Physiological integrity; CNS: Pharmacological and parenteral therapies; CL: Analyze

25. 1. Sperm continues to be produced as a male ages; however, the rate of sperm cell production slows. Decreased size and increased firmness of the testes, a decrease in sexual potency, and decreased production of testosterone and progesterone are normal age-related changes.
CN: Physiological integrity; CNS: Physiological adaptation; CL: Apply

CN: Client needs category   CNS: Client needs subcategory   CL: Cognitive level

26. A client is being treated for chronic prostatitis. Which comment indicates to the nurse that further teaching is necessary?
1. "I miss not being able to have sex."
2. "I enjoy soaking in a hot tub of water."
3. "Cutting down on coffee hasn't been as hard as I expected."
4. "I'm used to getting up and moving, not just sitting for long periods."

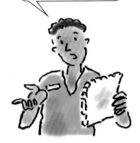

Client teaching includes making sure your client understands your instructions.

26. 1. Ejaculation can aid in the treatment of chronic prostatitis by decreasing the retention of prostatic fluid. Coffee should be eliminated from the diet because it can increase prostate secretion. Warm sitz baths and not sitting for long periods at a time promote comfort.
CN: Physiological integrity; CNS: Physiological adaptation; CL: Apply

27. A male client reports perineal pain without any observable cause. What condition does the nurse suspect?
1. Endometriosis
2. Internal hemorrhoids
3. Prostatitis
4. Renal calculus

27. 3. Prostatitis can cause prostate pain, which is felt as perineal discomfort. Endometriosis can cause pain low in the abdomen, deep in the pelvis, or in the rectal or sacrococcygeal area, depending on the location of the ectopic tissue. Hemorrhoids cause rectal pain and pressure. Renal calculi typically produce flank pain.
CN: Health promotion and maintenance; CNS: None; CL: Analyze

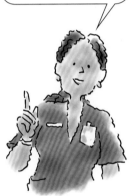

Which assessment finding is cause for alarm? Here's a hint: I think it's a waste.

28. A client is taking finasteride. The nurse is **most** concerned when this client manifests:
1. azotemia.
2. breast enlargement.
3. decreased prostate size.
4. flushing.

28. 1. Azotemia, a buildup of nitrogenous waste products in the blood, indicates impaired renal function. Finasteride, an antiandrogenic agent, is prescribed for chronic urinary retention secondary to benign prostatic hypertrophy (BPH). Azotemia in a client on finasteride therapy can indicate that the drug is not effective in relieving the urinary symptoms associated with BPH, or that an unrelated renal problem has occurred. Breast enlargement, decrease in prostate size, and flushing are expected effects of finasteride.
CN: Physiological integrity; CNS: Pharmacological and parenteral therapies; CL: Apply

29. A client with cervical polyps has been treated with cryosurgery? What would be the **best** nursing intervention?
1. Daily douche
2. Oral antibiotics
3. Intravaginal antibiotic cream
4. Use of tampons for 72 hours

29. 3. Intravaginal antibiotic cream is commonly used to aid healing and prevent infection. Oral antibiotics are used for clients with acute cervicitis or perimetritis. Douching and tampons are generally avoided for two weeks following cryotherapy.
CN: Physiological integrity; CNS: Reduction of risk potential; CL: Apply

30. A client is having intracavitary radiation for cancer of the cervix? What would be an appropriate nursing intervention?
1. High-residue diet
2. Fowler's position when in bed
3. Intermittent urinary catheterization
4. Bed rest

30. 4. Clients having intracavitary radiation therapy will be on strict bed rest, with the head of the bed elevated no more than 10 to 15 degrees to avoid displacing the radiation source. A low-residue diet is used to prevent diarrhea during treatment. Placing the client in Fowler's position while in bed is incorrect. An indwelling urinary catheter, not intermittent urinary catheterization, is used to prevent urine from distending the bladder and changing the position of tissues relative to the radiation source.
CN: Physiological integrity; CNS: Physiological adaptation; CL: Analyze

CN: Client needs category   CNS: Client needs subcategory   CL: Cognitive level

31. The nurse is caring for several clients. Which client would be required to identify sexual partners for treatment?
  1. The client with bartholinitis
  2. The client with candidiasis
  3. The client with chlamydia
  4. The client with endometriosis

31. 3. Chlamydia is a common sexually-transmitted disease for which all sexual partners need identified for treatment to prevent reinfection. Bartholinitis results from obstruction of a duct. Sexual partners may become infected, and affected men can usually be treated with over-the-counter products. Candidiasis is a yeast infection that typically occurs as a result of antibiotic usage. Endometriosis occurs when endometrial cells are seeded throughout the pelvis and is not a sexually transmitted disease.
CN: Health promotion and maintenance; CNS: None; CL: Apply

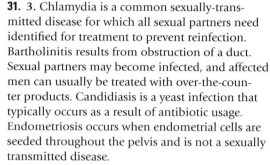

Drugs and alcohol typically don't mix.

32. What is the **most** important information for the nurse to include when teaching a client about metronidazol?
  1. Breathlessness and cough are common adverse effects.
  2. Urine may develop a greenish tinge while the client is taking this drug.
  3. Mixing this drug with alcohol causes severe nausea and vomiting.
  4. Heart palpitations may occur and should be immediately reported.

32. 3. When mixed with alcohol, metronidazole causes a disulfiram-like effect involving nausea, vomiting, and other unpleasant symptoms. Urine may turn reddish brown, not greenish, from the drug. Cardiovascular or respiratory effects are not associated with this drug.
CN: Physiological integrity; CNS: Pharmacological and parenteral therapies; CL: Apply

33. Hydrocodone with acetaminophen has been prescribed for a client with metastatic prostate cancer. What information is essential for the nurse to include in the teaching plan?
  1. "You may develop blurred vision."
  2. "Constipation may develop with constant use."
  3. "You may feel more relaxed and calm."
  4. "Nausea may occur."

33. 2. Constipation commonly develops with constant use of hydrocodone. The nurse should teach the client about constipation, and tell the client ways to decrease this risk, such as increasing fiber and liquids in the diet. Nausea may occur on occasion, however, it is not a severe problem, and could be related to constipation. Blurred vision and diarrhea are not associated with the use of hydrocodone with acetaminophen. Feeling relaxed and calm is a common side effect does not need medical attention. As the body adjusts to the medicine during treatment these side effects may go away.
CN: Physiological integrity; CNS: Pharmacological and parenteral therapies; CL: Apply

34. The nurse is planning care for a client having a hysterosalpingography. What is the **most** important intervention for the nurse to provide?
  1. Give the client a perineal pad to wear after the procedure
  2. Give the client nothing by mouth after midnight the night before the procedure
  3. Position the client in the knee-chest position during the procedure
  4. Keep the client in a dorsal recumbent position for four hours after the procedure

34. 1. A perineal pad is needed after hysterosalpingography because the contrast medium may leak from the vagina for several hours and stain the clothing. The bowel needs to be cleaned before the procedure, but the client does not have to refrain from having anything by mouth after midnight. The procedure is performed with the client in the lithotomy position, and no special positioning is required after the procedure.
CN: Physiological integrity; CNS: Basic care and comfort; CL: Apply

CN: Client needs category   CNS: Client needs subcategory   CL: Cognitive level

35. The nurse is instructing a client with vulvovaginal candidiasis on the use of the prescribed nystatin vaginal tablets. Which statement indicates that the client requires additional teaching?
   1. "I will need to refrigerate the nystatin tablets."
   2. "I can get up to do other activities after inserting the medicine."
   3. "I will finish all the tablets even if I am feeling better."
   4. "I should report increased skin irritation to my doctor."

35. 2. The client will need to lay down for at least 30 minutes after insertion of the vaginal tablets. Refrigerating nystatin tablets, finishing all the tablets, and reporting increased skin irritation to the health care provider are all important interventions concerning this medication.
CN: Physiological integrity; CNS: Pharmacological and parenteral therapies; CL: Apply

36. A 36-year-old client who never had the measles, mumps, and rubella (MMR) immunization reports that a child, with whom he recently stayed, has been diagnosed with mumps. Which treatment should the client receive?
   1. Intravenous antibiotics
   2. The MMR vaccine
   3. Application of a scrotal support
   4. Administration of gamma globulin

36. 4. Gamma globulin provides passive immunity to mumps. Antibiotic therapy is used in the treatment of bacterial orchitis. Ice and the use of a scrotal support are used as comfort measures in the treatment of orchitis. The client should not receive the MMR vaccine at this point in time.
CN: Health promotion and maintenance; CNS: None; CL: Apply

37. A client scheduled for a vasectomy. Which statement by the client indicates that further teaching is required?
   1. "I'm glad I won't have to worry about contraception as soon as this procedure is done."
   2. "I'll need to place an ice pack over the incision several times a day when I first go home."
   3. "I know this procedure can be reversed, but the success rate is low."
   4. "I'll have to limit my usual activities for about one week."

37. 1. After vasectomy, the client remains fertile for several weeks until sperm stored distal to the severed vas deferens are evacuated. After this occurs, sperm are still produced, but they do not enter the ejaculate, and are absorbed by the body. The other statements are accurate.
CN: Physiological integrity; CNS: Physiological adaptation; CL: Analyze

38. What should the nurse teach an uncircumcised client to prevent phimosis?
   1. Proper cleaning of the prepuce
   2. Importance of regular ejaculation
   3. Technique of testicular self-examination
   4. Proper hand washing before touching the genitals

38. 1. Proper cleaning of the preputial area to remove secretions is critical to the prevention of noncongenital phimosis. Regular ejaculation can decrease the symptoms of chronic prostatitis, but it has no effect on the development of phimosis. Testicular self-examination is important in the early detection and treatment of testicular cancer but is unrelated to phimosis. Hand washing is important in preventing the spread of infection.
CN: Health promotion and maintenance; CNS: None; CL: Apply

CN: Client needs category   CNS: Client needs subcategory   CL: Cognitive level

39. What is the most accurate information a nurse can teach a newly-diagnosed client with testicular cancer?

1. Testicular cancer isn't responsive to chemotherapy, but it is highly curative with surgery.
2. Radiation therapy is never used, so the unaffected testicle remains healthy.
3. Testicular self-examination is important because there is an increased risk for a second tumor.
4. Taking testosterone after orchiectomy prevents changes in appearance and sexual function.

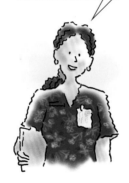

You can ease your client's worries through effective teaching efforts.

39. 3. A history of a testicular malignancy puts the client at increased risk for a second tumor. Testicular self-examination allows for early detection and treatment. Chemotherapy is added for clients who have evidence of metastasis after irradiation. Radiation therapy is used on the retroperitoneal lymph nodes. Testosterone usually is not needed because the unaffected testis usually produces sufficient hormone.

CN: Physiological integrity; CNS: Reduction of risk potential; CL: Apply

40. The nurse is teaching a client about penile hygiene. What is the **most** important information for the nurse to include?

1. Use warm water without soap
2. Dry all areas of the penis thoroughly
3. Wash from the base of the shaft to the tip
4. Avoid retracting the foreskin if not circumcised

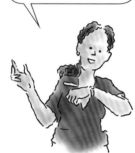

You've made it through 40 questions in no time!

40. 2. Careful drying is essential to avoid maceration of the penis. To decrease the risk of genitourinary infection, wash the penis from the tip to the base to reduce the risk of introducing pathogens into the urethral meatus. Effective cleaning requires soap and thorough rinsing. It is also essential to remove secretions that accumulate under the foreskin because they can lead to inflammation, and are associated with the development of penile cancer. The foreskin in uncircumcised men must be retracted for cleaning and then replaced to prevent paraphimosis.

CN: Health promotion and maintenance; CNS: None; CL: Apply

41. A client underwent an orchiectomy for testicular cancer and now has a persistent elevation in alpha-fetoprotein levels. Which statement by the nurse is **most** accurate?

1. "You are still fertile."
2. "This is related to the surgical procedure."
3. "You need further testing to determine the cause of this elevation."
4. "When testosterone decreases, alpha fetoprotein increases."

41. 3. Alpha-fetoprotein is a tumor marker elevated in nonseminomatous malignancies of the testicle. After the tumor is removed, the level should decrease. A persistent elevation after orchiectomy may indicate that a tumor may still be present outside the testicle that was removed. The nurse should tell the client that further testing is necessary. The level of alpha-fetoprotein is not related to fertility or testosterone level. A recurrence of the cancer is indicated by a postsurgical decrease in alpha-fetoprotein level followed by an elevation as a new tumor starts to grow.

CN: Physiological integrity; CNS: Physiological adaptation; CL: Analyze

42. Which discharge instruction should the nurse give to a client after a prostatectomy?

1. Avoid straining at stool
2. Report clots in the urine right away
3. Soak in a warm tub daily for comfort
4. Return to your usual activities in three weeks

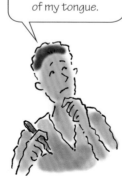

I know the answer. It's right on the tip of my tongue.

42. 1. Straining at stool after prostatectomy can cause bleeding. Small blood clots or pieces of tissue are commonly passed in the urine for up to two weeks postoperatively. Tub baths are prohibited because they cause dilation of pelvic blood vessels. Other activities are resumed based on the guidance of the health care provider. Sexual intercourse and driving are usually prohibited for about three weeks. Exercising and returning to work are usually prohibited for about six weeks.

CN: Physiological integrity; CNS: Reduction of risk potential; CL: Apply

CN: Client needs category   CNS: Client needs subcategory   CL: Cognitive level

43. Which symptom should the nurse instruct a client to report following a biopsy of the prostate?
1. Pain on the following day
2. Discolored semen
3. Difficulty urinating
4. Temperature greater than 99° F (37.2° C)

43. 3. Difficulty urinating suggests urethral obstruction. Mild pain is expected for one to three days after the biopsy. Semen may be discolored for up to a month after the biopsy. Temperature higher than 101° F (38.3° C) should be reported because it suggests infection.
CN: Physiological integrity; CNS: Reduction of risk potential; CL: Analyze

44. Two days after a transrectal biopsy of the prostate, the client calls the clinic to report that his stool is streaked with blood. Which response by the nurse is appropriate?
1. Tell the client to take a laxative
2. Tell the client to come in for examination
3. Reassure the client that this is an expected occurrence
4. Ask the client to collect a stool specimen for testing

44. 3. After a transrectal prostatic biopsy, blood in the stool is expected for a number of days. Because blood in the stool is expected, testing the stool or examining the client isn't necessary. Stool softeners are prescribed if the client reports constipation. Straining at stool can precipitate bleeding, but laxatives generally are not necessary.
CN: Physiological integrity; CNS: Reduction of risk potential; CL: Apply

45. A nurse is caring for clients who have a history of genital herpes infection. Which client is **most** at risk for an outbreak of genital herpes?
1. A client who reports headache and fever
2. A client who reports vaginal and urethral discharge
3. A client who reports dysuria and lymphadenopathy
4. A client who reports genital pruritus and paresthesia

45. 4. Pruritus and paresthesia as well as redness of the genital area are prodromal symptoms of recurrent herpes infection. These symptoms occur 30 minutes to 48 hours before the lesions appear. Headache and fever are symptoms of viremia associated with the primary infection. Vaginal and urethral discharge are also a local sign of primary infection. Dysuria and lymphadenopathy are localized symptoms of a primary infection that may also occur with recurrent infection.
CN: Physiological integrity; CNS: Physiological adaptation; CL: Analyze

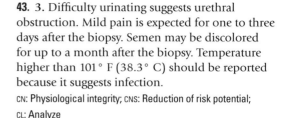

Cheers to you! You're doing a great job.

46. Which instruction should the nurse give to a female client newly diagnosed with genital herpes?
1. Obtain a Papanicolaou (Pap) test every year
2. Have your partner use a condom when lesions are present
3. Use a water-soluble lubricant for relief of pruritus
4. Limit stress and emotional upset as much as possible

46. 4. Stress, anxiety, and emotional upset seem to cause recurrent outbreaks of genital herpes. Because a relationship has been found between genital herpes and cervical cancer, a Pap test is recommended every six months. Sexual intercourse should be avoided during outbreaks, and a condom should be used between outbreaks. It is unknown if the virus can be transmitted at this time. During an outbreak, creams and lubricants should be avoided because they may prolong healing.
CN: Physiological integrity; CNS: Physiological adaptation; CL: Apply

47. A client newly diagnosed with genital herpes is crying and wringing her hands as the nurse approaches her. What is the **priority** nursing intervention?
1. Assess the client's pain
2. Teach the client about genital herpes
3. Assess the client's anxiety level
4. Ask the client about her significant other

47. 3. The client is demonstrating anxiety. This problem needs to be incorporated into the plan of care. The client is not demonstrating a pain response, or require teaching at this point. This would not be an appropriate time to ask the client about her significant other. When anxiety is high, the client is unable to focus on other things such as teaching.
CN: Psychosocial integrity; CNS: None; CL: Apply

48. A client is describing how she palpates her breasts for breast self-examination. Which statement indicates a need for further teaching?
1. "I put lotion on my breasts before I begin to palpate them."
2. "I palpate both breasts standing up and then lying on my back."
3. "I'm careful to only palpate under each arm and up to two inches below my collarbone."
4. "I start at the outer edge of the breast and work in to the nipple in smaller and smaller circles."

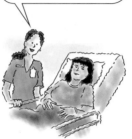

Make sure your client understands the proper technique for breast self-examination.

48. 3. Breast self-examination requires palpation of all breast tissue. This includes checking the area above the breast up to the collarbone, over to the shoulder, as well as between the breast and the underarm, including the underarm itself. Lotion or powder helps the fingers glide over the skin and facilitates palpation. Breasts should be palpated in both standing and lying positions. Any pattern of palpation may be used in performing breast self-examination as long as each quadrant of the breast, tail, and axilla are examined.
CN: Health promotion and maintenance; CNS: None; CL: Apply

49. During a routine physical examination, a firm mass is palpated in the right breast of a 35-year-old client. Which finding suggests cancer of the breast rather than fibrocystic disease?
1. Mass located in upper, outer quadrant
2. Cyclic change in mass size
3. History of anovulatory cycles
4. Increased vascularity of the breast

49. 4. Increase in breast size or vascularity is consistent with cancer of the breast. Masses associated with fibrocystic disease of the breast are firm, most commonly located in the upper outer quadrant of the breast, and increase in size prior to menstruation. They may be bilateral, and are typically well demarcated and freely moveable.
CN: Health promotion and maintenance; CNS: None; CL: Apply

50. Which client does the nurse evaluate as having the **highest** risk of developing a postoperative wound infection?
1. A postsurgical client following a radical prostatectomy
2. The client who had a perineal prostatectomy
3. A postsurgical client following a suprapubic prostatectomy
4. The client who had a transurethral resection of the prostate

50. 2. The incision in a perineal prostatectomy is close to the rectum, which normally contains gram-negative organisms that can cause infection if introduced into other areas of the body. Therefore, a perineal incision can become contaminated more easily than those of the other procedures.
CN: Physiological integrity; CNS: Reduction of risk potential; CL: Analyze

51. A client with pneumonia requires mechanical ventilation, and is being transferred to the intensive care unit. Blood pressure is 70/40 mmHg, heart rate is 115 bpm, and respiratory rate is 32 breaths/min using accessory muscles. Intravenous fluids are infusing at 150 ml/hr. Urinary output has been 50 ml for the past four hours. This client is most at risk for:
1. postrenal failure.
2. prerenal failure.
3. intrarenal failure.
4. dehydration.

51. 2. Prerenal refers to renal failure due to an interference with renal perfusion. Decreased cardiac output causes a decrease in renal perfusion, which leads to a lower glomerular filtration rate. There is no indication that this client has a problem that would indicate post renal failure or intrarenal failure. The infusion of fluid would prevent dehydration.
CN: Physiological integrity; CNS: Physiological adaptation; CL: Analyze

52. A client admitted for acute pyelonephritis is about to start antibiotic therapy. Which symptom would the nurse expect this client to present?
1. Hypertension
2. Flank pain on the affected side
3. Bradycardia
4. Inability to walk

52. 2. The client may report pain on the affected side because the kidney is enlarged and might have formed an abscess. Hypertension is associated with chronic pyelonephritis. The client would have tenderness with deep palpation over the costovertebral angle. Tachycardia would be expected with pain, not bradycardia. The client may have pain when walking, but should still be able to walk.
CN: Physiological integrity; CNS: Physiological adaptation; CL: Apply

53. The nurse is providing discharge instructions for a client treated for acute pyelonephritis. What is the **most** important information for the nurse to include?
1. Avoid taking any dairy products
2. Return for follow-up urine cultures
3. Stop taking the prescribed antibiotics when the symptoms subside
4. Recurrence is unlikely because you've been treated with antibiotics

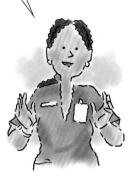

Here's another question about client teaching, an essential topic on NCLEX examinations.

53. 2. The client needs to return for follow-up urine cultures because bacteriuria may be present but asymptomatic. Intake of dairy products won't contribute to pyelonephritis. Antibiotics need to be taken for the full course of therapy regardless of symptoms. Pyelonephritis typically recurs as a relapse or new infection within two weeks of completing therapy.
CN: Health promotion and maintenance; CNS: None; CL: Apply

54. A client reports severe flank and abdominal pain. A flat plate of the abdomen shows urolithiasis. Which intervention does the nurse determine is appropriate?
1. Strain all urine
2. Limit fluid intake
3. Enforce strict bed rest
4. Encourage a high-calcium diet

54. 1. Urine should be strained for calculi and sent to the laboratory for analysis. Fluid intake of 3 to 4 qt (3 to 4 L) per day is encouraged to flush the urinary tract, and prevent further calculi formation. Ambulation is encouraged to help pass the calculi through gravity. A low-calcium diet is recommended to help prevent the formation of calcium calculi.
CN: Physiological integrity; CNS: Reduction of risk potential; CL: Apply

55. A client is receiving a radiation implant for the treatment of bladder cancer. Which nursing intervention is **most** appropriate?
1. Flush all urine down the toilet
2. Restrict the client's fluid intake
3. Place the client in a semiprivate room
4. Monitor the client for signs and symptoms of cystitis

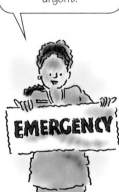

Question 56 asks you to prioritize responses according to which is most urgent.

55. 4. Cystitis is the most common adverse reaction of clients undergoing radiation therapy. Symptoms include dysuria, frequency, urgency, and nocturia. Urine of clients with radiation implants should be sent to the radioisotopes laboratory for monitoring. It is recommended that fluid intake be increased. Clients with radiation implants require a private room.
CN: Physiological integrity; CNS: Physiological adaptation; CL: Apply

56. The nurse is assessing a client who has undergone a radical cystectomy and ileal conduit for the treatment of bladder cancer. Which finding would prompt the nurse to provide immediate intervention?
1. A red, moist stoma
2. A dusky colored stoma
3. Urine output more than 30 ml/hr
4. Slight bleeding from the stoma when changing the appliance

56. 2. The stoma should be red and moist, indicating adequate blood flow. A dusky or cyanotic stoma indicates insufficient blood supply, and requires prompt intervention. Urine output less than 30 ml/hr, or no urine output for more than 15 minutes should be reported. Slight bleeding from the stoma when changing the appliance may occur because the intestinal mucosa is fragile.
CN: Physiological integrity; CNS: Reduction of risk potential; CL: Apply

57. The nurse is providing instruction about skin care at the stoma site for a client with an ileal conduit. What is the **most** important information for this nurse to provide?
1. Change the appliance at bedtime
2. Leave the stoma open to air while changing the appliance
3. Clean the skin around the stoma with mild soap and water and dry it thoroughly
4. Cut the faceplate or wafer of the appliance no more than four mm larger than the stoma

57. 3. Cleaning the skin around the stoma with mild soap and water and drying it thoroughly helps keep the area free of urine, which can irritate the skin. The appliance should be changed in the early morning when urine output is low to decrease the amount of urine in contact with the skin. The stoma should be covered with a gauze pad when changing the appliance to prevent urine from contacting the skin. The faceplate or wafer of the appliance should not be more than three mm larger than the stoma to reduce the skin area in contact with urine.
CN: Physiological integrity; CNS: Basic care and comfort; CL: Apply

CN: Client needs category   CNS: Client needs subcategory   CL: Cognitive level

58. What is the **most** important information for the nurse to include when teaching a male client diagnosed with overflow incontinence? Select all that apply:
1. How to perform self-catheterization
2. The purpose of medication therapy
3. How to perform Kegel exercises
4. Elimination of caffeine in the diet
5. Increasing acidic fluids in daily diet

58. **1, 2.** Overflow incontinence occurs when the detrusor muscle fails to contract. The bladder becomes over distended. Causes for the underactive bladder may, or may not, be determined. An alpha adrenergic blocker medication may be used for male clients with an enlarged prostate to relax the muscle at the base of the urethra and allow urine to pass. Self catheterization may also be needed to empty the bladder. Kegel exercises are not utilized by men with this problem. Caffeine is not thought to be a cause of this condition and acidic fluids are not thought to be a cure.
CN: Health promotion and maintenance; CNS: None; CL: Apply

59. When performing a physical assessment, the nurse discovers the client's urinary drainage bag lying on the bed. Based on this finding, the nurse identifies which problem as the **priority**?
1. Risk for infection
2. Reflex urinary incontinence
3. Risk for pain
4. Potential for ruptured bladder

59. **1.** Placing the drainage bag beside the client will allow the urine to flow back into the bladder, potentially causing an infection. This does not place the client at risk for incontinence or pain or a ruptured bladder.
CN: Safe, effective care environment; CNS: Management of care; CL: Apply

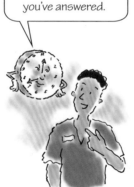

Time is flying! Look how many questions you've answered.

60. A urine culture has been ordered for a male client. What information should the nurse teach the client?
1. Void in a clean container
2. Clean the foreskin of the penis if uncircumcised before specimen collection
3. Void into a urinal and then pour the urine into the specimen container
4. Begin the stream of urine in the toilet and catch the urine in a sterile container midstream

60. **4.** Catching urine midstream reduces the amount of contamination by microorganisms at the meatus. Voiding in a clean container is done for a random specimen, not a clean-catch specimen for urine culture. When cleaning an uncircumcised male, the foreskin should be retracted and the glans penis should be cleaned to prevent specimen contamination. Voiding in a urinal does not allow for an uncontaminated specimen because the urinal isn't sterile.
CN: Physiological integrity; CNS: Reduction of risk potential; CL: Apply

61. A client with a history of chronic renal failure missed a scheduled dialysis treatment, and is now being admitted to the hospital with pulmonary edema. The client's lab results include serum potassium 6.0 mEq/L (mmol/L), serum sodium 130 mEq/L (mmol/L), serum bicarbonate 18 mEq/L (mmol/L). What is this client's **greatest** risk?
1. Hypoxemia
2. Cardiac dysrhythmia
3. Fluid overload
4. Pericardial effusion

61. **1.** The client has developed pulmonary edema, which will decrease the client's air exchange. Airway and breathing are the priority. Elevated potassium can result in cardiac dysrhythmias. Fluid overload is possible due to missing a dialysis appointment. The client needs to be dialyzed as quickly as possible. Pericardial effusion occurs in advanced heart failure, pericarditis, metastatic carcinoma, cardiac surgery or trauma.
CN: Physiological integrity; CNS: Physiological adaptation; CL: Analyze

62. A client with acute renal failure has a serum potassium level of 7.0 mEq/L (mmol/L). What is the nurse's **priority** action for this client?
1. Urine specific gravity
2. Electrocardiogram (ECG) results
3. Mental status
4. Blood pressure

62. **2.** Acute renal failure can result in hyperkalemia, which can manifest in widening of the PR and QRS intervals on the ECG as well as irregular heartbeats, such as premature ventricular contractions. Urine specific gravity, mental status, and blood pressure are not a priority for this client.
CN: Safe, effective care environment; CNS: Management of care; CL: Apply

CN: Client needs category   CNS: Client needs subcategory   CL: Cognitive level

63. A client has just received a renal transplant, and has started cyclosporine therapy. What is the **most** important information for the nurse to share with this client?
1. "You may have a decreased appetite."
2. "Dizziness is common."
3. "Report any fever, a flushed feeling, or lethargy."
4. "Report any stomach discomfort or dyspepsia."

64. A client received a transplanted kidney two months ago. He's admitted to the hospital with the diagnosis of acute rejection. Which assessment finding should the nurse anticipate?
1. Hypotension
2. Normal body temperature
3. Decreased white blood cell (WBC) counts
4. Elevated blood urea nitrogen (BUN) and creatinine levels

65. A client is diagnosed with chronic renal failure and is told to start hemodialysis. What is the **priority** teaching for the nurse to provide?
1. Follow a high-potassium diet
2. Strictly follow the hemodialysis schedule
3. There will be few changes in your lifestyle
4. Increase your fluid intake

66. A client is to undergo kidney transplantation with a living donor. What is the **most** important preoperative assessment by the nurse?
1. Urine output
2. Signs of graft rejection
3. Signs and symptoms of infection
4. Client's support system and understanding of lifestyle changes

67. A client is undergoing peritoneal dialysis. The dialysate dwell time is completed, and the clamp is opened to allow the dialysate to drain. The nurse notes 1,500 ml was instilled, but only 500 ml has drained. Which intervention should be done **first**?
1. Change the client's position
2. Call the health care provider
3. Assess the catheter for kinks or obstruction
4. Clamp the catheter and instill more dialysate at the next exchange time

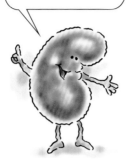

Cyclosporine suppresses the immune system to prevent rejection of a transplanted organ. This puts the client at risk for …

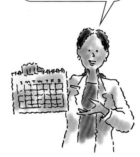

It's important that your client follow scheduled treatment.

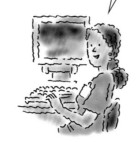

This question is asking for the first thing you should do.

63. 3. Fever, a flushed feeling, or lethargy suggest an infection. The nurse should closely monitor these symptoms in clients taking cyclosporine because it is an immunosuppressive drug. This medication should not cause decreased appetite, dizziness or stomach discomfort.
CN: Physiological integrity; CNS: Pharmacological and parental therapies; CL: Apply

64. 4. A client with acute renal graft rejection, will show evidence of deteriorating renal function. Elevated BUN and creatinine levels are expected. The client would most likely have acute hypertension. The nurse would see fever and elevated WBC counts because the body is recognizing the graft as foreign and is attempting to fight it.
CN: Physiological integrity; CNS: Reduction of risk potential; CL: Analyze

65. 2. To prevent life-threatening complications, the client must follow the dialysis schedule. The client should follow a low-potassium diet, because potassium levels increase in chronic renal failure. The client should know that hemodialysis is time-consuming and will cause a change in current lifestyle. The client does not need to increase fluid intake.
CN: Physiological integrity; CNS: Reduction of risk potential; CL: Apply

66. 4. A client undergoing renal transplantation will need vigilant follow-up care and must adhere to the medical regimen. The client is most likely anuric or oliguric preoperatively. Postoperatively this client will need to closely monitor urine output to make sure the transplanted kidney is functioning optimally. Rejection can occur postoperatively. Although the client will always need to be monitored for signs and symptoms of infection, it is a priority during the immediate postoperative period because of the initiation of immunosuppressive therapy.
CN: Psychosocial integrity; CNS: None; CL: Apply

67. 3. The first intervention should be to check for kinks and obstructions because that could be preventing drainage. After checking for kinks, the client should change position to promote drainage. Don't give the next scheduled exchange until the dialysate is drained because abdominal distention will occur, unless the output is within the parameters set by the health care provider. If unable to get more output despite checking for kinks and changing the client's position, the nurse should then call the health care provider to determine another intervention.
CN: Physiological integrity; CNS: Reduction of risk potential; CL: Analyze

68. A client receiving hemodialysis treatments arrives at the hospital with a blood pressure of 200/100 mmHg, a heart rate of 110 bpm, and a respiratory rate of 36 breaths/min. Oxygen saturation on room air is 89%. The client reports shortness of breath, and has + 2 pedal edema. The last hemodialysis treatment was yesterday. Which intervention should be done **first**?
1. Administer oxygen
2. Elevate the foot of the bed
3. Restrict the client's fluids
4. Prepare the client for hemodialysis

69. A client with renal insufficiency is being treated with intravenous antibiotics. Which laboratory value should be monitored closely?
1. Blood urea nitrogen (BUN) and creatinine levels
2. Arterial blood gas (ABG) levels
3. Platelet count
4. Potassium level

70. A client had a transurethral prostatectomy for benign prostatic hypertrophy, and is currently being treated with continuous bladder irrigation. The client reports an increase in the severity of his bladder spasms. Which intervention is **most** important for the nurse to implement?
1. Administer an oral analgesic
2. Stop the irrigation and call the health care provider
3. Administer a belladonna and opium suppository as ordered by the health care provider
4. Check for the presence of clots, and make sure the catheter is draining properly

71. A client has returned from surgery with continuous bladder irrigation. Which assessment finding indicates the bladder irrigation is successful?
1. The urine flow is red.
2. The irrigant flow is pink.
3. The bladder feels distended.
4. The irrigant outflow is half of the intake.

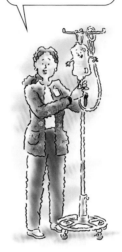

A client with renal insufficiency is vulnerable to drugs affecting kidney function. Which lab values measure that?

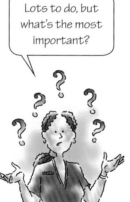

Lots to do, but what's the most important?

68. 1. Airway and oxygenation are always the first priority. Because the client is reporting shortness of breath, and his oxygen saturation is only 89%, the nurse needs to try to increase the partial pressure of arterial oxygen by administering oxygen. The foot of the bed should not be elevated at this time as this may increase venous return to the heart and worsen pulmonary edema. The client is in pulmonary edema from fluid overload and will need to be dialyzed and have fluids restricted.
CN: Physiological integrity; CNS: Physiological adaptation; CL: Analyze

69. 1. BUN and creatinine levels should be monitored closely to detect elevations due to nephrotoxicity. ABG determinations are inappropriate in this situation. Platelets and potassium levels should be monitored according to routine.
CN: Physiological integrity; CNS: Reduction of risk potential; CL: Analyze

70. 4. Blood clots and blocked outflow of the urine can increase spasms. The irrigation shouldn't be stopped as long as the catheter is draining because clots will form. A belladonna and opium suppository should be given to relieve spasms per order, but only after assessment of the drainage. Oral analgesics should be given if the spasms are unrelieved by the suppository.
CN: Physiological integrity; CNS: Physiological adaptation; CL: Analyze

71. 2. The irrigant should be infused at a rate fast enough to maintain pink urine. Red urine indicates inadequate irrigation and possible clot formation. Bladder distention should not occur as long as the system is draining properly, and no clots are obstructing the outflow of urine. The outflow should be almost the same as the intake.
CN: Physiological integrity; CNS: Physiological adaptation; CL: Apply

CN: Client needs category   CNS: Client needs subcategory   CL: Cognitive level

72. A client has an indwelling urinary catheter. Urine is leaking from a hole in the collection bag. Which nursing intervention would be **most** appropriate?
1. Cover the hole with tape
2. Remove the catheter and insert a new one using sterile technique
3. Disconnect the drainage bag from the catheter and replace it with a new bag
4. Place a towel under the bag to prevent spillage of urine on the floor, which could cause the client to slip and fall

72. 2. The system is no longer a closed system, and bacteria might have been introduced. A new sterile catheter should be inserted. Taping the hole and placing a towel under the bag leave the system open, which increases the risk of infection. Replacing the drainage bag by disconnecting the old one from the catheter opens up the entire system and increases the risk of infection. It is not recommended.
CN: Safe, effective care environment; CNS: Safety and infection control; CL: Analyze

73. A client is admitted with a diagnosis of hydronephrosis secondary to calculi. The calculi have been removed, and post-obstructive diuresis is occurring. What is the nurse's **most** important intervention?
1. Take vital signs every eight hours
2. Weigh the client every other day
3. Assess the urine output every shift
4. Monitor the client's electrolyte levels

73. 4. Post-obstructive diuresis, seen in hydronephrosis, can cause electrolyte imbalances. Laboratory values must be checked so electrolytes can be replaced as needed. Vital signs should initially be taken every 30 minutes for the first four hours and then every two hours. Urine output should be assessed hourly. The client's weight should be taken daily to closely monitor fluid status.
CN: Physiological integrity; CNS: Reduction of risk potential; CL: Analyze

74. An older adult has developed a urinary tract infection, and is at risk for urosepsis. Which signs or symptoms should the nurse monitor? Select all that apply.
1. Decreased temperature
2. Increased heart rate
3. Decreased urinary output
4. Increased respiratory rate
5. Change in level of consciousness

74. 2, 3, 4, 5. Symptoms of sepsis include low grade fever (in the older adult), rapid breathing, fast heart rate, weak pulse, profuse sweating, unusual anxiety, changes in mental status or level of consciousness, and decreased, or absent, urinary output.
CN: Physiological integrity; CNS: Physiological adaptation; CL: Analyze

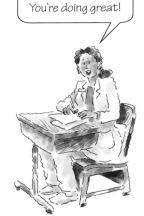

Don't give up now. You're doing great!

75. What should the nurse include when prioritizing care for a client with polycystic kidney disease (PKD)? Select all that apply.
1. Pain management
2. Prevention of infection
3. Prevention of constipation
4. Monitoring of electrocardiogram (ECG)
5. Monitoring of electrolytes

75. 1, 2, 3. Interventions for the client with PKD include pain management and prevention of infection, constipation, hypertension, and chronic kidney disease. Monitoring electrolytes is not necessary unless the disease progresses to kidney failure. If kidney failure is imminent, the client's ECG and electrolytes would be closely monitored.
CN: Physiological integrity; CNS: Physiological adaptation; CL: Apply

76. The nurse is obtaining a health history on a client. Which client statement indicates a risk of renal calculi?
1. "I've been drinking a lot of cola soft drinks lately."
2. "I've been jogging more than usual."
3. "I've had more stress since we adopted a child last year."
4. "I'm a vegetarian and eat cheese two or three times each day."

76. 4. Renal calculi are commonly composed of calcium. Diets high in calcium may predispose a person to renal calculi. Milk and dairy are high in calcium. Soft drinks don't contain ingredients that would increase the risk of renal calculi. Jogging and increased stress are not considered risk factors for renal calculi formation.
CN: Health promotion and maintenance; CNS: None; CL: Analyze

CN: Client needs category   CNS: Client needs subcategory   CL: Cognitive level

77. The nurse is assessing a client who reports having pain during and after urination. The nurse suspects that this client may have a problem with the:
1. bladder.
2. kidneys.
3. ureters.
4. urethra.

77. 1. Pain during or after voiding indicates a bladder problem. Kidney and ureter pain would be in the flank area. Problems with the urethra would cause pain at the urinary meatus, and are commonly felt at the start of voiding.
CN: Health promotion and maintenance; CNS: None; CL: Apply

78. A client is ordered diuretics. When should the nurse schedule this medication?
1. Anytime
2. Nighttime
3. Morning
4. Noon

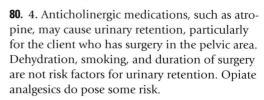

This is the best time of day.

78. 3. A diuretic given in the morning has time to work throughout the day. Diuretics given at nighttime will cause the client to get up to go to the bathroom frequently, interrupting sleep.
CN: Physiological integrity; CNS: Pharmacological and parenteral therapies; CL: Apply

79. Which nursing intervention would be the **most** appropriate for a client with postoperative urinary retention?
1. Give a diuretic
2. Pour warm water over the perineum
3. Consider inserting a bladder catheter
4. Lay the client flat in bed

79. 2. Urinary retention reflects bladder distention from urine. Sitting the client upright and pouring warm water over the perineum may help the client void. A diuretic is not necessary. If these measures aren't successful, the nurse should consider getting an order from the provider to insert a bladder catheter.
CN: Physiological integrity; CNS: Basic care and comfort; CL: Apply

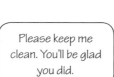

I never meant to put anyone at risk.

80. A client has not voided for 10 hours following an inguinal hernia repair. What would the nurse consider as the cause of this problem?
1. Dehydration
2. History of smoking
3. Duration of surgery
4. Preoperative atropine

80. 4. Anticholinergic medications, such as atropine, may cause urinary retention, particularly for the client who has surgery in the pelvic area. Dehydration, smoking, and duration of surgery are not risk factors for urinary retention. Opiate analgesics do pose some risk.
CN: Physiological integrity; CNS: Reduction of risk potential; CL: Apply

81. What is **most** important for the nurse to teach a client with urinary retentions about self-catheterization?
1. "You must keep the catheter clean as it is inserted."
2. "Catheterization is not something clients can perform alone."
3. "You will need to keep a catheter in at all times."
4. "The catheter is used to put fluid into the bladder."

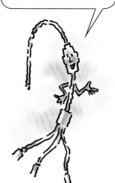

Please keep me clean. You'll be glad you did.

81. 1. The catheter must be kept clean as it is inserted. In an inpatient setting, nurses generally perform sterile catheterization. In the home setting the client utilizes clean technique. Clients can be taught to perform clean intermittent self-catheterization. The client does not have to keep the catheter in at all times. The catheter will not be used for irrigation as this is not an intervention for urine retention.
CN: Physiological integrity; CNS: Basic care and comfort; CL: Apply

82. An 80-year-old male client reports urinary retention. Which factor may contribute to this client's problem?
1. Benign prostatic hyperplasia (BPH)
2. Diabetes
3. Diet
4. Hypertension

82. 1. BPH is common among older adult men, and typically results in urinary retention, frequency, dribbling, and difficulty starting the urine stream. Diabetes, diet, and hypertension usually do not affect urinary retention.
CN: Physiological integrity; CNS: Reduction of risk potential; CL: Apply

CN: Client needs category   CNS: Client needs subcategory   CL: Cognitive level

83. A 75-year-old client is admitted with dehydration. The client's laboratory results are serum sodium 145 mEq/L, serum potassium 5.0 mEq/L, and serum creatinine 1.2 mg/dl and a BUN of 28 mg/dl. Based on these results, the nurse determines that the client is at risk for developing:
1. cancer.
2. urinary retention.
3. acute renal failure.
4. cardiac arrhythmias.

84. A client with an overactive neurogenic bladder reports a dry mouth caused by oxybutynin. The nurse is aware that this adverse effect is commonly found with:
1. anti-infectives.
2. corticosteroid.
3. urinary antiseptics.
4. spasmolytics.

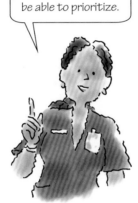

A nurse needs to be able to prioritize.

85. A client is injected with radiographic contrast medium and immediately shows signs of dyspnea, flushing, and pruritus. What is the nurse's **priority** intervention?
1. Check vital signs
2. Make sure the airway is patent
3. Apply a cold pack to the IV site
4. Call the health care provider

86. A client is admitted for a cystoscopy with biopsy of the bladder. After obtaining the client's history, surgery was postponed. What would cause this surgery to be postponed?
1. The client stopped taking his anticoagulant three days ago.
2. The client has a urinary tract infection.
3. The client was previously been treated for carcinoma of the bladder.
4. The client took an antibiotic prior to the procedure.

87. A client who underwent a cystoscopy is scheduled to be discharged to home within 24 hours. What is the **most** important information for the nurse to give the client?
1. Expect bloody urine for about a week
2. Drink eight to ten glasses of water every eight hours
3. Try to urinate frequently and measure your output
4. Check the color, consistency, and amount of urine in the indwelling urinary catheter bag every four to eight hours

83. 3. The laboratory results indicate an elevated serum blood urea nitrogen (normal ranges are from 10-20 mg/dl), which is reflective of dehydration. Volume depletion or dehydration is a risk factor for developing acute renal failure due to decreased perfusion of the kidneys. The serum potassium, sodium, and creatinine levels are within -normal range. A normal creatinine level and elevated BUN suggest intravascular fluid volume deficit.
CN: Physiological integrity; CNS: Reduction of risk potential; CL: Apply

84. 4. Oxybutynin belongs to the spasmolytic drug classification. A common side effect is dry mouth. The other drug classifications do not commonly have an adverse effect of dry mouth.
CN: Physiological integrity; CNS: Pharmacological and parenteral therapies; CL: Apply

85. 2. The client is showing symptoms of an allergy to the iodine in the contrast medium. The priority action is to make sure the client's airway is patent. Checking vital signs and calling for the health care provider are important nursing actions, but are not the priority. A cold pack is not indicated.
CN: Physiological integrity; CNS: Physiological adaptation; CL: Analyze

86. 2. Bladder biopsies should not be done when an active urinary tract infection is present because sepsis may result. Anticoagulants should be discontinued for three to five days before the procedure. The client who has been treated for bladder cancer may still require a biopsy to check effectiveness of treatment. Antibiotics are sometimes given prophylactically prior to the procedure.
CN: Physiological integrity; CNS: Reduction of risk potential; CL: Analyze

87. 3. The bladder needs to be emptied frequently, and output should be measured to make sure the bladder is emptying. Blood in the urine is not normal except for small amounts for the first 24 hours following the procedure. Large amounts of fluids help flush microorganisms out of the body, but eight to ten glasses every eight hours may not be reasonable. This client may not have an indwelling urinary catheter.
CN: Physiological integrity; CNS: Reduction of risk potential; CL: Apply

CN: Client needs category   CNS: Client needs subcategory   CL: Cognitive level

88. Before a renal biopsy, which information is **most** important to tell the health care provider?
1. The client signed a consent form.
2. The client understands the procedure.
3. The client has normal urinary elimination.
4. The client regularly takes aspirin or nonsteroidal anti-inflammatory drugs (NSAIDs).

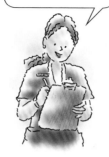

It is important to share vital client information.

88. 4. Aspirin and NSAIDs can increase bleeding times, and commonly result in hemorrhaging when biopsies are performed. It is the health care provider's responsibility to make sure the client understands the procedure, which is needed for informed consent. It is not necessary to report that this client has normal urinary elimination.
CN: Physiological integrity; CNS: Reduction of risk potential; CL: Apply

89. Which instruction would help the client perform Kegel exercises?
1. Completely empty the bladder
2. Do the exercise 200 times per day
3. Sit or stand with your legs together
4. Drink small amounts of fluid frequently

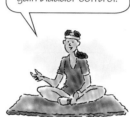

Kegel exercises can help the client gain bladder control.

89. 2. Exercises begin with tightening and relaxing the vagina, rectum, and urethra two or three times a day. Depending on the strength of the pelvic musculature, anywhere from 10-30 repetitions can be done petitions during each session, and gradually increased.. The client stops the flow of urine during urination to practice holding the flow. Standing or sitting with the legs apart will facilitate the exercises. Clients should drink 2-3L of fluids to prevent urinary problems.
CN: Physiological integrity; CNS: Physiological adaptation; CL: Apply

90. A client with chronic pyelonephritis is preparing to be discharged from the hospital. What is the **most** important information for the nurse to tell the client?
1. Stay on bed rest for up to two weeks
2. Use analgesia on a regular basis for up to six months
3. Have a urine culture every two weeks for up to six months
4. Antibiotic treatment may be needed for several weeks or months

90. 4. Chronic pyelonephritis can be a long-term condition requiring antibiotic treatment for several weeks or months, as well as close monitoring to prevent permanent damage to the kidneys. Bed rest and analgesia may be used during the acute stage but usually are not required long-term. A urine culture is done two weeks after stopping antibiotics to make sure the infection has been eradicated.
CN: Physiological integrity; CNS: Reduction of risk control; CL: Apply

91. Which client does the nurse determine as being at **greatest** risk for developing acute renal failure?
1. A dialysis client who gets influenza
2. A teenager who has an appendectomy
3. A pregnant woman who has a fractured femur
4. A client with diabetes who has a heart catheterization

91. 4. Clients with diabetes are prone to renal insufficiency and renal failure. The contrast used for heart catheterization must be eliminated by the kidneys, causing stress, and may produce acute renal failure. A dialysis client already has end-stage renal disease and would not develop acute renal failure. A teenager who has an appendectomy and a pregnant woman who fractures a femur are not at increased risk for renal failure.
CN: Health promotion and maintenance; CNS: None; CL: Analyze

92. The nurse is caring for a client who is receiving hemodialysis treatments. Which intervention would be the **most** appropriate for this client?
1. Palpate for a thrill on the arm with the fistula
2. Palpate for a thrill on the arm without the fistula
3. Document the absence of a bruit as a normal finding
4. Take the blood pressure on the arm with the fistula

92. 1. The nurse would palpate for a thrill, and auscultate for a bruit on the arm with the fistula. No procedures should be done on the arm with a fistula because it could damage the fistula. The absence of a thrill or bruit should be reported promptly to the health care provider because it indicates an occlusion and is not a normal finding.
CN: Physiological integrity; CNS: Reduction of risk potential; CL: Apply

93. A client has passed renal calculi. The nurse sends the specimen to the laboratory so it can be analyzed for:
1. antibodies.
2. type of infection.
3. composition of calculus.
4. size and number of calculi.

93. **3.** The calculus should be analyzed for composition to determine appropriate interventions such as dietary restrictions. Calculi do not result from infections. The size and number of calculi are not relevant. Calculi do not contain antibodies.
CN: Physiological integrity; CNS: Reduction of risk potential; CL: Apply

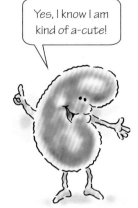

Yes, I know I am kind of a-cute!

94. Which symptom may indicate acute rejection of a transplanted kidney?
1. Increased urine output
2. Hypotension
3. Pain at the graft site
4. Decreased white blood cell (WBC) count

94. **3.** Signs and symptoms of acute rejection of a transplanted kidney include pain at the graft site, decreased urine output, hypertension, elevated WBC count, fever, and elevated creatinine level.
CN: Physiological integrity; CNS: Physiological adaptation; CL: Analyze

95. A client has been placed on prednisone therapy. The client asks the nurse if any adverse reactions can occur when taking the medication. What is the nurse's **most** appropriate response?
1. Decreased appetite
2. Sodium loss and constipation
3. Hypotension
4. Increased blood glucose levels and decreased wound healing

95. **4.** Steroid use tends to increase blood glucose levels, particularly in clients with diabetes and borderline diabetes. Steroids cause retention of sodium, increased appetite and hypertension. Steroids don't affect bleeding tendencies, constipation, or thermoregulation.
CN: Physiological integrity; CNS: Pharmacological and parenteral therapies; CL: Analyze

This side effect of prednisone is especially important to communicate to clients with diabetes.

96. Steroids, such as prednisone and methylprednisolone, are used to suppress the inflammatory immune response following a kidney transplant. Which information should the nurse provide to a client with a transplant?
1. Alopecia may occur.
2. Weight loss is common.
3. Cholesterol levels may become elevated.
4. Hypokalemia may result.

96. **4.** Steroids may decrease serum potassium levels but do not increase cholesterol levels. Hirsutism may occur but not alopecia. Weight gain is commonly reported, not weight loss.
CN: Physiological integrity; CNS: Pharmacological and parenteral therapies; CL: Analyze

97. A nurse suspects that a client with polyuria is experiencing water diuresis. The nurse assesses the laboratory values for which finding?
1. High urine specific gravity
2. High urine osmolarity
3. Normal to low urine specific gravity
4. Elevated urine pH

97. **3.** Water diuresis causes low urine specific gravity, low urine osmolarity, and a normal to elevated serum sodium level. High urine specific gravity indicates dehydration. Elevated urine pH can result from potassium deficiency, a high-protein diet, or uncontrolled diabetes.
CN: Physiological integrity; CNS: Physiological adaptation; CL: Apply

98. A client with bladder cancer has had his bladder removed, and an ileal conduit created for urine diversion. While changing this client's pouch, the nurse observes that the area around the stoma is red, weeping, and painful. What is the nurse's conclusion?
 1. The skin wasn't lubricated before the pouch was applied.
 2. The pouch faceplate doesn't fit the stoma.
 3. A skin barrier was applied properly.
 4. Stoma dilation wasn't performed.

98. 2. If the pouch faceplate doesn't fit properly, the skin around the stoma will be exposed to continuous urine flow from the stoma, causing excoriation, redness, weeping, and painful skin. A lubricant should not be used because it would prevent the pouch from adhering to the skin. When properly applied, a skin barrier prevents skin excoriation. Stoma dilation is not performed with an ileal conduit.
CN: Physiological integrity; CNS: Basic care and comfort; CL: Analyze

99. A client is diagnosed with prostate cancer. Which test should the nurse anticipate to monitor this client's progress?
 1. Serum creatinine
 2. Complete blood count (CBC)
 3. Prostate-specific antigen (PSA)
 4. Serum potassium

99. 3. The PSA test is used to monitor prostate cancer progression. Higher PSA levels indicate a greater tumor burden. Serum creatinine levels may suggest blockage from an enlarged prostate. CBC is used to diagnose anemia and polycythemia. Serum potassium levels identify hypokalemia and hyperkalemia.
CN: Physiological integrity; CNS: Physiological adaptation; CL: Apply

100. When teaching a client about cystitis, a nurse explains that females are more prone to the disorder than males. Which factor explains a female's increased susceptibility?
 1. Higher estrogen levels
 2. Inadequate fluid intake
 3. Urethral proximity to the rectum
 4. Continuous nature of the mucosa

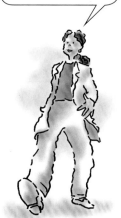

You're making great strides. Keep going!

100. 3. In females, the urethra and rectum are in close proximity, posing a greater risk for urethral contamination with feces after a bowel movement. Decreased estrogen levels may reduce vaginal and urethral lubrication, increasing the chance of irritation during coitus. Males and females can have equivalent fluid intake. The mucosa is continuous in both males and females.
CN: Physiological integrity; CNS: Physiological adaptation; CL: Apply

101. A client presents with a possible urinary tract infection. Which urine characteristic should the nurse assess **first**?
 1. Urine clarity
 2. Urine specific gravity
 3. Urine acetone
 4. Urine protein

101. 1. The nurse should first assess urine clarity. Cloudy urine usually indicates drainage, which may indicate an infection. Urine specific gravity provides information about fluid balance. Neither urine acetone nor urine protein indicates infection.
CN: Health promotion and maintenance; CNS: None; CL: Analyze

102. A 70-year-old male client is diagnosed with syphilis in the secondary stage. Which finding should the nurse expect during assessment?
 1. Chronic bone and joint irritation
 2. Tender lymphadenopathy
 3. Generalized rash on the palms and soles
 4. Personality changes and mental confusion

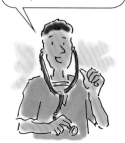

Location. It's a hint to help you answer question 102.

102. 3. In secondary syphilis, a maculopapular non-pruritic rash appears on the palms and soles. Chronic bone and joint irritation are not related to secondary syphilis. During the second stage of syphilis, non-tender lymphadenopathy occurs. Personality changes occur during the late stage of syphilis.
CN: Physiological integrity; CNS: Basic care and comfort; CL: Apply

103. A client has received ceftriaxone for the treatment of gonorrhea. What is the **most** important information for the nurse to teach this client?
1. "Take this medication with food or milk."
2. "Report pain, tenderness or warmth at the injection site."
3. "Take the medication every other day."
4. "Call your health care provider if you have diarrhea and cramping."

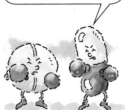

Sometimes meds can do a number on your tummy.

103. 4. Diarrhea and cramping can cause the client to have fluid and electrolyte disturbances and should be reported to the provider immediately. The nurse should also teach the client that pain and tenderness can develop at the injection site. Though not a priority, this should be monitored. The medication is not taken orally, and is taken daily.
CN: Physiological integrity; CNS: Pharmacological and parenteral therapies; CL: Apply

104. Which assessment finding would indicate that a client with renal failure is experiencing hypocalcemia?
1. Headache
2. Increased urinary output
3. Increased blood coagulation
4. Diarrhea

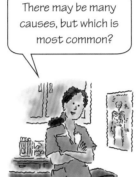

There may be many causes, but which is most common?

104. 4. In renal failure, calcium absorption from the intestine declines, leading to increased smooth-muscle contractions, causing diarrhea. Central nervous system changes in renal failure rarely cause headache. As renal failure progresses, bleeding tendencies increase.
CN: Health promotion and maintenance; CNS: None; CL: Apply

105. A client who became paraplegic after a swimming accident, is experiencing autonomic dysreflexia. Which condition is the **most** common cause of autonomic dysreflexia?
1. Upper respiratory infection
2. Incontinence
3. Bladder distention
4. Diarrhea

105. 3. Autonomic dysreflexia is a potentially life-threatening complication of spinal cord injury, occurring from obstruction of the urinary system or bowel. An upper respiratory infection could obstruct the respiratory system but not the urinary or bowel system. Incontinence and diarrhea do not result in obstruction of the urinary system or bowel.
CN: Physiological integrity; CNS: Physiological adaptation; CL: Analyze

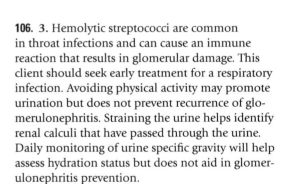

106. When teaching a client how to prevent recurrences of acute glomerulonephritis, which instruction should the nurse include?
1. Avoid physical activity
2. Strain all urine
3. Seek early treatment for respiratory infection
4. Monitor urine specific gravity every day

106. 3. Hemolytic streptococci are common in throat infections and can cause an immune reaction that results in glomerular damage. This client should seek early treatment for a respiratory infection. Avoiding physical activity may promote urination but does not prevent recurrence of glomerulonephritis. Straining the urine helps identify renal calculi that have passed through the urine. Daily monitoring of urine specific gravity will help assess hydration status but does not aid in glomerulonephritis prevention.
CN: Physiological integrity; CNS: Reduction of risk potential; CL: Analyze

107. After radical prostatectomy for prostate cancer, a client has an indwelling catheter removed. He then begins to have periods of incontinence. During the postoperative period, which intervention should be implemented **first**?
1. Kegel exercises
2. Fluid restriction
3. Artificial sphincter use
4. Self-catheterization

107. 1. Kegel exercises are noninvasive and are recommended as the initial intervention for incontinence. Fluid restriction is useful for a client with increased detrusor contraction related to acidic urine. Artificial sphincter use is not a primary intervention for post-prostatectomy incontinence. Self-catheterization may be used as a temporary measure but is not a primary intervention.
CN: Physiological integrity; CNS: Physiological adaptation; CL: Apply

CN: Client needs category   CNS: Client needs subcategory   CL: Cognitive level

108. When providing discharge teaching for a client with uric acid calculi, the nurse should include an instruction to avoid:
1. cottage cheese.
2. beets.
3. spinach.
4. organ meats.

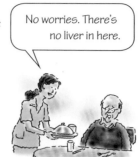

No worries. There's no liver in here.

108. 4. To control uric acid calculi, the client should avoid high-purine foods such as organ meats. Beets and spinach are high in oxalate. Cottage cheese is high in calcium.

CN: Physiological integrity; CNS: Reduction of risk potential; CL: Apply

109. A client with nephrotic syndrome has developed anasarca. Which abnormally low laboratory value would indicate this assessment finding?
1. Cholesterol
2. Prothrombin time
3. Albumin
4. Calcium

109. 3. When the glomeruli are damaged, the kidneys are excessively permeable to plasma protein, causing proteinuria and hypoalbuminemia. This leads to a decreased oncotic pressure, which results in anasarca.

CN: Physiological integrity; CNS: Physiological adaptation; CL: Apply

110. After a retropubic prostatectomy, a client requires continuous bladder irrigation. The client has an IV of dextrose 5% in water infusing at 40 ml/hr, and a triple-lumen urinary catheter with normal saline solution infusing at 200 ml/hr. The nurse empties the urinary catheter drainage bag three times during an 8-hour period for a total of 2,780 ml. How many milliliters does the nurse calculate as urine? Record your answer using a whole number.

_____ ml

110. 1,180.
During 8 hours, 1,600 ml of bladder irrigation has been infused:

$$200\ ml \times 8\ hours = 1,600\ ml$$

The nurse then subtracts this amount of infused bladder irrigation from the total volume in the drainage bag to determine urine output:

$$2,780\ ml - 1,600\ ml = 1,180\ ml$$

CN: Physiological integrity; CNS: Basic care and comfort; CL: Analyze

111. A nurse is caring for a client with chronic renal failure. The laboratory results indicate hypocalcemia and hyperphosphatemia. Which signs and symptoms should the nurse expect to find in this client? Select all that apply.
1. Trousseau's sign
2. Cardiac arrhythmias
3. Constipation
4. Decreased clotting time
5. Drowsiness and lethargy
6. Fractures

111. 1, 2, 6. Hypocalcemia is a calcium deficit that causes nerve fiber irritability and repetitive muscle spasms. Signs and symptoms of hypocalcemia include Trousseau's sign, cardiac arrhythmias, diarrhea, increased clotting, anxiety, and irritability.

CN: Physiological integrity; CNS: Reduction of risk potential; CL: Apply

CN: Client needs category   CNS: Client needs subcategory   CL: Cognitive level

112. A client with chronic renal failure plans to receive a transplanted kidney. The health care provider recently told the client that he is a poor candidate for transplant because of chronic uncontrolled hypertension and type 1 diabetes mellitus. The client tells the nurse, "I want to go off dialysis. I'd rather not live than be on this treatment for the rest of my life." How should the nurse respond to this client? Select all that apply.

1. Say nothing. Sit quietly next to the client.
2. Tell the client, "We all have days when we don't feel like going on."
3. Leave the room to allow the client to collect his thoughts.
4. Say to the client, "You're feeling upset about the news you got about the transplant."
5. Tell the client, "Your treatments are only three days a week. You can live with that."

112. 1, 4. Silence is a therapeutic communication technique that allows the nurse and client to reflect on what has taken place or what has been said. By waiting quietly and attentively, the nurse encourages the client to initiate and maintain conversation. By reflecting the client's implied feelings, the nurse also promotes communication. Using platitudes such as "We all have days when we don't feel like going on," the nurse fails to address this client's needs. The nurse should not leave the client alone because he may harm himself. Reminding the client of the treatment frequency does not address his feelings.

CN: Psychosocial integrity; CNS: None; CL: Analyze

113. The radiology nurse is reviewing a list of home medications of a client scheduled for an outpatient intravenous pyelogram (IVP) at 10:00 am. The client took the following medications at home with sips of water at 8:00 am. Which medication would prompt the nurse to contact the health care provider?

1. Metoprolol 25 mg by mouth
2. Sitagliptin 100 mg by mouth
3. Metformin 500 mg by mouth
4. Lorazepam 0.5 mg by mouth

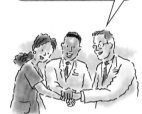

Interdisciplinary care means everyone works toward the same goal.

113. 3. Metformin, a biguanide oral hypoglycemic agent, should be held 24 hours before and 48 hours after IVP to reduce the potential of lactic acidosis and renal failure. Sitagliptin, metoprolol, and lorazepam do not produce harmful effects when IV contrast is administered.

CN: Physiological integrity; CNS: Pharmacological and parenteral therapies; CL: Apply

114. The nurse is caring for a client with acute glomerulonephritis. Which signs and symptoms would the nurse anticipate? Select all that apply.

1. Fatigue
2. Periorbital edema
3. Thromboemboli
4. Cola-colored urine
5. Hypertension
6. Proteinuria

114. 1, 2, 4, 5, 6. Fatigue, periorbital edema, hematuria (cola-colored urine), hypertension, and proteinuria are common manifestations of acute glomerulonephritis. Thromboemboli are common manifestations of nephrotic syndrome.

CN: Physiological integrity; CNS: Physiological adaptation; CL: Apply

115. The nurse is reviewing admission orders for a client with a diagnosis of pneumonia. The client has no known drug allergies. The client's laboratory results consist of blood urea nitrogen (BUN) 29 mg/dl, and creatinine 2.8 mg/dl. Which of the health care provider's orders would the nurse question?

1. Gentamicin 150 mg intravenous piggyback (IVPB) q24h
2. Doxycycline 100 mg IVPB q12h
3. Rocephin 1 g IVPB q24h
4. Zithromax 500 mg IVPB q24h

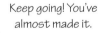

Keep going! You've almost made it.

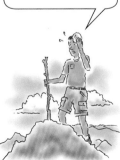

115. 1. The aminoglycoside gentamicin may be nephrotoxic when administered to a client with altered renal function. This client's BUN and creatinine are elevated. The client is elderly, placing them at increased risk for the nephrotoxic effects of medications.

CN: Physiological integrity; CNS: Pharmacological and parenteral therapies; CL: Analyze

116. The spouse of a client diagnosed with acute glomerulonephritis asks the nurse to clarify foods that are a complete source of protein. Which foods should the nurse include in this list? Select all that apply.
1. Nuts
2. Eggs
3. Fish
4. Legumes
5. Soy

116. 2, 3, 5. Eggs, fish, soy, meat, poultry and dairy all contain essential amino acids, and are considered a source of complete protein. When renal function is impaired, urea accumulates in the body as a result of impaired protein metabolism. Complete proteins are efficiently metabolized by the body, reducing urea accumulation.

CN: Physiological integrity; CNS: Basic care and comfort; CL: Apply

117. A client diagnosed with acute renal failure voided 260 ml of urine on Tuesday. What is the maximum amount of fluid the client may consume PO on Wednesday?
1. 360 ml
2. 500 ml
3. 740 ml
4. 760 ml

117. 4. The nurse adds the client's urine output for the previous 24 hours (260 ml) to 500 ml, which is the standard amount for insensible losses.
260 ml + 500 ml = 760 ml

CN: Physiological integrity; CNS: Basic care and comfort; CL: Apply

118. The intensive care unit nurse is explaining the procedure for continuous renal replacement therapy (CRRT) to a client with acute renal failure. Which statement **best** describes how CRRT will be initiated?
1. "I will attach the machine to the central venous catheter the health care provider placed in your upper chest."
2. "I will attach the machine to the catheter the health care provider placed in your abdomen."
3. "I will attach the machine to the fistula the health care provider placed in your arm."
4. "I will attach the machine to the shunt the health care provider placed in your arm."

118. 1. Through CRRT, blood from a double-lumen central venous line is slowly filtered and returned to the client. The slow filtration promotes hemodynamic stability and minimizes complications related to changes in extracellular fluid composition. The peritoneal catheter is used for peritoneal dialysis. The fistula and shunt are used for hemodialysis.

CN: Physiological integrity; CNS: Physiological adaptation; CL: Apply

119. The nurse is reviewing the urinalysis results on four different adult clients. Which client would the nurse anticipate receiving an IV fluid bolus?
1. A client with a specific gravity of 1.005
2. A client with a specific gravity of 1.022
3. A client with a specific gravity of 1.030
4. A client with a specific gravity of 1.045

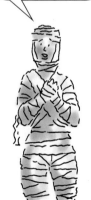

Looks like you've almost wrapped it up.

119. 4. Specific gravity measures the ratio of the density of urine compared to the density of an equal volume of water, and is a reflection of the client's hydration status. Normal specific gravity in adults ranges between 1.016 and 1.030. An elevated specific gravity indicates that the client is dehydrated.

CN: Physiological integrity; CNS: Reduction of risk potential; CL: Analyze

120. A male client tells the nurse he has been taking saw palmetto by mouth twice a day for the past three years as treatment for urinary hesitancy due to an enlarged prostate. What is the **priority** nursing assessment for this client?
1. Hypertension
2. Jaundice
3. Joint pain
4. Dry mouth

120. 2. Saw palmetto is used by more than two million men to treat benign prostatic hypertrophy, and may cause damage to the liver and pancreas. The nurse should assess for signs of jaundice as an adverse effect of using saw palmetto.

CN: Physiological integrity; CNS: Pharmacological and parenteral therapies; CL: Apply

CN: Client needs category   CNS: Client needs subcategory   CL: Cognitive level

121. A female client is at the clinic for her yearly gynecological evaluation. She expresses concern about a family friend who recently had a hysterectomy due to cancer, and asks the nurse how she can prevent this type of cancer. Which statements describe how to prevent this type of cancer? Select all that apply.
1. Not smoking reduces risk for cervical cancer.
2. A high-fat diet decreases risk for ovarian cancer.
3. Using condoms reduces risk for cervical cancer.
4. Limiting your number of sexual partners reduces risk for cervical cancer.
5. A human Papillomavirus quadrivalent (types 6, 11, 16, and 18) vaccine, given as an injection two times over a six-month period, can reduce risk for cervical cancer.

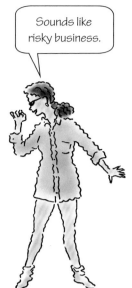

Sounds like risky business.

121. 1, 3, 4. Not smoking, using condoms, and limiting the number of sexual partners can reduce the risk for cervical cancer. A high-fat diet increases the risk for ovarian cancer. A human Papillomavirus quadrivalent (types 6, 11, 16, and 18) vaccine is given as three intramuscular injections over a six-month period.
CN: Physiological integrity; CNS: Reduction of risk potential; CL: Apply

122. The nurse is to prepare a client diagnosed with acute kidney injury (AKI) for a renal radiologic study. The health care provider orders the client to have the bowel evacuated before the study. Which orders for bowel evacuation would the nurse question? Select all that apply.
1. Soap suds cleansing enema until clear
2. Fleet enema until clear
3. Bisacodyl 15 mg po
4. Magnesium citrate 240 ml po
5. Castor oil 30 ml po

122. 2, 4. Fleet enema and magnesium citrate are hyperosmolar solutions, which are contraindicated for those with renal problems. The salt content in these solutions can cause toxicity. Soap suds enema, bisacodyl, and castor oil may be used.
CN: Physiological integrity; CNS: Pharmacological and parental therapies; CL: Apply

123. A client who is alert and oriented has been receiving hemodialysis three times per week for the last five years. The client's condition has gradually declined, and the client tells the dialysis nurse, "I don't want to do this anymore. I'm tired and ready to let my body shut down. I know that I'll die, but I'm ready." What is the **most** appropriate response by the nurse?
1. "I understand. My grandmother decided to give up too."
2. "You are just having a really bad day. You will feel better tomorrow."
3. "Have you thought about how your children will react?"
4. "Are you saying you no longer want to receive dialysis treatments?"

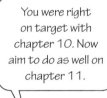

You were right on target with chapter 10. Now aim to do as well on chapter 11.

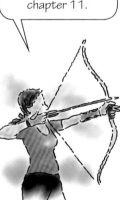

123. 4. Clarification is a therapeutic communication technique that is helpful in validating the intended meaning of the client's statement. Insinuating that the client decided to "give up" is judgmental. Telling the client he is having a "bad day" invalidates his feelings. Asking how his children will react places guilt on the client.
CN: Psychosocial integrity; CNS: None; CL: Apply

Chapter 11

Integumentary Disorders

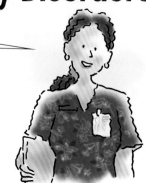

So you think the care of the client with a skin disorder isn't your strong suit, eh? Maybe you'd like to check out this Web site before taking on this chapter: **www.aad.org**. Enjoy!

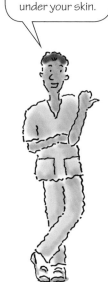

Don't let this chapter get under your skin.

1. Which statement **most** appropriately identifies the nutritional needs of a client related to the physiologic processes that occur following a burn injury?
1. The client needs 100 cal/kg during hospitalization.
2. The hypermetabolic state after a burn injury contributes to poor healing.
3. Keeping the environment cool decreases caloric demand.
4. Maintaining a hypermetabolic rate decreases the client's risk of infection.

2. The nurse is assessing a client admitted to the emergency department with a deep partial-thickness burn on his arm. What is the **most** accurate way for the nurse to document this finding?
1. Pain and redness
2. 10% damage to the epidermis
3. Necrotic tissue through all layers of skin
4. Necrotic tissue through most of the dermis

3. The nurse is caring for a client who was bitten by a brown recluse spider. Which assessment supports this finding?
1. Bull's-eye rash
2. Painful rash around a necrotic lesion
3. Patch of oval lesions
4. Line of papules and vesicles

1. 2. A burn injury causes a hypermetabolic state that results in protein and lipid catabolism which affects wound healing. Calories should be one-and-a-half to two times the basal metabolic rate, with at least 1.5 to 2 g of protein/kg of body daily. An environmental temperature within normal range allows the body to function efficiently, and devote caloric expenditure to healing and normal physiologic processes. If the temperature is too warm or too cold, the body uses its energy on temperature regulation rather than tissue repair. High metabolic rates increase the risk of infection.
CN: Physiological integrity; CNS: Basic care and comfort; CL: Apply

2. 4. A deep partial-thickness burn causes necrosis of the epidermal and dermal layers. Redness and pain are characteristics of a superficial injury. Superficial burns cause slight epidermal damage. Necrosis through all skin layers is seen with full-thickness injuries.
CN: Physiological integrity; CNS: Physiological adaptation; CL: Apply

3. 2. A necrotic, painful rash is associated with the bite of a brown recluse spider. A bull's-eye rash is a classic sign of Lyme disease. A slightly raised, oval lesion about two to six cm in diameter on the body is indicative of pityriasis rosea. A linear, popular, vesicular rash is characteristic of exposure to poison ivy.
CN: Physiological integrity; CNS: Physiological; CL: Apply

CN: Client needs category   CNS: Client needs subcategory   CL: Cognitive level

4. Which statement indicates that a client understands the administration of a Mantoux test?
  1. "You will use my deltoid muscle."
  2. "I will rub the site to help absorption."
  3. "I will come to get it read within 72 hours."
  4. "If there is a rash, it is positive."

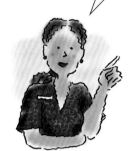

Your most important skill is assessment.

5. The nurse performs an assessment and determines that a client has head lice. Which finding is conclusive of head lice?
  1. Diffuse pruritic wheals
  2. Oval, white dots stuck to the hair shafts
  3. Pain, redness, and edema of the scalp
  4. Pruritic papules and pustules

6. A client is admitted with a suspected superficial fungal infection of the skin. How should the nurse collect the laboratory specimen?
  1. Aspirate fluid from the lesion with a sterile needle
  2. Scrape scales into a clean container
  3. Swab the area with a culturette culture swab
  4. Wash the site with sterile saline

7. A client visits the clinic with intensely itchy, dark red lesions on his hands, wrist, and waistline. Some of the lesions have been scratched open and are bleeding. What is the **first** intervention the nurse should teach this client to decrease his itching?
  1. Blow on the lesions
  2. Place the lesions under a heat lamp
  3. Place ice on the lesions
  4. Press on the lesions

8. A client with a skin infection is prescribed linezolid 400 mg/po/q8h. What is a **priority** nursing intervention?
  1. Teach the client to take the mediation on an empty stomach
  2. Have the client take a stool softener daily
  3. Teach the client to report diarrhea
  4. Have the client monitor their urine for a dark color

4. 3. Mantoux test results should be read 48 to 72 hours after placement by measuring the diameter of the induration at the site of the injection. The Mantoux test is injected intradermally on the volar surface of the forearm. It is not injected into muscle. Rubbing the site could cause leakage, and should be avoided. An induration develops, not a rash.
CN: Physiological integrity; CNS: Reduction of risk potential; CL: Apply

5. 2. Nits, the eggs of lice, are seen as oval, white dots on the hair shafts. Diffuse pruritic wheals are associated with an allergic reaction. Lice does not cause pain, and redness. Pruritic papules, with vesicles may be caused by scabies.
CN: Physiological integrity; CNS: Physiological; CL: Apply

6. 2. Cultures for fungal infections are obtained by using a tongue blade. The skin should be scraped into a clean container and sent to the laboratory. Lesions do not typically have fluid. Biopsies are performed for deep fungal infections, or for lesions suspected of being cancerous. Washing the site will not assist in the diagnosis of a fungal infection.
CN: Physiological integrity; CNS: Physiological; CL: Apply

7. 4. Pressing the skin stimulates nerve endings, and can reduce the sensation of itching. Blowing on the lesions will not decrease the sensation of itching. Heat and ice may further damage the skin.
CN: Physiological integrity; CNS: Physiological; CL: Apply

8. 3. This medication is an antibiotic, and may cause diarrhea. The client should understand that the healthcare provider should be called if diarrhea develops, as this may indicate pseudomembranous colitis. The medication does not have to be administered on an empty stomach, and this medication does not turn the urine dark.
CN: Physiological integrity; CNS: Pharmacological and parenteral therapies; CL: Apply

CN: Client needs category   CNS: Client needs subcategory   CL: Cognitive level

9. A nurse is teaching a female client about the use of isotretinoin. The client understands this teaching when she states:
   1. "I will take precautions so I do not become pregnant."
   2. "I will take an antiemetic."
   3. "I may need to take analgesics due to side effects."
   4. "I may need to take an antidiarrheal medication with this medication."

10. A hospitalized client is diagnosed with scabies. What is the **most** appropriate nursing intervention?
   1. Administer an antibiotic
   2. Administer an opioid
   3. Place the client on contact precautions
   4. Place the client in isolation

11. A client is receiving a low dose of methotrexate for psoriasis. Which nursing intervention is **essential**?
   1. Administer with food
   2. Assess hemoglobin and hematocrit.
   3. Assess liver function tests
   4. Administer at bedtime

12. The nurse is teaching a client about nystatin oral solution. The client understands the usage of this medication when she states:
   1. "I need to take the drug right after meals."
   2. "I need to take the drug right before meals."
   3. "I need to mix the drug with small amounts of food"
   4. "I need to take half the dose before and half after meals."

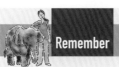

Remember

"Iso*tret*inoin is a 'threat' to pregnant women."

This drug is a retinoid and thus closely resembles retinoic acid, or vitamin A, which plays an instrumental role in skin development in fetuses. Because of this similarity, isotretinoin can cause birth defects and should be strictly avoided by any woman who is pregnant or at risk of becoming pregnant.

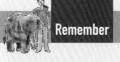

Remember

"Nystatin causes fungi to 'stand still.'"

This antifungal drug name is partly derived from the Greek word *statos*, meaning "standing." The drug is also named after the New York State Department of Health, which is where the chemist who developed the drug worked.

9. 1. Even small amounts of isotretinoin are associated with severe birth defects. Most female clients are prescribed an adjunct oral contraceptive while taking this medication. There is no reason for the client to take antimetics, analgesics or antidiarrheals.
CN: Physiological integrity; CNS: Pharmacological and parenteral therapies; CL: Apply

10. 3. Scabies are caused by a transmittable mite, and should be placed on contact precautions to prevent spreading it to others. Pain is not typically an issue, and opioids are not used. Antibiotics do not cure the infestation. Isolation is not necessary.
CN: Physiological integrity; CNS: Physiological; CL: Apply

11. 3. This medication can cause damage to the liver. Liver function tests must be done prior to starting therapy, and yearly while on the medication. The medication does not have to be administered with food or at bedtime, and hemoglobin and hematocrit does not have to be routinely assessed.
CN: Physiological integrity; CNS: Pharmacologic and parenteral therapy; CL: Apply

12. 1. Nystatin oral solution should be swished around the mouth after eating for the best contact with mucous membranes. Taking the drug before, or with, meals does not allow for the best contact with the mucous membranes.
CN: Physiological integrity; CNS: Pharmacological and parenteral therapies; CL: Apply

13. A client has a pilonidal cyst. Which intervention should the nurse perform **first**?
1. Keep the area clean
2. Teach the client about surgery
3. Assess for infection
4. Teach the client signs of infection

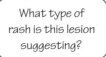

What type of rash is this lesion suggesting?

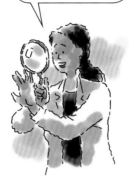

13. 3. The nurse should first assess for infection. A pilonidal cyst forms at the end of the sacral area and can easily become infected. The area should be kept clean, and the client should be taught the signs of infection and about surgery. If the infection is recurrent, the best intervention may be surgical removal.
CN: Physiological integrity; CNS: Physiological; CL: Apply

14. The nurse is admitting a client who has alopecia. What is the **most** appropriate assessment question to ask this client?
1. "Do you take medications to stimulate hair growth?"
2. "Do you have hair loss elsewhere?"
3. "What is your past medical history?"
4. "Do you shave your head?"

14. 3. Alopecia is the correct term for hair loss. Hair loss often occurs with other chronic diseases, such as cancer, arthritis, or lupus. It is most appropriate to assess this client for other conditions that may have caused the hair loss. The other questions would yield the appropriate information.
CN: Physiological integrity; CNS: Physiological; CL: Apply

15. A client is diagnosed with atopic dermatitis. What is the **best** information for the nurse to include in the teaching plan?
1. Stay away from people who have bacterial infections
2. Take antibiotics daily
3. Avoid going out in the sun
4. Keep your skin lubricated

15. 4. Atopic dermatitis is a chronic rash which worsens if the skin is dry and irritated. Clients often have respiratory allergies or diseases associated with this condition. Food allergies and stress may also prompt this condition.
CN: Physiological integrity; CNS: Physiological; CL: Apply

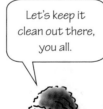

Let's keep it clean out there, you all.

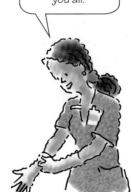

16. A client has been diagnosed with plantar warts. What information should the nurse teach this client?
1. "Keep your feet clean."
2. "Take your antibiotics daily."
3. "Notify your healthcare provider if painful."
4. "Do not walk on the warts."

16. 3. Plantar warts are rough papules commonly found on the soles of the feet, and are caused by the human papillomavirus (HPV). This client should be instructed to notify her healthcare provider if the warts are painful, as they can be surgically removed. Antibiotics are not prescribed for this condition. Keeping feet clean will not cure the condition. Walking on the warts will not make them worse.
CN: Physiological integrity; CNS: Physiological; CL: Apply

17. A client has recently been diagnosed with tinea corporis. What is the **primary** nursing intervention for this client?
1. Teach the client how this infection is spread
2. Administer routine immunizations
3. Teach the client how to take antibiotics
4. Establish dietary restrictions

17. 1. Tinea corporis, or ringworm is caused by mold-like fungi called dermatophytes that thrive in warm, moist areas. Tinea corporis is easily spread. It is transmittable by direct contact with clothing, combs, shower walls, or floors that have the fungus on them, or by direct contact with an area of ringworm on someone's body. A tinea infection is more likely if you have wet skin for long periods of time, or do not bathe or wash your hair often. Immunizations do not prevent the infection. Antibiotics do not cure the infection. Diet does not modify the condition.
CN: Physiological integrity; CNS: Physiological adaptation; CL: Apply

CN: Client needs category   CNS: Client needs subcategory   CL: Cognitive level

18. The nurse is caring for a client who has been diagnosed with psoriasis. Which intervention will hasten this client's recovery?
  1. Apply antibiotic cream daily to lesions
  2. Increase exposure to sunlight
  3. Wash lesions with antibacterial soap
  4. Keep cold and utilize air conditioning

18. **2.** Psoriasis is a chronic skin condition that often occurs without family history. Exposure to warmer climates and sunlight will decrease the severity and likelihood of a psoriasis breakout. Antibiotic cream or antibacterial soap does not cure or improve lesions. Cold temperatures and air-conditioning are not proven to ease lesions.
CN: Physiological integrity; CNS: Physiological adaptation; CL: Apply

19. What information is important for the nurse to consider when planning care for a client diagnosed with squamous cell carcinoma of the face?
  1. The client will need to be taught about surgery.
  2. This type of cancer is very difficult to cure.
  3. Antibiotic therapy is necessary.
  4. Antifungal cream is often utilized on the lesions.

19. **1.** Squamous cell carcinomas of the face are cancers of the epidermis. They are firm nodular lesions with a crust or central ulcers on areas of the face, neck head and lower lip that have been exposed to sunlight. Rapid metastasis into the lymph system occurs in ten percent of cases. Clients should be informed that the lesions are potentially metastatic, and that surgical intervention may be necessary. Antibiotic and antifungal cream is not generally used on the lesions unless there is an identified secondary infection.
CN: Physiological integrity; CNS: Physiological adaptation; CL: Analyze

20. What is the **best** information for the nurse to share with a client who has tinea capitis?
  1. Keep the area clean and dry
  2. Do not share combs or brushes
  3. Use antibacterial soap
  4. Spend time in the sun

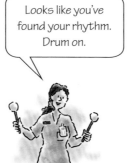

Looks like you've found your rhythm. Drum on.

20. **2.** Tinea capitis is a fungal infection of the scalp. Dermatophyte infections can differ in lesion appearance, body location, and species of the infecting organism. Infections are spread by direct contact. The client should not share combs or brushes. Keeping the scalp clean and dry does not stop the spread of tinea capitis. Antibacterial soap will not have an effect on this fungal infection. Being in the sun will not cure the infection. Antifungal agents are needed to cure tinea capitis.
CN: Physiological integrity; CNS: Physiological adaptation; CL: Apply

21. A client has been diagnosed with secondary syphilis. What does the nurse expect to find on assessment?
  1. Chancre ulcers
  2. No significant symptoms
  3. Nodular, pustular, annular lesions
  4. Destructive lesions involving many organs and tissues

21. **3.** Nodular, pustular, annular lesions and generalized lymphadenopathy occur in secondary syphilis. The chancre, a painless, shallow ulcer, develops in primary syphilis and appears three weeks after exposure. The latent phase occurs between the secondary and tertiary stages. Tertiary syphilis has destructive lesions involving many organs and tissues.
CN: Physiological integrity; CNS: Physiological adaptation; CL: Apply

CN: Client needs category   CNS: Client needs subcategory   CL: Cognitive level

22. A client with full-thickness, circumferential burns to the chest has been intubated and is experiencing pressure from edema that is inhibiting chest wall expansion. What is the nurse's **priority** intervention for this client?
1. Cricothyrotomy
2. Escharotomy
3. Thoracentesis
4. Chest tube insertion

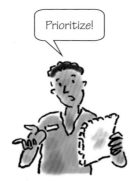

Prioritize!

22. 2. Escharotomy is a surgical incision used to relieve the pressure from edema. It is sometimes needed with circumferential burns that prevent chest expansion or circulatory compromise. Cricothyrotomy is an emergency procedure that involves puncturing the trachea through the cricothyroid membrane to create an airway. This client is already intubated. Needle thoracentesis and insertion of a chest tube are performed to relieve a pneumothorax.
CN: Physiological integrity; CNS: Physiological adaptation; CL: Analyze

23. What is the nurse's **priority** assessment for a client during the first 48 hours following a major burn injury?
1. Hyponatremia and hypokalemia
2. Hyponatremia and hyperkalemia
3. Hypernatremia and hypokalemia
4. Hypernatremia and hyperkalemia

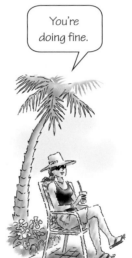

You're doing fine.

23. 2. During the first 48 hours after a burn, capillary permeability increases, allowing fluids to shift from the plasma to the interstitial spaces. This fluid is high in sodium, causing a decrease in serum sodium levels. Potassium also leaks from the cells into the plasma, causing hyperkalemia.
CN: Physiological integrity; CNS: Physiological adaptation; CL: Analyze

24. A client sustained partial-thickness burns to his trunk and both lower extremities. Which IV fluid will the nurse initiate?
1. Albumin
2. 5% dextrose in water
3. Lactated ringer's solution
4. 0.9% normal saline with 20 mEq potassium

24. 3. Lactated ringer's solution replaces lost sodium, and corrects metabolic acidosis, which commonly occurs following a burn. Albumin may be used as supportive therapy, but is not the primary fluid for replacement. Dextrose is not given to clients with burns during the first 24 hours as it may cause pseudodiabetes. The client is hyperkalemic due to the potassium shift from intracellular space to the plasma. Potassium would not be administered.
CN: Physiological integrity; CNS: Pharmacological and parenteral therapies; CL: Apply

25. The nurse is planning care for a client requiring a dressing change. What action should the nurse take?
1. Change dressing per providers order
2. Place a sign above the client's bed
3. Communicate the treatment plan at end of shift report
4. Document the dressing change in the narrative note

25. 1. Following the provider's order will ensure consistency and patient safety. Posting a sign above the bed is a good reminder, but does not ensure that the treatment will be performed. Verbally reporting to the nurse on the upcoming shift does not clearly ensure the dressing change will be completed. Although the intervention should be documented in the narrative note, this will not guarantee the treatment will be continued consistently by the next nurse.
CN: Safe, effective care environment; CNS: Management of care; CL: Apply

26. A client has a reddened sacral area that is unrelieved by changing his position. Which intervention should the nurse begin?
1. Develop an updated turning schedule for the client
2. Massage the reddened area
3. Place a pillow under the client's sacrum
4. Wash the area with hot water

26. 1. A client who has been sitting, and has a reddened sacral area that is unrelieved by a position change has been in that position for too long. The nurse should turn the client more frequently. Although every two hours is the routine to turn clients, pressure can start to decrease blood flow after only twenty minutes. Clients at high risk should most likely be turned every hour. The areas should never be rubbed or massaged as this can further destroy tissue. A pillow will not decrease pressure on the area. Luke warm water can be used for cleansing, but never hot water.
CN: Physiological integrity; CNS: Basic care and comfort; CL: Apply

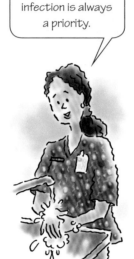

Preventing infection is always a priority.

27. The client is experiencing the initial phase of a burn injury. What is the nurse's **priority** intervention?
1. Decrease anxiety
2. Promote hygiene
3. Turn frequently
4. Prevent infection

27. 4. Because the body's protective barrier is damaged, and the immune system is compromised, preventing infection is the primary action. Decreasing anxiety, promoting hygiene, and turning frequently are important but are not the primary focus. Physiologic needs take precedence.
CN: Physiological integrity; CNS: Physiological adaptation; CL: Apply

28. Which client would be at **highest** risk for impaired wound healing following surgery?
1. An adult with hypertension
2. An adult with a BMI of 25
3. An older adult in general good health
4. An older adult with poorly controlled type 1 diabetes mellitus

28. 4. Poorly controlled type 1 diabetes is a serious risk factor for impaired wound healing. Hypertension, in itself, does not put a client at high risk of impaired skin integrity. A BMI of 25 is within normal range. A BMI over 30 may be associated with increased health risks. Older adults are at higher risk than younger clients, however, other factors can increase the risk.
CN: Physiological integrity; CNS: Physiological adaptation; CL: Analyze

29. The nurse teaches a client about how a wound culture will be completed. Which action demonstrates correct procedure?
1. Thoroughly irrigate the wound before collecting the culture
2. Use a sterile swab to wipe the crusty area around the outside of the wound
3. Gently roll a sterile swab from the center of the wound outward to collect drainage
4. Use one sterile swab to collect drainage from several possible infected sites along the incision

29. 3. Rolling a swab from the center outward is the correct way to culture a wound. Irrigating the wound washes away drainage, debris, and many of the microorganisms colonizing or infecting the wound. The outside of the wound may be colonized with microorganisms from various sources on the client's skin. These may grow in culture and yield inaccurate sensitivity. Each swab should be used on only one site to prevent the spread of microorganisms from one site to another.
CN: Safe, effective care environment; CNS: Safety and infection control; CL: Apply

30. Which documentation indicates that a client with an abdominal incision has delayed wound healing?
1. Wound edges red
2. Edema around sutured area
3. Purulent drainage on soiled wound dressing
4. Sanguineous drainage in wound collection drainage bag

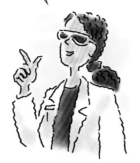

You're a rock star. Keep on rocking.

31. The nurse is planning care to prevent pressure ulcers in a client who is at high risk. Which interventions should the nurse include in the plan of care? Select all that apply.
1. Rub bony prominences each time the client changes position
2. Turn the client by pulling the client on the sheet.
3. Elevate the head of the bed 90 degrees
4. Assess nutritional status
5. Keep skin clean and dry

32. What is the **best** nursing intervention for a client with a Braden scale score of 10?
1. Continue to assess client each shift
2. Implement interventions for a high risk client
3. Notify the healthcare provider
4. Assess client for malnutrition

33. A client has recently had a skin graft. What is the **most** important instruction for the nurse to give this client?
1. Attend physical therapy
2. Protect the graft from direct sunlight
3. Use cosmetics to cover the area
4. Apply lubricating lotion to the graft site

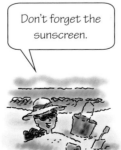

Don't forget the sunscreen.

34. The nurse is teaching the client how to prevent the development of basal cell carcinoma. Which **priority** instruction should the nurse give this client?
1. Avoid drying out your skin
2. Avoid exposure to the sun
3. Avoid immunosuppressive drugs
4. Avoid exposure to radiation

30. 3. Purulent drainage contains white blood cells, which fight infection, and indicate a possible delay in wound healing. Red edges of a wound are typical due to irritation and trauma. Slight edema is also typical after the trauma of a surgical incision. Sanguineous drainage indicates bleeding, not infection, which is expected after surgery.
CN: Physiological integrity; CNS: Physiological adaptation; CL: Analyze

31. 4, 5. The client should have their nutritional status assessed, as decreased nutrition can contribute to skin breakdown. Skin should be kept clean and dry to prevent maceration and skin breakdown. Bony prominences should not be rubbed. The client should not be pulled on a sheet as this causes shearing force. The head of the bed should not be elevated 90 degrees because this increases pressure on the client's back and sacral area.
CN: Safe, effective care environment; CNS: Safety and infection control; CL: Analyze

32. 2. A client with a Braden score less than 11 is at high risk. The nurse should assess a client every two hours who is at high risk. There is no emergent reason to call the healthcare provider. Assessment is completed during initial Braden score assessment. There is no need to reassess for malnutrition.
CN: Physiological integrity; CNS: Basic care and comfort; CL: Analyze

33. 2. To avoid burning and sloughing, the client must protect the graft from direct sunlight. The other three interventions are all helpful to the client and his recovery, but not the most important.
CN: Physiological integrity; CNS: Physiological adaptation; CL: Analyze

34. 2. The sun is the best known and most common cause of basal cell carcinoma. Dry skin is not noted to be a cause. Immunosuppressive drug therapy and radiation are less common causes of carcinoma.
CN: Physiological integrity; CNS: Reduction of risk potential; CL: Apply

35. The nurse is assessing an older client's skin turgor. The client's skin shows poor elasticity and tents. How does the nurse interpret this finding?
1. The client is overhydrated.
2. It indicates normal skin turgor.
3. These findings are a normal part of the aging process.
4. The findings indicate dehydration and electrolyte imbalance.

35. 3. Inelastic skin turgor is a normal part of aging. Over hydration causes the skin to appear edematous and spongy. Normal skin turgor is dry and firm. Dehydration can cause inelastic skin with tenting in younger clients.
CN: Health promotion and maintenance; CNS: None;
CL: Apply

36. A client has a stage-two sacral pressure ulcer that is being treated with a transparent-film dressing. What is the purpose of this intervention?
1. The dressing keeps the wound moist.
2. The dressing dries out and debrides the wound.
3. The film works best on wounds that have large amounts of thick exudate.
4. The transparent film dressing should be tightly packed into the wound.

36. 1. A transparent film dressing keeps the wound moist and enhances autolysis of necrotic tissue. It helps to provide a barrier to external contaminants. The dressing does not dry out. The dressing creates a barrier over the wound but is not packed into the wound. Transparent film is indicated for partial-thickness wounds with little or no exudate.
CN: Physiological integrity; CNS: Physiological adaptation;
CL: Analyze

37. A client presents to a clinic with a second-degree sunburn on her face and arms. What is the **first** intervention by the nurse?
1. Administer analgesic medication as ordered
2. Apply cold, moist towels to the burns
3. Apply sterile, dry towels to the burns
4. Apply vitamin A, D, and E ointment to the burns

37. 2. Cold, moist towels help stop the burning process. Analgesics should be administered as ordered after the burning process has been controlled. Dry towels would retain the heat and aren't used. Ointments are applied during the healing phase but not initially.
CN: Physiological integrity; CNS: Basic care and comfort;
CL: Apply

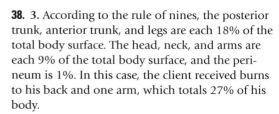
One back and one arm equal …

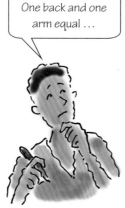

38. A client received burns to his entire back and left arm. The nurse uses the rule of nines to calculate the percentage of his body that is burned. What percentage of the client's body is burned?
1. 9%
2. 18%
3. 27%
4. 36%

38. 3. According to the rule of nines, the posterior trunk, anterior trunk, and legs are each 18% of the total body surface. The head, neck, and arms are each 9% of the total body surface, and the perineum is 1%. In this case, the client received burns to his back and one arm, which totals 27% of his body.
CN: Physiological integrity; CNS: Reduction of risk potential;
CL: Apply

39. The nurse is performing a sterile dressing change. What is the nurse's **most** important intervention?
1. Change the sterile field after sterile water is accidentally spilled on it
2. Put on sterile gloves, then open a container of sterile saline
3. Place a sterile dressing 1/20 in (1.3 cm) from the edge of the sterile field
4. Clean the wound with a circular motion, moving from outer circles toward the center

39. 1. A sterile field is considered contaminated when it becomes wet. Moisture can act as a wick, allowing microorganisms to contaminate the field. The outside of containers such as sterile saline bottles aren't sterile. The containers should be opened before sterile gloves are put on, and the solution poured over the sterile dressings placed in a sterile basin. The outer inch of a sterile field is not considered sterile. Wounds should be cleaned from the least contaminated area to the most contaminated area, for example, from the center outward.
CN: Safe, effective care environment; CNS: Safety and infection control; CL: Apply

CN: Client needs category   CNS: Client needs subcategory   CL: Cognitive level

40. The client has sustained a burn. Which intervention will help to decrease hypertrophied scarring during the later stages of healing?
1. Remove all tissue in the wound area
2. Apply continuous pressure using elastic wraps
3. Wear clothing to protect the burn from the sun
4. Maintain wound dressing changes

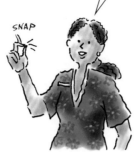

You're doing very well. The remaining questions should be a snap.

SNAP

40. 2. Using elastic wraps and bandages to apply continuous pressure during the early stages of wound healing can help prevent keloid scar formation. Removing tissue, especially eschar, promotes wound healing as do dressing changes, but neither directly decreases scar formation. Wearing clothing prevents sunburn but doesn't decrease scar formation.
CN: Physiological integrity; CNS: Physiological adaptation; CL: Apply

41. The home healthcare nurse is teaching a client's family about measures to prevent skin breakdown. The nurse determines that teaching was effective when the family members avoid:
1. placing the client the client on a waterbed.
2. using a rubber ring to support the sacral area.
3. using a gel flotation pad.
4. placing the client on a polyurethane foam mattress.

41. 2. Rings or donuts shouldn't be used because they restrict circulation. The waterbed distributes pressure over the entire surface. Gel pads give with weight. Foam mattresses distribute pressure evenly.
CN: Physiological integrity; CNS: Reduction of risk potential; CL: Apply

42. The nurse enters the room of a postoperative client and notes a wound evisceration. What is the **most** important action by the nurse?
1. Give prophylactic antibiotics as ordered
2. Place the client on nothing-by-mouth (NPO) status
3. Explain to the client what's happening and give support
4. Cover the protruding internal organs with sterile gauze moistened with sterile saline

42. 4. Covering the wound with moistened gauze is the priority to prevent the organs from drying. Both the gauze and the saline must be sterile to reduce the risk of infection. Because evisceration usually requires emergency surgery, the nurse should place the client on NPO status. Evisceration is a frightening situation for any client. While the nurse works quickly to get the client treated, she can provide support to reduce the client's anxiety. Antibiotics will usually be ordered, and should be started as soon as possible.
CN: Physiological integrity; CNS: Physiological adaptation; CL: Analyze

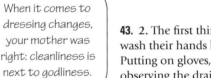

When it comes to dressing changes, your mother was right: cleanliness is next to godliness.

43. The nurse is teaching a client's family how to do a dressing change when the client is discharged. The nurse should teach the family that the first step should be to:
1. put on gloves.
2. wash hands thoroughly.
3. slowly remove the soiled dressing.
4. observe the dressing for the amount, type, and odor of drainage.

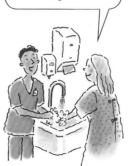

43. 2. The first thing that someone must do is wash their hands before changing a dressing. Putting on gloves, removing the dressing, and observing the drainage are all parts of the procedure for a dressing change.
CN: Safe, effective care environment; CNS: Safety and infection control ; CL: Apply

44. The nurse is teaching an unlicensed assistive personnel (UAP) about the importance of preventing pressure ulcers. Which action by the UAP indicates that teaching was successful?
1. Placing the patient in an upright position
2. Turning the client hourly
3. Applying lotion to the client's buttocks
4. Positioning the client on his back during the day

44. 2. Turning the client every one to two hours will prevent pressure areas from developing, and help prevent atelectasis and other pulmonary complications. The client should spend time on his back according to the turning schedule, but not remain on his back throughout the day. Lotion may cause increased skin breakdown due to maceration.
CN: Physiological integrity; CNS: Basic care and comfort; CL: Apply

45. What is the **most** important information for the nurse to teach a client about hypersensitivity skin test results?
  1. Wash the sites daily with a mild soap
  2. Have the sites read on the correct date
  3. Keep the skin test areas moist with a mild lotion
  4. Stay out of direct sunlight until the tests are read

46. The nurse is reviewing lab results of a client diagnosed with disseminated herpes zoster. The client is receiving hydrocortisone. Which laboratory value does the nurse anticipate will be elevated?
  1. Calcium
  2. Glucose
  3. Magnesium
  4. Potassium

47. A client is admitted to the burn unit with extensive full-thickness burns. What is the nurse's **priority** during the early phases of treatment?
  1. Fluid status
  2. Body image
  3. Level of pain
  4. Risk of infection

48. A nurse is performing an assessment on a recently admitted client. What assessment findings place the client at high risk for skin breakdown? Select all that apply.
  1. A family history of pressure ulcers
  2. A history of leukemia
  3. Being 50 years old
  4. Taking corticosteroids daily for asthma
  5. Taking aspirin daily

49. A client with burns has a new donor site. What is the **most** important intervention by the nurse?
  1. Keep the site dependent
  2. Avoid pressure on the site
  3. Keep the site tightly covered
  4. Covered the site with antibiotic cream

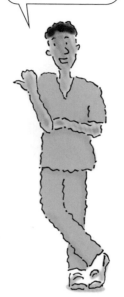

It's most important that you read this question carefully.

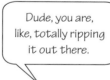

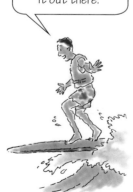

Dude, you are, like, totally ripping it out there.

45. 2. An important facet of evaluating skin tests is to read the skin test results at the proper time. Evaluating the skin test too late or too early will give inaccurate and unreliable results. Both the gauze and the saline must be sterile to reduce the risk of infection. There is no need to wash the site with soap. The site should be kept dry. Direct sunlight is not prohibited.
CN: Health promotion and maintenance; CNS: None; CL: Apply

46. 2. Corticosteroids increase blood sugar and tend to lower serum potassium and calcium levels. Their effect on magnesium isn't substantial.
CN: Physiological integrity; CNS: Pharmacological and parenteral therapies; CL: Analyze

47. 1. In early burn care, the client's greatest need is fluid resuscitation, as a large-volume of fluid is lost through the skin. Body image, pain, and infection are important concerns in the nursing care of a burn client, but they do not take precedence over fluid management in the early phase of care.
CN: Safe, effective care environment; CNS: Management of care; CL: Analyze

48. 2, 4, 5. A history of leukemia places the client at risk for pressure ulcers and skin breakdown. The systemic inhibition of leukocytic response, results in impaired resistance to infections increasing the risk of skin breakdown. Taking corticosteroid daily and aspirin daily also places the client at risk for skin breakdown. A family history of pressure ulcers is not relevant as there is no genetic predisposition for skin breakdown. A 50-year-old client is not old to be at risk for skin breakdown.
CN: Safe, effective care environment; CNS: Management of care; CL: Analyze

49. 2. A universal concern in the care of donor sites for burn care is keeping the site away from sources of pressure. Placing the site in a position of dependence is not a justified aspect of donor site care. Tightly covering the site is not recommended. Covering the site with antibiotic cream is not recommended.
CN: Physiological integrity; CNS: Physiological adaptation; CL: Apply

CN: Client needs category   CNS: Client needs subcategory   CL: Cognitive level

50. A client has been diagnosed with late-stage Lyme disease. What is the **priority** nursing assessment?
1. Fever
2. Malaise
3. Urinary output
4. Neurologic status

50. 4. The nurse should assess for neurological problems as a priority. Late stage Lyme disease symptoms can occur weeks, months, and even years after a tick bite as the infection spreads throughout the body and infiltrates the central nervous system. Fever and malaise are early symptoms of Lyme disease. Change in urinary output is not typically a complication of Lyme disease.
CN: Physiological integrity; CNS: Physiological adaptation; CL: Apply

> Color can be a classic sign of some conditions.

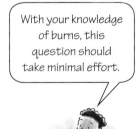

51. A client is admitted with suspected malignant melanoma on his left shoulder. Which assessment finding assists the nurse in confirming this diagnosis?
1. A brown birthmark that has lightened in color
2. A brown or black mole with red, white, or blue areas
3. Petechiae
4. A red birthmark that has recently become darker

51. 2. Melanomas have an irregular shape and lack uniformity in color. They may appear brown or black with red, white, or blue areas. Melanoma lesions don't appear as petechiae or as birthmarks that have changed color.
CN: Health promotion and maintenance; CNS: None; CL: Apply

52. A nurse educator is teaching a group of clients about hygiene. Which client statement indicates the need for further teaching?
1. "The skin absorbs fluids."
2. "The skin serves as the body's first line of defense."
3. "The skin excretes waste products."
4. "The skin changes vitamin D into a form the body can use."

52. 4. The skin doesn't change vitamin D into a form the body can use. The sun helps to convert vitamin D. The skin absorbs fluids, serves as the body's first line of defense, and excretes waste products.
CN: Physiological integrity; CNS: Physiological adaptation; CL: Analyze

53. The nurse is teaching a client how to care for his skin. The nurse determines that the client understands teaching about sebum when the client states:
1. "It is the most superficial layer of the skin."
2. "It is the oil secreted by the skin."
3. "It is a pouch-like depression from which a hair grows."
4. "It is the deepest layer of the skin."

53. 2. Sebum is the oil secreted by the skin. The epidermis and dermis are skin layers. A follicle is a pouch-like depression from which a hair grows.
CN: Physiological integrity; CNS: Physiological adaptation; CL: Apply

> With your knowledge of burns, this question should take minimal effort.

54. The nurse is planning care for a client with a late-stage burn. What is the **most** important intervention for the nurse to include to promote healing?
1. Removing eschar from the skin
2. Applying continuous-compression wraps
3. Wearing clothing to protect the burn from the sun
4. Maintaining wound care irrigation

54. 2. Applying continuous-compression wraps promotes skin healing, and prevents hypertrophied tissue from forming. The other interventions are appropriate for the client with a burn wound but don't necessarily help minimize scarring.
CN: Physiological integrity; CNS: Reduction of risk potential; CL: Apply

55. A client has an inflamed area on the right fore-arm that's causing considerable discomfort. Which intervention should the nurse implement?
1. Apply warm, moist compresses
2. Wrap the forearm with elastic bandage
3. Apply hydrocortisone cream
4. Apply a non-adherent dressing

55. 1. Warm, moist compresses increase circulation to the area, reducing discomfort and redness. An elastic bandage decompresses the area but doesn't ease inflammation. Hydrocortisone cream is useful on an inflamed area that itches. A non-adherent dressing does not relieve inflammation or pain.
CN: Physiological integrity; CNS: Basic care and comfort; CL: Apply

56. An older adult states that the sore on the inside of his ankle "won't heal." After noting varicosities and coarse discoloration around the sore, the nurse assesses for:
1. acute venous insufficiency.
2. chronic venous insufficiency.
3. acute arterial occlusive disease.
4. chronic arterial occlusive disease.

56. 2. Classic signs of chronic venous insufficiency include skin discoloration and stasis ulcers, usually found on the ankle's medial aspect. Asymmetric moderate edema, normal pulses, and deep muscle pain relieved by elevation are signs of acute venous insufficiency. Acute or chronic arterial occlusive disease usually cause intermittent claudication and severe burning pain.
CN: Physiological integrity; CNS: Physiological adaptation; CL: Apply

57. A nurse prepares a client for a shave biopsy of a skin lesion. What is the **priority** information for the nurse to include in the teaching plan?
1. How to care for the suture line
2. The need for a skin graft
3. The need for sedation
4. How to care for the dressing

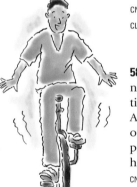

I had no idea how talented you are!

57. 4. Dressing care should be included in the teaching plan. A shave biopsy removes only the first or second layer of skin, causing a superficial wound with no suture line, and minimal scarring. There is no need for a skin graft or sedation with a shave biopsy.
CN: Physiological integrity; CNS: Physiological adaptation; CL: Apply

58. The health care provider orders a wet-to-dry dressing for a client who has a pressure ulcer with infected, necrotic tissue. What should the nurse teach the client about this intervention?
1. This intervention prevents extension of the infection.
2. This will help to debride the wound.
3. This intervention keeps the wound moist.
4. The dressing reduces pain.

58. 2. A wet-to-dry dressing placed over a necrotic area adheres to tissue as it dries, and tissue is debrided when the dressing is removed. Antibiotics, not dressings, help prevent extension of the infection. Keeping the wound moist would prevent the necessary debridement. The dressing has no analgesic effect.
CN: Physiological integrity; CNS: Physiological adaptation; CL: Apply

59. Which assessment finding would indicate to the nurse that treatment with moist saline dressings has been effective in healing a wound?
1. Red, swollen tissue
2. Dry, crusted scab
3. Deep, wide keloid
4. Warm, painful tissue

59. 2. Ten days into healing, a wound should be at the end of the lag phase of healing, as indicated by a dry, crusted scab. Tissue will be red, swollen, warm, or painful during the inflammatory phase, which occurs two to seven days after the ulcer develops. A deep, wide keloid may appear three weeks to two years after ulcer development, but does not indicate healing.
CN: Physiological integrity; CNS: Physiological adaptation; CL: Apply

60. When changing the dressing on a pressure ulcer, a nurse notes necrotic wound tissue. What is the **most** appropriate nursing intervention?
1. Apply antibiotic cream to the area
2. Culture the wound
3. Notify the health care provider
4. Prepare to irrigate the wound

60. 3. The priority is to notify the healthcare provider of the findings and obtain appropriate interventions. Wound cultures are done when an infection is present or suspected. Wound irrigation with an antiseptic may damage sensitive tissue and prevent healing.
CN: Physiological integrity; CNS: Physiological adaptation; CL: Apply

61. After a traumatic injury, a client's wound heals. A smooth, pink, thickened, rubbery lesion forms over the wound. What is the nurse's **best** intervention?
1. Notify the healthcare provider
2. Teach the client about dietary measures to dissolve keloids
3. Apply anti-inflammatory cream to the area
4. Teach the client about the condition

61. 4. The nurse should teach the client about keloids. A keloid results from a defect in the healing process in which excess collagen develops at the healing site. There is no need to call the healthcare provider at this time. There is no research showing that any particular dietary measures can resolve keloids. The client does not need anti-inflammatory medications.
CN: Physiological integrity; CNS: Physiological adaptation; CL: Analyze

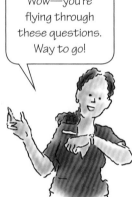

Wow—you're flying through these questions. Way to go!

62. A client is diagnosed with urticaria. What is the **priority** nursing intervention?
1. Administer antibiotics
2. Assess for a cause
3. Administer an antihistamine
4. Assess respiratory system

62. 4. Urticaria or hives herald an allergic event. This allergic reaction may advance to include the respiratory system. The priority is to assess the client for an impaired airway. The nurse needs to assess the respiratory system. Once the nurse determines the client's airway and breathing is alright, the nurse should assess for a cause of the allergy. An antihistamine is often administered, but an antibiotic is not.
CN: Physiological integrity; CNS: Physiological adaptation; CL: Apply

63. A client has multiple blisters from a superficial burn. What intervention will the nurse perform when the blisters break?
1. Remove the raised skin
2. Wash the area vigorously with soap and water
3. Apply silvadene cream
4. Clean the area with normal saline solution and cover it with a dressing

63. 4. To maintain asepsis, the nurse should clean the area with normal saline solution and cover it with a dressing. Removing the raised skin would cause further skin damage. Washing the area vigorously with soap and water would damage the tissue and cause drying. Silvadene cream is used as an antimicrobial, and not currently needed.
CN: Safe, effective care environment; CNS: Safety and infection control; CL: Apply

64. A client undergoes cryosurgery to remove a cancerous skin lesion. Which assessment finding indicates to the nurse that the surgery was successful?
   1. Dry, itchy skin patches
   2. Purulent drainage at the site
   3. Pain without edema
   4. Edema, blistering, and tenderness

64. 4. Cryosurgery leaves a wound resembling a burn, with edema, blistering, and tenderness. Purulent drainage and pain suggest a possible infection. The wound from cryosurgery is not dry or itchy.
CN: Physiological integrity; CNS: Physiological adaptation; CL: Analyze

65. The nurse assesses a client who has scabbed lacerations. Based on this assessment, in which phase of wound healing are these wounds?
   1. Contraction
   2. Inflammatory
   3. Proliferative
   4. Remodeling

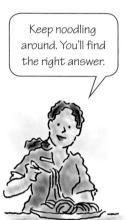

Keep noodling around. You'll find the right answer.

65. 3. During the proliferative phase of wound healing, which lasts from the 4th to the 21st day after injury, granulation tissue appears, and the wound edges start to pull together. Contraction, the third phase of wound healing, may begin around the 7th day and involves a significant decrease in the wound surface. The inflammatory phase is the first healing phase. It immediately follows the injury and lasts four to six days. It involves the control of bleeding and the release of chemicals needed for healing. The remodeling phase, the final phase, may lead to scar flattening and correction of any deformities that occurred during the third phase.
CN: Physiological integrity; CNS: Basic care and comfort; CL: Analyze

66. An elderly client who has spent a great deal of time outdoors tells the home health nurse that her skin is "dry and itchy." What is the **most** important information for the nurse to give this client?
   1. Soak in a bubble bath once per day
   2. Bathe with antimicrobial soap once per day
   3. Bathe with mild soap and water or with water only
   4. Scrub the skin vigorously to remove dead skin cells

66. 3. Bathing with mild soap and water, or with water only can relieve itching and dryness. Bubble baths and antimicrobial soap can be very drying to an elderly person's sensitive skin. Scrubbing vigorously may worsen skin dryness.
CN: Physiological integrity; CNS: Basic care and comfort; CL: Apply

67. The nurse is caring for a client diagnosed with pityriasis rosea. What is the **most** appropriate nursing intervention?
   1. Teach the client about antibiotic therapy
   2. Teach the client about antifungal therapy
   3. Keep the client comfortable
   4. Have the client take daily hot showers

67. 2. Pityriasis rosea is a rash of unknown origin that might be related to a virus. It will resolve in six to eight weeks. The nurse should treat symptoms, such as itching, to keep the client comfortable. The client will not be on antibiotic or antifungal therapy. Hot showers will exacerbate the condition.
CN: Physiological integrity; CNS: Physiological adaptation; CL: Analyze

68. At an outpatient clinic, a medical assistant interviews a client and documents findings as follows:

Progress notes	
2/10/17	Client is new, and very anxious.
0900	Black mole with shades of brown
	noted on upper, outer, right thigh.
	Asymmetric inshape, with an irregular
	border. ———— *M. Rosenfeld, MA*

After reading the chart note, a nurse begins planning this client's care based on the:

1. client's need for information about the potential diagnosis of basal cell carcinoma.
2. client's concern over the potential diagnosis of malignant melanoma.
3. potential for skin breakdown from squamous cell carcinoma.
4. client's misunderstanding about preventive measures.

69. The nurse is examining the back of a client and notes a rash with a discrete lesion configuration. Which graphic shows a discrete lesion configuration?

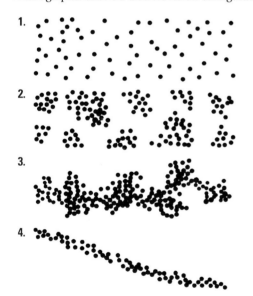

1.
2.
3.
4.

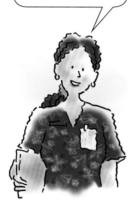

Read that note again. Which word jumps out at you?

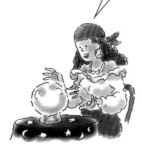

Hooray! You've finished Part II. I see your future success in Part III.

68. **2.** Documentation reveals that the client is anxious about her symptoms. These symptoms (asymmetry, variable color, and border irregularity) most closely resemble malignant melanoma. The nursing note contains no indication that the client currently has a lack of knowledge regarding the diagnosis or a misunderstanding of preventative measure. The characteristics of the lesion aren't consistent with basal or squamous cell carcinoma or a benign nevus. There is no indication that the client has squamous cell carcinoma. or has any risk of skin breakdown.

CN: Physiological integrity; CNS: Physiological adaptation; CL: Analyze

69. **1.** In a discrete pattern, individual lesions are separate and distinct. Graphic two shows a grouped pattern, in which lesions are clustered together. Graphic three shows a confluent pattern. In this configuration, lesions merge so that individual lesions aren't visible or palpable. Graphic four shows a linear pattern, in which lesions form a line.

CN: Physiological integrity; CNS: Physiological adaptation; CL: Analyze

Part III

Care of the Psychiatric Client

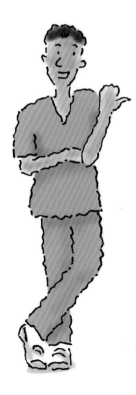

Chapter 12

Essentials of Psychiatric Care

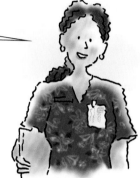

Before you take the tests relating to psychiatric care, take this test relating to tests (and treatments, too) in psychiatric care.

1. The preceptor is teaching a graduate nurse about electroconvulsive therapy (ECT). The preceptor determines that teaching has been effective when the graduate nurse states that ECT is commonly used for clients with:
1. major depression.
2. antisocial personality disorder.
3. schizophrenia.
4. somatoform disorders.

1. 1. ECT is commonly used for the treatment of major depression in clients who have not responded to antidepressants, or who have medical problems that contraindicate the use of antidepressants. ECT is uncommon for the treatment of personality disorders, chronic schizophrenia or somatoform disorders.
CN: Psychosocial integrity; CNS: None; CL: Apply

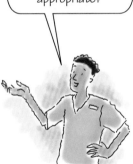

All of these options might be acceptable, but which is most appropriate?

2. A client diagnosed with bipolar disorder becomes verbally aggressive during group therapy. The client states, "I hate all of you." Which response by the nurse is **best**?
1. "You are behaving in an unacceptable manner."
2. "If you continue to talk like that, I will dismiss you from the group."
3. "Other people are not comfortable with your statement. Please, stop it."
4. "You are frightening people. We will walk down the hall to release some energy."

2. 4. This response indicates that the behavior is unacceptable, and that the client deserves help. The other responses are nontherapeutic and accusatory.
CN: Safe, effective care environment; CNS: Management of care; CL: Apply

3. A client has just met the nursing staff and is expressing hostility. The nurse should interpret this behavior as:
1. intellectualization.
2. transference.
3. triangulation.
4. splitting.

3. 2. Transference is the unconscious assignment of negative or positive feelings evoked by a significant person in the client's past to another person. Intellectualization is a defense mechanism in which the client avoids dealing with emotions by focusing on facts. Triangulation refers to conflicts involving three family members. Splitting is a defense mechanism commonly seen in clients with personality disorders, in which the world is perceived as all good or all bad.
CN: Psychosocial integrity; CNS: None; CL: Analyze

CN: Client needs category   CNS: Client needs subcategory   CL: Cognitive level

4. The nurse is aware that cognitive-behavioral therapy is most appropriate for a client experiencing low self-esteem. Which intervention **best** facilitates this therapy?
1. Conditional positive regard
2. Analysis of free association of thoughts
3. Classical conditioning
4. Examination of negative thought patterns

5. A client in group therapy states, "I didn't think anyone else felt like I did as a child." The nurse interprets this statement as:
1. altruism.
2. universality.
3. catharsis.
4. existential factor.

6. The nurse is teaching a group of students about the benefits of using group psychotherapy. Which statement **best** describes the advantage of group psychotherapy?
1. "It decreases the focus on the individual."
2. "It fosters the health care provider–client relationship."
3. "It confronts individuals with their shortcomings."
4. "It fosters a new learning environment."

7. A client whose wife recently died in an automobile accident is being treated at an outpatient psychiatric clinic. Which treatment should the nurse anticipate to be **most** effective?
1. Electroconvulsive therapy
2. Group therapy
3. Hypnotherapy
4. Individual therapy

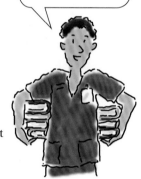

Let's see … interventions. Which one is best?

This question reminds me that I'm not alone in the universe.

4. 4. Cognitive-behavioral approaches examine the validity of habitual patterns of negative thinking and belief systems that influence feelings and behaviors. In Conditional positive regard, people are valued only when they live up to certain conditions assigned by others. Analysis of free associations is characteristic of Freudian psychoanalysis. Classical conditioning is characteristic of a pure behavioral intervention.
CN: Psychosocial integrity; CNS: None; CL: Apply

5. 2. One of the 11 curative factors of group therapy identified by Irvin D. Yalom, a contemporary psychiatrist and educator is universality, which assists participants in recognizing common experiences and responses. This action helps reduce anxiety, and allows other members to provide support and understanding. Altruism, catharsis, and existential factors are other curative factors Yalom described, but they don't describe this particular statement. Altruism refers to finding meaning through helping others. Catharsis is an open expression of previously suppressed feelings. Existential factors describe the recognition that a person has control over the quality of their life.
CN: Psychosocial integrity; CNS: None; CL: Apply

6. 4. In a group, the individual has an opportunity to learn that others experience problems and needs similar to their own. The group can also provide an arena in which individuals can relate to others in new ways. Decreasing focus on the individual is not a key advantage in group psychotherapy. Groups do not, by themselves, foster the health care provider–client relationship, and are not always used to confront individuals.
CN: Psychosocial integrity; CNS: None; CL: Analyze

7. 2. The client's history suggests that he is experiencing complicated mourning. Group therapy is most effective with this condition. Electroconvulsive therapy is effective in treating depression. Hypnotherapy is not indicated for the treatment of grief and bereavement.
CN: Psychosocial integrity; CNS: None; CL: Apply

8. An adolescent client verbalizes to the nurse that he is fat and ugly and states, "Everybody makes fun of me." How does the nurse interpret this statement?
1. Fear of the unknown
2. Fear of losing respect
3. Anxiety related to guilt
4. Anxiety related to body image

9. The nurse assesses a client who recently lost his spouse. The nurse determines that this client is experiencing a normal grief response when he:
1. abuses drugs or alcohol.
2. becomes an overachiever.
3. demonstrates hyperactivity.
4. displays lack of warmth toward others.

10. The nurse observes two clients playing basketball during exercise activity. The clients are engaged in aggressive communication and begin to fight. Which nursing intervention is **most** appropriate?
1. Remove the clients to separate areas and set limits
2. Remind each client that fighting is not allowed
3. Demonstrate how they should play basketball
4. Obtain an order to place both clients in seclusion

11. A client has been prescribed sertraline. Which adverse effects are **most** important for the nurse to communicate to this client? Select all that apply.
1. Agitation
2. Agranulocytosis
3. Sleep disturbance
4. Intermittent tachycardia
5. Dry mouth
6. Seizures

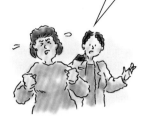

In psychiatric care, the nurse needs to recognize clues.

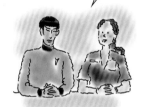

Your reaction is a normal part of the grief response.

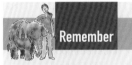

Remember

"Sertraline intervenes in depression."

A selective serotonin reuptake inhibitor (SSRI), sertraline treats depression. It also treats the following:
• Generalized anxiety disorder
• Major depressive disorder
• Obsessive-compulsive disorder
• Panic disorder
• Post-traumatic stress disorder
• Premenstrual dysphoric disorder
• Social anxiety disorder

8. **4.** Anxiety about body image and changes in physical appearance are a common fear for adolescents. Fear of the unknown is associated with toddlerhood. The fear of losing respect, and anxiety related to guilt, are associated with the developmental phase of school-aged children.
CN: Psychosocial integrity; CNS: None; CL: Apply

9. **4.** Hostile reactions, such as the loss of warmth when interacting with others, occurs during normal grieving. Chemical use, overachieving, and hyperactivity commonly occur with complicated grieving.
CN: Psychosocial integrity; CNS: None; CL: Apply

10. **1.** Setting limits and removing the clients from the situation are the best ways to handle aggression. Reminders of appropriate behavior are not likely to be effective. Seclusion and restraints are reserved for more serious situations. It is inappropriate for the nurse to provide a demonstration at this time.
CN: Psychosocial integrity; CNS: None; CL: Apply

11. **1, 3, 5.** Common adverse effects of sertraline include agitation, sleep disturbance and dry mouth. Agranulocytosis, intermittent tachycardia and seizures are adverse effects of clozapine.
CN: Physiological integrity; CNS: Pharmacological and parenteral therapies; CL: Apply

CN: Client needs category   CNS: Client needs subcategory   CL: Cognitive level

12. The nurse is preparing discharge instructions for a client with bipolar disorder who has been prescribed lithium. Which information is **most** important for the nurse to provide to this client? Select all that apply.

1. The potential for addiction
2. The signs and symptoms of drug toxicity
3. The risk for tardive dyskinesia
4. The restrictions of a low-tyramine diet
5. The need to consistently monitor blood levels
6. The expected time frame for improvements in mood

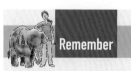

Remember

"Lithium licks bipolar disorder."

In bipolar disorder, mania, caused by excessive stimulation of catecholamines, alternates with depression, caused by decreased catecholamine stimulation. Lithium treats the manic phases of bipolar disorder.

12. **2, 5, 6.** Client education should cover the signs and symptoms of drug toxicity, as well as the need to report them to the health care provider. The importance of monitoring lithium levels on a regular basis to avoid toxicity should be included. The nurse should explain that seven to 21 days may pass before a change in mood is noticed. Lithium does not have addictive properties. Tardive dyskinesia is not associated with lithium. Tyramines in the diet are a potential concern for clients taking monoamine oxidase inhibitors.

CN: Physiological integrity; CNS: Pharmacological and parenteral therapies; CL: Apply

13. A nurse is administering haloperidol to a client experiencing psychosis. What are the **most** appropriate nursing interventions to manage potential adverse effects? Select all that apply.

1. Review subcutaneous drug administration with the client
2. Monitor vital signs, especially temperature
3. Provide the client an opportunity to pace
4. Monitor blood glucose levels
5. Provide the client with hard candy
6. Monitor for urticaria

13. **2, 3, 5.** Neuroleptic malignant syndrome is a life-threatening adverse effect of haloperidol. It is characterized by a rapid increase in body temperature. Extrapyramidal effects, such as akathisia, are also common. Pacing provides an outlet for the symptoms of akathisia. Haloperidol, and the anticholinergic medications provided to alleviate extrapyramidal effects, can cause dry mouth. Hard candy can increase salivation which moistens the mouth. Haloperidol is not given subcutaneously, and does not affect blood glucose levels. Urticaria is an uncommon side effect of haloperidol.

CN: Physiological integrity; CNS: Pharmacological and parenteral therapies; CL: Analyze

14. A nurse is caring for an adolescent whose best friend died in a car accident. The driver of the vehicle was under the influence of alcohol. The adolescent says, "It can't be possible. It's not true." Which stage of grief is the adolescent experiencing according to Kübler-Ross?

1. Denial
2. Anger
3. Bargaining
4. Acceptance

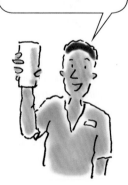

Here's to you! You've just zipped through another important NCLEX topic.

14. **1.** During the denial phase an individual has difficulty believing that a loss has occurred. This client's statements do not reflect the stages of anger, bargaining, or acceptance.

CN: Psychosocial integrity; CNS: None; CL: Apply

Chapter 13

Somatic Symptom & Related Disorders

Can't remember much about a particular somatic symptom disorder? Medline Plus can help. Type this address into your Web browser: **www.nlm.nih.gov/medlineplus**. Then search for the disorder.

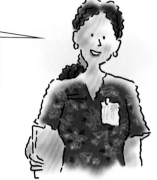

1. The nurse is teaching a student nurse about somatoform disorders. Which statement **most** accurately describes an individual with a somatoform disorder?
1. Physical symptoms have no organic cause
2. Should attend brief, intense, short-term psychotherapy sessions
3. Considered to have somatic symptom disorder
4. Become frustrated about the inability to find a source of symptoms

2. The nurse is preparing a teaching plan for the family of a loved one diagnosed with somatoform disorder. Teaching has been effective if the family describes somatoform disorder as:
1. limited to a single organ system.
2. a disorder that only occurs after a recent physical illness.
3. one with an organic pathologic cause.
4. one that occurs in the absence of an organic finding.

3. A nurse and nursing student are caring for a client with somatoform disorder. The student tells the nurse that associated physical symptoms occur because the client is delusional. What is the nurse's **best** response?
1. "Physical symptoms are associated with psychological symptoms."
2. "Help me to understand more about your rationale."
3. "We will review the symptoms of delusional disorders."
4. "Tell me more about the symptoms of somatoform disorder."

1. 1. A client with a somatization disorder has a history of multiple physiologic symptoms without associated organic pathologic causes. The etiology of this disease takes priority over a focus on the physical symptoms. These clients are frequently very patient and unconcerned with the persistence of the symptoms. If psychotherapy is prescribed, it would not be brief, intense, or short term.
CN: Health promotion and maintenance; CNS: None;
CL: Apply

2. 4. The essential feature of somatoform disorder is that the report of multiple physical symptoms over an extended period can have no organic etiology. Symptoms are not limited to one organ or system. There is no relationship to other physical illnesses.
CN: Psychosocial integrity; CNS: None; CL: Apply

3. 2. The nurse should respond using therapeutic language to encourage dialogue. The correct response includes the rationale, which will help the nurse understand the student's reasoning. Giving a short response about physical symptoms is not helpful. Reviewing the symptoms is too vague, and does not help the nurse detect faulty thinking.
CN: Psychosocial integrity; CNS: None; CL: Analyze

CN: Client needs category   CNS: Client needs subcategory   CL: Cognitive level

4. A nurse is caring for a client with somatization disorder. The client demonstrates an ego defense mechanism. Which finding supports the nurse's observations?
  1. Repression of anger
  2. Suppression of grief
  3. Denial of depression
  4. Preoccupation with pain

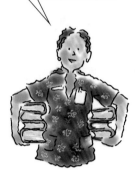

Remember, you're looking for a defense mechanism.

4. 1. One psychodynamic theory states that somatization transforms the aggressive and hostile feelings a client has toward others into physical complaints. Repressed anger originating from past disappointments and unfilled needs for nurturing and caring are expressed by soliciting other people's concern and rejecting them as ineffective. Denial, suppression, and preoccupation are not defense mechanisms underlying the dynamics of somatization disorder.
CN: Psychosocial integrity; CNS: None; CL: Apply

5. The nurse is caring for an 86-year-old client in an extended care facility. The client is anxious most of the time, and frequently reports vague symptoms that interfere with his ability to eat. With which disorder are these symptoms associated?
  1. Functional neurological symptom disorder
  2. Somatic symptom disorder
  3. Generalized anxiety disorder
  4. Sublimation defense mechanisms

5. 2. Reports of vague physical symptoms that have no apparent medical causes are characteristic of clients with somatic symptom disorder. In many cases, the gastrointestinal system is affected. Functional neurological symptom disorders are characterized by one or more neurological symptom. The client's symptoms do not suggest unusual anxiety. A client who displays the defense mechanism of sublimation channels maladaptive feelings or impulses into socially acceptable behavior.
CN: Psychosocial integrity; CNS: None; CL: Analyze

6. The nurse is preparing a care plan for a client experiencing somatic symptom disorder. What is the **most** appropriate intervention for this client?
  1. Initiate a special watch to monitor for injury
  2. Assist the client to process his sense of loss and grief
  3. Develop interventions to address situational low self-esteem related to feelings of worthlessness
  4. Encourage the client to participate in activities to increase social skills

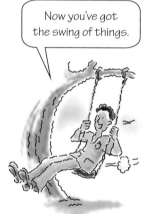

Now you've got the swing of things.

6. 3. Somatic symptom disorder is manifested by fear, situational low self-esteem, and feelings of worthlessness. Therapeutic interventions must be developed to address these symptoms. The risk for injury, grief resolution work, and impaired social skills have no direct correlation to the disorder.
CN: Safe, effective care environment; CNS: Management of care; CL: Apply

7. A college student frequently visits the campus health center with multiple vague reports of gastrointestinal symptoms before taking examinations. Physical causes have been eliminated, but the student continues to express a belief that she has a serious illness. How should the nurse interpret this student's symptoms?
  1. Functional neurological symptom disorder
  2. Depersonalization-derealization disorder
  3. Somatic symptom disorder
  4. Generalized anxiety disorder

7. 3. Somatic symptom disorder is shown by this client's belief that she has a serious illness, though pathologic causes have been eliminated. The disturbance usually lasts at least six months, and the gastrointestinal system is commonly affected. Exacerbations are usually associated with identifiable life stressors such as course examinations. Functional neurological symptom disorders are characterized by one or more neurological symptom. Depersonalization-derealization disorder refers to persistent, recurrent episodes of feeling detached from one's self or body. Anxiety disorders generally have stages that may not be associated with somatic symptom disorder.
CN: Psychosocial integrity; CNS: None; CL: Analyze

8. What is a **priority** nursing goal for a client diagnosed with somatic symptom disorder?
1. Determine the cause of the sleep disturbance
2. Relieve the fear of a serious illness
3. Recover the lost or altered function
4. Improve low self-esteem

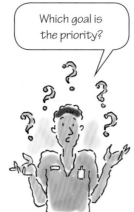

Which goal is the priority?

8. 2. Relieving fear is the priority nursing goal for somatic symptom disorder. For insomnia, the goal is focused on determining the cause of the sleep disturbance. The nursing goal for a functional neurological symptom disorder would focus on the recovery of lost or altered function. An appropriate goal for body dysmorphic disorder focuses on positive reinforcement related to physical appearance.
CN: Psychosocial integrity; CNS: None; CL: Apply

9. A client with somatic symptom disorder is seen in the outpatient clinic. Which intervention should the nurse implement?
1. Assess prior coping strategies and teach new adaptive skills
2. Help the client eliminate, rather than reduce, stress in her life
3. Inform the client that it's all in her head
4. Encourage the client to focus on physical symptoms

9. 1. Because of weak ego strength, a client with somatic symptom disorder is unable to use coping mechanisms effectively. Assessing prior coping strategies is essential prior to teaching new adaptive skills. It is not realistic to eliminate all stress. A client should never be told something is all in her head. This would not facilitate a long-term therapeutic relationship. It is necessary to offer reassurance that no physical disease is present. Focusing on physical symptoms is counterproductive to treatment.
CN: Health promotion and maintenance; CNS: None; CL: Apply

10. After repeated office visits and diagnostic tests for assorted medical symptoms, a client is referred to a psychiatrist. The client states, "I cannot imagine why I should see a psychiatrist." Which statements would explain this client's comment? Select all that apply.
1. Psychiatrists are only for mentally ill people
2. There is no correlation between physical symptoms and stress
3. Health care provider is unable to figure out what's wrong
4. Health care provider no longer wants me as a client
5. Psychiatric treatment can resolve physical symptoms

10. 1, 2, 3. The preoccupation in somatic symptom disorder is related to bodily functions or physical sensations. Repeated physical examinations, diagnostic tests, and reassurance from the health care provider won't allay the clients concerns about physiologic disease. Many clients falsely believe that there is no relationship between psychological and physiologic issues, and many don't understand the benefit of psychiatric care for medical illnesses. The client may believe that his health care provider has misdiagnosed him. Unless paranoid thinking is present, it is unlikely that the client would believe that his health care provider no longer wishes to treat him. This client most likely does not believe that psychiatric treatments can influence or resolve physical symptoms.
CN: Psychosocial integrity; CNS: None; CL: Analyze

11. Which therapeutic modality would be used to treat an individual diagnosed with somatic symptom disorder?
1. Suicide precautions
2. Relaxation exercises
3. Electroconvulsive therapy (ECT)
4. Aversion therapy

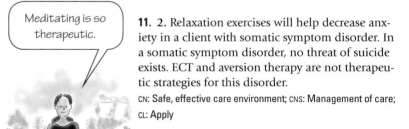

Meditating is so therapeutic.

11. 2. Relaxation exercises will help decrease anxiety in a client with somatic symptom disorder. In a somatic symptom disorder, no threat of suicide exists. ECT and aversion therapy are not therapeutic strategies for this disorder.
CN: Safe, effective care environment; CNS: Management of care; CL: Apply

12. A new medication has been prescribed for a client with a sleep disorder. The nurse is teaching the precautions associated with this type of medication. The nurse determines that teaching has been successful when the client states:
1. "I must avoid drinking alcohol while taking this medication."
2. "I can double the dose if I feel I need more."
3. "I will need to take this medication for a long time."
4. "It is acceptable to smoke while I take this medication."

12. 1. Alcohol is contraindicated when most prescribed medications, but especially with sedating medications. Sedation may be magnified by the use of alcohol. These medications include those prescribed for hypnotic sleep or antidepressants and antipsychotics that may also cause sedation. It is especially risky to increase the dosage of sedating medications without first consulting your provider. Sedative-hypnotic medications should only be used for a limited time because of the risk of dependence. Smoking reduces drug effectiveness.
CN: Physiological integrity; CNS: Pharmacological and parenteral therapies; CL: Analyze

13. A nurse is developing a teaching plan for sleep hygiene. Which interventions should the nurse include? Select all that apply.
1. Keep the room very warm
2. Eat a large meal and drink fluids before bedtime
3. Schedule bedtime when you feel tired
4. Avoid caffeine, alcohol, and nicotine before bedtime
5. Prepare the room for sleep and turn off distracting noise
6. Participate in a bedtime routine

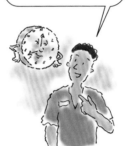

Looks like it's almost bedtime. How can we ensure a good night's sleep?

13. 4, 5, 6. Caffeine, alcohol, and substances such as nicotine act as stimulants, avoiding them should help promote sleep. Maintaining a cool temperature in the room will facilitate optimal sleep. Excessive fullness or hunger can disrupt or interfere with sleep. A regular sleep-wake time facilitates physiologic patterns, rather than waiting until an individual begins to feel tired. The room should be conducive to sleep. Eliminate distractions such as a television or radio. Participation in a relaxation, prayer, or meditation routine can help prepare an individual for a restful night.
CN: Health promotion and maintenance; CNS: None; CL: Apply

14. A nurse is interviewing a client newly admitted to the unit. The client falls asleep while reporting the list of his medications. Which disorder is this client most likely exhibiting?
1. Hypersomnolence disorder
2. Insomnia disorder
3. Narcolepsy
4. Parasomnias

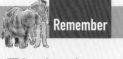

Remember

"Triazolam slams insomnia."

Triazolam is a benzodiazepine that is used as a short-term treatment of insomnia.

14. 3. Narcolepsy is also known as sleep attacks. Hypersomnolence disorder refers to excessive sleepiness, or seeking excessive amounts of sleep. An individual has difficulty initiating or maintaining sleep with insomnia disorder. Parasomnias refer to unusual or undesired behavior that occurs during sleep, such as nightmares, night terrors, or sleepwalking.
CN: Physiological integrity; CNS: Physiological adaptation; CL: Analyze

15. During group therapy a client states, "I just can't seem to sleep in this place." What is the nurse's **best** response?
1. Television, music, or a sound machine can block distractions at night
2. Psychopharmacology is one way to treat a variety of sleep difficulties
3. Group therapy is helpful to manage stress and feelings
4. Psychotherapy is required to improve disturbed sleep

15. 2. Biofeedback, relaxation therapy, and psychopharmacology are appropriate treatments for sleep disorders. While television, music, and sound machines can provide background distractions and white noise, they can be very disruptive to sleep. Cell phones and computers in the bedroom can disrupt sleep hygiene. Behavior therapy, group therapy, and insight-oriented psychotherapy are treatments related to somatoform disorders.
CN: Physiological integrity; CNS: Basic care and comfort; CL: Apply

16. A client with depression is experiencing symptoms of insomnia. What is the **most** appropriate nursing intervention?
  1. Ask the health care provider to prescribe a bedtime sleep medication
  2. Invite the client to sit at the nurses' station to chat
  3. Allow the client to watch television until he is sleepy
  4. Encourage the client to take a warm bath before retiring

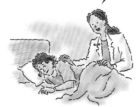

Hope you enjoyed your warm bath. It should help you sleep better.

16. 4. Sleep-inducing activities, such as a warm bath, help promote relaxation and sleep. Although consulting the health care provider about prescribing a bedtime sleep medication is possible, it would not be the best nursing intervention for this client. Encouraging the client to watch television or sit at the nurses' station may provide too much stimulation, and would not necessarily promote sleep.
CN: Physiological integrity; CNS: Basic care and comfort; CL: Apply

17. The nurse is observing an individual who is sleeping, and determines the client is in rapid eye movement (REM) sleep when he has:
  1. restless legs with frequent night cramps.
  2. jerky limb movements and position changes.
  3. decreased physiologic activity and a slowed pulse rate.
  4. increased physiologic activity levels, rapid eye movements.

17. 4. Highly active brain and physiologic activity levels characterize the REM stage of sleep. During REM sleep, body movement, except eyes, ceases. The pulse rate slows during non-REM sleep. Restless legs and night leg cramps are unrelated to sleep stage.
CN: Physiological integrity; CNS: Physiological adaptation; CL: Analyze

18. A client with sleep terror disorder might have autonomic signs of intense anxiety. What is the nurse's **priority** assessment for this client?
  1. Tachycardia
  2. Pupil constriction
  3. Cool, clammy skin
  4. Decreased muscle tone

18. 1. Autonomic arousal includes tachycardia, which should be closely monitored by the nurse to prevent the occurrence of further complications such as arrhythmia. Sweating, increased muscle tone, and pupillary dilation are responses that may also occur, but aren't considered a priority.
CN: Physiological integrity; CNS: Physiological adaptation; CL: Apply

19. Which considerations are important in planning the care for individuals experiencing sleep deprivation? Select all that apply.
  1. Sleep is influenced by biological rhythms.
  2. The natural body clock follows a 24-hour cycle.
  3. Long sleepers have more rapid eye movement (REM) periods.
  4. Sleep deprivation can result in alterations in mental status.
  5. Sleep is of one quality, whether day or night, naps or single session.

19. 1, 2, 4. All sleep is not equal. Uninterrupted sleep as well as the quality of sleep is an important nursing consideration in planning care. Sleep is influenced by biological rhythms and the natural body clock, which follows a 24-hour cycle. Both of these can be quite problematic and disrupt sleep. Sleep deprivation can lead to hallucinations and delusions. Environment encompasses shift workers, young mothers, and traffic among other things, and plays a tremendous role in sleep hygiene. Genetics also play a role in sleep deprivation. Assessment of REM does not contribute to treatment of sleep deprivation. During sleep, we usually pass through five phases of sleep: stages 1, 2, 3, 4, and REM (rapid eye movement) sleep. These stages progress in a cycle from stage 1 to REM sleep, then the cycle starts over again with stage 1. Almost 50% of our total sleep time in stage 2 sleep, about 20% in REM sleep, and the remaining 30% in the other stages.
CN: Physiological integrity; CNS: Physiological adaptation; CL: Apply

20. A nurse is providing instruction to a 38-year-old male client undergoing treatment for anxiety and insomnia. The practitioner has prescribed lorazepam 1 mg/po/tid. The nurse determines that teaching has been effective when the client states:
1. "I'll avoid coffee."
2. "I can drink red wine."
3. "I'll avoid sunlight."
4. "I must eat enough salt."

21. A client diagnosed with a sleep disorder suddenly awakens with a piercing scream. With which condition is this behavior **most** often seen?
1. Hypersomnolence disorder
2. Nightmare disorder
3. Sleep terror disorder
4. Sleepwalking

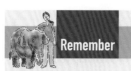

Remember

"No caffeine on benzodiazepines."

Caffeine should be avoided by clients taking benzodiazepines, which are used to treat anxiety and insomnia, because it is a stimulant and increases anxiety.

20. 1. Lorazepam is a benzodiazepine used to treat various forms of anxiety and insomnia. Caffeine is contraindicated because it is a stimulant and increases anxiety. A client taking lorazepam should avoid alcoholic beverages. Clients taking certain antipsychotic medications should avoid sunlight. Salt intake has no effect on lorazepam.
CN: Physiological integrity; CNS: Pharmacological and parenteral therapies; CL: Analyze

21. 3. Sleep terror disorder refers to an abrupt arousal from sleep with a piercing scream or cry. Nightmares are frightening dreams that wake the client, and are severe enough to interfere with social or occupational functioning. Nightmares can also cause screaming during sleep, or upon awakening, but not as frequently as with sleep terror disorder. Hypersomnia is excessive sleepiness or seeking excessive amounts of sleep. Sleepwalking refers to motor activity initiated during sleep in which the individual leaves the bed and walks around.
CN: Psychosocial integrity; CNS: None; CL: Analyze

22. Which complications are the client with a sleep disorder at risk of developing? Select all that apply.
1. Lowered resistance to illness
2. Increased potential for injury
3. Reduced ability to concentrate
4. Disturbed sensory perception
5. Isolation from social activities

22. 1, 2, 3, 5. A client with a sleep disorder may be at risk for injury due to drowsiness and decreased concentration. The client may experience difficulty socializing due to disorganized thinking because of disrupted sleep patterns. Sleep deprivation can lead to reduced immune defense against physical illness and accidents. Sleep deprivation can also result in cognitive distortions such as hallucinations.
CN: Safe, effective care environment; CNS: Management of care; CL: Analyze

23. An individual is experiencing a functional neurologic symptom disorder presenting as paralysis of the legs. What information is important for the nurse to discuss with the client?
1. "Describe how this paralysis has hindered your lifestyle."
2. "Tell me what you understand about the diagnostic test results."
3. "Please show me how much you can move each of your legs."
4. "Explain how you plan to manage when you return home."

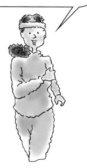

You've made it through 23 questions. You're almost there.

23. 4. The paralysis serves as the client's inappropriate way of expressing unmet psychologic needs. The nurse should avoid talking about the paralysis to shift the client's attention to the secondary gains of the disorder. Patients achieve secondary gain by avoiding activities that are particularly offensive to them, thereby gaining support from family and friends, which otherwise may not be offered The other options focus on the paralysis, which does not allow the client to recognize his underlying psychological motivation.
CN: Psychological integrity; CNS: None; CL: Apply

24. Which statement **best** describes functional neurologic symptom disorders?
  1. The physical symptoms can be controlled.
  2. The psychological conflicts are repressed.
  3. The client is aware of psychologic conflicts.
  4. The client should not be confronted.

24. 2. In functional neurological symptom disorders, physical symptoms are manifestations of a repressed psychological conflict. The client is unable to control or produce symptoms, and is unaware of the psychological conflict. Understanding the principles and conflicts behind the symptoms can provide insight during a client's therapy.
CN: Psychosocial integrity; CNS: None; CL: Analyze

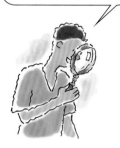

In question 25, you should focus on what exacerbates the client's symptoms.

25. A client is admitted for the abrupt onset of paralysis in his left arm. Although no physiologic causes have been found, the symptoms are exacerbated when he speaks of losing custody of his children in a recent divorce. Which disorder is characterized by these symptoms?
  1. Body dysmorphic disorder
  2. Functional neurologic symptom disorder
  3. Delusional disorder
  4. Malicious malingering

25. 2. Functional neurologic symptom disorders are characterized by neurologic symptoms associated with psychological conflict which is exacerbated by multiple stressors. Body dysmorphic disorder is an imagined belief that there is a defect in the appearance of the body. The client does not exhibit a delusion which is the sole manifestation of a delusional disorder. Malingering is the intentional production of symptoms to avoid obligations or obtain rewards.
CN: Psychosocial integrity; CNS: None; CL: Analyze

26. A client has been hospitalized with a diagnosis of functional neurologic symptom disorder blindness, and displays a lack of concern about this diagnosis. Which statement **best** describes the client's reaction?
  1. The client is suppressing feelings.
  2. The client's anxiety is relieved through physical symptoms.
  3. The client is acting indifferent.
  4. The client is not anxious because her basic needs have been met.

26. 2. Functional neurologic symptom disorder reduces anxiety by manifesting physical symptoms symbolically linked to an underlying conflict. This, in part, explains this client's indifference about a serious symptom such as blindness. The client is not aware of her internal conflict. Hospitalization does not remove the source of the conflict.
CN: Psychosocial integrity; CNS: None; CL: Analyze

27. A client with somatic symptom disorder reports new pain in his right side. The nurse should reply by saying:
  1. "It's time for group therapy now. You shouldn't miss this session."
  2. "Tell me about your new pain. You will miss group therapy today."
  3. "I'll contact your health care provider, but you must leave now to be on time for group."
  4. "I'll call your health care provider to ask him to order pain medication. You should rest now."

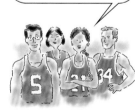

Interdisciplinary care makes sure all staff works as a team!

27. 3. The amount of time spent discussing physical symptoms should be decreased. Lack of positive reinforcement may help stop the maladaptive behavior. However, avoiding the statement altogether demeans the client and does not address the underlying problem. Asking the client to further explain the pain emphasizes physical symptoms, and prevents this client from attending group therapy. All physical complaints need to be evaluated for physiologic causes.
CN: Safe, effective care environment; CNS: Management of care; CL: Apply

28. What nursing intervention can assist a client with functional neurologic symptom disorder blindness with meals?

1. Direct the client to independently locate items on the tray and feed himself
2. Address the needs of other clients in the dining room and feed this client last
3. Establish a buddy system with other clients who can feed the client at each meal
4. Expect the client to feed himself after explaining the location of food on the tray

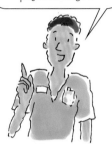

A client with a disorder of psychologic origin may need the same interventions as one with a disorder of physical origin.

28. 4. The nurse should provide direction and allow this client to maintain some level of independence by feeding himself. Feeding the client leads to dependence. It is inappropriate to expect other clients to feed this client, or for this client to feed himself without some direction.
CN: Physiological integrity; CNS: Basic care and comfort; CL: Apply

29. A client diagnosed with functional neurologic symptom disorder is experiencing left-sided paralysis. The client tells the nurse that he received a lot of attention in the hospital, and that it's unfortunate others outside the hospital don't understand him. Which is the nurse's **best** response?

1. "How difficult that must be for you."
2. "How much help do you receive at home?"
3. "Describe a typical day at home."
4. "I'm glad that you are comfortable here."

29. 3. This client cannot express his internal conflicts in appropriate ways. Asking him to describe a typical day at home will help reveal social isolation as a likely factor in this disorder. Observing how difficult circumstances are could encourage this client to focus on the disorder. Asking directly how much help he receives at home also places the focus back on the disorder. Answer four dismisses the client's concern.
CN: Psychosocial integrity; CNS: None; CL: Apply

30. Which nursing intervention would **best** increase the self-esteem of a client with functional neurologic symptom disorder?

1. Focus attention on the client as a person rather than on the symptom
2. Discuss the client's childhood to link present behaviors with past traumas
3. Encourage the client to use avoidant-interactional patterns rather than assertive patterns
4. Assist the client in developing short-term goals

30. 1. Focusing on the client directs attention away from the symptom. This approach eventually reduces the client's need to gain attention through physical symptoms. Discussing the client's childhood has no correlation with self-esteem. Avoiding interactional situations does not foster self-esteem. Small goals ensure success and reinforce self-esteem.
CN: Safe, effective care environment; CNS: Management of care; CL: Apply

31. A nurse is teaching the family of a client with functional neurologic symptom disorder about signs and symptoms. Which sign or symptom is **most** important for the nurse to teach?

1. Expression of complex delusions
2. Feelings of deep depression or strong euphoria
3. A feeling of dread accompanied by physical symptoms
4. Neurologic symptoms related to psychological conflict or need

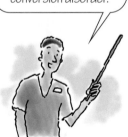

Don't be paralyzed with fear or blind to the client's needs when you teach about signs and symptoms of conversion disorder.

31. 4. Symptoms of functional neurologic symptom disorder are neurologic in nature. Delusional disorders are characterized by delusions. Mood disorders are characterized by abnormal feelings of depression or euphoria. Anxiety is characterized by a feeling of dread, with or without associated physical symptoms.
CN: Health promotion and maintenance; CNS: None; CL: Apply

32. A client with functional neurologic symptom disorder reports having a lack of energy and little interaction with friends. How should the nurse respond?
  1. "How would you describe your health?"
  2. "Are you getting enough sleep?"
  3. "How stressful is your life?"
  4. "Do you maintain a healthy diet?"

32. **3.** When clients focus their mental and physical energy on somatic symptoms, they have little energy to expend on social or diversional activities. It would be most helpful to understand the presence and extent of life stressors for this client. Although the other questions reflect concerns common with functional neurological symptom disorder, the information given in the question doesn't support them.
CN: Psychosocial integrity; CNS: None; CL: Apply

33. A client is diagnosed with functional neurologic symptom disorder. The client reports overwhelmingly stressful family conflicts. Which discharge planning goal should the nurse include for this client?
  1. Resume former roles and routine tasks
  2. Assume roles of other family members
  3. Depend on family members to meet all client needs
  4. Focus attention on problems occurring in the family

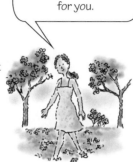

Looks like this test is a walk in the park for you.

33. **1.** The client who uses somatization has adopted a sick role in the family, typically characterized by dependence. Increasing independence and resuming former roles is necessary to change this pattern. The client should not be expected to take on the roles or responsibilities of other family members. It is not therapeutic for this client to depend on, or allow family members to meet all of his needs. Focusing attention and energy on problems occurring in the family does not support the client or his recovery.
CN: Health Promotion and Maintenance; CNS: None; CL: Apply

34. A new client admitted to a psychiatric unit is diagnosed with functional neurologic symptom disorder. The client shows a lack of concern for his sudden paralysis, although his athletic abilities have always been a source of pride. The nurse understands that the client is demonstrating:
  1. acute dystonia.
  2. La belle indifference.
  3. malingering.
  4. secondary gain.

34. **2.** La belle indifference is a lack of concern about a present illness. Acute dystonia refers to muscle spasms. Malingering is the voluntary production of symptoms. Secondary gain refers to the unconscious benefits of an illness.
CN: Psychosocial integrity; CNS: None; CL: Apply

35. Which nursing intervention is the **most** appropriate for a client diagnosed with functional neurologic symptom disorder who has experienced pseudoseizures?
  1. Explain that the pseudoseizures are not a real seizure
  2. Promote dependence so that unfilled dependency needs are met
  3. Encourage the client to discuss his feelings about the pseudoseizures
  4. Promote independence and withdraw attention from the pseudoseizures

35. **4.** Successful performance of independent activities enhances self-esteem. Telling the client that the symptoms are imaginary may jeopardize the nurse-client relationship. Positive reinforcement encourages the use of maladaptive responses. The focus should not be on the disability because it may provide positive gains for the client.
CN: Psychosocial integrity; CNS: None; CL: Apply

36. A client is attempting to effectively cope with life stress without experiencing conversion disorder symptoms. Which therapeutic intervention should the nurse use to help this client reach this goal?

1. Focus on the symptoms to obtain necessary details
2. Ask for clarification and history of the symptoms
3. Listen to the client's symptoms in a nonjudgmental manner
4. Reinforce that symptoms are an escape from dealing with conflict

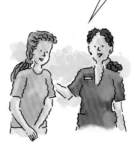

Focus on what the client is saying.

36. 3. Active listening in a nonjudgmental manner allows the nurse to engage the client in a therapeutic dialogue and redirect the focus away from the client's symptoms. The other interventions focus on the client's physical symptoms, not the underlying cause.

CN: Health promotion and maintenance; CNS: None; CL: Apply

37. The nurse teaches a client with a pain disorder a progressive relaxation exercise. The goal of stress management was attained when the client states:

1. "My arm hurts more than ever."
2. "Everyone here is so nice to me."
3. "I don't really understand why I'm here."
4. "My pain is better, and now I feel relaxed."

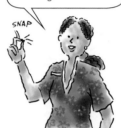

That's it! You got the right answer.

SNAP

37. 4. This statement demonstrates that the client is experiencing positive results from the relaxation exercise. All other responses alert the nurse that the client needs further interventions.

CN: Physiological integrity; CNS: Basic care and comfort; CL: Analyze

38. A nurse is discharging a client with somatic symptom disorder. What is the nurse's **priority** goal?

1. Reduce the sense of hopelessness
2. Increase self-esteem
3. Reduce the fear of illness
4. Prevent violence toward self and others

38. 3. A client with somatic symptom disorder has a preoccupying fear of having a serious disease. Although hopelessness may be present, it is not the primary focus. While all persons can benefit from a goal to increase self-esteem, this is not a priority goal for these clients. Clients with this disorder are not prone to violence toward themselves or others.

CN: Safe, effective care environment; CNS: Management of care; CL: Apply

39. A nurse is teaching the family of a client diagnosed with a somatoform pain disorder. Which statement by the nurse most accurately describes this disorder?

1. A preoccupation with pain in the absence of physical disease
2. A physical or somatic report without any demonstrable organic findings
3. A morbid fear or belief that one has a serious disease where none exists
4. One or more neurologic symptom associated with psychological conflict or need

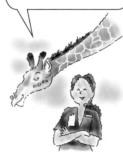

It's not a stretch to say you've come a long way on this test.

39. 1. Somatoform pain disorder is a preoccupation with pain in the absence of physical disease. A physical or somatic report refers to somatoform disorders in general. A morbid fear of serious illness is a somatic symptom disorder. Neurological symptoms are associated with functional neurologic symptom disorder.

CN: Psychosocial integrity; CNS: None; CL: Apply

CN: Client needs category   CNS: Client needs subcategory   CL: Cognitive level

40. The nurse is caring for a client with a pain disorder. The client is very secretive and reluctant to share pain-related information when asked what he thinks, does, or feels. Which defense mechanism is this client exhibiting?
1. Displacement
2. Rationalization
3. Regression
4. Substitution

40. 2. Rationalization is a process by which an individual deals with emotional conflict or stressors by concealing the true motivations for his thoughts, actions, and feelings. He accomplishes this by creating false explanations that are reassuring or self-serving. This process is not a usual defense mechanism related to pain disorders. Displacement, substitution, and regression are defense mechanisms that would be expected from a client with a pain disorder.
CN: Psychosocial integrity; CNS: None; CL: Apply

41. What is the **most** appropriate nursing goal for a client with a pain disorder?
1. Acknowledge reduced fear
2. Demonstrate increased independence
3. Report improvement in pain level
4. Adapt coping skills to manage stress

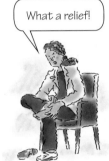

What a relief!

41. 3. Relief of pain is a priority for clients experiencing pain. Expression of less fear applies to a client with somatic symptom disorder. A focus on independence is appropriate for a client diagnosed with functional neurological symptom disorder. The development of coping strategies would be beneficial for a client with a somatization disorder.
CN: Physiological integrity; CNS: Physiological adaptation; CL: Apply

42. Which conditions or situations are most likely to result in difficulty sleeping? Select all that apply.
1. Shift work
2. Sleep apnea
3. Reduction of external stimuli
4. Caffeine intake in the evening
5. Consistent bedtime routine
6. Excessive worry or anxiety

42. 1, 2, 4, 6. Shift work can disrupt the circadian rhythm. Sleep apnea can cause a reduction in oxygen to the brain, which can reduce the quality of rest. Caffeine is a stimulant and, if taken too close to bedtime, can interfere with falling asleep. Excessive worry or anxiety causes an increase in adrenaline, which enhances alertness and reduces sleepiness. A consistent bedtime routine and reduction of external stimuli promote good sleep.
CN: Health promotion and maintenance; CNS: None; CL: Analyze

43. A nurse is working with a client with somatoform pain disorder who displays ineffective coping skills. Which goal is **most** realistic for this client?
1. To be free from injury
2. To recognize sensory impairment
3. To discuss beliefs about spiritual issues
4. To reduce the focus on physical symptoms

43. 4. Expression of feelings enables the client to vent emotions. This expression decreases anxiety and draws attention away from physical symptoms. This client is not experiencing a safety issue. There is no apparent correlation with any sensory-perceptual alterations. Spiritual issues are related to spiritual distress, and no evidence exists to support such distress.
CN: Physiological integrity; CNS: Basic care and comfort; CL: Analyze

CN: Client needs category   CNS: Client needs subcategory   CL: Cognitive level

44. Which client statement best meets the diagnostic criteria for a pain disorder?
1. "I cannot move my right leg."
2. "I have stomach and leg pain."
3. "I am afraid I have cancer."
4. "I have crushing chest and jaw pain."

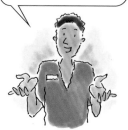

Remember, diagnostic criteria for psychologic problems come from the latest edition of the Diagnostic and Statistical Manual of Mental Disorders, currently known as DSM-5.

44. 2. The diagnostic criteria for a pain disorder states a client feels pain in one or more site and that the pain is severe enough to warrant clinical attention. A client with a functional neurologic symptom disorder can experience a motor neurological symptom such as paralysis. Somatic symptom disorder is a morbid fear or belief that one has a serious disease where none exists. Pain disorder is chronic pain experienced by a patient in one or more areas, and is thought to be caused by psychological stress. Unremitting chest pain with radiation to the jaw is symptomatic of a myocardial infarction and would be considered an acute situation

CN: Psychosocial integrity; CNS: None; CL: Apply

45. A client with somatoform pain disorder describes a chaotic home and work environment. Which nursing intervention is **most** appropriate?
1. Participate in relaxation techniques
2. Demonstrate conflict management skills
3. Engage in assertiveness role playing
4. Schedule daily family meetings

45. 2. A somatoform pain disorder is closely associated with the client's inability to handle stress and conflict. The client's home and work life is chaotic, making conflict management the correct priority. Since this client did not specifically identify stress, relaxation would not be the most appropriate choice. There is no need for assertiveness training or role playing. A family meeting may be indicated prior to discharge, but would be premature at this time.

CN: Safe, effective care environment; CNS: Management of care; CL: Apply

46. A newly admitted client is diagnosed with somatoform pain disorder. Which statement, by the nurse, would promote independence in self-care?
1. "I will call you for all the group activities."
2. "I will assist you each day with your care."
3. "The staff will help you with everything today."
4. "You should be pain-free before you participate in activities."

46. 3. Limited assistance will help this client develop independence. All other options would promote dependence on the staff. It is inappropriate to advise a client to remain inactive until they are pain-free.

CN: Safe, effective care environment; CNS: Management of care; CL: Apply

47. Which **initial** therapeutic intervention is appropriate for a client exhibiting ineffective coping to a pain disorder?
1. An accurate assessment
2. Encourage the expression of feelings
3. Promote insight into the pain disorder
4. Develop alternate coping strategies.

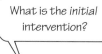

What is the initial intervention?

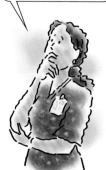

47. 1. It is essential to accurately assess the client before any interventions take place. Promoting the expression of feelings, development of insight, and helping the client to develop coping strategies are appropriate interventions that can be implemented after the initial assessment.

CN: Psychosocial integrity; CNS: None; CL: Apply

48. A client with a somatoform pain disorder may receive both primary and secondary gain from symptoms. Which statement **best** describes secondary gain?
1. It brings much needed stability to the client's family.
2. It decreases the preoccupation with the physical illness.
3. It enables the client to avoid some unpleasant activity.
4. It promotes emotional support or attention for the client.

48. 4. Secondary gain refers to the benefits of an illness that allow the client to receive emotional support or attention. An unstable family may disregard the real issue, although some conflict is relieved. Somatoform pain disorder is a preoccupation with pain in the absence of physical disease. Primary gain enables the client to avoid some unpleasant activity.

CN: Psychosocial integrity; CNS: None; CL: Analyze

49. Which nursing intervention is **most** appropriate for a client diagnosed with a somatoform pain disorder?
1. Reinforce behavior when it is not focused on pain
2. Encourage verbalization of anxieties related to body image
3. Validate expressed fears related to the illness
4. Support recovery of the lost or altered function of a body part

49. 1. Help the client get attention and see himself as valuable without using pain. Verbalization of anxieties related to body image may be beneficial in a client with body dysmorphic disorder. Fear of illness is related to somatic symptom disorder. The recovery of a lost or altered function of a body part is related to functional neurologic symptom disorder.

CN: Psychosocial integrity; CNS: None; CL: Apply

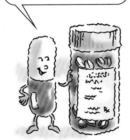

Remember to use the correct formula when calculating the appropriate drug dose.

50. A client has primary insomnia and requires pharmacological assistance to sleep. The health care provider prescribes secobarbital sodium 75 mg/po/hr. The nurse has secobarbital sodium 25 mg tablets on hand. How many tablets should the nurse administer to the client? Record your answer using a whole number.

_____ tablets

50. 3.
Each tablet contains 25 mg of the medication. The correct formula to calculate this drug dose is:

$$X = 75 \div 25$$
$$X = 3$$

CN: Physiological integrity; CNS: Pharmacological and parenteral therapies; CL: Analyze

51. A home health nurse is caring for a client diagnosed with a functional neurologic symptom disorder manifested by paralysis of the left arm. An organic cause for the deficit has not been found. Which nursing intervention is **most** appropriate for this client?
1. Perform all physical tasks for the client to maintain safety
2. Schedule an hour each day to discuss the paralysis and its cause
3. Identify primary or secondary gains that the physical symptom provides
4. Allow the client to withdraw from physical activities

51. 3. Primary or secondary gains should be identified because they're etiological factors used in problem resolution. The nurse should encourage the client to be as independent as possible, and should intervene only when the client requires assistance. The nurse should not focus on the disability. The nurse should encourage this client to perform physical activities to the greatest extent possible.

CN: Psychosocial integrity; CNS: None; CL: Apply

52. A client with somatoform disorder states that her frequent headaches result from a brain tumor. A tumor has not been detected on any of her diagnostic tests. The nurse interprets this client's form of somatization as which disorder?

1. Functional neurologic symptom disorder
2. Adjustment disorder
3. Somatic symptom disorder
4. Body dysmorphic disorder

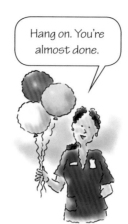

Hang on. You're almost done.

52. 3. A client with somatic symptom disorder, interprets a physical symptom as severe, or life threatening, and will worry incessantly about these symptoms. In functional neurologic symptom disorder, the client loses a motor or sensory function, but lacks appropriate concern about the loss. Adjustment disorder is not a type of somatization disorder. In body dysmorphic disorder, the client is preoccupied with a perceived defect in appearance.

CN: Psychosocial integrity; CNS: None; CL: Apply

53. A college student visited the health center almost daily during the second half of the semester, before course examinations. Physical causes for these visits have been eliminated. Based on the following progress note entry in the client's chart, which disorder should the nurse suspect?

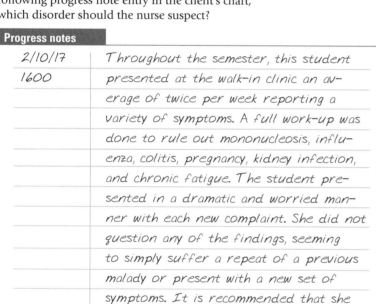

Progress notes	
2/10/17 1600	Throughout the semester, this student presented at the walk-in clinic an average of twice per week reporting a variety of symptoms. A full work-up was done to rule out mononucleosis, influenza, colitis, pregnancy, kidney infection, and chronic fatigue. The student presented in a dramatic and worried manner with each new complaint. She did not question any of the findings, seeming to simply suffer a repeat of a previous malady or present with a new set of symptoms. It is recommended that she have a consult to mental health services.

1. Functional neurologic symptom disorder
2. Depersonalization-derealization disorder
3. Somatic symptom disorder
4. Generalized anxiety disorder

53. 3. Somatic symptom disorder, in this case, is shown by the client's belief that she has a serious illness, although pathologic causes have been eliminated. The disturbance usually lasts at least six months, and the gastrointestinal system is commonly affected. Exacerbations are usually associated with identifiable life stressors, in this case the client's examinations. Functional neurologic symptom disorder is characterized by one or more neurologic symptom. Depersonalization-derealization disorder refers to persistent, recurrent episodes of feeling detached from one's self or body. Generalized anxiety disorder presents with persistent, overwhelming anxiety unrelated to life stressors.

CN: Psychosocial integrity; CNS: None; CL: Analyze

54. A 26-year-old client is diagnosed with somatoform disorder. How should the nurse instruct this client's wife to manage his symptoms?

1. Tell him that his symptoms are all in his head to force him to deal with reality
2. Remind him that his symptoms are an attempt to get attention, and reassure him that you'll be more attentive
3. Accept the reality of his symptoms as he presents them, and do not challenge his perception of those symptoms
4. Understand that your husband is creating these symptoms for a specific purpose

54. 3. For a client with somatoform disorder, caregivers should accept the symptoms and avoid disputing them. The symptoms are not contrived or all in the client's head. They are neither an attempt to get attention nor created on purpose.

CN: Psychosocial integrity; CNS: None; CL: Apply

55. A client, with a diagnosis of somatoform disorder, has been admitted to the psychiatric unit and has difficulty breathing, numbness, and loss of movement in his left arm. The client seems unusually calm and unconcerned about his symptoms. These symptoms are associated with:

1. functional neurological symptom disorder.
2. somatic symptom disorder.
3. body dysmorphic disorder.
4. somatic symptom disorder with predominant pain.

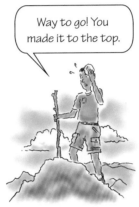

Way to go! You made it to the top.

55. 1. Functional neurologic symptom disorder is characterized by a loss of motor, sensory, or visceral functions accompanied by a client's indifference to the loss. In somatic symptom disorder, the client interprets a physical symptom as severe or life threatening, and worries about it excessively. Body dysmorphic disorder is a preoccupation with a perceived defect in appearance. In somatic symptom disorder with predominant pain, pain is the dominant physical symptom.

CN: Psychosocial integrity; CNS: None; CL: Apply

Chapter 14

Anxiety & Mood Disorders

Want more information on anxiety and mood disorders to help you prepare for the NCLEX? Check out the Web site of the National Alliance on Mental Illness at **www.nami.org**.

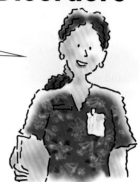

1. A client experiences periodic panic attacks. Which statement **best** reflects this client's experiences?
  1. "Yesterday, I sat up in bed and just felt so scared."
  2. "I have difficulty sleeping because I'm so anxious."
  3. "Sometimes, I have nausea that makes me feel dizzy."
  4. "When I drink beer, I fall asleep without any problems."

Listen carefully to how your client describes his or her symptoms.

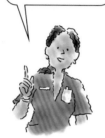

2. A client with generalized anxiety disorder states, "I'm worried about my health and afraid that someday I'm going to die from cancer." What is the nurse's **most** appropriate response?
  1. "We all live in fear of dying from cancer."
  2. "People think the worst and it usually doesn't happen."
  3. "You are healthy so don't worry yet."
  4. "Has something happened that is causing you to worry?"

3. A client with a history of panic attacks tells the nurse, "I feel so trapped right after an attack." The nurse determines that this client is **most** likely expressing loss of:
  1. control.
  2. identity.
  3. memory.
  4. maturity.

You're in control, so read the question carefully and choose the most likely response.

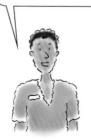

1. **3.** A person who has periodic panic attacks often experiences nausea and abdominal distress, accompanied by dizziness or lightheadedness. These symptoms can occur at various times and last for several minutes. The other responses refer to people who experience generalized anxiety disorder. They tend to worry excessively, become fearful and be unable to sleep. People with an anxiety disorder may use alcohol to self-medicate. CN: Psychosocial integrity; CNS: None; CL: Analyze

2. **4.** By inquiring about the source of the client's worry, the nurse can determine the cause of the anxiety. The other responses deflect and minimize the client's concerns. CN: Psychosocial integrity; CNS: None; CL: Analyze

3. **1.** People who fear loss of control during a panic attack commonly make statements about feeling trapped, getting hurt, or having little or no control over their situations. They don't tend to have a loss of identity or memory impairment, and don't regress or become immature. CN: Psychosocial integrity; CNS: None; CL: Apply

CN: Client needs category CNS: Client needs subcategory CL: Cognitive level

4. Alprazolam has been prescribed for a client who has been experiencing panic attacks. The nurse reviews the client's records and determines further intervention is needed when the health history includes:

1. intermittent insomnia.
2. acute-angle glaucoma.
3. seizure disorder.
4. tartrazine hypersensitivity.

4. 2. Acute-angle glaucoma is a medical problem that contraindicates the use of alprazolam. Alprazolam causes drowsiness and sedation, so the client should not experience insomnia. Seizure disorder isn't a contraindication for the use of alprazolam. Tartrazine hypersensitivity is associated with yellow dye used in some foods, and is not a contraindication for the use of alprazolam.

CN: Physiological integrity; CNS: Pharmacological and parenteral therapies; CL: Apply

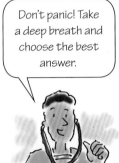

Don't panic! Take a deep breath and choose the best answer.

5. Which intervention is **most** important for the nurse to include in the plan of care for a client experiencing a panic attack?

1. Instruct the client to take deep breaths
2. Have the client talk about the anxiety
3. Encourage the client to verbalize feelings
4. Ask the client about the cause of the attack

5. 1. During a panic attack, the nurse should remain with the client and attempt to change the physiologic response with actions such as taking deep breaths. During an attack, the client is unable to talk about anxious situations, and isn't able to address feelings, especially uncomfortable feelings and frustrations. While having a panic attack, the client is focused on the symptoms, and won't be able to discuss the cause of the attack.

CN: Safe, effective care environment; CNS: Management of care; CL: Apply

6. The nurse is teaching a client and family about the management of panic attacks. What is the **most** important information for the nurse to include?

1. Identify when anxiety is escalating
2. Determine how to stop a panic attack
3. Address strategies to reduce physical pain
4. Prevent the client from depending on others

6. 1. By identifying the presence of anxiety, it's possible to take steps to prevent its escalation. A panic attack cannot be stopped. The nurse can take steps to assist the client safely through the attack, and later, focus on alleviating the precipitating stressors. Clients who experience panic disorder don't tend to be in physical pain, but do experience uncomfortable and distressing symptoms. The client experiencing a panic disorder may need to depend on other people when having a panic attack.

CN: Psychosocial integrity; CNS: None; CL: Apply

7. What is the **most** important question for a nurse to ask a client with agoraphobia?

1. "How realistic are your goals?"
2. "Are you able to go shopping?"
3. "Do you struggle with impulse control?"
4. "Who else in your family has panic disorder?"

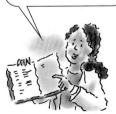

For the NCLEX, you should memorize the definitions of common fears such as agoraphobia.

7. 2. The client with agoraphobia typically isolates himself at home, and can't carry out normal socializing and life-sustaining activities. Clients with panic disorder are able to set realistic goals, and tend to be cautious and reclusive rather than impulsive. Although there's a familial tendency toward panic disorder, information about the client's needs must be obtained to determine how agoraphobia affects his life.

CN: Psychosocial integrity; CNS: None; CL: Apply

8. The nurse has been working with a client who is interested in making lifestyle changes and behavior modification to treat panic attacks. What is the **most** important information for the nurse to tell the client?
 1. Cigarettes can trigger panic attacks.
 2. Fermented foods can cause panic attacks.
 3. Hormonal therapy can induce panic attacks.
 4. Tryptophan can predispose a person to panic attacks.

8. **1.** Cigarettes contain nicotine, which can be a stimulant, a depressant, or a tranquilizer, and can trigger panic attacks. None of the other options causes panic attacks.
CN: Psychosocial integrity; CNS: None; CL: Apply

9. What is the **priority** nursing intervention when caring for a client with a panic disorder?
 1. Encourage the client to role-play panic attacks
 2. Assist the client to develop an exercise program
 3. Train the client to identify cognitive distortions
 4. Teach the client to identify sources of anxiety

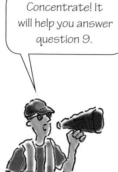

Concentrate! It will help you answer question 9.

9. **4.** The client must understand the connection between the sources of anxiety and the symptoms of a panic attack. Role-playing a panic attack isn't useful. Role-playing coping strategies would be useful for the client. Later in treatment, the client can develop an exercise program as part of the overall plan to handle stress. Learning to identify cognitive distortions will help the client after he's begun to work on identifying sources of anxiety.
CN: Psychosocial integrity; CNS: None; CL: Analyze

10. The nurse is planning care for a client with panic disorder. What is the **priority** nursing intervention?
 1. Identify childhood trauma
 2. Supervise nutritional intake
 3. Evaluate for depression
 4. Monitor episodes of disorientation

10. **3.** Clients with panic disorder are at risk for suicide when they are experiencing depression and other mental health disorders. It is imperative that they be evaluated for depression. Childhood trauma is associated with many comorbid conditions, including post-traumatic stress disorder, not panic disorder. Nutritional problems don't typically accompany panic disorder. Clients are not disoriented, but may temporarily have an altered sense of reality, that lasts the duration of the attack.
CN: Psychosocial integrity; CNS: None; CL: Analyze

11. Which statement indicates a positive response to treatment from the client diagnosed with panic disorder and agoraphobia?
 1. "I went to the mall with my friend last Saturday."
 2. "I only hyperventilate when I have a panic attack."
 3. "Today, I decided that I can stop taking my medication."
 4. "Last night, I decided to eat more than a bowl of cereal."

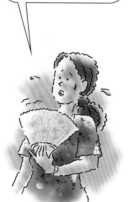

On second thought, maybe I'll just stay home and watch a movie.

11. **1.** Clients with panic disorder and agoraphobia tend to be socially withdrawn. Going to the mall indicates progress in overcoming avoidant behaviors. Hyperventilation is a key symptom of panic disorder. Teaching breath control is a major intervention for clients with panic disorder. The client taking anti-anxiety or antidepressant medications for panic disorder, must be gradually weaned off these drugs. Most clients with panic disorder and agoraphobia don't have nutritional problems.
CN: Psychosocial integrity; CNS: None; CL: Analyze

CN: **Client needs category**   CNS: **Client needs subcategory**   CL: **Cognitive level**

12. Which group therapy intervention is of **primary** importance to a client with panic disorder?
   1. Explore how secondary gains are derived from the disorder
   2. Discuss new ways of thinking and feeling about panic attacks
   3. Work to eliminate manipulative behavior used to meet needs
   4. Provide safe exposure to factors that trigger anxiety attacks

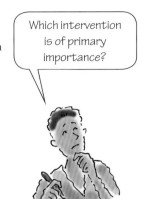

Which intervention is of primary importance?

12. 2. Restructuring an anxiety-producing event allows the client to gain control over the situation. Discussing new ways of thinking and feeling about panic attacks can enable others to learn and benefit from a variety of intervention strategies. There are usually no secondary gains from having a panic disorder. People with panic disorder aren't using the disorder as a way to manipulate others. Providing safe exposure to factors that trigger anxiety is used for clients experiencing a specific phobic reaction.
CN: Psychosocial integrity; CNS: None; CL: Analyze

13. The nursing team members are evaluating the care of a client with social anxiety disorder. Which statement informs the nurse that the client is appropriately addressing this disorder?
   1. "I exercise two times a week even though I do not feel like doing it.
   2. "Sometimes I cannot stop myself when I don't get what I want."
   3. "There are times that I change my thoughts from negative to positive."
   4. "I'm not so concerned about being laughed at by the people at work."

13. 4. Clients with social anxiety disorder are fearful about public and social situations. They fear being humiliated, embarrassed or laughed at by others. Exercise is a healthy coping strategy for all clients, not just clients with social anxiety disorder. It is common to become irritable, especially when desires are not fulfilled, but this behavior is associated with clients with bipolar disorder, not clients with social anxiety disorder. Changing one's thoughts from negative to positive reflect the client's use of strategies that are helpful in handling a depressive disorder, not a social anxiety disorder.
CN: Psychosocial integrity; CNS: None; CL: Apply

14. Which statement is a client with social anxiety disorder **most** likely to make?
   1. "Without people around, I just feel so lost."
   2. "There's nothing wrong with my behavior."
   3. "I know that I can't accept the award for my brother."
   4. "I like to be the center of attention."

14. 3. People who have a social phobia usually undervalue themselves and their capabilities. They don't like to be in feared social situations or around many people. They tend to stay away from situations in which they may feel humiliated or embarrassed. They fear social gatherings and dislike being the center of attention. They're very critical of themselves and believe that others also will be critical.
CN: Psychosocial integrity; CNS: None; CL: Apply

15. The nurse is aware that clients with social anxiety disorder typically fear:
   1. dental procedures.
   2. meeting strangers.
   3. a dog bite.
   4. a car accident.

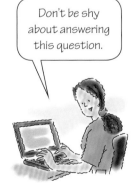

Don't be shy about answering this question.

15. 2. Fear of meeting strangers is an example of social anxiety disorder. Fears of having a dental procedure, being bitten by a dog, or having a car accident are not related to social anxiety disorder, but to a specific phobia.
CN: Psychosocial integrity; CNS: None; CL: Apply

CN: Client needs category   CNS: Client needs subcategory   CL: Cognitive level

16. The nurse is assessing a client for blood-injection-injury phobia. Which finding is **most** predictive of this phobia?
1. Episodes of fainting
2. Gregarious personality
3. Difficulty managing anger
4. Dramatic, over reactive personality

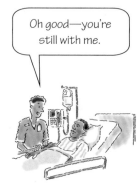

Oh good—you're still with me.

16. 1. Many people with a history of a specific phobia, such as blood-injection-injury, report frequent fainting when exposed to this type of situation. Personality type doesn't provide information for assessing phobias anyone can develop phobias. Information about a client's anger management are not related to a specific phobia disorder. Individuals with blood-injection-injury phobias aren't being dramatic or over reactive.
CN: Psychosocial integrity; CNS: None; CL: Analyze

17. A client with a specific phobia disorder would benefit **most** from which individual counseling approach?
1. Have the client write in a journal each evening
2. Help the client identify the source of the anxiety
3. Teach the client effective ways to problem solve issues
4. Develop strategies to prevent the client from using substances

17. 2. By understanding the anxiety source, the client will understand how the anxiety has been displaced by a specific phobia. Keeping a journal is an effective method in many situations; however, its use is limited in the treatment of phobias. Problem solving is a more useful technique for clients with obsessive-compulsive disorder than for clients with a specific phobia. People with a specific phobia don't tend to self-medicate like clients with other psychiatric disorders.
CN: Psychosocial integrity; CNS: None; CL: Apply

Along with assessment, you also need to familiarize yourself with common treatments.

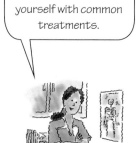

18. The health care team is planning interventions to modify the behaviors of clients with social anxiety disorder. What would be the **most** appropriate intervention to include?
1. Aversion therapy
2. Imitation or modeling
3. Positive reinforcement
4. Systematic desensitization

18. 4. Systematic desensitization is a common behavior modification technique used to help treat social anxiety disorder. Aversion therapy and positive reinforcement are not behavior modification techniques used with treatment of social anxiety disorder. Imitation and modeling are social learning techniques, not behavior modification techniques.
CN: Psychosocial integrity; CNS: None; CL: Apply

19. The nurse is teaching the client and her family about social anxiety disorder. Which statement **best** describes the role of the family?
1. Family support system is only temporary.
2. The family should reinforce the client's need to be assertive.
3. The family should set limits on the client's inappropriate behaviors.
4. The family can participate in promoting client independence.

19. 4. The family plays a vital role in supporting the client in treatment, and preventing her from using the disorder to obtain secondary gains. Family support must be ongoing, not temporary. It is more helpful if the family focuses on effectively handling anxiety, rather than focusing on developing assertiveness skills. People with social anxiety disorder are already restrictive in their behavior. More restrictions are not necessary.
CN: Psychosocial integrity; CNS: None; CL: Analyze

20. The nurse is caring for a client who is receiving paroxetine for a major depressive disorder. What is the nurse's **most** important intervention?
1. Monitor thyroid function.
2. Determine electrocardiogram (ECG) changes
3. Assess for sleeping difficulties
4. Observe for extrapyramidal symptoms

20. 3. Clients taking paroxetine may experience insomnia and abnormal dreams. Clients do not tend to experience thyroid dysfunction when taking paroxetine. Paroxetine does not adversely affect the heart. Extrapyramidal symptoms are not seen with paroxetine.
CN: Physiological integrity; CNS: Pharmacological and parenteral therapies; CL: Analyze

CN: Client needs category   CNS: Client needs subcategory   CL: Cognitive level

21. The nurse suspects that a client may have posttraumatic stress disorder (PTSD). It would be **most** important for the nurse to assess the client for:
1. an eating disorder.
2. schizophrenia.
3. suicide.
4. sundowner's syndrome.

21. 3. Clients who experience PTSD are at risk for suicide and often have unstable behaviors. Eating disorders are possible, but are not a common complication of PTSD. The anxiety experienced with PTSD does not usually manifest itself as schizophrenia. Sundowner's syndrome usually affects people with dementia or cognitive impairment, and manifests as agitation accompanied by confusion.
CN: Psychosocial integrity; CNS: None; CL: Apply

22. A client is prescribed a tricyclic antidepressant after other medications were ineffective. What outcome would indicate that this medication is effective?
1. Prevented purposeless movements
2. Increased in the client's ability to concentrate
3. Helped prevent the re-experience of the trauma
4. Facilitated the client's normal grieving process

22. 3. Tricyclic antidepressant medications will decrease the frequency of trauma reenactment for the client. It will help memory problems, sleeping difficulties, and will decrease numbing. The medication won't prevent purposeless movements or increase the client's concentration. No medication will facilitate the grieving process.
CN: Physiological integrity; CNS: Pharmacological and parenteral therapies; CL: Apply

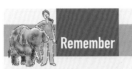

Remember

"-ine drugs help you feel more serene."

Tricyclic antidepressants and selective serotonin uptake inhibitors (SSRIs) are antidepressants. Many of them end in "-ine."

Tricyclic antidepressants:
- Amitriptyline
- Amoxapine
- Clomipramine
- Desipramine
- Imipramine
- Nortriptyline
- Protriptyline
- Trimipramine

SSRIs:
- Fluoxetine
- Fluvoxamine
- Paroxetine
- Sertraline

23. The nurse is planning care for a client with post traumatic stress disorder (PTSD) who stated that the experience was "bad luck." What intervention is the **most** important for the nurse to include?
1. Encourage the client to verbalize his feelings about the experience
2. Assist the client in defining the experience as a trauma
3. Work with the client to take steps to move on with life
4. Help the client accept positive and negative feelings

23. 2. The client must define the experience as traumatic, and realize that it wasn't under his personal control. Encouraging the client to verbalize his feelings about the trauma experience should be done after acknowledging the reality of the traumatic event. The client can move on with life after acknowledging the trauma and processing the experience. Acknowledgment of the actual trauma and verbalization of the event should come before the acceptance of feelings.
CN: Psychosocial integrity; CNS: None; CL: Analyze

24. The nurse is teaching a client with post traumatic stress disorder (PTSD) about relationships. What is the **most** important information for the nurse to provide?
1. Encourage the client to resume former roles as soon as possible
2. Discuss the client's discomfort when talking to others about his feelings
3. Explain that avoiding emotional attachment protects against anxiety
4. Alert the client of his tendency to be over-dependent in relationships

24. 3. The client may tend to avoid interpersonal relationships as a way to protect himself against unrelieved anxiety. Because relationships tend to be avoided, the client won't express his feelings to others at this time, and won't resume roles and responsibilities for a while. Clients with PTSD don't tend to become over-dependent in relationships, but they do tend to withdraw from them.
CN: Psychosocial integrity; CNS: None; CL: Apply

Don't deny it. You're doing great!

CN: Client needs category   CNS: Client needs subcategory   CL: Cognitive level

25. The nurse is caring for a client diagnosed with post traumatic stress disorder (PTSD). The client tells the nurse, "My family doesn't believe anything about PTSD." What is the **most** appropriate intervention by the nurse?
1. Provide the family with information
2. Teach the family about problem solving
3. Discuss the family's view of the problem
4. Assess for the presence of family violence

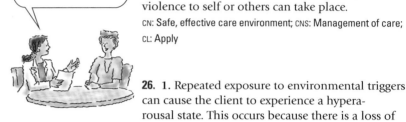

Caring for clients commonly means working with their families—a skill you can expect the exam to test.

25. 1. If the family understands PTSD, they can be supportive, and more readily participate in the client's care. Learning problem-solving skills doesn't help clarify PTSD. Only after being given information about PTSD can the family then ask questions and present its views. The family must first have information about PTSD, then a discussion about violence to self or others can take place.
CN: Safe, effective care environment; CNS: Management of care; CL: Apply

26. While caring for a client with post traumatic stress disorder (PTSD), the family notices that loud noises cause a serious anxiety response. What is the **best** explanation the nurse can give to this family?
1. Environmental triggers can cause the client to become hyper aroused.
2. Clients commonly experience extreme fear about normal environmental stimuli.
3. After a trauma, the client can't respond to stimuli in an appropriate manner.
4. The anxiety response indicates that another emotional problem needs investigation.

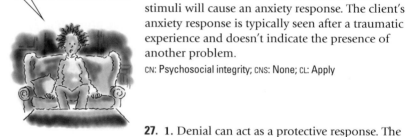

Scary movies always make me jump.

26. 1. Repeated exposure to environmental triggers can cause the client to experience a hyperarousal state. This occurs because there is a loss of physiologic control over incoming stimuli. After experiencing a trauma, the client may have strong reactions to stimuli similar to those that occurred during the traumatic event; however, not all stimuli will cause an anxiety response. The client's anxiety response is typically seen after a traumatic experience and doesn't indicate the presence of another problem.
CN: Psychosocial integrity; CNS: None; CL: Apply

27. What primary psychologic symptom should a nurse expect to find in a client who is the lone survivor of a multiple-car collision, and was recently hospitalized?
1. Denial
2. Indifference
3. Perfectionism
4. Trust

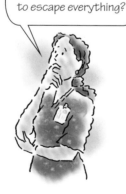

What is the greatest risk for someone who is trying to escape everything?

27. 1. Denial can act as a protective response. The client tends to be overwhelmed and disorganized by the trauma, not indifferent to it. Perfectionism is more commonly seen in clients with eating disorders, not in clients with post traumatic stress disorder. Clients who have had a severe trauma commonly experience an inability to trust others.
CN: Psychosocial integrity; CNS: None; CL: Analyze

28. A client who is suffering from post traumatic stress disorder (PTSD) tells the nurse, "I've decided to just avoid everything and everyone." The client is at **greatest** risk for:
1. becoming malnourished.
2. exhausting his finances.
3. being terminated from employment.
4. substance use.

28. 4. The use of substances is a way for the client to deny problems and self-medicate the feelings of distress. People with PTSD, who isolate themselves, do not tend to become malnourished. Most clients with PTSD can manage money and maintain employment.
CN: Psychosocial integrity; CNS: None; CL: Apply

29. What is the nurse's **best** intervention while speaking to a client with posttraumatic stress disorder (PTSD) about the trauma?
1. Obtain validation of what the client says from another party
2. Request that the client write down what's being said
3. Ask questions to convey an interest in the details
4. Listen attentively and remain with the client

29. 4. An effective communication strategy for a nurse to use with a PTSD client is listening attentively and staying with the client. There's no need to obtain validation about what the client says by asking for information from another party, asking the client to write down what's being said, or distracting the client by asking questions.
CN: Psychosocial integrity; CNS: None; CL: Apply

CN: Client needs category   CNS: Client needs subcategory   CL: Cognitive level

30. Which statement **best** expresses a client's survivor guilt?
 1. "I think I can see the purpose of my survival."
 2. "I can't help but feel that everything was their fault."
 3. "I now understand why I'm not able to forgive myself."
 4. "I wish I could stop sabotaging my family relationships."

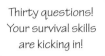

Thirty questions! Your survival skills are kicking in!

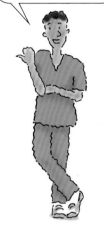

31. What is the **best** nursing action for a client with post traumatic stress disorder (PTSD), and his family, with interpersonal conflicts at home?
 1. Encourage the family to teach the client how to identify defensive behaviors
 2. Discuss ways to change dysfunctional patterns with the family
 3. Have the family agree not to tell the client what to do about problems
 4. Teach the family how to arrange social activities for the client

32. The family members of a client diagnosed with post traumatic stress disorder (PTSD) tell the nurse that they cannot understand why the client has this disorder, because the client did not directly experience personal trauma. What is the **most** appropriate intervention by the nurse?
 1. Advise them to obtain a second psychiatric evaluation
 2. Ask them what they perceive as the client's problem
 3. Explain the effect of learning about another's experience
 4. Identify the time period the client manifested symptoms

33. The effectiveness of selective serotonin reuptake inhibitor (SSRIs) therapy, in a client with post traumatic stress disorder (PTSD), can be verified when the client states:
 1. "I'm sleeping better now."
 2. "I'm not losing my temper."
 3. "I've lost my craving for alcohol."
 4. "I've lost my phobia for water."

30. 3. Survivor guilt occurs when the person has almost constant thoughts about the other people who perished in an event. The survivor doesn't understand why he survived, but a friend or loved one didn't. Blaming self, not others, is a component of survivor guilt. Survivor guilt and impaired interpersonal relationships are two different categories of responses to trauma.
CN: Psychosocial integrity; CNS: None; CL: Analyze

31. 2. Discussing dysfunctional family patterns will allow the family to determine why these patterns are maintained. Encouraging family members to point out the defensive behaviors of the client may inadvertently produce more defensive behavior. Families can be a source of support and assistance; therefore, inflexible rules are not useful to either the client or the family. The family should not be encouraged to arrange social activities for the client. Social activities outside of the home do not help the family handle conflict within the home.
CN: Psychosocial integrity; CNS: None; CL: Apply

32. 3. Post traumatic stress disorder can occur if a client has experienced the traumatic event, witnessed the event, or learned that trauma has happened to a family member or close friend. After educating the family about PTSD, a second evaluation may not be necessary. Encouraging family members to discuss the situation and share their perceptions can be helpful, but it isn't their responsibility, or within their abilities, to diagnose the health problem. Symptoms of PTSD usually appear after the event has occurred and last for at least one month. This information isn't as important as an explanation of what constitutes a traumatic event.
CN: Psychosocial integrity; CNS: None; CL: Analyze

33. 1. Selective serotonin reuptake inhibitors are used to treat sleep problems, nightmares, and intrusive thoughts in individuals with PTSD. Selective serotonin reuptake inhibitors are not used to control flashbacks, to treat a specific phobia, or to decrease the craving for alcohol.
CN: Physiological integrity; CNS: Pharmacological and parenteral therapies; CL: Analyze

34. What is the major purpose of group therapy for adolescents who have witnessed the violent death of a peer?
1. To learn violence prevention strategies
2. To focus on ways to suppress anger
3. To discuss the effect of this trauma on their lives
4. To develop trusting relationships among their peers

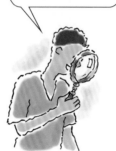

The term major purpose indicates that there may be more than one right answer. You need to choose the best answer.

35. Which symptom of post traumatic stress disorder (PTSD) can be treated with hypnosis?
1. Addiction
2. Confabulation
3. Dissociation
4. Hallucinations

36. A nurse is assigned a client with generalized anxiety disorder. How can the nurse **best** demonstrate appropriate caring for this client?
1. Verbalize concern to the client during an interaction
2. Arrange weekly group activities for the client
3. Have the client sign the treatment plan
4. Hold psychoeducational groups on medications

37. The nurse is talking about school to a child with generalized anxiety disorder. Which information would the child share with the nurse during their interaction?
1. There has been fighting with peers for the past month.
2. The child can't stop lying to parents and teachers.
3. In the last month the child has gained 10 lb (4.53 kg).
4. School grades are a major concern for the child.

38. The nurse is aware that a client, who has generalized anxiety disorder, may also have:
1. bipolar disorder.
2. gender identity disorder.
3. panic disorder.
4. schizoaffective disorder.

34. 3. By discussing the effect of the trauma on their lives, the adolescents can grieve and develop effective coping strategies. Learning violence prevention strategies is not the most immediate concern after a trauma occurs, nor is working on developing healthy relationships. It's appropriate to talk about how to express anger constructively after the trauma is addressed.
CN: Psychosocial integrity; CNS: None; CL: Apply

35. 3. Hypnosis is one of the therapies used with clients who dissociate. Hypnosis isn't a treatment of choice for clients with addictive disorders or hallucinations. Confabulation isn't a symptom of PTSD.
CN: Psychosocial integrity; CNS: None; CL: Apply

36. 1. The nurse, who verbally expresses concern about a client's well-being, is acting in a caring and supportive manner. The nurse has no direct client contact while arranging weekly group activities. Having a client sign the treatment plan may not be viewed as a sign of caring. Having a psychoeducational group on medications may be viewed, by clients, as a teaching experience and not interpersonal contact.
CN: Psychosocial integrity; CNS: None; CL: Apply

37. 4. Children with generalized anxiety disorder will worry about how well they're performing in school. They don't tend to be involved in conflict. They're more oriented toward good behavior. Children with generalized anxiety disorder don't tend to lie to others, and would want to do their best to please others. A weight gain of 10 lb (4.53 kg) isn't a typical characteristic of a child with anxiety disorder.
CN: Psychosocial integrity; CNS: None; CL: Analyze

38. 3. Approximately 75% of clients with generalized anxiety disorder may also have a diagnosis of specific phobia, panic disorder, or substance abuse. Clients with generalized anxiety disorder don't tend to have a coexisting diagnosis of gender identity disorder, bipolar disorder, or schizoaffective disorder.
CN: Psychosocial integrity; CNS: None; CL: Apply

39. The nurse determines that nutritional teaching, for a client with generalized anxiety disorder, was successful when the client states:
1. "I've stopped drinking so much cola."
2. "I've reduced my intake of carbohydrates."
3. "I eat less at dinner and before bedtime."
4. "My use of dairy products has decreased."

40. A client with generalized anxiety disorder is refusing the prescribed anxiolytic medication. What is the **most** likely explanation for this refusal?
1. "I don't think the psychiatrist likes me."
2. "I want to solve my problems on my own."
3. "The voices say I don't have to take the medication."
4. "I think my family wants me to be medicated."

41. The nurse is helping a client with generalized anxiety disorder verbalize her feelings. What tendencies are important for the nurse to consider?
1. The client may intellectualize feelings of anxiety.
2. The problem is seen as due to genetics.
3. The client feels that talking about feelings isn't beneficial.
4. The client may believe that only medications are useful.

42. An adult client with a long-standing history of generalized anxiety disorder would **most** likely state:
1. "I was, and still am, an impulsive person."
2. "I've always been hyperactive but not in useful ways."
3. "When I was in school, I never thought I would finish."
4. "I've had intrusive dreams and scary nightmares all my life."

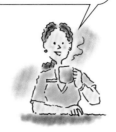

What do you know about the relationship between anxiety and caffeine?

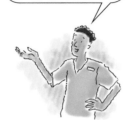

40 questions done, 58 questions left to finish!

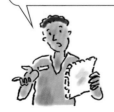

Certain psychological disorders tend to appear at particular ages—that's information to know for the NCLEX.

39. 1. Clients with generalized anxiety disorder can decrease anxiety by eliminating caffeine from their diets. It isn't necessary for clients with generalized anxiety to decrease their carbohydrate intake, eat less at dinner or before bedtime, or cut back on their use of dairy products.
CN: Physiological integrity; CNS: Basic care and comfort; CL: Apply

40. 2. It's common for a client with generalized anxiety disorder to refuse medication because he believes the medication is a sign of personal weakness, and that he can't solve problems by himself. Fear that the psychiatrist dislikes him reflects paranoid thinking that isn't usually seen in a client with generalized anxiety disorder. Auditory hallucinations and paranoia about the motives of friends and family members aren't characteristic of clients with generalized anxiety disorder.
CN: Psychosocial integrity; CNS: None; CL: Analyze

41. 1. Clients who experience generalized anxiety disorder commonly need assistance acknowledging their anxiety instead of denying or intellectualizing it. Although scientists believe that there may be a tendency for anxiety to be familial, the problem isn't regarded as genetic. A client who is unwilling to express feelings may not view therapy as helpful. The most effective treatment of generalized anxiety disorder combines psychotherapy and pharmacotherapy.
CN: Psychosocial integrity; CNS: None; CL: Analyze

42. 3. For many people who have a generalized anxiety disorder, there is concern about not accomplishing routine tasks and expected activities during the life cycle. The symptoms of impulsiveness and hyperactivity aren't commonly associated with a diagnosis of generalized anxiety disorder. Intrusive dreams and nightmares are associated with post traumatic stress disorder rather than generalized anxiety disorder.
CN: Psychosocial integrity; CNS: None; CL: Analyze

43. The nurse is assessing a client with generalized anxiety disorder for signs of muscle tension. Which symptom might the client display?
1. Disturbed sleep
2. Restless periods
3. Startle response
4. Tachycardia intervals

43. 2. Restlessness is a symptom associated with muscle tension. Difficulty sleeping and a startle response are considered symptoms of vigilance and scanning of the environment. Tachycardia at intervals is classified as a symptom of autonomic hyperactivity.
CN: Physiological integrity; CNS: Physiological adaptation; CL: Apply

44. The chart entry reads:

Progress notes	
2/10/17 1000	The client is pacing the hallway and stated, "I'm feeling so bad that I could jump out of my skin." Vital sign: T 97.8, P 124, R 24. The client is sweating and trying to hold back tears. The client refuses to participate in relaxation exercises or to do deep breathing with the nurse.

What is the **best** action for the nurse to initiate based on the information in this record?
1. Place the client in bed in a reclining position
2. Call the family and request them to visit now
3. Contact the provider for a PRN medication
4. Establish a social conversation to distract the client

44. 3. It would be most helpful to obtain an order and administer a PRN medication to assist the client with this intense anxiety. It is not helpful to decrease the client's anxiety by putting the client in bed. It may not be feasible for the family to come to the unit, and there is no guarantee that they can calm the client if they are able to visit. A therapeutic intervention is necessary, rather than a social conversation which minimizes the client's present situation.
CN: Psychosocial integrity; CNS: None; CL: Apply

45. The nurse is caring for a client who has a history of escalating anxiety. What is the **most** appropriate intervention by the nurse?
1. Explore the client's feelings about current life stressors
2. Have the client discuss the need to flee from painful situations
3. Encourage the client to develop a realistic view of self
4. Provide appropriate phone numbers for hotlines and clinics

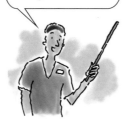

Thorough teaching plans typically include ways to contact support organizations.

45. 4. By having information on hotlines and clinics, this client can pursue help when the anxiety escalates. Discussing current life stressors isn't helpful when focusing on ways to alleviate the client's escalating anxiety. Fleeing from painful situations and discussing views of self aren't the best strategies, neither allows for problem solving.
CN: Psychosocial integrity; CNS: None; CL: Apply

46. The nurse is teaching the family of an adult client about generalized anxiety disorder. What is the nurse's **most** important action?
1. Explain how the family can handle the confusion related to memory loss
2. Teach the family to assist the client with coping strategies as needed
3. Address ways to cope with the client's unexpected travel behavior with the family
4. Have the family determine the reasons why the client should take medication

46. 2. The family can be there for support, but they negate the client's ability to function if they take control of the situation and don't allow the client to use his own coping skills. A client who has confusion related to memory loss is commonly struggling with dissociative amnesia, not a generalized anxiety disorder. Unexpected travel behavior is a problem for families who have members with dissociative identity disorder, not generalized anxiety disorder. The client must learn to use medication as prescribed.
CN: Psychosocial integrity; CNS: None; CL: Apply

CN: Client needs category   CNS: Client needs subcategory   CL: Cognitive level

47. A client with generalized anxiety disorder tells the nurse that he wants to stop taking his lorazepam. What is the nurse's **most** appropriate response?
1. "Be aware that stopping the drug may cause depression to occur."
2. "Sometimes the drug increases cognitive abilities if stopped."
3. "There may be a decrease in sleeping difficulties after the drug is stopped."
4. "If you just stop the drug it can cause withdrawal symptoms."

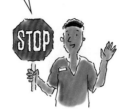

You should be familiar with the symptoms that discontinuing key medications may cause.

47. 4. Stopping antianxiety drugs such as benzodiazepines can cause the client to have withdrawal symptoms. Stopping a benzodiazepine doesn't tend to cause depression, increase cognitive abilities, or decrease sleeping difficulties.
CN: Physiological integrity; CNS: Pharmacological and parenteral therapies; CL: Apply

48. Five days after running out of medication, a client taking clonazepam tells the nurse, "I know I shouldn't have just stopped the drug like that, but I'm OK." What is the nurse's **most** appropriate response?
1. "Let's monitor you for problems, in case something else happens."
2. "You could go through withdrawal symptoms for up to two weeks."
3. "You have handled your anxiety, and now you know how to cope with stress."
4. "If you're fine now, chances are you won't experience withdrawal symptoms."

48. 2. Withdrawal symptoms can appear after one or two weeks because the benzodiazepine has a long half-life. Looking for another problem unrelated to withdrawal isn't the nurse's best strategy. The act of discontinuing an antianxiety medication doesn't indicate that a client has learned to cope with stress. Every client taking medication needs to be monitored for withdrawal symptoms when the medication is abruptly stopped.
CN: Physiological integrity; CNS: Pharmacological and parenteral therapies; CL: Analyze

49. A client taking alprazolam reports light-headedness and nausea every day while getting out of bed. What is the **most** important action by the nurse?
1. Take the client's blood pressure
2. Monitor body temperature
3. Teach the Valsalva maneuver
4. Obtain a blood chemistry profile

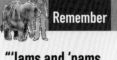

Remember

"'lams and 'pams have a calming effect."

Benzodiazepines are medications used to sedate and treat anxiety and panic disorders. Many of them end in "-lam" and "-pam":
- Alprazolam
- Clonazepam
- Diazepam
- Flurazepam
- Lorazepam
- Oxazepam
- Quazepam
- Temazepam
- Triazolam

49. 1. The nurse should take a blood pressure reading to validate orthostatic hypotension. A body temperature reading or chemistry profile won't yield useful information about hypotension. The Valsalva maneuver is performed to lower the heart rate and isn't an appropriate intervention.
CN: Physiological integrity; CNS: Reduction of risk potential; CL: Apply

50. A client with generalized anxiety disorder reports having a headache and upset stomach to the nurse. What else might this client report to the nurse during their conversation?
1. A variety of somatic concerns
2. An alteration in self-care skills
3. Unhealthy binge eating episodes
4. Secondary gains from mental illness

50. 1. Clients with generalized anxiety disorders commonly experience somatic symptoms. They don't usually experience problems with self-care. Eating problems aren't a typical part of the diagnostic criteria for anxiety disorders. Not all clients obtain secondary gains from mental illness.
CN: Psychosocial integrity; CNS: None; CL: Apply

51. The nurse needs to communicate with a client experiencing mania. How should the nurse address this client?
1. In a light and joking manner
2. Focus and redirect the conversation as necessary
3. Allow the client to talk about several different topics
4. Ask only open-ended questions to facilitate conversation

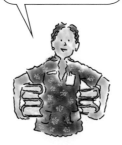

Stay focused on the topic at hand.

51. 2. To decrease stimulation, the nurse should attempt to redirect and focus the client's communication. Addressing the client in a light and joking manner may make the client feel out of control. For a manic client, it's best to ask closed questions that help maintain focus and a feeling of control.
CN: Psychosocial integrity; CNS: None; CL: Apply

52. A nurse is providing teaching for a client with major depressive disorder. The client is scheduled for electroconvulsive therapy (ECT), and asks the nurse, "What are the adverse effects of this therapy?" What is the nurse's **best** response?
1. Cholestatic jaundice
2. Hypertensive crisis
3. Mouth ulcers
4. Respiratory distress

52. 4. Respiratory distress or even respiratory arrest may occur as a complication of the anesthesia used with ECT. Cholestatic jaundice, hypertensive crisis, and mouth ulcers don't occur during, or as a result of, ECT.
CN: Physiological integrity; CNS: Physiological adaptation; CL: Apply

53. A client who has just had electroconvulsive therapy (ECT) asks the nurse for a drink of water. What is the **most** important intervention by the nurse?
1. Take client's blood pressure
2. Monitor the gag reflex
3. Obtain a body temperature
4. Determine level of consciousness

53. 2. The nurse must check the client's gag reflex before allowing the client to drink water after an ECT procedure. Blood pressure and body temperature don't determine the client's ability to swallow after the procedure. The client would be conscious if he's requesting a glass of water.
CN: Physiological integrity; CNS: Reduction of risk potential; CL: Analyze

54. The nurse is assessing the behavior of a client with hypomania. What behavior would the nurse expect from this client?
1. On the verge of depression and the potential for a crisis
2. Indecisive and vacillating, with a diminished ability to think
3. Irritable, with an elevated mood and increased motor activity
4. Disorganized, tending to exhibit impaired judgment

54. 3. When a client is hypomanic, there's evidence of an elevated and irritable mood, along with mild or beginning symptoms of mania such as excessive motor movement. A hypomanic client is experiencing a period of mild elation, not a depression or crisis. Indecision and vacillation with a diminished ability to think are symptoms more likely seen in a major depressive episode than in a hypomanic episode. A client with hypomania may tend to be creative and more productive than usual, rather than disorganized with impaired judgment.
CN: Psychosocial integrity; CNS: None; CL: Apply

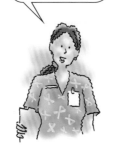

The words most likely can help you focus on the answer.

55. A client with bipolar disorder is reporting insomnia, restlessness, and clouded thinking. The nurse understands that this client is **most** likely experiencing:
1. depression.
2. cyclothymia.
3. hypomania.
4. mania.

55. 4. Headache, insomnia, restlessness, and the feeling unclear thinking are symptoms suggestive of mania in a client with a history of bipolar disorder. These symptoms are not suggestive of depression, cyclothymia, or hypomania.
CN: Physiological integrity; CNS: Physiological adaptation; CL: Apply

56. The nurse is teaching a client with major generalized anxiety disorder progressive relaxation exercises. Prioritize these relaxation techniques.

> **1.** Tense the muscles in your face for five seconds and then release and relax

> **2.** Place feet flat on floor, close your eyes, rest hands on lap, and take five deep breaths

> **3.** Inhale through nose and exhale through mouth as you tense and relax the muscles

> **4.** Tense and relax a muscle group, noticing the rise and fall of the abdomen with each breath

56. Ordered Response:

> **2.** Place feet flat on floor, close your eyes, rest hands on lap, and take five deep breaths.

> **4.** Tense and relax a muscle group, noticing the rise and fall of the abdomen with each breath

> **1.** Tense the muscles in your face for five seconds and then release and relax

> **3.** Inhale through nose and exhale through mouth as you tense and relax the muscles

CN: Safe, effective care environment; CNS: Management of care; CL: Apply

57. A client who is experiencing a manic episode has been admitted to an inpatient unit. The most important intervention to ensure adequate nutrition for this client would be to:
1. determine the client's metabolic rate.
2. make the client sit down for each meal and snack.
3. give the client foods to be eaten while he's active.
4. have the client interact with a dietician twice a week.

Keep it up! You're answers are sounding great.

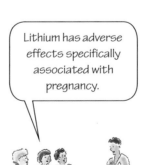

57. 3. By giving the client high-calorie foods that can be eaten while he's active, the nurse facilitates the client's nutritional intake. Determining the client's metabolic rate isn't useful information when the client is experiencing mania. During a manic episode, the client can't be still or focused long enough to interact with a dietitian or eat a relaxed meal.
CN: Physiological integrity; CNS: Basic care and comfort; CL: Apply

58. The nurse is providing discharge teaching for a client who will be taking lithium. Which condition would necessitate a call to the client's health care provider?
1. Development of black tongue
2. Increased lacrimation.
3. Periods of excitability.
4. Persistent gastrointestinal upset.

58. 4. Persistent gastrointestinal upset indicates a mild-to-moderate toxic reaction to lithium. Black tongue is an adverse reaction of mirtazapine, not lithium. Increased lacrimation and periods of excitability aren't adverse effects of lithium.
CN: Physiological integrity; CNS: Pharmacological and parenteral therapies; CL: Apply

59. A client with bipolar disorder tells the nurse that she just found out she is pregnant, and is concerned because she takes lithium. What is the **most** important information for the nurse to provide to this client?
1. Use of lithium usually results in serious congenital problems.
2. Thyroid problems can occur in the first trimester of the pregnancy.
3. Lithium causes severe urine retention and increased risk of toxicity.
4. Women who take lithium are very likely to have a spontaneous abortion.

Lithium has adverse effects specifically associated with pregnancy.

59. 1. Use of lithium during pregnancy will result in congenital defects, especially cardiac defects. Thyroid problems don't occur in the first trimester of the pregnancy. In lithium toxicity, a condition called nontoxic goiter may occur. An adverse effect of lithium is polyuria, not urine retention. The rate of spontaneous abortion for women taking lithium is no greater than for nonusers.
CN: Physiological integrity; CNS: Pharmacological and parenteral therapies; CL: Apply

60. A nurse is teaching a client with bipolar disorder about the drug carbamazepine. The nurse determines teaching was effective when the client states:
1. "My hair will fall out after I take this drug for a few months."
2. "I will drink plenty of water so I don't develop kidney problems."
3. "I need to have my blood counts checked periodically."
4. "I can't take any other drugs while I am taking this one."

60. 3. The most dangerous adverse effect of carbamazepine is bone marrow depression. Other medications may be taken with carbamazepine. Hair loss doesn't occur in clients taking carbamazepine. Clients who take lithium, not carbamazepine, must be closely monitored for nephrogenic diabetes insipidus. The interactions of all drugs must be monitored because some can either increase or decrease the blood level of carbamazepine.
CN: Physiological integrity; CNS: Pharmacological and parenteral therapies; CL: Analyze

61. The nurse is developing a plan of care for a newly-admitted client with bipolar disorder. What is **most** important for the nurse to include in this client's plan of care?
1. Obtain medication for sleep
2. Work on solving a problem
3. Exercise before bedtime
4. Develop a sleep ritual

61. 1. The client with bipolar disorder demonstrates extreme hyperactivity and a disturbed sleep pattern manifested by difficulty falling asleep and staying asleep. In addition to decreasing environmental stimuli, the use of an appropriate sleep medication is essential for this client until the prescribed medications have a therapeutic effect. Working on problem solving may excite the client rather than tire him. Exercise before retiring is inappropriate. Developing a sleep ritual is appropriate after the mood is stabilized.
CN: Physiological integrity; CNS: Reduction of risk potential; CL: Analyze

62. Family members of a client with bipolar disorder tell the nurse that they are distressed about the client's increasing episodes of mania. They are unsure of what to do. What is the **most** important information for the nurse to give this family?
1. "Learn ways to protect yourself from the client's behavior."
2. "Know how to proceed with a voluntary client commitment."
3. "Establish ways to confront the client about the reckless behavior."
4. "Know when to safely increase medication during manic periods."

Great job! Everything's going purr-fectly.

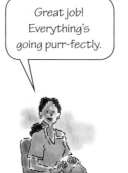

62. 1. Family members need to assess their needs and develop ways to protect themselves. Clients with symptoms of impulsive or reckless behavior that might endanger others, is a candidate for involuntary hospitalization. Confronting a client during a manic episode may escalate the behavior. The family must never increase the dosage of prescribed medication without first consulting the primary health care provider.
CN: Safe, effective care environment; CNS: Safety and infection control; CL: Analyze

63. A client, who is taking lithium, asks the nurse why she has to have her blood drawn for a lithium level. What is the nurse's **most** appropriate response?
1. Lithium levels are obtained to determine if you have any liver and renal damage."
2. Lithium levels demonstrate whether you are taking a therapeutic dose range of the drug."
3. Lithium levels indicate whether the drug has passed through your blood-brain barrier."
4. Lithium levels are unnecessary if you commit to taking the drug as ordered."

63. 2. Lithium levels determine if lithium dosage is adequate to maintain a therapeutic level of the drug. The drug is contraindicated for clients with renal, cardiac, or liver disease. Lithium levels aren't drawn for the purpose of determining whether the drug passes through the blood-brain barrier. Taking the drug as ordered doesn't eliminate the need for blood work.
CN: Physiological integrity; CNS: Pharmacological and parenteral therapies; CL: Apply

64. What is the **most** important information for the nurse to include when providing nutritional counseling for family members of a client with bipolar disorder?
   1. If sufficient roughage isn't eaten while taking lithium, bowel problems will occur.
   2. If the intake of carbohydrates increases, the lithium level will increase.
   3. If the intake of calories is reduced, the lithium level will increase.
   4. If the intake of sodium increases, the lithium level will decrease.

64. 4. Any time the level of sodium increases, such as with a change in dietary intake, the level of lithium will decrease. The intake of roughage and carbohydrates in the diet isn't related to the metabolism of lithium. Reducing the number of calories the client eats doesn't affect the lithium level in the body.
CN: Physiological integrity; CNS: Reduction of risk potential; CL: Analyze

65. The nurse teaches a client with bipolar disorder effective coping strategies. The nurse determines that teaching was successful when the client states:
   1. "I can decide what to do to prevent family conflict."
   2. "I can handle problems without asking for any help."
   3. "I can stay away from my friends when I feel distressed."
   4. "I can ignore things that go wrong instead of getting upset."

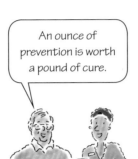

An ounce of prevention is worth a pound of cure.

65. 1. The client should be focusing on his strengths and abilities to prevent family conflict. Not being able to ask for help is problematic, and is not a good coping strategy. Avoiding problems also is not a good coping strategy. It's better to identify and handle problems as they arise. Ignoring situations that cause discomfort won't facilitate solutions or allow the client to demonstrate effective coping skills.
CN: Psychosocial integrity; CNS: None; CL: Analyze

66. The nurse is developing a plan of care for a client with major depressive disorder. This client has been admitted to the inpatient unit because of an attempted suicide. What is the **priority** goal for this client?
   1. The client will seek out the nurse when feeling sad and self-destructive.
   2. The client will identify and discuss actual and perceived losses.
   3. The client will learn strategies to promote relaxation and self-care.
   4. The client will establish healthy and mutually caring relationships.

66. 1. By seeking out the nurse when feeling sad and self-destructive, the client can feel safe, and begin to see that there are coping skills to assist in dealing with self-destructive tendencies. Discussion of losses and depression is also important, but the priority intervention is the client's immediate safety. Although relationship building and learning strategies to promote relaxation and self care are important goals, safety is the priority intervention.
CN: Safe, effective care environment; CNS: Management of care; CL: Analyze

67. A nurse is caring for a client with major depressive disorder who reports that he thinks about suicide every day. The nurse anticipates that the client's care will include:
   1. a no-suicide contract.
   2. weekly outpatient therapy.
   3. a second psychiatric opinion.
   4. intensive inpatient treatment.

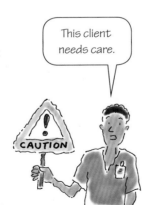

This client needs care.

CAUTION

67. 4. For a client thinking about suicide on a daily basis, inpatient care would be the best intervention. Although a no-suicide contract can be an important strategy, it is important to remember that they do not work with all clients, and most importantly, this client needs additional care. The client needs a more intensive level of care than weekly outpatient therapy. Immediate intervention is paramount, not a second psychiatric opinion.
CN: Safe, effective care environment; CNS: Management of care; CL: Apply

68. The nurse is developing short-term goals for a client who repeatedly makes statements about not deserving things. Which short-term goal is appropriate for this client?
1. Identify distorted thoughts
2. Describe self-care patterns
3. Discuss family relationships
4. Explore communication skills

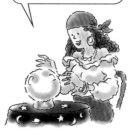

You're doing great in the short term, and your long-term goal is in sight.

68. 1. It's important to identify distorted thinking because self-deprecating thoughts lead to depression. Self-care patterns don't necessarily reflect distorted thinking. Family relationships might not influence distorted thinking patterns. A form of communication called negative self-talk would be explored after distorted thinking patterns were identified.
CN: Psychosocial integrity; CNS: None; CL: Apply

69. A client with major depressive disorder is making self-derogatory statements during interactions with the nurse. What is the nurse's **most** appropriate intervention?
1. Encourage the client to discuss spiritual matters
2. Help the client learn problem solving techniques
3. Help the client explore issues related to loss
4. Have the client identify positive aspects of self

69. 4. A priority nursing intervention is identify positive aspects of self, and address self-derogatory statements, beliefs and criticisms that can escalate the client's depression. Discussion of spiritual matters does not address the need to change negative self-statements. Learning how to problem solve will not modify the client's self-derogatory statements. If the client dwells on the negative and focuses on loss, it will be natural to continue this path of negativity.
CN: Psychosocial integrity; CNS: None; CL: Apply

70. The nurse is concerned that a client admitted with major depressive disorder may be suicidal. What is the **most** important action by the nurse?
1. Speak to family members to ascertain whether the client is suicidal
2. Talk to the client to determine whether the client is an attention seeker
3. Arrange for the client to be placed on immediate suicidal precautions
4. Ask a direct question such as, "Do you ever think about killing yourself?"

70. 4. The best approach is to ask about thoughts of suicide in a direct and caring manner. Assessing for attention-seeking behaviors doesn't deal directly with the problem. The client should be assessed directly, not through family members. Assessment must be performed before determining whether suicide precautions are necessary.
CN: Psychosocial integrity; CNS: None; CL: Apply

71. A client diagnosed with major depressive disorder has been admitted to an inpatient unit. The client's family members are upset, and tell the nurse they don't understand what is wrong. What is the nurse's **best** response?
1. Explain that depression is a lifelong illness
2. Explain that depression is an illness and can be treated
3. Describe how depression masks a person's true feelings
4. Teach how depression causes frequent disorganized thinking

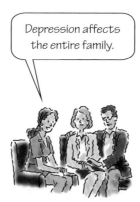

Depression affects the entire family.

71. 2. The nurse must help the family understand depression, its impact on the family, and the recommended treatments. Depression doesn't need to be a lifelong illness. It's important to help families understand that depression can be successfully treated and that, in some situations, depression can reoccur during the life cycle. The feelings expressed by the client are genuine, they reflect cognitive distortions and disillusionment. Disorganized thinking is more commonly associated with schizophrenia rather than with depression.
CN: Psychosocial integrity; CNS: None; CL: Apply

72. A client with major depressive disorder is participating in outpatient group therapy. Prioritize the events that the nurse would anticipate as the group organizes.

1. The group members may experience difficulties and regress

2. Members give feedback on other group members' progress

3. The rules and expectations for the group are established

4. Decision making and problem solving begin to occur

72. Ordered Response:

3. The rules and expectations for the group are established

4. Decision making and problem solving begin to occur

1. The group members may experience difficulties and regress

2. Members give feedback on other group members' progress

CN: Safe, effective care environment; CNS: Management of care; CL: Analyze

73. A nurse is planning interventions to enhance the self-esteem of a client with major depressive disorder. What is the **most** appropriate intervention for this client?
1. Playing cards
2. Praying daily
3. Taking medication
4. Writing poetry

73. 4. Writing poetry or engaging in some other creative outlet will enhance self-esteem. Playing cards and praying don't necessarily promote self-esteem. Taking medication will decrease symptoms of depression after a blood level is established, but it won't promote self-esteem.

CN: Psychosocial integrity; CNS: None; CL: Apply

74. An adolescent who is depressed and reportedly having difficulty in school is brought to the community mental health center by his parents for evaluation. The nurse performs an assessment and suspects the client may also be experiencing:
1. delusional thinking.
2. behavioral difficulties.
3. cognitive impairment.
4. labile moods.

74. 2. Adolescents tend to demonstrate severe irritability and behavioral problems rather than simply a depressed mood. Delusional thinking is usually associated with the diagnosis schizophrenia. Serious delusional thinking rarely occurs in the client experiencing depression. Cognitive impairment is typically associated with delirium or dementia. Labile mood is characteristic of a client with cognitive impairment or bipolar disorder.

CN: Psychosocial integrity; CNS: None; CL: Analyze

75. The nurse is developing a plan of care for a hospitalized client who is at risk for suicide. What is the **most** important intervention for the nurse to include?
1. Use a caring approach to maintain close observation of the client
2. Develop a strong and healthy relationship with the client
3. Obtain an order for an antianxiety medication to keep the client calm
4. Encourage the client to avoid over-stimulating group activities

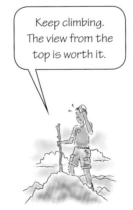

Keep climbing. The view from the top is worth it.

75. 1. Close observation, using a caring and therapeutic approach, is essential in order to decide the level of suicide precautions needed. Merely developing a strong relationship with the client isn't addressing the client's potential for self harm. Although antianxiety medication is sometimes used, the efficacy of antianxiety medications in lowering suicide risk is limited. Encouraging the client to stay away from group activities could cause isolation that would be detrimental to the client's well-being.

CN: Psychosocial integrity; CNS: None; CL: Apply

CN: Client needs category   CNS: Client needs subcategory   CL: Cognitive level

76. The nurse is working with a client who experiences a specific animal-type phobia. Which long-term goal will the nurse and client develop?
  1. Sustain a clear and realistic perception of one's self
  2. Develop self-understanding on how to maintain personal health
  3. Engage in appropriate verbal communication when agitated
  4. Learn to function with the stimulus without experiencing severe anxiety

76. 4. A client experiencing a phobic stimulus manifests severe anxiety which prevents that person from performing the usual activities of daily living. An appropriate long-term goal would be to function in the presence of the phobic object without having severe anxiety. The other long term goals are associated with clients who have been diagnosed with schizophrenia.
CN: Psychosocial integrity; CNS: None; CL: Analyze

77. The nurse is teaching a client with a specific phobia to verbalize fears and anxiety related to the phobia. Which statement, by the client, indicates progress in understanding the nurse's teaching?
  1. "I'm worried that I didn't outgrow my phobia from childhood."
  2. "Today I realized that my fear is the result of unresolved grief."
  3. "If I forget about this fear by distracting myself I'll feel better."
  4. "It is good to know that I have a choice on how to handle things."

77. 4. Clients with a specific phobia may make a decision to avoid the stimulus or work to eliminate the fear associated with it. A specific phobia is not outgrown. Specific phobias are not related to unresolved grief. Distracting one's self from a specific fear may only provide temporary relief from the anxiety.
CN: Psychosocial integrity; CNS: None; CL: Analyze

78. A client with a natural environment type of specific phobia is participating in a behavior modification technique called systematic desensitization. Prioritize the steps of the systematic desensitization process?

| 1. The client experiences a relaxation intervention |
| 2. The client is slowly exposed to the least fear-producing stimulus, and then progresses to more intense stimuli |
| 3. There is identification of fear producing stimuli from the most to the least fear arousing |
| 4. The nurse and the client establish a therapeutic rapport |

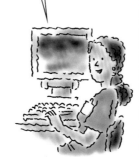

Don't be afraid. Just take it one step at a time.

78. Ordered Response:

| 4. The nurse and the client establish a therapeutic rapport |
| 1. The client experiences a relaxation intervention |
| 3. There is identification of fear producing stimuli from the most to the least fear arousing |
| 2. The client is slowly exposed to the least fear-producing stimulus, and then progresses to more intense stimuli |

CN: Safe, effective care environment; CNS: Management of care; CL: Analyze

79. The nurse has provided teaching for a client who will be taking lorazepam upon discharge. The nurse determines that teaching was effective when the client states the need to avoid:
  1. shellfish.
  2. alcohol.
  3. coffee.
  4. cheese.

79. 2. Alcohol should be avoided because of the added depressive effects. Ingestion of shellfish, coffee, and cheese is not problematic.
CN: Physiological integrity; CNS: Pharmacological and parenteral therapies; CL: Apply

80. A client describes her unpredictable episodes of acute anxiety and states, "I feel really awful, like I'm about to die, and I can hardly breathe." The nurse interprets these symptoms as:
1. agoraphobia.
2. dissociative disorder.
3. post traumatic stress disorder.
4. panic disorder.

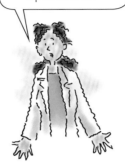

Don't panic if the answer isn't immediately clear—read through the question carefully and eliminate the obviously incorrect options first.

80. 4. This client is describing the characteristics of panic disorder. Agoraphobia is characterized by fear of public places. Dissociative disorder is characterized by lost periods of time, and post traumatic stress disorder, by hypervigilance and sleep disturbance.
CN: Psychosocial integrity; CNS: None; CL: Apply

81. A client who was diagnosed with major depressive disorder three weeks ago tells the nurse that he is feeling better since he started taking the prescribed antidepressant medication. The nurse is aware that it is **most** important to assess this client for:
1. manic depression.
2. violent behavior.
3. substance abuse.
4. suicidal ideation.

81. 4. After a client has been on antidepressants and is feeling better, he commonly has the energy to harm himself. Manic depression isn't treated with antidepressants. Nothing in the client's history suggests violent behavior. There are no signs or symptoms suggesting substance abuse.
CN: Safe, effective care environment; CNS: Safety and infection control; CL: Analyze

82. The nurse is performing an initial admission assessment on a 40-year-old client with a diagnosis of major depressive disorder. The client was brought to the hospital by her husband who states, "My wife has refused to get out of bed for two days, has not eaten, and is tired all the time." What is the **most** important question for the nurse to ask the client at this time?
1. "What has been troubling you?"
2. "Why do you dislike yourself?"
3. "How do you feel about your life?"
4. "What can we do to help?"

82. 3. The nurse must develop nursing interventions based on the client's perceived problems and feelings. Asking the client to draw a conclusion may be difficult for her at this time. Questions that ask "why" can place the client in a defensive position. Requiring the client to find possible solutions is beyond the scope of her present abilities.
CN: Psychosocial integrity; CNS: None; CL: Analyze

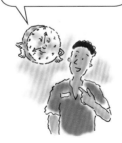

Timing is critical here. Read the question again if you have any doubts about what's being asked.

83. A client with bipolar disorder has been receiving lithium for two weeks. He also takes chemotherapeutic drugs that cause him to feel nauseated and anorexic. It is **most** important for the nurse to assess this client for:
1. hyperpyrexia with double vision.
2. marked arthritis with joint tenderness.
3. hypotonic reflexes with muscle weakness.
4. oliguria and cardiac dysrhythmias.

83. 3. Lithium alters sodium transport in nerve and muscle cells, slowing the speed of impulse transmission. Hypotonic reflexes and muscle weakness can be an adverse effect of lithium. Lithium has no known effect on body temperature, does not cause double vision or arthritis with joint tenderness. Oliguria and symptoms of cardiac dysrhythmias occur late in severe lithium toxicity.
CN: Physiologic integrity; CNS: Pharmacological and parenteral therapies; CL: Analyze

84. A client with a history of bipolar disorder was admitted to the psychiatric unit two days ago. The client stopped taking her lithium two weeks ago and now is in a manic phase. The nurse would anticipate the client's assessment to include:
1. flight of ideas.
2. echolalia.
3. clang associations.
4. neologism.

84. 1. Flight of ideas is a speech pattern, common in mania, characterized by rapid transition from topic to topic, typically without finishing one idea. Echolalia, clang associations, and neologism aren't seen in mania states.
CN: Psychosocial integrity; CNS: None; CL: Apply

85. A client with bipolar disorder is working with the nurse to establish a healthy sleep pattern before discharge. What is the **most** appropriate sleep strategy for the nurse to teach this client?
1. Effective use of medication for sleep
2. Perform mild exercise prior to bedtime
3. Identify factors that influence the sleep pattern
4. Engage is conversation with a peer before going to sleep

85. 3. The client must become aware of the factors that influence the sleep-wake pattern in order to successfully deal with them. Medication is a temporary intervention which can be used until a healthy sleep pattern is restored. The performance of exercise prior to bedtime is counterproductive, and will not promote relaxation and rest. Engaging in a conversation with another person will stimulate the client rather than promote a calm environment needed for sleep.
CN: Psychosocial integrity; CNS: None; CL: Apply

86. The nurse is preparing discharge instructions for a client taking lithium. What is the **most** important information for the nurse to give the client?
1. Limit fluids to 1,500 ml daily
2. Maintain a consistent fluid intake
3. Exercise outside whenever possible
4. Take over-the-counter remedies for cold symptoms

86. 2. Clients taking lithium need to maintain a consistent fluid intake. The client should not limit fluids. Exercising outside may not be safe. Photosensitivity occurs with lithium use, and activity in warm weather can increase sodium loss, predisposing the client to lithium toxicity. The client shouldn't take over-the-counter drugs without the health care provider's approval.
CN: Physiological integrity; CNS: Pharmacological and parenteral therapies; CL: Apply

87. A client with obsessive-compulsive disorders is in treatment. Which behaviors would indicate an improvement in this client's condition? Select all that apply.
1. The client refrains from performing rituals during stress
2. The client verbalizes using the "thought-stopping" strategy
3. The client identifies situations promoting anxiety and ritualistic behaviors
4. The client avoids stressful situations
5. The client rationalizes ritualistic behavior
6. The client performs ritualistic behaviors in private

87. 1, 2, 3. Refraining from rituals demonstrates that the client manages stress appropriately. Using the "thought-stopping" strategy demonstrates the client's ability to employ appropriate interventions for obsessive thoughts. Identifying situations that promote anxiety and precipitate ritualistic behavior help the client cope with the anxiety as well as understand the disease process. Avoiding, rationalizing, and hiding behaviors demonstrate maladaptive methods for managing stress and anxiety.
CN: Psychosocial integrity; CNS: None; CL: Analyze

88. A depressed client, who is taking fluoxetine, tells the nurse that he has difficulty sleeping at night, is often sleepy during the day, and does not feel like doing anything. What is the nurse's **best** response?
1. Tell the client to stop taking the drug until he sees his health care provider
2. Advise the client to continue taking the drug to see whether these effects wear off
3. Ask the prescriber whether the medication can be given early in the day
4. Advise the client to see another provider to obtain another opinion

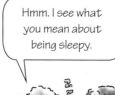

Hmm. I see what you mean about being sleepy.

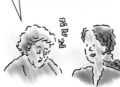

88. 3. A common side effect of fluoxetine is insomnia, which is best addressed by administering this medication early in the day. It is inappropriate for the nurse to tell the client to stop taking the drug, to continue taking it until the undesired effects wear off, or to seek a second opinion.
CN: Physiological integrity; CNS: Pharmacological and parenteral therapies; CL: Apply

CN: Client needs category   CNS: Client needs subcategory   CL: Cognitive level

89. A depressed client has been taking a selective serotonin reuptake inhibitor (SSRI) in the evening, and is upset because he cannot perform sexually due to erectile problems. What is the nurse's best response?
1. Stop taking the drug and notify the prescriber
2. Engage in sexual activity prior to taking the drug
3. Monitor for low blood pressure on a daily basis
4. Take the drug with food or 8 oz of water

89. 2. A viable option is for the client to engage in sexual activity before taking his daily antidepressant medication. It is not appropriate to suggest stopping the medication. Monitoring the client's blood pressure and taking the drug with food or 8 oz of water will not address the erectile dysfunction experienced by the client.
CN: Physiological integrity; CNS: Pharmacological and parenteral therapies; CL: Apply

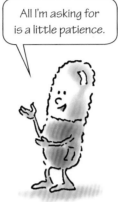

All I'm asking for is a little patience.

90. A nurse is teaching a client about tricyclic antidepressants. The nurse determines that teaching has been effective when the client states:
1. "This drug causes weight loss so I need to eat properly."
2. "I should avoid all milk and dairy products."
3. "I need to call the prescriber if I get a sore throat."
4. "Improvement in my mood will take up to 28 days."

90. 4. The client's mood may not improve until the third or fourth week of tricyclic antidepressant therapy. The client needs to be reassured that the drug works slowly. The drug does not cause weight loss. It does not interact with milk and dairy products. Tricyclic antidepressants do not cause symptoms of infection.
CN: Physiological integrity; CNS: Pharmacological and parenteral therapies; CL: Apply

91. The nurse is developing interventions for a client newly diagnosed with type 1 diabetes who has a blood-injection-injury phobia. What is the **most** appropriate intervention for this client?
1. Teach the client to avoid fainting by tensing the muscles of the legs and abdomen
2. Quickly expose the client to feared situations through systematic desensitization
3. Have the client do self-monitoring to avoid medical care whenever possible
4. Focus on treating the client's current symptoms with an antianxiety medication

91. 1. The client may be able to avoid fainting and relieve hypotension by tensing the larger muscle groups. Desensitization by slowly, not quickly, exposing the client to blood injection is indicated to reduce fear. Clients with blood-injection-injury phobia may avoid all medical care, which is dangerous to their health. Antianxiety medications may help on a short-term basis only.
CN: Psychosocial integrity; CNS: None; CL: Apply

92. The nurse is developing a plan of care for a client with social anxiety disorder. The client tells the nurse that he is embarrassed while in the presence of others. What would be the **most** important goals for this client? Select all that apply.
1. Manage his fear in group situations
2. Develop a plan to avoid situations that may cause stress
3. Verbalize feelings that occur in stressful situations
4. Develop a plan for responding to stressful situations
5. Deny feelings that may contribute to irrational fears
6. Use suppression to deal with underlying fears

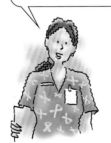

Remember to plan adaptive goals for responding to stress, not maladaptive ones.

92. 1, 3, 4. Improving stress-management skills, verbalizing feelings, and anticipating and planning for stressful situations are adaptive responses to stress. A client with social anxiety disorder is usually aware that the fear is out of proportion to the actual threat and causes impairment in overall functioning. Avoidance, denial, and suppression are maladaptive defense mechanisms.
CN: Psychosocial integrity; CNS: None; CL: Apply

93. A nurse is teaching a client who was diagnosed with persistent depressive disorder about her condition. What is the **most** appropriate information for the nurse to include?
   1. It involves a mood problem related to a concurrent medical condition.
   2. It involves a series of repeating manic episodes and depression.
   3. It's a form of depression that occurs in the fall and winter.
   4. It's a mood disorder with poor concentration and difficulty making decisions.

93. 4. Persistent depressive disorder is similar to major depressive disorder, and is characterized by poor concentration and difficulty making decisions. A persistent depressive disorder is different from a depressive disorder due to a medical condition. Bipolar I disorder with rapid cycling is characterized by a series of manic episodes. Seasonal affective disorder is a form of depression occurring in the fall and winter.

CN: Psychosocial integrity; CNS: None; CL: Apply

94. After interviewing a client diagnosed with major depressive disorder, the nurse determines the client's potential to commit suicide. What factors contribute to the client's suicide potential? Select all that apply.
   1. Psychomotor retardation
   2. Impulsive behaviors
   3. Criminal involvement
   4. Chronic, debilitating illness
   5. Decreased physical activity
   6. Substance use

94. 2, 3, 4, 6. Impulsive behavior, criminal activity and involvement with a law enforcement agencies, chronic illness, and substance use are factors that contribute to suicide potential. Psychomotor retardation and decreased activity are symptoms of depression, but don't typically lead to suicide because the client doesn't have the energy to harm himself.

CN: Psychosocial integrity; CNS: None; CL: Analyze

95. A client with bipolar disorder tells the nurse that he has suddenly stopped taking his medication. The nurse assesses the client. What finding would indicate a manic episode?
   1. Binge eating
   2. Relationship avoidance
   3. Sudden relocation
   4. Thoughtless spending

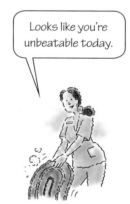

Looks like you're unbeatable today.

95. 4. Thoughtless or reckless spending is a common symptom of a manic episode. Binge eating isn't a behavior characteristic of a client during a manic episode. Relationship avoidance doesn't occur in a client experiencing a manic episode. During episodes of mania, a client may in fact interact with many people and participate in unsafe sexual behavior. Sudden relocation isn't a common characteristic of impulsive behavior demonstrated by a client with bipolar disorder.

CN: Psychosocial integrity; CNS: None; CL: Apply

CN: Client needs category   CNS: Client needs subcategory   CL: Cognitive level

96. What is the **priority** nursing action for a client with generalized anxiety disorder who is working to develop coping skills?

1. Determine whether the client has fears or obsessive thinking
2. Monitor the client for overt and covert signs of anxiety
3. Teach the client how to use effective communications skills
4. Assist the client to identify coping mechanisms used in the past

96. 4. To help a client develop effective coping skills, the nurse must know the client's baseline functioning. Determining whether the client has fears or obsessive thinking, monitoring for signs of anxiety, and teaching about effective communications skills are later priorities.
CN: Safe, effective care environment; CNS: Management of care; CL: Apply

97. A chart entry reads:

Progress notes	
2/10/17	The client presents with a sad affect,
1700	stooped posture, limited eye contact, and
	slow, but clear speech. The client is oriented
	and stays away from peers. During a one-to-
	one interaction the client stated," I'm not
	worth it. It won't do me any good to talk
	about it."

Based on the progress note shown here, which is the **best** intervention for the nurse to initiate?

1. Talk about community resources that may be of use to the client
2. Gently question the negative self-statements made by the client
3. Have the client identify spiritual needs to develop comfort and strength
4. Address how building social skills will prevent escalation of anxiety

97. 2. Gently challenging the client's negative self-statements will help this client begin to look at self-criticism and negative feelings. Talking about community resources is premature when the client sees little value in addressing personal issues and feelings. Identifying spiritual needs can lead to obtaining spiritual support to assist with this anxiety. Obtaining resources is premature until the client starts to acknowledge self-worth. Building social skills is a premature action when the client isolates, feels unworthy and lacks self-acceptance.
CN: Psychosocial integrity; CNS: None; CL: Apply

98. The note on the chart of a client with post traumatic stress disorder reads:

Progress notes	
2/10/17	During the group therapy session, the client
1300	spoke about facts related to the train
	accident, but did not express his feelings
	related to the trauma experienced.

Based on this chart entry, what is the **best** strategy for the nurse to use to prompt further discussion during the next group therapy session?

1. Encourage the client to explore feelings of survivor guilt and self-blame
2. Address the client's struggle to develop coping skills and sources of support
3. Determine if a history of child abuse prevents discussion of concerns and life events
4. Discuss if the family or other people hold him responsible for what happened

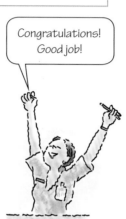

Congratulations! Good job!

98. 1. The client needs to recognize that his survival may have been due to chance and not due to a personal action or inaction. Developing coping skills and sources of support do not assist this client with his feelings. Determining if the client has a history of being abused as a child is best asked in a one-on-one interaction, or done in an assessment session prior to a group session. Prior to discussing the involvement and feelings of other people, the client needs to express his feelings about the trauma.

CN: Psychosocial integrity; CNS: None; CL: Apply

CN: Client needs category   CNS: Client needs subcategory   CL: Cognitive level

Chapter 15

Cognitive Disorders

This chapter covers a host of cognitive disorders. Are your own cognitive powers ready? OK, let's go!

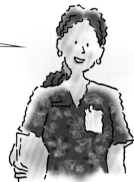

1. The nurse is asking a client in the psychiatric crisis unit specific questions about recent substance use. Which assessment finding could indicate, to the nurse, that this client is experiencing mild to moderate delirium?
1. Time and place disorientation
2. Impaired abstract thinking
3. Persistent memory disturbance
4. Changes in personality

2. The nurse is explaining the symptoms of dementia to a family member who has not seen his mother in 15 months. Which characteristics of neurocognitive disorder due to Alzheimer's disease would the nurse address in the teaching session? Select all that apply.
1. Experiences an impending sense of doom
2. Forgets that food is cooking on the stove
3. Becomes lost walking on her own street
4. Unable to write and to sign her name
5. Begins to fear using public transportation
6. Unable to understand new information

1. 1. Clients with delirium experience disorientation to time, place, and person. Impaired abstract thinking, and noted changes in personality are characteristics of dementia. Persistent memory disturbance is associated with an amnestic disorder.
CN: Physiological integrity; CNS: Physiological adaptation;
CL: Analyze

2. 2, 3, 4, 6. Common symptoms of neurocognitive disorder due to Alzheimer's disease include forgetting things such as cooking food, and where specific items were placed, becoming lost in a familiar neighborhood, being unable to write or sign a document, and the inability to understand new information. A client experiencing an impending sense of doom and fearing public transportation is most likely dealing with a panic attack with agoraphobia.
CN: Health promotion and maintenance; CNS: None;
CL: Apply

CN: Client needs category   CNS: Client needs subcategory   CL: Cognitive level

3. During an interaction with the spouse of a client with neurocognitive disorder due to Alzheimer's disease, the nurse is asked, "What exactly is Alzheimer's disease?" Which is the correct explanation of this disease?

1. Alzheimer's disease is often a combination of several common autoimmune diseases that attack and shrink brain tissue.
2. It is a brain disease that results from the development of abnormal structures called neurofibrillary tangles found in the person's brain.
3. Alzheimer's is a genetic disease that changes a person's brain tissue, causing it to deteriorate due to an accumulation of excessive fluid.
4. A biological and psychosocial component of undiagnosed moderate depression is causing a steady decline in daily performance.

4. A home health nurse notices that the older adult client with diabetes, who she sees weekly, is starting to demonstrate some difficulty answering questions about her chronic disease strategies and self-management activities. Which action would the nurse take to validate her suspicion that her client is experiencing cognitive changes, and may be showing the early stages of dementia?

1. Speak to the health care provider about ordering cardiac diagnostic studies
2. Have a social worker arrange for a weekly home health aide
3. Request that another nurse visit and perform a mental status exam
4. Arrange to speak to a consistent family caregiver as soon as possible

5. A nurse is caring for a client with delirium. Which nursing interventions are important to implement after establishing a safe client environment? Select all that apply.

1. Talking about self-care needs
2. Offering recreational activities
3. Providing a structured environment
4. Instituting measures to promote sleep
5. Distracting the focus away from others

6. A client with dementia is about to eat his dinner. He picks up his spoon, looks at it, puts it down, and then picks up his fork, looks at it, and puts it back on the table. He sits staring at the utensils and his dinner. How should the nurse interpret this behavior?

1. A risk for altered nutrition
2. A disruption in metabolic functioning
3. A disturbance in executive functioning
4. A potential sensory-motor deficit

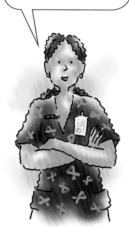

The answer is on the tip of my tongue, but I just can't remember.

3. 2. People with neurocognitive disorder due to Alzheimer's disease have abnormal structures composed of twisted protein fibers called neurofibrillary tangles found within the nerve cells of the brain. These neurofibrillary tangles attack the inside of the neurons. The possible link to autoimmune diseases, as well as the genetic errors identified on chromosomes 14, 19, and 21, and biological and neurochemical problems are currently being investigated.
CN: Physiological integrity; CNS: Physiological adaptation; CL: Analyze

4. 4. By speaking to the consistent family caregiver, that person may be able to validate the presence of the slow and progressive changes that occur in the early stages of dementia. In these stages, the client will have recurrent memory impairment and will attempt to hide these cognitive losses. The nurse should communicate these changes to a provider, not to request a cardiac workup. The need for a home health aide can be addressed when speaking to the caregiver, rather than having a social worker act independently without family consultation. There is no need to request a different home health nurse to perform a mental status assessment.
CN: Safe, effective care environment; CNS: Management of care; CL: Apply

5. 2, 3, 4. After providing a safe environment for the client with delirium, it would be appropriate for the nurse to offer recreational activities, provide a structured environment, and institute measures to promote sleep.
CN: Safe, effective care environment; CNS: Management of care; CL: Analyze

6. 3. The client's inability to initiate activities or perform routine tasks are examples of loss of the ability to think and reason abstractly. A disturbance or interference in this client's executive functioning has occurred. This behavior does not indicate a problem with nutrition or with metabolic or sensory-motor functioning.
CN: Physiological integrity; CNS: Physiological adaptation; CL: Analyze

CN: Client needs category   CNS: Client needs subcategory   CL: Cognitive level

7. The family of a client with increasing dementia asks the nurse, "How can we convince our sibling that dementia is causing our mother's personality to change?" Which information would help this sibling understand the personality changes that occur with dementia? Select all that apply.
1. Loss of interest in surroundings
2. Lack of consideration for others
3. Difficulty learning new things
4. Disregard for the concept of time
5. Inability to do things in sequence
6. Decreased performance of daily activities

8. Which intervention should help a client, diagnosed with neurocognitive disorder due to Alzheimer's disease, perform activities of daily living?
1. Have the client perform all basic care without help
2. Tell the client that morning care must be completed by 9 am
3. Give the client a written list of activities he is expected to do
4. Encourage the client, and give ample time to complete basic tasks

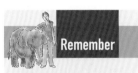

A gentle, calm approach is comforting and nonthreatening.

9. The nurse has taught a family about the medication donepezil. The nurse determines that teaching has been successful when the family states:
1. "We'll need to figure out a schedule to get dad's weekly blood work done."
2. "When dad's Alzheimer's disease worsens, he will need to stop taking this drug."
3. "This drug may slow dad's pulse, since he has pre-existing heart disease."
4. "Donepezil acts like a diuretic, so dad should take it in the morning."

10. The home health nurse is speaking to the wife of a client with neurocognitive disorder due to Alzheimer's disease. The client has been taking donepezil. The nurse is **most** concerned when the caregiver states:
1. "In the last few days, the main thing that my husband wants to eat is bread."
2. "Yesterday, I managed to weigh my husband, and he has lost 8 lbs this month."
3. "Somehow, this medication has been making my husband sleep longer in the morning."
4. "My husband no longer has any interest in listening to the radio with me."

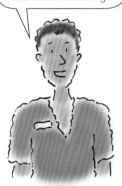

Remember

"Donepezil helps solve the puzzle of dementia."

This drug is an anticholinesterase that is used to treat mild to moderate dementia in patients with Alzheimer disease. Other drugs in this class include the following:
• Ambenonium
• Galantamine
• Edrophonium
• Neostigmine
• Physostigmine
• Pyridostigmine
• Rivastigmine
• Tacrine

7. 1, 2. Clients with dementia often manifest a loss of interest in their surroundings, a lack of consideration for others, and a tendency to be self-absorbed. Having difficulty learning new things and the loss, or disregard, for the concept of time are cognitive changes that occur in dementia. The inability to do things in an orderly sequence, and the decreased performance of daily activities indicate the functional changes seen in clients with dementia.
CN: Physiological integrity; CNS: Physiological adaptation; CL: Apply

8. 4. Clients with Alzheimer's disease respond to the effect of those around them. A gentle, calm approach is comforting and nonthreatening. A tense, hurried approach may agitate the client. This client has problems performing independently. The inherent expectations of deadlines and activity lists may lead to frustration.
CN: Physiological integrity; CNS: Basic care and comfort; CL: Apply

9. 3. Donepezil has the potential to cause bradycardia in clients with cardiac disease. Weekly blood work is not necessary. Donepezil can be used for mild, moderate, or severe Alzheimer's disease. It does not act like a diuretic, and can cause urinary retention.
CN: Physiological integrity; CNS: Pharmacological and parenteral therapies; CL: Apply

10. 2. A side effect of donepezil is weight loss, and it would be important to discuss the weight loss with the primary care provider. The desire to eat bread, the ability to sleep longer, and the lack of interest in listening to the radio are not changes related to the use of donepezil.
CN: Physiological integrity; CNS: Pharmacological and parenteral therapies; CL: Analyze

CN: Client needs category   CNS: Client needs subcategory   CL: Cognitive level

11. Which nursing intervention would help a client with progressive memory deficit function in his environment?
1. Help the client do simple tasks by giving step-by-step directions
2. Avoid frustrating the client by performing basic care routines for her
3. Stimulate the client's intellectual functioning by discussing new topics daily
4. Promote the client's sense of humor by discussing cartoons in a magazine

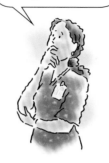

Mmmmm? Let me think about what you said.

11. 1. Clients with cognitive impairment should do tasks within their capabilities. By receiving simple directions in a step-by-step fashion, the client can better process information and perform tasks. Stimulation of intellect can be accomplished by discussing familiar topics with the client. Discussing of new topics may add to the client's confusion. Clients with cognitive impairment may not be able to understand cartoons, and this may add to their confusion.
CN: Psychosocial integrity; CNS: None; CL: Apply

12. Which intervention is a **priority** for the nurse who is providing care to a client diagnosed with neurocognitive disorder due to Alzheimer's disease?
1. Avoid physical contact with the client
2. Confine the client to his room after 8:00 pm
3. Provide a high level of sensory stimulation
4. Monitor the client's activities carefully

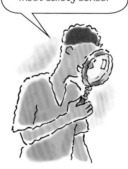

Look for the answer that makes the most safety sense.

12. 4. Whenever a client's safety is at risk, careful observation and supervision are of ultimate importance to avoid injury. Physical contact is implemented during basic care. Confining the client may cause agitation and combativeness. A high level of sensory stimulation may be too stimulating and distracting.
CN: Safe, effective care environment; CNS: Management of care; CL: Apply

13. Which nursing intervention is **most** important while caring for a client diagnosed with neurocognitive disorder due to Alzheimer's disease?
1. Provide the client with a balanced schedule for sleep, rest and activity
2. Supervise favorite food selections for the client's enjoyment of meals
3. Initiate client meetings with other clients for social interactions
4. Encourage the client to independently perform daily physical care

13. 1. After meeting safety concerns, it is important for the nurse to provide the client with a balanced schedule for sleep, rest and activity. The other options may be part of care for a client with Alzheimer's disease, but they are not the priority.
CN: Safe, effective care environment; CNS: Physiological integrity; CL: Apply

14. The nurse administered haloperidol to a client with dementia. The client was experiencing severe agitation. Which adverse effects should the nurse to assess this client for? Select all that apply.
1. Photosensitivity
2. Bradycardia
3. Urinary output
4. Skin irritations
5. Insomnia
6. Dizziness

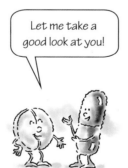

Let me take a good look at you!

14. 1, 3, 6. A client taking haloperidol must be monitored for photosensitivity reactions to sunlight, urinary retention, dizziness, and drowsiness. Haloperidol does not cause bradycardia, dermatological problems, or disturbances in sleep.
CN: Physiological integrity; CNS: Physiological adaptation; CL: Apply

15. A client, diagnosed with neurocognitive disorder due to Alzheimer's disease, tells the nurse that today she has a luncheon date with her daughter. The daughter is, in fact, not visiting that day. Which response, by the nurse, would be **most** appropriate?
1. "Where and when are you planning on having your lunch?"
2. "You're confused and don't know what you're saying."
3. "I think you need some more medication, and I'll bring it to you."
4. "Today is Monday, March 8, and you'll eat lunch in the dining room today."

15. 4. The nurse should reorient the client to the date and environment. Humoring the client isn't therapeutic. Medication won't provide immediate relief for memory impairment. Confrontation can provoke an outburst.
CN: Psychosocial integrity; CNS: None; CL: Apply

16. During a visit to the outpatient clinic, a wife asks the nurse if she should be concerned that her 80-year-old husband consistently refers to items as "whatchamacallits." What is the nurse's **best** response?
1. "Sometimes, a change in cognitive functioning is occurring when a person has difficulty finding the right word to say."
2. "You need to write down the word you think your husband wanted to say when he says whatchamacallit."
3. "Tell me if he also has periods of dizziness, balance problems, and walks leaning forward with an unsteady gait."
4. "I don't think you need to worry about this, as it is an unpleasant but normal behavior associated with aging."

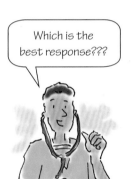

Which is the best response???

16. 1. Many people with dementia experience changes in cognitive functioning, such as increasing and persistent forgetfulness, difficulty finding the right word to say, and trouble with abstract thinking. Writing down forgotten words, asking about other physical problems, and minimizing the caregiver's concern do not address the caregiver's question.
CN: Physiological integrity; CNS: Physiological adaptation; CL: Apply

17. A 65-year-old man recovering from a mild stroke questions the nurse about his risk for vascular dementia. What is the nurse's **best** response?
1. "It is hard to predict the risk factors for vascular dementia, since anything that affects your heart and your circulation also increases your risk for vascular dementia."
2. "The factors that increase your risk of stroke, such as hypertension, high cholesterol, and smoking, will also increase your risk for vascular dementia."
3. "Usually, only the people who suffer from traumatic brain injuries are the ones who will develop vascular dementia as they age."
4. "I suggest that you request a diagnostic workup and a brain magnetic resonance imaging study from your primary care provider."

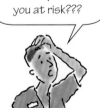

What places you at risk???

17. 2. Controlling hypertension, high cholesterol levels, and not smoking will decrease the risk for vascular dementia. The other options present incorrect information. Risk factors are known. Other people, in addition to those with brain injuries, can develop vascular dementia. Talking to your provider about a diagnostic workup does not address lifestyle risks.
CN: Physiological integrity; CNS: Physiological adaptation; CL: Apply

CN: Client needs category   CNS: Client needs subcategory   CL: Cognitive level

18. A nurse is teaching the family of a client with who has progressed to mid stage dementia. What is the **most** appropriate way for the nurse to explain the progression of dementia to this family?
   1. Increased forgetfulness, slight difficulty concentrating, decreased work performance
   2. Difficulty concentrating, decreased memory of recent events, and difficulties managing finances or traveling alone to new locations.
   3. No ability to speak or communicate
   4. Loss of intellectual abilities sufficient to impair the ability to perform basic care

18. 4. Clients in mid stage dementia require extensive assistance to carry out daily activities and self care. They start to forget names of close family members and have little memory of recent events. Mild cognitive decline occurs when a client has increased forgetfulness, slight difficulty concentrating, and decreased work performance. Early stage dementia is difficulty concentrating, decreased memory of recent events, and difficulties managing finances or traveling alone to new locations. In late stage dementia the client may have no ability to speak or communicate
CN: Physiological integrity; CNS: Physiological adaptation; CL: Apply

19. While interacting with a client who is suspected of having a dementia disorder, the nurse asks, "What was on your tray for breakfast?" This question allows the nurse to assess:
   1. food preferences.
   2. recent memory.
   3. remote memory.
   4. speech clarity.

19. 2. A person with dementia will have difficulty with recent memory or learning, which may be a key to early detection. Assessing food preferences may be helpful in determining what the client likes to eat, but this assessment has no direct correlation in assessing dementia. Speech difficulties, such as rambling, irrelevance, and incoherence, may be related to delirium.
CN: Health promotion and maintenance; CNS: None; CL: Apply

20. The client states, "Just because I get a little confused at times, my doctor told my wife that I have the beginnings of Alzheimer's disease!" What is the nurse's **most** appropriate response?
   1. "Anyone who has struggled with health problems can easily have periods of confusion, but it may be premature to be diagnosed with Alzheimer's disease."
   2. "The symptoms of Alzheimer's disease occur over time and in stages. In the beginning, forgetfulness and confusion are often experienced."
   3. "A diagnosis of Alzheimer's disease is a serious health concern. I suggest that you and your wife meet to discuss this with the health care provider."
   4. "You should be worried about this, and your health care provider should not have had this discussion with only your wife."

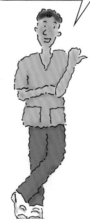

You're already at question 20 and doing great. Keep going!

20. 2. Loss of short-term memory, forgetfulness, and increasing levels of confusion are the characteristics of the early phases of Alzheimer's disease. As the symptoms progress, they become more obvious, and the person can become more defensive and depressed. The other options do not give the client information about Alzheimer's disease, or help to explain the disease process.
CN: Health promotion and maintenance; CNS: None; CL: Analyze

CN: Client needs category   CNS: Client needs subcategory   CL: Cognitive level

21. The nurse is teaching a client and his family about cognitive vascular impairment that occurs when a person has vascular dementia. Which comment, by a family member, would indicate the need for additional teaching?

1. "The vision and speech problems that dad has are part of his vascular dementia."
2. "Now I know that inadequate blood flow to the brain affects the ability to think."
3. "It's good to know that vascular dementia is nothing like Alzheimer's disease."
4. "I understand how regular strokes and small strokes can cause changes in the brain."

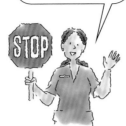

This question is asking specifically about vascular dementia.

21. 3. Vascular dementia and Alzheimer's disease are both types of dementias. Vascular dementia is ranked as the second most common cause of dementia after Alzheimer's disease. The other statements are all true about vascular dementia.
CN: Physiological integrity; CNS: Physiological adaptation; CL: Analyze

22. The family of a client recently admitted with vascular dementia asks the nurse about the cause of the client's condition. What would be the **most** accurate response by the nurse?

1. It is caused by high blood pressure.
2. It is caused by low oxygen levels.
3. It is caused by an infection.
4. It is caused by toxins.

22. 1. Vascular dementia is a result of small strokes that can either destroy or damage cerebral tissue. Strokes may be caused by high blood pressure, high cholesterol levels, heart disease, or diabetes. Hypoxia, infection, and toxins are not causes of dementia.
CN: Physiological integrity; CNS: Physiological adaptation; CL: Apply

23. During the admission assessment, the nurse focuses on the client's reflexes, muscle strength, coordination, eye movements, and mental status. What symptoms would the nurse identify as suggestive of vascular dementia? Select all that apply.

1. Swinging leg
2. Losing bladder control
3. Laughing inappropriately
4. Shuffling gait
5. Hyperextending the head
6. Aching joint deformities

23. 2, 3, 4. The typical symptoms of vascular dementia are confusion, memory deficits, wandering, shuffling gait, loss of bladder and bowel control, and inappropriate laughter. Leg swinging, head hyperextension, and joint deformities are not symptoms associated with vascular dementia.
CN: Physiological integrity; CNS: Physiological adaptation; CL: Analyze

24. The spouse of a client diagnosed with vascular dementia asks the nurse how this disorder differs from neurocognitive disorder due to Alzheimer's disease. Which response is **most** appropriate?

1. Vascular dementia can have an insidious onset, or a more abrupt onset, depending on the change in blood flow to the brain.
2. Vascular dementia can be treated with medications to improve the prognosis and prevent further circulatory decline.
3. Personality change is a common characteristic seen in vascular dementia, and frequently occurs in the final stages of the disease.
4. The inability to perform motor activities, and language difficulties occur in the severe stage of vascular dementia.

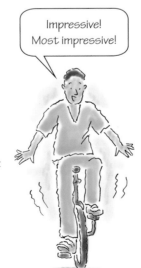

Impressive! Most impressive!

24. 1. Vascular dementia differs from Alzheimer's disease because it can have either an abrupt, or insidious, onset depending on the disruption of blood flow to the brain. Vascular dementia has a poor prognosis and can shorten the client's lifespan. Personality change is common in Alzheimer's disease. The inability to carry out motor activities and language difficulties are common in Alzheimer's disease.
CN: Health promotion and maintenance; CNS: None; CL: Analyze

CN: Client needs category   CNS: Client needs subcategory   CL: Cognitive level

25. Which type of dementia occurs as series of small strokes over a long period of time?
1. Alzheimer's dementia
2. Parkinson's dementia
3. Substance-induced dementia
4. Vascular dementia

25. 4. Vascular dementia is caused by a series of small strokes over a long period. Vascular dementia is also called multi-infarct dementia. Vascular dementia differs from Alzheimer's disease in that vascular dementia has a more abrupt onset and progresses in steps. At times, the vascular dementia seems to ease, and the individual shows fairly lucid thinking. Alzheimer's has a slow onset with a progressively deteriorating course. Dementia of Parkinson's sometimes resembles the dementia of Alzheimer's disease. Substance-induced dementia is related to the persisting effects of the substance.
CN: Physiological integrity; CNS: Physiological adaptation; CL: Analyze

26. A client's grandson, a biology major in college, asks the nurse what pathologic change in the brain causes Alzheimer's disease. What is the nurse's **best** response?
1. Impairment in glucose metabolism
2. Atrophy of the frontal lobe of the brain
3. Degeneration of the cholinergic system
4. Intracranial bleeding in the limbic system

26. 3. Research related to Alzheimer's disease indicates that the enzyme needed to produce acetylcholine is dramatically reduced. The other pathophysiologic changes don't cause the symptoms of Alzheimer's disease.
CN: Physiological integrity; CNS: Physiological adaptation; CL: Analyze

27. An elderly client has experienced memory and attention deficits that have developed over a three-day period. The nurse is aware that these symptoms are characteristic of:
1. Alzheimer's disease.
2. amnesia syndrome.
3. delirium.
4. dementia.

27. 3. Delirium is characterized by an abrupt onset of fluctuating levels of awareness, clouded consciousness, perceptual disturbances, and disturbed memory and orientation. Alzheimer's disease is a progressive dementia. Amnesia refers to recent short- and long-term memory loss. Dementia is characterized by a general impairment in intellectual functioning, and occurs in a progressive, irreversible course.
CN: Physiological integrity; CNS: Physiological adaptation; CL: Apply

28. An extended family is composed of children in elementary school and high school, grandparents, and an unmarried adult brother. Which age group is at **highest** risk for developing a state of delirium?
1. Adolescent
2. Elderly
3. Middle-aged
4. School-aged

Age is an important factor when assessing a client.

28. 2. The elderly population, is highly susceptible to delirium because of normal physiologic changes.
CN: Health promotion and maintenance; CNS: None; CL: Apply

29. An elderly client is experiencing visual and auditory hallucinations. Which assessment finding would the nurse document in the client's health care record?
1. Conflict with family members
2. Feelings of role inadequacy
3. Inability to communicate
4. Misinterpreting environmental stimuli

30. The nurse is teaching a group of caregivers, who live with family members who have mild to moderate changes in their cognitive functioning. Which goal will the nurse identify as a **priority** of care for the family members?
1. Promote frequent socialization
2. Maintain optimal physical health
3. Provide frequent changes in caregivers
4. Provide a stimulating environment

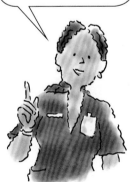

Sometimes we're not a good combination.

31. A newly admitted client, diagnosed with delirium, has a history of hypertension and anxiety. The client had been taking digoxin, furosemide, and diazepam. The nurse suspects that this client's impairment may be the result of:
1. opportunistic infection.
2. metabolic acidosis.
3. drug intoxication.
4. hepatic encephalopathy.

32. A client who has experienced cerebral hypoxia demonstrates sensory-perceptual alterations. Which environment would the nurse create for this client?
1. A softly lit room around the clock with the curtains kept open
2. A brightly lit room around the clock with the curtains closed
3. A low-lit room situated near the nurses' station with soft background music
4. A well-lit room without glare during the day and a darkened room for sleeping

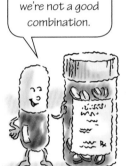

Your clients depend on you for meeting their environmental needs as well as their physical ones.

29. 4. The client is experiencing visual and auditory hallucinations related to an inaccurate perception of sensory stimulation associated with the environment. The other options don't address the hallucinations the client is experiencing.
CN: Safe, effective care environment; CNS: Psychosocial integrity; CL: Analyze

30. 2. A client's cognitive impairment may hinder self-care abilities. More socialization, frequent changes in caregivers, and a stimulating environment would only increase anxiety and confusion.
CN: Health promotion and maintenance; CNS: None; CL: Apply

31. 3. Digoxin, furosemide, and diazepam have a propensity for producing delirium.
CN: Physiological integrity; CNS: Physiological adaptation; CL: Analyze

32. 4. A quiet, shadow-free environment produces the fewest sensory-perceptual distortions for a client with cognitive impairment associated with delirium.
CN: Psychosocial integrity; CNS: None; CL: Apply

33. As a nurse enters a client's room, the client says, "They're crawling on my sheets! Get them off my bed!" The nurse interprets this assessment finding as:
1. aphasia.
2. dysarthria.
3. illusions.
4. hallucinations.

33. 4. The presence of a false sensory stimulus correlates with the definition of a hallucination. Aphasia refers to a communications problem. Dysarthria is difficulty in speech production. Illusions are incorrectly perceived sensory stimuli.
CN: Psychosocial integrity; CNS: None; CL: Apply

34. A delirious client is shouting for someone to get the bugs off her. Which response by the nurse is the **most** appropriate?
1. "Don't worry. I'll stay here and talk to you while I brush the bugs away for you."
2. "You need to try and relax. The crawling sensation will go away sooner if you can relax."
3. "There are no bugs on your legs or in the bed. It's just your imagination playing tricks on you."
4. "I see that you are frightened, and I will stay with you. I don't see any bugs crawling on you."

34. 4. Never argue about hallucinations with a client. Instead, promote an environment of trust and safety by acknowledging the client's perceptions.
CN: Physiological integrity; CNS: Basic care and comfort; CL: Apply

35. The nurse is discussing the goal of learning social skills with a client who has bipolar disorder. Which statements indicate the client is making positive progress? Select all that apply.
1. "Last night I didn't make excuses about not being able to pay for the food."
2. "What I did yesterday was impulsive, but he made me so angry and upset."
3. "I gave my friend a compliment and didn't talk about my needs."
4. "At the party this person was getting all the attention, so I just went home."
5. "Sometimes it isn't worth the effort to be friendly and to try to please people."

35. 1, 3. Not making excuses, and not giving compliments attached to requests for favors are indicative of the client attempting to stop his manipulative behavior. Saying that it was just luck is an example of disqualifying the positive. Being impulsive and losing control indicate that more work on developing social skills is needed. Feeling jealous of others and leaving a social situation is indicative of needing to develop additional social skills. Not wanting to be friendly and feeling like one has to please people indicates that additional social skills are needed.
CN: Health promotion and maintenance; CNS: None; CL: Analyze

36. The nurse explains to the client and his family that the changes occurring in Alzheimer's disease are irreversible. Which is/are an expected neurological change of aging?
1. Widening of the central sulci
2. Depletion of neurotransmitters
3. Neurofibrillary tangles and plaques
4. Degeneration of the temporal lobes

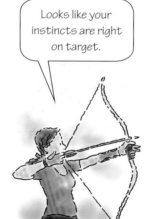

Looks like your instincts are right on target.

36. 3. Aging isn't necessarily associated with significant decline, but neurofibrillary tangles and plaques are expected age-related changes. These occurrences are sometimes referred to as benign senescent forgetfulness, or age-associated memory impairment.
CN: Physiological integrity; CNS: Physiological adaptation; CL: Apply

37. The nurse is teaching a caregiver how to effectively interact with her older adult parent who suffers from impaired memory and judgment. What is the **most** important information for the nurse to provide? Select all that apply.
1. "Perform all your parent's care and activities of daily living."
2. "Speak slowly and use understandable words and phrases."
3. "Keep music playing to promote environmental stimulation."
4. "Allow ample time for your parent to respond to a question."
5. "Orient and re-orient your parent as needed throughout the day."
6. "Approach your parent from the front when beginning a conversation."

37. 2, 4, 5, 6. When interacting with a parent who has cognitive impairment, a person should speak slowly and use simple, understandable language, allow ample time for a reply, orient and re-orient as needed, and approach the parent from an angle where the speaker can be seen. The caregiver must not provide care and activities that the parent can perform. The caregiver should provide a low-stimulus environment, so continuous music would cause agitation.
CN: Physiological integrity; CNS: Physiological adaptation; CL: Apply

38. During morning care, a nurse asks a client with dementia, "How was your night?" The client replies, "My husband and I went out to dinner and a movie and had a wonderful evening!" The nurse interprets the client's statement as:
1. interpretation.
2. perseveration.
3. confabulation.
4. disorientation.

38. 3. Confabulation is the process in which an individual makes up stories to answer questions. It's considered a defensive tactic to protect the individual's self-esteem and prevent others from noticing the memory loss. Interpretation is assigning meaning and understanding to a question in order to reply appropriately. Perseveration is persistent repetition of the same word or idea in response to different questions. Disorientation is a state of mental confusion characterized by incorrect perceptions of time, place, or person.
CN: Psychosocial integrity; CNS: None; CL: Apply

39. A nursing student tells the nurse that a client with amnesia looks fine, but responds to questions in a vague, distant manner. The nursing student then asks how she should take care of this client. Which response is the **most** appropriate?
1. "Give her ample time and plenty of space to test her independence."
2. "Keep her busy and make sure she doesn't take naps during the day."
3. "Whenever you think she needs direction, use short, simple sentences."
4. "Spend as much time talking as you can with her and ask her questions."

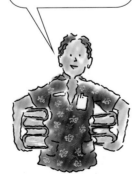

Teaching nursing students helps to improve the quality of care they provide.

39. 3. Confusion, anxiety, and disruptions in the ability to perform basic care are often apparent in clients with amnesia. Offering simple directions to promote daily functions and reduce confusion may help to increase feelings of safety and security. Giving this client ample time and plenty of space may make her feel insecure. Excessive talking, and asking questions that she won't be able to answer will intensify her anxiety level. There is no significant rationale for keeping this client busy all day with no rest periods. This action will make the client tired and less functional at performing other basic tasks.
CN: Safe, effective care environment; CNS: Management of care; CL: Apply

40. The nurse is assessing an older adult client diagnosed with amnestic disorder related to a traumatic head trauma. Which assessment finding can be expected during the nurse's interaction with this client?

1. Speech patterns are altered and difficult to understand.
2. The inability to concentrate occurs since diagnosis.
3. There is a noted disruption in intellectual functioning.
4. Recent recall of life events is severely impaired.

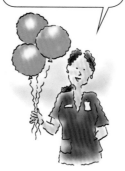

Well done! You made it to question 40.

40. 4. The primary area affected in an amnestic disorder is memory. The client cannot recall previously learned information or learn new information. All other areas of cognition will be normal.

CN: Physiological integrity; CNS: Physiological adaptation; CL: Analyze

41. A client with mild neurocognitive disorder due to Alzheimer's disease would like to continue living at home with his extended family. What is the **most** appropriate nursing intervention?

1. Provide mandated written directions for all activities of daily living
2. Obtain a provider's order for either a mild anxiolytic or sleeping pill
3. Advise the client to attend occupational therapy three times a week
4. Maintain a stable, predictable environment and daily routine

41. 4. Clients in the early stages of Alzheimer's disease remain fairly functional with familiar surroundings and a predictable routine. They become easily disoriented with surprises and social overstimulation. Requiring that a client in the early stages of Alzheimer's disease follow mandated written directions for daily activities is unnecessary and disempowering. Anxiolytics or sleeping medication can impair memory and worsen the problem. Advising the client to attend occupational therapy is nonproductive and will serve to frustrate and fatigue the client.

CN: Safe and effective care environment; CNS: Management of care; CL: Apply

42. The nurse is providing care to a client with Alzheimer's-type dementia. Which nursing intervention is the **priority**?

1. Establish a routine that reinforces memories and supports former habits
2. Maintain an environment with cheerful and pleasant surroundings
3. Structure a daily and precise routine that can be used after discharge
4. Control the environment by providing structure and consistent boundaries

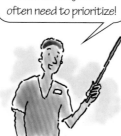

As a nurse, you will often need to prioritize!

42. 4. By controlling the environment and providing structure and consistent boundaries, the nurse is helping to keep the client safe and secure. Establishing a routine that reinforces memories, supports former habits, maintains pleasant surroundings, and structures a daily routine fosters a supportive environment; however, keeping the client safe and secure is the priority.

CN: Safe, effective care environment; CNS: Management of care; CL: Apply

43. The wife of a client with neurocognitive disorder due to Alzheimer's disease reports that she often finds her husband wandering in the backyard in the middle of the night looking for their dog who died 10 years ago. The wife states, "I haven't had a good night's sleep in months." What is the nurse's **most** appropriate response?

1. "Let's talk about having a caregiver look after your husband at night."
2. "Do you know that sleep deprivation may cause you to develop Alzheimer's disease?"
3. "This is a sign that your husband can no longer be cared for in your home."
4. "Learning how to communicate with your husband will keep him calm at night."

43. 1. This wife needs to get uninterrupted sleep while feeling secure that her spouse is safe. Obtaining a night time caregiver is an important option to discuss. Sleep deprivation does not cause Alzheimer's disease, but it can temporarily impair memory, and contribute to cognitive changes. Wandering behavior is not a sign that care can no longer be given at home. It is a sign that the client's safety and security needs must be met, and that the needs of the caregiver must also be met. Effective couple communication will not stop the spouse's wandering behavior.

CN: Safe, effective care environment; CNS: Management of care; CL: Analyze

CN: Client needs category   CNS: Client needs subcategory   CL: Cognitive level

44. A client experiencing delirium makes inaccurate interpretations of the hospital environment. What is the **most** appropriate nursing intervention?

1. Obtain an order for soft restraints to use as needed
2. Discuss the positive and negative aspects of being on the hospital unit
3. Identify the client's emotional needs and find strategies to meet them
4. Talk to the client about the place where he is and the people there

44. 4. Talking about real people, and where the client currently is, will orient and assist this client. It also alleviates the frustration and confusion associated with a loss of contact with reality. Obtaining an order to use soft restraints can confuse and anger the client. The client's thought process is impaired with delirium, so it is non-productive to discuss the hospital unit with him. Safety and maintaining physiologic integrity are the most important needs for this client. Once the client's physical needs are met, his emotional needs can be addressed.

CN: Safe, effective care environment; CNS: Management of care; CL: Analyze

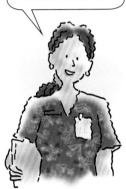

Be sure to pick all of the interventions that are needed.

45. The nurse institutes measures to prevent accidental injury for a client with neurocognitive disorder due to Alzheimer's disease. Which interventions should the nurse perform? Select all that apply.

1. Stay with the client when he is ambulating
2. Monitor one-to-one interactions to prevent conflict
3. Have client wear a medical identification bracelet
4. Prevent the client from accessing cigarettes and matches
5. Encourage the client to verbalize feelings of anger

45. 1, 3, 4. The actions that the nurse will take are based on promoting well-being and safety. Accompany the client during ambulation ensures safety. Wearing a medical identification bracelet provides client safety information if it is needed. Prevention of access to cigarettes and matches eliminates the possibility of sustaining a burn or starting a fire. Social interactions are usually limited, as this client exhibits deficits in executive functioning and in language, and has difficulty verbalizing feelings.

CN: Safe and effective Care; CNS: Safety; CL: Apply

46. The nurse is reviewing the chart of a man admitted with an amnestic disorder. Which medical condition may be associated with an amnestic disorder?

1. Drug overdose
2. Cerebral anoxia
3. Anticonvulsant medication
4. Environmental toxins

46. 2. A variety of medical conditions are related to amnestic disorders, such as head trauma, stroke, cerebral neoplastic disease, herpes simplex, encephalitis, poorly-controlled insulin-dependent diabetes, and cerebral anoxia. The other three options are substance induced.

CN: Physiological integrity; CNS: Physiological adaptation; CL: Apply

47. The nurse is preparing to teach a group of caregivers about medication management for family members with Alzheimer's disease. What is the **most** important information for the nurse to include? Select all that apply.

1. Determine if the client is able to safely self-medicate
2. Visually inspect the mouth after giving a pill
3. Use one pharmacy for all of the client's prescriptions
4. Be certain that this client can swallow a pill
5. Consult with the pharmacy about altering the dosage
6. Know what to do if the client refuses to take the medication.

47. 1, 2, 3, 4, 6. A teaching plan would include evaluating whether the client is able to safely self-medicate, performing a visual mouth inspection after giving a pill, using only one pharmacy for all of the client's prescriptions, checking that the client can swallow a pill, and knowing what to do if the client refuses to take the medication. The caregiver should consult with the pharmacist about obtaining an alternative form of the drug if the client can no longer swallow a pill or capsule. The health care provider would be consulted to change the medication dose.

CN: Health promotion and maintenance; CNS: None; CL: Analyze

CN: Client needs category   CNS: Client needs subcategory   CL: Cognitive level

48. The home health nurse is consulting with a family about creating a safe environment in their home for a person who has Alzheimer's disease. What is the **most** important information for the nurse to provide? Select all that apply.

1. Keep all household cleaning products in a locked cabinet
2. Supervise the client when cooking or fixing a snack
3. Place all matches and cigarette lighters in a safe place
4. Install locks on places where garden equipment is kept
5. Monitor the use of stoves, ovens, and heating appliances
6. Mount heat sensors or smoke detectors in each room

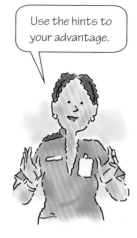

Use the hints to your advantage.

48. 1, 2, 3, 4, 5. To create a safe home environment, the nurse should discuss keeping all household cleaning products in a locked cabinet, supervising the client when cooking or fixing a snack, placing all matches and cigarette lighters in a safe place, installing locks on places where garden equipment is kept, and monitoring the use of stoves, ovens, and heating appliances. Some people place heat sensors beside a stove or oven, but they are not needed in every room. Extra smoke detectors are not required. Smoke detectors are typically placed on each floor of the house, not in each room.

CN: Safe, effective care environment; CNS: Management of care; CL: Apply

49. The client's daughter tells the nurse, "I don't understand the doctor's explanation of my father's transient global amnesia." What are appropriate responses by the nurse? Select all that apply.

1. "Your father will draw a blank when asked about things that happened a day, a month, or a year ago."
2. "Transient global amnesia is usually harmless, and a recurrence is unlikely."
3. "After this type of amnesia, your father will undergo a period of depression and feelings of hopelessness."
4. "Your dad may have a lack of insight and permanent memory problems."
5. "A stroke caused your father's transient global amnesia and sudden, temporary memory loss."
6. "Even though there is memory loss, your dad remembers you, and recognizes the people he knows well."

49. 1, 2, 5, 6. Transient global amnesia is a sudden, temporary episode of memory loss that can be attributed to a more common neurological condition, such as a stroke. During an episode of transient global amnesia, a person's recall of recent events vanishes. The person also draws a blank when asked to remember things that happened a day, a month, or even a year ago. However, the person does recognize familiar people. Transient global amnesia is rare, usually harmless, and unlikely to happen again. Episodes are usually short lived, and returns after the event. After an episode of transient global amnesia, a person does not have a lack of insight, does not experience feelings of depression and hopelessness, and does not have permanent memory problems.

CN: Physiological integrity; CNS: Physiological adaptation; CL: Analyze

50. During a conversation with a client, the nurse observes that he shifts from one topic to the next on a regular basis. Which condition is the client **most** likely experiencing?

1. Flight of ideas
2. Concrete thinking
3. Ideas of reference
4. Loose associations

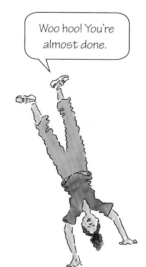

Woo hoo! You're almost done.

50. 4. Loose associations are conversations that constantly shift in topic. Loose associations don't necessarily start in a disorganized way. The conversations can begin cogently, and then become loose. Flight of ideas is characterized by conversation that is disorganized from the onset. Concrete thinking implies a highly definitive thought processes. Ideas of reference are characterized by a delusional belief that things irrelevant to the client, such as newspaper headlines, are referring to the client directly.

CN: Psychosocial integrity; CNS: None; CL: Apply

CN: Client needs category CNS: Client needs subcategory CL: Cognitive level

51. A daughter tells the nurse that she thinks her mother's dementia is becoming worse. Which assessment finding would indicate that this client's dementia is worsening?
1. The client resists logical explanations.
2. The client stops redirecting negative energy.
3. The client maintains a non-defensive position.
4. The client becomes increasingly agitated.

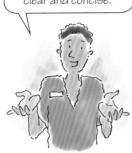

For effective communications, think clear and concise.

52. One goal for the family of a client with Alzheimer's disease is improved communication. What is the **best** way to reach this goal?
1. Don't use humor when communicating with this client
2. Speak to the client in a loud voice
3. Give this client one-step commands
4. Don't touch the client while speaking

53. Immediately following visiting hours, the nurse monitors a client with neurocognitive disorder due to Alzheimer's disease for wandering behaviors. What would cue the nurse that wandering is about to occur?
1. Needing to walk after eating a complete meal
2. Feeling tense due to an uncomfortable situation
3. Demonstrating eccentric behavior
4. Having difficulty following directions

54. Which is the nurse's **priority** goal for a client with dementia who lives in a long-term care facility?
1. Maintaining the client's optimal level of functioning
2. Having the client identify coping methods to handle stress
3. Facilitating client conversation with five people each day
4. Having the client use physical activity to work off aggressive energy

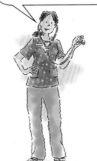

What symptoms should I assess for in a client who may have dementia?

55. A nurse is assessing a client for dementia. What history would the nurse expect to find in a client with dementia? Select all that apply.
1. There's a slow progression of symptoms.
2. The client admits to feelings of sadness.
3. The client acts apathetic and pessimistic.
4. The family can't determine when the symptoms first appeared.
5. There are changes in the client's basic personality.
6. The client has great difficulty paying attention to others.

51. 4. A client with dementia, who becomes increasingly agitated, may be unable to perform expected tasks. Communication must be clear and concise. Giving logical explanations is inappropriate. This client may revert to old ways of coping, and trying to change the client rarely proves successful. The nurse should try to decrease the source of negativity. The client with dementia is rarely defensive.
CN: Psychosocial integrity; CNS: None; CL: Apply

52. 3. Giving this client one-step commands will keep communication simple, clear, concise, and pleasant. Humor must be used judiciously to avoid confusing the client. Speaking in a loud voice may be interpreted as shouting and cause the client agitation. The use of touch may be appropriate, and may reassure and soothe the client.
CN: Psychosocial integrity; CNS: None; CL: Apply

53. 2. Tension and stress may cause a client with Alzheimer's disease to want to flee an uncomfortable situation. Exercise is an important health promotion activity, but it doesn't help explain wandering behavior. Eccentric behavior is rarely related to wandering. Many clients with dementia have difficulty following directions; however, wandering typically results from disorientation.
CN: Psychosocial integrity; CNS: None; CL: Apply

54. 1. The priority goal is to maintain the client's optimal level of functioning. Reducing the client's stress is the nurse's responsibility. Having a conversation with five people each day is unrealistic for this client. Expecting a client with dementia to use physical activity to decrease aggressive energy is also unrealistic.
CN: Safe, effective care environment; CNS: Management of care; CL: Apply

55. 1, 4, 5, 6. Common characteristics of dementia are a slow onset of symptoms, progressing to noticeable changes in the client's personality, and impaired ability to pay attention to other people. Feelings of sadness, apathy, and pessimism are symptoms of depression.
CN: Health promotion and maintenance; CNS: None; CL: Analyze

56. The nurse and client are discussing examples of negative thinking, and how to eliminate negative thought patterns. Which statements indicate cognitive distortions often seen in depressed clients? Select all that apply.

1. The client responds that it was just luck when a peer compliments his success.
2. The client believes that the manager overlooked the mistake that he made.
3. The client knows his parents are angry at him for not getting into a specific college.
4. The client is convinced that he will not get through the interview successfully.
5. The client decides to never drive a car again after he was in an accident.
6. The client reported that there was positive group feedback from all but one person.

56. 1, 3, 4, 5. Saying that it was just luck is an example of disqualifying the positive. Stating that his parents are angry at him for not getting into a specific college is an example of mind reading. Knowing in advance that he will not have a successful interview is fortune telling. Saying he will never drive again because of an accident is an example of catastrophizing. The statement that the manager overlooked a mistake is a positive response to a factual experience. Commenting on the feedback from his peers reflects a realistic appraisal of the situation.
CN: Health promotion and maintenance; CNS: None; CL: Apply

57. The chart entry for a client with bipolar disorder reads:

Progress notes	
2/10/17 1300	The client reported a rash on his chest and back. He denies food, environmental or other allergies. Vital signs: T 98.2, P 88 R 22, BP 128/78.

Based on this chart entry, the nurse reviews the client's current medications. Which medication would the nurses suspect as the cause of the rash?

1. Trazadone
2. Lamotrigine
3. Quetiapine
4. Diphenhydramine

57. 2. Lamotrigine is the drug most likely to cause a rash. Lamotrigine has a warning that it has caused serious, life-threatening rashes, including rash-related deaths. Although any of the other medications can cause an allergic reaction, such as skin rash, hives or other distress, lamotrigine is the drug with the highest hypersensitivity reaction.
CN: Physiological integrity; CNS: Pharmacological and parenteral therapies; CL: Analyze

58. A client with major depressive disorder is grieving a recent loss, and is assessed as having experienced spiritual distress. Prioritize the ways that the nurse integrate spiritual practices into the client's care.

1. Address what can be done to implement practices that may be helpful
2. Ask if the client has participated in past spiritual practices
3. Talk about the client's values and spiritual beliefs
4. Have the client determine if any spiritual practices provide support

58. Ordered Response:

3. Talk about the client's values and spiritual beliefs
2. Ask if the client has participated in past spiritual practices
4. Have the client determine if any spiritual practices provide support
1. Address what can be done to implement practices that may be helpful

CN: Safe, effective care environment; CNS: Management of care; CL: Analyze

---

CN: Client needs category   CNS: Client needs subcategory   CL: Cognitive level

59. The nurse in an outpatient community mental health center is monitoring the effects of a new antidepressant medication administered to a client with a diagnosis of major depressive disorder. Prioritize the steps the nurse would take to monitor this client's medication.

1.	The client is monitored, and a determination of effectiveness is made
2.	The medication is administered and monitored for adverse effects
3.	The duration of the medication regimen is determined
4.	Education is provided about the prescribed medication

59. Ordered Response:

2.	The medication is administered and monitored for adverse effects
4.	Education is provided about the prescribed medication
1.	The client is monitored, and a determination of effectiveness is made
3.	The duration of the medication regimen is determined

CN: Physiological integrity; CNS: Pharmacological and parenteral therapies; CL: Analyze

60. The chart entry for a client in the psychiatric emergency department reads:

Progress notes	
2/10/17 1200	The client was cooperative and cheerful during the first part of the assessment. The client then responded strongly and arrogantly to questions, and became excessively talkative about "needing a new car to be an effective salesman." The family reported that the client was loud, pacing, gesturing frantically, and verbally threatening the client's father for refusing to buy him a car. The client admitted to "not taking my medications for the last three days." Client is admitted to the psychiatric hospital unit. Vital signs: T 98.6, P 100 R 22, BP 128/78.

Based on this chart entry, what additional behaviors might the nurse observe after admission to the unit? Select all that apply.
1. During unit orientation, the client may become easily distracted by others.
2. The client tries to speak to each staff member and other clients on the unit.
3. Non-acceptance and negativity are apparent during the client's interactions.
4. When the nurse sets a limit, the client laughs and interrupts the nurse.
5. The client requires more sleep than usual.

60. **1, 2, 4.** In this hypomanic phase, the client is easily distracted, talks to the staff and other clients, and laughs loudly and interrupts when limits are set for inappropriate behavior. A client who is depressed would verbalize negativity and non-acceptance of self in his interactions. A client experiencing hypomania requires less than the usual amount of sleep.

CN: Safe, effective care environment; CNS: Safety and infection control; CL: Apply

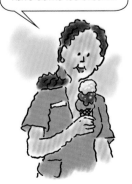

Congratulations, you finished! Now have some ice cream.

CN: Client needs category   CNS: Client needs subcategory   CL: Cognitive level

Chapter 16

Personality Disorders

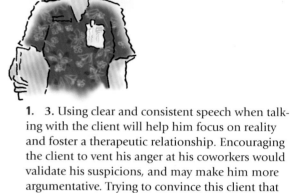

No, this chapter doesn't cover quirks of the rich and famous. It's all about mental disorders affecting the personality. Have a blast!

1. A client tells the nurse that his coworkers are sabotaging his computer. When the nurse asks questions, the client becomes argumentative. What is the **most** appropriate intervention for the nurse to implement?
  1. Encourage the client to vent his anger about his coworkers.
  2. Tell the client that his coworkers haven't touched his computer
  3. Use clear and consistent speech when talking to the client
  4. Tell the client to go to his room and stay there until he calms down

2. A family member of a client with schizoid personality disorder asks the nurse, "Why doesn't my brother want any contact with his family?" Which responses are accurate? Select all that apply.
  1. A person often struggles with their emotions and can become emotional detached.
  2. Due to the chaotic relationships in your brother's early life, he has become irresponsible and asocial.
  3. Clients like your brother are very objective, with no room to consider the emotions of others.
  4. Your brother doesn't obtain pleasure from social encounters.
  5. Your brother gets pleasure from being the center of attention.

1. 3. Using clear and consistent speech when talking with the client will help him focus on reality and foster a therapeutic relationship. Encouraging the client to vent his anger at his coworkers would validate his suspicions, and may make him more argumentative. Trying to convince this client that his coworkers haven't touched his computer, or telling him to go to his room, may make him more defensive.

CN: Psychosocial integrity; CNS: None; CL: Apply

2. 1, 4. Emotional detachment, difficulty in experiencing emotions, and the lack of pleasure derived from social interactions are common characteristics of a person with a schizoid personality disorder. Experiencing chaotic relationships during childhood, and becoming irresponsible and asocial, are characteristic of a person with antisocial personality disorder. A person with paranoid personality disorder is very objective and has no tolerance for the emotions of other people. A person with schizoid personality disorder lacks interest in social relationships and tends toward a solitary lifestyle, not toward being the center of attention.

CN: Psychosocial integrity; CNS: None; CL: Analyze

3. The nurse is assessing a new client who was just admitted to the psychiatric unit. Which assessment questions, by the nurse, would determine if this client has a schizotypal personality disorder? Select all that apply.
1. "Do you often feel that people want to reject you, or think that you're odd?"
2. "Does anxiety make you want to hurt or injure yourself?"
3. "Do you feel that that everyone of the opposite sex finds you extremely attractive?"
4. "Do you feel that other people take advantage of you?"
5. "Have you ever felt like you had special powers or magical influence over others?"
6. "Do you tend to stay by yourself, even though you would like to be with others?"

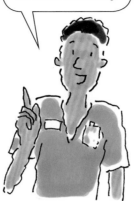

Understanding a client's traits will help you deal with the client effectively.

3. 1, 5, 6. People with schizotypal personality disorder have odd thinking and strange mannerisms, magical thinking, ideas of reference, and they tend to isolate from others. Self-mutilation describes borderline personality disorders. Extreme craving of attention of the opposite sex describes histrionic personality disorders. Histrionic personality disorder is characterized by a long-standing pattern of attention seeking behavior and extreme emotionality. Feelings that others take advantage describes paranoid personality disorder.
CN: Psychosocial integrity; CNS: None; CL: Analyze

4. While planning the care of a client with a schizotypal personality disorder, the nurse recognizes that this client has serious difficulty interacting socially. Which is a **priority** nursing intervention for this client?
1. Encourage the client to compose and write a list of social rules
2. Role play a troublesome social dilemma and have the client work through the scenario
3. Discuss the client's thoughts and feelings about engagement in peer conversations
4. Talk about how and why the client becomes absorbed in negative self-labeling

4. 3. The priority intervention is to begin a dialog with this client regarding his thoughts and feelings about having social interactions. People with a schizotypal personality disorder can become highly distressed if made to compose a list of rules for socializing, to role play a problematic situation, or to explain negativity.
CN: Safe, effective care environment; CNS: Management of care; CL: Analyze

5. A nurse is caring for a client with schizotypal personality disorder. How should the nurse approach care for this client?
1. Expect the client to participate in all classes offered on the unit
2. Allow the client to work on assigned work sheets in her room
3. Ask the client to conduct the daily community meeting
4. Have the client assist the instructor of a group medication class

5. 2. Clients with schizotypal personality disorders tend to isolate, and the nurse should respect this. The other answer choices would cause a client with schizoid personality disorder to interact with a group. The nurse may receive quite a bit of resistance from the client when there is a tone of control from the nurse.
CN: Safe, effective care environment; CNS: Management of care; CL: Apply

6. Which behaviors should the nurse anticipate from a client with a personality disorder? Select all that apply.
1. Compliance with the rules of the unit
2. Tendency to provoke interpersonal conflict
3. Inflexibility toward unit change
4. Maladaptive responses to stress
5. Trouble in social and professional relationships
6. Blurred personal boundaries

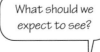

What should we expect to see?

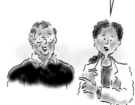

6. 2, 3, 4, 5, 6. These behaviors are common in all types of personality disorder. The nurse will not see compliance with the unit rules with any personality disorder.
CN: Psychosocial integrity; CNS: None; CL: Analyze

7. Which response would **best** facilitate communication with a client who has a personality disorder?
1. "What would you like to do today after you have finished your breakfast?"
2. "After you attend the morning community meeting, you may work on your homework."
3. "You remind me of a friend that I was very close to in high school."
4. "We may get comfortable on the unit before you do your therapy homework."

7. 2. This response reflects a firm yet supportive approach. Answers one and four leave the nurse open for manipulation by the client. The client could suggest any activity that might not be therapeutic. This client may never become comfortable on the unit. Comfort is not the reason for their admission. Answer three is an example of countertransference. The nurse may discuss countertransference with other staff, but not with the client.
CN: Safe, effective care environment; CNS: Management of care; CL: Analyze

8. A client with paranoid personality disorder is discussing his current problems with a nurse. Which intervention is **most** important for the nurse to implement?
1. Have the client explore personal sources of frustration
2. Have the client focus on ways to interact with others
3. Have the client discuss the use of defense mechanisms
4. Have the client clarify his thoughts and beliefs about an event

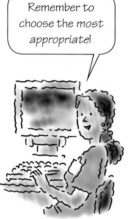

Remember to choose the most appropriate!

8. 4. Clarifying thoughts and beliefs will help this client avoid misinterpretations. Clients with a paranoid personality disorder tend to mistrust people, and don't see interacting with others as a way to handle problems. These clients tend to be aggressive and argumentative rather than frustrated. A paranoid client will focus on defending self rather than acknowledging the use of defense mechanisms.
CN: Safe, effective care environment; CNS: Management of care; CL: Analyze

9. A client with paranoid personality disorder makes an inappropriate and unreasonable report to the nurse. What is the **most** appropriate intervention by the nurse?
1. Use logic and a strong rationale to address the client's concern
2. Immediately confront the client about the stated misperception
3. Use nonverbal communication in the group setting to address the issue
4. Matter-of-factly tell the client that you don't share his interpretation

9. 4. Telling the client that you don't share his interpretation will help the client differentiate between realistic and emotional thoughts and conclusions. When the nurse uses logic to respond to a client's inappropriate statement, the nurse risks creating a power struggle. The use of nonverbal communication will likely be misinterpreted and arouse the client's suspicion. It's unwise to confront a client with a paranoid personality disorder, as the client will immediately become defensive.
CN: Psychosocial integrity; CNS: None; CL: Analyze

10. What is the **most** appropriate short-term goal for a client with paranoid personality disorder and impaired social skills?
1. Obtain feedback from other people and staff on the unit
2. Discuss anxiety-provoking situations and possible solutions
3. Address positive and negative feelings the client has about self
4. Identify personal feelings that hinder the client's social interaction

10. 4. The client must address feelings that impede social interactions before developing ways to manage impaired social skills. Feedback can only be obtained after action has been taken to improve or change the situation. Discussing anxiety-provoking situations is important, but does not help the client with impaired social skills. Addressing the client's positive and negative feelings about self will not directly influence impaired social skills.
CN: Psychosocial integrity; CNS: None; CL: Apply

11. A nurse is caring for a client with schizotypal personality disorder. Which behavior would the nurse anticipate from this client?
1. Exhibitionism
2. Impulsiveness
3. Bodily illusions
4. Repetitive behaviors

12. A nurse is assessing a client to determine if he has an avoidant personality disorder. What are the **most** appropriate questions for the nurse to ask the client? Select all that apply.
1. "Are you worried that people won't like you?"
2. "Do you drive yourself pretty hard, and frequently feel that you need to do more?"
3. "Are you a perfectionist in the things that you do at home?"
4. "Would it be easier for you to lie, or to tell the truth?"
5. "Are wary of opening yourself to others because other have hurt you in the past?"
6. "Do you carefully select your friends, and prefer just one or two close friends?"

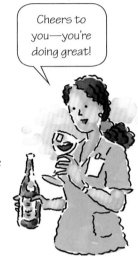

Cheers to you—you're doing great!

13. A client with paranoid personality disorder responds aggressively to another client during a psychoeducational group therapy session. How should the nurse interpret this client behavior? Select all that apply.
1. This client prefers individual therapy to group therapy.
2. This client took the statement as a personal criticism.
3. This client is impulsive and was acting out of frustration.
4. This client was attempting to handle emotional distress.
5. This client likes the attention received.

14. A client with avoidant personality disorder tells the nurse, "There is not a person in this world who likes me, and I don't know what to do." What is the nurse's **most** appropriate intervention?
1. Discuss ways to think of others instead of focusing on your personal needs
2. Explore the client's personal feelings about relationship distress
3. Discuss ways to form peer relationships that are warm and empathetic
4. Identify ways the client seeks immediate gratification despite the consequences

11. 3. Clients with schizotypal personality disorders tend to have bodily illusions. Clients with histrionic personality disorder tend to be exhibitionists. Those with borderline personality disorders are impulsive, and those with obsessive-compulsive tend to engage in repetitive behaviors.
CN: Psychosocial integrity; CNS: None; CL: Apply

12. 1, 5, 6. People with avoidant personality disorder are timid, sensitive to criticism, and fear not being accepted. They are often hesitant to enter into relationships. People with an obsessive-compulsive personality disorder feel the need to check things repeatedly, or have certain thoughts or perform routines and rituals over and over. The thoughts and rituals associated with OCD cause distress and get in the way of daily life. People with an antisocial personality disorder are described as dishonest and manipulative.
CN: Psychosocial integrity; CNS: None; CL: Apply

13. 1, 2. Clients with paranoid personality disorder tend to be hypersensitive and take the comments of others as a personal attack. This client is driven by the suspicion that others will inflict harm. The aim of treatment is to help the person to get rid of feelings of mistrust, resentment, jealousy and anxiety. Clients with a paranoid personality tend to be rigid and guarded rather than expressive and acting out. Group therapy sessions along with individual therapy are the best treatment options for people with paranoid personality disorder symptoms. The client with a paranoid personality disorder is acting to defend himself, not handle emotional distress.
CN: Psychosocial integrity; CNS: None; CL: Analyze

14. 2. Clients with avoidant personality disorder fear criticism, disapproval, and rejection. This client needs to discuss the stress felt when attempting to form relationships. A client with narcissistic personality disorder has an inflated sense of self and is focused on personal needs rather than those of others. An intervention for a narcissistic client would include forming peer relationships that are warm and empathetic because they struggle to care about others. A person with an antisocial personality disorder tends to seek immediate gratification at the expense of other people.
CN: Safe, effective care environment; CNS: Management of care; CL: Analyze

15. A client with avoidant personality disorder is in treatment. What is an appropriate outcome for this client?
1. Demonstrates an ability to use constructive criticism
2. Participates in impulse control training
3. Demonstrates a reduction in clinging, splitting, and manipulation behaviors
4. Demonstrates a decrease in attention-seeking behaviors

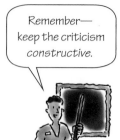

Remember—keep the criticism constructive.

15. 1. Clients with avoidant personality disorder fear rejection and criticism. They are very reluctant to participate in social situations because of this fear. Answer choices two, three and four describe a borderline, antisocial, histrionic, or narcissistic personality disorder.
CN: Safe, effective care environment; CNS: Management of care;
CL: Analyze

16. The nurse is caring for a client with an avoidant personality disorder. Which characteristics define this client's behavior? Select all that apply.
1. Vigilant and suspiciousness
2. Distant personal relationships
3. Unstable relationships
4. View themselves as inferior to others
5. Inflexible, rigid, and needs to be in control
6. Social phobias

16. 5, 7. Avoidant personality disorder is characterized by feelings of extreme social inhibition, inadequacy, and sensitivity to negative criticism and rejection Suspiciousness is characteristic of paranoid personality disorder. Distant personal relationships are characteristic of schizoid personality disorder. Unstable relationships are characteristic of borderline personality disorder. Those with obsessive-compulsive disorder tend to be inflexible, rigid, and controlling.
CN: Psychosocial integrity; CNS: None; CL: Apply

17. A nurse, caring for a client with an avoidant personality disorder. The nurse would like this client to demonstrate her newly acquired social skills in social situations. Which intervention would **best** facilitate this outcome?
1. Discuss the factors that interfere with the client's social interactions
2. Identify social skills that the client currently performs well
3. Go to the hospital cafeteria, purchase lunch, and dine in a group setting
4. Complete a work sheet on social skills

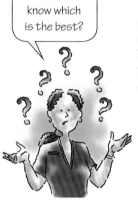

How do I know which is the best?

17. 3. This activity demonstrates the desired outcome. The other selections address social skills, but no performance skills are associated with them.
CN: Psychosocial integrity; CNS: None; CL: Apply

18. The nurse is teaching a client with paranoid personality disorder about ways to address behaviors that negatively affect relationships. Which statement, made by the client, **best** demonstrates that teaching has been effective?
1. "I won't abide by social rules as long as I live."
2. "Sometimes, I can see what causes my relationship problems."
3. "I will learn from other's problems so that I won't repeat them."
4. "I have never had problems in social relationships."

18. 2. Progress is shown when the client addresses behaviors that negatively impact relationships. Clients with paranoid personality disorder tend to have impaired social relationships and are very uncomfortable in social settings. Clients with paranoid personality disorder struggle to understand and express their feelings about social rules. Knowing other people's problems is not useful. This client must focus on his own issues. Not recognizing the problem indicates that the client is in denial.
CN: Psychosocial integrity; CNS: None; CL: Apply

CN: Client needs category   CNS: Client needs subcategory   CL: Cognitive level

19. The nurse is developing long-term goals, for a client with paranoid personality disorder, who is trying to improve peer relationships. What is the **most** appropriate goal?

1. The client will verbalize a realistic view of self.
2. The client will take steps to address disorganized thinking.
3. The client will become appropriately interdependent on others.
4. The client will become involved in activities that foster social relationships.

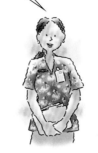

The word long-term is a clue to the correct choice.

20. A client with a history of social inhibition, agoraphobia, the fear of criticism, feelings of inferiority, and feelings of being extremely unattractive to others has been admitted to the hospital. With which disorder would the nurse associate these behaviors?

1. Dependent personality disorder
2. Histrionic personality disorder
3. Narcissistic personality disorder
4. Avoidant personality disorder

21. A client with antisocial personality disorder is trying to convince the nurse that he deserves special privileges, and that an exception to the rules should be made for him. What is the nurse's **best** response to this client's requests?

1. "I believe we need to sit down and talk about this."
2. 'Don't you know better than to try to bend the rules?"
3. "Your requests are unacceptable."
4. "Let's discuss your requests at the community meeting tomorrow."

22. The chart documentation of a client with paranoid personality disorder reads:

Progress notes	
10/15/16 1830	The client stays by himself as much as possible during the afternoon. He paced the hallway at times at times and was irritated if approached by staff or other clients. The client questioned another male client and accused him of lying. At the beginning of the shift the nurse spoke to the client accused of lying.

Which statement, from the client accused of lying, would require further intervention?

1. "Now I know not to trust, or even speak to that person."
2. "I do not know what his problem is, but I know it is his issue."
3. "I'm upset, but I'm not doing anything to lose my privileges."
4. "If I have an opportunity, I will not let him get away with this."

19. 4. An appropriate long-term goal is for this client is to increase interactions and social skills, and make a commitment to become involved with others on a long-term basis. Verbalizing a realistic view of self is a short-term goal. The client with a paranoid personality disorder doesn't tend to have disorganized thinking. A client with paranoid personality disorder won't allow himself to be interdependent on others.
CN: Psychosocial integrity; CNS: None; CL: Analyze

20. 4. These behaviors are characteristic of avoidant personality disorder. Histrionic and narcissistic behaviors are typical of cluster B. Clients with dependent personality disorders generally cling to others in their personal relationships.
CN: Psychosocial integrity; CNS: None; CL: Apply

21. 3. These clients often try to manipulate the nurse to gain special privileges, or create exceptions to the rules on their behalf. By directly informing the client that their actions are inappropriate, the nurse helps the client learn to control unacceptable behaviors by setting limits. Offering to discuss the problem creates the illusion that the rules are negotiable. Answer two humiliates the client. This client's behavior is unacceptable and should not be brought to a community meeting.
CN: Psychosocial integrity; CNS: None; CL: Apply

22. 4. Clients with paranoid personality disorder can be frustrating to staff and other clients. It is appropriate for the nurse to ask the person accused of lying if he is feeling rebuffed and retaliatory. Answer four indicates that the client is considering retaliation. The other options indicate that the accused client has a cautionary approach, and is able to set boundaries concerning the person with paranoid personality disorder.
CN: Safe and effective care environment; CNS: Safety and infection control; CL: Analyze

CN: Client needs category   CNS: Client needs subcategory   CL: Cognitive level

23. Which assessment questions would determine if the client has a histrionic personality disorder? Select all that apply.
  1. "Do you frequently feel let down by people?"
  2. "If a friend hurts you, do you sometimes feel like hurting yourself?"
  3. "Do you find that most people aren't quite up to your standards?"
  4. "Do you think that you would make a good actor?"
  5. "Compared to other people, do you feel that a very special person?"
  6. "Do people of the opposite sex frequently find you attractive?"

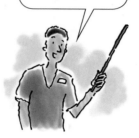

Which of these questions pertain specifically to histrionic personality disorder?

23. 4, 6. Histrionic personality disorder is characterized by a long-standing pattern of attention seeking behavior and extreme emotionality. Answers one and two assess borderline personality disorders. Answers three and five assess narcissistic personality disorder.
CN: Psychosocial integrity; CNS: None; CL: Apply

24. When reviewing a client's chart, the nurse reads the progress note.

Progress notes	
10/15/16 1130	Client, age 28, admitted to unit with diagnosis of antisocial personality disorder and suicide attempt after cutting his right wrist. Right wrist dressing appears dry and intact. Client states, 'I don't want to be here and I'm not following your treatment plan or any of your rules. I'm going to tell everyone here not to follow your rules.' —Barbara Jones, RN

Which statement, about the client's condition, is **most** accurate?
  1. The client is refusing the required psychotropic drugs used to treat his condition.
  2. The client manipulates others, but not his family.
  3. The client is not be motivated to change his behavior or his lifestyle.
  4. The client can quickly make behavior changes if motivated

24. 3. Clients with antisocial personality disorder feel nothing is wrong with their behavior, and they have no desire to change. These clients don't benefit from psychotropic drug therapy. They attempt to manipulate the people around them. A quick behavior change isn't a realistic expectation for clients with this disorder.
CN: Psychosocial integrity; CNS: None; CL: Apply

25. Which behavior would the nurse observe in a client who has a histrionic personality disorder?
  1. Manipulates others to meet their own needs
  2. Portrays an attitude of grandiosity
  3. Demonstrates highly provocative behaviors
  4. Expresses feelings of emptiness and boredom

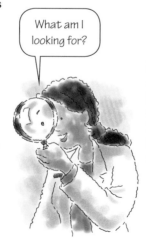

What am I looking for?

25. 3. People with histrionic personality disorders tend to display highly provocative behaviors. Manipulation of others and grandiosity are descriptions of narcissistic personality disorder. Feelings of emptiness and boredom are descriptions of borderline personality disorder.
CN: Psychosocial integrity; CNS: None; CL: Apply

26. Which behavioral pattern is characteristic of individuals with histrionic personality disorders?
1. Berating themselves and their abilities
2. Overreacting to frustrations and annoyances
3. Suspicious and mistrustful of others
4. Social withdraw, and distant in relationship

27. A nurse notices that other clients on the unit are avoiding a client diagnosed with antisocial personality disorder. During group therapy, the topic of appropriate behavior is being discussed. Which behavior does the group associate with the client who is being avoided?
1. Lacks honesty
2. Believes in superstitions
3. Has frequent temper tantrums
4. Constantly craves attention

28. The nurse is caring for a client with histrionic personality disorder. The client's family member asks, "How do I handle the drama that occurs when she doesn't get her own way?" What information should the nurse provide this family? Select all that apply.
1. "Do not argue or try to rationalize things with the person."
2. "Talk about the trauma to show that you understand."
3. "State your responses in a non-emotional manner."
4. "Sit in the person's visual field, but avoid having much eye contact."
5. "Remember to give positive feedback whenever possible."
6. "Maintain a serious and personal interest in the person."

29. A client with antisocial personality disorder has a high risk for violence directed at others. What is an appropriate goal for this client?
1. The client will discuss the desire to hurt others rather than act.
2. The client will be given something to destroy to displace the anger.
3. The client will develop a list of resources to use when anger escalates.
4. The client will understand the difference between anger and physical symptoms.

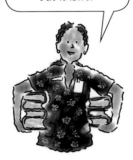

Read this question carefully. It seems to be asking you for a positive response, but it isn't.

26. 2. Clients with a histrionic personality disorder are emotional and overreact to stimuli. Berating themselves describes an avoidant personality disorder. Suspiciousness describes a paranoid personality disorder. Socially withdrawn and distant relationships describe schizotypal personality disorder.
CN: Psychosocial integrity; CNS: None; CL: Apply

27. 1. Clients with antisocial personality disorder tend to engage in acts of dishonesty. Clients with schizotypal personality disorder tend to be superstitious. Clients with histrionic personality disorders tend to overreact to frustrations and disappointments, have temper tantrums, and seek attention.
CN: Psychosocial integrity; CNS: None; CL: Apply

28. 1, 3, 5, 6. Communication with clients with histrionic personality disorders needs to be firm and calm, without bargaining or rationalizing with the person. The family member needs to refrain from engaging in emotional responses. Appropriate positive feedback and verbalized care and concern for the person is useful. People with this personality disorder are dramatic, and discussing their trauma will increase dramatic responses. It's not helpful to sit near the person and avoid eye contact.
CN: Safe, effective care environment; CNS: Management of care; CL: Analyze

29. 1. By discussing the desire to be violent toward others, the nurse can help the client get in touch with the pain associated with angry feelings. It isn't helpful to have the client destroy something. The client needs to talk about strong feelings in a non-violent manner, rather than refer to a list of crisis references. Helping the client understand the relationship between feelings and physical symptoms can be done after discussing the desire to hurt others.
CN: Psychosocial integrity; CNS: None; CL: Analyze

CN: Client needs category   CNS: Client needs subcategory   CL: Cognitive level

30. Which nursing intervention is the **priority** while caring for a client with antisocial personality disorder who shows defensive behaviors?
   1. Help the client accept responsibility for his own decisions and behaviors
   2. Work with the client to feel better about himself by taking care of basic needs
   3. Teach the client to identify the defense mechanisms used to cope with distress
   4. Confront the client about the disregard of social rules or the feelings of others

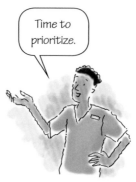

Time to prioritize.

30. 1. Clients with antisocial personality disorder tend to blame other people for their behaviors, and should learn how to take responsibility for their actions. Clients with antisocial personality disorder don't tend to have problems with self-care or meeting their basic needs. Clients with antisocial personality disorder will deny that they're defensive or distressed. These clients frequently feel justified with retaliatory behavior. Confronting the client would only cause him to become even more defensive.
CN: Psychosocial integrity; CNS: None; CL: Analyze

31. The nurse is developing outcomes for a client with a histrionic personality disorder. What is the **most** appropriate outcome for this client?
   1. The client agrees to contracts for safety, and is free of self-inflicted injury.
   2. The client participates in impulse control training.
   3. The client participates in anger management classes.
   4. The client participates in group session without being the center of attention.

31. 4. A client with histrionic personality disorder thrives on being the center of attention. The use of contracts facilitates the therapeutic alliance, and aids in the avoidance of excessive regression and acting out Contracting for safety and impulse control training would be appropriate for a client with borderline personality disorder. Anger management class would be appropriate for antisocial personality disorder.
CN: Safe, effective care environment; CNS: Management of care; CL: Apply

32. A client with antisocial personality disorder says, "I always want to blow things off." Which response, by the nurse, is **most** appropriate?
   1. "Try to focus on what needs to be done and just do it."
   2. "Let's work on considering some options and strategies."
   3. "Procrastinating is a part of your illness that we'll work on."
   4. "The best thing to do is decide on some useful goals."

Teach the client skills to overcome ineffective behaviors.

32. 2. By considering options or strategies, the client gains skills to overcome ineffective behaviors. The client tends to be irresponsible and needs guidance on what to focus on to change behavior. Clients with an antisocial personality disorder don't tend to struggle with procrastination. They typically show reckless and irresponsible behaviors. It's premature to decide on goals when the client needs to address the mental mind-set, and work to change the irresponsible behavior.
CN: Psychosocial integrity; CNS: None; CL: Apply

33. A client with antisocial personality disorder is trying to manipulate the health care team. What is the staff's **best** strategy?
   1. Focus on teaching the client more effective behaviors to meet basic needs
   2. Help the client verbalize underlying feelings of hopelessness and learn coping skills
   3. Remain calm and don't respond in an emotional manner to the client's manipulative actions
   4. Help the client eliminate the intense desire to have everything in life turn out perfectly

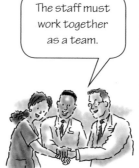

The staff must work together as a team.

33. 3. The best strategy is to stay calm and refrain from responding in an emotional manner. The negative reinforcement of inappropriate behavior would increase the chance of repeat behavior. Though not the priority, it may be possible, to address how this client addresses their basic needs. Clients with antisocial personality disorder don't tend to experience feelings of hopelessness or desire life events to turn out perfectly.
CN: Psychosocial integrity; CNS: None; CL: Analyze

34. A client with dependent personality disorder is working to increase self-esteem. Which statement, by the client, shows teaching was successful?
  1. "I'm not going to look at the negative things about myself."
  2. "I'm most concerned about my level of competence and progress."
  3. "I'm not as envious of other peoples' things as I used to be."
  4. "I can't stop myself from taking over tasks others should be doing."

34. **1.** As the client makes progress on improving self-esteem, self-blame and negative self-evaluations will decrease. Clients with dependent personality disorder tend to feel fragile and inadequate, and most likely would not discuss their level of competence and progress. These clients focus on self, and aren't envious or jealous. Individuals with dependent personality disorders don't take over situations because they see themselves as inept and inadequate.
CN: Psychosocial integrity; CNS: None; CL: Apply

35. The nurse is reviewing the behaviors of a client with a histrionic personality disorder. The nurse determines that a change in behavior may be occurring when the client:
  1. draws attention to themselves, and dresses provocatively.
  2. becomes easily influenced by others or circumstances.
  3. shows concern about hurting someone else's feelings.
  4. describes intimate relationships with casual acquaintances.

35. **3.** A client with a histrionic personality disorder is typically insensitive to anyone else's experience. Exhibiting concern for another's feelings would indicate a change in this client's behavior. Answers one, two, and four describe typical behaviors of a client with a histrionic personality disorder.
CN: Psychosocial integrity; CNS: None; CL: Apply

36. A client with antisocial personality disorder talks about personal life changes that need to occur. Which client statement shows that group therapy is having a positive therapeutic effect?
  1. "I'm not doing as bad as I thought I was."
  2. "I wish I could believe I can change, but it's probably too late."
  3. "I see all the problems, but I'm not sure there are good solutions."
  4. "I'm finally learning how to live my life without living on the edge."

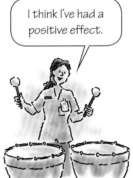

I think I've had a positive effect.

36. **4.** This statement indicates that the client is becoming aware of risky behaviors and how problematic they are. Answer one indicates denial, and that the client is somewhat defensive about making a change. Answer two indicates defeat, and that the client seems to feel stuck. Answer three indicates that the client can identify the problem, but is uncertain or ambivalent that a change can be made.
CN: Psychosocial integrity; CNS: None; CL: Analyze

37. A nurse tells a client, with a personality disorder, that he must clean his room before he can go to the dayroom. The client asks if he can play one game of pool first. What is the nurse's **most** appropriate response?
  1. "You can play one quick game. Then you have to clean your room."
  2. "No, you may not."
  3. "No, you may not play pool first. The rules were explained to you."
  4. "Yes, you may play a quick game. But don't tell the other clients about this."

37. **3.** This response is firm and reinforces the rules. Allowing the client to play one game before cleaning his room and then not to tell anyone else, encourages manipulative behavior. Saying "no" to the client without an explanation doesn't outline or reinforce the rules.
CN: Psychosocial integrity; CNS: None; CL: Analyze

CN: Client needs category   CNS: Client needs subcategory   CL: Cognitive level

38. The sibling of a client with schizoid personality disorder doesn't understand why his brother doesn't care about him or want to be his friend. Which statement, by the nurse, explains the client's behavior?
1. "Someday your brother will become your best friend."
2. "Your brother does not enjoy having relationships with others."
3. "When your brother is able to trust, then you and he can be friends."
4. "After his medication starts to work, he will become your brother again."

38. 2. A client with schizoid personality disorder is indifferent to interpersonal relationships and does not derive pleasure from social or personal relationships. Answer one does not answer the question, and gives false hope. Answer three refers to a client with paranoid personality disorder. Taking medication does not guarantee that a healthy relationship will form between the brothers.
CN: Psychosocial integrity; CNS: None; CL: Analyze

39. The nurse is assessing a client who was just admitted to the psychiatric unit. Which questions should the nurse ask to help determine if this client has an obsessive-compulsive personality disorder? Select all that apply.
1. "Do you tend to drive yourself pretty hard, then frequently feel like you need to do just a little more?"
2. "Is it hard for you to argue with your spouse, because you are worried that they will get angry with you and start to dislike you?"
3. "Does anxiety make you want to self-mutilate?"
4. "Do you keep things to yourself to be sure the wrong people don't get the right information?"
5. "Do you keep lists, or sometimes feel a need to keep repeatedly check things?"
6. "Do you tend to be a perfectionist?"

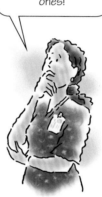

Questions, questions. I want to ask the correct ones!

39. 1, 5, 6. These questions describe the obsessive-compulsive personality disorder. Answer two describes a dependent personality disorder. Self-mutilation describes borderline personality disorders. Keeping things to yourself so the wrong people don't get the right information describes paranoid personality disorder.
CN: Psychosocial integrity; CNS: None; CL: Apply

40. A client with an obsessive-compulsive personality disorder is in the community room. Which behavior pattern would a nurse expect to observe from this client?
1. Discussing people who are viewed as superior versus those viewed as inferior
2. Questioning others about their mastery of marital arts and self-defense skills
3. Telling another client about making drugs like methamphetamine in the garage
4. Ridiculing law enforcement officials, and saying that they are out to get people

40. 1. Clients with obsessive-compulsive personality disorder are very conscious of a person's rank, and will focus on people who are authority figures. A client with an antisocial personality disorder is likely to talk about fighting and self-defense skills, making synthetic and illegal drugs, and ridiculing law enforcement officials.
CN: Psychosocial integrity; CNS: None; CL: Apply

41. A nurse is working with a client at a community mental health center who has an antisocial personality disorder. What behavior, exhibited by the client, would require **immediate** intervention from the nurse?
1. Remaining quiet during the meeting
2. Suppressing laughter at the end of the meeting
3. Starting an argument with a peer at the meeting
4. Chewing gum while attending the meeting

41. 3. The client with an antisocial disorder has great difficulty developing relationships with peers, and can often be intimidating, manipulative and argumentative. Although client participation is the desired behavior during a community meeting, being quiet does not require immediate intervention. Suppressing laughter and chewing gum at the meeting are behaviors that can be addressed after the meeting is completed.
CN: Psychosocial integrity; CNS: None; CL: Apply

CN: Client needs category   CNS: Client needs subcategory   CL: Cognitive level

42. A client with an antisocial personality disorder is court-mandated to receive counseling after being detained by law enforcement officials. The chart entry reads:

Progress notes	
10/15/16	The client came to the group therapy
1130	session and was verbally aggressive to other
	clients. The group leader set limits on his
	behavior, reinforced the group rules and
	guidelines. At two different times the client
	made excuses for his behavior, stating, 'I
	really don't have to be here,' and minimized
	the comments of other group members.

Which **priority** action, by the nurse group leader, must be initiated?
1. Obtain an order for medication to be given every morning
2. Role-play social skills with client before the next group meeting
3. Arrange for a coach to be present with the client at each meeting
4. Formulate an individual contract for appropriate behavior during the group

42. 4. The documented client behavior indicates a need for limits during group. Formulating a contract that addresses the appropriate behavior, and the consequences for violating the contract, is the priority strategy. Medication for a client with antisocial personality disorder is only used to manage the symptoms of depression or disordered thinking. The first action to be taken is setting limits on inappropriate behavior, not role playing skills and arranging for a coach.
CN: Psychosocial integrity; CNS: None; CL: Analyze

43. The nurse is developing outcomes for a recently-admitted a client with an obsessive-compulsive personality disorder. What is the **most** appropriate outcome for this client?
1. Participating in training classes
2. Demonstrating a reduction in manipulative behavior
3. Demonstrating decreased suspicion and increased security
4. Participating in recreational therapy on the unit

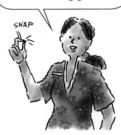

That's it! You got it. You're doing great.

SNAP

43. 4. The obsessive-compulsive personality over-emphasizes work to the exclusion of participating in pleasurable leisure activities. For the client to be able to participate in recreational therapy on the unit is a good first step. Assertiveness training is useful for clients with cluster B personality disorders. Splitting and manipulation, and distancing behaviors describe borderline personality disorder. A decrease in suspicion and increased security would be outcomes for a client with paranoid personality disorder.
CN: Psychosocial integrity; CNS: None; CL: Apply

44. A nurse is providing care for a client who has obsessive-compulsive disorder. What is the **priority** nursing intervention?
1. Use a friendly, gentle, reassuring approach because it is the best way to treat clients with an obsessive-compulsive disorder
2. Avoid engaging in a power struggle with these clients. Their need for control is very high
3. Be aware that clients with this personality disorder can instill guilt when they are not getting what they want
4. Use teaching and role model assertiveness

44. 2. Guarding against involvement in power struggles is the approach the nurse should take with a client who has obsessive-compulsive personality disorder. A friendly, gentle, reassuring approach is the best way to treat clients with an avoidant personality disorder. Antisocial personality disorder clients instill guilt when they don't get what they want. Teaching and role modeling assertiveness are strategies for dependent and histrionic personality disorders.
CN: Safe, effective care environment; CNS: Management of care; CL: Apply

CN: Client needs category   CNS: Client needs subcategory   CL: Cognitive level

45. What behaviors would a nurse expect to see in a client who has an obsessive-compulsive personality disorder? Select all that apply.
1. Meticulous in their work area
2. Unresponsive to social cues
3. Refuses to bend the rules
4. Have a strong job loyalty
5. Tries to hide anger

45. 1, 3, 4, 5. The client with an obsessive-compulsive disorder is meticulous at work, and tries to be accurate and diligent in their responsibilities. This client will refuse to bend the rules and will show no desire to be flexible with others. This client sees himself as a conscientious employee who is very loyal to his company. This client will often feel very angry at others for not being dependable or responsible, but will hide his anger. A client with schizotypal personality disorder is frequently unable to recognize or respond to social cues.
CN: Psychosocial integrity; CNS: None; CL: Apply

46. The nurse is assessing a new client who was just admitted to the psychiatric unit. Which assessment questions should the nurse ask to determine if the client has a schizoid personality disorder? Select all that apply.
1. "Do you tend to be a perfectionist?"
2. "Have you found yourself being worried that people won't like you?"
3. "Do you enjoy making the decisions in your house, or would you prefer that others make decisions for you?"
4. "During the course of your life, have you had only one or two friends?"
5. "Over the years, have you been able to physically defend yourself?"
6. "Do you prefer to be alone?"

46. 4, 6. Clients with schizoid personality disorders will only one or two friends throughout their life, and prefer to be alone. Clients with obsessive-compulsive personality disorders are perfectionists. Clients with avoidant personality disorders are worried that people won't like them. Clients with dependent personality disorders would prefer that others make decisions. Clients with antisocial personality disorders can take care of themselves in a physical fight.
CN: Psychosocial integrity; CNS: None; CL: Apply

47. Which behavior patterns would a nurse expect to observe in a client with a schizoid personality disorder?
1. Emotional coldness and flattened affect
2. Submissive and clinging
3. Impulsive and unstable emotionally
4. Cheerful and carefree

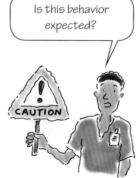
Is this behavior expected?

47. 1. Clients with schizoid personality disorder are emotionally cold and have a flattened affect. Submissive and clinging behaviors describe the dependent personality disorder. Impulsivity and unstable emotions describe borderline personality disorder, and cheerful and carefree describe the narcissistic personality disorder.
CN: Psychosocial integrity; CNS: None; CL: Apply

48. A preceptor is orienting a new nurse who will be caring for clients with borderline personality disorder. What information should the preceptor share with the new nurse?
1. When problems emerge, calmly review the treatment goals.
2. Try to prevent or decrease the amount of time that the client is manipulative.
3. Remain neutral and avoid engaging in power struggles.
4. Respect the client's need for social isolation and privacy.

48. 1. Reminding the borderline client of established goals and boundaries of treatment will help maintain focus. Guarded behavior is an issue with clients who have paranoid personality disorder. Power struggles are an issue for the narcissistic client, and respecting the client's need for social isolation applies to a client with schizotypal personality disorder.
CN: Safe, effective care environment; CNS: Safety and infection control; CL: Apply

49. Which nursing intervention is a **priority** for the client with borderline personality disorder?
1. Maintain consistent, realistic limits
2. Give instructions for meeting basic self-care needs
3. Engage in daytime activities to stimulate wakefulness
4. Have the client attend group therapy on a daily basis

49. 1. Clients with borderline personality disorder who are needy, dependent, and manipulative will benefit from maintaining consistent, realistic limits. They don't tend to have difficulty meeting their self-care needs, and don't tend to have sleeping difficulties. They enjoy attending group therapy because they typically attempt to use the opportunity to become the center of attention.
CN: Safe, effective care environment; CNS: Management of care; CL: Apply

50. The nurse is working with a client who has been diagnosed with borderline personality disorder. Prioritize the nurse's interventions.

| 1. Anticipate and prepare for the first crisis |
| 2. Advocate for and validate client support |
| 3. Maintain a consistent level of contact and support |
| 4. Listen to the client's fears and feelings of anger |

You're making this test look as easy as a walk in the park.

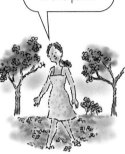

50. Ordered Response:

| 4. Listen to the client's fears and feelings of anger. |
| 3. Maintain a consistent level of contact and support |
| 1. Anticipate and prepare for the first crisis |
| 2. Advocate for and validate client support |

CN: Safe, effective care environment; CNS: Management of care; CL: Analyze

51. The nurse is identifying outcomes for a client with a schizoid personality disorder. What is the **most** appropriate outcome?
1. Demonstrates the ability to use constructive criticism
2. Participates in two of the four scheduled groups on the unit
3. Demonstrates a reduction in clinging, splitting, and manipulative behaviors
4. Demonstrates a decrease in attention-seeking behaviors

51. 2. Clients with a schizoid personality disorder prefer solitary activities and do not enjoy close relationships. Attending two out of four unit group meetings would be a step toward gaining comfort in a social setting. Avoidant personality disorder clients experience fear of rejection or criticism, and are very reluctant to participate in social situations. Answers three and four describe cluster B personality disorders.
CN: Safe, effective care environment; CNS: Management of care; CL: Apply

52. Which intervention would be **most** effective for client with a schizoid personality disorder?
1. Participates in impulse control training
2. Participates in anger management classes
3. Participates in group without being the center of attention
4. Participates in social skills training

52. 4. Clients with schizoid personality disorder will benefit from social skills training because they are detached from others and are loners. A client with histrionic personality disorder thrives on being the center of attention. Impulse control training would be appropriate for a client with borderline personality disorder. Anger management class would be appropriate for a client with antisocial personality disorder.
CN: Safe, effective care environment; CNS: Management of care; CL: Apply

53. The nurse is assessing a client for narcissistic personality disorder. What questions should the nurse ask the client? Select all that apply.
1. "Do you frequently feel let down by people?"
2. "Do you find that most people aren't quite up to your standards?"
3. "Do you feel that other people take advantage of you?"
4. "Do you find that people often have a tendency to be disloyal or dishonest?"
5. "If people give you a hard time, do you tend to put them in their place quickly?"
6. "Are you a very special person?"

53. 2, 5, 6. Clients with narcissistic personality disorders feel others are not up to their standards, they put people in their place quickly, and they feel that they are very special people. Clients with borderline personality disorders feel let down by people. Clients with paranoid personality disorders feel that others take advantage of them, and that people tend to be disloyal or dishonest.
CN: Psychosocial integrity; CNS: None; CL: Apply

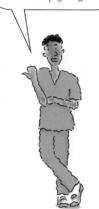

You've finished 54 questions. That should motivate you to keep going.

54. A nurse is assessing a client with a narcissistic personality disorder. Which characteristics would define client's personality?
1. Pleasant and encouraging to peers
2. Submissive and clinging with staff
3. Impulsive and emotional in groups
4. Provocative and seductive to visitors

54. 1. Although clients with a narcissistic personality disorder are grandiose and display a sense of entitlement, they are usually optimistic, cheerful and pleasant to others. Submissive and clinging behavior characterizes a client with a dependent personality disorder. Acting impulsively and being highly emotional are behaviors of a client with a borderline personality disorder. Provocative and seductive behaviors characterize a client with a histrionic personality disorder.
CN: Psychosocial integrity; CNS: None; CL: Analyze

55. A client with dependent personality disorder is working on goals for self-care with the nurse. Which short-term goal is **most** important for the client's activities of daily living?
1. Complete all self-care activities independently
2. Establish a schedule for each day of the week
3. Perform self-care activities in a minimal amount of time
4. Identify activities that can be performed independently

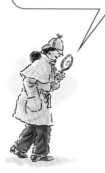

It's most important that you look for clues in this one.

55. 4. By determining activities that can be performed independently, the client can begin to practice them independently. If the nurse encourages a client to perform self-care activities without first identifying them, nothing may change. Writing a daily schedule does not help the client focus on what needs to be done to promote self-care. The amount of time needed to perform self-care activities is not important. If time pressure is put on the client, there may be more reluctance to perform self-care activities.
CN: Psychosocial integrity; CNS: None; CL: Apply

56. A nurse is caring for a client who has an avoidant personality disorder. Which statement is expected from a client who has this disorder?
1. "I'm scared that you're going to leave me."
2. "I'll go to group therapy if you'll let me smoke."
3. "I need to feel that everyone knows and likes me."
4. "I can sometimes feel better if I cut myself."

56. 1. Clients who have avoidant personality disorder often have a fear of abandonment. An "if you do this, then I'll do that" statement indicates manipulation, which is common for a client with borderline personality disorder. A statement which indicates the client's need for admiration is common with a client with a narcissistic personality disorder. When a client indicates a risk for self-injury, the client is frequently a person with a borderline personality disorder.
CN: Safe, effective care environment; CNS: Management of care; CL: Apply

57. The nurse reviews the health record of a client with a narcissistic personality. What assessment information, gained from the family, might explain the client's narcissistic personality disorder? Select all that apply.
1. Family history of autism
2. Very demanding parents
3. Delayed language development
4. Overly critical caregivers
5. Limited financial resources
6. Being overly-indulged in childhood

58. Which response would a nurse expect from a client with a narcissistic personality disorder?
1. "You owe me five more minutes of smoke break time since you let us out late from group."
2. "You're the only nurse that understands me. I don't like the other nurses at all. They're mean."
3. "I don't know what I should wear today, or what groups I should go to."
4. "I can't go to group today because one of the clients hurt my feelings in group yesterday."

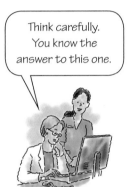

Think carefully. You know the answer to this one.

59. A client with dependent personality disorder is having trouble performing activities of daily living. Which nursing intervention would help facilitate the client's daily activities?
1. Have the client eat three meals a day
2. Work with the client to establish a budget
3. Make a chart to document hygiene practices
4. Discuss how the client can obtain a driver's license

60. A client with a dependent personality disorder is taking fluoxetine for depression. Which instruction should be included in client teaching?
1. Drink only wine and beer when taking this drug
2. Add as-needed doses if depression becomes worse
3. Expect three to four weeks to go by before the medication is effective
4. Be aware that you will sleep more when taking the medication

57. 2, 4, 6. The family of a client with narcissistic personality disorder would tend to be very demanding and critical. The parents may have over-indulged the client as a child, and failed to set limits on behavior. Typically, there is no family history of autism, language delays, or family economic problems.
CN: Psychosocial integrity; CNS: None; CL: Analyze

58. 1. Clients with narcissistic personality disorder have a sense of entitlement. Splitting staff is a typical response from a client who has a borderline personality disorder. Indecisiveness is a characteristic of a client with a dependent personality disorder. Holding grudges is a characteristic of a client with a paranoid personality disorder.
CN: Psychosocial integrity; CNS: None; CL: Apply

59. 2. Clients with dependent personality disorder tend to withdraw from adult responsibilities. Establishing a budget to help manage finances is a positive step toward assuming adult responsibilities. These clients don't tend to have problems with nutritional intake. Hygiene issues usually aren't a problem for clients with dependent personality disorder. Clients with a dependent personality disorder don't have any special reasons for not obtaining a driver's license.
CN: Psychosocial integrity; CNS: None; CL: Apply

60. 3. The client must take the drug for three to four weeks before therapeutic effects are seen. The nurse must caution the client against the use of alcohol, including wine and beer, when taking fluoxetine. The client is to take the drug as prescribed. Additional doses must not be self-administered. Insomnia is a major side effect of fluoxetine.
CN: Physiological integrity; CNS: Pharmacological and parenteral therapies; CL: Apply

61. The nurse is assigned to care for four clients. Which client should the nurse see **first**?
   1. A divorced client with a dependent personality disorder who is seeking care from another client
   2. A client with borderline personality disorder who continues to talk about wanting to cut her arms
   3. A client with an avoidant personality disorder who refuses to go to groups on the unit
   4. A client with paranoid personality disorder client who refuses to attend the community morning meeting

61. 2. The nurse has to address the physical safety of the borderline personality disorder client first. The behaviors of the other three clients with personality disorders affect the milieu of the unit and can be addressed later.
CN: Safe, effective care environment; CNS: Management of care; CL: Apply

62. The nurse plans care for a client with dependent personality disorder. Prioritize the short-term goals used to assist this client.

1.	Teach about the decision making process
2.	Discuss self reliance as much as possible
3.	Perform self-management activities
4.	Learn and practice assertiveness skills

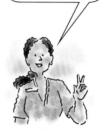

Ooh—a sequencing question. Those are tricky.

62. Ordered Response:

2.	Discuss self reliance as much as possible
3.	Perform self- management activities
1.	Teach about the decision making process
4.	Learn and practice assertiveness skills

CN: Safe, effective care environment; CNS: Management of care; CL: Analyze

63. Which personality disorder cluster would be the **most** challenging for the nurse to manage in the unit milieu?
   1. Cluster A
   2. Cluster B
   3. Cluster C
   4. Cluster D

63. 2. It would be most challenging to maintain a positive milieu with clients in cluster B. These clients are very labile emotionally and are quite dramatic. Clusters A and C avoid close relationships, and prefer to isolate in their rooms. There is no such cluster D nomenclature for personality disorders.
CN: Safe, effective care environment; CNS: Management of care; CL: Apply

64. Which client would require one-on-one contact with a staff member?
   1. A client with histrionic personality disorder who frequently faints when a male individual is near
   2. A client with antisocial personality disorder who steals food from other clients' meal trays
   3. A client with an obsessive-compulsive personality disorder who insists that all the rules of the unit be followed
   4. A client with borderline personality disorder who has acted on suicidal ideation, and has cut herself

64. 4. Because of the labile emotion and impulsivity characteristics of a client with borderline personality disorder, it is necessary to implement one-on-one staffing to ensure safety of the client. The other client behaviors do need to be addressed but do not require one-on-one staffing.
CN: Safe, effective care environment; CNS: Management of care; CL: Apply

CN: Client needs category   CNS: Client needs subcategory   CL: Cognitive level

65. A nurse is evaluating the effectiveness of an assertiveness group that a client with dependent personality disorder attended. Which client statement indicates that the group had therapeutic value?
  1. " I can't seem to do the things other people do."
  2. "I wish I could be more organized like other people."
  3. "I want to talk about something that's bothering me."
  4. "I just don't want people in my family to fight anymore."

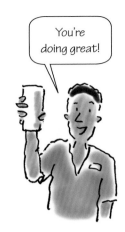

You're doing great!

65. 3. By initiating conversation, the client has taken the first step toward assertive behavior. To smooth over, or minimize, troubling events is not an assertive position. The first option reflects a lack of self-confidence, and is non assertive. Statements that express the client's wishes aren't assertive statements.

CN: Psychosocial integrity; CNS: None; CL: Analyze

66. Which factors contribute to a difficulty creating a therapeutic alliance among clients with personality disorders? Select all that apply.
  1. Client's suspiciousness
  2. Detachment from clients
  3. Secretive style and hostility of clients
  4. Transference from the nurse
  5. Setting limits

66. 1, 2, 3. When client's display behaviors of suspicion, detachment, secretive style, and hostility it becomes difficult to create a therapeutic alliance. . Setting limits is a crucial component of a therapeutic alliance with clients who have personality disorders. These limits will need to be repeated to maintain client responsibilities.

CN: Psychosocial integrity; CNS: None; CL: Analyze

67. The health care provider is preparing to write a plan of care for a client with borderline personality disorder. Which medication would the nurse anticipate for this client?
  1. Monoamine oxidase inhibitors (MAOIs) work best because the effects are felt very quickly
  2. Selective serotonin reuptake inhibitors (SSRIs), along with an atypical antipsychotic, are used to treat, mood instability and impulsivity
  3. Antipsychotics, along with an antidepressant, will treat illusions, ideas of reference, paranoid thinking, anxiety, and hostility in clients
  4. Anxiolytics will reduce the anxiety and cognitive distortions which frequently occur in these clients

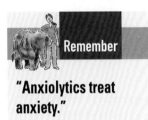

Remember

"Anxiolytics treat anxiety."

These include buspirone.

67. 2. Selective serotonin reuptake inhibitors and atypical antipsychotics are used to treat dysphoria, mood instability, and impulsivity in clients with borderline personality disorder. This is the best choice of medications for a client with borderline personality disorder. Monoamine oxidase inhibitors have food restrictions, and clients with borderline personality disorder would not comply with such restrictions. Antipsychotics are prescribed for psychotic behaviors such as illusions, ideas of reference, and paranoid thinking. Anxiolytics may be prescribed for clients with borderline personality disorder, but these medications are limited to addressing anxiety. Clients with borderline personality disorder experience symptoms other than anxiety.

CN: Safe, effective care environment; CNS: Management of care; CL: Analyze

68. A nurse notices that a client with dependent personality disorder is depressed. Which factor contributes to depression?
  1. Unmet needs
  2. Sense of smothering
  3. Messy, unkempt appearance
  4. Difficulty delaying gratification

I wonder what caused the change.

68. 1. Having unmet needs is a precursor to depression. Clients with dependent personality disorder don't experience a sense of smothering which is seen in clients with panic disorder. Poor hygiene is often a manifestation of depression. Clients with delayed gratification tend to have anxiety problems, not problems with depression.

CN: Psychosocial integrity; CNS: None; CL: Analyze

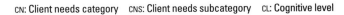

69. A client with dependent personality disorder states, "I'll never be able to take care of myself." What is the nurse's **best** response?
1. "You are perfectly capable of normal functioning."
2. "Let's talk about what makes you so fearful."
3. "I think we need to work on identifying your strengths."
4. "Can we talk about this tomorrow at the family meeting?"

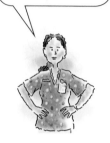

Keep in mind the type of personality this client has.

69. 2. The client with dependent personality disorder is afraid of abandonment and being unable to care for himself. Talking about his fears is a useful strategy. Answer one is inappropriate because the nurse doesn't recognize the client's feelings. When the client makes a desperate statement, the nurse must respond to the client's feelings, rather than insert her opinion. Identifying a client's strengths will add to his feelings inadequacy. Waiting to talk about his concern until the family meeting minimizes its importance.
CN: Psychosocial integrity; CNS: None; CL: Analyze

70. A client on your unit says, "There is a contract out on me." The client refuses to leave the semiprivate room, and insists on searching the roommate before allowing him to enter. Which action should the nurse take **first**?
1. Transfer the client to a private room on another floor
2. Acknowledge the client's fear of leaving his room
3. Transfer the roommate to another room on a different unit
4. Lock the client out of his room for a while

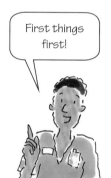

First things first!

70. 2. Acknowledging underlying feelings may help defuse the client's anxiety without promoting his delusional thinking. This, in turn, may help the client distinguish between his emotional state and external reality. Transferring either client to another room would validate the client's delusional thinking. Locking the client out of his room may further escalate the client's anxiety and stimulate aggressive behavior.
CN: Psychosocial integrity; CNS: None; CL: Apply

71. A client with schizotypal personality disorder is sitting in urine. He's playing in it, smiling, and softly singing a child's song. Which action would be **best**?
1. Ask the client why he didn't use the bathroom
2. Firmly tell the client that their behavior is unacceptable
3. Ask the client if they are ready to get cleaned up now
4. Help the client to the shower and change the bedclothes

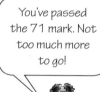

You've passed the 71 mark. Not too much more to go!

71. 4. A client with a schizotypal personality disorder can experience high levels of anxiety and regress to childlike behaviors. This client may require help meeting self-care needs. The client may not respond to the other options, or those options may generate more anxiety.
CN: Psychosocial integrity; CNS: None; CL: Apply

72. A client with avoidant personality disorder states that occupational therapy (OT) is boring, and she does not want to go. Which action by the nurse is **most** appropriate?
1. State firmly that you'll escort the client to OT
2. Arrange OT on the unit for this client
3. Ask the client to describe why OT is boring
4. Allow the client to skip OT until she feels better

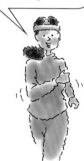

72. 1. If given the chance, a client with avoidant personality disorder will typically choose to remain immobilized. The nurse should insist that the client participate in OT. Arranging for OT on the unit validates and reinforces the client's desire to be immobile. Addressing the client's perceived boredom negates the client's real need for OT. There is no indication that the client is incapable of participating in OT.
CN: Psychosocial integrity; CNS: None; CL: Apply

73. A client with paranoid personality disorder is working toward the goal of increasing social interactions. Which behavior indicates that the client is meeting this goal?
1. The client develops and follows a schedule of group activities.
2. The client verbalizes aggressive feelings to the nurse.
3. The client visits the consumer center to use the internet.
4. The client explores somatic reports with the staff.

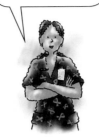

Which answer will help the client increase social interaction?

73. 1. By developing and following a schedule of group activities, the client increases their opportunity to develop social skills and increase interactions with others. Verbalizing aggressive feelings doesn't give the client an opportunity to increase social interaction. Using a computer at the consumer center is a solitary activity. Talking to the staff about somatic reports doesn't provide opportunities for social interaction.
CN: Psychosocial integrity; CNS: None; CL: Apply

74. A nurse is working with the family of a client diagnosed with schizoid personality disorder. The goal is to help the client with decision making. Which outcome indicates that the nurse's interventions have been successful?
1. The family prevents the client from experiencing disappointments.
2. The family encourages the client to talk about specific issues and concerns.
3. The family removes alcohol and unnecessary prescription drugs from the house.
4. The family does not let the client obtain secondary gains from illness

74. 2. A client with schizoid personality disorder is typically vague and has difficulty with self-expression. Goals of treatment most often are solution-focused using brief therapy approaches.. Encouraging the client to talk about specific issues and concerns shows that the nurse's interventions were successful. It is neither realistic nor helpful for the family to protect the client from disappointments. Clients with schizoid personality disorder are not at high risk for substance abuse, and don't seek secondary gains from illness.
CN: Psychosocial integrity; CNS: None; CL: Apply

75. A nurse discusses job opportunities with a client diagnosed with schizoid personality disorder. Which suggestion would be **most** helpful?
1. "You could work part time in a family restaurant."
2. "Maybe your friend could get you a customer service job where you work in the evenings."
3. "Your idea of applying for the position of filing and organizing records is worth pursuing."
4. "Being an introvert limits your employment opportunities."

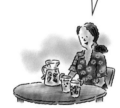

When trying to answer question 75, think about the type of activities this client prefers.

75. 3. Clients with schizoid personality disorder prefer solitary activities, such as filing. Working as a cashier or customer service representative would involve interacting with people.
CN: Psychosocial integrity; CNS: None; CL: Analyze

76. A client with borderline personality disorder is learning how to verbalize, rather than act on, a desire to hurt himself. What is the **most** appropriate nursing intervention?
1. Explain how pain triggers intense anger and causes the client to act out
2. Determine if problems with the client's family cause him to act aggressively
3. Teach the client that being volatile is a normal reaction to unfair events
4. Have the client work on identifying speech and behavior that accompany anger

76. 4. Aggressive speech and inappropriate behaviors indicate that the client is angry or upset. These feelings may trigger inappropriate behavior. Pain rarely triggers intense anger or causes a client to act out. Blaming family for inappropriate handling of anger is not helpful. Being volatile isn't a normal reaction to unfair life events. This client needs to express anger in safe and appropriate ways.
CN: Psychosocial integrity; CNS: None; CL: Analyze

CN: Client needs category   CNS: Client needs subcategory   CL: Cognitive level

77. A client with borderline personality disorder states that he doesn't know how to deal with his impulsive behavior. Which intervention should the nurse implement?
1. Teach the client that impulsive behavior is part of his illness
2. Explore how depression influences impulsive situations
3. Choose an example of an impulsive situation and explore it
4. Decrease interactions in which impulsive behavior occurs

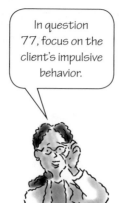

In question 77, focus on the client's impulsive behavior.

77. 3. By choosing an impulsive situation to explore with the client, the nurse can help him begin to understand the cause and consequences of his behavior and how to modify it. Although impulsive behavior is part of borderline personality disorder, the nurse's intervention needs to address ways to handle it. Anxiety, not depression, is strongly related to impulsive behavior. Decreasing social interactions is unrealistic. It is more useful to address the impulsive behavior.
CN: Psychosocial integrity; CNS: None; CL: Analyze

78. A nurse is monitoring a client who appears to be hallucinating. The nurse notes paranoid content in the client's speech, and increasing agitation. The client is gesturing at a figure on the television. Which nursing interventions are appropriate? Select all that apply.
1. In a firm voice, instruct the client to stop the behavior
2. Reinforce that the client is not in any danger
3. Acknowledge the presence of the hallucinations
4. Instruct other team members to ignore the client's behavior
5. Immediately implement physical restraint procedures
6. Use a calm voice and simple commands

78. 2, 3, 6. Using a calm voice, the nurse should reassure the client of his safety. The nurse should acknowledge his hallucinatory experience, and should not challenge the client. It's not appropriate to ask the client stop the behavior. Implementing restraints is not warranted at this time. Although the client is agitated, no evidence suggests that he is at risk of harming himself or others.
CN: Psychosocial integrity; CNS: None; CL: Apply

79. When assessing a client diagnosed with impulse control disorder, the nurse observes violent, aggressive, and assaultive behavior. Which assessment data will the nurse likely find? Select all that apply.
1. The client functions well in other areas of his life.
2. The degree of aggressiveness is out of proportion to the stressor.
3. The violent behavior is most often justified by the stressor.
4. The client has a history of parental alcoholism and a chaotic, abusive family life.
5. The client has no remorse about the inability to control his behavior.

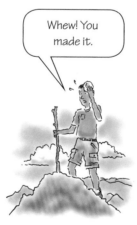

Whew! You made it.

79. 1, 2, 4. A client with an impulse control disorder who displays violent, aggressive, and assaultive behavior will generally function well in other areas of his life. The degree of aggressiveness is typically out of proportion to the stressor. This client commonly has a history of parental alcoholism and a chaotic family life, and will often verbalize sincere remorse and guilt for the aggressive behavior.
CN: Psychosocial integrity; CNS: None; CL: Apply

CN: Client needs category   CNS: Client needs subcategory   CL: Cognitive level

Chapter 17

Schizophrenic & Delusional Disorders

So I'm talking to Queen Elizabeth the other day, and she said you'd do spectacularly well on this chapter. (I'm kidding. What, do I look delusional?) Personally, I think you'll do even better than that. Go for it!

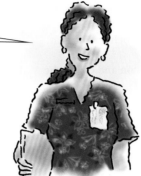

1. A client with schizophrenia tells his nurse that he is scheduled to meet the King of Samoa at a certain time, making it impossible for the client to leave his room for dinner. Which response by the nurse is **most** appropriate?
1. "It's mealtime. Let's go to the dining room so you can eat."
2. "The King of Samoa told me to take you to dinner until he arrives."
3. "The provider expects you to follow the unit schedule."
4. "People who do not eat on this unit are not being cooperative."

Therapeutic intervention is the key.

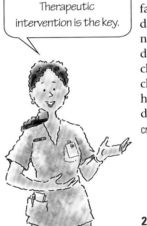

1. 1. A delusional client is so wrapped up in his false beliefs that he tends to disregard activities of daily living, such as nutrition and hydration. He needs clear, concise, firm directions to meet his daily needs. Answer two belittles and tricks the client, possibly evoking mistrust on the part of the client. Answer three evades the issue of meeting his basic needs. Answer four is demeaning and doesn't address the delusion.
CN: Health promotion and maintenance; CNS: None; CL: Apply

2. During breakfast, a client announces that he is the President of the United States. What is the nurse's **best** response?
1. "How are you feeling today, Mr. President?"
2. "What do you enjoy most about being President?"
3. "How is your breakfast this morning, sir?"
4. "What is the President having for breakfast today?"

2. 3. Asking about breakfast redirects the client, and sets his focus on a structured activity or reality-based task. The other responses focus attention on, or support, the client's delusion.
CN: Psychosocial integrity; CNS: None; CL: Apply

3. A 40-year-old client with schizophrenia lives in a rooming house. At the weekly nursing clinic he reports creatures eating at his skin while scratching vigorously. Which intervention should be done **first**?
1. Encourage him to discuss his delusions
2. Administer an anticholinergic medication
3. Assess the physical problems
4. Call the healthcare provider

3. 3. Clients with schizophrenia generally have poor visceral recognition because they live so fully in their fantasy world. They need to have an in-depth assessment of physical complaints that may spill over into their delusional symptoms. Talking with the client won't provide an assessment of his itching, and itching isn't an adverse reaction of antipsychotic drugs. The client's provider should be called if the assessment warrants.
CN: Safe, effective care environment; CNS: Management of care; CL: Apply

CN: Client needs category   CNS: Client needs subcategory   CL: Cognitive level

4. A 22-year-old client with schizophrenia was admitted to the psychiatric unit during the night. The next morning, he began to misidentify the nurse and call her by his sister's name. Which intervention is **best**?
1. Assess the client for impulse control and potential violence
2. Take the client to his room, where he will feel safer
3. Understand that the client believes he is at home
4. Correct the misidentification and orient the client to the unit and staff

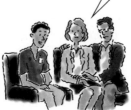

Orienting a new client to the staff and the surroundings can help the client feel in control.

4. 4. Misidentification can contribute to anxiety, fear, aggression, and hostility. Orienting a new client to the hospital unit, staff, and other clients, along with establishing a nurse–client relationship, can decrease these feelings and help the client feel in control. Assessing for impulse control and potential violence are important nursing functions for any psychiatric client, but is not a first priority in this situation. A perceived supportive environment reduces the risk for violence. Withdrawing to his room, unless interpersonal relationships have become nontherapeutic, encourages this client to remain in his fantasy world. There is no data to suggest that the client does not realize he is not at home.
CN: Psychosocial integrity; CNS: None; CL: Apply

5. A client with schizophrenia withdraws to his room and resists efforts to engage in activities. The nurse is aware that a client with schizophrenia, who is experiencing isolation, is at risk for developing:
1. delusions.
2. hallucinations.
3. anhedonia.
4. depression.

5. 2. Prolonged isolation can produce sensory deprivation, manifested by hallucinations. A delusion is a false, fixed belief that has no basis in reality. Anhedonia is the inability to find enjoyment in activities, a symptom typically associated with depression. Experiencing a mood disorder, such as depression, does not result from withdrawal to one's room or failure to engage in activities.
CN: Psychosocial integrity; CNS: None; CL: Apply

6. A client diagnosed with schizophrenia several years ago tells a nurse that he feels "very sad." The nurse observes that the client is smiling when he makes this statement. The nurse interprets the behavior as:
1. inappropriate affect.
2. extrapyramidal symptoms.
3. high level insight.
4. disguised depression.

6. 1. Affect refers to behaviors, such as facial expressions, that can be observed when a person is experiencing feelings. If the client's affect doesn't reflect the emotional content of the statement, the affect is considered inappropriate. This is a typical symptom of schizophrenia. Extrapyramidal symptoms are adverse effects of some categories of antipsychotic medication. Insight is a component of the mental status examination and is the ability to perceive oneself realistically and understand if a problem exists. Disguised depression is more subtle than the overt inappropriate, or conflicting affect, seen in clients with schizophrenia.
CN: Psychosocial integrity; CNS: None; CL: Apply

7. A client with schizophrenia exhibits extreme social withdrawal, odd mannerisms, and other regressive behaviors. What is the nurse's **most** appropriate intervention for this client?
1. Require that the client attend one group activity each day
2. Suggest that the client socialize with his same gender peer group
3. Interact with the client often and briefly, in a genuine manner
4. Allow the client to join the community when he is ready

7. 3. Plan to frequently interact with the client in a friendly, brief, undemanding manner. Clients with disorganized thinking related to schizophrenia require one-on-one non-threatening activities and should not remain in social isolation. There is no particular indication for socializing with a same gender peer group. Requiring a client to attend a group may create undue pressure and impede trust-building. Clients may feel threatened by group activities and are likely to be a poor judge of their own readiness to participate in the milieu.
CN: Psychosocial integrity; CNS: None; CL: Apply

8. A client on the psychiatric unit is copying and imitating the movements of his primary nurse. During recovery, he says, "I thought the nurse was my mirror. I only felt connected when I saw my nurse." How would the nurse interpret this behavior?
1. Modeling
2. Echopraxia
3. Ego-syntonicity
4. Ritualism

9. A teenager states, "My father has schizophrenia and I am afraid I have it too." Which behavior would prompt further evaluation by the nurse?
1. Changes in his mood
2. Preoccupation with his body
3. Spending more time away from home
4. Changes in sleep patterns

10. The nurse is teaching the family of a client with a psychiatric disorder about traditional antipsychotic drugs and their effect on symptoms. Which symptom would be **most** responsive to these types of drugs?
1. Apathy
2. Delusions
3. Social withdrawal
4. Attention impairment

11. A client was hospitalized after his son filed a petition for the involuntary hospitalization of the client for safety reasons. The son tells the nurse that his father is angry, and will not talk with him. This leaves the son feeling frustrated and guilty about his decision. What is the **most** appropriate response by the nurse?
1. "Your father is very sick and doesn't know he needs help."
2. "He will feel differently about this once he gets better."
3. "It sounds as if you are feeling guilty about bringing your father here."
4. "This is a stressful time for you, but you will feel better as he gets well."

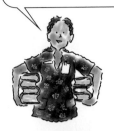

There's a fancy word that describes this behavior—I remember reading it somewhere.

Remember

"Typical" or traditional antipsychotics treat the "typical" positive symptoms associated with psychotic disorders, such as delusions, hallucinations, thought disorder, and disorganized speech. "Atypical" antipsychotics treat the negative symptoms, including affective flattening, restricted thought and speech, apathy, anhedonia, asociality, and attention impairment.

Typical antipsychotics
- Chlorpromazine
- Fluphenazine decanoate
- Fluphenazine
- Haloperidol
- Haloperidol decanoate
- Loxapine
- Molindone
- Perphenazine
- Perphenazine and amitriptyline
- Pimozide
- Thioridazine
- Thiothixene
- Trifluoperazine

Atypical antipsychotics
- Aripiprazole
- Clozapine
- Olanzapine
- Quetiapine
- Risperidone
- Ziprasidone

8. 2. Echopraxia is the involuntary copying of another's behaviors, and is the result of the loss of ego boundaries. Modeling is the conscious copying of someone's behaviors. Ego-syntonicity refers to behaviors that correspond with the individual's sense of self. Ritualistic behaviors are repetitive and compulsive.
CN: Psychosocial integrity; CNS: None; CL: Apply

9. 4. In conjunction with other signs, such as changes in personal care habits and social isolation, changes in sleep patterns are distinctive initial signs of schizophrenia. A change in sleep pattern by itself could be a normal adolescent behavior. Moodiness, preoccupation with the body, and spending more time away from home are normal adolescent behaviors.
CN: Health promotion and maintenance; CNS: None; CL: Apply

10. 2. Positive symptoms, such as delusions, hallucinations, thought disorder, and disorganized speech, respond to traditional antipsychotic drugs. The other options belong in a category of negative symptoms, including affective flattening, restricted thought and speech, apathy, anhedonia, asociality, and attention impairment. Negative symptoms are more responsive to the new atypical antipsychotics, such as clozapine risperidone, and olanzapine.
CN: Physiological integrity; CNS: Pharmacological and parenteral therapies; CL: Apply

11. 3. This response focuses on the son and helps him discuss, and deal, with his feelings. Unresolved feelings of guilt, shame, isolation, and loss of hope can impact a family's ability to manage the crisis and be supportive to the client. The other options offer premature reassurance and cut off the opportunity for the son to discuss his feelings.
CN: Psychosocial integrity; CNS: None; CL: Apply

12. A client has been compliant with her prescribed antipsychotic medication regimen for a number of years. With the addition of an antibiotic, the client reports distressing new symptoms. What is the **most** appropriate intervention by the nurse?

1. Arrange for the client to be hospitalized
2. Have a community nurse administer the medication
3. Assess the client's symptoms and reinforce medication teaching
4. Direct the client immediately to the health care provider

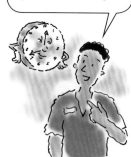

Looks like you are flying through these questions. Great job!

12. 3. This client has been successful and reliable in carrying out her current medication regimen. The nurse should assume that competency includes self-administration of antibiotics if the instructions are understood. The nurse should assess the client's symptoms and reinforce all medication teaching. No evidence exists that the client is experiencing relapse, so hospitalization would not be indicated. Having a community nurse give the medication encourages dependency as opposed to self-care. It is premature to direct the client to a provider without the results of the nursing assessment.

CN: Physiological integrity; CNS: Pharmacological; CL: Apply

13. A client calls the clinic worried about experiencing new symptoms after taking antipsychotic medicine. The client reports persistent, uncontrollable restlessness of the limbs and head despite improvement in psychotic symptoms. What is the **most** appropriate intervention by the nurse?

1. Inform the client to ignore these symptoms because they will go away
2. Advise the client to experiment with different dosages to see how he feels
3. Tell the client to go to the emergency room if blurred vision or fever develops
4. Direct the client to see the provider for medication to address these side effects

13. 4. Symptoms of tardive dyskinesia include tongue protrusion, lip smacking, chewing, blinking, grimacing, choreiform movements of limbs and trunk, and foot tapping. Primary prevention of tardive dyskinesia is achieved by using the lowest effective dose of a neuroleptic for the shortest time. However, with diseases of chronic psychosis such as schizophrenia, this strategy must be balanced with the fact that increased dosages are more beneficial in preventing recurrence of psychosis. If tardive dyskinesia is diagnosed, the causative drug should be discontinued. Blurred vision is a common adverse reaction of antipsychotic drugs and usually disappears after a few weeks of therapy. Restlessness is associated with akathisia. Sudden fever is a symptom of a malignant neurological disorder. The prescribing provider will make appropriate changes to meet the client's need. Clients should not ignore such symptoms, or adjust their own medication dosage.

CN: Physiological integrity; CNS: Reduction of risk potential; CL: Apply

14. A client approaches a nurse and tells her that he hears voices telling him that he is evil and deserves to die. Which response, by the nurse, is **most** appropriate?

1. "The voices are not real, so ignore them."
2. "I do not see anyone in the room."
3. "I do not hear any voices, but I understand that you do."
4. "Tell the voices you will not listen to them."

14. 3. The nurse should let the client know that although she cannot hear the voices, she understands that they are real to him. She should keep communication open and encourage him to talk. Telling the client that the voices are not real may make him hold tighter to his belief and does not promote trust. Telling him to talk back to the voices validates their reality.

CN: Psychosocial integrity; CNS: None; CL: Apply

15. A 49-year-old client is admitted to the emergency department frightened and reporting that he hears voices telling him to do bad things. Which intervention should be the nurse's **priority**?
1. Reassure the client that he is safe and that the voices are not real
2. Tell the client he is safe now and promise the staff will protect him
3. Assess the nature of the commands by asking what the voices are saying
4. Administer a neuroleptic medication before speaking with the client

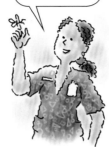

Remember to prioritize!

15. 3. Safety is the priority. The nurse should ask the client directly about the nature of the auditory commands to ensure the safety of the client and staff. The nurse should never make promises to the client that she may not be able to fulfill. The provider may order a neuroleptic, but the nurse's priority is to address safety.

CN: Safe, effective care environment; CNS: Management of care; CL: Apply

16. A client newly admitted to an inpatient unit approaches a nursing student and states, "I am the leader of a super race!" What is the nursing student's **most** appropriate response?
1. Smile, and walk into the nurses' station without responding to the client
2. Immediately challenge the client's false belief to address his denial
3. Listen for hidden messages in themes of delusion, indicating unmet needs
4. Introduce herself, shake hands, and sit down with the client in the dayroom

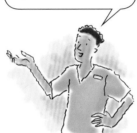

Teach nursing students the importance of genuine interest and concern for the client's needs.

16. 4. The first goal is to establish a trusting relationship with the client. Ignoring the client and walking into the nurses' station would indicate disinterest, and lack of concern about the client's feelings. The student should sit, and make herself available, reflecting concern and interest. After establishing a trusting relationship and easing the client's anxiety, the student can then orient the client to reality, listen to his concerns and fears, and try to understand the feelings reflected in the delusions. Delusions are firmly maintained false beliefs, and attempts to dismiss or dispute them do not work.

CN: Safe, effective care environment; CNS: Management of care; CL: Apply

17. A client is admitted with an acute schizophrenic reaction after a home rampage that ended with an assault on local police. Which medication should the nurse anticipate if these aggressive symptoms persist?
1. Diphenhydramine
2. Paroxetine
3. Haloperidol
4. Fluoxetine

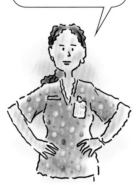

Often a combination of medications is needed to address a problem.

17. 3. Haloperidol is the classic drug of choice to treat symptoms of acute psychosis. Diphenhydramine may be indicated in conjunction with other medications for its sedating effect, but is not a primary drug of choice. Paroxetine and Fluoxetine are antidepressant medications, and not indicated to treat acute schizophrenia.

CN: Physiological integrity; CNS: Pharmacological and parenteral therapies; CL: Analyze

18. A nurse is assisting with morning care when a client suddenly throws off her covers and starts shouting, "My body is changing and disintegrating because I am of the other world." The nurse describes this behavior as:
1. depersonalization.
2. ideas of reference.
3. looseness of association.
4. paranoid ideation.

18. 1. Depersonalization is a state in which the client feels unreal, or believes parts of the body are being distorted. Ideas of reference involve the belief that casual events, people's remarks, etc. are referring to oneself when, in fact, they are not. The term *loose associations* refers to sentences that have vague connections to each other. Paranoid ideations are beliefs that others intend to harm the client in some way.

CN: Psychosocial integrity; CNS: None; CL: Analyze

19. A 16-year-old client with a diagnosis of schizophrenia has become very clingy and begins sucking her thumb while interacting with the nurse. The nurse interprets this behavior as:
1. repression.
2. regression.
3. rationalization.
4. projection.

20. The nurse is interviewing a client with paranoid ideation. Which assessment technique is **most** appropriate for the nurse to use?
1. Indirect questions
2. Direct questions
3. Lead-in remarks
4. Open-ended sentences

21. A nurse on a psychiatric unit observes a client in the corner of the room moving his lips as if he were talking to himself. What is the **most** appropriate intervention?
1. Ask him why he is talking to himself
2. Leave him alone until he stops talking
3. Tell him it is not good for him to talk to himself
4. Invite him to join in a card game with the nurse

22. A client makes vague statements with no logical connections and asks whether the nurse understands. What is the **best** response by the nurse?
1. "Why not wait until later to talk about it?"
2. "I cannot talk about this with you until you are able to make sense."
3. "Yes, I understand exactly what you mean."
4. "I want to understand what you are saying, but I am confused."

23. A client asks the nurse if she hears the voice of a nonexistent man speaking to him. What is nurse's **most** appropriate response?
1. "There is no one is in your room except you."
2. "Yes, I hear him, but we will not listen to him."
3. "What has he told you? Is it helpful advice?"
4. "No, I don't hear him, but I know you do. What is he saying?"

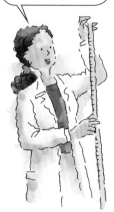

Any way you measure it, you're doing great.

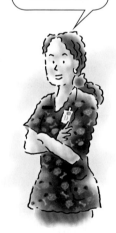

I'm trying to understand but sometimes it's difficult.

19. 2. Regression, a return to earlier behavior in order to reduce anxiety, is the basic defense mechanism in schizophrenia. Repression is the blocking of unacceptable thoughts or impulses from the consciousness. Rationalization is a defense mechanism used to justify one's behavior. Projection is a defense mechanism in which one blames others and attempts to justify actions.
CN: Psychosocial integrity; CNS: None; CL: Apply

20. 2. Direct questioning is the most appropriate technique to use when interviewing a client with paranoid ideation. Specific questions provide the nurse with useful information. The other forms of communication may be misunderstood by the client, and his responses may be vague.
CN: Psychosocial integrity; CNS: None; CL: Apply

21. 4. Being with the nurse provides stimulation that competes with the hallucinations. The client doesn't think he is talking to himself. He thinks that he is responding to the voices he hears. Being alone keeps the client in his fantasy world. Telling the client that he should not talk to himself fails to understand how real his fantasy world and hallucinations are.
CN: Psychosocial integrity; CNS: None; CL: Apply

22. 4. The nurse needs to communicate that she wants to understand without blaming the client for the lack of understanding. Asking the client to wait cuts off an attempt to communicate and asks the client to do what he cannot at present. Telling the client that he is not making sense is judgmental and could impair the therapeutic relationship. Pretending to understand is a violation of trust and can damage the therapeutic relationship.
CN: Psychosocial integrity; CNS: None; CL: Apply

23. 4. This response points out reality and shows concern and support. Attempting to convince the client that no voice exists could deepen his misbelief, and make him feel more out of control due to the negative and fearful nature of hallucinations. The other two options violate the trust of the therapeutic relationship.
CN: Safe, effective care environment; CNS: Management of care; CL: Apply

24. The nurse is providing information to a client who is taking chlorpromazine. What is the **most** important information for the nurse to provide?
1. Reduce the dosage if feeling better
2. Stop taking medication when sunbathing
3. Stop taking the drug if adverse reactions develop
4. Schedule routine medication checks

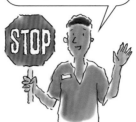

Checking the client's medications regularly is always a good idea.

24. 4. It is important to continually assess for adverse reactions and continued therapeutic effectiveness. The dosage should be changed if ordered by the primary care provider. While chlorpromazine can exacerbate serious sunburns, medication should not be discontinued without an order from the provider. Adverse reactions should be immediately reported to the provider.
CN: Physiological integrity; CNS: Pharmacological and parenteral therapies; CL: Apply

25. A 34-year-old male, who is single and employed, has been referred to a mental health clinic by the court. The man has accused his next-door neighbor's wife of being in love with him. He states that she, "Writes love notes and calls me constantly throughout the week." The clinic nurse suspects that this client has:
1. major depression.
2. paranoid schizophrenia.
3. delusional disorder.
4. bipolar affective disorder.

25. 3. This client has a delusional disorder with erotomanic delusions as his primary symptom. He believes that he is loved intensely by a married person who shows no interest in him. No symptoms of major depression exist. The client does not believe someone is trying to harm him, the hallmark characteristic of paranoia. Bipolar affective disorder is characterized by cycles of mania and depression.
CN: Psychosocial integrity; CNS: None; CL: Apply

26. A homebound client taking clozapine tells the nurse that he has been feeling tired for five days. His temperature is 99.6° F (37.5° C); pulse, 110 bpm; and respirations, 20 breaths/min. What is the **best** information for the nurse to tell the client?
1. Take the medication with milk, fruit juice, soda or coffee
2. Stop the medication at once and see the provider immediately
3. Understand that the symptoms will disappear as soon as you get more rest
4. Stop the medication gradually and see the provider next week

Do the client's symptoms suggest an emergency situation?

26. 2. The client should stop the medication and see his provider immediately. Fever can be a sign of agranulocytosis, which is a medical emergency. Taking antipsychotic medication with milk, nicotine, and caffeine will decrease the effectiveness. Rest will have no effect on this client's symptoms. Drowsiness and fatigue usually disappear with continued therapy.
CN: Physiological integrity; CNS: Pharmacological and parenteral therapies; CL: Apply

27. A client who is delusional approaches the nurse and states, "You are my aunt and you live with my family." What is the **most** appropriate response by the nurse?
1. "I work here; I am not your aunt."
2. "I do not live in your town."
3. "I am honored to be your aunt."
4. "My name is Anne. What is your name?"

27. 4. By the nurse stating her name and asking the name of the client's aunt, the nurse acknowledges the client is speaking about a family member. The nurse's response is based on reality orientation. The other responses all focus on and respond directly to the client's fixed delusional system.
CN: Psychosocial integrity; CNS: None; CL: Apply

28. A client tells the nurse that he can only drink bottled water because his tap water has been poisoned. The nurse understands that this client is exhibiting:
1. paranoid ideation.
2. auditory hallucinations.
3. delusions of grandeur.
4. perseveration.

28. 1. Paranoid ideation is a baseless or excessive suspicion of the motives of others. This suspicion sometimes progresses to disturbances of consciousness or acts of aggression believed to be performed in self-defense. This client is extremely suspicious and distrustful of others. Auditory hallucinations occur when a client hears voices that are often threatening or violent. Delusions of grandeur are an exaggerated sense of self-importance. A client with perseveration involuntarily repeats words.
CN: Psychosocial integrity; CNS: None; CL: Apply

29. A client diagnosed with schizophrenia is receiving an antipsychotic medication. His provider has just prescribed benztropine. Which adverse reaction was this medication **most** likely prescribed for?
1. Tardive dyskinesia
2. Hypertensive crisis
3. Acute dystonia
4. Orthostatic hypotension

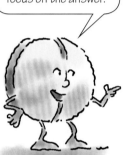

The words *most likely* can help you focus on the answer.

29. 3. Benztropine is used as an adjunctive therapy in parkinsonism, and for all conditions and medications that produce extrapyramidal symptoms except tardive dyskinesia, which is permanent and untreatable. Its anticholinergic action reduces the extrapyramidal effects associated with antipsychotic drugs. Hypertensive crisis and orthostatic hypotension are not associated with extrapyramidal symptoms.
CN: Physiological integrity; CNS: Pharmacological and parenteral therapies; CL: Analyze

30. What is the **most** appropriate nursing intervention for a client experiencing hallucinations?
1. Restrict the client to his room to help reduce all stimulation
2. Engage him in an activity that distracts from the hallucinations
3. Discourage attempts to understand what precipitates his hallucinations
4. Support perceptual distortions until he gives them up of his own accord

30. 2. Providing distracting activities acknowledges the presence of the hallucination and teaches the client ways to decrease the frequency or intensity of hallucinations. The other options support and maintain hallucinations or deny their existence.
CN: Psychosocial integrity; CNS: None; CL: Apply

31. A client with schizophrenia reports that her hallucinations have decreased in frequency. Which client statement indicates an understanding of her illness and medication?
1. "I am happy I can read and watch television again."
2. "I like to be in my room where it is quiet."
3. "Now that the voices are leaving, I can stop my medicine."
4. "The new medicine is really helping to quiet the voices."

31. 4. The client reports an understanding of the relationship between her symptoms and her medication. In addition she implies that this healing is an ongoing process. Being able to read and watch television does not indicate a reduction of her symptoms. A pattern of isolating herself in her room may exacerbate symptoms again. Further, a reduction of symptoms is supportive of continuation of the medication rather than stopping it.
CN: Physiological integrity; CNS: Pharmacological; CL: Apply

CN: Client needs category   CNS: Client needs subcategory   CL: Cognitive level

32. A single, 24-year-old client is admitted to the hospital for the first time with an acute schizophrenic reaction. What therapy should the nurse anticipate for this client?
1. Counseling
2. Biofeedback
3. Drug therapy
4. Electroconvulsive therapy

32. 3. Drug therapy is usually successful in normalizing behavior and reducing, or eliminating, hallucinations, delusions, thought disorder, affect flattening, apathy, and asociality. Counseling is not appropriate at this time. Electroconvulsive therapy might be considered for schizoaffective disorder, which has a mood component, and is a treatment of choice for clinical depression. Biofeedback reduces anxiety and modifies behavioral responses, but isn't a major component in the treatment of schizophrenia.
CN: Psychosocial integrity; CNS: None; CL: Apply

33. A client tells a nurse that voices are telling him to do "terrible things." What is the nurse's **best** response?
1. Find out what the voices are telling him
2. Let him go to his room to decrease his anxiety
3. Begin talking to the client about an unrelated topic
4. Tell the client the voices are not real

33. 1. For safety purposes, the nurse must find out whether the voices are directing this client to harm himself or others. Further assessment can help identify appropriate therapeutic interventions. Isolating a person during this intense sensory confusion often reinforces the psychosis. Changing the topic indicates that the nurse isn't concerned about the client's fears. Dismissing the voices shuts down communication between the client and the nurse.
CN: Psychosocial integrity; CNS: None; CL: Apply

34. A client insistently reports that the CIA has been planning to recruit him for a secret mission. This delusion is a defense against the feeling of:
1. aggression.
2. guilt.
3. inferiority.
4. persecution.

34. 3. This example of a delusional system contains grandiose ideation that allows the client to feel important rather than inferior. Feelings of aggression will appear as violent or hostile thoughts. Guilt results in beliefs that the person deserves to be punished. Persecution is the fear that others are trying to harm you.
CN: Psychosocial integrity; CNS: None; CL: Apply

35. A client has started taking haloperidol. What is the **most** important instruction for the nurse to give the client?
1. "You should report feelings of restlessness or agitation at once."
2. "Use a sunscreen outdoors on a year-round basis."
3. "Be aware you will feel increased energy taking this drug."
4. "This drug will help control high blood pressure."

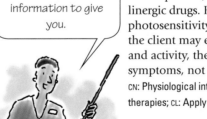

I have important information to give you.

35. 1. Agitation and restlessness are adverse effects of haloperidol, and can be treated with anticholinergic drugs. Haloperidol isn't likely to cause photosensitivity or control hypertension. Although the client may experience increased concentration and activity, these effects are due to a decrease in symptoms, not the medication itself.
CN: Physiological integrity; CNS: Pharmacological and parenteral therapies; CL: Apply

36. A 45-year-old client experiencing delusions has been admitted to the crisis center. When assessing the content of her delusions, the nurse should look for:
  1. logic.
  2. religious beliefs.
  3. themes.
  4. true experiences.

36. 3. A delusion is a false, fixed belief that misrepresents perceptions or experiences and isn't open to rational discussion. Understanding the themes inherent in the client's psychotic symptoms may help the nurse learn what stresses trigger the symptoms. Assessing for logic, religious beliefs, or true experiences will draw the nurse into the delusional thinking and therefore is not therapeutic.
CN: Psychosocial integrity; CNS: None; CL: Analyze

37. The nurse is caring for a 58-year-old male client with schizophrenia. The client says, "The earth and the roof of the house rule the political structure with particles of rain." The nurse interprets this statement as:
  1. tangentiality.
  2. perseveration.
  3. loose association.
  4. thought blocking.

37. 3. Loose association refers to a client's changing ideas from one unrelated theme to another. Tangentiality is the wandering from topic to topic. Perseveration is the involuntary repetition of an answer to a question, in response to a new question. Thought blocking is a client's difficulty articulating a response or stopping midsentence.
CN: Psychosocial integrity; CNS: None; CL: Apply

38. Clients with schizophrenia often experience non-adherence to prescribed medication protocols. Nurses collaborate with these clients to develop a program of successful adherence. How are long-acting decanoate injections a helpful treatment option for these clients?
  1. Clients who decline or miss their scheduled injection can receive a double dose the next time.
  2. Clients generally do not recognize or report the side effects of injected medications.
  3. Decanoate injections improve adherence and sustained therapeutic drug levels despite possible client ambivalence.
  4. Clients report significantly fewer side effects from decanoate injections than from oral versions of the same medicine.

38. 3. Long-acting decanoate injections are a good treatment option for clients with a known pattern of non-adherence, ambivalence about their treatment, and limited insight into their illness. These injections share the same side effects as oral forms of the drug. Injections are not implemented until oral medication tolerance and effectiveness is established. Clients do not necessarily recognize side effects or realize that they are related to medications or dosage. Decanoate injections have the same side effect profile as the oral version of the medication.
CN: Physiological integrity; CNS: Pharmacology; CL: Analyze

39. A client with schizophrenia tells the nurse that the President consults with him before making major decisions. What is the nurse's **best** response?
  1. "How long have you known the President?"
  2. "You are fortunate to know the President."
  3. "Will the President visit you at the hospital?"
  4. "You must feel important. Now let's make your bed."

39. 4. Acknowledging that the client feels important addresses the underlying reason for the delusion. The other options reinforce the reality of the delusion.
CN: Psychosocial integrity; CNS: None; CL: Analyze

40. A client is admitted to the hospital after being found in a parking lot, kicking cars and yelling at passersby. When approached by the nurse, the client shouts, "You're the one who stole my husband from me!" How does the nurse interpret this behavior? Select all that apply.

1. Hallucinatory
2. Delusional
3. Disorientation
4. Fearful
5. Confusion
6. Paranoia

40. 2, 6. A delusion is a false, fixed belief manufactured without appropriate or sufficient evidence to support it. Paranoid ideation reflects baseless or excessive suspicion of others. The client's statements don't represent hallucinations because they are not perceptual disorders. No information in the question addresses orientation. The client's statements do not reflect fearfulness.

CN: Psychosocial integrity; CNS: None; CL: Apply

41. The nurse is teaching the family of a client with schizophrenia about the symptoms of remission. Which response would be the **most** accurate?

1. The disease is in the prodromal phase.
2. Symptoms of psychosis are no longer disruptive to the client.
3. There is no longer a need for medication as the disease is cured.
4. The client can best decide how to take medication for his symptoms.

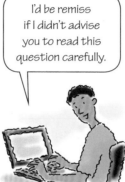

I'd be remiss if I didn't advise you to read this question carefully.

41. 2. The prodromal phase is the precursor to an exacerbation. Schizophrenia is a chronic disorder with periods of remission and exacerbation. The symptoms may dramatically improve, then lesson or worsen, creating the need for continued monitoring and possible adjustments to treatment. Clients are usually treated over time with case management, medication, symptom management skills, social skill training, network support, vocational training, and health-promoting practices. Few clients are able to independently determine their need for medication.

CN: Psychosocial integrity; CNS: None; CL: Apply

42. A client with schizophrenia is alone on the bed in his room and appears to be interacting with someone beside him. The nurse notes that the client appears afraid. What is the **most** likely explanation for this client's behavior?

1. Hallucinations
2. Suicidal ideations
3. Nightmares
4. Delusions

42. 1. This client appears to be experiencing auditory hallucinations, and is interacting with a nonexistent person. There is no evidence that the client is having suicidal ideations, nightmares, or delusions.

CN: Psychosocial integrity; CNS: None; CL: Analyze

43. A nurse is talking with a client, who has schizophrenia, about the inpatient activity schedule. The client randomly begins to describe a volunteer who assists at the client's home. The nurse interprets the client's response as reflecting which symptom?

1. Circumstantiality
2. Loose associations
3. Referential
4. Tangentiality

43. 4. Tangentiality describes thought patterns loosely connected but not directly related to the topic. In circumstantiality, the person digresses with unnecessary details. Loose associations are rapid shifts in ideas, from one subject to another, in an unrelated manner. Referential thinking is when an individual incorrectly interprets neutral incidents and external events as having a particular or special meaning.

CN: Psychosocial integrity; CNS: None; CL: Apply

44. While talking to a client with schizophrenia, the nurse notes that the client frequently uses unrecognizable words with no common meaning. How would the nurse interpret this behavior?
1. Echolalia
2. Clang association
3. Neologisms
4. Word salad

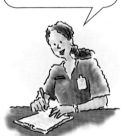

That's a word I've never heard before.

44. 3. Neologisms are newly coined words with personal meanings to the client with schizophrenia. Echolalia is the echoing of spoken words or sounds. Clang association is the linking of words by sound rather than meaning. A word salad is the stringing of words in sequence that have no connection to one another.
CN: Psychosocial integrity; CNS: None; CL: Apply

45. While caring for a hospitalized client diagnosed with schizophrenia, the nurse observes the client watching television. The client reports that the television is speaking directly to him. Which type of thinking **best** describes this belief?
1. Autistic
2. Concrete
3. Paranoid
4. Referential

45. 4. Referential, or primary process thinking, is a belief that incidents or events in the environment have special meaning for that client. Autistic thinking is a disturbance in thought due to the intrusion of an internally stimulated, private-fantasy world, resulting in an abnormal response. Concrete thinking is the literal interpretation of words and symbols. Paranoid thinking is the misbelief that others are trying to harm you.
CN: Psychosocial integrity; CNS: None; CL: Apply

46. A nurse is talking with the family of a client diagnosed with schizophrenia. The mother asks, "What causes this disorder?" What is the nurse's **best** response?
1. Prenatal or postpartum central nervous system damage
2. Bacterial infections in the mother during pregnancy or delivery
3. A biological predisposition exacerbated by environmental stressors
4. Lack of bonding and attachment during infancy, which leads to depression in later life

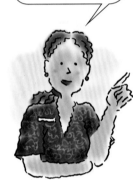

Pay attention to the key words.

46. 3. The holistic theory states that an interaction between biological predisposition and environmental stressors is the cause of schizophrenia. The biological explanation states that schizophrenia is caused by a brain disease, a bacterial infection in utero, or early brain damage. The psychoanalytic perspective involves the belief that the mother-infant bond is the source of the schizophrenia. The biological and psychoanalytic theories are no longer scientifically supported. There is no evidence that the lack of bonding and attachment during infancy cause the development of schizophrenia.
CN: Physiological integrity; CNS: Physiological adaptation; CL: Apply

47. What is the **most** appropriate action for a nurse to implement while caring for a client who is experiencing a delusion?
1. Ask the client to describe his delusion in detail
2. Explain to the client that the delusion isn't real
3. Act as if the delusion is real to reduce the client's anxiety
4. Engage the client in an organized activity

47. 4. Engaging the client in an organized activity reinforces reality. Asking the client to describe the delusion and acting as if the delusion is real reinforces the delusion's reality. Explaining that the delusion isn't real won't help, and may make the client hold tighter to the delusion.
CN: Psychosocial integrity; CNS: Physiological adaptation; CL: Apply

48. A client with schizophrenia reports to the admitting nurse, "I don't enjoy things anymore. I used to love to read mystery books, but even that isn't enjoyable now." The nurse determines the client is experiencing:
1. avolition.
2. anhedonia.
3. alogia.
4. flat affect.

49. A client diagnosed with schizophrenia was taught symptom self-management, as part of a relapse prevention program, in preparation for discharge. Which statement indicates to the nurse that the client understands symptom monitoring?
1. "When I hear voices, I become afraid I will relapse."
2. "My parents are afraid to be near me when I am sick."
3. "My family is better off if I keep them out of my treatment."
4. "When I'm feeling stressed, I will practice stress reduction techniques."

50. A client diagnosed with schizophrenia has been taking haloperidol for one week when a nurse observes that the client's gaze is fixed on the ceiling. Which specific condition is the client exhibiting?
1. Akathisia
2. Neuroleptic malignant syndrome
3. Oculogyric crisis
4. Tardive dyskinesia

51. The nurse notes that a client taking antipsychotic medications becomes agitated, fearful, and panicky when his neck twists to one side and his eyes forcefully draw upward toward the ceiling. Which medication should be administered to the client?
1. Benztropine
2. Haloperidol
3. Paliperidone
4. Diazepam

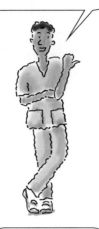

Here's a tip—hedonism means taking pleasure in something. So, a lack of pleasure would be described as . . .

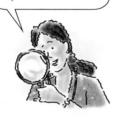

Keep your eye on question 50. It's asking for a specific condition.

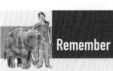

Remember

"Anticholinergics address adverse effects of antipsychotics."

Antipsychotics such as haloperidol can cause agitation, restlessness, and dystonic reactions. Anticholinergics such as benztropine can reduce these symptoms.

Anticholinergics
- Benztropine
- Trihexyphenidyl
- Diphenhydramine

48. 2. Anhedonia is the loss of pleasure in things that are usually pleasurable. Avolition is the lack of motivation. Alogia, also called poverty of speech, is a decrease in the amount of richness of speech. A flat affect is the absence of emotional expression.
CN: Physiological integrity; CNS: None; CL: Apply

49. 4. This statement indicates the client has learned stress reduction techniques. The other options don't show an understanding of symptom self-monitoring, and may result in social withdrawal, symptom intensification and possible relapse.
CN: Psychosocial integrity; CNS: None; CL: Apply

50. 3. An oculogyric crisis involves the eyes fixated in one direction, typically in an upward gaze. Neuroleptic malignant syndrome causes increased body temperature, muscle rigidity, and altered consciousness. Akathisia is a restlessness that can cause pacing and tapping of the fingers or feet. Stereotyped involuntary movements, such as tongue protrusion, lip smacking, chewing, blinking, and grimacing characterize tardive dyskinesia.
CN: Physiological integrity; CNS: Pharmacological and parenteral therapies; CL: Apply

51. 1. Benztropine is an anticholinergic drug used to counteract the dystonic reactions and adverse reactions of antipsychotic drugs. If the client experiences difficulty swallowing, benztropine may be administered by injection. Haloperidol is an antipsychotic medication used to control tics and vocal utterances that are part of Tourette's syndrome. Paliperidone is used to treat mania, and at low dosage, is used as a maintenance medication for bipolar disorder, schizophrenia and schizoaffective disorder. Diazepam is a benzodiazepine. Each of these medications require a provider's order.
CN: Physiological integrity; CNS: Pharmacological and parenteral therapies; CL: Apply

52. A 50-year-old client with schizophrenia becomes agitated and confronts the nurse with clenched fists. What is the nurse's **most** appropriate intervention?
1. Lead the client by the hand to the activity room for cards
2. Step up to the client and tell him his behavior is inappropriate
3. Call for security to take him to a seclusion room
4. Speak to him quietly and offer medication to help him calm down

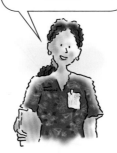

For question 52, you're looking for the most appropriate action.

52. 4. Always use the least restrictive means to calm a client. Never touch an agitated client. Touch can be misinterpreted as a threat and can further escalate the situation. Stepping up to an agitated client can be seen as an aggressive act. Seclusion is a last resort.
CN: Physiological integrity; CNS: Reduction of risk potential; CL: Apply

53. A client with schizophrenia has been admitted to an inpatient unit. The client lives alone and has recently lost a full-time job. The client is unkempt, avoidant, and isolative on the unit. What is the **priority** nursing intervention for the client?
1. Encourage social interactions with staff and others on the unit
2. Assist the client to bathe daily and eat all meals
3. Limit visitors until the client requests they come to the hospital
4. Establish rapport, build trust, and maintain client safety

53. 4. A client with schizophrenia typically experiences mistrust, suspicion, fear, and anxiety. It is critical for the nurse to address these concerns. The deterioration of the client experiencing a schizophrenic crisis is manifested in multiple self-care deficits. These other problems can be addressed after the client has been stabilized. Insisting the client eat or bathe establishes a power struggle and will reduce trust. There is no justification for limiting visitors, the client may not request them for a long period, and can benefit from caring visits.
CN: Safe, effective care environment; CNS: Management of care; CL: Apply

54. A nurse walks down the hall as she returns from lunch. A client with delusional disorder shouts, "You're following me. What do you want?" Which is the nurse's **best** response?
1. "Who did something to frighten you?"
2. "You know I am not following you."
3. "You must go to seclusion if you threaten me."
4. "I didn't intentionally frighten you."

54. 4. Being clear in communication, remaining calm, and showing concern will increase client cooperation, and decrease the potential for violence. Answer one tries to identify the client's feelings but does not convey warmth and concern. Answer two is not empathic, and shows no indication of trying to reach the client at a level beyond content of communication. Answer three may trigger a competitive power struggle with the client, and increase anxiety, fear, and mistrust.
CN: Psychosocial integrity; CNS: None; CL: Apply

55. A client with schizophrenia has been stable for some time. What action is **most** important for preventing relapse?
1. Attending group therapy sessions
2. Participating in family support meetings
3. Going to social skills training sessions
4. Consistently taking prescribed medications

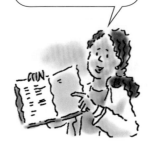

The words most important in question 55 indicate the need to prioritize. As a matter of fact, there's lots of prioritizing in this chapter.

55. 4. Although all of the choices are important for preventing relapse, compliance with the medication regimen is the priority in the treatment of schizophrenia.
CN: Safe, effective care environment; CNS: Management of care; CL: Apply

56. A client approaches the nurse and points at the sky. The client states, "This is where the men, who are coming to get me, are coming from." What is the nurse's **best** response?
1. "What makes you think the men are coming here to get you?"
2. "You are safe here. We will not let them in to harm you."
3. "It seems like the world is pretty scary for you, but you are safe here."
4. "There are no bad men coming here because no one lives in the sky."

56. 3. This response acknowledges the client's fears, listens to his feelings, and offers a sense of security as the nurse tries to understand the concerns behind the symbolism. She reflects these concerns to the client, along with reassurance of safety. Answer one validates the delusion, not the feelings or fears, and does not orient the client to reality. Answer two gives false reassurance. Because the nurse is not sure of the symbolism, she cannot make this promise. Answer four rejects the client's feelings and does not address the client's fears.
CN: Safe, effective care environment; CNS: Management of care; CL: Apply

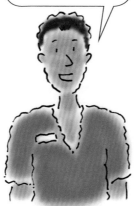

They're all important, but which one is *most* important?

57. A client is brought to the crisis response center by her family. During evaluation, the client reports being depressed for the last month and that voices are telling her to hurt herself. Which intervention is **most** important for the nurse to implement?
1. Social interactions
2. Distraction strategies
3. Relaxation techniques
4. Suicide precautions

57. 4. A client with a major depressive episode, who begins to experience command hallucinations, is at great risk for self-injury. Nonpharmacological strategies such as music can be a helpful distraction for someone experiencing auditory hallucinations, but will not address the danger of command hallucinations. Social interactions and relaxation techniques are two opposing poles of treatment. Both extremes would be inappropriate primary interventions in the face of active suicidal ideation.
CN: Psychosocial integrity; CNS: Safety; CL: Analyze

58. A client with schizophrenia experiences suspicion, mistrust, and paranoia. What is the **most** appropriate nursing intervention for this client?
1. Defend yourself when the client is verbally hostile toward you
2. Provide a warm approach by touching the client
3. Explain everything you are doing before you do it
4. Clarify the content of the client's delusions

58. 3. Explaining everything you do will prevent misinterpretation of your actions. A non-defensive stance provides an atmosphere in which the client's angry feelings can be explored. Touching a paranoid client should be avoided because it can be interpreted as a threat. The content of delusions should not be the focus of your care because the content is illogical.
CN: Psychosocial integrity; CNS: Safety; CL: Analyze

59. The nurse is interviewing a client with a delusional disorder. Which condition would the nurse anticipate from this client?
1. Bizarre behavior
2. Agitation
3. Impaired short-term memory
4. Intact psychosocial skills

59. 4. The psychosocial functioning of the person with a delusional disorder may be relatively unimpaired. Another common characteristic of the client with a delusional disorder is the apparent normality of his behavior and appearance when his delusional ideas are not being discussed or acted on. The client with delusional disorder does not have symptoms such as concrete thinking, bizarre or agitated behavior, or impaired memory, typical in a client with schizophrenia who functions at a lower level.
CN: Psychosocial integrity; CNS: None; CL: Apply

60. A client admitted with a delusional disorder reports that his friends avoid him because they know he is secretly working for the CIA. This client does not exhibit impairment in psychosocial functioning. Which condition would the nurse suspect?
1. Non-bizarre delusions
2. Fragmentary delusions
3. Regressive behavior
4. Regressive delusions

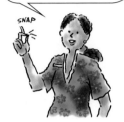

You've finished 60 questions. The rest should be a snap.

SNAP

60. 1. The essential feature of delusional disorder is the presence of one or more non-bizarre delusions that persist for at least one month. The most common delusions by subtypes are erotomanic, grandiose, jealousy, persecutory, and somatic. Bizarre delusions are patently absurd beliefs with no foundation in reality. Fragmentary delusions are unconnected delusions not organized around a coherent theme. Regressive behaviors revert back to a less mature state and are not associated with a mental disorder.
CN: Psychosocial integrity; CNS: None; CL: Apply

61. A client is taking fluphenazine. The nurse understands that teaching and discharge instructions are understood when the client states:
1. "I need to stay out of the sun."
2. "I need to double my fluids."
3. "I can't eat cheese or eggs."
4. "I need to plan frequent naps."

I didn't intend to cause any adverse reactions.

61. 1. Fluphenazine is an antipsychotic drug that can cause photosensitivity and sunburn. Clients taking this drug don't need to increase fluid intake, avoid cheese or eggs, or plan rest periods.
CN: Physiological integrity; CNS: Pharmacological and parenteral therapies; CL: Analyze

62. The nurse is teaching a client who has been prescribed thiothixene. Which adverse reaction is **most** important for the nurse to discuss with this client?
1. Akinesia
2. Hypotension
3. Sedation
4. Weight gain

62. 1. Thiothixene is a high-potency agent with a high affinity for dopamine-2 receptors. This affinity increases the likelihood of akinesia, a form of extrapyramidal symptoms. Although thiothixene targets other neurotransmitters responsible for hypotension, sedation, and weight gain, their affinity to these receptors is weak, and more likely to occur with lower-potency psychotropics.
CN: Physiological integrity; CNS: Pharmacological and parenteral therapies; CL: Apply

63. The inability to carry out daily responsibilities will typically occur during the prodromal phase of schizophrenia. Which symptom may also occur during this phase?
1. Increased energy and social interaction
2. Improved mood and attention span
3. Impaired functioning and neglect of personal hygiene
4. Stable sleep and work performance

63. 3. Prodromal signs and symptoms of schizophrenia can occur one month to one year before the first psychotic break, and represent a clear deterioration in functioning. They may include impaired role functioning and neglect of personal hygiene as well as social withdrawal and depression. Increases in energy, social interaction, mood, and attention span don't occur during the prodromal phase. Sleep and work performance are more likely to deteriorate than improve or remain stable.
CN: Psychosocial integrity; CNS: None; CL: Apply

64. The daughter of a client with schizophrenia states, "I'm afraid that I may develop this disease too." The nurse explains that schizophrenia is associated with:
1. physical or sexual abuse.
2. a combination of genetic and other factors.
3. both parents having schizophrenia.
4. emotional trauma during childhood.

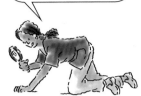

Families often search for the link to their loved one's disease.

64. 2. Experts believe schizophrenia results from a combination of genetic, environmental, and other factors, such as viruses, birth injuries, and nutrition. Schizophrenia incidence is higher among relatives of a person with the disease. It can occur even if both parents don't have schizophrenia. Emotional trauma and physical and sexual abuse during childhood have not been linked to schizophrenia.
CN: Psychosocial integrity; CNS: None; CL: Apply

65. A nurse teaches a class of caregivers about the positive and negative behaviors of schizophrenia. The nurse explains positive behaviors as:
1. a pattern of limited spontaneous speech.
2. the inability to initiate and maintain goal-directed activities.
3. the misinterpretation of experiences and altered sensory input.
4. a style of extremely brief replies to questions.

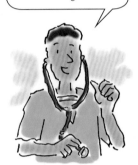

Which pattern of speech is the client using?

65. 3. Positive behaviors of schizophrenia include attention-getting, which can result from misinterpretation of experiences and altered sensory input. Negative behaviors are those that render the client inert and unmotivated, such as lack of spontaneous speech, poverty of thought, apathy, and poor social functioning.
CN: Psychosocial integrity; CNS: None; CL: Apply

66. The nurse is facilitating a group when a client with schizophrenia says, "I like to drive my car, bar, tar, far." This pattern of speech is known as:
1. clang association.
2. echolalia.
3. echopraxia.
4. neologisms.

66. 1. Linking together words based on their sounds rather than their meanings is called clang association. Echolalia is the involuntary repetition of words spoken by others. Echopraxia refers to meaningless imitation of others' motions. Neologisms are words that a person invents.
CN: Psychosocial integrity; CNS: None; CL: Apply

67. A client with schizophrenia, who is receiving antipsychotic medication, reports that he feels nervous. The client paces, fidgets, and can't seem to stay still. Which disorder is the **most** likely cause?
1. Akathisia
2. Tardive dyskinesia
3. Akinesia
4. Anxiety

67. 1. Akathisia is an extrapyramidal adverse effect of some antipsychotic medications. It manifests as restlessness and an inability to stay still. Tardive dyskinesia refers to involuntary abnormal movements of the mouth, tongue, face, and jaw. Akinesia is absence of movement. Anxiety is an unpleasant state of inner turmoil, often accompanied by nervous behavior, somatic complaints, and rumination.
CN: Physiological integrity; CNS: Pharmacological and parenteral therapies; CL: Analyze

68. What side effects are important for the nurse to mention when teaching a client about long-term use of antipsychotics? Select all that apply.
1. Constipation
2. Sedation
3. Headaches
4. Blurred vision
5. Nausea

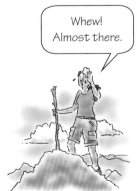

Whew! Almost there.

68. 2, 1, 4. The most persistently reported side effect by clients is that of sedation in a variety of forms. This frequently includes difficulty waking, needing naps, or feeling heavy or weighed down physically or mentally. A persons who has been prescribed antipsychotic medications is at risk for constipation, sedation, blurred vision, dry mouth, and akathisia. Headaches and nausea can be associated with some antidepressants, but are not typically a side effect of antipsychotic medications.
CN: Physiological integrity; CNS: Pharmacological; CL: Analyze

CN: Client needs category   CNS: Client needs subcategory   CL: Cognitive level

69. A client with schizophrenia tells the nurse that two people, talking in the hall, are planning to kidnap and kill him. The client's thought pattern reflects:
1. auditory hallucinations.
2. delusions of grandeur.
3. ideas of reference.
4. echolalia.

69. 3. A client with ideas of reference mistakenly believes that other people's thoughts, speech, and behaviors refer to them. Auditory hallucinations are sounds or voices that aren't based in reality. Delusions of grandeur are false beliefs that arise without appropriate external stimuli. Echolalia refers to involuntary repetition of words spoken by others.

CN: Psychosocial integrity; CNS: None; CL: Apply

70. A client with schizophrenia is taking clozapine. Which adverse effects would the nurse anticipate from this medicate? Select all that apply.
1. Sore throat
2. Pill-rolling movements
3. Polyuria
4. Fever
5. Polydipsia
6. Orthostatic hypotension

70. 1, 4. Sore throat, fever, and sudden onset of flulike symptoms are signs of agranulocytosis. This condition is caused by a lack of sufficient granulocytes, which cause the client to be susceptible to infection. The client's white blood cell count should be monitored weekly throughout the course of treatment. Pill-rolling movements can occur in those experiencing extrapyramidal adverse effects associated with antipsychotic medication that have been prescribed for a much longer duration of time. Polydipsia and polyuria are common adverse effects of lithium. Orthostatic hypotension is an adverse effect of tricyclic antidepressants.

CN: Physiological integrity; CNS: Pharmacological and parenteral therapies; CL: Apply

71. Adult or older adult clients with schizophrenia can present with petulance and temper tantrums. How would the nurse interpret these behaviors in a person diagnosed with psychoses?
1. Malingering to seek attention
2. Being intellectually challenged
3. Employing regression to reduce anxiety
4. Being spoiled and angry

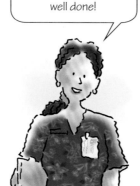

You finished! Job well done!

71. 3. Clients who have impaired or ineffective communication skills may communicate instead through behavior. A sense of powerlessness may be related to perceived, or real, threats that they are unable to express. The behavior exhibited may relate to the level of Maslow's Hierarchy of Needs that they perceive as being threatened. Having this need met, even temporarily or briefly, reduces the anxiety for these persons. None of the remaining answers speak to addressing the client's needs or reducing anxiety.

CN: Psychosocial integrity; CNS: None; CL: Apply

CN: Client needs category   CNS: Client needs subcategory   CL: Cognitive level

Chapter 18

Substance Related & Addictive Disorders

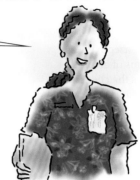

About the only substance use this chapter doesn't cover is my personal weakness—chocolate mousse! Think of me as you work through this chapter. I'll be the one with chocolate smudges on her fingers. Tee-hee!

1. Family members of an alcoholic client ask the nurse to help them intervene. Which action is essential for a successful intervention?
   1. All family members must tell the client they're powerless.
   2. All family members must describe how the addiction affects them.
   3. All family members must come up with their share of financial support.
   4. All family members must become caregivers during the detoxification period.

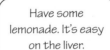

Have some lemonade. It's easy on the liver.

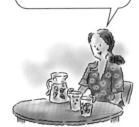

1. 2. After the family is taught about addiction, they must write down examples of how the addiction has affected each of them, and use this information during the intervention. It isn't necessary to tell the client the family is powerless. The family is empowered through this intervention experience. In many cases, a third-party payer will help with treatment costs. Doing an intervention doesn't make family members responsible for financial support, or client care and support during the detoxification period.
CN: Psychosocial integrity; CNS: None; CL: Analyze

2. A client who uses alcohol tells a nurse, "I'm sure I can become a social drinker." What is the **most** appropriate response by the nurse?
   1. "When do you think you can become a social drinker?"
   2. "What makes you think you'll learn to drink normally?"
   3. "Can you tell me how the use of alcohol affects your life?"
   4. "How many alcoholic beverages can a social drinker consume?

The words most appropriate help clarify the correct answer.

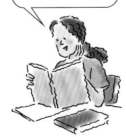

2. 3. This question may help the client recall the problematic results of using alcohol, and the reasons the client began treatment. Asking when he can become a social drinker will only encourage the addicted person to deny the problem and develop an unrealistic, self-defeating goal. Asking how many alcoholic beverages a social drinker can consume, and why the client thinks he can drink normally will encourage the addicted person to defend himself and deny the problem.
CN: Psychosocial integrity; CNS: None; CL: Apply

3. An adult client asks the nurse not to tell his parents about his alcohol problem. What is the **most** appropriate response by the nurse?
   1. "It would be dishonest not to tell them."
   2. "Don't you think you'll need to tell them someday?"
   3. "Does alcoholism run in either side of your family?"
   4. "What do you think will happen if you tell your parents?"

3. 4. Clients who struggle with addiction often believe people will be judgmental, rejecting, and uncaring if their history of alcohol use is revealed. Answer one challenges the client and will put him on the defensive. Answer two will make the client defensive and cause rationalizations about his parents need to know. Answer three is not a good assessment question. It takes the focus off of the client.
CN: Psychosocial integrity; CNS: None; CL: Analyze

CN: Client needs category   CNS: Client needs subcategory   CL: Cognitive level

4. The nurse is caring for a client who is experiencing alcohol withdrawal. The nurse would be **most** concerned if the client exhibited:
1. hallucinations.
2. nervousness.
3. diaphoresis.
4. nausea.

5. A client is receiving chlordiazepoxide as needed for signs and symptoms of alcohol withdrawal. The nurse assesses the client and determines the need for medication when the client displays:
1. mild tremors, hypertension, tachycardia.
2. bradycardia, hyperthermia, sedation.
3. hypotension, decreased reflexes, drowsiness.
4. hypothermia, mild tremors, slurred speech.

6. A client who uses alcohol tells a nurse, "Alcohol helps me sleep." What is the **most** appropriate response by the nurse?
1. Alcohol doesn't help promote sleep.
2. Continued alcohol use causes insomnia.
3. One glass of alcohol at dinnertime can induce sleep.
4. Sometimes, alcohol can make one drowsy enough to fall asleep.

7. A client, who is withdrawing from alcohol, is being given lorazepam. The client's family asks the nurse about the medication. What is the nurse's **best** response?
1. Short-term use of lorazepam can lead to dependence.
2. The lorazepam will reduce the symptoms of withdrawal.
3. The lorazepam will make a client forget about symptoms of withdrawal.
4. The lorazepam will also help with heart disease.

8. A client who uses alcohol tells the nurse that everyone in his family has an alcohol problem, and nothing can be done about it. What is the nurse's **most** appropriate response?
1. "You're right, it's much harder to recover from alcoholism."
2. "This is just an excuse so you don't have to work on your sobriety."
3. "Sometimes, nothing can be done, but you may be the exception in your family."
4. "Alcohol problems can occur in families, but sobriety is your choice."

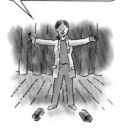

A disease can have many "stages," each with its own symptoms.

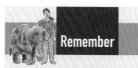

Remember

"Chlordiazepoxide provides relief from alcohol withdrawal."

A benzodiazepine, this drug helps treat such symptoms of alcohol withdrawal as the following:
• Tremors
• Hypertension
• Tachycardia
• Elevated body temperature

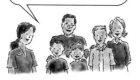

It's important to teach the family *and* the client.

4. 1. Hallucinations are a sign of late alcohol withdrawal. The nurse should stay with this client, have someone notify the provider, and institute seizure precautions. Nervousness, diaphoresis, and nausea are signs of early withdrawal.
CN: Physiological integrity; CNS: Reduction of risk potential; CL: Analyze

5. 1. Chlordiazepoxide is given during alcohol withdrawal. Symptoms that indicate a need for this drug include tremors, hypertension, tachycardia, and elevated body temperature. Bradycardia, sedation, hypotension, decreased reflexes, hypothermia, and slurred speech aren't symptoms of alcohol withdrawal.
CN: Physiological integrity; CNS: Pharmacological and parenteral therapies; CL: Apply

6. 1. Alcohol use may initially promote sleep, but with continued use, it causes insomnia. Evidence shows that alcohol doesn't facilitate sleep. One glass of alcohol at dinnertime won't induce sleep. Answer four doesn't give information about how alcohol affects sleep.
CN: Physiological integrity; CNS: Physiological adaptation; CL: Analyze

7. 2. Lorazepam is a short-acting benzodiazepine usually given for one week to ease the effects of alcohol withdrawal. Long-term use of lorazepam can lead to dependence. The medication isn't given to help forget the experience. Lorazepam isn't used to treat coexisting cardiovascular problems.
CN: Physiological integrity; CNS: Pharmacological and parenteral therapies; CL: Apply

8. 4. This statement challenges the client to become proactive and take the steps necessary to maintain a sober lifestyle. Answer one agrees with the client's denial and isn't a useful response. Answer two confronts the client and may make him more adamant in defense of his position. Answer three agrees with the client's denial and isn't a useful response.
CN: Psychosocial integrity; CNS: None; CL: Apply

CN: Client needs category   CNS: Client needs subcategory   CL: Cognitive level

9. The nurse is caring for a client with a history of chronic alcoholism and is aware that the client may be predisposed to:
1. arteriosclerosis.
2. heart failure.
3. heart valve damage.
4. pericarditis.

10. A client with a history of alcohol use has been diagnosed with nutritional deficits. What is the nurse's **best** intervention?
1. Encourage the client to eat a diet high in calories
2. Help the client recognize and follow a balanced diet
3. Have the client drink liquid protein supplements daily
4. Have the client monitor the calories consumed each day

11. A client with a history of alcohol use tells the nurse that he refuses to take his thiamine vitamin. The client won't share the reason for refusing the medication with the nurse. What is the **most** appropriate response by the nurse?
1. "It's important to take vitamins to stop your craving."
2. "Prolonged use of alcohol can cause vitamin depletion."
3. "For every vitamin you take, you'll help your liver heal."
4. "By taking vitamins, you don't need to worry about your diet."

12. The nurse determines further teaching about nutrition is necessary when a client who uses alcohol states:
1. "I should avoid foods high in fat."
2. "I should only eat one balanced meal per day."
3. "I should take vitamin and mineral supplements."
4. "I should eat large portions of food containing fiber."

13. A client tells the nurse, "I have been drinking ever since they told me I had learning disabilities." How does the nurse interpret this response?
1. The client is self-medicating.
2. The client has an excuse to drink.
3. The client isn't a productive person.
4. The client will be unable to stop drinking.

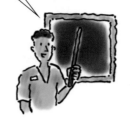

Teach the client to be proactive in his recovery.

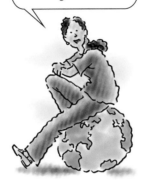

I am the best at taking this test.

9. 2. Heart failure is a severe cardiac consequence associated with long-term alcohol use. Arteriosclerosis, heart valve damage, and pericarditis aren't medical consequences of alcoholism.
CN: Physiological integrity; CNS: Reduction of risk potential; CL: Apply

10. 2. Clients who use alcohol are usually malnourished, and need help to follow a balanced diet. Increasing calories may cause the client to eat empty calories. The client must be involved in the decision to supplement the daily dietary intake. The nurse can't force the client to drink liquid protein supplements. Having the client monitor calorie intake could only be done if the client recognizes the need to maintain a balanced diet. Calorie counts usually aren't needed in most recovering clients who begin to eat from the basic food groups.
CN: Physiological integrity; CNS: Basic care and comfort; CL: Apply

11. 2. Chronic alcoholism interferes with the metabolism of many vitamins. Vitamin supplements can prevent deficiencies from occurring. Taking vitamins won't stop a person from craving alcohol or help a damaged liver heal. A balanced diet is essential in addition to taking multivitamins.
CN: Health promotion and maintenance; CNS: None; CL: Apply

12. 2. If the client only eats one adequate meal each day, there will be a deficit of essential nutrients. It's appropriate for the client to take vitamin and mineral supplements to prevent deficiency in these nutrients. Avoiding foods high in fat content, and consuming large portions of foods containing fiber, indicate the client has good knowledge of nutrition.
CN: Health promotion and maintenance; CNS: None; CL: Analyze

13. 1. A client with learning disabilities may experience frustration, depression, or overall feelings of low self-esteem, and may self-medicate with alcohol. Many people with learning disabilities don't resort to alcohol, but develop other coping skills to handle the disability. People with learning disabilities can be very productive. A person with a learning disability can successfully recover from alcohol addiction.
CN: Psychosocial integrity; CNS: None; CL: Apply

CN: Client needs category   CNS: Client needs subcategory   CL: Cognitive level

14. A nurse is caring for a client undergoing treatment for acute alcohol dependence. The client tells the nurse, "I don't have a problem. My wife made me come here." Which defense mechanisms do this client's statement represent?
1. Projection and suppression
2. Denial and rationalization
3. Rationalization and repression
4. Suppression and denial

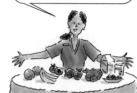

Three square meals a day, please.

14. 2. The client is using denial and rationalization. Denial is the unconscious disclaimer of unacceptable thoughts, feelings, needs, or certain external factors. Rationalization is the unconscious effort to justify intolerable feelings, behaviors, and motives. The client isn't using projection, suppression, or repression.
CN: Psychosocial integrity; CNS: None; CL: Apply

15. During a family therapy session, a client who uses alcohol tells a family member, "You made it easy for me to use alcohol. You always made excuses for my behavior." What should the nurse encourage this family to do?
1. Give up enabling behaviors
2. Manage the client's self-care
3. Deal with negative behaviors
4. Evaluate the home environment

15. 1. Enabling behaviors from family members allow this client to continue his addiction by rationalizing, denying, or otherwise excusing the problem. Based on the client's statement, managing self-care isn't an issue that needs to be addressed. Dealing with negative behaviors and evaluating the home environment don't address the client's statement about his family.
CN: Psychosocial integrity; CNS: None; CL: Apply

16. What is the **most** important short-term goal for a client who is curious about the effects of alcohol on her body?
1. Have blood chemistries tested daily
2. Verbalize the results of substance use
3. Meet with a pharmacist to discuss alcohol ingestion
4. Attend a weekly aerobic exercise program

16. 2. It is important for the client to talk about the health consequences of the continued use of alcohol. Testing blood chemistries daily gives the client minimal knowledge of the effects of alcohol on her body. A pharmacist isn't the appropriate health care professional to educate the client about the effects of alcohol on her body. Although exercise is an important goal of self-care, it doesn't address the client's knowledge deficit.
CN: Safe, effective care environment; CNS: Management of care; CL: Apply

17. A client who uses alcohol tells the nurse, "I feel so depressed about what I've done to my family that I feel like giving up." It is **most** important for the nurse to assess the client for:
1. family support.
2. a plan for self-harm.
3. a sponsor for the client.
4. other ambivalent feelings.

17. 2. When a client talks about giving up, the nurse must explore the potential for suicidal behavior. Although questioning the client about family support, the availability of a sponsor or ambivalent feelings is important, the priority action is to assess for suicide.
CN: Psychosocial integrity; CNS: None; CL: Apply

18. A client, withdrawing from alcohol, tells the nurse that he is worried about periodic hallucinations. What is the **most** appropriate intervention by the nurse?
1. Point out that the sensation doesn't exist
2. Ask the client to talk about the experience
3. Encourage the client to wash all body areas well
4. Determine if the client has a cognitive impairment

18. 2. The client needs to talk about the periodic hallucinations to prevent them from becoming triggers to acting out behaviors and possible self-injury. The client's experience of sensory-perceptual alterations must be acknowledged; therefore, denying that the client's hallucinations exist is not a helpful strategy. Determining if the client has a cognitive impairment, and encouraging the client to wash all body areas well does not address the problem of periodic hallucinations.
CN: Psychosocial integrity; CNS: None; CL: Apply

CN: Client needs category   CNS: Client needs subcategory   CL: Cognitive level

19. A client, who has been drinking alcohol for 30 years, asks a nurse if permanent damage has occurred to his immune system. What is the nurse's **best** response?

1. "There is often less resistance to infections."
2. "Sometimes, the body's metabolism will increase."
3. "Put your energies into maintaining sobriety for now."
4. "Drinking puts you at high risk for disease later in life."

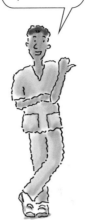

You need to know how to prioritize!

19. 1. Chronic alcohol use depresses the immune system and causes increased susceptibility to infections. A nutritionally well-balanced diet, that includes foods high in protein and B vitamins, will help develop a strong immune system. The potential damage to the immune system doesn't increase the body's metabolism. Answer three negates the client's concern, and isn't an appropriate or caring response. Drinking alcohol may put the client at risk for immune system problems at any time in life.
CN: Psychosocial integrity; CNS: None; CL: Analyze

20. A client experiencing alcohol withdrawal tells the nurse that she is upset about going through detoxification. Which goal is the **priority** for this client?

1. Committing to a drug-free lifestyle
2. Working with the nurse to remain safe
3. Drinking plenty of fluids on a daily basis
4. Making a personal inventory of strengths

20. 2. The priority goal is for client safety. Although drinking enough fluids, identifying personal strengths, and committing to a drug-free lifestyle are important goals, the nurse's first priority must be to promote client safety.
CN: Safe, effective care environment; CNS: Management of care; CL: Apply

21. A client recovering from alcohol use needs to develop effective coping skills to handle daily stressors. What is the **most** appropriate nursing intervention for this client?

1. Determine the client's level of verbal skills
2. Help the client avoid areas that cause conflict
3. Discuss examples of successful coping behavior
4. Teach the client to accept uncomfortable situations

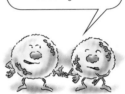

I've been feeling a little depressed lately. How about you?

21. 3. This client needs help identifying successful coping behavior and developing ways to incorporate that behavior into daily functioning. There are many skills for coping with stress. Determining the client's level of verbal skills may not be important. Encouraging the client to avoid conflict prevents him from learning skills to handle daily stressors.
CN: Psychosocial integrity; CNS: None; CL: Analyze

22. The nurse is caring for a client struggling with alcohol dependence. It is most important for the nurse to:

1. speak briefly and directly.
2. avoid blaming or preaching to the client.
3. confront feelings and examples of perfectionism.
4. determine if nonverbal communication will be more effective.

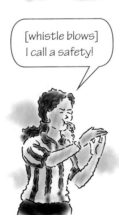

[whistle blows] I call a safety!

22. 2. Blaming or preaching to the client causes negativity and prevents the client from hearing what the nurse has to say. Speaking briefly to the client may not allow time for adequate communication. Perfectionism doesn't tend to be an issue. Determining if nonverbal communication will be more effective is better suited to a client with cognitive impairment.
CN: Psychosocial integrity; CNS: None; CL: Analyze

23. A nurse is working with a client on recognizing the relationship between alcohol use and interpersonal problems. What is the nurse's **priority** intervention for this client?

1. Help the client recognize personal strengths
2. Have the client identify compulsive behaviors
3. Encourage the client's use of defense mechanisms
4. Have the client work with peers who can serve as role models

23. 3. Defense mechanisms can impede the development of healthy relationships and cause the client pain. After identifying barriers to relationship problems, it would be appropriate to identify or clarify personal strengths. Compulsive behavior doesn't tend to be a problem for alcoholic clients who struggle with interpersonal problems. Working with peers who are role models would be useful after the client recognizes, and gains, some insight into the problems.
CN: Safe, effective care environment; CNS: Management of care; CL: Analyze

CN: Client needs category   CNS: Client needs subcategory   CL: Cognitive level

24. The nurse has just completed the assessment of a client, recovering from alcohol addiction, who has limited coping skills. During the assessment, the nurse also identified that the client is experiencing relationship problems. Which assessment finding would indicate relationship difficulties?
1. The client is prone to panic attacks.
2. The client doesn't pay attention to details.
3. The client has poor communication skills.
4. The client ignores the need to relax and rest.

24. 3. To have satisfying relationships, a person must be able to communicate and problem solve. Relationship problems don't predispose people to panic attacks more than other psychosocial stressors. Paying attention to details isn't a major concern when addressing the client's relationship difficulties. Although ignoring the need for rest and relaxation is unhealthy, it shouldn't pose a major relationship problem.

CN: Psychosocial integrity; CNS: None; CL: Analyze

25. A nurse suggests to a client, struggling with alcohol addiction, that keeping a journal may be helpful. What is the goal for this intervention?
1. Identify stressors and the client's responses to them
2. Understand the diagnosis
3. Help others by reading the journal to them
4. Develop an emergency plan for use in a crisis

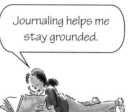

Journaling helps me stay grounded.

25. 1. Keeping a journal enables the client to identify problems and patterns of coping. From this information, the difficulties the client faces can be addressed. A journal isn't necessarily kept to promote better understanding of the client's illness, but it helps the client understand himself better. Journals aren't read to other people unless the client wants to share a particular part. Journals aren't typically used to identify an emergency plan for use in a crisis.

CN: Psychosocial integrity; CNS: None; CL: Apply

26. The nurse is preparing a teaching plan for a client who used alcohol. What is the **most** important information for the nurse to include?
1. Personal needs
2. Illness exacerbation
3. Cognitive distortions
4. Communication skills

26. 4. Addicted clients typically have difficulty communicating their needs in an appropriate way. Learning appropriate communication skills is a major goal of treatment. Behavior that focuses on self and meeting personal needs will be addressed next. The identification of cognitive distortions would be difficult if the client has poor communication skills. Teaching about illness exacerbation isn't a skill, but it is essential for relaying information about relapse.

CN: Psychosocial integrity; CNS: None; CL: Analyze

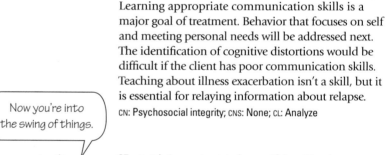

Now you're into the swing of things.

27. What is the **most** important assessment for a nurse to implement before starting a teaching session for a client who uses alcohol?
1. Sleep patterns
2. Decision making
3. Note-taking skills
4. Readiness to learn

27. 4. It's important to know if the client's current situation helps or hinders the potential to learn. Decision making and sleep patterns aren't factors that must be assessed before teaching about addiction. Note-taking skills aren't a factor in determining whether the client will be receptive to teaching.

CN: Psychosocial integrity; CNS: None; CL: Apply

28. The nurse is developing interventions to prevent a client, who used alcohol, from relapsing. What is the **most** important intervention for this client?
1. Avoid taking over-the-counter medications
2. Limit monthly contact with the family of origin
3. Refrain from becoming involved in group activities
4. Avoid people, places, and activities from the former lifestyle

28. 4. Changing the client's old habits is essential for sustaining a sober lifestyle. Certain over-the-counter medications that don't contain alcohol will probably need to be used by the client at certain times. It's unrealistic to have the client abstain from all such medications. Contact with the client's family may not trigger a relapse, so limiting contact wouldn't be useful. Refraining from group activities isn't a good strategy to prevent relapse. Going to Alcoholics Anonymous and other support groups will help prevent relapse.

CN: Psychosocial integrity; CNS: None; CL: Analyze

CN: Client needs category   CNS: Client needs subcategory   CL: Cognitive level

29. A client recovering from alcohol use tells the nurse, "I get nothing out of Alcoholics Anonymous (AA) meetings." What is the nurse's **best** response?
  1. "What were you told about going to AA meetings?"
  2. "What do you want to get out of the AA meetings?"
  3. "When do you think you'll stop going to the meetings?"
  4. "Do you think you can control what happens in a meeting?"

29. 2. This response puts some of the responsibility for staying sober on the client, and encourages the client to take a more active role. Asking what the client was told about AA meetings opens up a discussion that allows the client to express disappointments rather than taking a proactive stand to support the value of AA meetings. Answer three condones the client's desire to stop going to the meetings. Answer four changes the issue from being responsible for staying sober to focusing on what the client can't control.
CN: Psychosocial integrity; CNS: None; CL: Analyze

30. A client asks the nurse, "Why does it matter if I talk to my peers in group therapy?" What is the nurse's **most** appropriate response?
  1. "Group therapy lets you see what you're doing wrong in your life."
  2. "Group therapy acts as a defense against your disorganized behavior."
  3. "Group therapy provides a way to ask for support as well as to support others."
  4. "In group therapy, you can vent your frustrations and others will listen."

30. 3. The best response addresses how group therapy provides opportunities to communicate, learn, and give and get support. Group members will offer a client feedback, not just point out what a client is doing wrong. Group therapy isn't a defense against disorganized behavior. People can express a variety of feelings, and discuss many topics in group therapy. Interactions are goal oriented rather than vehicles to vent frustrations.
CN: Psychosocial integrity; CNS: None; CL: Apply

31. The nurse is facilitating a family meeting for a client who uses alcohol. During the meeting, the nurse observes the communication and determines an unhealthy pattern of:
  1. using descriptive jargon.
  2. disapproving of others' behavior.
  3. avoiding conflicting issues.
  4. limitless expression of nonverbal communication.

31. 3. The interaction pattern of a family with a member who uses alcohol often revolves around denying the problem, avoiding conflict, or rationalizing the addiction. Health care providers are more likely to use jargon. The family might have a problem setting limits and expressing disapproval of the client's behavior. Nonverbal communication often gives the nurse insight into family dynamics.
CN: Psychosocial integrity; CNS: None; CL: Analyze

32. A client, addicted to alcohol, is scheduled to begin individual therapy with the nurse. What is the **most** appropriate nursing intervention for this client?
  1. Help the client learn to express feelings
  2. Have the client establish new roles in the family
  3. Encourage the client to determine strategies for socializing
  4. Have the client decrease preoccupation with physical health

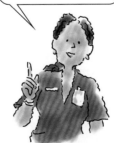

All answers may seem right, but choose the most appropriate one.

32. 1. The client must address issues, learn ways to cope effectively with life stressors, and express his needs appropriately. After the client establishes sobriety, the possibility of taking on new roles can become a reality. Determining strategies for socializing isn't the priority intervention for an addicted client. Usually, these clients need to change former socializing habits. Clients addicted to alcohol don't tend to be preoccupied with physical health problems.
CN: Safe, effective care environment; CNS: Management of care; CL: Analyze

33. A client recovering from alcohol addiction asks the nurse how to talk to his children about how his addiction has impacted them. What is the nurse's **best** response?
1. "Try to limit references to the addiction and focus on the present."
2. "Talk about all the hardships you've had in working to remain sober."
3. "Tell them you're sorry and emphasize that you're doing so much better now."
4. "Talk to them by acknowledging the difficulties and pain your drinking caused."

33. 4. Part of the healing process for the family is to acknowledge the pain, embarrassment, and overall difficulties the client's drinking problem has caused family members. Answer one facilitates the client's ability to deny the problem. Answer two prevents the client from acknowledging the difficulties the children endured. Answer three leads the client to believe only a simple apology is needed. The addiction must be addressed and the children's pain acknowledged.
CN: Psychosocial integrity; CNS: None; CL: Apply

34. The nurse is preparing a client with the diagnosis of alcohol dependency for discharge from the hospital. What is the **most** important goal for the client?
1. Find a way to drink socially
2. Allow self to grieve recent losses
3. Work to bring others into treatment
4. Develop relapse-prevention strategies

34. 4. The primary goal for a client in outpatient treatment is to focus on strategies that prevent relapse. Finding ways to drink socially and working to bring others into treatment aren't goals of outpatient therapy. Allowing self to grieve the losses that the addiction has caused is a part of the early work of inpatient therapy, and may be continued in outpatient therapy.
CN: Safe, effective care environment; CNS: Management of care; CL: Analyze

35. A client addicted to alcohol tells a nurse, "Making friends used to be hard for me." The nurse determines that client teaching about relationships has been successful when the client states:
1. "I am trying to set boundaries with others."
2. "I need to be judgmental of others."
3. "I won't become intimately involved with others."
4. "I can't bear to see myself hurt again in a relationship."

35. 1. When the client can set personal limits and maintain boundaries, the ability to have successful interpersonal relationships can occur. Being judgmental is contraindicated if a client wants to have successful relationships. Setting arbitrary limits on relationships indicates the client needs to learn more interpersonal relationship skills. The universal truth about relationships is that they bring both joy and pain. The last statement indicates a need to learn more about relationships.
CN: Psychosocial integrity; CNS: None; CL: Apply

36. A client tells a nurse, "I'm not going to incur problems from smoking marijuana." What is the nurse's **most** appropriate response?
1. Evidence shows it can cause major health problems.
2. Marijuana produces physical and psychological dependence.
3. Smoking marijuana isn't as dangerous as smoking cigarettes.
4. Some people have minor or no reactions to smoking marijuana.

36. 2. Marijuana causes cardiac, respiratory, immune, and reproductive health problems. All people who smoke marijuana have symptoms of intoxication. The residues from marijuana are more toxic than those from cigarettes.
CN: Psychosocial integrity; CNS: None; CL: Apply

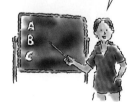

Clients with addictions often need help learning how to set boundaries in relationships.

37. The nurse is performing an assessment of a client with a history of polysubstance use. What is the **most** important information for the nurse to obtain?
1. Oral administration of any drug
2. Time of last use of each drug
3. How the drug was obtained
4. The place the drug was used

CN: Client needs category   CNS: Client needs subcategory   CL: Cognitive level

37. 2. The time of last use gives information about expected withdrawal symptoms of the drugs, and what immediate treatment is necessary. How the drugs were obtained and the places the drugs were used aren't essential information for treatment, nor is the administration.
CN: Psychosocial integrity; CNS: None; CL: Apply

38. A client says, "I started using cocaine as a recreational drug on weekends, and now I can't seem to get through a weekend without it." The nurse interprets the client's statement as **most** consistent with:
1. toxic dose.
2. dual diagnosis.
3. cross-tolerance.
4. compulsive use.

39. A client tells the nurse that he uses amphetamines to be productive at work. The nurse is aware that abrupt discontinuation of the drug will produce:
1. severe anxiety.
2. increased yawning.
3. altered perceptions.
4. amotivational syndrome.

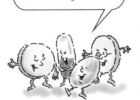

Tablet: "How long have you been in the bloodstream?" Capsule: "A couple of hours—how about you?"

40. A 20-year-old client is admitted with bone marrow depression. He tells the nurse he's been using drugs since age 13. Which drug should the nurse anticipate finding in this client's history?
1. Amphetamines
2. Cocaine
3. Inhalants
4. Marijuana

Way to go! You're almost halfway done.

41. A client has stopped using phencyclidine (PCP). It is **most** important for the nurse to monitor the client's behavior for:
1. fatigue and feelings of being overwhelmed.
2. agitation and mood swings.
3. bizarre behavior leading to a psychotic episode.
4. memory loss and forgetfulness.

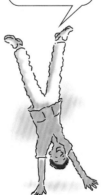

42. A nurse is caring for a client who is experiencing amphetamine withdrawal. The nurse should assess the client for:
1. disturbed sleep.
2. increased yawning.
3. psychomotor agitation.
4. an inability to concentrate.

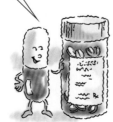

You should know which drugs cause which adverse effects!

43. A client has been admitted to the emergency department and states that he just used cocaine. The nurse should monitor this client for:
1. tachycardia.
2. hypothermia.
3. hypotension.
4. bradypnea.

38. 4. Compulsive drug use involves taking a substance for a period of time significantly longer than intended. A toxic dose is the amount of a drug that causes a poisonous effect. Dual diagnosis is the coexistence of a drug problem and a mental health problem. Cross-tolerance occurs when the effects of a drug are decreased and the client takes larger amounts to achieve the desired drug effect.
CN: Psychosocial integrity; CNS: None; CL: Apply

39. 1. When amphetamines are abruptly discontinued, the client may experience severe anxiety or agitation. Increased yawning is a symptom of opioid withdrawal. Altered perceptions occur when a client is withdrawing from hallucinogens. Amotivational syndrome is seen with clients using marijuana.
CN: Psychosocial integrity; CNS: None; CL: Apply

40. 3. Inhalants cause severe bone marrow depression. Marijuana, cocaine, and amphetamines don't cause bone marrow depression.
CN: Physiological integrity; CNS: Pharmacological and parenteral therapies; CL: Apply

41. 3. Bizarre behavior and speech are associated with PCP withdrawal, and can indicate psychosis. Fatigue isn't necessarily a problem when a client stops using PCP. Agitation, mood swings, memory loss, and forgetfulness don't tend to occur when a client has stopped using PCP.
CN: Psychosocial integrity; CNS: None; CL: Analyze

42. 1. It's common for a person withdrawing from amphetamines to experience disturbed sleep and unpleasant dreams. Increased yawning is seen with clients withdrawing from opioids. Psychomotor agitation is seen in cocaine withdrawal, and the inability to concentrate is seen with caffeine withdrawal.
CN: Psychosocial integrity; CNS: None; CL: Apply

43. 1. Tachycardia is common because cocaine increases the heart's demand for oxygen. Cocaine causes hyperthermia. Cocaine doesn't cause hypothermia, hypotension, or bradypnea.
CN: Psychosocial integrity; CNS: None; CL: Apply

CN: Client needs category   CNS: Client needs subcategory   CL: Cognitive level

44. What is the **most** important teaching information for the nurse to provide a client who uses prescription drugs without a prescription?
1. Herbal substitutes are safer to use.
2. Medication should be used only for the reason prescribed.
3. The client should consult a provider before using a drug.
4. Consider if family members influence the client's drug use.

44. 2. People often take prescribed drugs for reasons other than those intended, primarily to self-medicate or experience a sense of euphoria. The safety and efficacy of most herbal remedies haven't been established. Sometimes, over-the-counter medications are necessary for minor problems. There may be a family history of substance use, but it isn't a priority when planning nursing care.
CN: Psychosocial integrity; CNS: None; CL: Apply

45. A pregnant client is thinking about stopping cocaine use. The nurse determines that teaching about drug use and pregnancy has been effective when the client states:
1. "Right after birth, I'll give my baby up for adoption."
2. "I'll help the baby get through the withdrawal period."
3. "I don't want the baby to have withdrawal symptoms."
4. "It's scary to think the baby may have Down syndrome."

45. 3. Neonates born to mothers addicted to cocaine have withdrawal symptoms at birth. If the client says she'll give the baby up for adoption after birth or help the baby get through the withdrawal period, the teaching was ineffective because the mother doesn't see the impact of her drug use on the child. Use of cocaine during pregnancy doesn't contribute to the baby having Down syndrome.
CN: Psychosocial integrity; CNS: None; CL: Analyze

46. A client with a history of cocaine use exhibits behavior changes following return from a weekend pass to visit his family. Which diagnostic screening should the nurse anticipate the health care provider will order?
1. Antibody
2. Glucose
3. Hepatic
4. Urine

Which drug is most likely to produce these symptoms?

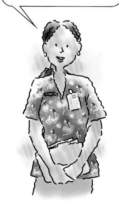

46. 4. A urine toxicology screen would show the presence of cocaine in the body. Glucose, hepatic, or antibody screening wouldn't show the presence of cocaine in the body.
CN: Psychosocial integrity; CNS: None; CL: Apply

47. A nurse is assessing a client with a history of substance use. The client has pinpoint pupils, a heart rate of 56 bpm, a respiratory rate of 6 breaths/min, and temperature of 96.4° F (35.8° C). What is the **most** likely cause of this client's symptoms?
1. Opioids
2. Amphetamines
3. Cannabis
4. Alcohol

47. 1. Opioids, such as morphine and heroin, can cause pinpoint pupils and a reduced heart rate, respiratory rate, and body temperature with intoxication. Amphetamine intoxication can lead to tachycardia, euphoria, and irritability. Cannabis intoxication can cause slowed reflexes, lethargy, and tachycardia. Alcohol intoxication leads to slurred speech, unsteady gait, and incoordination.
CN: Psychosocial integrity; CNS: None; CL: Apply

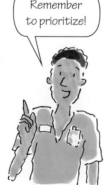
Remember to prioritize!

48. A nurse is caring for a client recovering from cocaine use. Which is the **priority** intervention for this client?
1. Skin care
2. Suicide precautions
3. Frequent orientation
4. Nutrition consultation

48. 2. Clients recovering from cocaine use are prone to post-coke depression, and have a likelihood of becoming suicidal if they can't take the drug. Frequent orientation and skin care are routine nursing interventions but aren't the most immediate considerations for this client. Nutrition consultation isn't the most pressing intervention for this client.
CN: Safe, effective care environment; CNS: Management of care; CL: Analyze

CN: Client needs category   CNS: Client needs subcategory   CL: Cognitive level

49. The nurse is assessing a client who repeatedly uses cocaine. It is important for the nurse to observe the client for:
1. panic attacks.
2. bipolar cycling.
3. attention deficits.
4. expressive aphasia.

49. 2. Clients who frequently use cocaine will experience the rapid cycling effect of excitement and then severe depression. They don't tend to experience panic attacks, expressive aphasia, or attention deficits.
CN: Psychosocial integrity; CNS: None; CL: Analyze

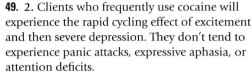

What would have the opposite effect?

50. A client who uses cocaine finally admits that he has also used other drugs to equalize the effect of cocaine. The nurse is aware that the client's drug history may include:
1. alcohol.
2. amphetamines.
3. caffeine.
4. phencyclidine.

50. 1. A cocaine addict will commonly use alcohol to decrease or equalize the stimulating effects of cocaine. Caffeine, phencyclidine, and amphetamines aren't used to equalize the stimulating effects of cocaine.
CN: Psychosocial integrity; CNS: None; CL: Apply

51. A group of teenagers tell the school nurse that they used cocaine because they were bored. What is the **most** important goal for the nurse?
1. Prepare a drug lecture
2. Restrict school privileges
3. Establish an activity schedule
4. Report the incident to their parents

51. 3. Having an activity schedule enables the adolescents to develop coping skills to make better choices about what to do with their free time. Preparing a drug lecture or restricting school privileges won't be seen as useful by the adolescents, and may inadvertently contribute to their inappropriate behavior. As the nurse works with the adolescents, it would be most effective to have the children tell their parents about the drug use.
CN: Psychosocial integrity; CNS: None; CL: Apply

52. The nurse determines that teaching about cocaine has been effective when the client states:
1. "I wasn't using cocaine to feel better about myself."
2. "I started using cocaine more and more until I couldn't stop."
3. "I'm not addicted to cocaine because I don't use it every day."
4. "I only use it on holidays, and am not a chronic user."

52. 2. This statement reflects the trajectory or common pattern of cocaine use and indicates successful teaching. Answer one reflects the client's denial. People gravitate to the drug and continue its use because it gives them a sense of well-being, competency, and power. Cocaine users tend to be binge users and can be drug free for days or weeks between uses, but they still have a drug problem. Answer four indicates the client is in denial about the drug's potential to become a habit. Effective teaching didn't occur.
CN: Psychosocial integrity; CNS: None; CL: Analyze

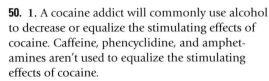

Don't panic. Read the question again, and I'm sure you'll catch the drift.

53. A client who formerly used lysergic acid diethylamide (LSD) is seeking counseling. The nurse anticipates that the assessment of the client will include:
1. a lack of trust.
2. panic attacks.
3. recurrent depression.
4. a loss of ego boundaries.

53. 2. Clients who used LSD typically have a history of panic attacks or psychotic behavior. This is often referred to as a "bad trip." Loss of ego boundaries, recurrent depression, and lack of trust don't tend to be problems for this type of client.
CN: Psychosocial integrity; CNS: None; CL: Analyze

CN: Client needs category   CNS: Client needs subcategory   CL: Cognitive level

54. A client who smoked marijuana daily for 10 years tells the nurse, "I don't have any goals, and I just don't know what to do." What is the **most** appropriate nursing intervention for this client?
1. Focus the interaction
2. Use nonverbal methods
3. Use reflection techniques
4. Ask open-ended questions

55. A nurse is performing a physical assessment on a client who uses heroin. It is **most** important for the nurse to assess the client for:
1. hepatitis.
2. peptic ulcers.
3. hypertension.
4. chronic pharyngitis.

56. The family of a client in rehabilitation following heroin withdrawal asks a nurse why the client is receiving naltrexone. What is the nurse's **best** response?
1. To help reverse withdrawal symptoms
2. To keep the client sedated during withdrawal
3. To take the place of detoxification with methadone
4. To decrease the client's memory of the withdrawal experience

57. What is the **priority** nursing intervention for a client recovering from cocaine addiction?
1. Help the client find ways to be happy and competent
2. Foster the creative use of self in community activities
3. Teach the client to handle stresses in the work setting
4. Help the client acknowledge the current level of dependency

58. A client tells a nurse, "I've been clean from drugs for the past five years, but my life really hasn't changed." The nurse determines that further discussion should include:
1. further education.
2. conflict resolution.
3. career development.
4. personal development.

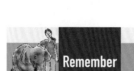

Remember

"Naltrexone avoids opioid dependency."

An opioid antagonist, naltrexone blocks the effects of opioids in clients with opioid dependence.

54. 1. A client with amotivational syndrome from chronic use of marijuana tends to talk in tangents and needs the nurse to focus the conversation. Nonverbal communication or reflection techniques wouldn't be useful as this client must focus and learn to identify and accomplish goals. Using only open-ended questions won't allow the client to focus and establish specific goals.
CN: Psychosocial integrity; CNS: None; CL: Apply

55. 1. Hepatitis is the most common medical complication of heroin use. Peptic ulcers are more likely to be a complication of caffeine use. Hypertension is a complication of amphetamine use, and chronic pharyngitis is a complication of marijuana use.
CN: Physiological integrity; CNS: Physiological adaptation; CL: Apply

56. 1. Naltrexone is an opioid antagonist and helps the client stay drug free. Keeping the client sedated during withdrawal isn't the reason for giving this drug. The drug doesn't decrease the client's memory of the withdrawal experience, and isn't used in place of detoxification with methadone.
CN: Psychosocial integrity; CNS: None; CL: Apply

57. 1. The major component of a treatment program for a client with cocaine addiction is to have the client feel happy and competent. Cocaine addiction is difficult to treat because the drug actions reinforce its use. There are often perceived positive effects. Clients often credit the drug with giving them creative energy instead of looking within themselves. Fostering the creative use of self may inadvertently reinforce the client's drug use. Teaching the client to handle stress is appropriate, but isn't the most immediate nursing action. Examining the client's level of dependency isn't the immediate choice, as this client needs to remain drug free.
CN: Safe, effective care environment; CNS: Management of care; CL: Apply

58. 4. True recovery involves changing the client's distorted thinking and working on personal and emotional development. Before the client pursues further education, career development, or conflict resolution skills, it is imperative that the client devote energy to emotional and personal development.
CN: Psychosocial integrity; CNS: None; CL: Analyze

59. A client discusses with the nurse how drug addiction has made life unmanageable. The nurse determines that coping methods for this client should include:
1. how peers have committed to sobriety.
2. how to accomplish family of origin work.
3. how to understand the addiction process.
4. how environmental stimuli can serve as a drug trigger.

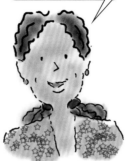

You're almost to question 60. That should motivate you to keep moving!

59. 3. When the client admits life has become unmanageable, the best strategy is to teach the client about the addiction, how to obtain support, and how to develop new coping skills. Information about how peers committed to sobriety would be shared with the client as the treatment process begins. Identification of how environmental stimuli serve as drug triggers would be a later part of the treatment process and family of origin work. "Family of origin work" in it's simplest form is, "healing from our past to be able to move forward in the present." Initially, the client must commit to sobriety and learn skills for recovery.
CN: Psychosocial integrity; CNS: None; CL: Analyze

60. A nurse is assessing a client with a history of cocaine use. The nurse is aware that the assessment may include:
1. glossitis.
2. pharyngitis.
3. bilateral ear infections.
4. a perforated nasal septum.

60. 4. When cocaine is frequently snorted, the client often develops a perforated nasal septum. Bilateral ear infections, pharyngitis, and glossitis aren't common physical findings for a client with a history of cocaine use.
CN: Psychosocial integrity; CNS: None; CL: Apply

61. A client recovering from cocaine use is participating in group therapy. The nurse determines that the client has benefited from the therapy when the client makes states:
1. "I think the laws about drug possession are too strict in this country."
2. "I'll be more careful about talking about my drug use to my children."
3. "I finally realize the short high from cocaine isn't worth the depression."
4. "I can't understand how I could have all the problems that we talked about in group."

61. 3. This is a realistic appraisal of a client's experience with cocaine and how harmful the experience is. Answer one indicates that the client was distracting self from personal issues and isn't working on goals in the group setting. Talking about drugs to children must be reinforced with nonverbal behavior, and not talking about drugs may give children the wrong message about drug use. Answer four indicates the client is in denial about the consequences of cocaine use.
CN: Psychosocial integrity; CNS: None; CL: Analyze

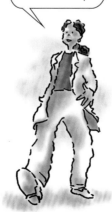

A journey of a thousand miles starts with one step.

62. A family tells the nurse that they are concerned about a sister who stopped using amphetamines three months ago and is now acting paranoid. What is the nurse's **best** response?
1. A person gets symptoms of paranoia with polysubstance use.
2. When a person uses amphetamines, paranoid tendencies may continue for months.
3. Sometimes, family dynamics and a high suspicion of continued drug use make a person paranoid.
4. Amphetamine users may have severe depression and paranoid thinking.

62. 2. After a client uses amphetamines, there may be long-term effects that exist for months after use. Two common effects are paranoia and ideas of reference. Even with polysubstance use, the paranoia comes from the chronic use of amphetamines. Answer three blames the family for the paranoia rather than the drug use. Severe depression isn't typically manifested in paranoid thinking.
CN: Psychosocial integrity; CNS: None; CL: Analyze

63. The nurse is trying to determine if a client, who uses heroin, has any drug-related problems. What is the **most** appropriate question for the nurse to ask?
1. "When did your spouse become aware of your use of heroin?"
2. "Do you have a probation officer that you report to periodically?"
3. "Have you experienced any legal violations while being intoxicated?"
4. "Do you have a history of frequent visits with the employee assistance program manager?"

63. 3. This question focuses on obtaining direct information about drug-related legal problems. When a spouse becomes aware of a partner's substance use, the first action isn't necessarily to institute legal action. Even if the client reports to a probation officer, the offense isn't necessarily a drug-related problem. Asking if the client has a history of frequent visits with the employee assistance program manager isn't useful. It assumes any visit to the employee assistance program manager is related to drug issues.
CN: Psychosocial integrity; CNS: None; CL: Analyze

64. A nurse is caring for a heroine-addicted client who is experiencing withdrawal symptoms. The nurse is aware that the withdrawal symptoms may be affected by:
1. ego strength.
2. liver function.
3. seizure history.
4. kidney function.

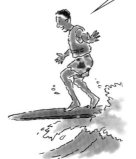

Ride that wave, dude! Cowabunga!

64. 2. Liver function status is an important variable that can be used to indicate the severity of a client's drug withdrawal. Ego strength, seizure history, and kidney function aren't variables that can be used to predict the severity of withdrawal symptoms.
CN: Physiological integrity; CNS: Reduction of risk potential; CL: Analyze

65. A client who uses cocaine denies that drug use is a problem. What is the **best** intervention by the nurse?
1. 1. State ways to cope with stress
2. 2. Repeat the drug facts as needed
3. 3. Identify the client's ambivalence
4. 4. Use open-ended, factual questions

65. 4. The use of open-ended, factual questions will help the client acknowledge that a drug problem is present. Stating ways to cope with stress and identifying the client's ambivalence won't be effective for breaking through a client's denial. Repeating drug facts won't be effective, as the client will perceive it as preaching or nagging.
CN: Psychosocial integrity; CNS: None; CL: Apply

66. A nurse is working with the parents of an adolescent client who uses inhalants. What is the **most** important information for the nurse to provide?
1. Specific consequences must be enforceable
2. Everything can become a consequence
3. When setting consequences, be verbally forceful
4. Consequences are seldom needed with adolescents

66. 1. Consequences must be specific and enforceable. Sometimes, parents are prone to make consequences that are too difficult to enforce or that actually become a punishment for the parents. Everything can't be made into a consequence. Being verbally forceful isn't appropriate because the consequence can occur in a civil tone of voice. A consequence can be used with every person regardless of their developmental stage.
CN: Psychosocial integrity; CNS: None; CL: Analyze

67. A nurse is caring for a very pessimistic client undergoing treatment for cocaine use. Which statement would the nurse anticipate from this client?
1. "I'll never get better. This is useless."
2. "I don't think I want to see my family anymore. They're not supportive."
3. "I'm fatigued all the time. My energy is low."
4. "I want to get better now. Can't we rush the treatment?"

67. 1. Clients withdrawing from drugs such as cocaine frequently experience depression. It's common for drug-addicted clients to experience fatigue without becoming pessimistic. Being impulsive or having feelings of estrangement aren't necessarily related to a client pessimism.
CN: Psychosocial integrity; CNS: None; CL: Analyze

68. A nurse is working with a client, addicted to cocaine, who is in denial. What is the **most** appropriate intervention for the nurse to implement?
1. Ask if the client sees the drug use as a problem
2. Focus on the pain the client is having during withdrawal
3. Reinforce the connection between drug use and harmful results
4. Help the client recognize reality by pointing out withdrawal symptoms

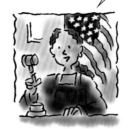

And the verdict is—the *most appropriate* answer.

68. 3. To deal with the client's denial, the nurse must confront the drug use and point out the results of the behavior. Asking if the client sees the drug use as a problem will only reinforce the client's denial and provide a forum to intellectualize the problem, or provide excuses for it. Pain isn't associated with withdrawal from cocaine. Pointing out withdrawal symptoms may not be the most effective strategy, as the client often downplays the significance of the problem.
CN: Psychosocial integrity; CNS: None; CL: Analyze

69. The nurse is caring for a client who uses cocaine and has been admitted to an intensive outpatient rehabilitation program. For which is it **most** important for the nurse to assess the client?
1. Gastrointestinal distress
2. Blurred vision
3. Perceptual distortions
4. Increased appetite

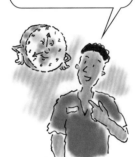

Time for a little therapeutic communication.

69. 4. Increased appetite is typical during cocaine or nicotine withdrawal. Gastrointestinal distress occurs during alcohol or opioid withdrawal. Blurred vision isn't typical in cocaine withdrawal. Perceptual distortions are common during withdrawal from phencyclidine, amphetamines, and hallucinogens.
CN: Physiological integrity; CNS: Physiological adaptation; CL: Apply

70. A client who uses alcohol is admitted to an outpatient drug and alcohol treatment facility. What is the **most** objective way for the nurse to determine if the client is still using alcohol?
1. Having the client walk a straight line
2. Smelling the client's breath
3. Giving the client a breath alcohol test
4. Asking the client if he has been drinking

70. 3. A breath alcohol test is the most objective way to determine if the client is still using alcohol. Having him walk a straight line and smelling his breath aren't objective tests. Asking him if he has been drinking may not elicit an honest answer.
CN: Psychosocial integrity; CNS: None; CL: Apply

71. The nurse anticipates that a client undergoing nicotine withdrawal may state:
1. "I sometimes feel like I'm seeing things."
2. "I feel lousy, and I'm grumpy with everybody."
3. "I can't believe I feel fine after just having stopped smoking."
4. "I'm always yawning now."

71. 2. During nicotine withdrawal, the client is typically irritable and nervous. Hallucinations aren't linked to nicotine withdrawal. A client going through nicotine withdrawal is unlikely to feel fine. Yawning is associated with withdrawal from opioids, not nicotine.
CN: Physiological integrity; CNS: Physiological adaptation; CL: Apply

72. A client with polysubstance use is hospitalized for withdrawal complications. What is the **most** important goal for this client?
1. Remain safe during the detoxification period
2. Develop an accurate perception of his drug problem
3. Abstain from mood-altering drugs
4. Learn coping strategies to help decrease reliance on drugs

72. 1. Client safety takes highest priority during detoxification. During this time, it's unrealistic to expect clients to perceive their drug problems accurately; typically, they will experience cognitive impairment or deny their addiction. In the hospital, the client usually doesn't have access to drugs, and should be drug free. The goal of abstaining from mood-altering drugs takes highest priority after discharge. Learning coping strategies is an appropriate goal immediately after withdrawal and when medical care is completed.
CN: Safe, effective care environment; CNS: Management of care; CL: Apply

73. A client with an alcohol addiction requests a prescription for disulfiram. To determine the client's ability to take the drug appropriately, the nurse should assess whether:
1. the client is capable of maintaining a medication regimen.
2. the client's family accepts the use of this treatment strategy.
3. the client is willing to follow the necessary dietary restrictions.
4. the client is motivated to maintain sobriety.

73. 4. A client with a strong craving for alcohol, and a lack of impulse control, isn't a good candidate for disulfiram therapy. Accepting the treatment strategy is a decision that the client and health care provider make. Although family input may be welcome, family members don't make the final decision. Alcohol must not be consumed, but significant dietary restrictions aren't necessary during disulfiram therapy.
CN: Psychosocial integrity; CNS: None; CL: Analyze

74. A nurse has developed a therapeutic relationship with a client who has an addiction problem. The nurse determines that their interactions are in the working stage when the client: Select all that apply.
1. addresses how the addiction has contributed to family distress.
2. reluctantly shares the family history of addiction.
3. verbalizes difficulty identifying personal strengths.
4. discusses financial problems related to the addiction.
5. expresses uncertainty about meeting with the nurse.
6. acknowledges the addiction's effects on the children.

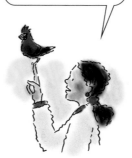

Feeling stressed? Take a minute to be thankful for the little things.

74. 1, 3, 6. These statements are indicative of the nurse-client working phase, in which the client explores, evaluates, and determines solutions to identified problems. The remaining statements address what happens during the introductory phase of the nurse-client interaction.
CN: Psychosocial integrity; CNS: None; CL: Analyze

75. A client has received an ordered dose of chlordiazepoxide to control the symptoms of alcohol withdrawal. Which symptoms would indicate that this client should receive an additional dose of the prescribed medication? Select all that apply.
1. Tachycardia
2. Mood swings
3. Elevated blood pressure and temperature
4. Piloerection
5. Tremors
6. Increasing anxiety

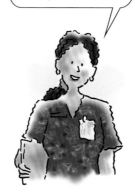

Use your nose to sniff out the answer to question 75.

75. 1, 3, 5, 6. Benzodiazepines are usually administered based on elevations in heart rate, blood pressure, and temperature as well as on the presence of tremors and increasing anxiety. Mood swings are expected during the withdrawal period, and are not an indication for further medication administration. Piloerection is not a symptom of alcohol withdrawal.
CN: Physiological integrity; CNS: Pharmacological and parenteral therapies; CL: Analyze

76. A client, newly admitted to the inpatient unit, has incurred physical health problems due to the long-term use of cannabis. What should the nurse expect to assess?
1. Brain and liver changes
2. Euphoria followed by depression
3. Slurred speech and diplopia
4. Tachycardia and orthostatic hypotension

76. 4. Long term use of cannabis causes tachycardia and orthostatic hypotension. With a decrease in blood pressure, oxygen supply to myocardial tissue is decreased, and tachycardia then increases the oxygen demand. Long-term use of alcohol can cause brain and liver damage. Frequent use of cocaine causes euphoria followed by depression and feelings of letdown. The frequent use of inhalants causes slurred speech and diplopia.
CN: Safe, effective care environment; CNS: Management of care; CL: Analyze

77. A client, who is in recovery from years of alcohol use, is trying to decrease his excessive use of caffeine. The nurse educates the client on his caffeine consumption. Which response, by the client, indicates the nurse's teaching was effective?
1. "Caffeine must be the cause of my awful dreams and disrupted sleep."
2. "Now I know why I sometimes have tremors and feel nervous."
3. "I'm glad to hear that I won't have any problems when I stop drinking coffee."
4. "Having nasal drainage occur when I stop drinking caffeine may not be worth it."

77. 2. Common withdrawal symptoms of caffeine withdrawal are tremors, irritability and nervousness. Common withdrawal symptoms of amphetamines are unpleasant dreams and disturbed sleep. Rhinorrhea, lacrimation, and yawning are symptoms of withdrawal from opioids.
CN: Health promotion and maintenance; CNS: None; CL: Analyze

78. The nurse is working with a client who has a diagnosis of gambling, and is developing strategies to encourage the client to participate in treatment. Prioritize these strategies, used by the nurse, in the order that they should be implemented.
1. Help the client learn strategies to delay gratification, and ways to select desirable social behaviors
2. Discuss the client's focus on gambling and its connection to feeling a sense of power and control
3. Address how gambling has effected the client, family members, and peers when the client minimizes involvement and denies the problem.
4. Have a conversation about how the urge to gamble increases when the client feels stressed

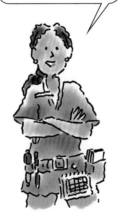

Maybe we should be called priority engineers instead of nurses.

78. **Ordered Response:**
2. Discuss the client's focus on gambling and its connection to feeling a sense of power and control
4. Have a conversation about how the urge to gamble increases when the client feels stressed
3. Address how gambling has effected the client, family members, and peers when the client minimizes involvement and denies the problem.
1. Help the client learn strategies to delay gratification, and ways to select desirable social behaviors
CN: Psychosocial integrity; CNS: None; CL: Analyze

79. A client requests help developing a plan to stop drinking ten, 12-ounce cups of coffee a day. Prioritize the interventions that will help this client decrease caffeine intake?
1. Address how to handle uncomfortable feelings that may occur
2. Reinforce the need to obtain assistance, when a relapse is imminent
3. Discuss how physiologic discomfort and other health conditions can increase the risk of injury
4. Educate the client about the signs and symptoms of caffeine withdrawal

79. **Ordered Response:**
4. Educate the client about the signs and symptoms of caffeine withdrawal
1. Address how to handle uncomfortable feelings that may occur
3. Discuss how physiologic discomfort and other health conditions can increase the risk of injury
2. Reinforce the need to obtain assistance, when a relapse is imminent
CN: Health promotion and maintenance; CNS: None; CL: Analyze

80. The nurse is caring for a client who was admitted to the hospital unit after experiencing an overdose of cocaine. What is the **most** important symptom to monitor after this client is admitted to the unit?
1. Hypertension
2. Hypothermia
3. Hyperglycemia
4. Seizures

80. 4. Seizures are a major sign of cocaine overdose as they can cause extreme physiologic instability. Hypertension is a normal side effect of cocaine use along with a rise in body temperature and heart rate. Clients with cocaine overdose often experience hyperthermia. Clients with an overdose of cocaine may present with hypoglycemia.
CN: Safe, effective care environment; CNS: Management of care; CL: Apply

81. The nurse is reviewing the results of diagnostic studies for a client who used an excessive amount of steroids. What lab value would the nurse expect to be abnormal?
1. Decreased low-density lipoprotein (LDL)
2. Increased blood urea nitrogen (BUN)
3. Increase high density lipoprotein (HDL)
4. Decreased prothrombin time/international normalized ratio (INR)

81. 2. Steroid use is a non-renal indication for an elevated blood urea nitrogen lab value. Steroids, particularly oral steroids, increase the level of low-density lipoprotein (LDL) and decrease the level of high-density lipoprotein (HDL). Steroids can also increase the clotting time of blood. There is a risk of blood clots forming in the blood vessels, potentially disrupting blood flow.
CN: Safe, effective care environment; CNS: Management of care; CL: Analyze

82. The nurse is working with a client diagnosed with a heroin overdose. What are the **most** important symptoms to monitor after establishing and maintaining a stable airway?
1. Hypertension and seizures
2. Incoordination and slurred speech
3. Nausea and vomiting
4. Psychosis and hypervigilance

82. 1. A client with a heroin overdose is at risk for hypertension and seizures. Clients with alcohol intoxication are at risk for incoordination, slurred speech, nausea and vomiting. Clients with an overdose of amphetamines are at risk for psychosis and hypervigilance.
CN: Safe, effective care environment; CNS: Management of care; CL: Apply

83. A college student, in the emergency department, was raped at a party after someone slipped Ecstasy into her drink. The client tells the nurse, "I think something was put into my drink without my knowing, but how did this happen?" What would be the nurse's **best** response?
1. "Unfortunately rape happens to female, college students with, or without, the use of drugs."
2. "Ecstasy makes a person become a little wild, and puts the person at risk for violent behavior."
3. "The drug is tasteless, odorless and colorless, so you wouldn't have known that you were ingesting it."
4. "You're not alone. This happens all over the world to many young, female, college students."

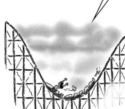

This test has been a wild ride, but we're almost over the last hill.

83. 3. A client, who was given Ecstasy in a beverage, has no way of knowing that the drug is present since it is colorless, tasteless, and odorless. Saying that rape happens is a minimizing statement that does not show compassion, or answer the client's question. The drug Ecstasy makes one empathetic, verbal, and excessively friendly. Consequently, males may take sexual advantage of a woman under the influence of Ecstasy. Answer four is not a sensitive or compassionate response to the client's situation.
CN: Psychosocial integrity; CNS: None; CL: Apply

84. A client is experiencing problems from the excessive use of caffeine. Prioritize these withdrawal symptoms from earliest to latest.

| **1.** Nausea and muscle pain |
| **2.** Fatigue and drowsiness |
| **3.** Headache |
| **4.** Irritability and depression |

85. The nurse reads the chart entry for a client who attends group therapy, and who uses cannabis daily:

| **Progress notes** |
| 2/10/17 1700 | The client is congested, with a dry hacking cough. He could not verbalize his treatment goals when asked in the group session. He laughed when the therapist gave each participant a worksheet to fill out and bring back to the next group, and stated, "I'm not doing that." |

What health problem is this client experiencing because of extended cannabis use?
1. Amotivational syndrome
2. Delirium tremens
3. Vascular dementia
4. Cognitive distortions

84. **Ordered Response**

| **3.** Headache |
| **2.** Fatigue and drowsiness |
| **4.** Irritability and depression |
| **1.** Nausea and muscle pain |

CN: Safe, effective care environment; CNS: Management of care; CL: Apply

85. **1.** Long-term use of cannabis is associated with amotivational syndrome. Amotivational syndrome is a psychological health condition that is characterized by losing interest in cognitive and social activities. The client will display a sense of apathy. Delirium tremens is associated with alcohol withdrawal. Vascular dementia is associated with an alteration in a person's thought processes caused by disrupted blood flow to the brain. Cognitive distortions are inaccurate thoughts used to reinforce negative thoughts or feelings, and are common in clients with depression.

CN: Psychosocial integrity; CNS: None; CL: Apply

86. A young adult client who uses cannabis multiple times a day, has just participated in a family meeting at a community mental health center. The chart entry reads:

Progress notes	
2/10/17 0900	The family meeting began by the client's family demanding that the client "stop using marijuana at once, or there will be severe consequences, including no support to attend college." The drug, and the problems associated with its use, were explained to the family.

What educational topic should the nurse address with this family during the next teaching session?

1. Talk about how things were prior to the client's substance use
2. Address how the substance use has effected each member of the family
3. Discuss the possibility of the client developing violent tendencies
4. Encourage the family to be more flexible with their thoughts and feelings

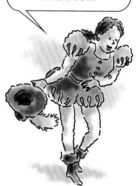

You made it to question 86! Now take a bow.

86. 2. As the client continues to use a substance, it is common for the family members to develop anxiety, depression, anger, and physical symptoms to help them to cope with the distress. Talking about how things were for this client in the past may, or may not, be effective. Clients who use cannabis do not tend to become violent. It is unrealistic to expect an immediate and dramatic shift in a person's thinking about substance use.

CN: Psychosocial integrity; CNS: None; CL: Analyze

Chapter 19

Dissociative Disorders

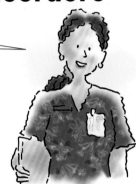

For more information on dissociative disorders, check the International Society for the Study of Trauma and Dissociation's Web site at **www.isst-d.org**.

1. The nurse is assessing a client experiencing dissociative identify disorder (DID). The nurse anticipates the client to make which statement?
1. "My father wasn't around much when I was growing up."
2. "I feel good about myself and my childhood."
3. "I have many childhood memories, both good and bad."
4. "My father loved me one day and hit me the next day."

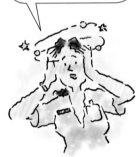

Sometimes I just can't remember anything.

1. 4. Repeated exposure to a childhood environment that alternates between highly stressful and loving and supportive can be a factor in the development of DID. Many children grow up in a household without a father, but don't develop DID. Clients with DID commonly have low self-esteem. Because of dissociation from the trauma, a client with DID usually can't recall childhood memories or traumatic events.
CN: Psychosocial integrity; CNS: None; CL: Apply

2. Which nursing intervention is **most** important for a client experiencing dissociative identity disorder (DID)?
1. Give medications to enhance memories
2. Maintain consistency when interacting with the client
3. Confront the client about the use of alter personalities
4. Discourage client interaction with others when an alter personality is in control

2. 2. Establishing trust and support is important when interacting with a client who has DID. This can be demonstrated through consistency in interactions. Many of these clients have had few healthy relationships. Medication hasn't proven effective in the treatment of DID. Confronting the client about the alter personalities would be ineffective because the client has little, if any, knowledge of the presence of these other personalities. Isolating the client wouldn't be therapeutically beneficial.
CN: Safe, effective care environment; CNS: Management of care; CL: Analyze

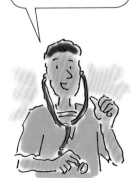

Which statement is consistent with dissociative identity disorder?

3. A nurse notes a change in the voice and mannerisms of a client experiencing dissociative identity disorders (DID) after learning that his wife has filed for divorce. What is the **most** appropriate nursing intervention?
1. Avoid discussing the client's feelings
2. Force the client to discuss his feelings
3. Challenge the client's feelings
4. Encourage the client to verbalize his feelings

3. 4. If a client with DID becomes upset, it is important that he be allowed to verbalize. The nurse should try to determine which personality is speaking, but remain supportive. Encouraging a client with DID to verbalize his feelings will help him cope with his anxieties Forcing the client to discuss his feelings can increase his level of anxiety. Avoiding discussion of feelings doesn't reduce anxiety, and avoids the issue. Challenging the client's feelings can erode the client's trust in the nurse.
CN: Psychosocial integrity; CNS: None; CL: Analyze

CN: Client needs category   CNS: Client needs subcategory   CL: Cognitive level

4. A client with dissociative identity disorder (DID) is demonstrating positive signs of progressing toward treatment goals. The nurse determines that therapeutic interventions have been successful when this client displays:
1. plans to confront the abuser.
2. attends the unit's milieu group meetings.
3. a lack of alter personalities.
4. no feelings of anger.

4. 2. Attending milieu meetings decreases feelings of isolation, and shows that the client has begun to trust the nurse. Often, the abuser was a part of the client's childhood, and confrontation in adulthood may not be possible or therapeutic. The client is often unaware of an alter personality and cannot prevent these alter personalities from emerging. Clients with DID have dissociated from painful experiences, so the host personality often doesn't have negative feelings about such experiences.
CN: Psychosocial integrity; CNS: None; CL: Analyze

5. Which behavior is **most** indicative of a client experiencing dissociative identity disorder (DID)?
1. Reporting physical health problems with no organic basis
2. Being unable to account for certain periods of time
3. Participating in discussions about previous abusive incidents
4. Forming an immediate therapeutic relationship with the nurse

5. 2. When alter personalities are in control, periods of amnesia are common for clients with DID. Reporting physical health problems with no organic basis describes clients with somatoform disorder. The client does not have memories of the abusive episodes, so he would be unable to participate in discussions. These clients typically are slow in forming trusting relationships because many past relationships have been hurtful.
CN: Psychosocial integrity; CNS: None; CL: Apply

6. A nurse is caring for a client experiencing a dissociative disorder. What is the nurse's **priority** intervention?
1. Plan activities in which the client will attain success
2. Offer praise regardless of the client's success
3. Engage the client in repetitive activities to reduce stress
4. Encourage journaling to recognize unsuccessful coping strategies

6. 1. The care plan should include activities that will help the client be successful and feel a sense of accomplishment. Offering false praise can harm the nurse–client relationship and erode any sense of trust that develops. While keeping a journal of successes helps promote the self-esteem of the individual, this is not a priority intervention. Engaging in repetitive activities may, or may not, reduce stress.
CN: Psychosocial integrity; CNS: None; CL: Apply

7. A client with dissociative identity disorder (DID) presents to the crisis clinic, and reports hearing voices. Which nursing intervention is **most** appropriate?
1. Instruct the client to lie down and rest
2. Administer a dose of haloperidol
3. Assist to continue with his daily activities
4. Notify the provider of this psychotic episode

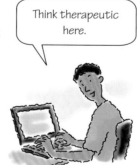

Think therapeutic here.

7. 3. Because many clients with DID hear voices, it's appropriate to have the client continue with daily activities. Having the client lie down and rest would have no therapeutic value. The voices that the client hears are probably alter personalities communicating. This doesn't indicate a psychotic episode, so the provider wouldn't be notified to prescribe an antipsychotic medication such as haloperidol.
CN: Safe, effective care environment; CNS: Management of care; CL: Apply

CN: Client needs category   CNS: Client needs subcategory   CL: Cognitive level

8. A client experiencing dissociative disorder (DID) has recently entered treatment. What is the nurse's **priority** goal?
1. Establish ways to manage periods of mania
2. Learn how to integrate the alternate personalities
3. Develop coping strategies to deal with a traumatic childhood
4. Determine the cause of having periods of lost time

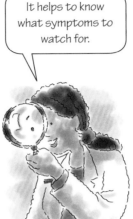

It helps to know what symptoms to watch for.

9. A client who is experiencing symptoms of dissociative identity disorder (DID) reports hearing voices. She asks the nurse, "Am I crazy?" Which response by the nurse is **best**?
1. "What do the voices say to you?"
2. "Why would you think you're crazy?"
3. "Clients with DID often report hearing voices."
4. "Hearing voices is a symptom of schizophrenia."

10. The nurse is preparing to admit a client with dissociative identity disorder (DID) to the inpatient psychiatric unit. The client is experiencing suicidal ideation after a suicide attempt. What is the nurse's **most** appropriate intervention?
1. Put the client on suicide precautions until fully assessed
2. Hold all visitors while the client is on suicide precautions
3. Maintain the client on elopement precautions
4. Place the client in a quiet room away from the nurse's station

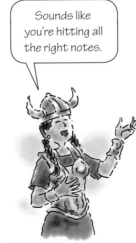

Sounds like you're hitting all the right notes.

11. A client is being treated at a community mental health clinic. The nurse has been instructed to observe for any behaviors that may indicate dissociative identity disorder (DID). Which behavior would **most** suggest DID?
1. Delusions of grandeur
2. Reports of frequently being very tired
3. Changes in dress, mannerisms, and voice
4. Resistance to make a follow-up appointment

8. 4. The initial symptom that prompts many clients with DID to seek health care is the sensation of lost time. These are times the alter personalities are in control. Before therapeutic interventions, clients with DID may not be aware of childhood trauma because of dissociation from the event. Initially, the client with DID isn't aware of the presence of alternate personalities. A long-term goal of treatment for this client is the integration of the various alter personalities. Depression, not mania, may be another early symptom of clients with DID.
CN: Psychosocial integrity; CNS: None; CL: Apply

9. 3. The most therapeutic answer is to give correct information. Asking what the voices tell the client would change topics without answering her question. Asking "why" questions can put the client on the defensive. Schizophrenia is not the only cause of hearing voices, and this response suggests the client may be experiencing schizophrenia.
CN: Psychosocial integrity; CNS: None; CL: Analyze

10. 1. Suicidal ideations or gestures are a common reason clients with DID are hospitalized. For the client's safety, frequent checks should be done. Family interactions might be therapeutic for the client, and the family may be able to provide a more thorough history because of the client's dissociation from traumatic events. Elopement is not an expected symptom of DID. Because of the possibility of suicide, the client's room should be close to the nurse's station.
CN: Safe, effective care environment; CNS: Management of care; CL: Apply

11. 3. When alter personalities are in control, the person will have complete personality changes. These personality shifts are often expressed through changes in dress, mannerism, and voice. Delusions of grandeur are more frequently associated with disorders such as manic states and schizophrenia. Reports of fatigue are not a primary symptom of DID. The refusal to make a follow-up appointment could indicate many problems, including lack of insight, motivation, or noncompliance.
CN: Psychosocial integrity; CNS: None; CL: Apply

CN: Client needs category   CNS: Client needs subcategory   CL: Cognitive level

12. When interacting with a client experiencing dissociative identity disorder (DID), a nurse observes that one of the alter personalities is in control. What is the **most** appropriate intervention?

1. Give recognition to the alter personality
2. Notify the health care provider as soon as possible
3. Stop interacting with the client immediately
4. Ask to speak to the host personality

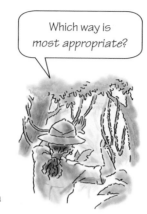

Which way is *most appropriate?*

12. 1. By giving recognition to the alter personality, the nurse conveys a belief that the alter personality exists. The health care provider does not need to be notified because this is an expected occurrence. Asking to speak to the host personality, or immediately stopping interaction with the client will not prevent the client from being controlled by an alter personality.

CN: Psychosocial integrity; CNS: None; CL: Apply

13. The family member of a client diagnosed with dissociative identity disorder (DID) asks a nurse if hypnotic therapy might help the client. How should the nurse respond?

1. "No, hypnosis is a controversial treatment."
2. "No, hypnosis is rarely used in the treatment of DID."
3. "Yes, but only after other types of therapy have failed."
4. "Yes, a client is often not consciously aware of alter personalities."

13. 4. Hypnosis is often a first-line treatment for a client with DID. Because of dissociation from painful events, hypnosis is often a very effective tool. Alter personalities may emerge when the client is under hypnosis.

CN: Psychosocial integrity; CNS: None; CL: Apply

14. Which nursing intervention is **most** appropriate when caring for a client with dissociative identity disorder (DID)?

1. Inform the alter personalities they are only a secondary part of the host's personality
2. Interact only when the host personality is in control, even if it means ending a session
3. Establish an empathetic relationship with each emerging personality, as each is part of the client
4. Provide positive reinforcement to the client only when calm alter personalities are present

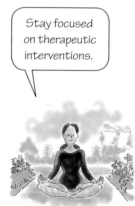

Stay focused on therapeutic interventions.

14. 3. Establishing an empathetic relationship with each emerging personality provides a therapeutic environment for the client. Interacting with the client only when the host personality is in control would be useless because the client has limited, if any, control or awareness of alter personalities. Because a client is not aware of, or in control of alter personalities, it is not helpful to offer a reward for the emergence of a specific alter. The goal of treatment is to work through complex issues represented by each personality, and to integrate them into a whole. The resulting predominant intact personality will be unknown until long-term therapy has concluded.

CN: Psychosocial integrity; CNS: None; CL: Apply

15. While interacting with a client experiencing dissociative identity disorder (DID), a nurse observes one of the alter personalities has taken over. The client goes from being very calm to angry and shouting. What is the nurse's **best** response?

1. "Is someone in the group upset?"
2. "Tell me why you have become angry?"
3. "Describe what you're feeling right now."
4. "Let me speak to someone who is not angry."

15. 3. This response encourages integration and discourages dissociation. When interacting with clients with DID, the nurse should remind the client that alter personalities are a component of one person. Asking close-ended questions may result in a single word answer, and do not encourage dialogue. Asking "why" can put the client on the defensive and impede further communication. Responses that reinforce interaction with only one alter personality rather than the individual as a whole are not appropriate.

CN: Psychosocial integrity; CNS: None; CL: Apply

16. A client with dissociative identity disorder (DID) has been in outpatient therapy for two years. This client has just learned that her father, who sexually abused her throughout childhood, has passed away. Which intervention should the nurse implement?

1. Suggest the support of inpatient therapy
2. Encourage the client to verbalize her feelings
3. Invite alter personalities to emerge during this stressful time
4. Emphasize that her healing process can now begin

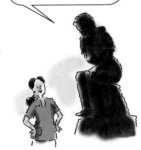

You can pick the right answer. Just think it over a little bit.

16. 2. The death of the abuser may cause the client to experience feelings of anger and guilt, or feelings of relief. Inpatient therapy will not be necessary unless the client becomes suicidal, or her status rapidly deteriorates. Encouraging the client's alter personalities to emerge could result in further dissociation. The death of the abuser can be a very stressful event, and can leave the client with unresolved feelings. The healing process is part of therapy, and does not begin with the death of an abuser.

CN: Health promotion and maintenance; CNS: None; CL: Analyze

17. The nurse is developing a teaching plan for a client experiencing dissociative identity disorder (DID). Which therapeutic activity is **most** appropriate?

1. Group therapy with clients who have DID
2. Group therapy with clients who have a variety of diagnoses
3. Attending an inpatient therapy groups led by a psychologist
4. Attending a support group with adult survivors of child abuse

17. 1. Homogenous group therapy has proven to be the most beneficial for clients with DID. In other groups, the members may find interacting, on an intimate level, with a client with DID overwhelming and frightening. Unless the client with DID is suicidal, hospitalization is not required. It is not required that group therapy sessions be led by any specific discipline. Not all victims of child abuse develop DID.

CN: Psychosocial integrity; CNS: None; CL: Apply

18. A client with dissociative identity disorder (DID) is sitting in the dayroom of an inpatient unit, interacting with others when a nurse observes that the client's alter personality is in control. The client's voice becomes louder and more intense, and the client is tearful and confused. What is the nurse's **priority** intervention?

1. Allow the client to continue interacting with other clients in the dayroom
2. Ask to speak to one of the adult alter personalities of the host personality
3. Redirect the client from the dayroom and allow the client to play with toys
4. Remove the client from the dayroom, and reorient the client, with the assurance of safety

18. 4. Removing the client at this time may protect him from future embarrassment. Reorienting the client discourages dissociation and encourages integration. Asking to speak to an alter personality encourages dissociation. Allowing the client to play with toys also reinforces and encourages dissociation.

CN: Safe, effective care environment; CNS: Safety and infection control; CL: Analyze

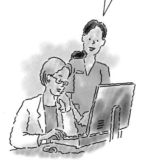

Take note: the question is asking which intervention has the priority.

19. A nurse on the psychiatric unit is caring for a 51-year-old male client who has suicidal ideations. What is the nurse's **priority** intervention?

1. Encourage the client to sleep in his bed and only at bedtime
2. Make a verbal contract with the client should suicidal thoughts return
3. Discourage isolation through client participation in group activities
4. Create a safe and supportive interpersonal environment

19. 4. Creating a safe environment, including the removal of obvious and non-obvious hazards, is the nurse's highest priorities. Other interventions, such as discouraging sleep except at bedtime, making a verbal contract, and encouraging participation in group activities, should be included in the client's plan, but are not the priority.

CN: Psychosocial integrity; CNS: None; CL: Apply

CN: Client needs category   CNS: Client needs subcategory   CL: Cognitive level

20. A unit manager is preparing an in-service meeting on the care of client's diagnosed with dissociative identity disorder (DID). What information should be included?
1. The unit seclusion and restraint protocol
2. Assignment of therapeutic group activities
3. Staff experience with clients with this disorder
4. Review of unique features and challenges of DID

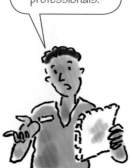

Know when to request a consultation from other medical professionals.

20. 4. If clients with DID are not frequently seen on an inpatient unit, a review of the disorder and its symptoms would be helpful. The review will address questions before assessment and treatment take place. Seclusion and restraint remain last resort options if other treatment interventions fail. Unless this client shows behaviors harmful to himself or others, seclusion and restraints are not required. Therapeutic activities are prescribed as part of milieu therapy. Clients with DID should not be excused from any activity based solely on their diagnosis. Depending on the staff, and experience levels, it may be important to identify nurses who have existing knowledge and experience with this type of client.
CN: Safe, effective care environment; CNS: Management of care; CL: Apply

21. A client has just been admitted to an inpatient psychiatric unit for confusion and agitation associated with an episode of dissociative fugue. What is the **most** important nursing intervention?
1. Encourage the client to verbalize his fear and anxiety
2. Allow the client to share his experiences during the episode
3. Have the client sign a contract stating he won't leave the premises
4. Calmly advise the client that his memory loss is irreversible

21. 1. During dissociative fugue the client will present with confusion and agitation. It can be a very frightening experience. There is typically amnesia for the fugue episode and the client rarely remembers, and therefore cannot share experiences. Signing a contract would have little effect, because an episode of dissociative fugue is involuntary. Dissociative fugue is a rare disorder but the associated amnesia is reversible.
CN: Psychosocial integrity; CNS: None; CL: Analyze

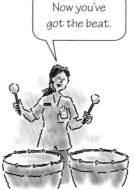

Now you've got the beat.

22. The nurse has provided teaching for family members of a client with a dissociative disorder. The nurse determines that teaching was effective when the family describes the occurrence of dissociative disorders as:
1. "The result of abuse or incest."
2. "A result of polysubstance abuse."
3. "Present in over 40% of people."
4. "A coping mechanism triggered by severe stress."

22. 4. Dissociative disorders are thought to be a coping mechanism triggered by an extreme stressor, or stressful event that has occurred in the client's life. Incest is only one of many reasons dissociative disorders occur. Typically, substance abuse is not a cause of a dissociative disorder. Dissociative disorders are uncommon.
CN: Psychosocial integrity; CNS: None; CL: Analyze

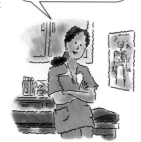

Helping the client help himself is an important aspect of teaching.

23. A client has recently experienced an episode of dissociative fugue. Which nursing intervention would likely prevent a similar recurrence?
1. Identify the client as a high risk for elopement
2. Identify resources to cope with stressful situations
3. Allow the client to share his experiences with the fugue episode
4. Confront the client about running away from his problems

23. 2. Dissociative fugue is precipitated by stressful situations. Helping the client identify resources could prevent recurrences. Following an episode of dissociative fugue, the client will return to normal functioning. He will not be an elopement risk. The client usually experiences amnesia about the events that occurred during the dissociative fugue episode, limiting his ability to share the experience. The client is unaware that he is running away from his problems.
CN: Psychosocial integrity; CNS: None; CL: Analyze

CN: Client needs category   CNS: Client needs subcategory   CL: Cognitive level

24. A 32-year-old client tells the nurse his home was lost in a flood last month. When questioned about his feelings about this loss, the client doesn't recall the flood or owning a home. This client most likely exhibiting:
1. depersonalization disorder.
2. dissociative amnesia.
3. dissociative fugue.
4. dissociative identity disorder.

24. 2. Dissociative amnesia commonly occurs after a person has been in a traumatic event. Depersonalization disorder is characterized by recurrent sensations of losing one's reality. Dissociative fugue usually involves unplanned travel or wandering, and is sometimes accompanied by the establishment of a new identity. Dissociative identity disorder is the presence of two or more personalities within the same individual.
CN: Psychosocial integrity; CNS: None; CL: Analyze

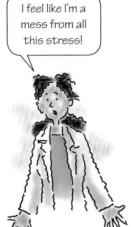

I feel like I'm a mess from all this stress!

25. The nurse is assessing a client with dissociative amnesia. Which circumstance would **most** likely contribute to this condition?
1. Binge drinking
2. A hostage situation
3. A closed head injury
4. Strenuous exercise

25. 2. Dissociative amnesia typically occurs after a person has experienced a very stressful, traumatic situation. Binge drinking doesn't cause dissociative amnesia. A closed head injury could result in physiologic, but not dissociative, amnesia. Strenuous exercise can contribute to transient global amnesia.
CN: Psychosocial integrity; CNS: None; CL: Apply

26. A three-year-old boy was killed in an automobile accident. A client, the driver of the vehicle, is diagnosed with dissociative amnesia following the accident. This client verbalizes an understanding of his treatment plan when making the statement:
1. "I won't drive a car alone again for at least a year."
2. "I will take my lorazepam anytime I feel upset about this situation."
3. "I will visit the child's grave as soon as I am released from the hospital."
4. "I will attend the therapy sessions prescribed by my psychiatrist."

26. 4. It is important for the client to attend all therapy sessions recommended by the psychiatrist. Hypnosis can be beneficial because it allows repressed feelings and memories to surface. The client may be ready to drive again before a year has passed. The client should learn non-pharmacological coping mechanisms to manage feelings. Visiting the child's grave on discharge may be too traumatic, and encourage continuation of the amnesia.
CN: Psychosocial integrity; CNS: None; CL: Apply

27. A client with dissociative amnesia shows an understanding of the condition when stating:
1. "I will probably never be able to regain my memories of the fire."
2. "I have problems with my memory due to my abuse of tranquilizers."
3. "If I concentrate hard enough, I will be able to remember the car accident."
4. "To protect my mental well-being, I am unable to remember details of the rape."

27. 4. One of the cardinal symptoms of dissociative amnesia is memory loss of a traumatic event. With therapy and time, the client will likely recall the traumatic event. This type of amnesia isn't related to substance abuse. Memory loss with a dissociative disorder is a protective function of the brain, and isn't within the client's conscious control.
CN: Psychosocial integrity; CNS: None; CL: Analyze

CN: Client needs category   CNS: Client needs subcategory   CL: Cognitive level

28. A client is admitted for a diagnostic workup for possible dissociative amnesia. What is the **most** appropriate nursing intervention for this client?
1. Restrain the client if he attempts to wander off the unit
2. Assess the client frequently for orientation to time, place, and person
3. Teach the client about the specific diagnostic tests ordered for him
4. Encourage the client not to dwell on events precipitating his memory loss

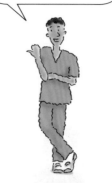

Hmm! Which intervention is the most appropriate?

28. 3. A client with memory loss will commonly have a diagnostic workup to rule out any physical basis. Providing information about prescribed tests and procedures would be most appropriate. Wandering is uncommon for clients with dissociative amnesia. Restraining a client is a last resort, after other treatment interventions have failed. Frequent attempts to assess the client's orientation level could make the client more distressed and agitated. In many cases, the client has no memory of the traumatic events that caused the amnesia.
CN: Health promotion and maintenance; CNS: None; CL: Apply

29. Amobarbital sodium has been prescribed for a client with dissociative amnesia. The nurse determines that teaching has been successful when the client states:
1. "This medication helps me sleep at night."
2. "This drug helps control my anxiety."
3. "This medication increases my ability to remember forgotten events during therapy sessions."
4. "I must take this drug daily at breakfast for it to be most effective."

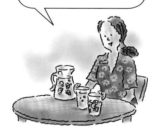

Remember

"Amobarbital helps recall of forgotten events."

Amobarbital, a sedative, is given to the client with dissociative amnesia to help remember forgotten events.

29. 3. This drug is prescribed to help a client with dissociative amnesia remember forgotten events. It is not prescribed as a sleep aid or antianxiety agent. This drug is given during therapy to promote recall, there would be no therapeutic benefit if taken at home.
CN: Physiological integrity; CNS: Pharmacological and parenteral therapies; CL: Analyze

30. A client experiencing dissociative amnesia says, "You must think I'm really stupid because I have no recollection of the accident." Which response by the nurse is **best**?
1. "Why would you say I think you're stupid?"
2. "Have I done something to make you think you're stupid?"
3. "What kind of academic record did you have in school?"
4. "To protect ourselves, we sometimes can't remember traumatic events."

Feeling stressed? Take a quick break and refresh yourself.

30. 4. A brief explanation of protective coping skills provides an understandable explanation to this client. The use of "why" questions can cause the client to be defensive. Taking the focus off of the client is not therapeutic, and discourages extended dialogue. Changing the subject does not establish rapport or maintain open communication.
CN: Psychosocial integrity; CNS: None; CL: Apply

31. What is the nurse's **priority** intervention when caring for a client with a dissociative disorder?
1. Encourage the client to participate in therapeutic activities and meetings
2. Question the client about the events triggering the dissociative disorder
3. Allow the client to withdraw anytime he is experiencing feelings of dissociation
4. Encourage the client to refrain from interaction with therapy group peers

31. 1. Attending therapeutic activities and meetings will help decrease the client's sense of isolation. The client frequently can't recall the events that triggered the dissociative disorder. Questioning would not be helpful.
CN: Safe, effective care environment; CNS: Management of care; CL: Apply

32. The nurse is performing an assessment on a client diagnosed with depersonalization disorder. The nurse should anticipate:
   1. disorientation to time, place, and person.
   2. a sensation of detachment from body or mind.
   3. sudden, unexpected travel to another location.
   4. a feeling that one's situation will never change.

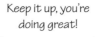

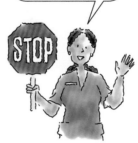

32. 2. In depersonalization disorder, the client feels detached from his body and mental processes. The client will experience this disorder as a fleeting, transitory experience, and will be able to describe the symptoms, but would not display them. The client is usually oriented to time, place, and person. Sudden, unexpected travel to another location is one of the characteristics of dissociative fugue. Feeling that one's situation will never change generally associated with depression.
CN: Psychosocial integrity; CNS: None; CL: Apply

33. A client with depersonalization disorder verbalizes understanding of some ways to decrease symptoms when stating:
   1. "I will avoid any stressful situation."
   2. "Meditation will help control my symptoms."
   3. "I will practice relaxation exercises regularly."
   4. "I have to keep taking antipsychotic medication."

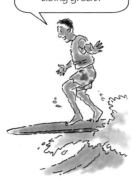

33. 3. Relaxation can lead to a decrease in maladaptive responses. Although stress can be a predisposing factor in depersonalization disorder, it is impossible to avoid all stressful situations. Meditation is the voluntary induction of the sensation of depersonalization, and therefore not an appropriate intervention. This is not a psychotic disorder, and antipsychotic medication would not be beneficial.
CN: Psychosocial integrity; CNS: None; CL: Analyze

34. A client tells the nurse that he frequently feels that he is floating above his body. During these times, he says he is aware of who he is and where he is located. The nurse determines that this client is experiencing:
   1. depersonalization disorder.
   2. dissociative amnesia.
   3. dissociative identity disorder.
   4. dissociative fugue.

34. 1. One of the cardinal symptoms of depersonalization disorder is the client's feeling of being detached from their body or mental processes. During the feelings of detachment, the client does not become disoriented. Dissociative amnesia is defined as one or more episodes of the inability to recall important information. Dissociative identity disorder is the existence of two or more personalities that take control of the client's behavior. Dissociative fugue is a rare condition in which a person suddenly leaves without planning or warning, travels far from home or work, and leaves a past life behind. Such persons show signs of amnesia, and have no conscious understanding or knowledge of the reason for their flight.
CN: Psychosocial integrity; CNS: None; CL: Analyze

35. The nurse is teaching the family of a client with depersonalization disorder. The family asks about an appropriate setting for the treatment of this disorder. What is the nurse's **best** response?
   1. "Inpatient psychiatric hospital"
   2. "Community mental health clinic"
   3. "Family practice physician's office"
   4. "Specialized support groups"

35. 2. Most clients with depersonalization disorder can be successfully treated as an outpatient. Clients with access to a setting close to their home and daily life have increased treatment adherence. Clients with depersonalization disorder only need to be hospitalized if they become suicidal, or have severe depression or anxiety. Because there is no organic basis for this disorder, clients are not treated in a family practice physician's office. The disorder is rare, and few support groups exist for clients who require treatment.
CN: Psychosocial integrity; CNS: None; CL: Apply

36. A client with depersonalization disorder tells the nurse, "I feel like such a freak when I have an out-of-body experience." What is the nurse's **most** appropriate response?
1. "How often do you experience these feelings?"
2. "Help me to understand what you mean by a freak."
3. "Please explain your out-of-body experiences."
4. "Does your husband know that you're having these experiences?"

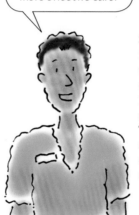

Understanding the client's problem allows you to provide more effective care.

36. 3. An open-ended response allows the client to focus, and expand on the topic. Asking how often the experiences occur is a closed-ended response that does not encourage extended discussion. Responding to the client's negative self-label could distract from the details of the actual topic. Inquiring about the husband's knowledge of these experiences is off topic.
CN: Psychosocial integrity; CNS: None; CL: Analyze

37. The nurse is assessing a client diagnosed with dissociative disorder. Which characteristics would the nurse likely observe?
1. Impairment of memory resulting from overwhelming, intrusive auditory and visual hallucinations
2. A very rapid or sudden disruption of the client's memory
3. Impairment of memory or identity due to the development of organic changes in the brain
4. Impairment of memory or identity due to an unconscious attempt to protect themselves from emotional pain

37. 4. Impairment of the client's memory or identity due to an unconscious attempt to protect themselves from emotional pain or traumatic experiences best describes dissociative disorders. Hallucinations do not directly impact memory, and are associated with schizophrenic disorders. The onset of dissociative disorders may be gradual, sudden, or chronic. There is no known organic cause for dissociative disorders.
CN: Psychosocial integrity; CNS: None; CL: Apply

38. A client diagnosed with depersonalization disorder tells the nurse, "I feel like my arm isn't attached to my body." Which response by the nurse is **most** appropriate?
1. "Do you know where you are right now?"
2. "What do you think makes you feel that way?"
3. "Don't worry, because I can clearly that see your arm is attached to your body."
4. "Your disorder causes you to feel that your arm isn't attached to your body."

38. 4. Explaining that what the client feels is part of the disease process would be most appropriate. Asking if the client knows where they are is off topic. Asking "why" puts the client on the defensive. Stating that his arm is attached to his body minimizes the client's feelings.
CN: Psychosocial integrity; CNS: None; CL: Apply

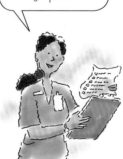

It's hard for me to associate this disorder with a symptom.

39. A nurse conducts an admission assessment on a client diagnosed with dissociative identity disorder. Which sign or symptom supports this diagnosis?
1. A sense of being in a dream
2. Frequent recall of a particular event
3. Having two or more personalities
4. Ritualistic behavior

39. 3. Dissociative identity disorder is characterized by having two or more distinct personalities, often in conflict with one another. A sense of being in a dream is common in depersonalization disorders. Selective amnesia refers to the inability to recall certain events that have occurred during a specified time period, and is more common in traumatic stress disorders. Ritualistic behavior is seen in obsessive-compulsive disorders.
CN: Psychosocial integrity; CNS: None; CL: Apply

CN: Client needs category   CNS: Client needs subcategory   CL: Cognitive level

40. The nurse has just completed an assessment of a client. Which findings place this client at the highest risk of suicide?
1. Having a suicide plan with the ability to implement the plan, and a history of previous attempts
2. Being preoccupied with morbid thoughts, and limited support system
3. Having suicidal ideation with an active suicide plan, and family history of suicide
4. Making threats of suicide, recent job loss, and intact support system

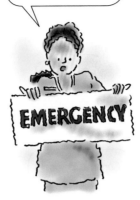

Which findings most indicate a person is ready to attempt suicide?

40. 1. A lethal plan with the means to carry it out poses the highest risk, and requires immediate intervention. Although all of the remaining risk factors can lead to suicide, they aren't considered the highest risk. A client exhibiting any of these risk factors should be taken seriously, and considered at risk for suicide.
CN: Safe, effective care environment; CNS: Safety and infection control; CL: Apply

41. A client is experiencing suicidal ideation. This client has previously attempted to hang himself. What is the nurse's **priority** intervention?
1. Place the client in seclusion with checks every 15 minutes
2. Assign nursing staff to remain with the client at all times
3. Have the client stay with the group at all times
4. Restrict the client from returning to his room

41. 2. Maintaining constant contact with this client is the nurse's highest priority. This allows the client to maintain his self-esteem and keeps him safe. Seclusion would damage the client's self-esteem. Forcing the client to stay with the group, and not allowing him in his room does not guarantee his safety.
CN: Psychosocial integrity; CNS: None; CL: Apply

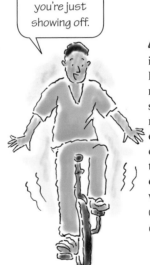

Okay—now you're just showing off.

42. After taking a potentially lethal drug overdose, a client with dissociative identity disorder tells the nurse that his alter did it. What is the nurse's **highest** priority?
1. Notify the health care provider immediately
2. Arrange seclusion for this client's safety
3. Initiate one-on-one suicide precautions
4. Administer a dose of haloperidol

42. 3. Taking a potentially lethal overdose indicates that the client poses a danger to himself. Because the alter personality may act again, the risk for self-directed violence remains. This risk is similar to that associated with command hallucinations, and one-on-one precautions should be enlisted. Seclusion is not indicated. The health care provider should be notified of the change in the client's condition, but this is not the highest priority. Haloperidol is an antipsychotic that would not be indicated for this client.
CN: Safe, effective care environment; CNS: Safety and infection control; CL: Analyze

43. A severely depressed client who has attempted suicide multiple times tells the nurse that her family life is normal and that she is unable to identify any stressors. The nurse should anticipate a diagnosis of dissociative identity disorder (DID) based on which findings? Select all that apply.
1. The inability to recall important personal information, and memory loss too severe to be dismissed as ordinary forgetfulness
2. The absence of the physiologic effects of a substance, such as alcohol or drugs
3. The ability to selectively and consciously choose to avoid certain painful topics
4. A sense of grandiosity, that she's special, and has a particular mission for mankind
5. Posttraumatic symptoms, such as flashbacks, nightmares, and an exaggerated startle response

43. 1, 2, 5. A dissociative disorder is a persistent state of being disconnected from the totality of one's self, and particularly painful emotions. With dissociative disorder, the inability to recall personal information is far more extensive than ordinary forgetfulness. The symptoms are not chemically induced, and the individual does not have the ability to consciously decide to separate from painful emotions or topics. Posttraumatic symptoms, such as flashbacks, nightmares, and an exaggerated startle response, are also symptoms of DID. A sense of grandiosity is not characteristic of this disorder, but more often is associated with schizophrenia.
CN: Safe, effective care environment; CNS: Safety and infection control; CL: Analyze

CN: Client needs category   CNS: Client needs subcategory   CL: Cognitive level

44. A client with dissociative identity disorder experiences frequent periods of memory loss. What is the **most** appropriate nursing intervention for this client?

1. Orient the client to time, place, person, and situation
2. Explain the circumstances surrounding the memory loss
3. Observe for cues that the client is ready to discuss his memory loss
4. Reassure him the memory loss has no physiologic basis

45. A client with dissociative identity disorder was admitted to the unit after a suicide attempt. Place the nursing interventions in priority order.

1. Explain unit policies and expectations, activity schedule, and therapeutic interventions

2. Assist the client to develop a schedule allowing him to manage this disorder in his daily life

3. Educate the client on medication usage, including therapeutic benefit, administration protocol, and possible side effects

4. Initiate a therapeutic relationship, establish trust and develop rapport

5. Assess suicide risk and implement a safety plan, to include a follow-up assessment

6. Teach the client specific aspects of his illness including symptoms and the treatment plan

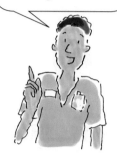

Which kinds of questions tend to encourage discussion?

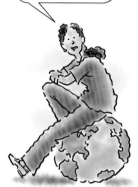

Congratulations! You should feel on top of the world!

44. 3. Memory loss serves as a protective mechanism for many clients with dissociative identity disorder. The nurse should discuss the problem when the client is ready. Orienting the client may force him out of the protective mechanism of the memory loss, and result in further harm. Explaining the circumstances surrounding the memory loss, and telling the client not to worry are not therapeutic interventions.

CN: Safe, effective care environment; CNS: Management of care; CL: Apply

45. Ordered Response:

5. Assess suicide risk and implement a safety plan, to include a follow-up assessment

4. Initiate a therapeutic relationship, establish trust and develop rapport

1. Explain unit policies and expectations, activity schedule, and therapeutic interventions

6. Teach the client specific aspects of his illness including symptoms and the treatment plan

3. Educate the client on medication usage, including therapeutic benefit, administration protocol, and possible side effects

2. Assist the client to develop a schedule allowing him to manage this disorder in his daily life

CN: Safe, effective care environment; CNS: Management of care; CL: Apply

Chapter 20

Sexual & Gender Identity Disorders

This chapter will test your knowledge of disorders of a highly sensitive nature. Remain professional at all times, and you'll do great. Good luck!

1. A client has undergone surgery for the repair of an abdominal aortic aneurysm. The client's wife asks the nurse if her husband will be impotent. What is the nurse's **most** appropriate response?
   1. "Don't worry, he will be all right in time."
   2. "He has more serious problems to worry about."
   3. "We will cross that bridge when we come to it."
   4. "There is a chance of impotence after this surgery."

Therapeutic communication involves demonstrating sensitivity to your client's and your client's family's concerns.

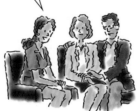

2. The nurse is preparing discharge instructions for a female client who has suffered a spinal cord injury at the C4 level. What is the **most** important information for the nurse to include?
   1. Women with a spinal cord injury usually remain fertile and can become pregnant.
   2. After a spinal cord injury, women usually are unable to conceive a child.
   3. Enjoyment of sexual intercourse will not change.
   4. After a spinal cord injury, menstruation usually stops immediately.

3. A nurse is caring for a 39-year-old male client who recently underwent surgery and is having difficulty accepting changes in his body image. What is the **most** appropriate nursing intervention?
   1. Actively listen as the client expresses both positive and negative feelings about his body image
   2. Restrict the client's opportunity to view his incision because it is upsetting
   3. Encourage the client to focus on future plans for his recovery
   4. Allow the client to repress anger while discussing changes in body image

Note that question 3 is asking you which action is most appropriate.

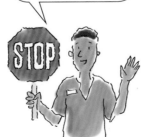

1. 4. Impotence and retrograde ejaculation are sexual dysfunctions commonly experienced by males after abdominal aortic aneurysm. Telling a family member that the client will be all right is offering false assurance. Stating that he has other problems isn't therapeutic and doesn't address the wife's concern. Telling the client's wife to "cross that bridge when we come to it" ignores her concerns, and isn't therapeutic.
CN: Psychosocial integrity; CNS: None; CL: Apply

2. 1. After a spinal cord injury, women remain fertile and can conceive and deliver a child. If a woman doesn't want to become pregnant, she must use contraception. Menstruation is not affected by a spinal cord injury, but sexual functioning may be altered.
CN: Physiological integrity; CNS: Physiological adaptation; CL: Apply

3. 1. The nurse must observe for any indication that the client is ready to address his body image change, this includes identifying and expressing both positive and negative changes to body image. The client should be allowed to look at the incision and dressing if he wants to do so. It is too soon to focus on the future with this client. The nurse should allow the client to express his feelings and not repress them because repression prolongs recovery.
CN: Psychosocial integrity; CNS: None; CL: Apply

CN: Client needs category   CNS: Client needs subcategory   CL: Cognitive level

4. A female client with chronic obstructive pulmonary disease (COPD) tells a nurse, "I no longer have enough energy to make love to my husband." What is the **most** appropriate nursing intervention?
1. Encourage the client to seek a sex therapist
2. Advise the client to schedule a gynecological consult
3. Suggest methods and measures that may facilitate sexual activity
4. Reassure the client that her husband will understand

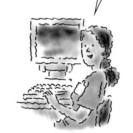

Several answers are possible. But which one is the most appropriate?

4. 3. Sexual dysfunction in COPD clients is the direct result of dyspnea and reduced energy levels. Measures to reduce physical exertion, enhance oxygenation, and accommodate decreased energy levels may aid sexual activity. If the problem persists, a consult with a sex therapist might be necessary. A gynecological consult is not indicated. Discussing this with her husband may not resolve the problem and offers false reassurance.
CN: Physiological integrity; CNS: Reduction of risk potential; CL: Apply

5. A client with an ileostomy tells the nurse that he is unable to have an erection. The nurse is aware that:
1. post-operative impotence is generally permanent.
2. impotence is common following abdominal surgery.
3. an immediate abdominal X-ray should be obtained.
4. impotence is uncommon following an ileostomy.

5. 4. Sexual dysfunction is uncommon after an ileostomy. Psychological causes of impotence should be explored. Impotence following abdominal surgery is neither common, nor generally permanent. An abdominal X-ray is not indicated for sexual dysfunction.
CN: Physiological integrity; CNS: Physiological adaptation; CL: Analyze

6. A 40-year-old client, who has completed radiation therapy for testicular cancer, tells the nurse that he is unable to achieve an erection. Which responses are appropriate? Select all that apply.
1. Impotence after testicular cancer is permanent.
2. Sexual dysfunction can be a side effect of radiation therapy.
3. Preoccupation and worry about sexual function can cause impotence.
4. Impotence can result from improper nutrition after radiation.
5. Impotence is the body's way of avoiding sex to allow healing.

6. 2, 3. Radiation or chemotherapy may cause sexual dysfunction. Libido may only be temporarily affected, and the client should be provided with emotional support. The client has not verbalized fear or concern related to the cancer. Impotence after cancer is not necessarily permanent. Impotence is not associated with imbalanced or improper nutrition. Impotence is not related to the body's capacity for healing.
CN: Physiological integrity; CNS: of Physiological adaptation; CL: Analyze

7. A nurse is preparing a teaching plan for a newly married female client with a cervical spinal cord injury. The client does not want to become pregnant at this time. What information would be important for the nurse to include? Select all that apply.
1. Provide brochures on adaptations for sexual practice
2. Provide her husband with a vasectomy referral
3. Encourage her to be patient and practice a variety of sexual techniques
4. Instruct the client's husband how to properly insert a diaphragm
5. Suggest she ask her husband substitute a vibrator in place of intercourse

7. 1, 3, 4. Because the client experienced a cervical spinal cord injury, she won't be able to insert any form of contraception protection by herself. If the couple does not use condoms, it is vital to provide her husband with instruction on insertion of a diaphragm. Providing the couple with literature on sexual practice will help to pave the way for discussion, but does not impact the need for an effective method to prevent conception. The couple doesn't wish to have children at this time, so providing a vasectomy referral is not appropriate. Suggesting that the couple suspend intercourse is an intimate decision that they should arrive at, on their own, after exploring multiple options. It's premature and inappropriate to advise this as a substitute for sexual intercourse for this newly married couple.
CN: Physiological integrity; CNS: None; CL: Apply

8. The nurse is caring for a female client who states, "I am having my menstrual period every two weeks and it lasts for one week. I am concerned because I want to get pregnant." How should the nurse respond? Select all that apply.
1. "You can get pregnant pretty easily."
2. "You may already be pregnant."
3. "Your health care provider should check your hormone levels."
4. "You should schedule an exam with your health care provider."
5. "Heavy bleeding means you have miscarried."

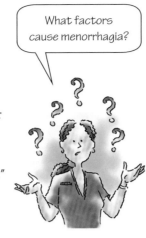

What factors cause menorrhagia?

8. 3, 4. Menorrhagia is an excessive menstrual period which can be caused by a number of factors. Medications and intrauterine devices can also contribute to menorrhagia. A gynecological exam can determine the presence of fibroids or polyps that may require surgical intervention. Excessive bleeding may result from an ectopic pregnancy, but this is a rare occurrence. There are also no additional indications that the client is already pregnant. There is no evidence that excessive bleeding or atypical menstrual cycles are related to one's ability to become pregnant. Frequent or regular excessive bleeding is not associated with miscarriage.
CN: Physiological integrity; CNS: Reduction of risk potential; CL: Apply

9. The nurse is caring for a couple being treated for infertility. What should the nurse identify as a major stressor for this couple?
1. Having frequent physical examinations
2. Producing on-demand semen specimens
3. Maintaining sexual intercourse schedule
4. Identifying the infertile spouse

9. 3. The major cause of stress in infertile couples is planning sexual intercourse to correlate to fertility cycles. The inconvenience and discomfort of producing specimens and receiving examinations isn't a major stressor. Most couples undergoing fertility treatment understand that one partner is usually infertile.
CN: Health promotion and maintenance; CNS: None; CL: Apply

10. The nurse is caring for a 38-year-old female client who is married, but nulliparous. The client has been diagnosed with uterine cancer and is scheduled for a hysterectomy. What is the nurse's **most** important intervention for this client?
1. Encourage her to verbalize her feelings
2. Advise her about adoption options
3. Refer her to a female psychotherapist
4. Avoid the cancer diagnosis and possible related fears of the client

10. 1. Encourage this client to verbalize her feelings because the loss of one's reproductive organs may produce feelings of lost sexuality. The loss of the ability to bear children may precipitate an emotional crisis, depression, or grieving. Advising this client about adoption is inappropriate and premature at this time. Referring this client to a psychotherapist may be premature. The client should be given time to work through her feelings. Avoidance of the cancer diagnosis and related fears is not a therapeutic nursing intervention.
CN: Psychosocial integrity; CNS: None; CL: Apply

11. A 50-year-old male client, who had a myocardial infarction eight weeks, ago tells a nurse, "My wife wants to make love, but I don't think I can. I'm worried that sex might kill me." What is the **most** appropriate response by this nurse?
1. "Let's increase your rehabilitation schedule."
2. "Does your wife's request cause you stress?"
3. "I will call the primary health care provider for you."
4. "Your wife must wait until your body is ready."

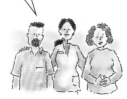

Let's put together a plan of care that will meet both of your needs.

11. 2. The nurse should address the client's concerns. Asking the client to identify stressors and verbalize his feelings will create insight into the problem. The rehabilitation schedule should not be increased until the nurse assesses the situation, and is sure no harm will come to the client. Calling the primary health care provider before a complete assessment is made is inappropriate. Telling the wife she must wait for the client to make love may place undue strain on the marriage.
CN: Psychosocial integrity; CNS: None; CL: Apply

CN: Client needs category   CNS: Client needs subcategory   CL: Cognitive level

12. A 55-year-old female client who is in cardiac rehabilitation tells a nurse that she is unable to make love to her husband because she often feels fatigued and feels a sense of doom. What is the **most** appropriate information for the nurse to provide?
  1. Advise her not to participate in intercourse until she is ready
  2. Instruct her to take a nitroglycerin tablet prior to intercourse
  3. Provide her information about new positions for sexual intercourse
  4. Encourage her to verbalize her feelings about these concerns

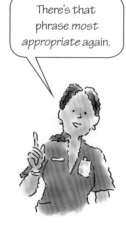

There's that phrase most appropriate again.

12. 4. A client in cardiac rehabilitation faces multiple life changes and can be confronted by a number of fears. The nurse should encourage her to verbalize her feelings and they should be explored. Encouraging her to talk about her concerns is vital because of the intimate nature of the complaint. Advising her not to have intercourse does not address her concerns. She shouldn't take nitroglycerin before intercourse unless recommended by her provider. Providing information on new positions for intercourse can be helpful, but it is more important to address this client's feelings at this time.
CN: Physiological integrity; CNS: Physiological adaptation; CL: Apply

13. A 33-year-old client tells the nurse that she has never had an orgasm. Her partner is upset that he is unable to meet her needs. Which interventions should the nurse implement? Select all that apply.
  1. Ask the client if she enjoys intercourse and if she feels there is a problem
  2. Assess the couple's sexual history and their perception of the problem
  3. Reassure her that most women don't reach orgasm
  4. Refer her to a therapist because she has sexual aversion disorder
  5. Discuss some ways that the client might fake orgasm to please her partner

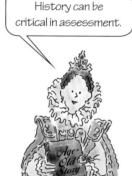

History can be critical in assessment.

13. 1, 2. In this case it is important to assess both partners to determine the perception and extent of the problem. When assessing the client, the nurse should be professional and matter-of-fact while discussing sexual activity and associated pleasure or possible difficulties. Assessing the couple's perception of the problem will help define it, and assist the couple and the nurse in understanding it. Most individuals can be taught to reach orgasm if there is no underlying medical condition. It is unethical and improper to direct the client to fake an orgasm with a sexual partner. A nurse cannot make a medical diagnosis such as sexual aversion disorder.
CN: Psychosocial integrity; CNS: None; CL: Apply

14. A 20-year-old female client is in the emergency department after being sexually assaulted by a stranger. Which nursing intervention is the **priority**?
  1. Assist her to identify which behaviors placed her at risk for the attack
  2. Make an appointment for her at a local sexual assault crisis center in six weeks
  3. Encourage discussion of her early childhood traumatic experiences
  4. Assist her to identify family or friends able to provide immediate support for her

14. 4. This client needs a lot of support to help her through this ordeal. Assisting the client in identifying behaviors that place her at risk for the attack places the blame on the client. Waiting six weeks to make an appointment is incorrect. The local crisis center must be called immediately. Some psychiatric disorders are related to early childhood experiences, but rape is not.
CN: Psychosocial integrity; CNS: None; CL: Apply

15. A 47-year-old client has been taking prescribed medication for an intestinal ulcer. During a routine office visit for blood pressure monitoring, the client tells the nurse that he is no longer able to have sexual intercourse with his wife. The nurse determines that this is most likely the result of his:
  1. advancing age.
  2. ulcer medication.
  3. stressful lifestyle.
  4. high blood pressure.

15. 2. Impotence in men is a lesser known side effect of ulcer medications prescribed for them. Impotence can occur at any time and is not age related. Elevated blood pressure itself doesn't cause impotence, but antihypertensive medication can produce this unwelcome side effect. It could contribute to the present difficulty in addition to possible side effects of the prescribed ulcer medication. Stress may cause erectile dysfunction, but there is no evidence that the client is under stress. Men are usually able to have an erection throughout their lives.
CN: Physiological integrity; CNS: Pharmacological and parenteral therapies; CL: Apply

CN: Client needs category   CNS: Client needs subcategory   CL: Cognitive level

16. For which signs and symptoms should an adult victim of childhood sexual abuse be monitored? Select all that apply.
1. Depression
2. Substance abuse
3. Narcissism
4. Posttraumatic stress
5. Enuresis

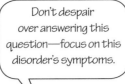

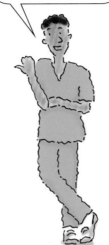

Don't despair over answering this question—focus on this disorder's symptoms.

16. 1, 2, 4. Childhood sexual abuse is closely linked to the development of depression and substance abuse disorders. It is also linked to the development of somatization and posttraumatic stress disorders. Victims of childhood sexual abuse aren't predisposed to developing narcissistic disorders. Enuresis is frequently seen in children who are victims of childhood sexual abuse. This is typically outgrown as the child ages.
CN: Psychosocial integrity; CNS: None; CL: Analyze

17. A 25-year-old client convicted of raping a female college student has been attending a sex offender recovery group for two years and very recently completed his parole. After group the client tells the nurse facilitator that he no longer wishes to attend group. What is the **most** important intervention by the nurse?
1. Insist that the client remain and continue therapy
2. Perform a self-evaluation to assess personal discomfort
3. Call the parole board to report the client's decision
4. Notify the client's family of his progress and decision

17. 2. If the client has successfully completed therapy, then the nurse must evaluate her own value system. Insisting that the client remain in therapy may not prove to be successful, as he must be motivated to continue therapy. Calling the parole board may be an inappropriate decision, especially if the client has met all of his court-ordered requirements. A nurse can't release confidential information to the client's family without his permission and consent.
CN: Psychosocial integrity; CNS: None; CL: Analyze

18. A 32-year-old client, recently arrested for voyeurism, has come to the hospital for treatment so that his family and friends don't find out. Which intervention should the nurse include in this client's plan of care?
1. Encourage the client to tell his family and friends the truth
2. Suggest individual therapy to discuss socially unacceptable behavior
3. Enroll the client in group therapy sessions
4. Direct the client to write his full history in a journal

18. 2. Discussing inappropriate sexual behavior with the client increases adherence with treatment and decreases the risk of relapse. Informing family and friends isn't an initial intervention. Disclosure to family and friends is usually delayed until the client can fully acknowledge his behavior. The treatment care plan should be shared with the client. In view of the client's reluctance to inform people of his voyeurism, it is unlikely that he is ready to write a detailed history of his behaviors in a journal.
CN: Psychosocial integrity; CNS: None; CL: Apply

19. A client is admitted to the psychiatric unit for depression after being arrested for exhibitionism. What are **most** likely the concerns of the client? Select all that apply.
1. Facing a criminal record as a sexual offender
2. The possible loss of his job as a bus driver
3. Embarrassment of people knowing his crime
4. Being imprisoned for a lengthy period
5. Fear of undergoing a chemical castration

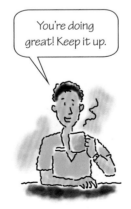

You're doing great! Keep it up.

19. 1, 2, 3. The client who has been arrested for exhibitionism is at risk of a number of consequences once his status becomes public information. He can expect to be registered as a sexual offender with public access to that information. A job serving the public is at increased risk of being terminated for the commission of sexual crimes. Embarrassment would most likely be associated with this situation. Without further information about the number of sexual offenses or arrests, it is not possible to determine whether this client is at risk of being incarcerated. Chemical castration is rarely a prescribed or court-ordered treatment, and is reserved for extreme cases.
CN: Psychosocial integrity; CNS: None; CL: Apply

20. A 38-year-old female client was sexually assaulted while returning home from the store late in the evening. She is brought to the emergency department and is crying. What is the nurse's **most** important intervention?
1. Help the police gather information for their report
2. Call the client's family to come to the hospital
3. Encourage the client to enroll in a self-defense class
4. Remain with the client and assist her through the crisis

20. 4. Sexual assault is treated as a medical emergency, and the client requires constant attention and assistance during the crisis period. Helping the police file their report would not take precedence over a medical emergency. Comforting the client by contacting family should be carried out after the client's injuries are treated, and only with permission. Encouraging the client to enroll in a self-defense class isn't appropriate during a crisis.
CN: Psychosocial integrity; CNS: None; CL: Apply

21. A client is admitted to the psychiatric unit as a condition of his probation period for exhibitionism and fetishism. The client seems to be adjusting well to the unit, but several clients report that their undergarments are missing. Which action would be **most** appropriate?
1. Notify the primary health care provider and local police
2. Search the entire unit, beginning with the client's room
3. Call a community meeting to let the clients settle the matter
4. Privately assess the client for sexual activities related to his diagnoses

21. 4. Meeting with the client privately establishes trust. This client needs to be assessed for what triggers might be present to prompt this behavior. Notification of the primary health care provider shouldn't be done before assessing the client. It is premature to notify any legal authority without full knowledge of events and intent. Searching the client's room without discussion is a violation of a trusting milieu. Searching the entire unit for a few missing items is exaggerated. It isn't therapeutic to encourage the unit to confront one member of the community.
CN: Psychosocial integrity; CNS: None; CL: Apply

22. A client is admitted to the hospital for frottage and tells the nurse that he doesn't want to talk about his problem. Which responses, from the nurse, would be appropriate? Select all that apply.
1. "I need to understand why you are here."
2. "It is your right not to answer my questions."
3. "I understand this must be difficult for you."
4. "It is important that you answer a few questions."
5. "You will have to be discharged right away."

22. 1, 3. 4. It is important to acknowledge the client's feelings in order to initiate open communication. The client may not realize that details are needed to complete the assessment and treatment plan. It is also helpful for the nurse to acknowledge the difficulties associated with the client being asked to share personal information and reassure him of the privacy in which it will be held. Clients have rights, but data collection is necessary so that help with the problem can be offered. It is not therapeutic and is demeaning to threaten a client with the pressure of facing immediate discharge.
CN: Psychosocial integrity; CNS: None; CL: Apply

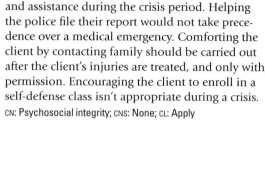

Acknowledging a client's difficulties can open communication.

23. Which type of therapy can serve as a vehicle of positive reinforcement for a client who admits to frottage?
1. Electroconvulsive therapy
2. Relaxation therapy
3. Psychotropic medications
4. Group therapy

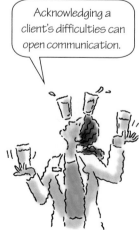

23. 4. Frottage involves rubbing against someone, typically a stranger, in a public place to elicit erotic feelings and sexual release. Positive reinforcement is an important component of group therapy and helps a client develop new sexual response patterns. Electroconvulsive therapy and relaxation therapy aren't indicated for this condition and do not emphasize positive reinforcement. Psychotropic medications are used for dangerous and compulsive practices and are not indicated for this condition.
CN: Psychosocial integrity; CNS: None; CL: Analyze

24. A client has been admitted to the psychiatric unit for transvestic fetishism. Which conditions, about this client, should the nurse acknowledge when planning care? Select all that apply.
1. Self-identifies as heterosexual
2. Existence of cross-dressing habits
3. Affects more men than women
4. Presence of gender identity disorder
5. Self-identifies as homosexual

24. 1, 2, 3. Transvestic fetishism is the existence of cross-dressing for the purpose of sexual arousal. It is most frequently found in heterosexual men, although some identify as gay or bisexual. It is identified in men more than women. Those with transvestic fetishism generally do not have difficulty with their assigned gender, although some may later develop gender dysphoria and the diagnosis of gender identity disorder.
CN: Psychosocial integrity; CNS: None; CL: Apply

25. The nurse is caring for a married client with a paraphilia disorder. What are important goals for this client? Select all that apply.
1. Attend a variety of meetings on the unit
2. Identify triggers that initiate sexual behaviors
3. Participate in a family meeting before discharge
4. Verbalize appropriate methods to meet sexual needs
5. Sign a contract to maintain sexual celibacy for one year

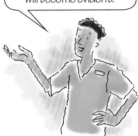

If you cross-examine this question, the answer will become evident.

25. 2, 3, 4. Upon discharge, this client should verbalize an appropriate alternative methods to meet his sexual needs, and effective strategies to prevent relapse. It isn't imperative that the client attend all meetings on the unit, but it is important that he attend the prescribed group sessions. A family meeting, in the hospital, can help support the client if it is therapeutically indicated and he is ready to share his illness with his spouse. It is unreasonable, and not therapeutically indicated, to discuss sexual celibacy.
CN: Psychosocial integrity; CNS: None; CL: Analyze

26. A client, admitted to the hospital with a diagnosis of pedophilia, tells his roommate about the symptoms of his illness. His roommate runs down the hall yelling, "I don't want to be in here with a child molester." What is the nurse's **most** appropriate response?
1. "What he told you is private information and shouldn't be shared."
2. "Calm down right now and go to the day room."
3. "I can see you're upset. Sit down so we can talk."
4. "Your roommate is not a child molester."

26. 3. Acknowledging that the roommate is upset and talking with him will allow the roommate to verbalize his feelings. If a client were agitated or anxious about his roommate, it wouldn't be therapeutic or safe to keep both clients together without intervention. Ordering the roommate to stop acting out or to calm down is demeaning rather than a therapeutic response. Replying that the information is private inadvertently reinforces it. Stating that the pedophile isn't a child molester doesn't acknowledge the client's feelings.
CN: Psychosocial integrity; CNS: None; CL: Apply

27. Which roommate assignment would a nurse question for a client with sexual sadism?
1. Sexual masochism
2. Voyeurism
3. Exhibitionism
4. Lesbianism

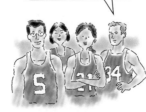

Effective care may involve managing interactions between clients.

27. 1. A client admitted with sexual masochism is aroused through suffering and, therefore, shouldn't be placed with a client diagnosed with sexual sadism. A voyeur is aroused by secretly observing someone who's naked or engaged in sexual activity. An exhibitionist is aroused through the exposure of one's genitals to an unsuspecting person. Similarly a voyeur and exhibitionist should not be paired together. A lesbian is a woman who enjoys sexual activities and relationships with someone of the same sex.
CN: Safe, effective care environment; CNS: Management of care; CL: Apply

CN: Client needs category   CNS: Client needs subcategory   CL: Cognitive level

28. A nurse is obtaining a health history from a client who states that he has been diagnosed with voyeurism. How would the nurse **most** accurately describe voyeurism?
1. Observing others while they disrobe
2. Wearing clothing of the opposite sex
3. Rubbing against a non-consenting person
4. Using rubber sheeting for sexual arousal

28. **1.** Voyeurism is sexual arousal from secretly observing someone disrobe. Transvestic fetishism describes someone who enjoys cross-dressing. Rubbing against someone who is non-consenting is frottage. Using objects for sexual arousal is fetishism.
CN: Psychosocial integrity; CNS: None; CL: Apply

29. The nurse is teaching the family of a client with a form of scatophilia about the disorder and causes of arousal. What would the nurse explain as a cause for this paraphilia?
1. Lewd language over the phone
2. Touching objects such as women's underwear
3. Having sexual contact with children
4. Rubbing against a non-consenting stranger

29. **1.** Telephone scatophilia is a paraphilia in which a person derives sexual arousal by engaging in lewd conversations on the telephone. Fetishism involves the use of non-living, or non-genital objects for sexual excitement. Pedophiles engage in fondling or sexual activities with children under 13 years of age. Frottage is rubbing against a non-consenting person for sexual arousal.
CN: Psychosocial integrity; CNS: None; CL: Apply

30. A female being treated for infertility confides to the nurse that she hasn't told her partner she had been treated for a sexually transmitted disease in the past. What is the nurse's **most** therapeutic response?
1. "Is withholding this information the basis for a trusting relationship?"
2. "Do you not think your partner deserves to know your past history?"
3. "What concerns you about sharing this information?"
4. "I understand why you would want to keep this information from him."

30. **3.** This response encourages the client to verbalize her concerns in a safe environment, and begin to choose a course of action to deal with this issue. Telling the client that she's withholding information that may cause distrust in her relationship, or that her partner deserves to know conveys negative judgments. Taking sides with the client is not therapeutic and does not encourage discussion or problem solving.
CN: Psychosocial integrity; CNS: None; CL: Apply

31. A client on the unit has learned that his gay roommate has tested positive for HIV. The client asks the nurse to be moved to another room on the psychiatric unit because he doesn't feel safe now. What is the nurse's **most** appropriate action?
1. Agree to move him to another room
2. Encourage him to discuss his fears
3. Move his roommate to a private room
4. Inform him that such a move is not therapeutic

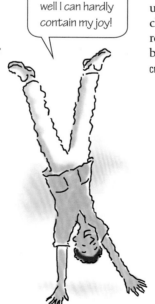

You're doing so well I can hardly contain my joy!

31. **2.** To intervene effectively, the nurse must first understand the client's fears. After exploring the client's fears, the nurse may move the client or his roommate, or explain why such a move would not be therapeutic for either clients.
CN: Psychosocial integrity; CNS: None; CL: Apply

CN: Client needs category   CNS: Client needs subcategory   CL: Cognitive level

32. The nurse is caring for a client being treated for pedophilia. The client discloses that his dose of medroxyprogesterone is not helping to reduce his sexual impulses. What is the nurse's **most** appropriate response?

1. "That is an off-label use for that medication."
2. "I will review your lab results and medication dosage."
3. "How are you tolerating that hormone therapy?"
4. "Have you registered yet as a sex offender?"

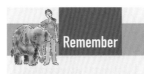

Remember

"Medroxyprogesterone tones down testosterone."

Medroxyprogesterone is a progestin that can be used to suppress testosterone levels and thus libido.

32. 2. The nurse should reinforce that testosterone suppression can take from three to ten months to realize symptom relief. It is important to understand serum levels as well as dosage before contacting the prescriber about a change in dosage. It is also helpful to learn how the client is tolerating the hormone, but this is not of primary importance. Hormone replacement therapy, as a treatment for this disorder, is not done universally. It is inappropriate to overreact about his disorder, or his provider's chosen treatment of this client.

CN: Physiological integrity; CNS: Pharmacological and parenteral therapies; CL: Analyze

33. The nurse is planning to discharge a 16-year-old adolescent with a diagnosis of autoerotic asphyxiation. The admission diagnosis was possible suicide attempt. What are concerns for this client? Select all that apply.

1. The risk of contracting an STI
2. Lack of knowledge related to diagnosis
3. Risk of accidental death
4. Risk of harming a sexual partner
5. The need for sexual celibacy

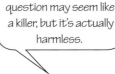

Don't worry—this question may seem like a killer, but it's actually harmless.

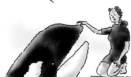

33. 2, 3. A person with autoerotic asphyxiation typically is a young person who acts alone. Masturbation with, and without, sexual toys and pornography is concluded with the act of deliberately hanging by the neck to increase sexual arousal. The nurse must emphasize, during discharge teaching, the need to avoid this risky behavior because it can end in accidental death. It is an opportunity to reinforce all disease, medication, and treatment planning. There little concern for contracting an STD or harming a sexual partner during this sexual act. Recommending celibacy is not an appropriate intervention.

CN: Health promotion and maintenance; CNS: None; CL: Analyze

34. Which statement, made by a client with paraphilia, indicates a potential for relapse?

1. "I am going to outpatient therapy."
2. "My goal is to attend all therapy sessions."
3. "I'm not getting any treatment here."
4. "The provider wants me to take leuprolide acetate."

34. 3. A lack of insight to the problem may indicate a potential for relapse. Attending all therapy sessions and outpatient therapy demonstrates adherence with the treatment plan. Leuprolide acetate is an antiandrogenic agent that lowers testosterone levels and decreases libido.

CN: Psychosocial integrity; CNS: None; CL: Analyze

35. A female client taking antidepressant medication discloses to the nurse that she has a decreased desire for sex, which is causing significant marital stress. What are appropriate responses by the nurse? Select all that apply.

1. "Have you stopped taking your antidepressant medication?"
2. "What are your thoughts on how you should handle this?"
3. "Does your husband understand you need this medication?"
4. "Have you spoken with your provider about this?"
5. "Are you able to discuss this with your husband?"

35. 1, 2, 4, 5. Encouraging the client to verbalize her thoughts will help the client identify feelings related to different choices. It may be helpful to understand if the conflict is greater for this client or her spouse. Confronting the client about continued adherence despite the side effects is a way to insure adherence despite her concerns. Focusing on the need for taking this medication does not encourage further communication about possible side effects or medication adjustments that may be indicated for the client. Referring to the client's husband is judgmental and blaming. It is appropriate to ask the client if she has spoken to her provider to gather as much information as possible.

CN: Psychosocial integrity; CNS: None; CL: Apply

CN: Client needs category   CNS: Client needs subcategory   CL: Cognitive level

36. A mother brings her 14-year-old son to a psychiatric crisis center. The mother privately states, "He's always dressing in female clothing. There must be something wrong with him." What is the nurse's **most** appropriate response?
1. "Why does your son think he is here today?"
2. "I will talk to him about this inappropriate behavior."
3. "You seem upset, tell me your concerns."
4. "I would not want my son to dress in girl's clothing either."

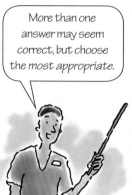
More than one answer may seem correct, but choose the most appropriate.

36. 1. It is most important for the nurse to talk with the client to determine what he understands about being brought in for evaluation, and what he perceives as the problem. Acknowledging the mother's feelings, and offering her an opportunity to verbalize her concerns provides a forum for open communication. Telling the client that dressing in female clothing is inappropriate, judgmental, and serves to destroy trust-building and open communication. The nurse should not offer a personal opinion about her own preferences.
CN: Psychosocial integrity; CNS: None; CL: Apply

37. A 17-year-old female client who enjoys playing ball with boys, and is most comfortable in jeans, tells her mother that she doesn't want to go to the prom if she has to wear a frilly dress. Her mother asks, "What should I do with my daughter?" What is the nurse's **best** response?
1. Tell the mother that she'll grow out of this phase
2. Offer to speak to the teen about her clothing preferences
3. Ask the client's mother to talk about her fears for her daughter
4. Tell the client's mother to make her go to the prom but not wear a dress

37. 3. Asking the client's mother to verbalize her fears will permit the nurse to accurately assess the mother's distress, which may not be about her daughter's sexual preference. The client's mother may be upset over her daughter's non-traditional behavior, or because her daughter doesn't wish to go to the prom. Telling the client's mother that her daughter will grow out of it may be offering the mother false reassurance. The nurse shouldn't speak to the client about her behavior, This implies a value judgment on the part of the nurse. Forcing her to go to the prom isn't therapeutic and doesn't address the mother's fears.
CN: Psychosocial integrity; CNS: None; CL: Apply

38. A 39-year-old client tells the nurse that he wants to undergo gender reassignment surgery because he feels trapped in his male body. What is the **priority** intervention for this client?
1. Telling his family and friends
2. Participating in psychotherapy
3. Visiting transsexual clubs
4. Scheduling a consult with a surgeon

38. 2. Before having gender reassignment surgery, this client should have several years of psychotherapy. Though not a priority, family and friends, should be told of the client's plans. Visiting transsexual clubs has no bearing on having gender reassignment surgery. Seeing a surgeon isn't usually done on a regular basis until after the completion of psychotherapy.
CN: Psychosocial integrity; CNS: None; CL: Analyze

39. Estrogen therapy has been prescribed for a male client who wishes to undergo gender reassignment surgery. The nurse determines that the client understands the purpose of therapy when he states:
1. "It will help me develop natural breasts."
2. "I will begin menstruating as a result of this therapy."
3. "The therapy will assist with cross-dressing."
4. "This therapy will prevent menstruation."

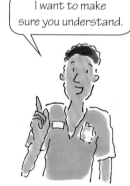
I want to make sure you understand.

39. 1. A male who receives long-term estrogen therapy will develop female secondary sexual characteristics such as breasts. A male on estrogen won't menstruate, because he doesn't have a uterus. Estrogen has no bearing on cross-dressing. Androgens would be taken by a female to stop menstruation.
CN: Physiological integrity; CNS: Pharmacological and parenteral Therapies; CL: Analyze

40. A nurse is caring for several clients with gender identity disorders. Which client is at greatest risk for anxiety related to transsexualism?
1. Older adult
2. Adolescent
3. Young adult
4. Prepubescent child

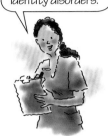

A client's age can affect his anxiety related to gender identity disorders.

40. 2. Adolescents who are transsexuals are usually very distraught over the changes occurring within their body. Elderly persons, young adults, and young children aren't experiencing fluctuating hormones and rapidly developing secondary sexual characteristics in their bodies. Therefore, they are not as high risk for anxiety as adolescents.
CN: Psychosocial integrity; CNS: None; CL: Analyze

41. In which gender identity disorder does the client identify as a person of the opposite gender?
1. Exhibitionism
2. Masochism
3. Transsexualism
4. Transvestitism

41. 3. A client who is diagnosed with transsexual disorder identifies as a person of the opposite gender. A masochist is sexually aroused by physical pain or humiliation. An exhibitionist is sexually aroused by displaying one's genitals in a public place. A transvestite enjoys cross-dressing.
CN: Psychosocial integrity; CNS: None; CL: Apply

42. A transsexual client wishes to have gender reassignment surgery and tells the nurse that he's ready to begin hormonal therapy. Which facts must be true before estrogen therapy is administered? Select all that apply.
1. He has cross-dressed and lived in the desired gender role for several years.
2. He remains undecided about undergoing the operation.
3. He understands that he no longer needs psychotherapy.
4. He has been functioning as a female within or outside of a relationship.
5. He has a full support system in place.

42. 1, 2, 4. Before gender reassignment surgery, the client should live as the desired gender after undergoing several years of psychotherapy. A client who takes hormonal therapy is in the final steps before having surgery, and hasn't decided for, or against, the surgery. Psychotherapy is an ongoing modality for someone requesting gender reassignment surgery, and it should not be interrupted or discontinued. Living as the desired gender can occur both within, and outside of, a relationship. While supportive people may be available, a full support system is evolving and is not a requirement to begin hormonal therapy.
CN: Psychosocial integrity; CNS: None; CL: Analyze

43. An adolescent is experiencing gender identity disorder. Which of Erikson's identified developmental tasks is this client unable to progress through?
1. Initiative versus guilt
2. Industry versus inferiority
3. Intimacy versus isolation
4. Identity versus role confusion

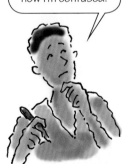

I remember reading about Erik Erikson. But now I'm confused.

43. 4. According to developmentalist Erik Erikson, adolescence is a time when role identity is found as a result of independence and sexual maturity. Role confusion would result from the inability to integrate all experiences. A child begins to conceptualize and interpersonalize relationships during the initiative versus guilt phase. A child incorporates and acquires social skills during the industry versus inferiority phase. Adolescents with gender identity disorder may be able to successfully progress through each of the latter two developmental tasks before encountering that of identity versus role confusion. Intimacy versus isolation is a stage in which the adult meets other adults and establishes relationships.
CN: Health promotion and maintenance; CNS: None; CL: Analyze

CN: Client needs category   CNS: Client needs subcategory   CL: Cognitive level

44. A 35-year-old married client is admitted to the psychiatric unit. During the nurse's interview the client states, "I can't live this lie anymore. I wish I were a woman. I can't live one more day feeling this way." What is the nurse's **priority** intervention?
1. Call the primary health care provider
2. Encourage the client to tell his wife
3. Initiate suicide precautions to ensure safety
4. Encourage him to talk about his feelings

44. 3. This client reveals that he is under severe stress with suicidal ideation. His arrival at the hospital for admission represents a true crisis situation. Sitting down with the client and exploring his feelings would allow the nurse to assess the client, and is a necessary next step. Assuring safety is the highest priority. Discussions should not focus on gender conflict issues as these are more long-term, and cannot be quickly assessed or resolved. The primary health care provider shouldn't be notified until an assessment is completed. The client should not speak to his wife until he has processed his feelings and is ready to face the associated challenges.
CN: Safe and effective care environment; CNS: Safety; CL: Apply

45. A 14-year-old female client admits to having transsexual feelings and states, "I would rather die than live in this body." What is the nurse's **priority** intervention?
1. Explain that she is too young to have these feelings
2. Call her parents to let them know about her feelings
3. Encourage her to verbalize her conflicting feelings.
4. Clarify her suicidal intention and plan

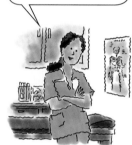

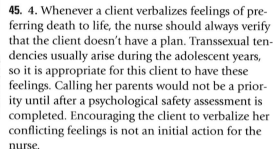

The NCLEX may include sexual identity questions for clients of different ages.

45. 4. Whenever a client verbalizes feelings of preferring death to life, the nurse should always verify that the client doesn't have a plan. Transsexual tendencies usually arise during the adolescent years, so it is appropriate for this client to have these feelings. Calling her parents would not be a priority until after a psychological safety assessment is completed. Encouraging the client to verbalize her conflicting feelings is not an initial action for the nurse.
CN: Psychosocial integrity; CNS: Safety; CL: Apply

46. A female client enjoys wearing men's clothing. Her sister tells the nurse that the client would like to have gender reassignment surgery. The client tells the nurse that she just wants to be left alone. Which nursing intervention should the nurse take **first**?
1. Tell the client that she is repressing her true feelings
2. Encourage the client to change her clothes
3. Inform the client's sister of medical privacy laws
4. Recommend that the client avoid her sister

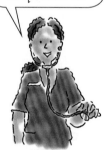

Prioritizing correctly is extremely important for question 46.

46. 3. The client's sister must understand that her sister's health care is private and cannot be discussed with her. The client needs to verbalize her feelings regarding wearing male attire, as well as her desire to be left alone. Telling the client that she is repressing her true feelings is judgmental. It's inappropriate for a nurse to have the client change her clothes for no safety or therapeutic reason, or to advise the client to avoid her sister.
CN: Psychosocial integrity; CNS: None; CL: Apply

47. A mother is concerned about her 10-year-old son, who has been playing with dolls since he was two. Which **initial** strategy should be included in this boy's care plan?
1. Provide counseling for his mother
2. Advise the mother throw the dolls away
3. Instruct the mother on age-appropriate play
4. Explore the child's feelings about the dolls

47. 4. It is important to assess the child's feelings, as well as explore his preference for dolls rather than sports. The mother may need to be instructed on methods to cope with his behaviors, but only after the child is permitted to verbalize. Until proper assessment is made, it is inappropriate to remove the dolls. There is no evidence of age-inappropriate play.
CN: Psychosocial integrity; CNS: None; CL: Apply

Sexual & Gender Identity Disorders **439**

48. During a hospital orientation class a graduate nurse expresses concern about working with clients who want to discuss sexual problems. What is the facilitator's **best** response?
1. "We should talk more about your concerns."
2. "You will get used to this part of your job."
3. "Refer those questions to other health care professionals."
4. "Every licensed nurse is qualified to discuss those problems."

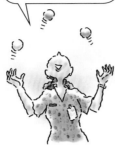

Keep going! Fewer than 10 questions to go!

48. 1. The nurse instructor should explore what the nurse's specific concerns are, and counsel her appropriately. Telling the nurse that "she will get used to it" does not allow the nurse to express her feelings or validate her concerns. Stating that "every nurse is qualified," or that these questions should be referred to other healthcare professionals are extremes that allow the nurse and nurse manager to avoid discussing the nurse's concerns.
CN: Safe effective care environment; CNS: Management of care; CL: Analyze

49. A 57-year-old male client, with a history of hypertension, expresses concern about his sexual functioning to the nurse. What should the nurse assess? Select all that apply.
1. Medication history
2. Sexual practices
3. Medical conditions
4. Family history
5. Alcohol consumption

49. 1, 3, 5. The nurse should first have the client clarify his concern. Obtaining a thorough medication history, and reviewing the effects of prescribed medications may alleviate misconceptions and identify the source of the problem. The client's medical conditions should be reviewed for new developments or unresolved issues that may contribute to his concern. Chronic or excessive alcohol use can contribute to alterations in sexual functioning. Family history and sexual practices are part of the nursing assessment, but would not be a priority at this time.
CN: Physiological integrity; CNS: Pharmacological and parenteral therapies; CL: Apply

50. A male client brings a list of his prescribed medications to the clinic. During the initial assessment, he tells the nurse that he has been experiencing delayed ejaculation. Which types of medication may contribute to this condition? Select all that apply.
1. Antihistamine drugs
2. Nonsteroidal anti-inflammatory drugs
3. Antihypertensive drugs
4. Steroidal drugs
5. Herbal diuretic

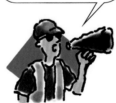

Remember: select all that apply.

50. 1, 2, 3. Antihypertensives are first-line agents known to cause or contribute to sexual dysfunction. Antihistamine and nonsteroidal anti-inflammatory agents may also contribute to sexual dysfunction. Steroids have no known effect on sexual function. Certain diuretics can contribute to delayed ejaculation. The nurse must also consider and explore non-prescription options such as over the counter medications, herbal remedies, and chronic or excess alcohol consumption.
CN: Physiological integrity; CNS: Pharmacological and parenteral therapies; CL: Apply

51. After a myocardial infarction (MI), a client tells the nurse that he is afraid he will have another heart attack if he attempts sexual intercourse. Which teaching points should the nurse emphasize? Select all that apply.
1. "You may have intercourse if your blood pressure is less than 140/90 mmHg."
2. "It is safe to resume sex when you can walk a quarter-mile."
3. "Sexual activity is considered a type of physical exercise."
4. "A good indicator of being ready is being able to climb two flights of stairs."
5. "You should be concerned about the stress sex puts on your heart."

51. 2, 3, 4. After an MI, many clients fear that engaging in sex will trigger another one; however, research indicates that this occurs in less than 1% of cases. Like other regular physical activity, sexual activity is heart-healthy, good for your circulation, metabolism, and reduces future risk of heart-disease. Clients should not automatically strive to resume activity levels previous to an MI. Strong benchmarks are being able to endure a quarter-mile walk or to climb two flights of stairs. Time frames may vary from two days to one month post MI.
CN: Physiological integrity; CNS: Physiological adaptation; CL: Apply

CN: Client needs category   CNS: Client needs subcategory   CL: Cognitive level

52. A 42-year-old female client reports dyspareunia. Which other information is **most** appropriate when accurately planning care for this client? Select all that apply.
1. The presence of other gynecological symptoms
2. A history of painful intercourse
3. A history of sexual abuse
4. A history of irregular or absent menstrual cycles
5. Previous radiation or chemotherapy treatments

52. 1, 2, 4, 5. It is important to know the history of the presenting symptoms, as well as other co-existing gynecological symptoms, to be able to thoroughly assess this client. Many gynecological conditions or surgeries, such as a hysterectomy, can contribute to dyspareunia. Having irregular or absent menstrual cycles is suggestive of perimenopause or early menopause. Dyspareunia is commonly reported by postmenopausal women. Radiation and chemotherapy can cause changes that make sex painful. Most women with dyspareunia do not have a history of sexual abuse, but, if present, might play a contributing role.
CN: Health promotion and maintenance; CNS: None; CL: Apply

I see you taking the NCLEX exam ... and passing it ... and jumping up and down with joy.

53. A 46-year-old female client is diagnosed with anorgasmia. Which nursing intervention takes **priority** when planning care for this client?
1. Clarifying changes in her sexual functioning
2. Assessing the client's role in her sexual relationship
3. Determining the nurse's own attitudes about this issue
4. Interviewing the client with her sexual partner

53. 3. The nurse must first identify her own beliefs and feelings about this issue and remain nonjudgmental. The other actions may be relevant in assessing and planning interventions, but risk being unconsciously influenced unless the nurse's comfort level with this intimate topic.
CN: Safe, effective care environment; CNS: Management of care; CL: Apply

54. A 35-year-old male client reports little or no sexual desire, which is causing marital discord. Which assessment information is appropriate for this client? Select all that apply.
1. Sexual history
2. History of decreased desire
3. Current list of medications
4. Medical history
5. Marital history

54. 2, 3. Clarifying the symptoms and their onset will provide an opportunity to gather useful information about the client's current condition. Many medications can have a profound effect on sexual desire. While a review of the client's medical history may provide helpful information, it is likely that only recent developments would contribute to his current concern. The client's sexual and marital history have no direct bearing on his lack of desire. Reporting previous problems is useful, but wouldn't provide a sufficient explanation for the lack of sexual desire.
CN: Psychosocial integrity; CNS: None; CL: Analyze

Time to celebrate! You finished Chapter 20!

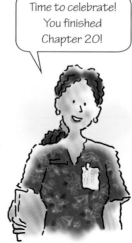

55. Pedophilia is diagnosed by the presence of specifically defined behaviors and characteristics. Which statements, regarding pedophilia, are correct? Select all that apply.
1. A person with pedophilia has strong sexual attraction to prepubescent children.
2. Male children are more commonly the focus of attention than female children.
3. A person with pedophilia is very attentive to a child's needs in order to win the child's trust.
4. Symptoms of pedophilia typically begin in early adulthood.
5. A person with pedophilia must be age 16 or at least five years older than the child.

55. 1, 3, 5. Pedophilia is a disorder characterized by a strong sexual attraction to prepubescent children that generally begins to manifest itself in adolescence, not early adulthood. By definition, the pedophile must be age 16 or older, or at least five years older than the child. The pedophile generally is attentive to the needs of children in order to gain their trust, loyalty, and attention. Female, not male, children are more commonly the focus of attention.
CN: Psychosocial integrity; CNS: None; CL: Apply

CN: Client needs category   CNS: Client needs subcategory   CL: Cognitive level

Chapter 21

Feeding & Eating Disorders

New information about feeding and eating disorders is released almost continuously. For the latest about disorders of critical importance for young people, check the Web site of the National Eating Disorders Association at **www.nationaleatingdisorders.org**.

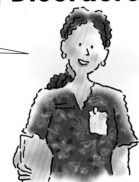

1. The parent of a daughter who was diagnosed with bulimia nervosa asks the nurse, "How can my child have an eating disorder when she isn't underweight?" What is the nurse's **most** appropriate response?
1. "A person with bulimia nervosa can maintain a normal weight."
2. "It's hard to face this type of problem in a person you love."
3. "At first, there is no weight loss; it comes later in the disease."
4. "This is a serious problem even though there is no weight loss."

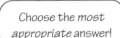

Choose the most appropriate answer!

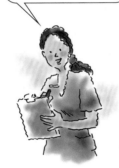

1. 1. A client with bulimia nervosa may be of normal weight, overweight, or underweight. Weight loss isn't a clinical criterion for bulimia nervosa. Answer two doesn't address the need for information about the relationship between weight change and bulimia nervosa. Answer three is incorrect because there may be little or no weight loss. Answer four doesn't address the issue of weight change in a client with bulimia nervosa.
CN: Psychosocial integrity; CNS: None; CL: Apply

2. A 29-year-old female comes to the clinic because of a significant weight loss in the past four months. The nurse suspects that the client may have anorexia nervosa. What sign or symptom would the nurse expect to find in this client?
1. Hypertension
2. Amenorrhea
3. Stress fractures
4. Primary diarrhea

2. 2. Anorexia nervosa is characterized by profound weight loss caused by severe restriction of food intake. If severe enough, it causes amenorrhea in females along with decreased body temperature. The presence of a stress fracture may be suggestive of an eating disorder, in conjunction with reduced caloric intake, associated reduced estrogen, and excessive exercise. It usually doesn't produce diarrhea, but it may produce constipation because decreased oral intake leads to decreased GI motility. If diarrhea is reported, the nurse should assess for laxative use.
CN: Physiological integrity; CNS: Reduction of risk potential; CL: Apply

Help your client understand her behavior.

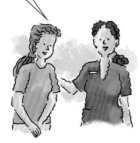

3. What is the **best** explanation of the binge–purge cycle of a client's bulimia nervosa?
1. There are emotional triggers connected to bingeing.
2. Over time, people usually grow out of binge-ing behaviors.
3. Bingeing isn't the problem; purging is the issue to address.
4. When a person gets too hungry, there is a tendency to binge

3. 1. It's important for the client to understand the emotional triggers of bingeing, such as disappointment, depression, and anxiety. People do not outgrow eating behaviors. It is not a normal part of the growth and development process. Answer three negates the seriousness of bingeing, and leads the client to believe that vomiting is the only problem. Physiologic hunger doesn't predispose a client to binge behaviors.
CN: Physiological integrity; CNS: Reduction of risk potential; CL: Apply

CN: Client needs category   CNS: Client needs subcategory   CL: Cognitive level

4. What would the nurse expect to find in the psychologic history of a client who has an eating disorder? Select all that apply.
1. Easy-going, laissez-faire attitude
2. Rigidity of thinking
3. Seeking to please others
4. Depressed Mood
5. Distorted body image

4. 2, 4, 5. Clients will typically be withdrawn, secretive, and isolative. Their thinking pattern will be black and white. They are often depressed and have a distorted sense of their body. An easy-going, laissez-faire attitude, and striving to please others are not in the psychologic profile of a client with an eating disorder.
CN: Psychosocial integrity; CNS: None; CL: Apply

5. A client, diagnosed with bulimia nervosa, is having trouble developing relationships. What is the **most** important nursing intervention?
1. Assist the client to develop social skills
2. Focus on how relationships cause bulimic behavior
3. Help the client identify feelings about relationships
4. Discuss ways to avoid getting overinvolved in relationships

5. 3. The client needs to address personal feelings, especially uncomfortable ones, because they may trigger bingeing behavior. Social skills are important to well-being, but they aren't typically a major problem for the client with bulimia nervosa. Relationships do not cause bulimic behaviors. It is the inability to handle stress or conflict that arises from interactions that cause the client to be distressed. The client isn't necessarily overinvolved in relationships, but they may lack satisfying relations in their life.
CN: Psychosocial integrity; CNS: None; CL: Apply

6. A young female client with bulimia nervosa tells the nurse that she wants to decrease her feelings of powerlessness. What is this client's **most** important short-term goal?
1. Learn problem-solving skills
2. Decrease symptoms of anxiety
3. Perform self-care activities daily
4. Verbalize how to set limits with others

6. 1. If the client can learn effective problem-solving skills, she will gain a sense of control and power in her life. Anxiety is commonly caused by feelings of powerlessness. Performing daily self-care activities will not reduce a sense of powerlessness. Verbalizing how to set limits and protect oneself from the intrusive behavior of others is a necessary life skill, but problem-solving skills are the priority.
CN: Psychosocial integrity; CNS: None; CL: Analyze

Question 7 is asking you to prioritize.

7. Which client's response should the nurse address **first**?
1. "My life is over if I gain weight."
2. "I feel dizzy and light-headed when I get up."
3. "I cannot eat because my teeth hurt."
4. "I do not have the same energy that I used to have."

7. 2. The priority intervention, by the nurse, would be to assess the client's vital signs to note any alterations. Answer one is an example of catastrophizing. Dental erosion and caries are commonly found in a client with an eating disorder. Muscle weakness is also commonly found in a client with an eating disorder.
CN: Safe, effective care environment; CNS: Management of care; CL: Apply

Read carefully! You need to select all.

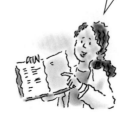

8. The nurse is developing interventions to prevent a client with an eating disorder from developing refeeding syndrome. Which interventions are appropriate? Select all that apply.
1. Monitor the client three times a week in an outpatient clinic.
2. Monitor serum electrolytes
3. Refeed the client over a period of three days
4. Administer fluid replacement as prescribed
5. Monitor the client's vital signs frequently

8. 2, 4, 5. It is important to monitor the electrolytes, fluid replacement, and vital signs. The client needs to be hospitalized during the refeeding phase of recovery from an eating disorder. The refeeding must be carried out over seven days.
CN: Physiological integrity; CNS: Reduction of risk potential; CL: Analyze

CN: Client needs category   CNS: Client needs subcategory   CL: Cognitive level

9. Which life-threatening complication of bulimia nervosa should the nurse closely monitor?
1. Serum calcium 10.1 mg/dl
2. Heart rate 56 bpm
3. Serum potassium 2.9 mEq/L
4. Respiratory rate 16 breaths/min

9. 3. Electrolyte imbalance such as hypokalemia can be a life-threatening complication of bulimia nervosa due to purging behaviors. A serum calcium level of 10.1 mg/dl is within normal range. A heart rate of 56 bpm indicates bradycardia, but is not life threatening. A respiratory rate of 16 breaths/min is within the normal range, and not life threatening.
CN: Physiological integrity; CNS: Reduction of risk potential; CL: Apply

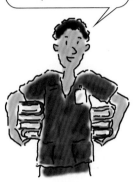

You're doing great! It looks like all your studying is paying off.

10. A nurse is talking to a client with bulimia nervosa about the complications of laxative abuse. Which client statement indicates an understanding of the risks?
1. "I don't really have much taste for food, so there's no loss in getting it out of my system more quickly."
2. "Laxatives help me get rid of extra calories before they are added to my body. I know I just shouldn't eat the extra calories to begin with."
3. "Laxatives are over-the-counter medications that have no harmful effect."
4. "Using laxatives prevents my body from absorbing essential nutrients, such as protein, fat, and calcium."

10. 4. A serious complication of laxative abuse is the malabsorption of nutrients, such as proteins, fats, and calcium. Laxative abuse doesn't tend to affect the client's sense of taste. Clients with bulimia nervosa need to change their negative thinking about calories and the use of laxatives.
CN: Physiological integrity; CNS: Reduction of risk potential; CL: Apply

11. How may the nurse distinguish between bulimia nervosa and binge-eating disorder?
1. Binge-eating disorder is not associated with the regular use of inappropriate compensatory behaviors, such as purging, fasting, and excessive exercise.
2. A client with bulimia nervosa will binge eat at least two time a week. A client with binge-eating disorder will not.
3. A client with bulimia nervosa will eat very large quantities of food in a relatively short amount of time.
4. A client with a binge-eating disorder will have a perceived lack of control of their food intake.

11. 1. In binge-eating disorder, there is no compensatory behavior associated with the binge eating. This client is at risk of developing obesity. The other listed characteristics are found in both disorders.
CN: Psychosocial integrity; CNS: None; CL: Analyze

12. A female client is talking to a nurse about her binge-purge cycle. What is the **most** appropriate question for the nurse to ask?
1. "How can you stop the binge-purge cycle?"
2. "Does the binge-purge cycle help you manage your weight?"
3. "Does the binge-purge cycle relieve your anxiety?"
4. "How often do you go through the binge-purge cycle?"

12. 4. Binge-purge cycles can vary greatly from client to client. Defining the frequency may alert the nurse to the degree of risk from fluid and electrolyte imbalances. Asking the client if she knows how to stop the binge-purge cycle is not appropriate. It will generate feelings of self-blame and shame. It's common for clients to experience daily fluctuations in weight. Although the binge-purge behavior may decrease anxiety initially, it tends to generate overall negative feelings about self.
CN: Psychosocial integrity; CNS: None; CL: Apply

CN: Client needs category   CNS: Client needs subcategory   CL: Cognitive level

13. A nurse is assessing a client with bulimia nervosa for possible substance abuse. What is the **most** important question for the nurse to ask this client?
1. "What drugs have you used to manage your weight and appetite?"
2. "What drugs have you used to help control anxiety?"
3. "How would you describe your alcohol use?"
4. "Do you participate in "pharm" parties?"

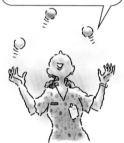

Consider all the answers. Then choose the most important one.

13. 1. Some clients with bulimia nervosa use, or have a history of using, amphetamines to control their weight. This is the most important question, as it asks about medications related to the eating disorder and the potential medical complications. The use of alcohol and street drugs is common. Direct questions about medications used for anxiety will likely elicit a direct response. Similarly, asking for a description of alcohol use might yield information about the pattern of drinking. Participation in *"pharm"* parties indicates a high-risk behavior that should be addressed during treatment.
CN: Psychosocial integrity; CNS: None; CL: Apply

14. A female client with bulimia nervosa is discussing her abnormal eating behaviors with the nurse. Which client statement would indicate an understanding of the disorder?
1. "When my loneliness gets to me, I start to binge."
2. "I know that when my life gets better, I'll eat right."
3. "I know I waste food and waste my money on food."
4. "After my parents' divorce, I'll talk about bingeing and purging."

14. 1. Binge eating is a way to handle the uncomfortable feelings of frustration, loneliness, anger, and fear. Answer two indicates the client is experiencing denial of the eating disorder. Answer three addresses the client's feelings of guilt. It does not reflect knowledge of her eating disorder. Answer four indicates that the client isn't ready to discuss her eating disorder.
CN: Psychosocial integrity; CNS: None; CL: Analyze

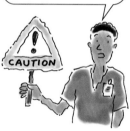

Remember to look closely for all that apply.

15. What would a nurse **most** likely observe in an anorexic client? Select all that apply.
1. Preoccupation with food
2. Amenorrhea
3. Body weight within normal range
4. Lanugo
5. Bradycardia
6. Hypertension

15. 1, 2, 4, 5. Body weight is below 85% of expected normal weight in anorexic clients. Amenorrhea, lanugo, hypotension and hypothermia are symptoms that the nurse could also expect to find in an anorexic client. Hypertension and hyperthermia are incorrect.
CN: Psychosocial integrity; CNS: None; CL: Apply

16. The mother of a female client with bulimia nervosa asks a nurse, "Will bulimia nervosa stop my daughter from menstruating?" What is the nurse's **best** response?
1. "Women with anorexia nervosa or bulimia nervosa stop menstruating in the first year."
2. "When your daughter is bingeing and purging, she will not have normal periods."
3. "The eating disorder must be ongoing for your daughter's menstrual cycle to change."
4. "Women with bulimia nervosa may have a normal or abnormal menstrual cycle, depending on the severity of the problem."

16. 4. The absence or presence of a menstrual cycle depends on the severity of the eating disorder. The eating disorder can disrupt the menstrual cycle at any point in the illness. Such disruptions are not directly associated with either the bingeing or purging cycles.
CN: Health promotion and maintenance; CNS: None; CL: Analyze

17. A 14-year-old client is admitted to an eating disorder clinic after the sudden death of her best friend. The client states that she and her friend had shared in bulimic behaviors since junior high school, and that she is now struggling to understand her friend's death. Which points should the nurse teach this client about the short-term and long-term effects of bulimic behaviors? Select all that apply.
1. Risk for malnutrition
2. Risk for dehydration
3. Risk for internal bleeding
4. Risk for severe tooth infection
5. Risk for stress fractures
6. Risk for fainting

18. A female client with bulimia nervosa reports that her major problem is eating too much food in a short period of time and then vomiting. Which short-term goal is the **most** important?
1. Help the client understand every person has a satiety level
2. Encourage the client to verbalize fears and concerns about food
3. Determine the amount of food the client will eat without purging
4. Obtain a therapy appointment to look at the emotional causes of bulimia nervosa

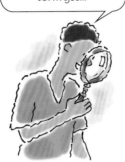

Help the client see the importance of reaching a short-term goal.

19. Which statement indicates to the nurse that a client, with bulimia nervosa, is successfully interrupting her binge-purge cycle?
1. "I called my friend the last two times I got upset."
2. "I purge only if I am alone at home."
3. "My sister watches me eat and writes it down."
4. "My boyfriend takes me out to eat if I want to purge."

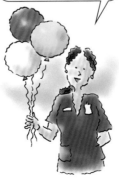

Congratulations! You've completed 20 questions. Have a balloon.

20. A client with bulimia nervosa asks the nurse, "How can I ask for help from my family?" What is the nurse's **most** appropriate response?
1. Instruct the client to ask for help after you have already purged
2. Ask the client if she has ever asked for help before
3. Have the client ask family members to spend time with you at every meal
4. Suggest that the client may want to think about how to handle the situation without help

17. 1, 2, 5, 6. Electrolyte imbalances caused by malnutrition and dehydration contribute to depletions severe enough to cause acute symptoms as well as more prolonged organ impairment. This can include fainting episodes and stress fractures associated with resulting osteoporosis. Chronic vomiting can lead to esophageal bleeding that results in severe blood loss and death. Dental infections can result from long-term vomiting, but may not present until an advanced stage of the illness.
CN: Safe, effective care environment; CNS: Management of care; CL: Analyze

18. 3. This client must meet her nutritional needs to prevent further complications. She must identify the amount of food she can eat without purging as her first short-term goal. Binge eaters cannot recognize their satiety level or their feelings of fullness. Obtaining knowledge, or verbalizing her fears and feelings about food are not priority goals for this client. After meeting immediate physiologic needs, therapy is an important of treatment for this disorder.
CN: Physiological integrity; CNS: Reduction of risk potential; CL: Apply

19. 1. A sign of progress is when the client begins to verbalize feelings and interact with people instead of going to food for comfort. The second option indicates that the client is in denial about the severity of her problem. Having another person watch the client eat or keep the client's food diary is not a helpful strategy, as it creates dependency on others to help control food intake. Answer four indicates the need for more information about the disorder.
CN: Psychosocial integrity; CNS: None; CL: Analyze

20. 2. Determine if the client has ever been successful in asking for help. Previous experiences affect the client's ability to ask for help now. The client needs to ask for help anytime, but it is most therapeutic before one has surrendered to the impulse to binge or purge. Having other people around at mealtime does not support developing independent self-control skills. Developing a support system is imperative for this client.
CN: Psychosocial integrity; CNS: None; CL: Analyze

21. A female client with bulimia nervosa tells a nurse that she doesn't eat during the day, and that she begins to binge and vomit after 5:00 p.m. What is the **most** appropriate nursing intervention?
1. Help the client stop eating the foods on which she binges
2. Discuss the effects of fasting on the client's pattern of eating
3. Encourage the client to become involved in food preparation
4. Teach the client to eat earlier in the day and decrease intake at night

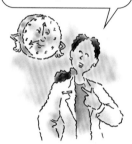

Twenty hours is a long time to go without eating. I wonder how that would affect someone's eating habits?

21. 2. If a person fasts for most of the day, it's common to become extremely hungry, over eat by bingeing, and then feel the need to purge. Restricting food intake can actually trigger the binge-purge cycle. In treatment, the client is taught to identify foods that trigger eating, discuss the feelings associated with these foods, and work to eat them in normal amounts. Involvement in food preparation will not promote changes in the client's behaviors. Answer four does not address how fasting can trigger the binge-purge cycle.
CN: Psychosocial integrity; CNS: None; CL: Apply

22. A female client with bulimia nervosa tells a nurse that she was doing well until last week, when she had a fight with her father. Which nursing intervention is **most** appropriate?
1. Examine the relationship between feelings and eating
2. Discuss the importance of therapy for the entire family
3. Encourage the client to avoid stressful relationships
4. Identify daily stressors and learn stress management skills

22. 1. The client needs to understand her feelings, and develop healthy coping skills to handle difficult feelings and unpleasant situations. Family therapy may be indicated, but should not be an immediate intervention. Avoidance isn't a useful coping strategy as relationship issues need to be explored. All clients can benefit from stress management skills, but for this client, care must focus on the relationship between feelings and eating behaviors.
CN: Psychosocial integrity; CNS: None; CL: Apply

23. Which statement, made by a bulimic, indicates that the client understands the concept of a relapse?
1. "If I can't maintain control over everything, I'll have problems with my food."
2. "I haven't healed much if I continue to experience difficulties."
3. "I will not be able to handle it if this illness becomes chronic."
4. "When I have problems, I can start over again and not feel hopeless."

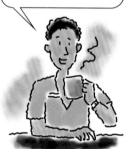

If at first you don't succeed, try again—to choose the correct answer.

23. 4. This statement indicates that the client knows a relapse is just a slip, and that positive gains made from treatment haven't been lost. Negative self-statements can lead to relapse. Control issues relate to powerlessness, which contributes to relapse.
CN: Psychosocial integrity; CNS: None; CL: Apply

24. What is the treatment team's **priority** in planning the care of a client with an eating disorder?
1. Preventing the client from performing any muscle-building exercises
2. Keeping the client on bed rest until she attains a specified weight
3. Meeting daily to discuss manipulation and countertransference
4. Monitoring the client's weight and vital signs daily

24. 3. Clients with eating disorders commonly use manipulative ploys and countertransference to resist weight gain, or to maintain purging practices if they are bulimic. Such clients commonly play staff members against one another. Muscle building is acceptable because it burns relatively few calories. Keeping the client on bed rest until a specified weight is reached may result in a power struggle, and prevent focusing on pertinent issues. Monitoring the client's weight and vital signs is important but not on a daily basis unless the client's condition warrants such attention..
CN: Psychosocial integrity; CNS: None; CL: Apply

25. A nurse is caring for a client with bulimia nervosa. For which is it **most** important for the nurse to assess the client? Select all that apply.
1. Severe electrolyte imbalances
2. Damaged teeth due to the eroding effects of gastric acids on tooth enamel
3. Pneumonia from aspirated stomach contents
4. Cessation of menses
5. Esophageal tears and gastric rupture
6. Intestinal inflammation

25. **1, 2, 4, 5.** Constant bingeing and purging behaviors can result in severe electrolyte imbalances, erosion of tooth enamel from constant exposure to gastric acids, menstrual irregularities, esophageal tears, and, in severe cases, gastric rupture. Aspiration pneumonia is unlikely because the vomiting is controlled. Intestinal inflammation isn't typically associated with bulimia nervosa.
CN: Physiological integrity; CNS: Physiological adaptation; CL: Apply

26. A client with anorexia nervosa attended psychoeducational sessions on the principles of adequate nutrition. Which client statement indicates that the teaching was effective?
1. "I eat while I am doing things to distract myself."
2. "I eat all my food at night right before I go to bed."
3. "I eat small amounts of food slowly, at every meal."
4. "I only eat when I am with my family as a way to be social."

26. **3.** Slowly eating small amounts of food facilitates adequate digestion and prevents distention. Healthy and mindful eating is best accomplished when a person isn't doing other things while they eat. Eating right before bedtime does not allow proper digestion to occur. If a client only eats when the family is present, or while trying to be social, eating will be tied to social or emotional cues rather than nutritional needs.
CN: Health promotion and maintenance; CNS: None; CL: Apply

27. A client with anorexia nervosa tells the nurse, "I'll never have the slender body that I want." What is the **most** appropriate intervention by the nurse?
1. Schedule a family meeting to get help from the parents
2. Help the client work on developing a realistic body image
3. Make an appointment to see the dietitian on a weekly basis
4. Allow the client to develop an intense exercise schedule

27. **2.** With anorexia nervosa, the client pursues thinness and has a distorted view of self. A family meeting may not help the client develop a more realistic view of the body. Although meeting with a dietitian might be helpful, it is not a priority. Clients with anorexia nervosa typically have difficulty determining a realistic exercise plan. It may be helpful to work with a fitness specialist. The inability to adhere to any plan can become another stressor or trigger for the client.
CN: Psychosocial integrity; CNS: None; CL: Apply

28. A client with anorexia nervosa tells a nurse, "My parents never hug me or say I've done anything right." What is the **most** appropriate nursing intervention?
1. Teach the family principles of assertive behavior
2. Discuss the difficulties the family has in social situations
3. Help the family convey a positive attitude toward the client
4. Explore the family's ability to express affection appropriately

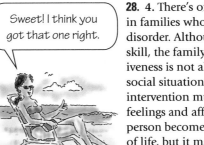

Sweet! I think you got that one right.

28. **4.** There's often a lack of affection and warmth in families who have a member with an eating disorder. Although assertiveness is an important skill, the family member needs to realize assertiveness is not always rewarded. Difficulties in social situations are important to address, but the intervention must focus on how to express positive feelings and affection. A positive attitude helps a person become better able to handle the pressures of life, but it may not change the family's display of affection.
CN: Psychosocial integrity; CNS: None; CL: Apply

29. Which communication strategy is the **best** choice for the nurse working with a client with anorexia nervosa who is experiencing difficulties with peer relationships?
1. Use concrete language and maintain a focus on reality
2. Direct the client to talk about what is causing the anxiety
3. Teach the client to communicate feelings and express self appropriately
4. Discuss the client's depression and focus on self

29. 3. Clients with anorexia nervosa often communicate on a superficial level, and avoid expressing feelings. Identifying feelings and learning to express them are initial steps in decreasing isolation. Clients with anorexia nervosa are usually able to discuss abstract and concrete issues. Discussions should not be limited to the client's feelings of anxiety as the client may not be aware of the cause of the anxiety, which may result in misdirected self-reflection. Discussing depression and focusing on self are not primary strategies used to assist the client with improving peer relationships.
CN: Psychosocial integrity; CNS: None; CL: Apply

30. A nurse plans to include the parents of a client with anorexia nervosa in therapy sessions along with the client. What is important for the nurse to consider about the parents?
1. They tend to overprotect their children.
2. They usually have a history of substance use.
3. They maintain emotional distance from their children.
4. They alternate between loving and rejecting their children.

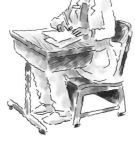

My plan to study all night is starting to seem unrealistic.

30. 1. Clients with anorexia nervosa typically come from a family with parents who are controlling and over protective. These clients eat to gain control of some aspect of their life. Having a history of substance abuse, maintaining an emotional distance, and alternating between love and rejection are not typical characteristics of parents of children who have anorexia nervosa.
CN: Psychological integrity; CNS: None; CL: Apply

31. The nurse has instructed a client with an eating disorder about fluoxetine, and determines that teaching has been effective when the client states:
1. "I can eat anything and anytime I want. This medication will control my eating."
2. "I cannot wait to get home so I can go for a drive in my car."
3. "I should call my provider if I have cravings for large amounts of food."
4. "It may take 1 to 3 weeks for this medication to be effective for me."

31. 4. It is important for the client to understand that fluoxetine can take 1 to 3 weeks to be effective. Fluoxetine does not control eating. Operating hazardous equipment, or driving may be hazardous, and should only be done only after the effects of this medication are determined. Cravings should be monitored in a food diary or discussed in treatment sessions. Providers should be notified if sexual dysfunction occurs, or is intolerable.
CN: Physiologic Integrity; CNS: Pharmacological and Parenteral Therapies; CL: Apply

32. A nurse is working with a female client, with anorexia nervosa, who has acrocyanosis in her extremities. Which short-term nursing goal is **most** important for this client?
1. Teach the client to do daily range-of-motion exercises
2. Encourage client to maintain adequate hydration
3. Perform neurological reflex checks
4. Assess the client for adequate circulation in each extremity

32. 4. Circulation changes will cause extremities to be cold, numb, and have dry, flaky skin. Exercise may help prevent contractures and muscle atrophy, but it may have a limited, secondary effect on promoting circulation. Adequate hydration is a long-term goal to impact her symptoms. Checking neurological reflexes will not necessarily assist with handling circulation problems.
CN: Physiological integrity; CNS: Reduction of risk potential; CL: Apply

CN: Client needs category   CNS: Client needs subcategory   CL: Cognitive level

33. A female client with anorexia nervosa is discharged from the hospital after gaining 12 lb (5.5 kg). Which client statement **best** indicates that the nurse's discharge teachings have been effective?
1. "I plan to eat two small meals a day."
2. "I feel that this is scary, but I'm not going to write about it in my journal."
3. "I have to diet because I've gained 12 lb (5.5 kg)."
4. "I'll need to attend therapy for support to stay healthy."

34. Fluoxetine has been prescribed for a client with an eating disorders. Which symptoms would alert the nurse to the development of serotonin syndrome? Select all that apply.
1. Sleepiness
2. Hallucinations
3. Fever
4. Anxiety
5. Tremors
6. Diaphoresis

35. Monoamine oxidase inhibitors (MAOIs) have been prescribed for a client with bulimia nervosa. What is the **most** important information for the nurse to give this client?
1. Drink several glasses of water with each dose. Do not drink water with meals.
2. Do not eat foods that contain tyramines, such as cheese, cottage cheese, pickled herring, and salami.
3. Watch for bleeding and bruising.
4. Call your provider if you have tremors or feel anxious or agitated.

36. A nurse is analyzing the need for health teaching in a female client with anorexia nervosa. The client lives in a chaotic family situation. What is the **most** important question for the nurse to ask this client?
1. "How long have you experienced irregular menstrual cycles?"
2. "How often do you think about food in a 24-hour period?"
3. "What were the circumstances before your eating disorder developed?"
4. "How much, and what kind of exercise do you engage in every day?"

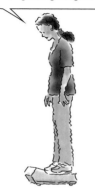

Clients with anorexia nervosa have an intense fear of gaining weight.

Remember

"No tyramine while on monoamines."

Eating foods that contain tyramine can result in a hypertensive crisis in clients taking monoamine oxidase inhibitors (MAOIs).

MAOIs
- Phenelzine
- Tranylcypromine

33. 4. The client is planning to attend therapy after discharge, which shows an understanding of the need for continued counseling. Eating only two small meals a day is an unrealistic plan for meeting nutritional needs. Feeling insecure when leaving a controlled environment is a common response to discharge, but such feelings are exactly what should be written about in a journal. Gaining 12 lb (5.5 kg) indicates that the client's nutritional needs are being met at the present caloric intake.
CN: Psychosocial integrity; CNS: None; CL: Analyze

34. 2, 3, 4, 5, 6. Other symptoms of serotonin syndrome include mental confusion, difficulty concentrating, agitation, hyperreflexia, and incoordination.
CN: Safe, effective care environment; CNS: Management of care; CL: Apply

35. 2. The ingestion of foods containing tyramines can result in a hypertensive crisis. Water and other fluids may be taken with meals, but can limit the amount of food that can be eaten. Bleeding and bruising is not related to taking MAOIs. Symptoms such as tremors, anxiety, or agitation are also unrelated to taking MAOIs.
CN: Safe, effective care environment; CNS: Management of care; CL: Analyze

36. 3. This question lets the nurse get information about the family and background situations that influenced the client's needs before the eating disorder developed. The other options deal with menstrual history, exercise patterns, and food obsessions. Although they are relevant, they do not provide information related to the family situation.
CN: Psychosocial integrity; CNS: None; CL: Analyze

37. An adolescent female client with anorexia nervosa tells a nurse about her feelings of insecurity and the poetry she reads about suicide. Which factor **must** the nurse consider when making a care plan for this client?
1. Safety
2. Physical illnesses
3. Paranoid delusions
4. Relationship avoidance

37. 1. Safety is the number one priority. The client lacks self-esteem, which contributes to her level of depression and feelings of personal ineffectiveness, which in turn may lead to suicidal thoughts. Physical illnesses are common with clients with anorexia nervosa, but they do not relate to this situation. Paranoid delusions refer to false ideas that others want to harm you. No evidence exists that this client is socially isolated.

CN: Safe, effective care environment; CNS: None; CL: Analyze

38. A nurse is developing a care plan for a family with a member who has anorexia nervosa. What is the **most** important information for the nurse to include?
1. Coping mechanisms that have been used in the past
2. Concerns about changes in lifestyle and daily activities
3. Rejection of feedback from family and significant others
4. Appropriate eating habits and social behaviors centering on eating

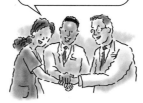

Care plans encourage staff to work toward the same goals.

38. 1. Examination of positive and negative coping mechanisms used by the family in the past will allow the nurse to build a new care plan specific to the family's strengths and weaknesses. The way this family copes with concerns is more important than the concerns themselves. Feedback from the family and significant others is vital when building a care plan. Eating habits and behaviors are symptoms of the way people cope with problems.

CN: Psychosocial integrity; CNS: None; CL: Apply

39. Which goal is **best** to help a client with anorexia nervosa recognize self-distortions?
1. Identify the client's misperceptions of self
2. Acknowledge immature and childlike behaviors
3. Determine the consequences of a faulty support system
4. Recognize the age-appropriate tasks to be accomplished

39. 1. Questioning the client's misperceptions and distortions will create doubt about how the client views himself. Acknowledging immature behaviors, or determining the consequences of a faulty support system will not promote client recognition of self-distortions. Recognizing the age-appropriate tasks to be accomplished will not help this client recognize distortions.

CN: Psychosocial integrity; CNS: None; CL: Analyze

40. Parents of a client with anorexia nervosa ask the nurse for information about the risk factors for this disorder. The nurse determines that the parents have a good understanding when they identify which risk factor?
1. Emotional lability, and the inability to be still
2. A high level of anxiety, and disorganized behavior
3. Low self-esteem, and problems with family relationships
4. A lack of life experience, and no opportunities to learn new skills

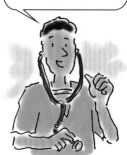

I don't doubt that you'll choose the correct answer.

40. 3. There are several risk factors for eating disorders, including low self-esteem, a history of depression, substance abuse, and dysfunctional family relationships. Anxiety and disorganized behavior could be signs of a psychotic disorder. Emotional lability and restlessness are symptoms of bipolar disorder. A lack of life experiences and an absence of opportunities to learn life skills may be a result of anorexia nervosa.

CN: Psychosocial integrity; CNS: None; CL: Analyze

CN: Client needs category   CNS: Client needs subcategory   CL: Cognitive level

41. A client with anorexia nervosa has started taking fluoxetine hydrochloride. Which adverse effect is **most** important for the nurse to monitor?
1. Drowsiness
2. Dry mouth
3. Light-headedness
4. Nausea

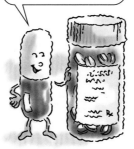

Knowing adverse reactions to key drugs is important.

41. 4. Nausea is an adverse reaction to fluoxetine hydrochloride that can compound the eating disorder problem, and the client should be closely monitored. Although the adverse reactions of drowsiness, dry mouth, or light-headedness may occur, they aren't likely to interfere with treatment, and are not the priority.
CN: Physiological integrity; CNS: Pharmacological and parenteral therapies; CL: Apply

42. A client who has been hospitalized during the past week for an eating disorder is quite concerned about being discharged today. Which responses, by the nurse, are appropriate? Select all that apply.
1. "I have set up a structured eating schedule for you to follow when you get home."
2. "You will need to have someone closely monitor you when you eat and right after you eat."
3. "I have set up follow-up treatment for you at the nearby outpatient clinic."
4. "I encourage you to participate in the eating disorder support group."
5. "We must create a maintenance food plan for you."

42. 3, 4, 5. Answers one and two are done while the client is still hospitalized.
CN: Psychosocial integrity; CNS: None; CL: Apply

43. A female client with anorexia nervosa tells a nurse that she has developed fine hair on most of her body. Which disorder would the nurse **most** likely expect to be associated with the client's anorexia nervosa?
1. Anemia
2. Osteoporosis
3. Dehydration
4. Electrolyte imbalance

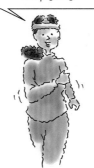

You're heading down the home stretch! Keep going!

43. 3. Lanugo is the growth of hair where it is not generally found, and is a result of severe malnutrition. Lanugo develops as an indication of dehydration due to starvation. When a client with anorexia nervosa has lanugo all over her body, the nurse should perform a more extensive assessment of the skin. Anemia is associated with hematological complications. While amenorrhea can contribute to osteoporosis, the resulting symptoms would be either hormonal or orthopedic in nature. Electrolyte imbalance is associated with body metabolism.
CN: Health promotion and maintenance; CNS: None; CL: Apply

44. A client with anorexia nervosa is talking to a nurse about group therapy. Which statement indicates that group therapy has helped this client?
1. "I feel I am different and I don't need a lot of friends."
2. "I will tell my parents it is not just me who has problems."
3. "I can see how to do things better and become my best."
4. "I think I have some unrealistic expectations of myself."

44. 4. A goal of group therapy is to provide methods to assess if personal expectations are unrealistic. Other goals are to learn to handle problems, not to blame parents or others, decrease perfectionist tendencies, decrease isolation, and learn to have healthy peer relationships.
CN: Psychosocial integrity; CNS: None; CL: Apply

45. A nurse is caring for a client with anorexia nervosa. The nurse and client are working on the goal of developing social relationships. The nurse determines that the client is meeting the goal when he:
   1. talks about the value of peer relationships.
   2. decides to talk to his parents about his friends.
   3. expresses the need to establish trusting relationships.
   4. attends an activity without prompting from others.

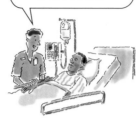

The client must agree to the goal or it won't work.

45. 4. When a client with anorexia nervosa attends an activity without prompting from others, it is a positive sign that the client is working toward developing social relationships. Talking about the value of relationships is also beneficial but is only the first step in establishing them. Talking to parents about friends is a start, but doesn't necessarily indicate that the client can establish relationships. Expressing the need to establish trusting relationships is a first step, but an indication of success would be actually initiating such a relationship.
CN: Psychosocial integrity; CNS: None; CL: Apply

46. What is the initial action a nurse should take when a young female client with anorexia nervosa says, "I need to eat something?"
   1. Provide a small portion of a healthy food
   2. Weigh the client before and after eating
   3. Ask the client what she thinks she can eat
   4. Suggest the client drink something before eating

46. 1. Small amounts of food will not overwhelm the client when given at frequent intervals. This will also not overtax the GI and cardiac systems. Weighing the client before and after meals is a useless, stress-provoking action. Asking the client questions may provoke anxiety. It's better to give the client food when she asks. Drinking something before eating isn't necessary. The fluid may prevent the client from being able to eat a sufficient amount of the food.
CN: Physiological integrity; CNS: Reduction of risk potential; CL: Apply

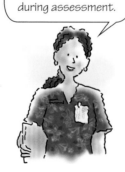

Redirection can be a helpful way to steer your client away from negative thinking.

47. A client with anorexia nervosa tells a nurse, "I feel so awful and inadequate." What is the nurse's **best** response?
   1. "You are just being too hard on yourself."
   2. "Someday, you will feel better about things."
   3. "Tell me something you like about yourself."
   4. "Maybe relaxing by yourself will help you feel better."

47. 3. This statement redirects the client to talk about positive aspects of self. The other options minimize her feelings, do not address the client's concerns, and do not help the client to change her self-image.
CN: Psychosocial integrity; CNS: None; CL: Apply

48. What is the **priority** nursing assessment of a client with an eating disorder?
   1. Cultural needs
   2. Substance abuse history
   3. Academic performance
   4. Level of danger to self

The term priority *indicates that you should select the answer which would be of first concern during assessment.*

48. 4. The priority assessment should be to determine if the client is a danger to herself. Cultural needs, substance abuse history, and academic performance are an important part of assessment, but not the priority.
CN: Safe, effective care environment; CNS: Management of care; CL: Analyze

49. An adolescent female client with anorexia nervosa starts outpatient treatment. Which client statement indicates an understanding of the eating disorder?
   1. "I am not worried because no one ever dies from anorexia."
   2. "I still feel fat even though I am told that I am not."
   3. "My old school friends are not important to me anymore."
   4. "I do not feel right unless I do an intense workout every day."

49. 2. A client with anorexia nervosa shows a basic understanding of the disorder if she can talk about feeling fat even though she's actually underweight, or if she expresses an intense fear of gaining weight. Anorexia nervosa has a mortality of approximately 10% to 15%. People with eating disorders tend to isolate themselves from friends and family members because of their intense focus on food, weight, and exercise. A client with anorexia nervosa may exercise compulsively to prevent weight gain. This behavior indicates continuing presence of the eating disorder.
CN: Psychosocial integrity; CNS: None; CL: Analyze

CN: Client needs category   CNS: Client needs subcategory   CL: Cognitive level

50. What is the **most** important question for a nurse to ask when assessing the self-esteem of a client with anorexia nervosa?
   1. "How would you describe yourself to others?"
   2. "What activities do you enjoy doing with your friends?"
   3. "Do you play any sports at school or in your community?"
   4. "How do you decide how to spend your free time?"

51. Which psychosocial finding should a nurse expect when assessing a client with anorexia nervosa?
   1. Avoidant behavior
   2. Antisocial behavior
   3. Introverted behavior
   4. Hypervigilant behavior

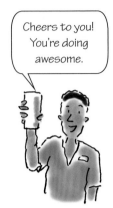

Cheers to you! You're doing awesome.

52. A nurse notes severe hypocalcemia in a client with anorexia nervosa. Which history finding supports a diagnosis of osteoporosis?
   1. Eating a vegetarian diet
   2. Drinking well water
   3. Going scuba diving
   4. Smoking cigarettes

53. A female client with anorexia nervosa is receiving care from her family after successfully completing the refeeding stage of treatment. Which nursing intervention takes **priority** at this time?
   1. Providing a strong support system and opportunities to do reality testing
   2. Teaching the family stress-reduction skills to help promote family harmony
   3. Promoting anticipatory grieving over the loss each family member is experiencing
   4. Assisting the family to work on the issues of autonomy and separation

54. A client with bulimia nervosa has a history of severe gastrointestinal problems caused by excessive purging. What is the client at risk of developing?
   1. Renal calculi
   2. Esophageal tears
   3. Focal seizures
   4. Muscle atrophy

50. 1. Clients with anorexia nervosa tend to have low self-esteem even if they are high achievers in school, activities, and sports. Asking for a self-description can uncover the client's distorted body image and low self-esteem. Questions about activities with friends, involvement in sports, or how the client decides to spend her free time do not elicit information about self-esteem.
CN: Psychosocial integrity; CNS: None; CL: Analyze

51. 3. Clients with anorexia nervosa typically demonstrate introverted behavior. Clients with bulimia tend to show avoidant and dependent behaviors. Clients with eating disorders do not necessarily demonstrate antisocial behavior. Hypervigilant behavior is common in clients with post-traumatic stress disorder, not eating disorders.
CN: Psychosocial integrity; CNS: None; CL: Analyze

52. 4. Hypocalcemia and cigarette smoking increase the risk for osteoporosis. Eating a vegetarian diet, drinking well water, and going scuba diving do not predispose the client to osteoporosis.
CN: Physiological integrity; CNS: Reduction of risk potential; CL: Analyze

53. 4. When a client with anorexia nervosa successfully completes the refeeding stage of treatment, the family must work on separation and individuation of the client, and on decreasing family rigidity and over protectiveness. Although the client needs a strong support system, developing a sense of self is more important at this time. Reality testing isn't a typical problem in clients with eating disorders. All families can benefit from learning stress-reduction skills; however, at this time, these skills take lower priority than developing client independence. Anticipatory grieving isn't relevant for family members of a client with an eating disorder.
CN: Psychosocial integrity; CNS: None; CL: Apply

54. 2. A bulimic client with severe gastrointestinal problems from excessive purging is at increased risk for esophageal tears and irritation or esophagitis. Although clients with eating disorders may develop renal calculi, this client is at greater risk for developing esophageal tears. Focal seizures and muscle atrophy are not related to severe gastrointestinal problems.
CN: Physiological integrity; CNS: Reduction of risk potential; CL: Analyze

55. A nurse is caring for a client with anorexia nervosa. Which interventions would be appropriate for this client? Select all that apply.
1. Provide small, frequent meals
2. Monitor weight gain
3. Allow the client to skip meals until the antidepressant levels are therapeutic
4. Encourage the client to keep a journal
5. Encourage the client to eat three substantial meals per day

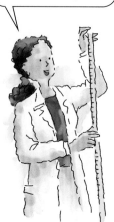

Good for you! It looks like you really measure up!

55. 1, 2, 4. Due to self-starvation, clients with anorexia can rarely tolerate large meals three times per day. Small, frequent meals may be tolerated better by the anorexic client, and they provide a way to gradually increase daily caloric intake. The nurse should monitor the client's weight carefully because a client with anorexia may try to hide weight loss. The client may be emotionally restrained and afraid to express her feelings; therefore, keeping a journal can serve as an outlet for these feelings. An anorexic client is already underweight and should not be permitted to skip meals.

CN: Health promotion and maintenance; CNS: None; CL: Analyze

Part IV

Maternal—Neonatal Care

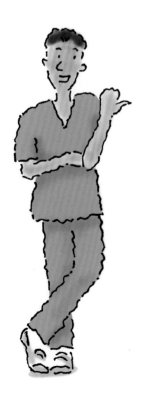

Chapter 22

Antepartum Care

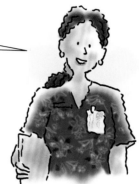

Looking for information about antepartum care before tackling this chapter? Visit **www.acog.org**, the American Congress of Obstetricians and Gynecologists' Web site.

1. During a routine prenatal examination, a client who is at 32 weeks' gestation becomes dizzy, lightheaded, and pale. After placing the client in a supine position, what is the **priority** nursing action?
 1. Listen to fetal heart tones
 2. Take the client's blood pressure
 3. Ask the client to breathe deeply
 4. Turn the client on her left side

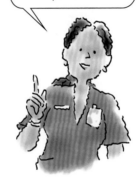

Which intervention is of primary importance?

1. 4. As the uterus gets larger, it increases pressure on the inferior vena cava. This inhibits venous return causing dizziness, lightheadedness, and pallor when the client is supine. Turning the client on her left side relieves the pressure on the vena cava and restores venous return. Although they're valuable assessments, listening to fetal heart tone and measuring maternal blood pressure don't alleviate the symptoms. Deep breathing has no effect on venous return, and will not relieve this client's symptoms.
CN: Safe, effective care environment; CNS: Management of care; CL: Analyze

2. A nurse is assessing a client at 33-weeks' gestation. Leopold's maneuvers indicate that the fetus is in a breech position. Where can fetal heart tones **best** be heard?
 1. Midway between the symphysis pubis and the umbilicus
 2. Right lower quadrant of the abdomen
 3. Right upper quadrant of the abdomen
 4. Above the level of the umbilicus

2. 4. When the fetus is in the breech position, fetal heart tones are best heard at or above the level of the umbilicus.
CN: Health promotion and maintenance; CNS: None; CL: Apply

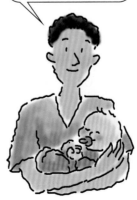

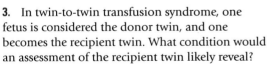

Careful. Question 3 asks about the recipient twin, not the donor.

3. In twin-to-twin transfusion syndrome, one fetus is considered the donor twin, and one becomes the recipient twin. What condition would an assessment of the recipient twin likely reveal?
 1. Anemia
 2. Oligohydramnios
 3. Polycythemia
 4. Small fetus

3. 3. The recipient twin in twin-to-twin transfusion syndrome is transfused by the donor twin. The recipient twin then becomes polycythemic, and often has heart failure due to circulatory overload. The donor twin becomes anemic. The recipient twin has polyhydramnios, not oligohydramnios. The recipient twin is usually large, whereas the donor twin is often small.
CN: Physiological integrity; CNS: Physiological adaptation; CL: Analyze

CN: Client needs category   CNS: Client needs subcategory   CL: Cognitive level

4. A client who reports painless vaginal bleeding at 28 weeks' gestation is diagnosed with placenta previa. The placental edge reaches the internal os. Which type of placenta previa should the nurse suspect?
1. Low-lying placenta previa
2. Marginal placenta previa
3. Partial placenta previa
4. Total placenta previa

5. Which procedure or treatment should the nurse anticipate for a client with a placenta implanted in the lower uterine segment?
1. Stat culture and sensitivity
2. Antenatal steroids after 34 weeks' gestation
3. A vaginal ultrasound examination every two to three weeks
4. Scheduled birth of the fetus before fetal maturity in a hemodynamically stable mother

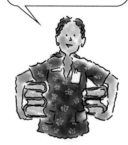

I feel like I'm attached at the hip to these books.

6. The nurse is teaching a client with painless vaginal bleeding at 28 weeks' gestation who has just been diagnosed with placenta previa. The nurse determines that teaching has been effective when the client states:
1. "I am still able to have sexual intercourse with my husband."
2. "I can continue to go to exercise class three times a week."
3. "I will still be able to fly to Florida for the holidays."
4. "I need to limit my activity and rest."

7. The nurse is teaching a client who has developed placenta accreta and a history of placenta previa. Which explanation of this condition would be the **most** correct?
1. The placenta invades the myometrium.
2. The placenta covers the cervical os.
3. The placenta penetrates the myometrium.
4. The placenta attaches to the myometrium.

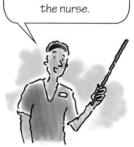

Client teaching is an important role for the nurse.

4. 2. A marginal placenta previa is characterized by implantation of the placenta in the margin of the cervical os, not covering the os. A low-lying placenta is implanted in the lower uterine segment but doesn't reach the cervical os. A partial placenta previa is the partial occlusion of the cervical os by the placenta. The internal cervical os is completely covered by the placenta in a total placenta previa.
CN: Physiological integrity; CNS: Physiological adaptation; CL: Analyze

5. 3. Placenta previa occurs when the placenta is implanted in the lower uterine segment. Fetal surveillance through ultrasound examination every two to three weeks is indicated to evaluate fetal growth, amniotic fluid, and placental location. A stat culture and sensitivity would be done for severe bleeding or maternal or fetal distress, and isn't part of anticipatory management. Antenatal steroids may be given to clients between 24 and 34 weeks' gestation to enhance fetal lung maturity. Birth of the fetus should be delayed until fetal lung maturity is attained if the mother is hemodynamically stable.
CN: Physiological integrity; CNS: Reduction of risk potential; CL: Analyze

6. 4. The client with placenta previa needs to restrict her activities, and may be placed on bed rest. She should avoid sexual intercourse, strenuous activity, and long-distance travel.
CN: Physiological integrity; CNS: Reduction of risk potential; CL: Analyze

7. 4. Placenta accreta is an abnormal attachment of the placenta to the myometrium of the uterus. When the placenta invades the myometrium, it's called placenta increta. When the placenta covers the cervical os, it's called placenta previa. Placenta percreta occurs when the villi of the placenta penetrate the myometrium to the serosa level.
CN: Physiological integrity; CNS: Physiological adaptation; CL: Apply

8. The nurse is caring for a client suspected of having a hydatidiform mole. Which signs and symptoms confirm this diagnosis? Select all that apply.
1. Heavy, bright red bleeding every 21 days
2. Fetal cardiac motion after six weeks' gestation
3. Benign tumors found in the smooth muscle of the uterus
4. Snowstorm pattern on an ultrasound with no fetus or gestational sac
5. Maternal hypertension early in the second trimester.

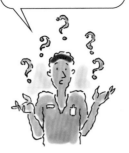

Sometimes it's hard to keep the symptoms straight, isn't it?

8. 4, 5. Ultrasound is the technique of choice used to diagnose a hydatidiform mole. The chorionic villi of a molar pregnancy resemble a snowstorm pattern on an ultrasound. Another sign of hydatidiform mole is development of hypertension early in the second trimester, which differs from the development of preeclamsia later in the pregnancy. Bleeding with a hydatidiform mole is often dark brown, and can occur erratically for weeks or months. There is no cardiac activity because there is no fetus. Benign tumors found in the smooth muscle of the uterus are leiomyomas or fibroids.
CN: Physiological integrity; CNS: Reduction of risk potential; CL: Analyze

9. A 21-year-old client who has just been diagnosed with having a hydatidiform mole asks the nurse about risk factors. What is the nurse's **best** response?
1. "Most prevalent in clients in their 20s or 30s"
2. "Clients with high socioeconomic status"
3. "Primigravida clients"
4. "Having a previous molar gestation"

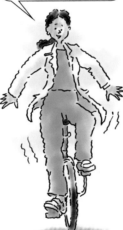

Now you're getting up to speed. Way to go!

9. 4. A previous molar gestation increases a woman's risk for developing a subsequent molar gestation by four to five times. Adolescents and women age 40 years and older are at increased risk for molar pregnancies. Multigravidas, especially women with a prior pregnancy loss, and women with lower socioeconomic status are at an increased risk for this problem.
CN: Health promotion and maintenance; CNS: None; CL: Analyze

10. A 21-year-old client arrives at the emergency department with a report of cramping, abdominal pain, and mild vaginal bleeding. A pelvic examination shows a left adnexal mass that is tender when palpated. Culdocentesis shows blood in the cul-de-sac. Which condition should the nurse suspect?
1. Abruptio placentae
2. Ectopic pregnancy
3. Hydatidiform mole
4. Pelvic inflammatory disease (PID)

10. 2. Most ectopic pregnancies don't appear as obvious life-threatening medical emergencies. Ectopic pregnancies must be considered in any sexually active woman of childbearing age who reports menstrual irregularity, cramping abdominal pain, and mild vaginal bleeding. The client with an ectopic pregnancy, who is experiencing blood loss, will have blood in the cul-de-sac. PID, abruptio placentae, and hydatidiform moles won't show blood in the cul-de-sac.
CN: Physiological integrity; CNS: Reduction of risk potential; CL: Analyze

11. The nurse assesses a client at 34 weeks' gestation who has arrived at the emergency department with severe abdominal pain, uterine tenderness, and increased uterine tone. The client denies vaginal bleeding. The external fetal monitor shows fetal distress with severe, variable decelerations. Which condition does this client mostly likely have?
1. Abruptio placentae
2. Ectopic pregnancy
3. Molar pregnancy
4. Placenta previa

11. 1. A client with severe abruptio placentae will often have severe abdominal pain. The uterus will have increased tone with little, or no, return to resting tone between contractions. The fetus will begin to show signs of distress, with decelerations in the heart rate, or even fetal death if the placental separation is large. An ectopic pregnancy, which usually occurs in the fallopian tubes, would rupture well before 34 weeks. A molar pregnancy generally would be detected before 34 weeks' gestation, and no fetal heart sounds would be present. Placenta previa usually involves painless vaginal bleeding without uterine contractions.
CN: Physiological integrity; CNS: Reduction of risk potential; CL: Analyze

CN: Client needs category   CNS: Client needs subcategory   CL: Cognitive level

12. During a routine visit to the clinic, a client tells the nurse that she may be pregnant. The health care provider orders a pregnancy test. Which indicator would most accurately confirm this client's pregnancy?
1. Increase in human chorionic gonadotropin (HCG)
2. Increased thyroxine level
3. Increase in luteinizing hormone (LH)
4. Elevated IgM

12. 1. HCG levels increase in a woman's blood and urine until the fifteenth week of pregnancy. Thyroxine and luteinizing hormone (LH) values aren't indicative of pregnancy. IgM antibodies are antibodies found in blood and lymph fluid and are the first type of antibody made in response to an infection

CN: Health promotion and maintenance; CNS: None; CL: Apply

13. A nurse is assessing a pregnant client in her second trimester. The nurse understands that this client's respiratory status should show:
1. increased tidal volume.
2. increased expiratory volume.
3. decreased inspiratory capacity.
4. decreased oxygen consumption.

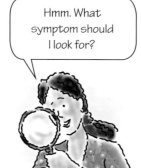

Hmm. What symptom should I look for?

13. 1. A pregnant client breathes deeper, which increases the tidal volume of gas moving in and out of the respiratory tract with each breath. The expiratory volume and residual volume decrease as the pregnancy progresses. The inspiratory capacity increases during pregnancy. Oxygen consumption is 15% to 20% greater in a pregnant client than in a non-pregnant client.

CN: Health promotion and maintenance; CNS: None; CL: Apply

14. A client is scheduled for amniocentesis. What **priority** intervention should the nurse implement?
1. Tell the client to drink 34 oz (1 L) of water
2. Have the client void
3. Instruct the client to fast for 12 hours
4. Place the client on her left side

14. 2. Before amniocentesis, the client should empty the bladder which reduces the risk of bladder perforation. This client doesn't need to drink fluids or fast before amniocentesis. A client would be placed in a supine position for an amniocentesis.

CN: Health promotion and maintenance; CNS: None; CL: Apply

15. The nurse is taking an initial history on a pregnant client, who asks about the chances of having dizygotic twins. The nurse correctly states:
1. "They occur most frequently in Asian women."
2. "There's a decreased risk with increased parity."
3. "There's an increased risk with increased maternal age."
4. "There's no increased risk with the use of fertility drugs."

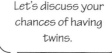

Let's discuss your chances of having twins.

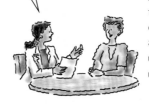

15. 3. The risk of dizygotic twinning is increased with maternal age. It is also most prevalent in black women, and least prevalent in Asian women. Multi parity, and the use of fertility drugs increase the risk of dizygotic twinning as well. The incidence of monozygotic twins is not affected by race, age, parity, heredity, or fertility medications.

CN: Health promotion and maintenance; CNS: None; CL: Apply

16. A client in her fifth month of pregnancy is having a routine clinic visit. Which common condition would the nurse asses for in the client's second trimester?
1. Mastitis
2. Metabolic alkalosis
3. Physiologic anemia
4. Hyperemesis

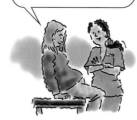

A pregnant client's needs may vary in each trimester.

16. 3. Hemoglobin and hematocrit values decrease during pregnancy as the increase in plasma volume exceeds the increase in red blood cell production. Mastitis is an infection characterized by a swollen tender breast and flulike symptoms. This condition is most frequently seen in breastfeeding clients. Alterations in acid-base balance during pregnancy result in a state of respiratory alkalosis, compensated by mild metabolic acidosis. Hyperemesis usually occurs during the first trimester of pregnancy.

CN: Health promotion and maintenance; CNS: None; CL: Apply

CN: Client needs category   CNS: Client needs subcategory   CL: Cognitive level

17. A 21-year-old client at six weeks' gestation is diagnosed with hyperemesis gravidarum. The nurse understands that this client is most at risk of developing:
  1. bowel perforation.
  2. electrolyte imbalance.
  3. miscarriage.
  4. gestational hypertension.

17. **2.** Excessive vomiting in clients with hyperemesis gravidarum often causes weight loss and fluid, electrolyte, and acid-base imbalances. Clients with severe hyperemesis may have a low-birth-weight infant, but the disorder generally isn't life threatening to the fetus. Gestational hypertension and bowel perforation aren't related to hyperemesis. The effects of hyperemesis on the fetus depend on the severity of the disorder.
CN: Physiological integrity; CNS: Reduction of risk potential; CL: Analyze

18. A 29-year-old client has gestational diabetes. The nurse is teaching her about managing glucose levels. Which therapy would be **most** appropriate for this client?
  1. Diet
  2. Long-acting insulin
  3. Oral hypoglycemic drugs
  4. Glucagon

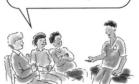

Clients with gestational diabetes need nutritional counseling.

18. **1.** Clients with gestational diabetes usually manage their glucose level by adjusting their diet. Long-acting insulin usually isn't needed for blood glucose control in the client with gestational diabetes. Oral hypoglycemic drugs are contraindicated in pregnancy. Glucagon raises blood glucose, and is used to treat hypoglycemic reactions.
CN: Health promotion and maintenance; CNS: None; CL: Apply

19. A client who is pregnant has developed preeclampsia. She asks the nurse why magnesium sulfate has been prescribed for her. What is the nurse's **best** response?
  1. "It prevents hemorrhage."
  2. "It prevents hypertension."
  3. "It prevents hypomagnesemia."
  4. "It prevents seizures."

19. **4.** The anticonvulsant mechanism of magnesium is believed to depress seizure foci in the brain and peripheral neuromuscular blockade. Magnesium does not help prevent hemorrhage in preeclamptic clients. Antihypertensive drugs, other than magnesium, are preferred for sustained hypertension. Hypomagnesemia is not a complication of preeclampsia.
CN: Physiological integrity; CNS: Pharmacological and parenteral therapies; CL: Analyze

20. While assessing a client in her 24th week of pregnancy, the nurse learns that the client has been experiencing signs and symptoms of pregnancy-induced hypertension, or preeclampsia. Which sign or symptom helps differentiate preeclampsia from eclampsia?
  1. Seizures
  2. Headaches
  3. Blurred vision
  4. Weight gain

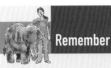

Remember

"Magnesium sulfate sidelines seizures."

The anticonvulsant mechanism of magnesium is believed to depress seizure foci in the brain.

20. **1.** The primary difference between preeclampsia and eclampsia is the occurrence of seizures, which occur when the client becomes eclamptic. Headaches, blurred vision, weight gain, increased blood pressure, and edema of the hands and feet are all indicative of preeclampsia.
CN: Physiological integrity; CNS: Physiological adaptation; CL: Apply

21. A pregnant client has a negative contraction stress test (CST). How does the nurse interpret this result?

1. Persistent late decelerations in fetal heart beat occurred, with at least three contractions in a 10-minute window
2. Accelerations of fetal heartbeat occurred, with at least 15 beats/min, lasting 15 to 30 seconds in a 20-minute period
3. Accelerations of fetal heartbeat were absent, or didn't increase by 15 beats/min for 15 to 30 seconds in a 20-minute period
4. Fetal heart rate (FHR) variability, and no decelerations from contraction in a 10-minute period in which there were three contractions.

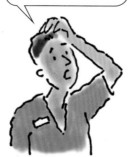

What does a contraction stress test measure?

21. 4. A CST measures the fetal response to uterine contractions. Normal test results are called negative. A negative CST shows good FHR variability with no decelerations from uterine contractions. If three contractions occur during a 10-minute period of stimulation or and there are no late decelerations in the baby's heart rate, the baby is expected to be able to handle labor. Persistent late decelerations with contractions indicate a positive CST. Positive results are abnormal and indicate the baby's heart rate gets slower (decelerates) and stays slow after the contraction (late decelerations).
CN: Physiological integrity; CNS: Reduction of risk potential;
CL: Analyze

22. A pregnant client with sickle cell anemia has an increased risk for having a sickle cell crisis during pregnancy. The nurse anticipates that aggressive management of a sickle cell crisis would include:

1. antihypertensive agents.
2. diuretic agents.
3. IV fluids.
4. acetaminophen for pain.

22. 3. A sickle cell crisis during pregnancy is usually managed by exchange transfusion, oxygen, and IV fluids. Antihypertensive drugs are not usually necessary. Diuretics wouldn't be used unless fluid overload resulted from administration of IV fluids. The client will usually require an analgesic stronger than acetaminophen to control the pain of a sickle cell crisis.
CN: Physiological integrity; CNS: Reduction of risk potential;
CL: Analyze

23. The nurse is performing a cardiac assessment on a pregnant client. Which finding would the nurse recognize as normal?

1. Fixed splitting of the second heart sound
2. Increased systemic vascular resistance
3. Endocarditis
4. Systolic murmur

23. 4. Systolic murmurs are heard in up to 90% of pregnant clients, and the murmur disappears soon after birth. Cardiac tamponade, which causes effusion of fluid into the pericardial sac, is not normal during pregnancy. Despite an increase in the heart's intravascular volume and workload associated with pregnancy, heart failure is not normal during pregnancy. Endocarditis is most often associated with a bacterial infection in the blood stream that invades the heart muscle and isn't a normal finding.
CN: Health promotion and maintenance; CNS: None;
CL: Apply

24. A 42-year-old client presents for her first prenatal visit at 16 weeks' gestation. She has severe morning sickness and no fetal heart tones. Her blood pressure is 150/100 mmHg. Her fundal height is 24 cm. Which condition is **most** likely indicated by these symptoms?

1. Abruptio placenta
2. Placenta previa
3. Normal pregnancy
4. Hydatidiform mole

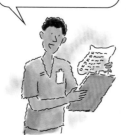

The words most likely can help you focus on the correct answer.

24. 4. The incidence of hydatidiform mole, also known as gestational trophoblastic disease, is higher in women over 35 years of age, who have low protein intake, and are of Asian heritage. Molar pregnancy should be suspected in clients who have bleeding during the first half of their pregnancy, hyperemesis, pregnancy-induced hypertension, an enlarged uterus, and absent fetal heart tones. These signs and symptoms do not pertain to the other conditions.
CN: Health promotion and maintenance; CNS: None;
CL: Apply

25. A client with gestational hypertension is receiving magnesium sulfate to prevent seizure activity. The nurse reviews the client's magnesium level and identifies a therapeutic level as:
1. 4 to 7 mEq/L.
2. 8 to 10 mEq/L.
3. 10 to 12 mEq/L.
4. greater than 15 mEq/L.

25. 1. The therapeutic level of magnesium for clients with gestational hypertension is 4 to 7 mEq/L. A serum level of 8 to 10 mEq/L may cause the absence of reflexes in the client. Serum levels of 10 to 12 mEq/L may cause respiratory depression, and a serum level greater than 15 mEq/L may result in respiratory paralysis.
CN: Physiological integrity; CNS: Pharmacological and parenteral therapies; CL: Apply

26. A client is receiving IV magnesium sulfate for severe preeclampsia. Which is the **priority** assessment for this client?
1. Anemia
2. Decreased urine output
3. Hyperreflexia
4. Increased respiratory rate

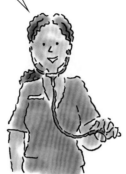
I think I hear the answer to question 26.

26. 2. Decreased urine output may occur in clients receiving IV magnesium. Urine output should be greater than 30 ml/hr because magnesium is excreted through the kidneys, and can easily accumulate to toxic levels. Anemia is not associated with magnesium therapy. Magnesium infusions may cause a depression of deep tendon reflexes or hyporeflexia. A client should be monitored for respiratory depression and paralysis when serum magnesium levels reach approximately 15 mEq/L.
CN: Physiological integrity; CNS: Pharmacological and parenteral therapies; CL: Analyze

27. The nurse is planning care for a client receiving IV magnesium sulfate for hypertension. Which medication should the nurse have available for an emergency?
1. Calcium gluconate
2. Hydralazine
3. Naloxone
4. Rho(D) immune globulin

27. 1. Calcium gluconate is the antidote for magnesium toxicity. Ten milliliters of 10% calcium gluconate is given IV push over three to five minutes to correct the effects of toxicity. Hydralazine is given for sustained elevated blood pressures in preeclamptic clients. Naloxone is used to correct narcotic toxicity. Rho(D) immune globulin is given to women with Rh-negative blood to prevent antibody formation from Rh-positive conceptions.
CN: Physiological integrity; CNS: Pharmacological and parenteral therapies; CL: Analyze

28. A client is screened for tuberculosis during her first prenatal visit. An intradermal injection of purified protein derivative (PPD) of the tuberculin bacilli is administered by the nurse. This client is considered to have a positive test when:
1. an indurated wheal under 10 mm in diameter appears in 6 to 12 hours.
2. an indurated wheal over 10 mm in diameter appears in 48 to 72 hours.
3. a flattened area under 10 mm in diameter appears in 6 to 12 hours.
4. a flattened area over 10 mm in diameter appears in 48 to 72 hours.

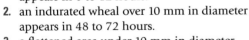
A mysterious wheal will appear within the next few days.

28. 2. A positive PPD result would be an indurated wheal over 10 mm in diameter that appears in 48 to 72 hours. The area must be a raised wheal, and not a flattened, to be considered positive.
CN: Physiological integrity; CNS: Reduction of risk potential; CL: Apply

29. A 23-year-old client who is at 27 weeks' gestation arrives at her health care provider's office with reports of fever, nausea, vomiting, malaise, unilateral flank pain, and costovertebral angle tenderness. Which diagnosis is **most** likely?
1. Interstitial cystitis
2. Bacterial vaginosis
3. Pyelonephritis
4. Urinary tract infection (UTI)

29. 3. The symptoms indicate acute pyelonephritis, a serious condition in a pregnant client. Interstitial cystitis causes bladder pressure and pain, not the symptoms listed. Bacterial vaginosis causes milky white vaginal discharge but no systemic symptoms. Symptoms of a UTI include dysuria, urgency, frequency, and suprapubic tenderness.
CN: Physiological integrity; CNS: Reduction of risk potential; CL: Analyze

30. Clients with which condition would be appropriate for trial of labor after cesarean section (TOLAC), after a prior cesarean birth?
1. Complete placenta previa
2. Invasive cervical cancer
3. Premature rupture of membranes
4. Prior classical cesarean birth

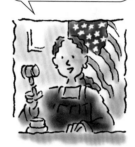

This isn't my kind of trial.

30. 3. TOLAC refers to attempted labor during a vaginal birth after cesarean (VBAC). Clients with a premature rupture of membranes are permitted a trial of labor after a previous cesarean birth. Clients with placenta previa, or a prior classical cesarean birth shouldn't be given a trial of labor due to the risk of uterine rupture or severe bleeding. In the absence of contraindications, a woman with one previous cesarean birth with a lower transverse uterine incision is a candidate. A woman who has had two or more previous cesarean deliveries with lower transverse uterine incisions, who has no contraindications is also a candidate. A client with invasive cervical cancer should be scheduled for a cesarean birth.
CN: Physiological integrity; CNS: Physiological adaptation; CL: Analyze

31. A nurse is teaching a client who received a dose of Rho(D) immune globulin at 28 weeks' gestation to prevent Rh isoimmunization. Which statement **most** accurately describes isoimmunization?
1. Rh-positive maternal blood crosses into fetal blood, stimulating fetal antibodies.
2. Rh-positive fetal blood crosses into maternal blood, stimulating maternal antibodies.
3. Rh-negative fetal blood crosses into maternal blood, stimulating maternal antibodies.
4. Rh-negative maternal blood crosses into fetal blood, stimulating fetal antibodies.

31. 2. Rh isoimmunization occurs when Rh-positive fetal blood cells cross into the maternal circulation and stimulate maternal antibody production. In subsequent pregnancies with an Rh-positive fetus, maternal antibodies may cross back into the fetal circulation and destroy the fetal blood cells.
CN: Physiological integrity; CNS: Reduction of risk potential; CL: Apply

32. The nurse is administering Rho(D) immune globulin to a pregnant client at 28 weeks' gestation. Which dose would be appropriate for this client?
1. 50 mcg in a sensitized client
2. 50 mcg in an unsensitized client
3. 300 mcg in a sensitized client
4. 300 mcg in an unsensitized client

32. 4. An Rh-negative unsensitized woman should be given 300 mcg of Rho(D) immune globulin at 28 weeks' gestation after an indirect Coombs test verifies that sensitization has not occurred. For a first trimester abortion or ectopic pregnancy, 50 mcg of Rho(D) immune globulin is given. The administration of Rho(D) immune globulin to a sensitized client is not effective.
CN: Physiological integrity; CNS: Pharmacological and parenteral therapies; CL: Analyze

33. A client hospitalized for preterm labor tells the nurse that she's having occasional contractions. Which nursing intervention would be the **most** appropriate?
1. Explain to the client the possible complications of preterm birth
2. Tell the client to ambulate in the hall to see if the contractions will lessen or stop
3. Encourage the client to empty her bladder, give IV fluids, and encourage oral fluids
4. Notify anesthesia for immediate epidural placement to relieve the pain associated with contractions

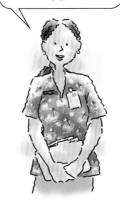

It may be premature. But I think you're doing great!

33. 3. An empty bladder and adequate hydration may help decrease or stop labor contractions. Teaching potential complications is likely to increase this client's anxiety rather than help with relaxation. Walking may cause contractions to become stronger. It would be inappropriate to call anesthesia and have an epidural placed because further assessment of contractions is necessary.
CN: Physiological integrity; CNS: Reduction of risk potential; CL: Apply

34. A client's prenatal history shows her to be a 23-year-old gravida 4, para 2. The nurse correctly interprets this history when she states:
1. "This client has been pregnant four times, and has had two miscarriages."
2. "This client has been pregnant four times, and has had two children born after 20 weeks' gestation."
3. "This client has been pregnant four times, and has had two cesarean deliveries."
4. "This client has been pregnant four times, and has had two spontaneous abortions."

34. 2. Gravida refers to the number of times a client has been pregnant. Para refers to the number of viable children born after 20 weeks' gestation. Therefore, the client who is gravida 4, para 2 has been pregnant four times and delivered two live infants.
CN: Health promotion and maintenance; CNS: None; CL: Analyze

35. A nurse is planning the care of a pregnant client. Which condition would require more frequent office visits?
1. Blood type O positive
2. A first pregnancy at 33 years of age
3. A history of allergy to honey bee pollen
4. A history of insulin-dependent diabetes mellitus

35. 4. A client with a history of diabetes has an increased risk for perinatal complications, including hypertension, preeclampsia, and neonatal hypoglycemia. This client should be closely monitored. A first pregnancy at 33-years-of-age, without other risk factors does not increase risk, nor do environmental allergens, or type O positive blood.
CN: Safe, effective care environment; CNS: Management of care; CL: Apply

36. To detect life-threatening complications as early as possible in a client receiving a tocolytic agent, the nurse should be alert for:
1. serum blood glucose level of 140 mg/dl.
2. maternal heart rate of 54 beats/min.
3. bilateral crackles on lung auscultation.
4. weakened carotid pulse.

Some complications require prompt action.

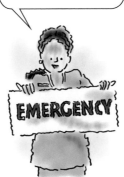

EMERGENCY

36. 3. Tocolytics are used to stop labor contractions. The most common adverse effect associated with the use of these drugs is pulmonary edema. Bilateral crackles on lung auscultation is a sign of pulmonary edema, and prompt action would be required. A serum glucose level of 140 mg/dl is elevated, and should be reported, but is not life threatening. Tocolytics may cause tachycardia and increased cardiac output with bounding arterial pulsations.
CN: Physiological integrity; CNS: Pharmacological and parenteral therapies; CL: Analyze

CN: Client needs category   CNS: Client needs subcategory   CL: Cognitive level

37. A client has been in early labor, with contractions ever 10 to 12 minutes, for the past 12 hours with no progression. What medication should the nurse anticipate to help stimulate this client's uterine contractions?
1. Estrogen
2. Magnesium sulfate
3. Oxytocin
4. Progesterone

37. 3. Oxytocin is the hormone responsible for stimulating uterine contractions. Pitocin, the synthetic form, has similar action, and may be given to some clients to induce or augment uterine contractions. Although estrogen plays a role in uterine contractions, it is not given in synthetic form to help uterine contractility. Progesterone has a relaxing effect on the uterus. Magnesium sulfate is used for maternal preeclampsia. It is not a tocolytic agent.
CN: Physiological integrity; CNS: Pharmacological and parenteral therapies; CL: Apply

38. A client asks the nurse when maternal and fetal blood are exchanged during a pregnancy. What is the nurse's **most** accurate response?
1. Conception
2. Nine-weeks' gestation, when the fetal heart is well developed
3. The third trimester (32 to 34 weeks' gestation)
4. Maternal and fetal blood are never exchanged

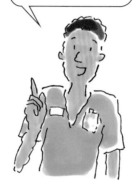

The resting or sleeping position is important in the later stages of pregnancy.

38. 4. Only nutrients and waste products are transferred across the placenta. Blood exchange never occurs between mother and fetus. No intermingling of maternal and fetal blood occurs in the placenta. Complications and some medical procedures can cause an accidental exchange of blood.
CN: Physiological integrity; CNS: Physiological adaptation; CL: Apply

39. A pregnant client asks the nurse why she should lie on her left side when resting or sleeping in the later stages of pregnancy. What is the **best** response by the nurse?
1. To facilitate digestion
2. To facilitate bladder emptying
3. To prevent compression of the inferior vena cava
4. To avoid the development of fetal anomalies

39. 3. The weight of the pregnant uterus is sufficiently heavy to compress the inferior vena cava, which can impair blood flow to the uterus, and decrease oxygen to the fetus. The side-lying position hasn't been shown to prevent fetal anomalies, nor does it facilitate bladder emptying or digestion.
CN: Physiological integrity; CNS: Reduction of risk potential; CL: Analyze

40. A pregnant client voices concerns about her perceived lack of fetal movement. How should the nurse **best** respond to this client?
1. "Start taking two prenatal vitamins."
2. "Take a warm bath to facilitate fetal movement."
3. "Eat foods that have a high sugar content to enhance fetal movement."
4. "Lie down once a day, and count the number of fetal movements for 15 to 30 minutes."

40. 4. Having the client lie down once a day will allow her to concentrate on detecting fetal movement. When the mother is actively walking around, it tends to soothe the fetus, and promote fetal sleep. Instructing this client to take additional prenatal vitamins is not recommended. Fat-soluble vitamins can be toxic when taken in excess. Taking a warm bath is also likely to soothe and relax the fetus. There is a risk for hyperthermia if bath water is too warm, or the client is immersed for too long. Eating sugary foods is not recommended, as some pregnant clients are more susceptible to cavities and hyperglycemia.
CN: Health promotion and maintenance; CNS: None; CL: Apply

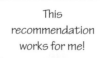

This recommendation works for me!

41. A pregnant client reports swelling in her feet and ankles. What is the **most** appropriate intervention for the nurse to recommend?
1. Limit fluid intake
2. Buy walking shoes
3. Sit and elevate the feet
4. Start taking a diuretic as needed daily

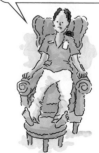

41. 3. Elevating the feet while seated will promote venous return and therefore decrease foot and ankle edema. Limiting fluid intake is not recommended unless there are additional medical complications such as heart failure. Buying walking shoes won't necessarily decrease edema. Diuretics are not recommended during pregnancy because it's important to maintain adequate circulatory volume.
CN: Physiological integrity; CNS: Basic care and comfort; CL: Apply

CN: Client needs category   CNS: Client needs subcategory   CL: Cognitive level

42. Which intervention should a nurse recommend to a client who has severe heartburn during her pregnancy?
1. Eat several small meals daily
2. Eat crackers on waking every morning
3. Drink large amounts of fluids with each meal
4. Drink orange juice frequently during the day

42. 1. Eating small, frequent meals will place less pressure on the esophageal sphincter, reducing the likelihood of stomach contents being regurgitated into the lower esophagus. None of the other suggestions have been shown to decrease heartburn.
CN: Physiological integrity; CNS: Basic care and comfort;
CL: Apply

43. Which maternal complication is **most** commonly associated with obesity in pregnancy?
1. Mastitis
2. Placenta previa
3. Preeclampsia
4. Rh isoimmunization

43. 3. The incidence of preeclampsia in obese clients is about seven times higher than that in non-obese clients. Mastitis, placenta previa, and Rh isoimmunization are not associated with obesity in pregnant clients.
CN: Physiological integrity; CNS: Reduction of risk potential;
CL: Analyze

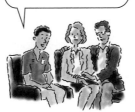

A careful explanation of all tests a pregnant client will be undergoing can alleviate concern.

44. A nonstress test (NST) is ordered for a client with preeclampsia. The nurse is aware that this test will be performed to assess:
1. anemia in the fetus.
2. fetal well-being.
3. intrauterine growth retardation (IUGR).
4. oligohydramnios.

44. 2. An NST is based on the theory that a healthy fetus will have transient fetal heart rate accelerations with fetal movement. A fetus with compromised uteroplacental circulation usually will not have these accelerations, which indicates a nonreactive NST. An NST cannot detect anemia in a fetus. Serial ultrasounds will detect IUGR and oligohydramnios in a fetus.
CN: Health promotion and maintenance; CNS: None; CL: Analyze

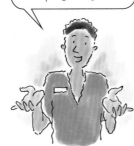

It's important to know the recommended fasting blood sugar level during pregnancy.

45. The nurse is checking the blood sugar level of a client who is at 33-weeks' gestation. This client has had type 1 diabetes since she was 12 years old. Which value would indicate to the nurse that this client's disease is controlled?
1. 45 mg/dl (2.5 mmol/L)
2. 85 mg/dl (4.7 mmol/L)
3. 120 mg/dl (6.7 mmol/L)
4. 136 mg/dl (7.6 mmol/L)

45. 2. The recommended fasting blood sugar level in a pregnant client with diabetes is 60 to 90 mg/dl (3.3 to 5.0 mmol/L). A fasting blood sugar level of 45 mg/dl (2.5 mmol/L) is low, and may result in symptoms of hypoglycemia. A blood sugar level below 120 mg/dl (6.7 mmol/L) is a recommended one-hour postprandial value. A blood sugar level above 136 mg/dl (7.6 mmol/L) in a pregnant client indicates hyperglycemia.
CN: Health promotion and maintenance; CNS: None; CL: Analyze

46. A client with diabetes who is late in her third trimester has a fetal non-stress test (NST) twice weekly. The 20-minute test showed three fetal heart rate accelerations that exceeded the baseline by 15 beats/min, and that lasted longer than 15 seconds. How should the nurse interpret these NST results?
1. Reactive test
2. Nonreactive test
3. Positive test
4. Negative test

46. 1. The NST is the preferred antepartum heart rate screening test for a pregnant client with diabetes. A reactive NST is two or more fetal heart rate accelerations that exceed the baseline by at least 15 beats/min, and last longer than 15 seconds within a 20-minute period. A nonreactive FST lacks accelerations in the fetal heart rate with fetal movement. The terms positive and negative aren't used to describe the interpretation of a NST.
CN: Physiological integrity; CNS: Reduction of risk potential;
CL: Analyze

47. A client is diagnosed with preterm labor at 28 weeks' gestation. At 32 weeks, this client comes to the emergency department saying, "I think I'm in labor." Which should the nurse expect during this client's physical examination?
1. Painful contractions with no cervical dilation
2. Regular uterine contractions with cervical dilation
3. Irregular uterine contraction with no cervical dilation
4. Irregular uterine contractions with cervical effacement

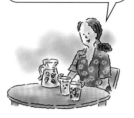

You're almost at question 50 and you're doing great.

47. 2. Regular uterine contractions (every 10 minutes or more), along with cervical dilation change before 36 weeks, is considered preterm labor. If there is no cervical change with uterine contractions it isn't considered preterm labor.

CN: Health promotion and maintenance; CNS: None; CL: Analyze

48. The nurse is teaching a client, who, at 18 weeks' gestation, reports a fluttering sensation in her abdomen. The nurse's teaching has been successful when the client states:
1. "This is my baby moving."
2. "I will seek prompt medical attention if this happens again."
3. "This is an early sign of labor."
4. "I will avoid spicy foods."

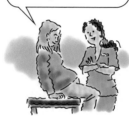

Oh my! I think my baby just moved.

48. 1. Fluttering in the abdomen, also called quickening, begins between 16 and 22 weeks' gestation, and is caused by fetal movement. It does not require medical attention, and is not a sign of early labor. Eating spicy foods has no effect on quickening.

CN: Health promotion and maintenance; CNS: None; CL: Analyze

49. A pregnant client is visiting the clinic and reports tiny, blanched, slightly raised-end arterioles on her face, neck, arms, and chest. The nurse explains that these are normal during pregnancy and referred to as:
1. epulis.
2. linea nigra.
3. striae gravidarum.
4. telangiectasias.

49. 4. The dilated arterioles that occur during pregnancy are called telangiectasias, and are due to an elevated level of circulating estrogen. An epulis is a red raised nodule on the gums that may develop at the end of the first trimester, and continue to grow as the pregnancy progresses. Linea nigra is a pigmented line extending from the symphysis pubis to the top of the fundus, and forms during pregnancy. Striae gravidarum, or stretch marks, are slightly depressed streaks that commonly occur over the abdomen, breast, and thighs during the second half of pregnancy.

CN: Health promotion and maintenance; CNS: None; CL: Apply

50. Which nursing intervention is **priority** for a pregnant adolescent during her first trimester?
1. Schedule the client for a screening glucose tolerance test
2. Refer the client to a dietitian for nutritional counseling
3. Tell the client that she will most likely need a cesarean birth due to the head size of the fetus
4. Assess the client for signs and symptoms of placenta previa

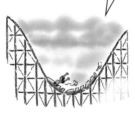

Knowing answers to questions is such a rush!

50. 2. Adolescents are at risk for delivering low-birth-weight neonates. Nutritional counseling should be a priority for these clients to ensure proper fetal development. A pregnant adolescent is not likely to deliver a macrosomic neonate. The final head size of the fetus is unknown at this time. Adolescents are not at increased risk for developing gestational diabetes or placenta previa.

CN: Health promotion and maintenance; CNS: None; CL: Analyze

51. A nurse is discussing a healthy diet with a prima gravida client. The client states that she doesn't consume much milk or other dairy, even though she knows they are important. What advice should the nurse give this client?
1. "The prenatal vitamins that are recommended will satisfy all dietary requirements."
2. "You could supplement your diet with 1,800 mg of over-the-counter calcium tablets."
3. "You should consume other non-dairy foods that are high in calcium."
4. "After the first trimester, calcium intake isn't significant because all fetal organ structures are formed."

51. 3. Milk and dairy aren't the only sources of calcium. Other foods that are high in calcium are considered an ideal source the mineral. While prenatal vitamins are generally recommended, they don't satisfy all nutrient requirements. The calcium requirement for a pregnant woman is 1,300 mg/day. Over-the-counter supplements are not always safe, and should be specifically recommended by the health care practitioner. While it's true that all fetal organs are formed by the end of the first trimester, body development continues throughout pregnancy.
CN: Health promotion and maintenance; CNS: None; CL: Apply

52. Which drug should a nurse choose as an antagonist for magnesium sulfate?
1. Oxytocin
2. Misoprostol
3. Calcium gluconate
4. Naloxone

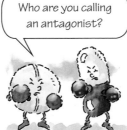

Who are you calling an antagonist?

52. 3. Calcium gluconate should be kept at the bedside while a client is receiving a magnesium infusion. If magnesium toxicity occurs, calcium gluconate is administered as an antidote. Oxytocin is the synthetic form of the naturally occurring pituitary hormone used to initiate or augment uterine contractions. Misoprostol is a labor-inducing drug that is administered vaginally to ripen the cervix and to cause uterine contractions. Naloxone is an opiate antagonist administered to reverse the respiratory depression that may follow administration of opiates.
CN: Physiological integrity; CNS: Pharmacological and parenteral therapies; CL: Analyze

53. A nurse receives an order to start an infusion of blood for a client who is hemorrhaging due to a placenta previa. Which equipment will the nurse need to initiate the infusion? Select all that apply.
1. Y tubing
2. 18-gauge catheter
3. Normal saline solution
4. Lactated Ringer's solution
5. 5% dextrose in water solution

53. 1, 2, 3. Blood transfusions require Y tubing, normal saline solution to mix with the blood product, and an 18-gauge catheter to avoid lysing the red blood cells. Lactated Ringer's solution is contraindicated.
CN: Physiological integrity; CNS: Pharmacological and parenteral therapies; CL: Apply

54. A nurse is assessing a client who is experiencing a normal pregnancy. Which assessment would the nurse find in a normal pregnancy?
1. A 10-beat/min drop in heart rate
2. A 2-breath/min increase in respiratory rate
3. A 15 mmHg increase in systolic blood pressure
4. A 2,000/∝l drop in leukocyte count

54. 2. During pregnancy there is a slight increase in respiratory rate. The heart rate may increase up to 15 beats/min by the end of pregnancy. Systolic and diastolic pressures may decrease by 5 to 10 mmHg. The leukocyte count rises in pregnancy, and may range from 10,000 to 12,000/∝l.
CN: Physiological integrity; CNS: Reduction of risk potential; CL: Apply

55. The nurse is teaching a student nurse about the GTPAL system. GTPAL documents a client's previous pregnancies. Which statement **most** accurately describes this system?
1. Total neonates, preterm neonates, anencephalic neonates, and live births
2. Total neonates, problem pregnancies, abortions, and living children
3. Term neonates, problem pregnancies, anencephalic neonates, and live births
4. Term neonates, Preterm neonates, Abortions, and Living children

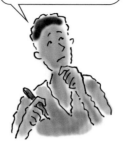

Hmm. Let me think. "G" is for gravida, "T" is for …

55. 4. In GTPAL, G stands for gravida, T denotes the number of term neonates born after 37-weeks' gestation, P is the number of pre-term neonates born before 37 weeks' gestation; A represents the number of pregnancies ending with spontaneous or therapeutic abortion, and L is the number of children currently living.
CN: Health promotion and maintenance; CNS: None;
CL: Apply

56. The nurse is reviewing the glucose tolerance test results of a client who is at 26 weeks' gestation. The nurse determines further intervention is necessary when the results identify:
1. a glucose level of 120 mg/dl (6.7 mmol/L) during a one-hour glucose tolerance test.
2. a one-hour glucose level of 160 mg/dl (8.9 mmol/L) during a three-hour glucose tolerance test.
3. a two-hour glucose level of 180 mg/dl (10.0 mmol/L) during a three-hour glucose tolerance test.
4. a three-hour glucose level of 130 mg/dl (7.2 mmol/L) during a three-hour glucose tolerance test.

56. 3. Gestational diabetes is diagnosed when a two-hour glucose level is 155 mg/dl (8.6 mmol/L) or greater
CN: Physiological integrity; CNS: Reduction of risk potential;
CL: Apply

57. A 32-year-old woman is at 15 weeks' gestation when she's admitted to the labor unit. According to the GTPAL system, she is a G5 P1212. Which description **best** describes this client?
1. Total of five pregnancies, one full-term pregnancy, two problem pregnancies, one spontaneous abortion, and two live births
2. Total of five children, one full-term pregnancy, two pre-term pregnancies, one abortion, and two live births
3. Total of five pregnancies, one full-term pregnancy, two pre-term pregnancies, one abortion, and two living children
4. Total of five pregnancies, one full-term pregnancy, two problem pregnancies, one abortion, and two living children

57. 3. This client has a total of five pregnancies, one full-term pregnancy, two pre-term pregnancies, one abortion, and two living children. In GTPAL, G stands for gravida, T denotes the number of term neonates born after 37 weeks' gestation, P is the number of pre-term neonates born before 37 weeks' gestation, A represents the number of pregnancies ending with spontaneous or therapeutic abortion, and L is the number of children currently living.
CN: Health promotion and maintenance; CNS: None;
CL: Apply

58. The nurse is assessing a 32-year-old woman who is 15 weeks' gestation, and has a history of hypertension. The nurse is aware that the client is most at risk for:
1. abruptio placentae.
2. preterm labor.
3. spontaneous abortion.
4. anemia.

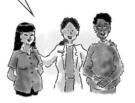

It's important to know the medical history of a pregnant client.

58. 1. A history of hypertension predisposes this client for developing abruptio placentae. She is not at risk for developing preterm labor, spontaneous abortion, or anemia.
CN: Physiological integrity; CNS: Reduction of risk potential;
CL: Analyze

59. A 32-year-old client has her first prenatal visit at 15 weeks' gestation. Her pre-pregnancy weight was 135 lb (61.2 kg). Which finding is abnormal during this visit?

1. Fundal height of 18 cm
2. Blood pressure of 124/72 mmHg
3. Urine negative for protein
4. Weight of 144 lb (65.3 kg)

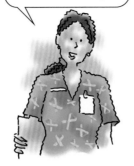

Question 59 is asking for an abnormal finding.

59. 1. The fundal height (in centimeters) should equal the number of weeks of gestation between 18 and 34 weeks. This indicator should not be used alone to determine weeks of gestation. This client should have a fundal height of 15 to 16 cm. The blood pressure, urine, and weight findings are within normal limits for the information given.
CN: Physiological integrity; CNS: Reduction of risk potential; CL: Analyze

60. A 25-year-old primiparous client arrives for her first prenatal visit at 10 weeks' gestation. She seems nervous and has many questions. What is the **most** important intervention by the nurse?

1. Address the client's concerns while taking a comprehensive history
2. Ask the client to undress to prepare for the physical examination
3. Reassure the client that all her questions will be answered during the visit
4. Tell the client there's nothing to worry about. The health care provider will take good care of her.

60. 3. Providing initial reassurance helps set the client's mind at ease. Assessing the client's concerns while taking a history would be appropriate only if the client wrote down her questions in advance. Asking this client to immediately disrobe could make the client even more nervous. The client should be treated as a partner in her care rather than being told that her health care provider will take care of everything.
CN: Safe, effective care environment; CNS: Management of care; CL: Apply

61. Accompanied by her father, a primiparous 15-year-old client arrives for her first prenatal visit at 30 weeks' gestation. Her father refuses to leave the room. He tells the nurse that the girl is shy, and that he will answer the questions for her. What should concern the nurse the **most** about this situation?

1. The possibility of preterm labor with an adolescent pregnancy
2. Lack of prenatal care until this visit
3. Possible child abuse or domestic violence
4. Difficulties of an overprotective parent in dealing with his daughter

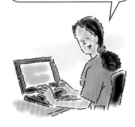

What should the nurse be most concerned about? Let me think.

61. 3. Generally, a father would be somewhat uncomfortable staying in a room while his pregnant daughter is examined. If he insists on staying during the history and physical examination, the nurse should gently but firmly ask him to wait in another room. If the nurse suspects possible child abuse or domestic violence, the father may not want the girl to be alone with the nurse, fearing that she might reveal the abuse or violence. The possibility of preterm labor and lack of prenatal care should be considered, but they are not the primary concerns in this situation. An overprotective parent can be supported and taught how to let go of a child as time goes by. Referral to a social worker may be warranted.
CN: Psychosocial integrity; CNS: None; CL: Analyze

62. What is the **best** way for a nurse to determine if a pregnant client is the victim of domestic abuse or violence?

1. Interview the client with her partner in the room
2. Interview the client with the health care provider present
3. Interview the client alone in a nonjudgmental way
4. Interview the client in a nonjudgmental way, with the partner present

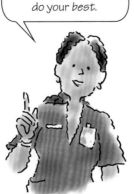

It's up to you to do your best.

62. 3. To help the client feel protected, and develop enough trust in the nurse to share her circumstance, the nurse should interview the client alone in a nonjudgmental way. If the partner is present, the client is likely to withhold information for fear of retaliation.
CN: Psychosocial integrity; CNS: None; CL: Apply

63. A client with gestational hypertension is experiencing abdominal pain and vaginal bleeding. Which assessment should the nurse perform **first**?
1. Fetal heart tones
2. Strength of contractions
3. Urinary output
4. Serum electrolytes

63. 1. Since the findings suggest that the client is experiencing abruptio placentae, fetal heart tones should be assessed immediately to determine fetal well-being. The other interventions should also be implemented after the fetus is assessed.
CN: Physiological integrity; CNS: Reduction of risk potential; CL: Analyze

64. Which assessment findings should the nurse expect to find in client, during the second and third trimesters of pregnancy? Select all that apply.
1. Ankle edema
2. Shortness of breath
3. Nausea and vomiting
4. Hypertension
5. Increased vaginal discharge

64. 1, 2. Leg cramps, ankle edema, and shortness of breath are normal during the second and third trimesters. The nurse should teach the client how to relieve these minor discomforts and what to report if they become unbearable. Nausea and vomiting should subside by the end of the first trimester, if they don't, the nurse should suspect an undiagnosed problem, such as hyperemesis gravidarum or emotional factors. Increased vaginal discharge generally occurs during the first trimester, and decreases by the end of this trimester. A yellow, curd-like, or malodorous discharge suggests an abnormal vaginal infection, and should be reported to the health care provider. Hypertension my indicate the development of preeclampsia and is not a normal occurrence.
CN: Health promotion and maintenance; CNS: None; CL: Apply

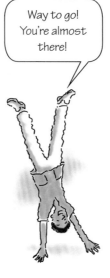

Way to go! You're almost there!

65. A client with mild preeclampsia is being prepared for discharge from the hospital. The client understands the discharge instructions when she states:
1. "I will lie on my left side."
2. "I should increase my sodium intake."
3. "I will take acetaminophen for a headache."
4. "I will monitor my weight each week."

65. 1. The client should lie on her left side to improve uterine and renal blood flow and enhance venous return. Sodium intake should be limited in a client with preeclampsia. A headache should be reported to the healthcare provider since it can signal a worsening of the eclampsia. Weight should be monitored daily to assess for fluid retention.
CN: Physiological integrity; CNS: Reduction of risk potential; CL: Analyze

66. The nurse describes the cardinal mechanisms of labor while teaching an antepartum client about the passage of the fetus through the birth canal during labor. Place these events in the proper sequence as they would occur.

| 1. Flexion |
| 2. External rotation |
| 3. Descent |
| 4. Expulsion |
| 5. Internal rotation |
| 6. Extension |

66. Ordered Response:

| 3. Descent |
| 1. Flexion |
| 5. Internal rotation |
| 6. Extension |
| 2. External rotation |
| 4. Expulsion |

CN: Health promotion and maintenance; CNS: None; CL: Apply

CN: Client needs category   CNS: Client needs subcategory   CL: Cognitive level

67. A nurse is palpating the uterus of a client who is at 20 weeks' gestation to measure fundal height. Identify the area of the abdomen where the nurse should expect to feel the uterine fundus.

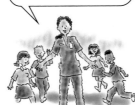

Hooray! You finished Chapter 22. Time for a party!

67. At 20-weeks' gestation, fundal height should be at about the umbilicus. Fundal height should be measured from the symphysis pubis to the top of the uterus. Serial measurements assess fetal growth over the course of the pregnancy. Between weeks 18 and 34, fundal height correlate roughly with the week of gestation.

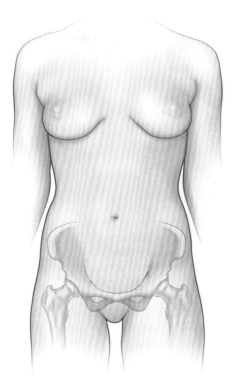

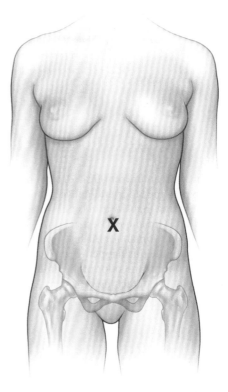

CN: Health promotion and maintenance; CNS: None;
CL: Apply

Chapter 23

Intrapartum Care

The prepartum and postpartum periods are important to know about. However, the intrapartum period—that's where the action is! This chapter covers the intrapartum period, perhaps the most critical of the three.

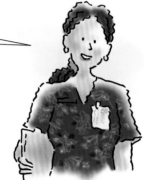

1. A client with an uncomplicated, term pregnancy arrives at the labor-and-delivery unit in early labor saying that she thinks her water has broken. What is the nurse's **best** action?
1. Prepare the woman for birth
2. Ask what time this happened and note the color, amount, and odor of the fluid
3. Immediately contact the provider
4. Collect a sample of the fluid for microbial analysis

1. 2. Gather more information. Noting the color, amount, and odor of the fluid, as well as the time of rupture, will help guide the nurse in her next action. There's no need to immediately call the client's provider or prepare this client for birth if the fluid is clear and birth isn't imminent. Rupture of membranes isn't unusual in the early stages of labor. Fluid collection for microbial analysis is not routine if there's no concern for infection.
CN: Physiological integrity; CNS: Reduction of risk potential; CL: Apply

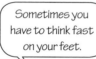

Sometimes you have to think fast on your feet.

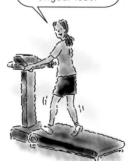

2. A client who is at 36 weeks' gestation comes into the labor and birth unit with mild contractions. The client reports that she has a history of placenta previa. The nurse should observe for which complication?
1. Sudden rupture of membranes
2. Vaginal bleeding
3. Precipitious birth
4. Fever

2. 2. Contractions may disrupt the microvascular network in the placenta of a client with placenta previa which can result in bleeding. If the separation occurs at the margin of the placenta, the blood will escape vaginally. Sudden rupture of the membranes and precipitious birth are not related to placenta previa. Fever would indicate an infectious process.
CN: Physiological integrity; CNS: Reduction of risk potential; CL: Apply

CN: Client needs category   CNS: Client needs subcategory   CL: Cognitive level

3. A client's labor is not progressing. After ruling out cephalopelvic disproportion, the provider orders 1,000 ml 0.9% normal saline with oxytocin 10 units to run at 2 milliunits/min. What is the correct infusion rate in milliliters per hour? Record your answer using one decimal place.

_____ ml/hr

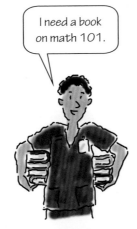

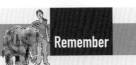

"Oxytocin is for inducin' labor."

Oxytocin stimulates the smooth muscle in the uterus and breast, inducing labor.

4. A client has been receiving oxytocin to augment her labor. The nurse notes that contractions are lasting 100 seconds. Which **immediate** action should the nurse take?
  1. Stop the oxytocin infusion
  2. Notify the provider
  3. Monitor fetal heart tones as usual
  4. Turn the client on her left side

5. A client at term arrives in the labor and delivery unit experiencing contractions every four minutes. After a brief assessment, the client is admitted, and an electronic fetal monitor is applied. Which assessment finding would be **most** concerning to the nurse?
  1. Total weight gain of 30 lb (13.6 kg)
  2. Maternal age of 32 years
  3. Blood pressure of 146/90 mmHg
  4. Treatment for syphilis at 15 weeks' gestation

3. 0.2
The answer is found by setting up a ratio and proportion. Each unit of oxytocin contains 1,000 milliunits. Therefore, 1,000 ml of IV fluid contains 10,000 milliunits (10 units) of oxytocin.

$$\frac{10,000}{1,000} = \frac{2}{X}$$

$$10,000\,X = 2,000$$

$$X = \frac{2,000}{10,000}$$

$$X = 0.2 \; ml$$

CN: Physiological integrity; CNS: Pharmacological and parenteral therapies; CL: Apply

4. 1. Oxytocin should be withheld immediately, as it stimulates contractions. A contraction that continues for more than 90 seconds signals tetany and could lead to decreased placental perfusion and possibly uterine rupture. The nurse should monitor the fetal heart tones, stop the oxytocin, and notify the provider. The client should be turned on her left side to increase blood flow to the fetus, which can be decreased with tetany. This decreased blood flow can potentially compromise the fetus.

CN: Physiological integrity; CNS: Reduction of risk potential; CL: Apply

5. 3. A blood pressure of 146/90 mmHg may indicate gestational hypertension. Over time, gestational hypertension reduces blood flow to the placenta and can cause intrauterine growth restriction, and other problems that reduce the fetus's ability to tolerate the stress of labor. A weight gain of 30 lb (13.6 kg) is within expected parameters for a healthy pregnancy. A woman over age 30 doesn't have a greater risk of complications if her general condition is healthy before pregnancy. Syphilis that has been treated does not pose an additional risk.

CN: Physiological integrity; CNS: Reduction of risk potential; CL: Apply

6. Which finding by the nurse would be most indicative of fetal distress during labor?
1. Fetal scalp pH of 7.14
2. Fetal heart rate of 144 beats/minute
3. Acceleration of fetal heart rate with contractions
4. Presence of long-term variability

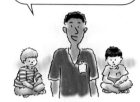

Relax. The questions in this chapter are child's play.

6. 1. A scalp pH below 7.25 indicates acidosis and fetal hypoxia. A fetal heart rate of 144 beats/min, acceleration of the fetal heart rate with contractions, and long-term variability are normal responses of a healthy fetus to labor.
CN: Physiological integrity; CNS: Reduction of risk potential; CL: Apply

7. The amniotic membranes rupture during the labor of a client with a breech presentation. Meconium is present in the amniotic fluid. The client asks the nurse what this means. What is an appropriate response by the nurse?
1. "This often happens during a prolonged birth."
2. "This indicates a blood incompatibility between the fetus and mother."
3. "This is a sign of fetal distress."
4. "This is normal in a breech birth."

7. 4. Meconium in a breech presentation may be caused by compression of the fetus's intestinal tract during descent. Meconium in the amniotic fluid is a sign of fetal distress in a cephalic presentation and is not a normal finding. Yellow-stained amniotic fluid is a sign of a possible blood incompatibility between fetus and mother, and is due to bilirubin from the breakdown of red blood cells.
CN: Physiological integrity; CNS: Reduction of risk potential; CL: Analyze

8. A client at 42 weeks' gestation is 3 cm dilated, 30% effaced, with membranes intact and the fetus at minus two station. The fetal heart rate (FHR) is 140 beats/min. After two hours, the nurse notes that the external fetal monitor indicates that, for the past 10 minutes, the FHR ranged from 160 to 190 beats/min. The client states that her baby has been extremely active. Uterine contractions are strong, occurring every three to four minutes and lasting 40 to 60 seconds. Which finding would indicate fetal hypoxia in this situation?
1. Abnormally long uterine contractions
2. Abnormally strong uterine intensity
3. Increased frequency of contractions, with rapid fetal movement
4. Excessive fetal activity and fetal tachycardia

8. 4. Fetal tachycardia and excessive fetal activity are the first signs of fetal hypoxia. The duration of uterine contractions is within normal limits. Uterine intensity can be mild to strong and still be within normal limits. The frequency of contractions is within the normal limits for the active phase of labor.
CN: Physiological integrity; CNS: Reduction of risk potential; CL: Analyze

9. A client who, at 33 weeks' gestation, is leaking amniotic fluid. She is placed on an external fetal monitor. The monitor indicates uterine irritability, and contractions are occurring every four to six minutes. The provider orders nifedipine 20 mg po now and every eight hours until birth or contractions cease. What is the **most** important information for the nurse to teach this client concerning nifedipine?
1. "This medicine will ensure that you do not deliver early."
2. "You will usually feel a fluttering or tight sensation in your chest."
3. "This will dry your mouth and make you feel thirsty."
4. "You may experience nausea and some dizziness."

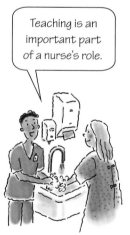

Teaching is an important part of a nurse's role.

9. 4. Common side effects of nifediine are feelings of dizziness, nausea and headache. The other side effects listed are very uncommon for this medications. Nifedipine is administered as an initial dose of 10 to 40 mg/po, then doses may continue to prevent ongoing contractions and early birth. Nifedipine relieves bronchospasm, but the client is receiving it to reduce uterine motility.
CN: Health promotion and maintenance; CNS: None; CL: Apply

CN: Client needs category   CNS: Client needs subcategory   CL: Cognitive level

10. A 17-year-old primigravida with severe hypertension of pregnancy has been receiving magnesium sulfate IV for three hr. The latest assessment reveals deep tendon reflexes (DTR) of +1, flushing, blood pressure of 150/100 mmHg, a pulse of 92 beats/min, a respiratory rate of 10 breaths/min, and urine output of 20 ml/hr. Which action would be **most** appropriate?

1. Continue monitoring per standards of care
2. Stop the magnesium sulfate infusion
3. Increase the infusion rate by 5 gtts/min
4. Decrease the infusion rate by 5 gtts/min

Remember

"Magnesium sulfate deflates hypertension."

Magnesium sulfate is the drug of choice to treat hypertension of pregnancy because it reduces edema by causing a shift from the extracellular spaces into the intestines. It also depresses the central nervous system, which decreases the incidence of seizures.

10. 2. Magnesium sulfate should be withheld if the client's respiratory rate or urine output falls, or if reflexes are diminished or absent, all of which are true for this client. The client also shows other signs of impending toxicity, such as flushing and feeling warm. Inaction will not resolve the client's suppressed DTRs, low respiratory rate and urine output. The client is already showing central nervous system depression because of excessive magnesium sulfate, so increasing the infusion rate is inappropriate. Impending toxicity indicates that the infusion should be stopped rather than just slowed down.
CN: Physiological integrity; CNS: Pharmacological and parenteral therapies; CL: Apply

11. A nurse administers oxytocin to a client to induce labor. Which finding would indicate to the nurse that this client requires an immediate intervention?

1. Contractions longer than 70 seconds, occurring every two minutes or less
2. Dry mucous membranes and decreased skin turgor
3. Fetal heart rate of 160 beats/min
4. Maternal heart rate of 56 beats/min

11. 1. Oxytocin, given to induce labor, may cause uterine tetany, which increases the risk of uterine rupture. Therefore, the infusion should be stopped and the provider notified if contractions last greater than 70 seconds and occur every two minutes or less. Oxytocin has an antidiuretic effect and can cause fluid overload, not dehydration as indicated by dry mucous membranes and decreased skin turgor. A normal fetal heart rate is 120 to 160 beats/min. Oxytocin may cause maternal tachycardia, not bradycardia.
CN: Physiological integrity; CNS: Pharmacologic parenteral therapies; CL: Apply

12. The cervix of a 26-year-old primigravida in labor is 5 cm dilated and 75% effaced, and the fetus is at zero station. The provider prescribes an epidural regional block. In which position should the nurse place this client to allow for an epidural regional block?

1. Lithotomy
2. Supine
3. Prone
4. Lateral

12. 4. The client should be placed on her left side or sitting upright, with her shoulders parallel and legs slightly flexed. Her back shouldn't be flexed because this position increases the possibility that the dura may be punctured and the anesthetic will accidentally be given as spinal, not epidural, anesthesia. None of the other positions allows proper access to the epidural space.
CN: Physiological integrity; CNS: Reduction of risk potential; CL: Apply

Be careful of the words will need to be in option 4. They indicate an absolute, a near rarity in health care.

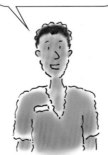

13. During the vaginal examination of a term, multiparous client in labor, the nurse palpates the fetus's larger, diamond-shaped fontanelle toward the anterior portion of the client's pelvis. The findings of this assessment would indicate that the:

1. client can expect a brief and intense labor with potential for lacerations.
2. client is at risk for uterine rupture and needs constant monitoring.
3. client may need interventions to ease back pain and change the fetal position.
4. fetus will need to be delivered using forceps or a vacuum extractor.

13. 3. The fetal position is occiput posterior, a position that commonly produces intense back pain during labor. Most of the time, the fetus rotates during labor to occiput anterior position. Positioning the client on her side can facilitate this rotation. An occiput posterior position would most likely result in prolonged labor. Occiput posterior alone doesn't create a risk of uterine rupture. The fetus would be delivered with forceps or vacuum extractor only if its presenting part doesn't rotate and descend spontaneously.
CN: Health promotion and maintenance; CNS: None; CL: Analyze

CN: Client needs category   CNS: Client needs subcategory   CL: Cognitive level

14. Which fetal position would be considered the most favorable for birth?
1. Vertex presentation
2. Transverse lie
3. Frank breech presentation
4. Posterior position of the fetal head

14. 1. Vertex presentation is the optimal presentation for passage through the birth canal. Transverse lie is an unacceptable fetal position for vaginal birth and requires a cesarean birth. Frank breech presentation, in which the buttocks present first, is a high-risk situation, and cesarean birth is recommended. If the fetal head is in the posterior position, it can be difficult to pass under the mother's symphysis pubis bone.
CN: Physiological integrity; CNS: Reduction of risk potential; CL: Analyze

15. The nurse is teaching a client admitted to the labor and delivery unit about the stages of labor. The client demonstrates an understanding of the instruction when she states that birth occurs during the:
1. first stage of labor.
2. second stage of labor.
3. third stage of labor.
4. fourth stage of labor.

Take the stage please!

15. 2. The second stage of labor begins with complete dilation, and ends with the expulsion of the fetus. The first stage of labor is the stage of dilation, which is divided into three distinct phases: latent, active, and transition. The third stage of labor follows the expulsion of the infant and ends with the expulsion of the placenta. The fourth stage of labor is the first four hours after placental expulsion, in which the client's body begins the recovery process.
CN: Health promotion and maintenance; CNS: None; CL: Apply

16. A nurse is reviewing laboratory data on a client admitted to the labor and delivery unit. What is the **most** important laboratory value for the nurse to obtain?
1. Blood type
2. Calcium
3. Iron
4. Oxygen saturation

16. 1. Blood type is a critical value to have because the risk of blood loss is always a potential complication during the labor and birth process. Approximately 40% of a woman's cardiac output is delivered to the uterus. Blood loss can occur quite rapidly in the event of uncontrolled bleeding. Calcium and iron aren't critical values, and oxygen saturation isn't a laboratory value.
CN: Physiological integrity; CNS: Reduction of risk potential; · CL: Analyze

17. The nurse is assessing the fetal heart rate of a laboring woman who is full term. Which finding should the nurse recognize as a normal value?
1. 80 to 100 beats/min
2. 100 to 120 beats/min
3. 120 to 160 beats/min
4. 160 to 180 beats/min

17. 3. A rate of 120 to 160 beats/min in the fetal heart is appropriate for filling the heart with blood and pumping it out to the system. Faster or slower rates do not accomplish perfusion adequately, and could indicate fetal compromise.
CN: Health promotion and maintenance; CNS: None; CL: Remember

18. A nurse connects a laboring client to an external electronic fetal monitor. The client asks the nurse the purpose of this intervention. What should the nurse tell this client about the external fetal monitor?
1. "It monitors fetal kicks."
2. "It assesses the fetal position."
3. "It determines how the labor is progressing."
4. "It monitors the baby's oxygenation by observing its heart rate."

18. 4. Oxygenation of the fetus may be indirectly assessed through fetal monitoring by closely examining the fetal heart rate strip. Accelerations in the fetal heart rate strip indicate good oxygenation, while decelerations in the fetal heart rate sometimes indicate poor fetal oxygenation. The fetal heart rate strip can't determine the number of fetal kicks or assess fetal position. Labor progress can be directly assessed only through cervical examination.
CN: Physiological integrity; CNS: Reduction of risk potential; CL: Apply

CN: Client needs category   CNS: Client needs subcategory   CL: Cognitive level

19. The nurse is preparing a client in labor for the administration of an epidural. What is the **most** important intervention by the nurse?
1. Give a fluid bolus of 500 ml
2. Administer IV pain medication prescribed by the provider
3. Elicit maternal reflexes
4. Insert a Foley catheter

19. 1. One of the major adverse effects of epidural administration is hypotension. Therefore, a 500-ml fluid bolus is usually administered to help prevent hypotension in the client who wishes to receive an epidural for pain relief. Eliciting maternal reflexes, inserting a foley catheter, administering IV pain medications are not necessary for the in insertion of an epidural.
CN: Physiological integrity; CNS: Reduction of risk potential; CL: Analyze

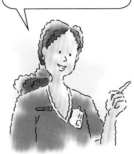
It's important to know the adverse effects of a procedure and how to offset them.

20. A client required an episiotomy for the birth of her baby. The nurse is aware that this client may experience:
1. excessive blood loss.
2. uterine disfigurement.
3. prolonged dyspareunia.
4. hormonal fluctuation postpartum.

20. 3. Prolonged painful intercourse (dyspareunia) may result when complications such as infection interfere with wound healing. Minimal blood loss occurs when an episiotomy is performed. The uterus isn't affected by episiotomy. Only the perineum is cut to accommodate the fetus. Hormonal fluctuations that occur during the postpartum period are not the result of an episiotomy.
CN: Physiological integrity; CNS: Reduction of risk potential; CL: Analyze

21. A client in early labor tells the nurse that she has a thick, yellow discharge from both of her breasts. What is the nurse's **most** appropriate intervention?
1. Tell her that her milk is starting to come in because she's in labor
2. Complete a thorough breast examination and document the results in the chart
3. Perform a culture on the discharge, and inform the client that she might have mastitis
4. Inform the client that the discharge is colostrum, and a normal finding

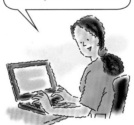
Pay attention to the words *most appropriate*. They're the key to the answer.

21. 4. After the fourth month, colostrum may be expressed. The breasts normally produce colostrum for the first few days after birth. Milk production begins one to three days postpartum. A clinical breast examination isn't usually indicated in the intrapartum setting. Although a culture may be indicated, it requires advanced assessment as well as a medical order.
CN: Physiological Integrity; CNS: Physiological Adaption; CL: Apply

22. While performing an admission nursing assessment of a client in early labor, the nurse observes a brown, raised lesion resembling a mole 2.5 in (5 cm) below the left breast. What would be the nurse's **most** appropriate response to this finding?
1. Ask the client if this is a new finding
2. Let the client know that this is abnormal, and that the nurse will notify the health care provider
3. Tell the client that it is a supernumerary nipple, a common finding
4. Inform the client that it is a skin tag, and is clinically insignificant

22. 3. Supernumerary nipples are common in men and women and are usually located 2.5 to 3 in (5 to 6 cm) below the breast near the midline. A supernumerary nipple resembles a mole, although closer inspection will reveal a small nipple and areola and is clinically insignificant. A mole may be macular or papular, tan to brown in color, and usually has smooth borders. Keratosis lesions are raised, thickened areas of pigmentation that look scaly and wart-like. They don't become cancerous. Skin tags are overgrowths of normal skin that form a stalk and are polyp-like.
CN: Health promotion and maintenance; CNS: None; CL: Analyze

23. A nurse is teaching a client in early labor about the pinkish stretch marks on her abdomen. Which client statement indicates that the nurse's teaching was effective?
1. "My stretch marks will completely fade within six weeks."
2. "My stretch marks will fade, but not disappear, after birth."
3. "An emollient cream will help fade my stretch marks."
4. "A regular exercise program will help my stretch marks go away."

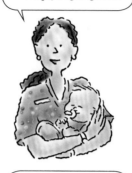

Stretch marks are yet another reminder of the joy of giving birth!

23. 2. Striae are wavy, depressed streaks that may occur over the abdomen, breasts, or thighs as pregnancy progresses. They fade with time to a silvery color, but won't disappear. Creams may soften the skin, but won't remove the striae. Regular exercise will not affect the stretch marks.
CN: Health promotion and maintenance; CNS: None; CL: Apply

24. The nurse wants to place a laboring client in the best position to increase her cardiac output and stroke volume. Which position would the nurse select?
1. Supine
2. Sitting
3. Side-lying
4. Semi-Fowler's

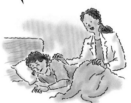

This position will help your heart pump better—I'm not lying!

24. 3. In the left side-lying position, cardiac output increases, stroke volume increases, and the pulse rate decreases. In the supine position, the blood pressure can drop severely, due to the pressure of the fetus and enlarged uterus on the vena cava, resulting in supine hypotensive or vena cava syndrome. Neither the sitting nor semi-Fowler's position increases cardiac output or stroke volume.
CN: Health promotion and maintenance; CNS: None; CL: Apply

25. A nurse is caring for a full-term pregnant client in active labor. The electronic fetal monitor reveals a fetal heart rate (FHR) of less than 70 beats for one minute. What is the nurse's **priority** intervention?
1. Position the mother in the lithotomy position
2. Place the mother on her left side and apply oxygen
3. Call the client's provider
4. Slow down the mother's IV rate

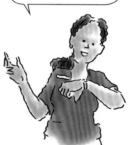

Things are sure getting slow around here.

25. 2. An FHR below 70 beats/min is considered severe fetal bradycardia, and immediate interventions are needed. The nurse would first apply oxygen after positioning the mother on her left side. Positioning the mother in the lithotomy position is not indicated. Although the provider would be notified of the status change in the client, the nurse would not wait on orders from the provider to act. Slowing the IV rate would reduce the circulating volume of blood and worsen the problem.
CN: Health promotion and maintenance; CNS: None; CL: Apply

26. A nurse is performing Leopold's maneuvers on a client who is in the early stages of labor. With which finding is the nurse **most** concerned?
1. Palpation of the upper fundus reveals a firm, round shape
2. Palpation of the upper fundus reveals a soft, less-defined shape
3. Palpation of the side of the fundus reveals a smooth, firm shape
4. Palpation of the left side of the fundus reveals a firm, round shape

26. 1. Palpation of the upper fundus reveals a firm, round head in a breech presentation, and a soft, less-defined shape in a cephalic birth. The firm, smooth back of the fetus is palpated on the side of the fundus, and may be palpated with cephalic and breech presentations. In a cephalic presentation, palpation of the lower fundus reveals a firm, round head.
CN: Health promotion and maintenance; CNS: None; CL: Apply

27. A client who is at 35 weeks' gestation arrives at a labor and delivery unit leaking clear fluid from her vagina. What is the **most** appropriate nursing intervention?
1. Perform a cervical examination and check dilation
2. Obtain a catheterized urine specimen to rule out urinary tract infection
3. Encourage the client to ambulate in the hall
4. Obtain a sterile speculum sample of the fluid for culture

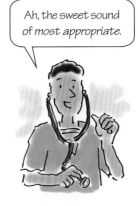

Ah, the sweet sound of most appropriate.

27. 4. A sterile speculum examination is performed to identify ruptured membranes. Confirmation is done with Nitrazine paper and a positive ferning test. With premature rupture of membranes in a client under 37 weeks' gestation, cervical examinations are contraindicated to reduce the incidence of infection. Clean catch urine specimens, not catheterized specimens, would be appropriate to rule out infection. The client should ambulate only after a thorough nursing assessment and examination to determine the safety of the client and fetus.

CN: Physiological integrity; CNS: Reduction of risk potential; CL: Apply

28. A client at 35 weeks' gestation tells the nurse she is worried because she is having irregularly occurring abdominal contractions that have remained irregular for the last few days. How should the nurse **best** explain these contractions to the client?
1. "These contractions will disappear when you walk."
2. "These contractions will increase in frequency and intensity."
3. "These contractions will become regular."
4. "These contractions will move to the lower back."

28. 1. Braxton Hicks contractions begin and remain irregular. They are felt in the abdomen, and remain confined to the abdomen and groin. They commonly disappear with ambulation. True contractions begin irregularly but become regular and predictable. They increase in frequency and intensity, causing cervical effacement and dilation. True contractions are felt initially in the lower back, and radiate to the abdomen in a wavelike motion.

CN: Physiological integrity; CNS: Physiological adaptation; CL: Analyze

29. A client with active genital herpes is admitted to the labor and delivery area in the first stages of labor. Her contractions are five to six minutes apart and she is dilated 2 to 3 cm, 40% effaced, at minus two station with intact membranes. What type of birth would the admitting nurse anticipate for this client?
1. Midforceps
2. Low forceps
3. Pitocin induction
4. Cesarean

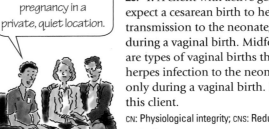

Take care to deliver sensitive news about your client's pregnancy in a private, quiet location.

29. 4. A client with active genital herpes should expect a cesarean birth to help avoid infection transmission to the neonate, which could occur during a vaginal birth. Midforceps and low forceps are types of vaginal births that could transmit the herpes infection to the neonate. Induction is used only during a vaginal birth. It is inappropriate for this client.

CN: Physiological integrity; CNS: Reduction of risk potential; CL: Apply

30. A nurse is monitoring a client in labor and notes that the fetal heart rate (FHR) slows with the start of each contraction on the external fetal monitor. What action should be taken by the nurse?
1. Turn the client to the left side
2. Continue to observe FHR
3. Administer oxygen by face mask
4. Place the client in Trendelenburg position

30. 2. Decelerations in FHR, called early decelerations, occur with the onset of uterine contractions. They are caused by head compression during the contraction, and are not a sign of fetal distress. No action is necessary, and the nurse should continue to monitor the FHR.

CN: Physiological integrity; CNS: Physiological Adaptation; CL: Apply

31. A nurse is assessing a laboring client who is in the second stage of labor. What findings would the nurse expect to note in this client?
1. Cervical dilation of 8 cm
2. Crowning of the fetal head
3. Contractions continuing to deliver the placenta
4. Contractions every 3 to 5 min lasting 60 seconds

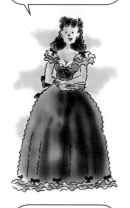

When is my crowning going to take place?

31. 2. The second stage of labor begins at full cervical dilation, and ends when the infant is born. Crowning is present during this stage as the fetal head, pushing against the perineum, causes the vaginal introitus to open, and the fetal scalp to be visible. The first stage begins with true labor contractions, and ends with complete cervical dilation. The third stage follows the birth and ends when the placenta is delivered.
CN: Health promotion and maintenance; CNS: None;
CL: Apply

32. A nurse suspects that the laboring client may have been physically abused by her partner. What is the **most** appropriate intervention by the nurse?
1. Confront the partner
2. Question the client in front of her partner
3. Contact hospital security to monitor the partner
4. Collaborate with the interprofessional team to make a referral to social services

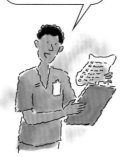

Did you notice the words *most appropriate* in question 32? Another hint!

32. 4. Collaborating with others in the health care team, and the provider to make a referral to social services will create a plan, and provide support for the client. Additionally, by law, the nurse or nursing supervisor must report the suspected abuse to the police, and follow up with a written report. Confrontation will most likely provoke anger in the suspected abuser. Questioning the woman in front of her partner doesn't allow her the privacy required to address this issue, and may place her in greater danger. If the woman is not in imminent danger, there is no need to call hospital security.
CN: Physiological integrity; CNS: Reduction of risk potential;
CL: Analyze

33. During a vaginal examination of a client in labor, it is determined that the biparietal diameter of the fetal head has reached the level of the ischial spines. How should the nurse document this finding?
1. −1
2. 0
3. +1
4. +2

33. 2. When the largest diameter of the presenting part is level with the ischial spines, the fetus is at station 0. A station of −1 indicates that the fetal head is 1 cm above the ischial spines. At +1, it's 1 cm below the ischial spines. At +2, it's 2 cm below the ischial spines.
CN: Health promotion and maintenance; CNS: None;
CL: Understand

34. 3A client who developed gestational diabetes mellitus during the pregnancy has just been admitted in the labor and delivery unit. What is the **priority** nursing action for this client?
1. Ask the client about her most recent blood glucose levels
2. Prepare oral hypoglycemic medications for administration during labor
3. Notify the neonatal intensive care unit that a client with diabetes has been admitted
4. Prepare the client for cesarean birth

34. 1. Asking about the client's most recent blood glucose levels will indicate how well her diabetes has been controlled. Oral hypoglycemic drugs are never used during pregnancy because they cross the placental barrier, stimulate fetal insulin production, and are potentially teratogenic. Plans to admit the infant to the neonatal intensive care unit are premature. Cesarean is not the preferred birth method for clients with diabetes. Vaginal birth is preferred and presents a lower risk to the mother and fetus.
CN: Physiological integrity; CNS: Reduction of risk potential;
CL: Apply

CN: Client needs category   CNS: Client needs subcategory   CL: Cognitive level

35. A client is admitted to the labor and delivery unit for birth of a known anencephalic fetus. What is the **most** appropriate intervention by the nurse?
1. Assess fetal heart tones via external monitor
2. Reassure the client that she'll get pregnant again soon
3. Avoid talking about the baby
4. Provide privacy and emotional support

35. 4. Providing privacy and support is an appropriate therapeutic intervention for the client and family to grieve their loss. Fetal heart tones are rarely assessed in a client with an anencephalic fetus. Most fetuses will not survive due to a lack of cerebral function. Reassuring the client that she will get pregnant again dismisses how she feels about her current loss, and also provides false reassurance.
CN: Psychosocial integrity; CNS: None; CL: Apply

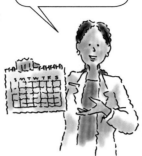

The estimated date of birth can be determined with the proper information.

36. A 30-year-old multiparous client in active labor is admitted to the labor and delivery unit. She has received no prenatal care for this pregnancy. Which data would the nurse obtain **first**?
1. Date of last menstrual period (LMP)
2. Family history of sexually transmitted infection (STIs)
3. Name of insurance provider
4. Number of and ages of previous children

36. 1. The date of the LMP is essential to estimate the date of birth, and should be obtained first. The nursing history would also include subjective information, such as personal history of STIs, gravidity, and parity. Although beneficial to the hospital for financial reimbursement, the insurance provider has no bearing on the nursing history. The number of siblings is not pertinent to the assessment.
CN: Health promotion and maintenance; CNS: None; CL: Analyze

37. The nurse is caring for a laboring client who presents with hypertension of pregnancy. The nurse is concerned that the client may be developing preeclampsia when she notes:
1. decreasing blood pressure.
2. increasing oliguria.
3. decreasing edema.
4. trace levels of protein in the urine.

37. 2. Renal plasma flow and glomerular filtration are decreased in gestational hypertension, so increasing oliguria indicates a worsening condition and potential preeclampsia. Blood pressure increases as a result of increased peripheral resistance. Increasing edema would suggest a worsening condition. Trace levels to +1 proteinuria are acceptable. Higher levels would indicate a worsening condition.
CN: Physiological Integrity; CNS: Physiological Adaption; CL: Apply

38. While performing a cervical examination on a client in labor, a nurse's fingertips feel pulsating tissue. What is the **most** appropriate nursing intervention?
1. Leave the client and call the provider
2. Put the client in a semi-Fowler's position
3. Ask the client to push with the next contraction
4. Leave the fingers in place and press the nurse call light

38. 4. When the umbilical cord precedes the fetal presenting part, it's known as a prolapsed cord. Leaving the fingers in place and calling for assistance is the safest intervention for the fetus. The nurse will need to keep the fetus off the cord to reduce cord compression. The nursing staff will contact the provider, and the client will probably require a cesarean birth to decrease the risk of fetal demise during birth. Placing the client in the semi-Fowler's position would increase the pressure of the fetus on the umbilical cord. Asking the client to push with the next contraction would force the presenting part against the cord, causing severe bradycardia and possible fetal demise.
CN: Physiological integrity; CNS: Reduction of risk potential; CL: Apply

CN: Client needs category   CNS: Client needs subcategory   CL: Cognitive level

39. A client is admitted to the labor and delivery unit in labor with blood flowing down her legs. What would be the **priority** nursing intervention?
1. Place an indwelling catheter
2. Monitor fetal heart tones
3. Perform a cervical examination
4. Prepare the client for cesarean birth

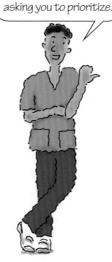

Question 39 is asking you to prioritize.

39. 2. Monitoring fetal heart tones would be the priority, due to a possible placenta previa or abruptio placentae. Although an indwelling catheter may be placed, it is not a priority intervention. Performing a cervical examination would be contraindicated because any agitation of the cervix with a previa can result in hemorrhage and death for the mother or fetus. Preparing the client for a cesarean birth may not be indicated. A sonogram will need to be performed to determine the cause of bleeding. If the diagnosis is a partial placenta previa, the client may still be able to deliver vaginally.
CN: Physiological integrity; CNS: Reduction of risk potential; CL: Apply

40. A client in labor is receiving magnesium sulfate to treat hypertension of pregnancy. How should this drug be administered?
1. As a loading dose of 4 g in Lactated ringers, followed by a continuous infusion of 1 to 2 g/hr
2. As a loading dose of 2 g in normal saline solution, followed by a continuous infusion of 2 g/hr
3. As a loading dose of 4 g in dextrose 5% in water (D5W), followed by a continuous infusion of 1 to 2 g/hr
4. As a loading dose of 4 g in dextrose 5%, followed by a continuous infusion of 4 g/hr

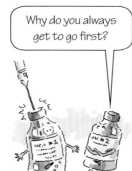

Why do you always get to go first?

40. 3. A loading dose of magnesium sulfate should be given as a 4 g bolus, followed by a continuous infusion of 1 to 2 g/hr in D5W for maintenance. Magnesium sulfate shouldn't be administered in normal saline solution.
CN: Physiological integrity; CNS: Pharmacological and parenteral therapies; CL: Apply

41. A multiparous client who has been in labor for two hours states that she feels the urge to move her bowels. What would the nurse do **first**?
1. Assist the client to get up to use the toilet
2. Allow the client to use a bedpan
3. Perform a pelvic examination
4. Check the fetal heart rate (FHR)

41. 3. A report of rectal pressure usually indicates a low presenting fetal part, and imminent birth. The nurse should perform a pelvic examination to assess the dilation of the cervix and station of the presenting fetal part. Do not let the client use the toilet or a bedpan before she's examined because she could deliver on the toilet or in the bedpan. Checking the FHR is important but comes after the nurse evaluates the client's report.
CN: Health promotion and maintenance; CNS: None; CL: Apply

42. The provider has ordered an IV of 5% dextrose in lactated Ringer's solution at 125 ml/hr. The IV tubing delivers 10 gtts/ml. How many gtts/min should fall into the drip chamber?
1. 10 to 11
2. 12 to 13
3. 20 to 21
4. 22 to 24

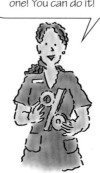

Your math skills are being tested on this one! You can do it!

42. 3. Multiply the number of ml to be infused by the drop factor:

$$125\,\frac{ml}{hr} \times 10\,\frac{gtts}{ml} = 1{,}250\,\frac{gtts}{hr}$$

Then divide the answer by the number of minutes to run the infusion:

$$1{,}250\,\frac{gtts}{hr} \div 60\,\frac{min}{hr} = 20.83\,gtts/min$$

This equates to 20 to 21 gtts/min.
CN: Physiological integrity; CNS: Pharmacological and parenteral therapies; CL: Apply

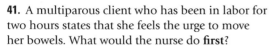

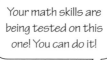

CN: Client needs category   CNS: Client needs subcategory   CL: Cognitive level

43. An amniotomy is performed on a client in labor. What is the **priority** nursing intervention following this procedure?
1. Encourage the client to use breathing exercises as contractions increase
2. Assess fetal heart tones
3. Assist the client to ambulate to promote labor
4. Position the client on her left side

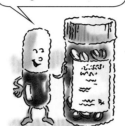

It's important to know how to measure a drug's effectiveness.

44. Which finding would indicate the effectiveness of magnesium sulfate for a client at 34 weeks' gestation with preeclampsia of pregnancy?
1. Absence of seizures
2. Weight gain of 4 lb/wk (1.8 kg/wk)
3. Blood pressure of 154/90 mmHg
4. Urinary output of 25 ml/hr

45. A laboring client in the latent stage of labor begins reporting pain in the epigastric area, blurred vision, and a headache. Which medication would the nurse anticipate for these symptoms?
1. Misoprostol
2. Oxytocin
3. Magnesium sulfate
4. Calcium gluconate

46. A nurse is assisting in monitoring a client in labor. Which monitoring data are indicative of fetal well-being?
1. Fetal heart rate of 145 to 155 bpm with 15-second accelerations to 160
2. Fetal heart rate of 130 to 140 bpm with late decelerations to 110
3. Fetal heart rate of 110 to 120 bpm with variable deceleration to 90
4. Fetal heart rate of 165 to 175 bpm with late decelerations to 140

43. 2. The nurse's priority is to assess fetal heart tones. When the amniotic membrane is ruptured, the umbilical cord may enter the birth canal with the gush of fluid and the presenting part may cause cord compression. Contractions may intensify after an amniotomy. Helping the client with her breathing should be done after fetal well-being is assessed. Ambulation may also promote labor, but should only be done after fetal well-being has been established. While the left lateral position enhances blood flow, it is not a priority until fetal heart tones have been assessed.
CN: Physiological integrity; CNS: Reduction of risk potential; CL: Apply

44. 1. Therapeutic effects of drugs, such as magnesium sulfate, used to treat hypertension of pregnancy, include an absence of seizures, a weight gain of 2 lb/wk (0.9 kg/wk), a normal blood pressure, and a urinary output greater than 30 ml/hr.
CN: Physiological integrity; CNS: Pharmacological and parenteral therapies; CL: Analyze

45. 3. Magnesium sulfate is the drug of choice to treat hypertension of pregnancy because it reduces edema by causing a shift from the extracellular spaces into the intestines. It also depresses the central nervous system, which decreases the incidence of seizures. Misoprostol is a labor-inducing drug that is administered vaginally to ripen the cervix and to cause uterine contractions. Oxytocin is the synthetic form of the pituitary hormone used to stimulate uterine contractions. Calcium gluconate is the antagonist for magnesium toxicity.
CN: Physiological integrity; CNS: Pharmacological and parenteral therapies; CL: Analyze

46. 1. Accelerations of up to 15 bpm above baseline for a duration of 15 seconds are signs of fetal well-being. Decelerations initiated 30 to 40 seconds after the onset of the contraction are termed late decelerations, and are due to uteroplacental insufficiency from decreased blood flow during uterine contractions. Variable decelerations are an indication of cord compression. Variable decelerations can occur with or without contractions.
CN: Physiological integrity; CNS: Physiological adaptation; CL: Analyze

47. A nurse is examining a client in active labor who has had spontaneous rupture of the amniotic membrane, and notes a protruding umbilical cord. What is the **priority** nursing action?
1. Push the umbilical cord back into the uterus
2. Place the client in knee-chest position
3. Instruct the client to begin to push
4. Wrap the cord in a dry sterile dressing

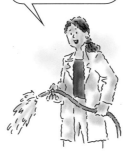

Looks like the water broke. What to do now?

47. 2. A Trendelenburg or knee-chest position takes the weight of the fetus off the umbilical cord, allowing blood to flow. The cord should never be pushed back into the uterus, as this could damage the cord, obstruct the flow of blood through the cord to the fetus, or introduce infection into the uterus. The client should not be instructed to push, as she is only in active labor, and emergency surgery may be necessary. The cord should be wrapped in a sterile saline-soaked gauze.
CN: Physiological integrity; CNS: Reduction of risk potential; CL: Apply

48. The first day of a client's last menstrual period (LMP) was October 10. Using Nägele's rule, what is the estimated date of birth?
1. July 10
2. July 17
3. August 10
4. August 17

Can you remember Nägele's rule? Subtract this, add that …

48. 2. After determining the first day of the LMP, the nurse would subtract three months and add seven days. If the client's LMP was October 10, subtracting three months is July 10, and adding seven days brings the date of birth to July 17.
CN: Health promotion and maintenance; CNS: None; CL: Analyze

49. At one minute of life, a neonate is crying vigorously, has a heart rate of 98, is active with normal reflexes and tone, and has a pink body and blue extremities. Which Apgar score would be correct for this neonate?
1. 6
2. 7
3. 8
4. 9

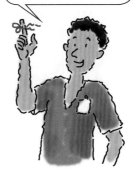

49. 3. Heart rate, respiratory effort, muscle tone, reflex irritability, and color are used to assess the Apgar score. Each of the signs is assigned a score of 0, 1, or 2. The highest possible score is 10. This neonate lost 1 point for a heart rate less than 100 bpm and 1 point for its acrocyanosis, a common finding in which the trunk is pink but the extremities are bluish.
CN: Health promotion and maintenance; CNS: None; CL: Analyze

50. A client in labor suddenly sits upright, clutches her chest, and develops acute shortness of breath. Which laboratory finding indicates that the client's condition is deteriorating?
1. Increased fibrinogen level
2. Increased platelet count
3. Prolonged prothrombin time
4. Reduced partial thromboplastin time

50. 3. The client most likely has an amniotic fluid embolism. Disseminated intravascular coagulation is a life-threatening complication of this condition, and is marked by a decreased platelet count and fibrinogen level, a prolonged prothrombin time, and partial thromboplastin time.
CN: Physiological integrity; CNS: Reduction of risk potential; CL: Analyze

51. Immediately after birth, a nurse assesses the neonate's respiratory effort as slow. The neonate is actively moving but grimaces in response to stimulation. His fingers and toes are bluish, and his heart rate is 130 bpm. Which step should the nurse take **next**?
1. Tell the provider that the neonate appears abnormal
2. Assign an Apgar score of 8
3. Wrap the infant in a warm blanket
4. Provide oxygen and stimulate the baby to cry

51. 4. The nurse should stimulate the baby to cry, provide oxygen, and call the provider to evaluate reflex irritability. It would be inappropriate to tell the provider that the neonate appears abnormal. The neonate's Apgar score is 7. Of a maximum possible Apgar score of 10, the nurse deducts one point for acrocyanosis, one point for slow respiratory effort, and one point for the grimace. Although keeping the infant warm is important, the infant clearly needs more aggressive interventions such as oxygen and stimulation.
CN: Safe, effective care environment; CNS: Management of care; CL: Apply

CN: Client needs category   CNS: Client needs subcategory   CL: Cognitive level

52. A pregnant client has a total hemoglobin level of 60 g/L. Which risk is **greatest** during the intrapartum period?
1. Small-for-gestational-age neonate
2. Fetal distress
3. Excessive postpartum bleeding
4. Shortness of breath

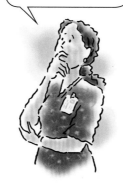

> What do you think is the greatest risk?

52. 2. Fetal distress is more common in women with anemia than in the general nonanemic population. A small-for-gestational-age neonate and excessive postpartum bleeding are diagnosed after the intrapartum period. Shortness of breath occurs more commonly antepartally. The risk for developing shortness of breath does not increase during the intrapartum period.
CN: Physiological integrity; CNS: Reduction of risk potential; CL: Apply

53. Which is the most reliable method for assessing fetal status throughout labor?
1. Fetal heart rate (FHR) auscultation using a stethoscope
2. FHR auscultation and recording using electronic fetal monitoring
3. Asking the client how she feels, and whether the fetus is moving
4. Pelvic examinations to check the location of the fetal presenting part

53. 2. The most reliable method for fetal assessment throughout labor is electronic monitoring, which records the FHR and maternal contractions, and shows how the fetus reacts to the stress of contractions. Although FHR auscultation can be done with a stethoscope, it's less common because it requires advanced skills. Asking the client how she feels, and whether the fetus is moving, are important but do not provide specifics about fetal well-being. A pelvic examination reveals cervical dilation and fetal station but doesn't reveal fetal well-being.
CN: Health promotion and maintenance; CNS: None; CL: Analyze

54. Which finding in a client who is at 36 weeks' gestation indicates that premature rupture of the membranes has occurred?
1. Fern-like pattern when vaginal fluid dries on a glass slide
2. Nitrogen paper indicates acidic pH of fluid
3. Cervical dilation of 8 cm
4. Contractions occurring every three minutes

54. 1. A fern-like pattern that forms when vaginal fluid is dried on a glass slide, called a ferning test, is a sign of ruptured membranes. Amniotic fluid is alkaline when tested with nitrogen paper. Cervical dilation and length of contractions do not indicate the condition of the membranes.
CN: Physiological integrity; CNS: Reduction of risk potential; CL: Apply

55. A nurse is precepting a student nurse in the intrapartum unit. The nurse realizes that the student has a clear understanding of the cardinal signs of fetal movement when the student places the signs in order of priority.

| 1. Flexion |
| 2. Extension |
| 3. Descent |
| 4. Internal rotation |
| 5. Engagement |
| 6. Expulsion |
| 7. External rotation |

55. Ordered Response:

| 5. Engagement |
| 3. Descent |
| 1. Flexion |
| 2. Extension |
| 4. Internal rotation |
| 7. External rotation |
| 6. Expulsion |

CN: Physiological integrity; CNS: Physiological adaptation; CL: Apply

56. A client with gestational diabetes has just delivered a 10 lb, 2 oz (4,601 g) neonate at 39 weeks' gestation. Which nursing intervention would be the **priority** in caring for the infant?
1. Teach the mother about the nutritional needs of the neonate
2. Obtain a serum neonatal glucose level
3. Feed the infant a D50W solution
4. Prepare to administer insulin to the neonate

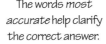

My, you're a big one!

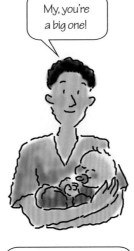

56. 2. The priority nursing intervention is to monitor the neonate's serum glucose level due to the increased risk of hypoglycemia. During pregnancy, the fetus secretes high levels of insulin to counteract the high maternal glucose levels. This elevated insulin secretion, in the neonate, can lead to severe hypoglycemia after birth. While it is important to discuss the neonate's nutritional needs with the mother, it is not an immediate priority. Infants birthed to diabetic mothers will probably require early feedings but determining the infant's blood glucose is a higher priority. Feeding the infant D50W would be inappropriate. The newborn of a mother with diabetes may develop hyperbilirubinemia, but not as quickly as hypoglycemia may develop. Since the neonate is at risk for hypoglycemia, insulin would not be appropriate.
CN: Safe, effective care environment; CNS: Management of care; CL: Apply

57. The nurse is caring for a client in active labor. Which components of labor contractions would be the **most** accurate for the nurse to assess?
1. Pelvic type, duration, contraction, and frequency
2. Contraction type and frequency and pelvic type
3. Contraction duration, frequency, and intensity
4. Contraction type, duration, and intensity

The words *most* accurate help clarify the correct answer.

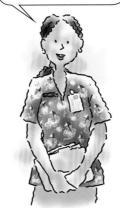

57. 3. The three components of a contraction that the nurse must evaluate are the duration, frequency, and intensity of each contraction. Pelvic type has no bearing on contractions, nor does the type of labor.
CN: Health promotion and maintenance; CNS: None; CL: Apply

58. A client in labor is using the Lamaze method of prepared birth. The nurse instructs the mother to use Level 2 breathing. Which client data would validate a need for this type of breathing?.
1. Cervical dilation of 2 to 4 cm, contractions occurring every 5 to 8 min
2. Cervical dilation of 1 cm, contractions occurring every 5 min
3. Cervical dilation of 4 to 6 cm, contractions occurring every 4 mins
4. Cervical dilation of 9 to 10 cm, contractions occurring 1 to 2 mins apart

The Lamaze method of prepared birth uses breathing techniques to ease birth.

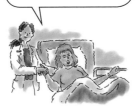

58. 3. Level 2 breathing techniques are useful when cervical dilation is between four and six cm. Level 1 breathing techniques are useful for early contractions. Level 3 and level 4 breathing techniques are used in the transition stage of labor.
CN: Health promotion and maintenance; CNS: None; CL: Apply

59. A client has received dinoprostone, intravaginally, for cervical ripening. For which adverse effect should the nurse assess?
1. Vomiting
2. Enuresis
3. Yellowing of the skin
4. Constipation

59. 1. Headache, nausea and vomiting, chills, fever, dizziness and flushing are the most common side effects of dinoprostone. Prostaglandin E does not cause enuresis and jaundice. Diarrhea, not constipation, is a possible adverse effect.

CN: Physiological integrity; CNS: Pharmacological and parenteral therapies; CL: Analyze

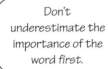

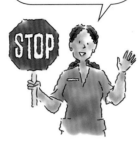

Don't underestimate the importance of the word first.

60. A nurse is caring for a client exhibiting mild contractions and a cervical dilation of 4 cm. Using an external fetal monitor, the nurse observes variable decelerations. Which action should the nurse take **first**?
1. Prepare for imminent birth
2. Place the client on her left side
3. Administer oxygen by face mask
4. Increase the IV rate

60. 2. Variable decelerations in fetal heart rate are caused by compression of the umbilical cord. Typically, variable decelerations are corrected by placing the client in a left lateral position to alleviate cord pressure. Since variable decelerations are usually transient and correctable, the nurse would not prepare for an imminent birth. Increasing the IV rate is not needed or ordered. If other measures have been ineffective in correcting the variable deceleration, oxygen may be administered.

CN: Physiological integrity; CNS: Reduction of risk potential; CL: Analyze

61. At 39 weeks' gestation, a primiparous client arrives at the labor and delivery unit reporting lower back pain that started six hours ago. A pelvic examination reveals that her cervix is dilated 3 cm and 75% effaced. Which action would be appropriate for the nurse to take?
1. Instruct the client to push
2. Send the client back home
3. Monitor the fetal heart rate
4. Assess the lochia

61. 3. This client is in the latent phase of the first stage of labor. The nurse should monitor the fetal heart in this stage and all stages of labor. Pushing is appropriate during the second stage of labor when the cervix is fully dilated. The nurse should keep the client for monitoring, and not send her back home. During the fourth stage, the nurse assesses the amount, color, and consistency of lochia.

CN: Health promotion and maintenance; CNS: None; CL: Apply

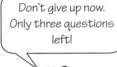

Don't give up now. Only three questions left!

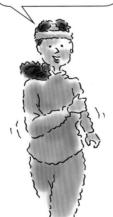

62. A nurse is assisting in monitoring a client who's receiving oxytocin to induce labor. Which maternal adverse reactions should the nurse should be alert to? Select all that apply.
1. Hypertension
2. Jaundice
3. Dehydration
4. Fluid overload
5. Uterine tetany
6. Hypoxia

62. 1, 4, 5. Adverse effects of oxytocin in the mother include hypertension, fluid overload, and uterine tetany. Oxytocin's antidiuretic effect increases renal reabsorption of water, leading to fluid overload, not dehydration. Jaundice and bradycardia are adverse effects that may occur in the neonate. Tachycardia, not bradycardia, is a maternal adverse effect.

CN: Physiological integrity; CNS: Pharmacology and parenteral therapies; CL: Apply

CN: Client needs category   CNS: Client needs subcategory   CL: Cognitive level

63. A client is admitted to the labor and delivery unit at 30 weeks' gestation. She has a history of cesarean birth, and reports severe abdominal pain that started less than one hour ago. When the nurse palpates tetanic contractions, the client again reports severe pain. After the client vomits, she states that the pain is better and then loses consciousness. The fetal heart rate is 100. What is the nurse's **priority** intervention?

1. Assess the client's level of pain
2. Place the client in a left lateral position
3. Administer IV antibiotics
4. Prepare the client for immediate surgery

64. Which illustration represents a right occiput posterior (ROP) fetal position?

1.   2.

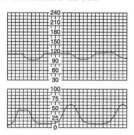

3.   4.

65. The nurse is evaluating an external fetal monitoring strip of a client in labor. What condition is the nurse concerned about?

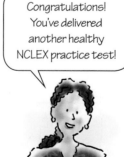

1. Cephalopelvic disproportion
2. Oligohydramnios
3. Uteroplacental insufficiency
4. Hydramnios

63. 4. Uterine rupture is a medical emergency that may occur before or during labor. Signs and symptoms typically include abdominal pain that may ease after uterine rupture, vomiting, vaginal bleeding, hypovolemic shock, and fetal distress. The client should be prepared for immediate surgery to save her life and that of the fetus. While assessing and relieving pain are important, they are not priorities in this life-threatening situation. Placing the client in a left lateral position will not affect her condition. Antibiotics may be administered but aren't the highest priority in this situation.

CN: Safe, effective care environment; CNS: Management of care; CL: Apply

64. 1. Fetal positioning is determined by how the fetus presents in relation to the mother's pelvis, which is divided into four quadrants: right anterior, left anterior, right posterior, and left posterior. In a ROP position, the fetus' occiput points to the maternal right posterior quadrant. Graphic two shows a right occiput anterior (ROA) position, graphic three shows a left occiput posterior (LOP), and graphic four shows a left occiput anterior (LOA).

CN: Health promotion and maintenance; CNS: None; CL: Apply

Congratulations! You've delivered another healthy NCLEX practice test!

65. 3. This fetal monitoring strip illustrates a late deceleration. The decrease in fetal heart rate begins after the peak of the contraction and doesn't return to baseline until the contraction is over. Late decelerations are associated with uteroplacental insufficiency, shock, or fetal metabolic acidosis. Cephalopelvic disproportion may cause early, not late, decelerations early in labor. Oligohydramnios be associated with variable decelerations. Hydramnios may be associated with uterine rupture.

CN: Physiological integrity; CNS: Reduction of risk potential; CL: Analyze

Chapter 24

Postpartum Care

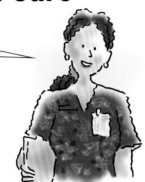

Before taking off through this chapter, why not spend a few minutes browsing the Internet for birthing stories. It'll get you in just the right mood to tackle care of the postpartum client. Enjoy!

1. While performing the morning postpartum assessment, the nurse notices that a client's perineal pad is completely saturated with lochia rubra. What action should the nurse take **first**?
   1. Vigorously massage the fundus
   2. Call the health care provider immediately
   3. Have the charge nurse review the assessment
   4. Ask the client when she last changed her perineal pad

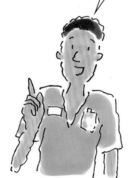

Question 1 is asking you what to do first! What a way to start!

1. 4. If the morning assessment is done relatively early, it's possible that the client hasn't yet been to the bathroom, and the perineal pad may have been in place all night. In addition, her lochia may have pooled during the night, resulting in a heavy flow in the morning. Vigorous massage of the fundus isn't recommended if heavy bleeding or hemorrhage is present. If the nurse were uncertain, and wanted a second opinion, it would be appropriate to call the health care provider or ask another qualified nurse after doing a complete assessment of the client's status.
CN: Safe, effective care environment; CNS: Management of care;
CL: Analyze

2. A postpartum mother is concerned about a noted decrease in her breast milk production. Which response by the nurse **best** addresses this mother's concern?
   1. Decrease supplemental feedings with formula
   2. Suggest the mother consume a diet high in vitamin C
   3. Have several alcoholic beverages for relaxation
   4. Feed the infant less frequently

2. 1. Routine formula supplementation may interfere with establishing an adequate milk volume because suckling the breast stimulates prolactin production. Prolactin is the hormone responsible for milk production. Vitamin C levels haven't been shown to influence milk volume. One alcohol beverage generally tends to relax the mother, and facilitate the milk let-down reflex. Excessive consumption of alcohol may block milk let-down, though supply isn't necessarily affected. Frequent feedings are likely to increase milk production.
CN: Health promotion and maintenance; CNS: None;
CL: Apply

CN: Client needs category   CNS: Client needs subcategory   CL: Cognitive level

3. A breastfeeding mother who is experiencing breast engorgement asks the nurse if there is anything she can do to get relief. What is the **best** intervention for the nurse to implement?
   1. Applying ice
   2. Applying a breast binder
   3. Teaching how to express the breasts
   4. Administering bromocriptine

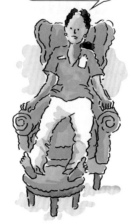

Which of these options would promote comfort best?

3. **3.** Teaching the client how to express her breasts will facilitate let-down, and provide temporary relief. Ice can promote comfort by decreasing blood flow numbing, and discouraging further let-down of milk. It is not recommended because it also causes the rebound reaction of more let-down once the ice is removed. Breast binders are not effective in relieving the discomforts of engorgement. Bromocriptine is no longer recommended for lactation suppression.
CN: Physiological integrity; CNS: Basic care and comfort; CL: Apply

4. A new graduate nurse is being oriented to care for clients on a postpartum unit. Which factor would the preceptor include as part of a routine maternal assessment?
   1. Antibody screen
   2. Babinski's reflex
   3. Homans' sign
   4. Gower sign

4. **3.** Homans' sign, or pain on dorsiflexion of the foot, may indicate deep vein thrombosis (DVT), and is this client's primary physiologic concern at this time. Postpartum women are at increased risk of DVT because of the changes in clotting mechanisms used to control bleeding during birth. Antibody screening is done during the first trimester and again during week 28 of pregnancy. The antibody screen is used to detect antibodies to Rh positive blood. A Babinski's reflex would not be routinely assessed in the postpartum woman. A positive Gower sign is associated with muscular dystrophy, and not a postpartum client.
CN: Health promotion and maintenance; CNS: None; CL: Analyze

5. A nurse is teaching a client about Kegel exercises. The nurse determines that teaching has been successful when the client states:
   1. "They assist with lochia removal."
   2. "They promote the return of normal bowel function."
   3. "They promote blood flow, and allow for healing and strengthening of the musculature."
   4. "They assist the mother in burning calories for rapid postpartum weight loss."

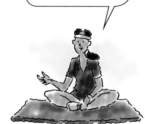

If you know what Kegel exercises are, you should get question 5 correct easily.

5. **3.** Relaxing and contracting the pubococcygeal (PCG) muscles four to five times per day for 10 to 20 minutes increases blood flow to the area. The increased blood flow brings oxygen and other nutrients to the perineal area to aid in healing. Additionally, these exercises help strengthen the musculature, thereby decreasing the risk of future complications. Performing Kegel exercises may assist with lochia removal, but that is not their main purpose. Bowel function isn't influenced by Kegel exercises. Kegel exercises don't expend sufficient energy to burn extra calories.
CN: Health promotion and maintenance; CNS: None; CL: Analyze

6. A nurse suspects that a client may have developed a pulmonary embolism. Which symptoms would validate the nurse's suspicion? Select all that apply.
   1. Sudden dyspnea and chest pain
   2. Chills and fever
   3. Bradycardia and hypertension
   4. Confusion and fainting
   5. Cough with bloody sputum

6. **1, 4, 5.** Signs of pulmonary embolus include sudden dyspnea and chest pain. There may also be a hacking cough with bloody sputum. Chills and fever signal an infection. The client with a pulmonary embolus would have fainting, tachycardia, hypotension, confusion, and tachypnea.
CN: Physiological integrity; CNS: Reduction of risk potential; CL: Analyze

CN: Client needs category   CNS: Client needs subcategory   CL: Cognitive level

7. The nurse is preparing a plan of care for a client who has had cesarean birth. What information should the nurse include in the discharge plan?
  1. Douche frequently after being discharged
  2. Do coughing and deep-breathing exercises
  3. Begin doing sit-ups two weeks postoperatively
  4. Do side-rolling exercises

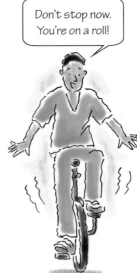

Don't stop now. You're on a roll!

7. 2. Coughing and deep-breathing exercises should be taught to any postoperative client to keep the alveoli open and prevent infection. Frequent douching is not recommended for women, and is contraindicated in women who have just given birth. Sit-ups at two weeks postpartum could potentially damage the incision. Side-rolling exercises are not an accepted medical practice.

CN: Physiological integrity; CNS: Reduction of risk potential; CL: Apply

8. A student nurse asks why a client would express disappointment after having a cesarean birth instead of a vaginal birth. What is the nurse's **best** response?
  1. Cesarean deliveries cost more.
  2. Depression is more common after a cesarean birth.
  3. The client is usually more fatigued after cesarean birth.
  4. The client may feel a loss after not experiencing a vaginal birth.

8. 4. Clients occasionally feel a loss after a cesarean birth, especially if it was unplanned. They may feel inadequate because they couldn't deliver their infant vaginally. The cost of cesarean birth doesn't generally apply because the woman isn't usually directly responsible for payment. No conclusive studies support the theory that depression is more common after cesarean birth. Although clients are usually more fatigued after a cesarean birth, fatigue hasn't been shown to cause feelings of disappointment over the method of birth.

CN: Psychosocial integrity; CNS: None; CL: Analyze

9. The nurse reviews the assessment findings of a postpartum client who has experienced a vaginal birth. Which finding should the nurse consider normal for this client?
  1. Redness or swelling in the calves
  2. A palpable uterine fundus beyond 10 days postpartum
  3. Vaginal dryness after the lochial flow has ended
  4. Dark red lochia for approximately six weeks after birth

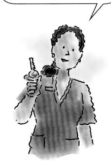

The word *normal* is the key to getting this one right.

9. 3. Vaginal dryness is a normal finding during the postpartum period due to hormonal changes. Redness or swelling in the calves may indicate thrombophlebitis. The fundus should not be palpable beyond 10 days. Dark red lochia should only last two to three days postpartum.

CN: Health promotion and maintenance; CNS: None; CL: Apply

10. On completing a fundal assessment, the nurse notes the fundus is firm and left of midline. What is the appropriate action?
  1. Ask the client to empty her bladder
  2. Straight catheterize the client immediately
  3. Call the client's health care provider for direction
  4. Vigorously massage the fundus

10. 1. A full bladder may push the uterine fundus to the side of the abdomen. A straight catheterization is unnecessarily invasive if the woman can urinate on her own. Nursing interventions should be completed before notifying the primary health care provider in a non-emergent situation. Fundal massage is not needed for this client.

CN: Physiological integrity; CNS: Reduction of risk potential; CL: Apply

CN: Client needs category   CNS: Client needs subcategory   CL: Cognitive level

11. A client who is HIV-positive tells the nurse that she would like to breastfeed. What is the nurse's **best** response?

1. "Breastfeeding will help reduce the risk of hemorrhage."
2. "Breast milk is better than formula for the baby."
3. "Breastfeeding will help with bonding."
4. "Breast milk can transmit HIV to your baby."

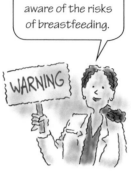

Make sure a client with HIV is aware of the risks of breastfeeding.

WARNING

11. 4. Because HIV is transmitted to the baby through breast milk, the client should not breast-feed. Breastfeeding does stimulate uterine contractions, but in this case, breastfeeding should be discouraged. It would be contradictory to tell a client who should not breastfeed that breast milk is best for her baby. In this case, formula is best. The client should be shown other ways to bond, such as holding, playing, and talking to her baby.
CN: Physiologic integrity; CNS: Reduction of risk potential; CL: Analyze

12. A client had a spontaneous vaginal birth after 18 hours of labor. Her vaginal bleeding is estimated to be 550 ml. Which nursing intervention should be a **priority** while caring for this client?

1. Avoid massaging the uterus
2. Monitor vital signs every hour
3. Empty the client's bladder
4. Elevate the head of the bed to increase blood flow

12. 3. Emptying the client's bladder will allow the uterus to contract and prevent displacement. The uterus should be palpated to determine if it's contracting, and should be massaged if it's boggy, or not contracting. Vital signs should be monitored continuously, or at least every 10 to 15 minutes until the client's condition stabilizes. The head of the bed should not be elevated because this will further lower the blood pressure.
CN: Safe, effective care environment; CNS: Management of care; CL: Analyze

13. A nurse is assessing a client with type 1 diabetes mellitus. The client's birth was complicated by polyhydramnios and macrosomia. The nurse is aware that this client is at risk for:

1. postpartum mastitis.
2. increased insulin needs.
3. postpartum hemorrhage.
4. gestational hypertension.

13. 3. The client is at risk for a postpartum hemorrhage from the over distention of the uterus because of the extra amniotic fluid and the large baby. The uterus may not be able to contract as well as it normally would. The mother with diabetes usually has decreased insulin needs for the first few days postpartum. Neither polyhydramnios nor macrosomia would increase the client's risk of mastitis or gestational hypertension.
CN: Physiological integrity; CNS: Reduction of risk potential; CL: Apply

14. The nurse is providing postpartum care for a client with type 1 diabetes mellitus. The client has developed an infection. The nurse should assess this client for:

1. anemia.
2. ketoacidosis.
3. respiratory acidosis.
4. respiratory alkalosis.

14. 2. Clients with diabetes who become pregnant tend to become sicker, and develop illnesses quicker, than pregnant clients without diabetes. A client with diabetes and a severe infection can quickly develop diabetic ketoacidosis. Anemia, respiratory acidosis, and respiratory alkalosis aren't generally associated with infections in clients with diabetes.
CN: Physiological integrity; CNS: Reduction of risk potential; CL: Analyze

15. The nurse is interviewing a client diagnosed with mastitis. Which information would require further intervention by the nurse?
   1. Breastfeeding every six hours
   2. Breastfeeding on the affected breast first
   3. Increasing daily fluid intake
   4. Emptying the affected breast completely with each feeding

15. 1. Mastitis is an infection of the breast characterized by flulike symptoms, along with redness and tenderness in the affected breast. Since mastitis may be due to milk stasis, the breastfeeding client should breastfeed every two to three hours. Other measures the client with mastitis should follow include breastfeeding on the affected side first, drinking plenty of fluids, and completely emptying the affected breast with each feeding.
CN: Physiological integrity; CNS: Physiological adaptation; CL: Analyze

16. A nurse is caring for a client on a postpartal unit following a vaginal birth. Within 24 hours following birth, the nurse finds there has been blood loss. Immediate intervention by the nurse is required if blood loss exceeds:
   1. 100 ml.
   2. 200 ml.
   3. 400 ml.
   4. 500 ml.

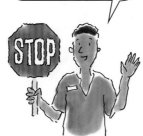

This question requires your immediate attention.

16. 4. Postpartum hemorrhage involves blood loss in excess of 500 ml. Most delayed postpartum hemorrhages occur between the fourth and ninth day postpartum. The most frequent causes of a delayed postpartum hemorrhage include retained placental fragments, intrauterine infection, and fibroids.
CN: Physiological integrity; CNS: Reduction of risk potential; CL: Apply

17. The nurse is prioritizing care of a client in the immediate postpartum period. What is the nurse's **priority** assessment? Select all that apply.
   1. Blood glucose level
   2. Electrocardiogram (ECG)
   3. Height of fundus
   4. Blood pressure
   5. Urinary output

First things first! The word *initial* is a clue in this one.

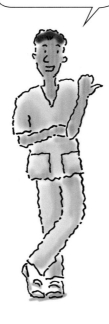

17. 3, 4, 5. A focused physical assessment should be performed every 15 minutes for the first one to two hours postpartum, including an assessment of the fundus, lochia, perineum, blood pressure, pulse, and bladder function. A blood glucose level needs to be obtained only if the woman has risk factors for an unstable blood glucose level, or if she has symptoms of an altered blood glucose level. An ECG would only be necessary if the woman is at risk for cardiac difficulty.
CN: Health promotion and maintenance; CNS: None; CL: Apply

18. A nurse is performing an assessment of a postpartum client two hours after birth, and notes heavy bleeding with large clots. What should be the nurse's **initial** action?
   1. Massaging the fundus firmly
   2. Performing bi-manual uterine compressions
   3. Administering ergonovine
   4. Notifying the health care provider

18. 1. Initial management of excessive postpartum bleeding is firm massage of the fundus along with a rapid infusion of oxytocin or lactated Ringer's solution. Bi-manual compression is performed by a health care provider. Ergonovine should only be used if the bleeding doesn't respond to massage and oxytocin. The health care provider should be notified if the client doesn't respond to fundal massage, but other measures should be taken in the meantime.
CN: Safe, effective care environment; CNS: Management of care; CL: Analyze

19. A nurse is about to give a client with type 2 diabetes mellitus her insulin before breakfast on her first day postpartum. Which client statement indicates an understanding of insulin requirements immediately postpartum?
  1. "I will need less insulin now than during my pregnancy."
  2. "I will need more insulin now than during my pregnancy."
  3. "I will need less insulin now than before I was pregnant."
  4. "I will need more insulin now than before I was pregnant."

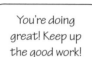

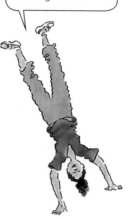

You're doing great! Keep up the good work!

19. 3. Postpartum insulin requirements are usually significantly lower than pre-pregnancy requirements. Occasionally, clients may require little or no insulin during the first 24 to 48 hours postpartum. Management of type 2 diabetes includes: healthy eating, regular exercise, possibly diabetes medication or insulin therapy, and blood sugar monitoring.
CN: Physiological integrity; CNS: Reduction of risk potential; CL: Analyze

20. Which finding in a postpartum client requires further nursing assessment?
  1. Fundus at the umbilicus one hour postpartum
  2. Fundus 3 cm below the umbilicus on postpartum day 3
  3. Fundus not palpable in the abdomen at two weeks postpartum
  4. Fundus slightly to right, and two cm above the umbilicus on postpartum day 2

20. 4. A uterus that isn't midline or is above the umbilicus on postpartum day 2 might be caused by a full, distended bladder or a uterine infection, requiring further assessment by the nurse. Within the first 12 hours postpartum, the fundus usually is at or below the umbilicus. The fundus should descend approximately 1 cm/day thereafter. The fundus shouldn't be palpated in the abdomen after day 10.
CN: Health promotion and maintenance; CNS: None; CL: Analyze

21. A client reports increasing severity of afterpains. What condition should the nurse look for in the client's history that may explain this symptom?
  1. Bottle feeding
  2. Diabetes
  3. Multiple gestation
  4. Primiparity

21. 3. Multiple gestation, breastfeeding, multiparity, and conditions that cause over distention of the uterus will increase the intensity of afterpains. Bottle feeding and diabetes aren't directly associated with increasing severity of afterpains, unless the client has delivered a macrosomic infant.
CN: Health promotion and maintenance; CNS: None; CL: Analyze

22. When giving a postpartum client self-care instructions, the nurse instructs the client to report heavy or excessive bleeding. Which client statement indicates that the nurse's teaching was effective?
  1. "I will call the doctor if I saturate a pad in one hour or less."
  2. "I will call the doctor if I if I have to change my pad at night."
  3. "I will call the doctor if I if I notice any blood clots in my pad."
  4. "I will call the doctor if bleeding continues beyond the fifth day post-birth."

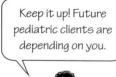

Keep it up! Future pediatric clients are depending on you.

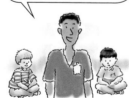

22. 1. Bleeding is considered heavy when a woman saturates a sanitary pad in one hour. Excessive bleeding occurs when a postpartum client saturates a pad in 15 minutes. Moderate bleeding occurs when the bleeding saturates less than 6 in (15 cm) of a pad in one hour. Having to change the pad during the night shortly after birth is normal and expected. Passing small blood clots and bleeding at five days after birth is a normal finding.
CN: Health promotion and maintenance; CNS: None; CL: Apply

CN: Client needs category   CNS: Client needs subcategory   CL: Cognitive level

23. The nurse is assessing a postpartum client who has lochia serosa. The client asks the nurse how long she should expect this type of bleeding to continue. The nurse's replies, "Your bleeding should stop on:
1. days 3 to 4 postpartum."
2. days 3 to 10 postpartum."
3. days 10 to 14 postpartum."
4. days 14 to 42 postpartum."

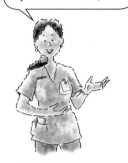

Remember: There are three types of lochia. Which type is this question referring to?

23. **2.** On the third and fourth postpartum days, the lochia becomes a pale pink or brown and contains old blood, serum, leukocytes, and tissue debris. This type of lochia usually lasts until postpartum day 10. Lochia rubra usually lasts for the first three to four days postpartum and consists of blood, decidua, and trophoblastic debris. Lochia alba, which contains leukocytes, decidua, epithelial cells, mucus, and bacteria, may continue for two to six weeks postpartum.
CN: Health promotion and maintenance; CNS: None; CL: Apply

24. A client and her neonate have a blood incompatibility. The neonate has had a positive direct Coombs' test. Which nursing intervention is appropriate?
1. Because the woman has been sensitized, give Rho(D) immune globulin
2. Because the woman hasn't been sensitized, give Rho(D) immune globulin
3. Because the woman has been sensitized, don't give Rho(D) immune globulin
4. Because the woman hasn't been sensitized, don't give Rho(D) immune globulin

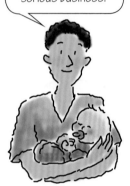

Blood incompatibility between a client and her neonate is serious business.

24. **3.** A positive Coombs' test means that the Rh-negative woman is now producing antibodies to the Rh-positive blood of the neonate. Rho(D) immune globulin shouldn't be given to a sensitized client because it won't be able to prevent antibody formation.
CN: Physiological integrity; CNS: Reduction of risk potential; CL: Analyze

25. The nurse is teaching a client with newly diagnosed mastitis about her condition. The client asks the nurse what caused her to develop mastitis. What is the nurse's **best** response?
1. "You are breastfeeding too frequently."
2. "Bacteria from the neonate's mouth has caused this."
3. "You are wearing a bra that did not provide adequate support."
4. "Expressing milk when your breasts become engorged causes this.""

25. **2.** The most common cause of mastitis is bacteria transmitted from the neonate's mouth. Mastitis isn't harmful to the neonate. Breastfeeding frequently lessens the chance of developing mastitis, as does expressing milk whenever the mother feels engorged. An ill-fitting bra may be uncomfortable but will not lead to mastitis.
CN: Health promotion and maintenance; CNS: None; CL: Apply

26. Which behavior should the nurse expect to observe in a client on the fourth postpartum day?
1. The client asks many questions about the baby's care.
2. The client wants to relate her birth experience.
3. The client asks the nurse to select her meals for her.
4. The client asks the nurse to help her bathe herself.

26. **1.** The taking-hold phase usually lasts from days 3 to 10 postpartum. During this stage, the mother strives for independence and autonomy. She also becomes curious and interested in the care of the baby, and is most ready to learn. During the taking-in phase, which usually lasts 2 to 3 days, the mother is passive and dependent and expresses her own needs rather than those of the neonate. During the taking-in phase, the client may ask the nurse to help with self-care, want to talk about her birth experience, and allow others to make decisions for her.
CN: Psychosocial integrity; CNS: None; CL: Apply

27. A nurse treating a postpartum client a few days after birth? Which verbalization should be cause for concern?
1. The client states that she is nervous about taking the baby home.
2. The client tells the nurse that she feels empty since she delivered the baby.
3. The client asks if she can watch the nurse give her baby the first bath.
4. The client says that she would like the nurse to take her baby to the nursery so she can sleep.

28. During the assessment of a postpartum client, the nurse notes a continuous flow of blood from the vagina and a firm uterus 1 cm below the umbilicus. Which complication does the nurse suspect this client may be experiencing?
1. Retained placental fragments
2. Urinary tract infection (UTI)
3. Cervical laceration
4. Uterine atony

29. The nurse determines further teaching is necessary when a client on anticoagulant therapy for deep vein thrombosis states:
1. "I will continue to take my iron replacement therapy."
2. "I will take aspirin for headaches."
3. "I will avoid restrictive clothing."
4. "I will report shortness of breath immediately."

30. A pregnant client is very confused when she hears that her TORCH panel has returned positive. She anxiously states, "This means the baby has HIV!" The nurse replies that the "H" in TORCH represents:
1. hemophilia.
2. hepatitis B virus.
3. herpes simplex virus.
4. human immunodeficiency virus.

31. The nurse is concerned that a client who experienced a perinatal loss three days ago may being exhibiting signs of dysfunctional grieving. Which sign should the nurse expect to see with this type of grieving?
1. Lack of appetite
2. Denial of the death
3. Blaming herself
4. Frequent crying spells

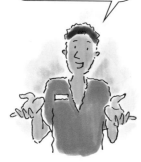

It's important to listen to the feelings and concerns of a postpartum client.

Anticoagulant therapy and I don't get along well together.

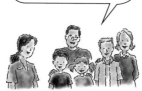

Remember to look out for the needs of the whole family, not just the client.

27. 2. A mother experiencing postpartum blues may say she feels empty now that the infant is no longer in her uterus. She may also verbalize that she feels unprotected now. Many first-time mothers are nervous about caring for their neonates following discharge. New mothers may want a demonstration before doing a task themselves. A client may want to get some uninterrupted sleep, so she may ask that the baby be taken to the nursery.
CN: Psychosocial integrity; CNS: None; CL: Analyze

28. 3. A continuous flow of blood may be due to cervical or vaginal lacerations if the uterus is firm and contracted. Retained placental fragments and uterine atony may cause subinvolution of the uterus, making it soft, boggy, and larger than expected. A UTI won't cause vaginal bleeding, although hematuria may be present.
CN: Physiological integrity; CNS: Reduction of risk potential; CL: Apply

29. 2. Discharge teaching should include informing the client to avoid salicylates, which may potentiate the effects of anticoagulant therapy. Iron won't affect anticoagulation therapy. Restrictive clothing should be avoided to prevent the recurrence of thrombophlebitis. Shortness of breath should be reported immediately because it may be a symptom of pulmonary embolism.
CN: Physiological integrity; CNS: Reduction of risk potential; CL: Analyze

30. 3. TORCH represents the following maternal infections: Toxoplasmosis, Others, such as gonorrhea, syphilis, varicella, hepatitis, and human immunodeficiency virus, Rubella, Cytomegalovirus, and Herpes simplex virus. Hemophilia is a clotting disorder in which factors VII and X are deficient. It is not a virus.
CN: Physiological integrity; CNS: Reduction of risk potential; CL: Apply

31. 2. Denial of the perinatal loss is a sign of dysfunctional grieving in the client. Lack of appetite, blaming oneself, and frequent crying spells are part of a normal grieving process.
CN: Psychosocial integrity; CNS: None; CL: Apply

CN: Client needs category   CNS: Client needs subcategory   CL: Cognitive level

32. A nurse is assessing the fundus of a client who is 12 hours postpartum, and finds that the fundus is boggy. Which action should the nurse take **first**?
1. Prepare the client for surgery
2. Administer blood replacement products
3. Massage the fundus
4. Administer methylergonovine, as ordered

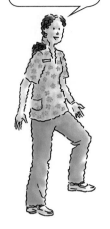

You're making great strides. Keep going!

32. 3. The nurse should first massage the boggy uterus to stimulate it to contract. The client may need surgery but only if other measures fail to cause the uterus to contract and control bleeding. Blood replacement products may be given if the client has a significant blood loss. Methylergonovine may be ordered if massage fails to firm the uterus.
CN: Physiological integrity; CNS: Reduction of risk potential;
CL: Analyze

33. An Rh-positive client has just delivered a 6 lb, 10 oz (3.03 kg) neonate vaginally, after 17 hours of labor. What factor would place this client at risk?
1. Length of labor
2. Maternal Rh status
3. Method of birth
4. Size of the baby

33. 1. A prolonged length of labor places the mother at increased risk for developing an infection. The size of the baby, vaginal birth, and Rh status of the client do not place the mother at increased risk.
CN: Physiological integrity; CNS: Physiological adaptation;
CL: Analyze

34. A nurse is caring for a breastfeeding client who delivered by cesarean. What is the **most** important information for the nurse to teach this client?
1. Delay breastfeeding until 24 hours after birth
2. Breastfeed frequently during the day and every four to six hours at night
3. Use the cradle hold position to avoid incisional discomfort
4. Use the football hold position to avoid incisional discomfort

34. 4. When breastfeeding after a cesarean birth, the client should be encouraged to use the football hold to avoid incisional discomfort. Breastfeeding should be initiated as soon after birth as possible. The mother should be encouraged to breastfeed her infant every two to three hours throughout the night as well as during the day to increase the milk supply.
CN: Health promotion and maintenance; CNS: None; CL: Analyze

35. Which client behavior indicates an understanding of the nurse's teaching plan for breastfeeding?
1. The client washes her nipples with soap and water.
2. The client lets her nipples air dry.
3. The client lets the baby attach to the nipple only.
4. The client pulls the baby off the nipple when feeding is done.

35. 2. The nipples should be allowed to air dry after breastfeeding to keep them dry and prevent irritation. Only water should be used to wash the nipples since soap removes natural oils and can be drying. When breastfeeding, the baby should grasp both the nipple and the areola. When the baby is done with a breast, the baby's grasp on the nipple should be released before removing the baby from the breast.
CN: Health promotion and maintenance; CNS: None;
CL: Apply

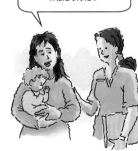

Is it OK to breastfeed with mastitis?

36. A client with mastitis tells the nurse she is concerned about breastfeeding her neonate. What is the nurse's **best** response?
1. Stop breastfeeding until completing the antibiotic
2. Supplement feeding with formula until the infection resolves
3. Do not use analgesics because they aren't compatible with breastfeeding
4. Continue to breastfeed; mastitis won't infect the infant

36. 4. The client with mastitis should be encouraged to continue breastfeeding while taking antibiotics for the infection. No supplemental feedings are necessary because breastfeeding encourages resolution of the infection, and doesn't need to be altered. Analgesics are safe and should be administered as needed.
CN: Health promotion and maintenance; CNS: None; CL: Analyze

CN: Client needs category   CNS: Client needs subcategory   CL: Cognitive level

37. The nurse is assessing a six-week postpartum client in the obstetrician's office. In the exam room, the nurse asks the client how she's feeling. The client bursts into tears and reports that she cries most of the time, feels like a failure and can barely get out of bed to dress. The nurse suspects the client is experiencing:
1. postpartum blues.
2. postpartum depression.
3. postpartum neurosis.
4. postpartum psychosis.

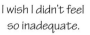

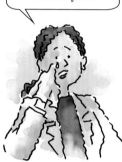

I wish I didn't feel so inadequate.

37. 2. Postpartum depression occurs in approximately 10% to 15% of all postpartum women. This depression is characterized by disabling feelings of inadequacy, and an inability to cope that can last up to three years. The client is often tearful and despondent. The client with postpartum blues experiences crying and sadness, generally between three and five days postpartum. This condition resolves itself quickly. Postpartum neurosis includes neurotic behavior during the initial six weeks after birth. Postpartum psychosis includes hallucinations, delusions, and phobias.
CN: Psychosocial integrity; CNS: None; CL: Apply

38. A client who is breastfeeding reports pain, redness, and swelling in her right breast. What is the **best** information for the nurse to give this client?
1. Wear a tight-fitting brassiere while breastfeeding
2. Breastfeeding should be stopped permanently
3. Continue antibiotics until pain, redness, and swelling subside
4. Apply moist heat compresses to the right breast

38. 4. Moist heat compresses reduce inflammation and swelling of the affected area and relieve pain. The client should avoid wearing a constrictive brassiere while breastfeeding so milk can flow freely. There is no need to stop breastfeeding permanently. Antibiotics should be taken for the prescribed cause of therapy and should not be stopped when symptoms subside.
CN: Health promotion and maintenance; CNS: None; CL: Apply

39. A six-week postpartum client is being assessed by the nurse at the obstetrician's office. The nurse notes that the uterus is soft and enlarged, and that the client is experiencing vaginal bleeding. The nurse is concerned that the client is experiencing:
1. cervical laceration.
2. clotting deficiency.
3. perineal laceration.
4. uterine subinvolution.

39. 4. Late postpartum bleeding is typically the result of subinvolution of the uterus. Retained products of conception or infection often cause subinvolution. Cervical or perineal lacerations can cause an immediate postpartum hemorrhage. A client with a clotting deficiency may also have an immediate postpartum hemorrhage, if the deficiency isn't corrected at the time of birth.
CN: Physiological integrity; CNS: Physiological adaptation; CL: Apply

40. A client states she needs to void three hours after a vaginal birth. Which risk factor would require the nurse to assist the client while getting out of bed?
1. Afterpains
2. Breast engorgement
3. Orthostatic hypotension
4. Painful episiotomy incision

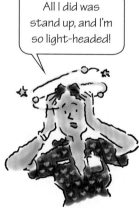

All I did was stand up, and I'm so light-headed!

40. 3. The rapid decrease in intra-abdominal pressure occurring after birth causes splanchnic engorgement. The client is at risk for orthostatic hypotension when standing due to the blood pooling in this area. Breast engorgement is caused by vascular congestion in the breast before true lactation, and occurs later in the postpartum period. The client may experience contractions, sometimes called afterpains, during the first few days after birth. These help prevent excessive bleeding by compressing the blood vessels in the uterus. Episiotomy pain is normal.
CN: Health promotion and maintenance; CNS: None; CL: Analyze

CN: Client needs category   CNS: Client needs subcategory   CL: Cognitive level

41. Prior to administering a rubella vaccine, what important information should the nurse share with the client?
1. "This vaccine is safe in clients with egg allergies.
2. "You should not breastfeed if you receive this vaccine."
3. "Expect to experience unusual tiredness or weakness after getting the vaccine."
4. "You should avoid getting pregnant for three months after receiving the vaccination."

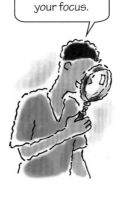

Don't lose your focus.

41. 4. The client must understand that she must not become pregnant for two to three months after the vaccination because of its potential teratogenic effects. The rubella vaccine is made from duck eggs so an allergic reaction may occur in clients with egg allergies. The virus isn't transmitted through breast milk, so clients may continue to breastfeed after vaccination. Unusual tiredness or weakness which may be sudden and severe is a symptom of an allergic reaction to the vaccine and not a normal response.
CN: Health promotion and maintenance; CNS: None; CL: Apply

42. A client is diagnosed with postpartum preeclampsia and asks the nurse what could have caused this to occur. Which causative factors should the nurse include in her teaching? Select all that apply.
1. Obesity
2. Prolonged labor
3. Fetal distress at birth
4. Poor diet
5. Damage to blood vessels during birth

42. 1, 4, 5. While preeclampsia occurs primarily during pregnancy, and is resolved at birth, it can occur up to six weeks postpartum. Identified risk factors are obesity, damage to uterine blood vessels during birth and poor maternal diet. Fetal distress and prolonged labor do not contribute to the occurrence of this disorder.
CN: Physiological integrity; CNS: Physiological Adaptation; CL: Apply

43. A client is receiving magnesium sulfate therapy. The nurse recognizes that this client must be monitored for:
1. hypotension.
2. postpartum depression.
3. postpartum hemorrhage.
4. uterine infection.

43. 3. Because magnesium sulfate relaxes smooth muscle, the uterus should be assessed for uterine atony, which would increase the risk of postpartum hemorrhage. Postpartum depression and uterine infection aren't associated with magnesium sulfate therapy. Magnesium sulfate is considered more of an anticonvulsant than an antihypertensive.
CN: Physiological integrity; CNS: Pharmacological and parenteral therapies; CL: Understand

44. A nurse is reviewing the plan of care on the third postpartum day for a client who has had an episiotomy. Which instructions should this plan include?
1. Apply ice to the perineum
2. Encourage the use of sitz baths
3. Avoid tightening the pelvic muscles
4. Massage the perineal area

44. 2. A sitz bath reduces inflammation and relaxes the perineum, promoting healing and reducing discomfort. Ice should only be used for the first 24 hours following birth. A client should begin, not avoid tightening and relaxing the pelvic muscles (known as Kegel exercise) during the postpartum period. Massaging the perineum may disrupt the suture line and cause more pain.
CN: Physiological integrity; CNS: Physiological adaptation; CL: Analyze

45. A mother with diabetes tells the nurse that she wants to breastfeed but is concerned about the effects of breastfeeding on her health. What is the nurse's best response?
1. "Mothers with diabetes will find it more difficult to control hyperglycemic episodes."
2. "Mothers with diabetes should not breastfeed because of potential complications."
3. "Insulin requirements are doubled for diabetic mothers who choose to breastfeed."
4. "Insulin requirements may decrease for diabetic mothers who choose to breastfeed."

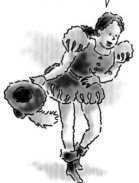

To breastfeed or not to breastfeed, that is the question.

45. 4. Breastfeeding has an antidiabetogenic effect. Insulin needs are decreased because carbohydrates are used in milk production. Breastfeeding mothers are at a higher risk of hypoglycemia in the immediate postpartum days because glucose levels are lowered. Mothers with diabetes should be encouraged to breastfeed.
CN: Physiological integrity; CNS: Pharmacological and parenteral therapies; CL: Apply

46. Which client activity would indicate that a nurse's teaching about perineal care has been effective?
1. The client uses a spray bottle to cleanse the perineum after urination and bowel movements.
2. The client wipes the perineum from back to front after urinating or a bowel movement.
3. The client douches after urination or a bowel movement.
4. The client changes perineal pads three times a day.

46. 1. The client should cleanse the perineal area using a spray or peri-bottle after urinating or a bowel movement. The client should wipe from front to back after voiding to avoid contaminating the perineal area. Perineal pads should be changed when they are soiled to keep the perineum clean. Douching is contraindicated for postpartum clients.
CN: Health promotion and maintenance; CNS: None; CL: Apply

47. A nurse is performing the morning assessment on a multiparous client on postpartum day 1. Which assessment finding would indicate that the client is at increased risk for hemorrhage?
1. Hemoglobin level of 12 g/dl (120 g/L)
2. Uterine atony
3. Thrombophlebitis
4. Moderate amount of lochia rubra

47. 2. Multiparous women often experience a loss of uterine tone due to frequent distention of the uterus from past pregnancies. This puts a multiparous client at higher risk for hemorrhage. Thrombophlebitis doesn't increase the risk of hemorrhage during the postpartum period. The hemoglobin level and lochia flow are within acceptable limits and do not indicate hemorrhage risk.
CN: Health promotion and maintenance; CNS: None; CL: Analyze

48. A client requests that her baby be sent back to the nursery on the first postpartum night, so she can get some sleep. Which postpartal phase is this client experiencing?
1. Depression phase
2. Letting-go phase
3. Taking-hold phase
4. Taking-in phase

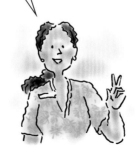

Remember, when you're dealing with a postpartum client, you've got two clients to think about.

48. 4. The taking-in phase occurs in the first 24 hours after birth. The mother is concerned with her own needs and requires support from staff and relatives. The depression phase isn't an appropriate answer. The letting-go phase begins several weeks later, when the mother incorporates the new infant into the family unit. The taking-hold phase occurs when the mother is ready to take responsibility for her care as well as her infant's care.
CN: Health promotion and maintenance; CNS: None; CL: Analyze

CN: Client needs category   CNS: Client needs subcategory   CL: Cognitive level

49. Four clients each gave birth 12 hours ago. Based upon report and assessment, which client should the nurse see **first**?
1. Gravida 2 Para 2002, cesarean birth, incisional site intact, hemoglobin level 9.8 g/dl
2. Gravida 2 Para 1011, cesarean birth, incisional site intact, pulse 84 beats/minute
3. Gravida 1 Para 1001, vaginal birth, midline episiotomy, temperature 99.8° F (37.7° C)
4. Gravida 1 Para 1001, vaginal birth, ruptured membranes 10 hours before birth

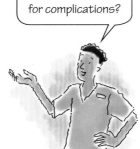

Which client is at the greatest risk for complications?

49. 1. Women who are anemic in pregnancy (defined as a hemoglobin <10 g/dl) may experience additional complications, such as poor wound healing, and the inability to tolerate activity. The vital signs in answers two and three are within normal limits. Dehydration can cause a slightly elevated temperature. The client with ruptured membrane is not displaying any symptoms. Women whose membranes are ruptured more than 24 hours before birth are more prone to developing chorioamnionitis Complications of chorioamnionitis may include high temperature, rapid heartbeat, sweating, a uterus that is tender to the touch, and discharge from the vagina that has an unusual smell.
CN: Health promotion and maintenance; CNS: None; CL: Analyze

50. Which client statement indicates an understanding of how to prevent breast engorgement while breastfeeding?
1. "I will apply moist heat to my breasts three times a day."
2. "I will breastfeed every one to three hours."
3. "I will use a breast pump to obtain milk for feedings."
4. "I will wear a tight bra continually."

50. 2. Frequent breastfeeding empties the breast, decreasing the risk of engorgement. Moist heat can stimulate the let-down reflex, leading to engorgement. A breast pump is not necessary if the breast-feed baby is emptying the breasts when fed. A tight brassiere may prevent the breasts from emptying completely when breastfeeding, increasing the risk of engorgement.
CN: Health promotion and maintenance; CNS: None;
CL: Apply

51. A client has delivered twins one hour ago. What is the **priority** nursing intervention?
1. Assess fundal tone and lochia flow
2. Apply a cold pack to the perineal area
3. Administer analgesics, as ordered
4. Encourage voiding by offering the bedpan

51. 1. Women who deliver twins are at a higher risk for postpartum hemorrhage due to over distention of the uterus, which causes uterine atony. Assessing fundal tone and lochia flow help to determine risks for hemorrhage. Applying cold packs to the perineum, administering analgesics as ordered, and offering the bedpan are all significant nursing interventions but not as important as preventing postpartum hemorrhage.
CN: Health promotion and maintenance; CNS: None;
CL: Apply

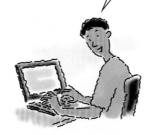

Question 52 is looking for a normal response.

52. Which finding would the nurse consider to be a normal physiologic response in the early postpartum period?
1. Urinary urgency and dysuria
2. Rapid diuresis
3. Decrease in blood pressure
4. Increased motility of the gastrointestinal system

52. 2. In the early postpartum period, there's an increase in the glomerular filtration rate and a drop in progesterone levels, which result in rapid diuresis. A client may feel anxious about voiding, but there should be no urinary urgency. There are minimal changes in blood pressure following birth, and a residual decrease in gastrointestinal motility.
CN: Physiological integrity; CNS: Physiological adaptation;
CL: Apply

53. On postpartum day 2, a client reports to the nurse that she is voiding more volume of urine than when she was pregnant. What is the nurse's **best** response?
1. "The IV fluids that you received while in labor are being excreted."
2. "The diuresis you are experiencing is the result of your body reducing the accumulated fluid you experienced during pregnancy."
3. "Your increased urinary output is caused by the amount of fluid you are drinking."
4. "Your kidneys were impaired while you were pregnant, and are now working normally."

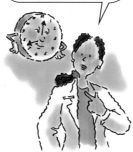

Note the reference to time in question 53. It's important to understanding the question.

53. 2. The excess water that was in the blood and which was retained in the body tissues during pregnancy is primarily excreted by the kidneys. Postpartum diuresis occurs when the body begins to reduce extracellular fluid volume that accumulated during the pregnancy. This causes marked increase in the daily output of urine (diuresis). It is not caused from IV fluid infusions since normal deliveries do not necessitate large amounts of IV fluids, and any infused or ingested fluids would have been eliminated. In healthy women, there is no renal impairment as part of pregnancy. There is an increase in glomerular filtration rate and renal blood flow following birth.
CN: Physiological Integrity; CNS: Physiological adaption; CL: Analyze

54. The nurse is aware that uterine atony that may lead to postpartum hemorrhage is most likely caused by:
1. hypertension.
2. cervical and vaginal tears.
3. urine retention.
4. endometritis.

Question 55 requires your *immediate* attention.

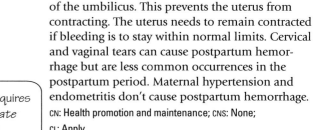

54. 3. Urine retention causes a distended bladder, or displaces the uterus above, and to the side of the umbilicus. This prevents the uterus from contracting. The uterus needs to remain contracted if bleeding is to stay within normal limits. Cervical and vaginal tears can cause postpartum hemorrhage but are less common occurrences in the postpartum period. Maternal hypertension and endometritis don't cause postpartum hemorrhage.
CN: Health promotion and maintenance; CNS: None; CL: Apply

55. The nurse is assessing a client 22 hours after a cesarean birth. Which assessment finding would require immediate action by the nurse?
1. Heart rate of 132 beats/min and blood pressure of 84/60 mmHg
2. Oral temperature of 100.2° F (37.9° C)
3. A gush of blood from the vagina when the client stands up
4. Reports of abdominal pain and cramping

55. 1. Tachycardia and hypotension may be signs of hemorrhage. An oral temperature of 100.2° F (37.9° C) may be due to dehydration, if it occurs on the first postpartum day. A gush of blood from the vagina when a client stands is a normal finding on the first postpartum day. Reports of abdominal pain and cramping are expected following cesarean birth.
CN: Physiological integrity; CNS: Reduction of risk potential; CL: Apply

Have you ever heard the postpartum blues?

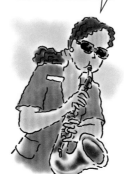

56. A nurse is talking to a client who delivered her baby five days ago, and suspects that the client is having the postpartum blues. Which client behavior is suggestive of this problem? Select all that apply.
1. Inability to care for the baby
2. Crying
3. Difficulty sleeping
4. Voicing feelings of worthlessness
5. Mood swings

56. 2, 3, 5. Postpartum blues are a transient mood alteration that arises during the first three weeks postpartum and are typically self-limiting. They affect 50% to 80% of postpartum clients. Postpartum depression, a more severe mood alteration, is seen in approximately 20% of clients. It involves changes that occur within a few days after birth, and may last for a few days to more than one year. Crying, difficulty sleeping and mood swings are commonly seen in clients with postpartum blues, while the inability to care for the infant and voicing feelings of worthlessness are more indicative of postpartum depression.
CN: Psychosocial integrity; CNS: None; CL: Analyze

57. A nurse is performing a comprehensive fundal check during a postpartum assessment. Which aspects of the fundus should the nurse assess?
  1. Fundal consistency, location, and height
  2. Fundal consistency and height
  3. Fundal location and potential fundal distention
  4. Fundal location and height

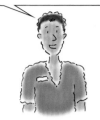

Check out the word comprehensive. Sounds important.

57. 1. A comprehensive fundal check includes evaluation of fundal consistency, height, and location. A firm fundus that is at the correct height for the postpartum day and located in the center of the pelvis is a normal finding. The other options don't reflect a comprehensive fundal check because they're missing valuable components.
CN: Physiological integrity; CNS: Physiological adaptation; CL: Analyze

58. A nurse is performing an assessment on a postpartum client. The assessment reveals that the fundus is firm. The nurse interprets this as:
  1. a firm tumor at the top of the uterus.
  2. contraction of the uterus.
  3. a uterus filled with blood.
  4. bladder distention.

58. 2. A firm postpartum fundus means that the uterus has contracted, and is constricting blood vessels, thereby decreasing lochial flow. A uterine tumor doesn't necessarily cause a firm fundus. A uterus filled with blood, and bladder distention will restrict the uterus from contracting downward, resulting in a soft, boggy uterus and increased vaginal bleeding.
CN: Physiological integrity; CNS: Physiological adaptation; CL: Analyze

59. A primipara who is Rho(D) negative has just given birth to a Rh-positive baby. The nurse is developing a plan of care. How should Rho(D) immune globulin be administered?
  1. To the neonate within three days
  2. To the client within three days
  3. To the client at her first postpartum visit in six weeks
  4. To the neonate at the first well-baby visit

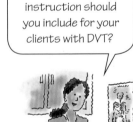

Discharge teaching is important. Which instruction should you include for your clients with DVT?

59. 2. Administering Rho(D) immune globulin to the client within 72 hours of birth prevents antibodies from forming that can destroy fetal blood cells in the next pregnancy. Rho(D) immune globulin isn't given to the baby. The client should not wait six weeks to receive Rho(D) immune globulin as antibodies will already have formed.
CN: Safe, effective care environment; CNS: Management of care; CL: Apply

60. A postpartum client is receiving enoxaparin at 1mg/kg every 12 hour subcutaneously for deep vein thrombophlebitis. What is the **most** important information for the nurse to include in discharge teaching?
  1. "Avoid heat compresses."
  2. "Keep legs crossed when sitting."
  3. "Avoid rubbing or massaging the legs."
  4. "You should experience numbness, tingling, or muscle weakness (especially in your legs and feet)."

60. 3. Discharge teaching should include a reminder to avoid rubbing or massaging the legs to lessen the chance of developing a pulmonary embolism. The client should avoid crossing their legs to prevent recurrence of thrombophlebitis. Heat compresses are advised for comfort. Numbness, tingling, or muscle weakness (especially in your legs and feet) are not expected results; they are serious side effects and need to be reported
CN: Health promotion and maintenance; CNS: Reduction of risk potential; CL: Apply

61. The nurse is assessing a breastfeeding client on the fourth postpartum day. Which findings would be expected?
  1. Soft, non-tender breasts
  2. Engorged breasts with inflamed, radiating areas that are sore to the touch
  3. Slightly tender, cracked nipples, slightly firm, non-tender breasts, and transitional milk
  4. Tender, intact nipples, firm, tender breasts, and transitional milk

61. 4. Tender, intact nipples, firm, tender breasts, and transitional milk are normal in a breastfeeding client on the fourth postpartum day. Engorged, inflamed breasts signal mastitis. Tender, cracked nipples are not a normal finding. They require intervention and client teaching to help the nipples heal, and allow this client to avoid the problem in the future.
CN: Physiological integrity; CNS: Physiological adaptation; CL: Apply

CN: Client needs category   CNS: Client needs subcategory   CL: Cognitive level

62. Which statement, made by a breastfeeding primiparous client, should alert the nurse to a potential problem?
   1. "I will consume an additional 500 calories/day."
   2. "I will increase my intake of protein."
   3. "I will limit my fluid intake."
   4. "I will eat foods high in vitamins and minerals."

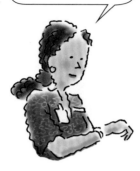

Uh oh. It's time to feed the baby again.

62. **3.** A breastfeeding client who states that fluid intake should be limited requires additional teaching. Increased fluids are needed for milk production. The breastfeeding client should consume an additional 500 calories/day, increase protein intake, and eat foods high in vitamins and minerals.
CN: Health promotion and maintenance; CNS: None; CL: Apply

63. A nurse is teaching a breastfeeding primiparous client how to prevent sore nipples. The nurse determines further teaching is necessary when the client states:
   1. "I should breastfeed for only three to four minutes at a time until my milk flow is established."
   2. "I should position the baby properly during feedings."
   3. "I should gently break the suction of the baby away from my nipple after the feeding."
   4. "I should prevent the baby from feeding after my breast has been emptied."

63. **1.** In some cases, it takes seven minutes for the let-down reflex to cause milk to fill the breast. The other answers indicate that the client understands the nurse's instructions.
CN: Physiological integrity; CNS: Reduction of risk potential; CL: Apply

64. A client is five days postpartum following a vaginal birth of a 7 lb 10 oz (3.48 kg) infant. She calls the clinic to inquire about her postpartum care. What information should the nurse share with this client? Select all that apply.
   1. "Douche daily to cleanse the vagina."
   2. "Use only sanitary pads, and avoid tampons."
   3. "Call your provider if you have any gushes of blood when stranding up."
   4. "Swimming may be resumed at two weeks postpartum."
   5. "Call your provider immediately if the bleeding increases, or if you are soaking a pad in one hour."

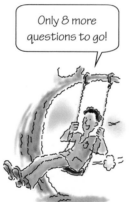

Only 8 more questions to go!

64. **2, 5, 3.** Postpartum clients must use sanitary pads instead of tampons to prevent infections and toxic shock syndrome. Clients must call their primary care provider if they experience increased blood flow, which would be abnormal. Douching and swimming are contraindicated for postpartum women, and it is normal for postpartum clients to have gushes of blood when standing up or changing positions.
CN: Physiological integrity; CNS: Physiological adaptation; CL: Apply

65. On examining a client who gave birth three hours ago, the nurse finds that the client has completely saturated a perineal pad within 15 minutes. Which actions should the nurse take? Select all that apply.
   1. Begin an IV infusion of lactated Ringer's solution
   2. Assess the client's vital signs
   3. Palpate the client's fundus
   4. Place the client in high Fowler's position
   5. Administer an ordered oral pain medication

65. **2, 3.** Assessing vital signs provides information about the client's circulatory status and identifies significant changes to report to the health care provider. By palpating the client's fundus, the nurse also gains valuable assessment data. A boggy uterus may lead to excessive bleeding. Starting an IV infusion requires an order by a health care provider. Placing the client in high Fowler's position may lower blood pressure and harm the client. Administration of a pain medication does not address the current problem.
CN: Physiological integrity; CNS: Reduction of risk potential; CL: Apply

CN: Client needs category   CNS: Client needs subcategory   CL: Cognitive level

66. A nurse is assessing a client who is two weeks postpartum. How should this client's normal lochia appear?
1. Creamy white to light yellow and may have a stale odor
2. Creamy white to light yellow, contains decidual cells, and may have a stale odor
3. Pinkish brown to red, and contains tissue fragments, and may have a foul odor
4. Brown to red, and contains residual cells and leukocytes

66. 2. Lochia alba occurs from one to three weeks postpartum. Lochia alba is creamy white to light yellow contains residual cells, and may have a stale odor. It also contains leukocytes. Lochia alba shouldn't contain tissue fragments or have a foul odor.

CN: Physiological integrity; CNS: Physiological adaptation; CL: Apply

67. Which condition would alert the nurse that a client who is one week postpartum has retained placental fragments?
1. Puerperal infection
2. Postpartum depression
3. Postpartum hemorrhage
4. Uterine tetany

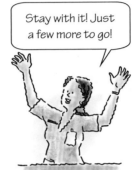

Stay with it! Just a few more to go!

67. 3. Retained placental fragments, which prevent the uterus from contracting properly, increase postpartum blood loss. This loss may be dramatic and lead to postpartum hemorrhage of 500 ml of blood or more. Although retained placental fragments may also lead to uterine subinvolution or infection, these are less common complications. Postpartum depression is a psychiatric disorder not related to retained placental fragments.

CN: Health promotion and maintenance; CNS: None; CL: Apply

68. Which interventions would the nurse implement to address pain issues related to a client's perineal sutures from her episiotomy? Select all that apply.
1. Sit on a cushion for comfort
2. Avoid the use of topical pain gels
3. Administer sitz baths three to four times per day
4. Discourage the client to do from doing Kegel exercises
5. Wash the stitches daily with soap and water

68. 1, 3. Sitting on a cushion will provide comfort for perineal pain from the birth. Sitz baths help decrease inflammation and tension in the perineal area. Kegel exercises improve circulation to the area and help reduce edema, and should be encouraged. Topical pain gels should be applied to the suture area to reduce discomfort, if ordered. Water is used to wash stitches and the perianal area but not soap. Soap will dry out the skin, increase pain and slow down healing.

CN: Physiological integrity; CNS: Basic care and comfort; CL: Apply

69. A nurse is palpating the uterine fundus of a client who delivered a baby eight hours ago. At what level in the abdomen would the nurse expect to feel the fundus?

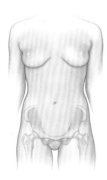

69. The uterus should be felt at the level of the umbilicus from one hour after birth and for the next 24 hours.

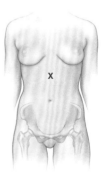

CN: Physiological integrity; CNS: Reduction of risk potential; CL: Apply

70. A client with a history of varicose veins has just delivered her first baby. A nurse suspects that the mother has developed pulmonary embolus. Which symptoms would confirm this suspicion? Select all that apply.
1. Sudden dyspnea
2. Chills, fever
3. Diaphoresis
4. Bradycardia
5. Confusion

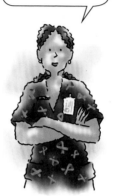

You did it! A star is born (no pun intended)!

71. A nurse observes several interactions between a mother and her neonate. Which maternal behaviors should the nurse identify as evidence of mother-infant attachment? Select all that apply.
1. Talks and coos to her son
2. Cuddles her son close to her
3. Doesn't make eye contact with her son
4. Requests that the nurse take the baby to the nursery for feedings
5. Encourages the father to hold the baby
6. Takes a nap when the baby is sleeping

70. 1, 3, 5. Sudden dyspnea along with diaphoresis and confusion are classic symptoms that develop when a thrombus from a varicose vein becomes an embolus that lodges in the pulmonary circulation. Chills and fever would indicate infection. A client with an embolus usually develops tachycardia.

CN: Physiological integrity; CNS: Physiological adaptation; CL: Analyze

71. 1, 2. Talking, cooing, and cuddling with her son are positive signs of mother-infant attachment. Avoiding eye contact is a non-bonding behavior. Eye contact, touching, and speaking help establish attachment with a neonate. Feeding a neonate is an important role of a new mother and facilitates attachment. Encouraging the father to hold the neonate will facilitate attachment. Resting while the neonate is sleeping will conserve needed energy and allow the mother to be alert.

CN: Psychosocial integrity; CNS: None; CL: Analyze

Chapter 25

Neonatal Care

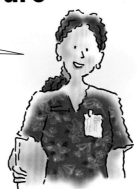

Neonates depend on you for everything. Let's show 'em you've got what it takes for neonatal care!

1. A client has given birth to an 8 lb 2.5 oz (3,700 g) male. The client tells the nurse that she wants to breastfeed her child. How many calories per day does this neonate require? Record your answer using a whole number.

_____ cal/day

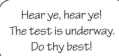

Hear ye, hear ye! The test is underway. Do thy best!

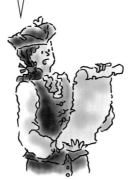

2. A neonate is admitted to the neonatal intensive care unit. The infant's parents ask why the health care provider has ordered surfactant replacement therapy. How should the nurse answer these parents' question?
  1. Surfactant therapy is given to all neonates.
  2. Surfactant therapy is used to prevent lung inflammation.
  3. Surfactant therapy is given to neonates with family history of chronic respiratory disorders.
  4. Surfactant helps in keeping the lungs expanded after the baby starts breathing on its own by keeping the lungs from sticking together.

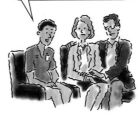

You need to keep the parents informed of the whats and whys of their baby's care.

1. 407.
A newborn infant requires 110 to 120 cal/kg/day. It is important in newborns to calculate fluid and caloric requirements exactly rather than rounding up or down. There are no differences in caloric requirements for males versus females.

Here are the calculations based on 110 cal/kg/day:

$$3,700 \text{ g} = 3.7 \text{ kg}$$

$$3.7 \text{ kg} \times 110 \text{ cal/kg/day} = 407 \text{ cal/day}$$

CN: Health promotion and maintenance; CNS: None; CL: Apply

2. 4. Surfactant works by reducing surface tension in the lungs. It allows the lungs to remain slightly expanded, decreasing the amount of work required for inspiration. It does not decrease inflammation. Surfactant is indicated for both prevention and treatment of Respiratory Distress Syndrome in premature infants. It is not given based on family history of respiratory disorders.

CN: Physiological integrity; CNS: Pharmacological and parental therapies; CL: Apply

CN: Client needs category   CNS: Client needs subcategory   CL: Cognitive level

3. While assessing a two-hour-old neonate, a nurse observes the neonate to have acrocyanosis. Which nursing action should be performed **first**?
1. Give the baby a warm bath
2. Do nothing different because acrocyanosis is normal in the early neonatal period
3. Take the neonate's temperature according to facility policy
4. Notify the health care provider of the need for a cardiac consult

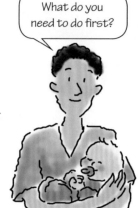

What do you need to do first?

3. **2.** Acrocyanosis, or bluish discoloration of the hands and feet in the early neonatal period is a normal finding and should not last more than 24 hours after birth. The other choices are inappropriate for this condition.
CN: Physiological integrity; CNS: Physiological adaptation; CL: Apply

4. A nurse teaches the parents of a neonate some home care strategies to reduce the risk of Sudden Infant Death Syndrome (SIDS). Which information should the nurse include when educating the parents? Select all that apply.
1. A pacifier may be used when putting the neonate down to sleep.
2. Use a cardiac monitor with all preterm neonates.
3. Place the neonate on their back for 12 months.
4. Co-share the room with the neonate.
5. Reposition the neonate if he or she has rolled over to his or her stomach.

4. **1, 3, 4.** Supine positioning is recommended to reduce the risk of SIDS in babies up to one year of age. Pacifiers have been shown to protect infants from SIDS. Co-sharing a room, rather than co-sharing a bed, allows for bonding and ease of breastfeeding at night. It also allows for frequent monitoring and reduces the risk of smothering the infant when the parent rolls over. Cardiorespiratory monitoring may be used with certain preterm infants with apnea. There is no evidence that repositioning the baby reduces the risk of SIDS.
CN: Health promotion and maintenance; CNS: None; CL: Apply

5. A nurse is caring for a client with gestational diabetes. Which complication is the neonate **most** at risk of developing?
1. Anemia
2. Hypoglycemia
3. Cardiomyopathy
4. Polycythemia

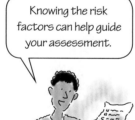

Knowing the risk factors can help guide your assessment.

5. **2.** Neonates of mothers with diabetes are most at risk for hypoglycemia due to increased insulin levels. During gestation, an increased amount of glucose is transferred to the fetus through the placenta. The neonate's liver cannot initially adjust to the changing glucose levels after birth. This may result in hypoglycemia in the neonate. Neonatal complications of having a mother with diabetes include anemia, polycythemia and cardiomyopathy. The neonate is most as risk for developing hypoglycemia.
CN: Physiological integrity; CNS: Physiological adaptation; CL: Analyze

6. The nurse is aware that preterm neonates who receive prolonged mechanical ventilation at birth are **most** at risk for which condition?
1. Chronic lung disease
2. Alveolar rupture
3. Bradycardia
4. Air-trapping

6. **1.** Chronic lung disease commonly results from the prolonged high pressures that must sometimes be used to maintain adequate oxygenation in preterm neonates. Alveolar rupture, bradycardia and air-trapping may be signs indicating the need for, or complications of, mechanical ventilation, but not as frequently as chronic lung disease.
CN: Physiological integrity; CNS: Physiological adaptation; CL: Analyze

7. The nurse assesses a three-week-old neonate to determine hydration status. Which assessment finding is the **best** indicator of adequate hydration?
1. Soft, smooth skin with good turgor
2. A 2 lb 3 oz (1 kg) weight gain
3. A heart rate of 120 bpm
4. 2 ml/kg/hr urine output

8. A nurse assesses the neuromuscular function of a neonate. Which finding should the nurse consider normal?

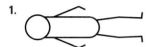
1.

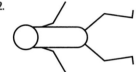
2.

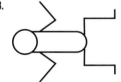
3.

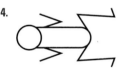
4.

9. A nurse is caring for four clients on an antepartum unit. What is the earliest gestational stage that a conceptus is considered viable?
1. 9 weeks
2. 14 weeks
3. 24 weeks
4. 30 weeks

10. A client's mother asks the nurse why her newborn grandson is getting an injection of vitamin K. What is the nurse's **best** response?
1. Vitamin K assists with coagulation.
2. Vitamin K assists the gut flora to manufacture more Vitamin K.
3. Vitamin K helps to decrease the effect of hemostatic process.
4. Vitamin K injections are easier to administer than oral preparations.

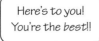

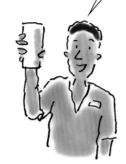

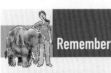

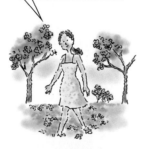

Remember

"Vitamin K is for klotting."

Vitamin K, deficient in the neonate, is needed to activate clotting factors. Thus, newborns are typically given an injection of vitamin K soon after birth.

7. 1. Soft, smooth skin with good turgor is the best sign of adequate hydration. Steady weight gain, normal heart rate and urine output are good signs but not the best sign of adequate hydration.
CN: Physiological integrity; CNS: Physiological adaptation; CL: Analyze

8. 4. Flexor tone tends to develop first in the lower extremities, and proceed toward the head and neck. A 28-week neonate will lie with minimally flexed limbs, and have minimal resistance to passive movement of all extremities. By 32 weeks, the neonate will develop flexor tone at the hips and knees, and be able to resist manipulation of the lower extremities. This progression correlates with increasing myelination of the subcortical motor pathways originating in the brainstem. By 36 weeks, the neonate will develop flexion at the elbows, and by term, the neonate will be able to flex all extremities.
CN: Health promotion and maintenance; CNS: None; CL: Apply

9. 3. At approximately 23 to 24 weeks, the lungs of the conceptus are sufficiently developed to maintain extrauterine life. The lungs are the most immature system during the gestational period. Medical care for premature labor begins much earlier (aggressively at 21 weeks' gestation).
CN: Health promotion and maintenance; CNS: None; CL: Apply

10. 1. Vitamin K is deficient neonates. This places the neonate at risk for excessive bleeding. This vitamin is needed to activate clotting factors II, VII, IX, and X. Vitamin K does not assist the gut flora to synthesize more Vitamin K. The route of administration is based on efficacy. Vitamin K injections as a onetime dose is more effective than oral vitamin K against bleeding. Vitamin K helps to achieve homeostatic process.
CN: Physiological integrity; CNS: Pharmacological and parenteral therapies; CL: Apply

CN: Client needs category   CNS: Client needs subcategory   CL: Cognitive level

11. A term neonate is born to a woman infected with hepatitis B. Which treatment would the nurse anticipate for this neonate?
1. Hepatitis B vaccine at birth and one month. No Hepatitis B immune globulin
2. Hepatitis B immune globulin at birth. No hepatitis B vaccine
3. Hepatitis B immune globulin within 48 hours of birth, and hepatitis B vaccine at one month
4. Hepatitis B immune globulin within 12 hours of birth, and hepatitis B vaccine at birth, 1 to 2 months, and six months

11. **4.** Hepatitis B immune globulin should be given as soon as possible, or within 12 hours of birth. Neonates should also receive hepatitis B vaccine at regularly scheduled intervals. This sequence of care has been determined as superior to the others provided.
CN: Health promotion and maintenance; CNS: None; CL: Analyze

12. The nurse is caring for a 1.2 kg neonate with anemia of prematurity. The health care provider orders a blood transfusion of 15 ml/kg red blood cells (RBCs) over four hours. At what rate and volume per hour should the nurse set the infusion pump? Record your answer using one decimal place.

_____ ml/hr

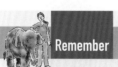

An ounce of prevention is worth a pound of cure!

12. **4.5.**
Neonatal blood transfusions, as with any blood transfusion, carry an increased risk. Smaller volumes are recommended to prevent complications. A maximum 5 ml/kg/h over a maximum time of four hours is recommended. Here are the calculations:

$$1.2 \; kg \times 15 \; ml/kg = 18 \; ml$$

$$18 \; ml \div 4 \; hours = 4.5 \; ml/hr$$

CN: Physiological integrity; CNS: Pharmacological and Parenteral Therapies; CL: Analyze

13. Which information regarding newborn eye care is true? Select all that apply.
1. The nurse examines the eyes to look for congenital cataracts.
2. Retinopathy of prematurity commonly occurs in late-preterm infants.
3. Erythromycin ointment is administered to help prevent infections due to *Neisseria gonorrhoeae* or *Chlamydia trachomatis*.
4. Strabismus is not seen until the neonate is over 12 weeks of age.
5. 1% silver nitrate is administered to help prevent infections due to *Treponema pallidum*.

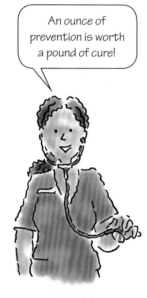

Remember

"Erythromycin in the eyes of every infant prevents infection."

Erythromycin ointment is administered to help prevent infections due to *Neisseria gonorrhoeae* or *Chlamydia trachomatis* (ophthalmia neonatorum).

13. **1, 3.** Erythromycin or silver nitrate eye prophylaxis is administered to the neonate immediately, or soon after birth, to prevent ophthalmia neonatorum often due to *N. gonorrhoeae* or *C. trachomatis*. It does not protect against *T. pallidum*. The risk for retinopathy of prematurity decreases with advancing gestational age, and is seen most often in neonates less than 32 weeks gestation. Cataracts are an opacity of the lens of the eye associated with children with congenital rubella, and can be discovered during an eye exam. Strabismus is neuromuscular incoordination of the eye alignment and affects many newborns. It is typically resolved by 6 to12 months of age.
CN: Physiological integrity; CNS: Reduction of Risk Potential; CL: Apply

14. The nurse is caring for a neonate whose mother has group AB blood, and whose father has group O blood. Which sign would initially indicate to the nurse ABO blood incompatibility in the neonate?
1. Anemia
2. Thrombocytopenia
3. Kidney failure
4. Jaundice

15. Which circumstance of delivery would place a neonate at **highest** risk of respiratory distress syndrome (RDS)?
1. Preterm birth
2. Infant of a diabetic mother
3. Twin gestation
4. Infant born through thick meconium

16. The nurse is caring for a recently circumcised newborn. Based on the progress note, what would be the **most** appropriate nursing intervention?

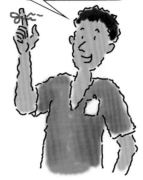

Progress notes	
2/10/17 0800	Three day old male, two days post-circumcision by Mogen clamp. Small amount of yellow-white exudate noted around glans. No bleeding or swelling noted. Axillary temp 36.4°C (97.5°F). Nursing eagerly, latching on well. Voided x1 post-circ.

1. Provide routine care to the circumcised area
2. Wrap the neonate in 2 additional blankets
3. Take the neonate's temperature every hour for the first 24 hours.
4. Give the neonate a pacifier to help soothe his pain

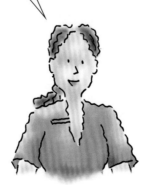

The color of an exudate helps determine its cause.

14. 4. The neonate with an ABO blood incompatibility will have jaundice within the first 24 hours of life. Anemia, thrombocytopenia and kidney failure are later signs of an ABO incompatibility.
CN: Physiological integrity; CNS: Reduction of risk potential; CL: Analyze

15. 1. Preterm birth is the single most important risk factor for developing RDS. The second born of twins, and neonates born by cesarean delivery, are also at increased risk for RDS. Infants of diabetic mothers, and those born through thick meconium, could develop respiratory problems.
CN: Physiological integrity; CNS: Physiological adaptation; CL: Apply

16. 1. The yellow-white exudate is part of the granulation process and is a normal finding for a healing penis following circumcision. Routine vital signs and normal layering would be recommended for this neonate as this temperature is normal in a newborn. It is not necessary to increase monitoring or covering of the neonate. Pacifiers do soothe pain in the neonate however, there is no indication in this progress note that the neonate is in pain.
CN: Health promotion and maintenance; CNS: None; CL: Analyze

17. The nurse assesses the Ballard score for a neonate delivered at 37 weeks' gestation. Using the chart and descriptions, what is the gestational age of this neonate?

Progress notes

2/10/17	Description:
1800	Neuromuscular exam: Wrist flexion 30 degrees; elbow flexion with arm recoil to the face; popliteal angel 90 degrees; elbow across the chest with resistance met at the ipsilateral nipple; and resistance of the pelvic girdle at the umbilicus. Physical exam; Skin peeling with parched appearance and cracking around the ankles; minimal lanugo on back and shoulders; planter creases 2/3 of the sole; 3 to 4 mm breast tissue; thick ear cartilage with stiffness of the pinna; scrotal skin thick with deep rugae; testes descended bilaterally.

_________ weeks' gestation

NEUROMUSCULAR MATURITY

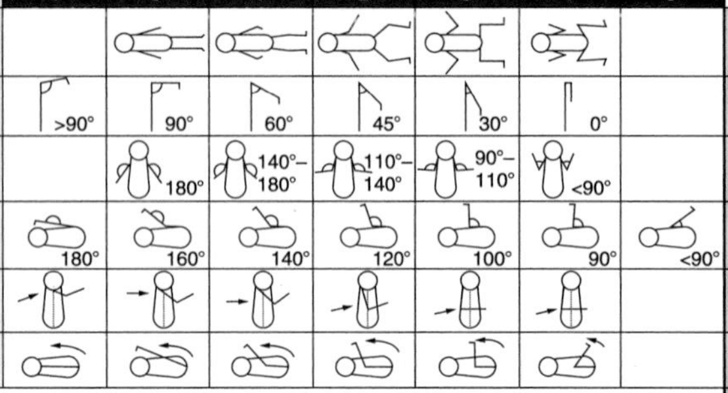

NEUROMUSCULAR MATURITY SIGN	SCORE −1	0	1	2	3	4	5	RECORD SCORE HERE
POSTURE								
SQUARE WINDOW (Wrist)	>90°	90°	60°	45°	30°	0°		
ARM RECOIL		180°	140°–180°	110°–140°	90°–110°	<90°		
POPLITEAL ANGLE	180°	160°	140°	120°	100°	90°	<90°	
SCARF SIGN								
HEEL TO EAR								
						TOTAL NEUROMUSCULAR MATURITY SCORE		

SCORE

Neuromuscular ___
Physical ___
Total ___

MATURITY RATING

Score	Weeks
−10	20
−5	22
0	24
5	26
10	28
15	30
20	32
25	34
30	36
35	38
40	40
45	42
50	44

PHYSICAL MATURITY

PHYSICAL MATURITY SIGN	SCORE −1	0	1	2	3	4	5	RECORD SCORE HERE
SKIN	sticky, friable, transparent	gelatinous, red, translucent	smooth, pink, visible veins	superficial peeling and/or rash, few veins	cracking pale areas, rare veins	parchment, deep cracking, no vessels	leathery, cracked, wrinkled	
LANUGO	none	sparse	abundant	thinning	bald areas	mostly bald		
PLANTAR SURFACE	heel-toe 40–50 mm: −1 <40 mm: −2	>50 mm no crease	faint red marks	anterior transverse crease only	creases ant. 2/3	creases over entire sole		
BREAST	impercep-tible	barely perceptible	flat areola no bud	stippled areola 1–2 mm bud	raised areola 3–4 mm bud	full areola 5–10 mm bud		
EYE-EAR	lids fused loosely: −1 tightly: −2	lids open pinna flat stays folded	sl. curved pinna; soft; slow recoil	well-curved pinna; soft but ready recoil	formed and firm instant recoil	thick cartilage, ear stiff		
GENITALS (Male)	scrotum flat, smooth	scrotum empty, faint rugae	testes in upper canal, rare rugae	testes descending, few rugae	testes down, good rugae	testes pendulous, deep rugae		
GENITALS (Female)	clitoris prominent and labia flat	prominent clitoris and small labia minora	prominent clitoris and enlarging minora	majora and minora equally prominent	majora large, minora small	majora cover clitoris and minora		
						TOTAL PHYSICAL MATURITY SCORE		

17. 42

Based on the description the infant scores the following on the New Ballard Score Sheet:
Posture = 4
Square Window = 3
Arm Recoil = 4
Popliteal angle = 4
Scarf sign = 3
Heel to ear = 3
Total Neuromuscular = 21
Skin = 4
Lanugo = 4
Plantar Surface = 3
Breast = 3
Eye/Ear = 4
Male genital = 3
Total score = 42. This score would be consistent with a gestational age between 40 and 42 weeks.

CN: Health promotion and maintenance; CNS: None; CL: Analyze

CN: Client needs category CNS: Client needs subcategory CL: Cognitive level

18. The nurse is assessing a newborn for incurvature of the trunk. Which illustration indicates the position in which the nurse should place the newborn?

1.

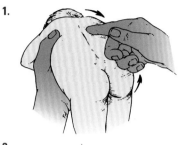

2.

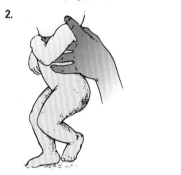

3.

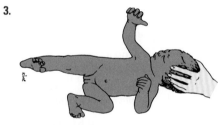

4.

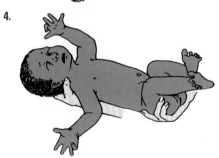

18. 1. The nurse would place the infant in a horizontal prone position with one hand, and stroke the side of the newborn's trunk, from shoulder to buttocks with the other hand. If the reflex is present, the newborn's trunk will curve toward the stimulated side. Answer two illustrates the position to test a stepping response. Answer three illustrates positioning to test for a tonic neck reflex. Answer four illustrates the position to test for a Moro reflex.

CN: Health promotion and maintenance; CNS: None;
CL: Apply

19. The nurse assesses a neonate for signs of infection. Which early finding would indicate the possibility of an infection?
1. Hypotension
2. Neurologic hyperactivity
3. Temperature instability
4. Thrombocytopenia

19. 3. Temperature instability, especially when it results in a low temperature, may be a sign of infection. Term infants with sepsis are more likely to be febrile, whereas preterm infants are more likely to show signs of hypothermia. Signs of neurologic hyperactivity are more likely late-onset. Hypotension and Thrombocytopenia are late signs.

CN: Physiological integrity; CNS: Physiological adaptation;
CL: Analyze

20. A full term neonate has just been delivered without complications. Which assessment findings would indicate successful adaptation to extrauterine life? Select all that apply.
1. Nasal flaring
2. Apgar scores of 9 at five minutes
3. A respiratory rate of 42
4. The infant nursed in the delivery room
5. Axillary temp 36.5°C (97.7°F)
6. Sleeping quietly

21. A neonate is born to a mother who received magnesium sulfate during labor. Which finding would be of **greatest** concern for the nurse?
1. Apgar score 7
2. Hypotonia
3. Respiratory rate of 10
4. Heart rate of 104

22. The nurse is caring for a newborn with neonatal abstinence syndrome. The practitioner has ordered methadone 2 mg/kg divided four times a day. The infant weighs 2,700 g. The medication comes prepared as 2 mg/ml. How many milliliters should the nurse administer per dose? Record your answer using three decimal places.

_____ ml

23. A client with gestational diabetes delivers a large-for-gestational-age neonate with mild grunting and jitteriness. Prioritize the nurse's care for this infant.

1. Check vital signs, including SaO_2, weight, length and occipital frontal circumference (OFC)
2. Obtain EKG and X-ray to evaluate cardio-pulmonary status
3. Start an IV
4. Obtain ordered labs for evaluation of electrolyte and metabolic abnormalities, including CBC with differential, glucose, electrolytes, bilirubin and possibly an arterial blood gas (ABG)
5. Give ordered glucose, magnesium and calcium
6. Give 40% FiO_2 at 1-2 lpm (liters per minute)

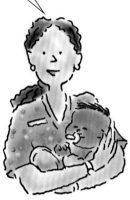

It's time to adapt to the "outside of the womb" world.

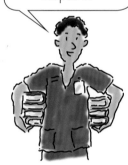

The test-taking expertise you're gaining from answering these questions will be well worth the effort you're putting in. Keep at it!

20. 2, 3, 4, 5. A respiratory rate of 30 to 60 breaths/min is normal for a neonate during the transitional period. Normal range of temperature: axillary: 36.5°C–37°C (97.5°F–98.6°F). Nasal flaring is a sign of respiratory distress. An Apgar score between 7 and 10 is considered excellent and indicates successful transition to extrauterine life. Nursing in the delivery room also shows a successful transition. Sleeping quietly may or may not be associated with a successful transition as sick neonates also sleep quietly at times.
CN: Health maintenance and promotion; CNS: None; CL: Analyze

21. 3. Magnesium sulfate crosses the placenta, and adversely affects the neonate. Common adverse effects are respiratory depression, hypotonia, and bradycardia. Respiratory depression would be the most critical assessment finding. An Apgar score of 7 to 10 is a sign that the newborn is transitioning well to extrauterine life. Bradycardia is defined as a heart rate less than 100 bpm.
CN: Physiological integrity; CNS: Pharmacological and parenteral therapies; CL: Analyze

22. 0.675.
Here are the calculations:

$$2{,}700\ g = 2.7\ kg$$
$$2\ mg/kg \div 4 = 0.5\ mg/kg/dose$$
$$2.7\ kg \times 0.5\ mg/kg = 1.35\ mg/dose$$
$$1.35\ mg \div 2\ mg/ml = 0.675\ ml$$

CN: Physiologic integrity; CNS: Pharmacological and parenteral therapies; CL: Analyze

23. Ordered Response:

1. Check vital signs, including SaO_2, weight, length and occipital frontal circumference (OFC).
6. Give 40% FiO_2 at 1-2 lpm (liters per minute)
4. Obtain ordered labs for evaluation of electrolyte and metabolic abnormalities, including CBC with differential, glucose, electrolytes, bilirubin and possibly an arterial blood gas (ABG)
3. Start an IV
5. Give ordered glucose, magnesium and calcium
2. Obtain EKG and X-ray to evaluate cardio-pulmonary status

CN: Health promotion and maintenance; CNS: None; CL: Analyze

24. The parents bring a two-day-old neonate, who was born at home without noticeable complications, to the hospital after noticing blood in the stool. The parents declined the administration of vitamin K for their neonate after birth. Based on the neonate's birth history and presenting symptom, which condition should the nurse suspect?
  1. Neonatal hemorrhagic disease
  2. Biliary atresia
  3. Intussusception
  4. Hepatitis

24. 1. Neonates have coagulation deficiencies because of a lack of organisms that help produce vitamin K in the intestines. Vitamin K helps the liver synthesize clotting factors II, VII, IX, and X. Infants born at home often do not receive vitamin K at birth. Blood in the stool may be one sign of neonatal hemorrhagic disease. Biliary atresia, intussusception and hepatitis may also be causes of bloody stools but the highest risk for the neonate is neonatal hemorrhagic disease.
CN: Health promotion and maintenance; CNS: None;
CL: Analyze

25. The nurse is attending the delivery of a neonate at 38 weeks' gestation. Prioritize the nurse's interventions for this neonate.

1.	Place a cap on the neonate's head
2.	Preheat the radiant warmer prior to delivery
3.	Obtain an axillary temperature
4.	Wrap the neonate in new blankets
5.	Dry the infant with new blankets

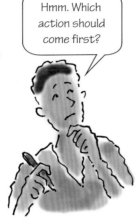

Hmm. Which action should come first?

25. Ordered Response:

2.	Preheat the radiant warmer prior to delivery
5.	Dry the infant with new blankets
4.	Wrapping the neonate in new blankets
1.	Place a cap on the neonate's head
3.	Obtain an axillary temperature

CN: Health promotion and maintenance; CNS: None;
CL: Apply

26. The nurse wraps a neonate in a blanket and keeps the ambient temperature warm. Which type of heat loss is this nurse trying to prevent?
  1. Conduction
  2. Convection
  3. Evaporation
  4. Radiation

26. 2. Heat loss from convection is the flow of heat from the body surface to cooler air. Conduction is the loss of heat from the body surface in direct contact with cooler surfaces. Evaporation is the loss of heat that occurs when a liquid is converted to a vapor. Radiation is the loss of heat from the body's surface not in direct contact with a cooler solid surfaces.
CN: Health promotion and maintenance; CNS: None;
CL: Apply

27. A nurse is explaining physiologic hyperbilirubinemia to the parents of a neonate. Which statement, made by the parents, would demonstrate a correct understanding?
  1. "The neonate usually has a medical problem."
  2. "In term neonates, it usually appears after 24 hours."
  3. "It is caused by elevated conjugated bilirubin levels."
  4. "It is usually progressive from the neonate's feet to his head."

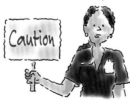

Be careful with this prefix. *Hyper* is almost identical to *hypo*, but its meaning, of course, is vastly different.

Caution

27. 2. Physiologic jaundice first appears after 24 hours. Neonates are otherwise healthy and have no medical problems. Hyperbilirubinemia is caused, almost exclusively, from unconjugated bilirubin. Jaundice usually appears in a cephalo-caudal progression from head to feet.
CN: Physiological integrity; CNS: Reduction of risk potential;
CL: Analyze

28. A neonate has been diagnosed with caput succedaneum. Which information should the nurse include while teaching the mother about this condition?
1. It usually resolves in three to six weeks.
2. It doesn't cross the cranial suture line.
3. It's a collection of blood between the skull and periosteum.
4. It involves swelling of the tissue over the presenting part of the fetal head.

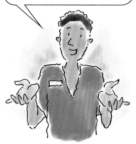

When you're teaching a new mom, it helps to know what to expect at each stage in a neonate's development.

29. A postpartum client expresses concern about the appearance of her baby's first stool, which she describes as "dark and slimy." What is the nurse's **best** response?
1. These types of stools may occur when the baby is dehydrated.
2. The health care provider will be notified about this when he examines the infant.
3. This bowel movement is called meconium and is considered normal.
4. The appearance of the baby's first stool is determined by your diet during pregnancy.

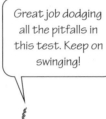

Great job dodging all the pitfalls in this test. Keep on swinging!

30. A three-day old infant has orders to begin phototherapy treatment for hyperbilirubinemia. The nurse teaches the parents how to use overhead phototherapy lights. Which information should the nurse include? Select all that apply.
1. Diuretics are given during treatment since bilirubin is excreted in the urine and stool.
2. Feed the neonate under phototherapy lights throughout the treatment to prevent dehydration.
3. A mask is placed over the eyes to prevent retinal damage.
4. The temperature is monitored frequently during phototherapy.
5. The neonate may develop loose green stools with phototherapy.
6. Place the bassinet near the window at home for sun exposure after discharge home.

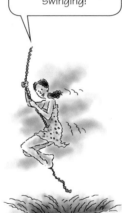

31. A nurse is caring for four neonates. Which neonate is most likely to develop hyperbilirubinemia?
1. The neonate of a black mother
2. The neonate of an Rh-positive mother
3. The neonate with ABO incompatibility
4. A neonate with Apgar scores of 8 and 9 at 1 and 5 minutes

28. 4. Caput succedaneum is the swelling of tissue over the presenting part of the fetal scalp due to sustained pressure. This boggy edematous swelling is present at birth, crosses the suture line, and most commonly occurs in the occipital area. A cephalohematoma is a collection of blood between the skull and periosteum that doesn't cross cranial suture lines and resolves in three to six weeks. Caput succedaneum resolves within three to four days.
CN: Physiological integrity; CNS: Physiological adaptation;
CL: Apply

29. 3. Meconium collects in the GI tract during gestation and is initially sterile. Meconium is greenish black and viscous because of occult blood. Dehydration would be rare in a neonate who is passing the first stool. Health care provider notification is not necessary, as this is a normal appearance. The stool of a neonate is not affected by the mother's antenatal diet.
CN: Health promotion and maintenance; CNS: None;
CL: Apply

30. 3, 4, 5. During overhead light phototherapy, a shield is placed over the infant's eyes to protect from retinal damage. The temperature is monitored frequently to prevent over or under heating. Phototherapy can cause dehydration. The neonate should be fed frequently, but not while under the phototherapy lights. Bilirubin is excreted in the urine and stool which may cause loose green stools. The use of photosensitizing medications should be avoided while infants are receiving phototherapy. Medications used in the newborn period that have been linked to phototoxic reactions include nonsteroidal anti-inflammatory, diuretics, and certain antibiotics. Exposure to sunlight was previously thought to be helpful, but currently is not recommended due to the risk of sunburn. Sunburn does not occur when phototherapy lights are properly used.
CN: Physiological integrity; CNS: Physiological adaptation;
CL: Apply

31. 3. The mother's blood type, which is different from the neonate's, has an impact on the bilirubin level because of the antigen-antibody reaction. Black neonates tend to have lower mean levels of bilirubin. Chinese, Japanese, Korean, and Greek neonates tend to have higher incidences of hyperbilirubinemia. Neonates of Rh-negative, not Rh-positive, mothers tend to have hyperbilirubinemia. Low Apgar scores indicate an increased risk of hyperbilirubinemia.
CN: Physiological integrity; CNS: Physiological adaptation;
CL: Analyze

CN: Client needs category   CNS: Client needs subcategory   CL: Cognitive level

32. A neonate has developed a major infection. Which bacteria **most** likely contributed to this problem?
1. *Escherichia coli*
2. Group B streptococci (GBS)
3. Klebsiella species
4. *Pseudomonas aeruginosa*

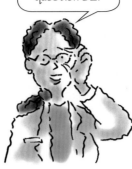

I'm *positive* you'll spot the right answer to question 32.

32. 2. GBS are gram-positive cocci that the neonate can be exposed to in the vaginal tract. *E. coli*, Klebsiella, and *P. aeruginosa* species are gram-negative rods that can produce bacterial infection in neonates. The incidence of early-onset GBS has declined by 80% with the use of intrapartum antibiotic prophylaxis (IAP). *E. coli* and GBS continue to account for approximately two-thirds of early-onset infection.

CN: Physiological integrity; CNS: Physiological adaptation; CL: Analyze

33. A neonate develops respiratory distress 18 hours after delivery. Which organism is the **most** likely cause of this problem?
1. *Candida albicans*
2. *Chlamydia trachomatis*
3. *Escherichia coli*
4. Group B beta-hemolytic streptococci

33. 4. Transmission of group B beta-hemolytic streptococci can result in respiratory distress that can rapidly lead to septic shock. It is the most common cause of sepsis in neonates. *E. coli* is the second most common cause. Candidiasis may be acquired from the birth canal, and can cause an infection after 24 hours. *C. trachomatis* infection causes neonatal conjunctivitis and pneumonia.

CN: Physiological integrity; CNS: Physiological adaptation; CL: Analyze

34. A mother tells the nurse she understands breastfeeding is the best, but will change to formula feedings when she returns to work in a few weeks. What should the nurse tell this mother about formula feedings? Select all that apply.
1. "All babies should be started on soy-based formulas because of the risk of future allergic reactions."
2. "When mixing the powdered formula, be sure to follow the manufacturer's directions on the container to ensure proper nutrition."
3. "All babies on formula should have an iron-fortified formula to ensure healthy brain growth."
4. "A brand-name formula should be used because it has the best nutritional value."
5. "Speak to your baby's health care provider about the best formula to use when you plan to change from breast to formula feeding."

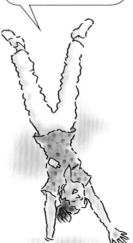

Hooray! You made it to question 35!

34. 2, 3, 5. Many different brands of formula are available, but all must meet strict U.S. Food and Drug Administration and Health Canada requirements. The American Academy of Pediatrics and the Canadian Pediatric Society recommend that all babies be fed iron-fortified formula unless contraindicated. It is vitally important that parents follow the directions on the package when mixing powdered formula to ensure proper nutrition. The baby's primary care provider, and the parents, should decide which formula is best for the baby. There has been no proven association of allergies for babies who begin with a cow-milk-based formula.

CN: Physiological integrity; CNS: Reduction of risk potential; CL: Apply

35. The nurse interacts with a neonate who is experiencing drug withdrawal. Which finding indicates to the nurse that the neonate has a problem with autonomic regulation?
1. Gaze aversion
2. Body arching
3. Sleep-wake disturbances
4. Yawning

35. 4. Yawning is a sign that the neonate is experiencing autonomic dysfunction. Gaze aversion indicates a problem with the neonate's state control capabilities. State control is the ability to process and respond to information from the caregiving environment. Sleep-wake disturbances and body-arching indicate a problem with sensory motor dysfunction.

CN: Psychosocial integrity; CNS: None; CL: Apply

CN: Client needs category   CNS: Client needs subcategory   CL: Cognitive level

36. A nurse is teaching neonate umbilical cord care to a new mother at a birthing center. Which information should the nurse include?
1. Apply alcohol to the cord with each diaper change until the infant is one week old
2. Clean the cord with chlorhexidine each time the diaper is changed until the neonate is discharged
3. Do nothing to the cord but keep it dry and open to air
4. Wash the cord with soap and water each day until the cord falls off

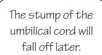

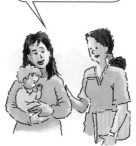

The stump of the umbilical cord will fall off later.

36. 3. Research has found that there is no difference in infection rates between cords treated with antiseptics or soap, and dry or natural cord care. In addition, antiseptics may prolong separation time. In developing countries, or in cases of a non-sterile delivery, the use of an antiseptic would be recommended.
CN: Health promotion and maintenance; CNS: None; CL: Apply

37. The nurse is teaching a group of parents about infant cardiopulmonary resuscitation prior to discharge of their newborns. Where should the nurse teach the parents to place their fingers to correctly perform chest compressions?

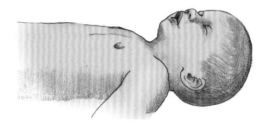

37. The correct position for the fingers is one fingerbreadth below the nipple line.

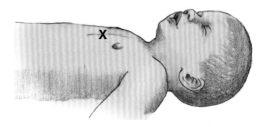

CN: Health promotion and maintenance; CNS: None; CL: Apply

38. The mother of a term neonate asks what the thick, white coating is on her baby's skin. Which statement by the nurse correctly describes the function of this coating?
1. It helps keep the neonate warm after birth.
2. It prevents neonatal dehydration after birth.
3. It serves as a protective coating in utero.
4. It decreases the development of birthmarks.

38. 3. Vernix caseosa is a thick, white coating on the neonate's skin at birth. The purpose of the vernix caseosa is to protect the fetus in utero. It does not prevent dehydration, or keep the neonate warm after birth. There is no association between vernix caseosa and birthmarks.
CN: Health promotion and maintenance; CNS: None; CL: Apply

39. Which medication is routinely given to the neonate within one hour of birth?
1. Erythromycin ophthalmic ointment
2. Hepatitis B vaccine
3. Glucose
4. Vitamin A

Check out that word *routinely*—I think it's important.

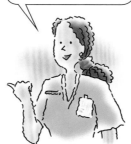

39. 1. Erythromycin ophthalmic ointment is given for prophylactic treatment of ophthalmic neonatorum. It is given within one hour of birth. Glucose would be given if the neonate is exhibiting signs of hypoglycemia. Many hospitals give the neonate the first dose of Hepatitis B vaccine prior to discharge.
CN: Physiological integrity; CNS: Pharmacological and parenteral therapies; CL: Apply

40. A client asks the nurse how fetal lung maturity is determined. What is the nurse's **best** response?
1. By gestational age by date
2. By the amount of stress the fetus experiences prior to delivery
3. By a lecithin-to-sphingomyelin (LS) ratio
4. By an elevated surfactant/albumin (SA) ratio

40. 3. Lecithin and sphingomyelin are phospholipids that help compose surfactant in the lungs. At 32 to 33 weeks gestation, lecithin and sphingomyelin concentrations are about equal. Subsequently, lecithin begins to increase, with an abrupt rise at 35 weeks. Lecithin continues to steadily increase until term. Sphingomyelin concentrations level off at 32 weeks and begin to decrease. There are currently no tests available for measuring the surfactant/albumin ratio. The amount of fetal stress, and gestational aging by date, are inaccurate measurements of fetal lung maturity.
CN: Physiological integrity; CNS: Physiological adaptation; CL: Apply

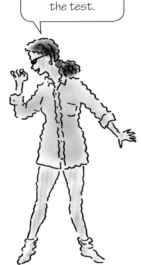

Rock on! You're halfway through the test.

41. Which neonate would be **least** likely to develop respiratory distress syndrome (RDS)?
1. Second born of twins
2. Neonate born at 34 weeks
3. Neonate of a diabetic mother
4. Chronic maternal hypertension

41. 4. Chronic maternal hypertension is an unlikely factor because chronic fetal stress tends to increase lung maturity. The second born of twins may be prone to a greater risk of asphyxia leading to RDS. Premature neonates, younger than 36 weeks, are associated with RDS. Even with a mature lecithin-to-sphingomyelin ratio, neonates of mothers with diabetes may still develop respiratory distress.
CN: Physiological integrity; CNS: Physiological adaptation; CL: Analyze

42. The nurse is performing an assessment on a term neonate. Which finding is considered common in the healthy neonate?
1. Single palmar crease
2. Subconjunctival hemorrhages
3. Lanugo over the back
4. Craniotabes

42. 2. Subconjunctival hemorrhages are commonly seen in neonates secondary to the cranial pressure applied during the birth process. Single palmar creases are present in approximately 5% of neonates. They can be associated with genetic abnormalities such as Trisomy 21. Lanugo, the soft downy hair often found on the back of neonates thins with increasing gestational age. Craniotabes, a softening of the skull bones, can be found in up to 30% of newborns. Recent evidence suggests that this may be an early sign of rickets.
CN: Health promotion and maintenance; CNS: None; CL: Apply

43. A nurse is providing care for a neonate during the first four hours following delivery. Which intervention should the nurse perform **first**?
1. Obtain a blood glucose sample
2. Give the initial bath
3. Give the vitamin K injection
4. Cover the neonate's wet head with a cap

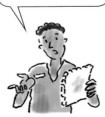

Which one of these is a priority right after birth?

43. 3. The American Academy of Pediatrics (AAP) and the Canadian Pediatric Society (CPS) recommend that vitamin K be given within one hour of birth (AAP) and by six hours of birth (CPS). Blood glucose tests, appropriate for neonates with risk factors, are obtained at 30 minutes to one hour of age. These are not routinely done in neonates without indication. Initial baths aren't given until the neonate's temperature is stable. The head should not be covered until the hair is dry.
CN: Safe, effective care environment; CNS: Management of care; CL: Apply

CN: Client needs category   CNS: Client needs subcategory   CL: Cognitive level

44. When assessing a neonate's skin, the nurse observes small, white papules surrounded by erythematous dermatitis. How should the nurse document this finding?

1. Milia
2. Epstein's pearls
3. Erythema toxicum
4. Neonatal acne

44. **3.** Erythema toxicum presents with lesions that come and go on the face, trunk, and limbs. They are small, white or yellow papules or vesicles with erythematous dermatitis and resemble flea bites. Milia are small white or yellow papules that are often found on the neonate's face and nose. They are not typically associated with erythema. Epstein's pearls, found in the mouth, are similar to facial milia. Neonatal acne typically consists of closed comedones on the forehead, nose and cheeks.

CN: Health promotion and maintenance; CNS: None; CL: Apply

45. The nurse is preparing to give a neonate the initial hepatitis B vaccine. Where should this injection be given?

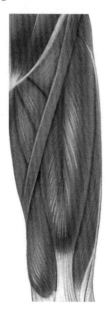

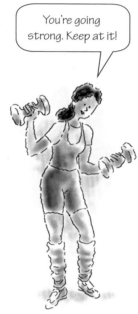

You're going strong. Keep at it!

45. The vastus lateralis should be used for infant IM injections.

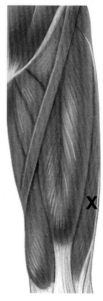

CN: Physiological integrity; CNS: Pharmacological and parenteral therapies; CL: Apply

46. The nurse is teaching the parents of a neonate about the Centers for Disease Control and Prevention (CDC), Health Canada, and the World Health Organization (WHO) recommendations for hepatitis B vaccine. Which information is **most** important for the nurse to provide?

1. It should be given to all neonates as soon as possible after birth.
2. It should be given to neonates at birth only if they are exposed to hepatitis B, otherwise wait until the infant is two months of age.
3. It should be given to neonates showing symptoms of hepatitis B.
4. It should be given to all neonates as soon as possible after birth along with the hepatitis B Immunoglobulin (HBIG).

46. **1.** The CDC, Health Canada and WHO recommend that the hepatitis B vaccine be given to all neonates, including those born to hepatitis B surface antigen-negative mothers, as soon as possible after birth, and before hospital discharge. HBIG should only be given to neonates born to a mother with Hepatitis B.

CN: Health promotion and maintenance; CNS: None; CL: Apply

47. A male neonate has just been circumcised. Which nursing intervention is part of the **initial** care of a circumcised neonate?
  1. Wash the circumcised penis with warm water
  2. Change the diaper as needed
  3. Keep a bandage on the site for 24 to 48 hours
  4. Apply petroleum jelly to the site for 24 to 48 hours

47. 4. Petroleum jelly should be applied to the site for the first 24 to 48 hours to prevent the skin edges from sticking to the diaper. A gauze or other type of bandage may or may not be used. Washing the area with warm water is indicated, but is not part of the initial care.
CN: Health promotion and maintenance; CNS: None;
CL: Apply

48. The nurse is performing an assessment on a neonate. Which assessment finding is suggestive of hypothermia?
  1. Bradycardia
  2. Hyperglycemia
  3. Metabolic alkalosis
  4. Shivering

48. 1. Hypothermic neonates become bradycardic proportional to the degree of core temperature. Hypoglycemia is seen in hypothermic neonates. Metabolic acidosis, not alkalosis, is seen as a result of slowed respirations. Neonates use non-shivering thermogenesis.
CN: Health promotion and maintenance; CNS: None;
CL: Apply

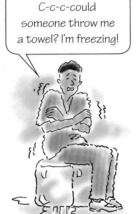

C-c-c-could someone throw me a towel? I'm freezing!

49. Which nursing intervention would help to prevent evaporative heat loss in the neonate immediately after birth?
  1. Administering warm oxygen
  2. Controlling the drafts in the room
  3. Immediately drying the neonate
  4. Placing the neonate on a warm, dry towel

49. 3. Immediately drying the neonate decreases evaporative heat loss from his moist body following birth. Controlling drafts in the room and administering warmed oxygen help reduce convective loss. Placing the neonate on a warm, dry towel decreases conductive losses.
CN: Health promotion and maintenance; CNS: None; CL: Analyze

50. A nurse is performing an assessment on a neonate. Which assessment findings would indicate a metabolic response to cold stress? Select all that apply.
  1. Arrhythmias
  2. Hypoglycemia
  3. Respiratory distress
  4. Jaundice
  5. Increase in blood pressure

50. 2, 3, 4. Hypoglycemia occurs as the consumption of glucose increases with the increase in metabolic rate. The increase in metabolic rate also leads to a decrease in surfactant production leading to hypoxemia and respiratory distress. Brown fat metabolism, as a result of the cold stress, can interfere with the transport of bilirubin to the liver for conjugation thus increasing the risk of jaundice. Arrhythmias and increases in blood pressure occur because of cardiorespiratory manifestations.
CN: Health promotion and maintenance; CNS: None; CL: Analyze

51. What is the nurse's **priority** to regulate the temperature of a neonate?
  1. Supply extra heat sources to the neonate
  2. Keep the ambient room temperature less than 100° F (37.8° C)
  3. Minimize the energy needed for the neonate to produce heat
  4. Block radiant, convective, conductive, and evaporative losses

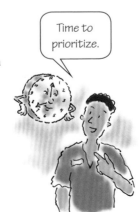

Time to prioritize.

51. 4. Prevention of heat loss is always the first goal in thermoregulation to avoid hypothermia. The second goal is to minimize the energy necessary for neonates to produce heat. Adding extra heat sources is a means of correcting hypothermia. The ambient room temperature should be kept at approximately 100° F (37.8° C).
CN: Safe, effective care environment; CNS: Management of care;
CL: Apply

CN: Client needs category   CNS: Client needs subcategory   CL: Cognitive level

52. Which neonate would be **most** at risk for a problem with thermoregulation?
1. A neonate born to a mother with diabetes
2. A neonate born at 36 weeks' gestation
3. A neonate born at 29 weeks' gestation
4. A neonate at 36 hours of age with signs of jaundice

52. 3. Preterm neonates are not able to thermoregulate due to the lack of brown fat. The more premature the infant, the more immature the thermoregulation system. With no other complications such as prematurity, infants born to mothers with diabetes and those with jaundice are not more at risk for problems with thermoregulation than a premature infant.
CN: Physiological integrity; CNS: Reduction of risk potential; CL: Apply

53. Which clinical finding does the nurse find **most** suggestive of physiologic hyperbilirubinemia in a neonate?
1. Clinical jaundice before 36 hours of age in a neonate with a family history of neonatal jaundice
2. Clinical jaundice in a breastfeeding neonate
3. Total bilirubin levels of 12 mg/dl (205.25 μmol/L) by three days of life
4. Serum total bilirubin levels increasing by more than 5 mg/dl/day (85.52 μmol/L/day)

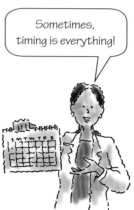

Sometimes, timing is everything!

53. 3. Increased bilirubin levels in the liver usually cause total bilirubin levels to rise to 12 mg/dl (205.25 μmol/L) by the third day of life. This is from the impaired conjugation and excretion of bilirubin, and difficulty of clearing bilirubin from plasma. A family history of neonatal jaundice or breastfeeding may increase the risk of jaundice, but further workup would be required to determine the type of jaundice seen. Rapidly rising levels suggest pathological jaundice.
CN: Physiological integrity; CNS: Reduction of risk potential; CL: Analyze

54. A nurse is caring for a full-term neonate who is receiving phototherapy for hyperbilirubinemia. The nurse determines immediate intervention is necessary when the neonate exhibits:
1. maculopapular rash.
2. absent Moro reflex.
3. greenish stools.
4. bronze-colored skin.

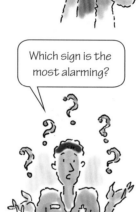

Which sign is the most alarming?

54. 2. An absent Moro reflex, lethargy, and seizures are symptoms of bilirubin encephalopathy, which can be life threatening. A maculopapular rash, greenish stools, and bronze-colored skin are minor side effects of phototherapy that should be monitored but do not require immediate intervention.
CN: Physiological integrity; CNS: Physiological adaptation; CL: Analyze

55. The nurse is aware that a neonate undergoing phototherapy treatment needs to be monitored for:
1. sunburn.
2. increased insensible water loss.
3. a decrease in platelet count.
4. the amount of light penetrating the tissue.

55. 2. Increased insensible water loss is due to absorbed photon energy from the phototherapy. Standard blue lights decrease the risk of sunburn. The amount of light penetrating the tissue is important; however, monitoring water loss is the priority. There may be a mild decrease in platelet count.
CN: Health promotion and maintenance; CNS: None; CL: Analyze

56. The nurse is counseling an expectant teen mother on the benefits of breastfeeding. What are the expected benefits of breastfeeding? Select all that apply
1. Decreased risk of prematurity
2. Increased chance of higher intelligence in the baby
3. Decreased risk of mastitis
4. Decreased risk of Sudden Infant Death Syndrome (SIDS)
5. Decreased risk of childhood obesity
6. Increased chance of return to pre-pregnant weight

56. 2, 4, 5. Studies have shown an increase in the intelligence scores of breastfed infants, and a decrease in the risk of SIDS and childhood obesity. The decision to breastfeed has no impact on the risk of delivering prematurely. Mastitis commonly occurs in breastfeeding mothers when bacteria enters the breast through a cracked nipple. Studies of the overall effect of breastfeeding on the return of the mothers to their pre-pregnancy weight are inconclusive.
CN: Health promotion and maintenance; CNS: None; CL: Apply

CN: Client needs category   CNS: Client needs subcategory   CL: Cognitive level

57. Which sign is the nurse's earliest indication of respiratory distress syndrome (RDS) in a neonate?
1. Bilateral crackles
2. Pale gray color
3. Tachypnea more than 60 breaths/min
4. Poor capillary filling time

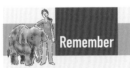

It's important to recognize the earliest clue.

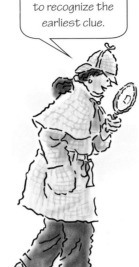

57. 3. Tachypnea and expiratory grunting occur early in RDS to help improve oxygenation. Crackles may occur as the respiratory distress progressively worsens. A pale gray skin color obscures earlier cyanosis as respiratory distress symptoms persist and worsen. Poor capillary filling time, a later manifestation, occurs if signs and symptoms are not treated.
CN: Health promotion and maintenance; CNS: None; CL: Analyze

58. A nurse is caring for a term neonate who has developed respiratory problems after being born by cesarean delivery for failure to progress during labor. Which condition is **most** likely causing this problem?
1. Neonatal respiratory distress syndrome (RDS)
2. Meconium aspiration
3. Pneumothorax
4. Transient tachypnea of a newborn

58. 4. Transient tachypnea of a newborn is caused by a delay in removing excess amounts of lung fluid. It is often seen in infants born by cesarean section. Neonatal RDS is caused by a surfactant deficiency, and is typically seen in preterm infants. Meconium is the first feces, or stool, of the newborn. Meconium aspiration syndrome occurs when a newborn breathes a mixture of meconium and amniotic fluid into the lungs around the time of deliver. Pneumothorax is a collection of air in the pleural space and can be a complication of respiratory disease.
CN: Physiological integrity; CNS: Physiological adaptation; CL: Analyze

59. A neonate is admitted to the neonatal intensive care unit with persistent pulmonary hypertension. Which medication should the nurse anticipate for this neonate?
1. Dobutamine
2. Isoproterenol
3. Prostaglandin E2
4. Inhaled nitric oxide

Remember

"Nitric oxide opens arteries wide."

Inhaled nitric oxide is a potent selective pulmonary vasodilator, which is administered in cases of persistent pulmonary hypertension.

59. 4. Inhaled nitric oxide is a potent selective pulmonary vasodilator. Dobutamine is a vasopressor, not a vasodilator. Isoproterenol dilates pulmonary arteries but does not decrease pulmonary vascular resistance. Prostaglandin E2 is an oxytocic substance used to induce labor and does not affect pulmonary vasodilation.
CN: Physiological integrity; CNS: Pharmacological and parenteral therapies; CL: Apply

60. The nurse is examining the neonate's fontanels and knows that the posterior fontanel lies along the sagittal and lambdoidal suture lines. Identify the lambdoidal sutures.

60. The lambdoidal suture is the line between the occipital and parietal skull bones. The sagittal suture is the line between the two parietal bones.

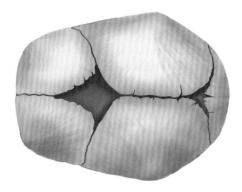

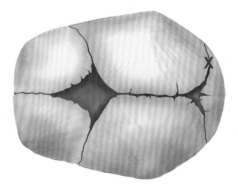

CN: Health promotion and maintanence; CNS: None; CL: Apply

61. Which procedure should be avoided in a neonate born with diaphragmatic hernia?
1. Chest X-ray
2. Mask ventilation
3. Placement of orogastric tube
4. Immediate endotracheal intubation

61. 2. Mask ventilation should be avoided to prevent air from being introduced into the GI tract by this technique. An emergency chest X-ray will help diagnose this defect. An orogastric tube is needed to decompress the bowel and stomach within the chest. Intubation is needed to ventilate the neonate because of the defect.

CN: Physiological integrity; CNS: Physiological adaptation; CL: Apply

62. A nurse is preparing to administer beractant to a preterm infant. The order is for 4 ml/kg. The neonate weighs 2,000 g. How many total milliliters will be used for one dose? Record your answer as a whole number.

_____ ml

62. 8.

First, convert the weight from grams to kilograms.

$$1,000 \ g = 1 \ kg$$

$$1,000 \ g/1 \ kg = 2,000 \ g/X \ kg$$

$$X = 2 \ kg$$

Then, determine how many milliliters are needed by using the following formula:

$$4 \ ml \times 2 \ kg = 8 \ ml \ total \ dose$$

CN: Physiological integrity; CNS: Pharmacological and parenteral therapies; CL: Apply

63. A nurse is caring for a neonate with fetal alcohol syndrome (FAS). Which finding is **most** indicative of FAS?
1. Delayed development
2. Smooth philtrum
3. Hearing loss
4. Growth retardation

63. 2. Distinctive facial dysmorphology of children with FAS most commonly includes small eyes with drooping upper lids, microcephaly, short palpebral fissures, thin lips, and a poorly developed philtrum. Delayed development, hearing loss and growth retardation may all be associated with FAS, but the distinctive facial features are most indicative.

CN: Physiological integrity; CNS: Physiological adaptation; CL: Analyze

64. A neonate is born after 36 weeks' gestation to a mother who used tobacco, alcohol and marijuana during her pregnancy. Which findings indicate the impact of substance abuse on the neonate? Select all that apply.
1. Birth weight of 1,800 g
2. Delayed passage of meconium
3. Facial abnormalities
4. Increase in sleep state
5. High-pitched cry

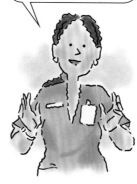

The mother's history may be the key to the neonate's current condition.

64. 1, 3. The most common effects of tobacco, alcohol and marijuana on fetal development are retarded growth in weight, length, and head circumference. Facial abnormalities are often seen with maternal alcohol use. Delayed meconium passage has not been correlated with maternal substance use. Marijuana exposure can cause difficulties with sleep. A high-pitched cry can signal neonatal abstinence syndrome which is associated with maternal narcotic use.

CN: Health promotion and maintenance; CNS: None; CL: Analyze

65. A nurse is providing care for a neonate with in utero alcohol exposure. Prioritize these infant care interventions.

1.	Dim the lights and decrease sound
2.	Monitor the neonate's blood glucose
3.	Educate the mother on the need for follow up appointments with therapy services
4.	Have the mother breastfeed the neonate every 2 to 3 hours
5.	Obtain a hearing screen

65. Ordered Response:

1.	Dim the lights and decrease sound
2.	Monitor the neonate's blood glucose
4.	Have the mother breastfeed the neonate every 2 to 3 hours
5.	Obtain a hearing screen
3.	Educate the mother on the need for follow up appointments with therapy services

CN: Physiological integrity; CNS: Physiological adaptation; CL: Analyze

66. A neonate is suspected to have a diagnosis of cystic fibrosis. Which symptoms would **most** likely indicate cystic fibrosis?
  1. Jaundice
  2. Undescended testicles
  3. Tachypnea
  4. Meconium ileus

66. 4. Meconium ileus is a luminal obstruction of the distal small intestine by abnormal meconium seen in neonates with cystic fibrosis. Jaundice, undescended testicles, and tachypnea may also be seen in cystic fibrosis but are not as likely to indicate that specific disease.
CN: Physiological integrity; CNS: Physiological adaptation; CL: Apply

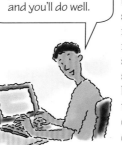

Keep reading each question carefully and you'll do well.

67. The nurse is providing discharge instructions to the parents of a neonate regarding safety. What information should the nurse include in these instructions? Select all that apply.
  1. "Cover your infant with heavy blankets when sleeping in the crib."
  2. "Never leave your infant alone in the tub."
  3. "Verify that your babysitter knows cardiopulmonary resuscitation (CPR)."
  4. "The car seat used should be a rear-facing model."
  5. "Dress the baby in two less layers than you are wearing."

67. 2, 3, 4. Infants should never be left alone in the tub, as they can easily drown. All caretakers should be trained in CPR. Car seats should be rear-facing until the infant is two years old or reaches the maximum height and weight for that seat. Heavy blankets in the crib increase the risk of sudden infant death syndrome. The infant should be dressed in only one layer more than the parent to prevent overheating.
CN: Health promotion and maintenance; CNS: None; CL: Apply

68. A neonate has an imperforate anus, tracheoesophageal fistula, and a single umbilical artery. Which congenital disorder would the nurse suspect as a cause?
  1. Beckwith-Wiedemann syndrome
  2. Trisomy 13
  3. Turner's syndrome
  4. VACTERL or VATER association

68. 4. VACTERL or VATER association clinically presents with three or more defects, including the three mentioned. VACTERL or VATER association includes vertebral anomalies, anal atresia, cardiac anomalies, tracheoesophageal fistula, renal anomalies, including a single umbilical artery, and limb anomalies. Beckwith-Wiedemann syndrome can have associated renal anomalies. Trisomy 13 can present with a single umbilical artery. Turner's syndrome (45XO) can have cardiac anomalies, but they do not typically have the other defects.
CN: Physiological integrity; CNS: Physiological adaptation; CL: Analyze

69. An initial assessment of a female neonate shows pink-streaked vaginal discharge. Which action should the nurse take?
1. Notify the practitioner, as this sign may be due to an early stage of cystitis
2. Notify the practitioner, as that this sign may be due to birth trauma
3. Do nothing different, as this sign may be due to urate acid crystals
4. Do nothing different, as this sign may be due to a withdrawal of maternal hormones

69. 4. Withdrawal of maternal estrogen can produce pseudomenstruation. No additional interventions are needed. Cystitis or a urinary tract infection in a neonate would show generalized signs of sepsis. Birth trauma may cause surface abrasions but not vaginal discharge. Urate acid crystals may cause a pink to orange tint to the diaper. They are harmless but could be a sign of dehydration.
CN: Health promotion and maintenance; CNS: None; CL: Apply

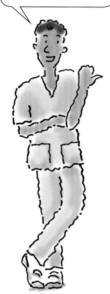

Question 70 asks which intervention should be performed first.

70. The nurse caring for a neonate observes excessive oral secretions, and suspects a tracheoesophageal atresia. Which **priority** intervention should the nurse perform?
1. Place a nasogastric (NG) tube
2. Stop PO feedings
3. Administer oxygen
4. Suction the secretions

70. 4. Accumulated secretions are copious in neonates with this disorder because the neonate cannot swallow. This places the neonate at risk for aspiration. Maintenance of the airway and suctioning the secretions would be the first priority. PO feedings would be withheld until further evaluation and treatment are completed. A NG tube would be placed after the initial evaluation. Oxygen would only be administered if indicated.
CN: Physiological integrity; CNS: Physiological adaptation; CL: Analyze

71. A new mother states, "My baby spits up after every feeding." Which interventions should the nurse teach to this mother **first**?
1. Feed the baby smaller, more frequent feeds
2. Change the infant to a soy formula
3. Elevate the head of the crib to 30°
4. Burp the infant more frequently during each feeding

71. 4. Frequent burping decreases the amount of air the infant has in her stomach and should be the first intervention. Feeding smaller more frequent may help if the infant is taking large amounts. Infants should be fed every 2 to 4 hours. Elevating the head of the bed 30° may help if the cause is gastroesophageal reflux. Formula may have to be changed if it is determined that the spitting is related to milk intolerance.
CN: Health promotion and maintenance; CNS: None; CL: Analyze

72. A new mother is on a chemotherapeutic agent, and is unable to breastfeed her newborn. She asks the nurse for guidance in feeding her neonate. What is the nurse's **most** appropriate response?
1. "Infant formula is a healthy alternative if you are unable to breastfeed."
2. "Neonates require less frequent feedings because formula is harder to digest."
3. "If you use infant formula, you don't have to worry about what you eat or drink."
4. "Formula feeding requires planning and organization to make sure that you have what you need."

72. 1. Although all the statements are true regarding formula feeding, only the first statement provides support for a mother who does not have the choice whether to formula or breastfeed her neonate.
CN: Physiological integrity; CNS: Physiological adaptation; CL: Analyze

CN: Client needs category   CNS: Client needs subcategory   CL: Cognitive level

73. Which nursing intervention **best** addresses the needs of a term neonate who has central cyanosis and adequate respiratory and heart rates?
1. Provide tactile stimulation
2. Give supplemental free-flow oxygen
3. Assist ventilation with a bag and mask
4. Intubate and suction the lower airway

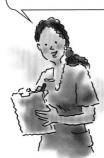

Question 74 asks about an expected finding, not necessarily an abnormal one.

73. 2. Central cyanosis indicates that room air is currently insufficient. Supplemental oxygen is required. Tactile stimulation is only needed if the neonate is apneic or gasping. Bag and mask ventilation is only indicated if the heart rate is less than 100 bpm. Intubation is only indicated in special circumstances, such as prematurity or a diaphragmatic hernia.

CN: Health promotion and maintenance; CNS: None; CL: Apply

74. A woman delivers a 3,250-g neonate at 42-weeks' gestation. Which physical finding is expected during an examination of this neonate's plantar creases?

74. 4. A neonate born at 42-weeks' gestation is considered postmature, and would have creases over the entire sole. An infant born after 37 weeks would have creases over the anterior two-thirds of the sole. Very premature infants have no creases or only very faint red lines over the anterior aspect of the foot.

CN: Health promotion and maintenance; CNS: None; CL: Analyze

1.

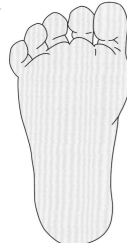

3.

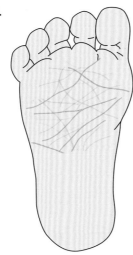

2.

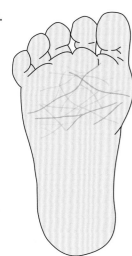

4.

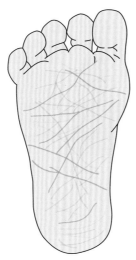

75. While performing an initial assessment on a term neonate, the nurse notes a bluish marking across the neonate's lower back. What information should the nurse share with the mother regarding this marking?
1. This marking is commonly found in babies born by caesarean delivery.
2. This resulted from poor nutrition during the pregnancy.
3. This marking is a "blue birthmark," and is typically found in dark-skinned races.
4. This will happen when the infant is cold.

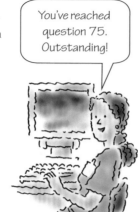

You've reached question 75. Outstanding!

75. 3. The marking is a Mongolian spot, commonly found over the lumbosacral area in neonates of Asian, Black, Latin, or aboriginal origin. They may be found on any part of the body. Mongolian spots may sometimes be confused with bruising, so thorough documentation of their presence is crucial. Prenatal nutrition, neonatal temperature or method of delivery are not causes of Mongolian spots.

CN: Health promotion and maintenance; CNS: None; CL: Apply

76. A nurse in the neonatal nursery is serving as preceptor for a student nurse. The student asks the nurse why a neonate's head is cone shaped. Which response is accurate?
1. It results from a fast delivery. The fast labor caused bruising and swelling of the neonate's head.
2. It results from molding. Overriding of the cranial sutures allows the neonate's head to pass though the birth canal.
3. It results from cephalohematoma. Some blood has collected between the skull bone and periosteum.
4. It results from hydrocephalus. Either too much cerebrospinal fluid (CSF) is being formed or too little is being absorbed.

76. 2. Molding refers to the overlapping of the cranial sutures, which causes the neonate's head to appear cone shaped. Cephalohematoma, and hydrocephalus do not result in a cone-shaped head. Cephalohematoma is a collection of blood between the skull bone and periosteum. Hydrocephalus is an increase in the size of the entire head as a result of increased CSF volume. The rate of delivery does not cause changes in head shape

CN: Health promotion and maintenance; CNS: None; CL: Apply

77. A neonate who has been receiving formula feedings is discharged from the neonate nursery. Twenty-four hours later, the mother calls the hospital, stating that the neonate is vomiting most of his feedings. The nurse determines further instruction is necessary when the mother makes states:
1. "Every time I feed him, he spits up about a teaspoonful of formula onto his bib."
2. "I'm using prepared formula, and he takes 1/2 oz (15 ml) to 1 oz (30 ml) every 3 to 4 hours."
3. "I feed him every time he cries. Sometimes, he eats 4 oz (120 ml) at a time every couple of hours."
4. "I burp him after each 1/2 oz (15 ml) of formula."

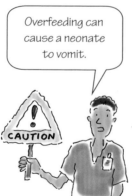

Overfeeding can cause a neonate to vomit.

77. 3. Feeding the neonate every time he cries will result in overfeeding. A neonate's crying doesn't always signal hunger. Sometimes, it means his diaper is wet, he needs to suck, or he wants to be held. A neonate who is spitting up should be burped after every ounce of formula or less. For the first few days, the neonate's normal stomach capacity is 15 ml, so he should be fed every 3 to 4 hours. All neonates spit up a small amount because of an immature cardiac sphincter.

CN: Physiological integrity; CNS: Basic care and comfort; CL: Apply

78. A healthy term neonate born by cesarean delivery was admitted to the transitional nursery 30 minutes ago and placed under a radiant warmer. The neonate has an axillary temperature of 99.5° F (37.5° C), a respiratory rate of 80 breaths/min, and a heel-stick glucose value of 60 mg/dl (3.33 mmol/L) Which action should the nurse take?
1. Wrap the neonate warmly and place him in an open crib
2. Administer an oral glucose feeding of dextrose 10% in water
3. Increase the temperature setting on the radiant warmer
4. Obtain an order for IV fluid administration

78. 4. Assessment findings indicate that the neonate is in respiratory distress, most likely from transient tachypnea, which is common after cesarean delivery. The normal respiratory rate is 30 to 60 breaths/min. A neonate with a rate of 80 breaths/min should not be fed, but should receive IV fluids until the respiratory rate returns to normal. To allow close observation for worsening respiratory distress, the neonate should be kept unclothed in the radiant warmer. Raising the warmer's temperature setting would cause overheating and worsen the neonate's respiratory distress.

CN: Physiological integrity; CNS: Basic care and comfort; CL: Apply

79. A home health nurse assesses a neonate who is 48 hours old, and was discharged from the hospital 24 hours ago. Which assessment finding indicates a potential problem?
1. The neonate cries but no tears appear.
2. Small papules appear all over the neonate's skin.
3. The neonate doesn't turn his head in the direction that his cheek is stroked.
4. The neonate produces a greenish-brown stool.

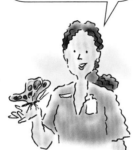

You're doing great! You've almost finished the chapter!

79. 3. A normal, healthy neonate turns in the direction that the cheek is stroked. Failure to do so may indicate a neurological problem, which the nurse should report to the health care provider. A neonate's lacrimal glands are immature, resulting in tearless crying for up to two months. Erythema toxicum neonatorum causes a transient maculopapular rash, which is normal in all neonates. Greenish-brown stools at 48 hours are normal, and indicate that the neonate is eliminating formula or breast milk instead of meconium.

CN: Health promotion and maintenance; CNS: None; CL: Apply

80. A nurse is administering vitamin K to a preterm neonate following delivery. The medication comes in a concentration of 2 mg/ml, and the ordered dose is 0.5 mg to be given subcutaneously. How many milliliters should the nurse administer? Record your answer using two decimal places.

_____ ml

80. 0.25.

Use the following formula to calculate drug dosages:

Dose on hand/Quantity on hand = Dose desired/X

The equation is as follows:

$$2 \text{ mg/ml} = 0.5 \text{ mg/X}; \quad X = 0.25 \text{ ml}$$

CN: Physiological integrity; CNS: Pharmacological and parenteral therapies; CL: Apply

81. A nurse is eliciting reflexes in a neonate during a physical examination. Identify the area the nurse would touch to elicit a plantar grasp reflex.

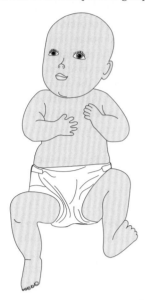

81. To elicit a plantar grasp reflex, the nurse should touch the sole of the foot near the base of the digits, causing flexion or grasping. This reflex disappears around 9 months of age.

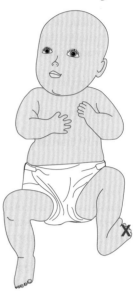

CN: Health promotion and maintenance; CNS: None;
CL: Apply

82. What information should a nurse include when teaching post-circumcision care to the parents of a neonate prior to discharge from the hospital? Select all that apply.

1. The infant must void before being discharged.
2. Petroleum jelly should be applied to the glans with each diaper change.
3. The infant can take tub baths while the circumcision heals.
4. Any blood noted on the front of the diaper should be reported.
5. The circumcision will require care for two to four days after discharge.

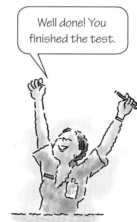

Well done! You finished the test.

82. **1, 2, 5.** It is necessary for the infant to void prior to discharge to ensure that the urethra isn't obstructed. Petroleum jelly is appropriate, and is applied with each diaper change. Typically, circumcision care is required for two to four days while the penis heals. To prevent infection, sponge baths should be given while the penis heals. A small amount of bleeding is expected following a circumcision. Parents should only report a large amount of bleeding.

CN: Health promotion and maintenance; CNS: None;
CL: Apply

Part V

Care of the Child

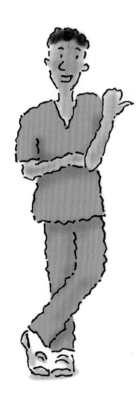

Chapter 26

Growth & Development

Here's a short but important chapter that covers growth and development of children. Enjoy!

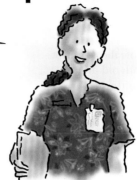

1. A mother tells a nurse that her 22-month-old child says "no" to everything. When scolded, the toddler becomes angry and starts crying loudly, then later wants to be held. How should the nurse **best** interpret this toddler's behavior?
  1. The toddler isn't effectively coping with the stress.
  2. The toddler's need for affection isn't being met.
  3. This is normal behavior for a two-year-old child.
  4. This behavior suggests the need for further assessment.

Question 1 wants you to read the rest but go with the best.

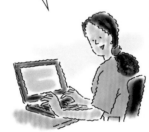

2. The mother of a 12-month-old infant expresses concern about the effects of frequent thumb sucking on her child's teeth. Which response indicates that effective teaching regarding thumb sucking?
  1. "Thumb sucking should be discouraged at 12 months of age."
  2. "I'll give my baby a pacifier instead."
  3. "Thumb sucking is important to my baby."
  4. "I'll wrap my baby's thumb in a bandage."

1. 3. Toddlers are confronted with the conflict of achieving autonomy, while relinquishing their dependence on, and affection of others. As a result, negativism becomes part of their growth and development. Negativism is a step toward autonomy. It is not related to their attachment to a parent, or their need for affection. This behavior does not indicate that the child is under stress, isn't receiving sufficient affection, or requires further assessment.
CN: Health promotion and maintenance; CNS: None; CL: Analyze

2. 3. Thumb sucking is a natural reflex for children. Sucking on thumbs, fingers, pacifiers or other objects may make the baby feel secure, happy, and help them learn about their world. Young children may also suck to soothe themselves and help induce sleep. Thumb sucking can cause malocclusion if it persists beyond age four. The intensity of the sucking determines dental problems. If a child rests his thumb passively in his mouth, he is less likely to have malocclusion than a child who vigorously sucks his thumb. If thumb sucking is aggressive the child may develop problems with their primary teeth. Many fetuses begin sucking their fingers in utero and, as infants, refuse a pacifier as a substitute. A young child is likely to chew on a bandage, which could lead to an airway obstruction.
CN: Health promotion and maintenance; CNS: None; CL: Analyze

CN: Client needs category   CNS: Client needs subcategory   CL: Cognitive level

3. An adolescent client has had surgery and now has a dressing on the abdomen. Which initial question should the nurse anticipate from this client?
  1. "When can I go swimming?"
  2. "Will I have a large scar?"
  3. "What complications can I expect?"
  4. "When can I return to school?"

3. 2. Adolescents are deeply concerned about body image, and how they appear to others. An adolescent probably wouldn't ask how the surgery went, or which complications she might expect. Although an adolescent may be curious about returning to school or swimming, this probably wouldn't be her primary concern.
CN: Health promotion and maintenance; CNS: None; CL: Apply

4. Which game would promote the cognitive development of an eight-month-old infant?
  1. Blocks to stack with the nurse
  2. Hide and seek with a toy behind the nurse's back
  3. Rolling a small rubber ball to the nurse
  4. A play gym strung across the crib

4. 2. According to Piaget's theory of cognitive development, an eight-month-old child will look for an object after it disappears from sight to develop the cognitive skill of object permanence. Small stacking blocks and balls are inappropriate because infants frequently put objects in their mouth. If stacking blocks are large enough, there is not a safety risk. A play gym is geared toward motor development. Anything strung across an infant's crib presents a safety hazard. The child may use it to pull themselves to a standing position.
CN: Health promotion and maintenance; CNS: None; CL: Apply

5. A toddler is admitted to the pediatric unit. Based on the progress notes, which developmental intervention should the nurse implement?

Progress notes	
2/10/17	History and Physical Tab
1000	14-month-old male with croup admitted at 1400. Temperature: 100.5° F (38.1° C), Heart rate: 126, regular, no murmur. Resp. rate 28. Lungs bilaterally clear. Frequent barky cough. Weight: 22.5 lb (10.24 kg) Height: 31.1 in (79 cm) Head circumference: 18.5 in (47 cm). Child is crying but easily consoled by the nurse. Smiles when he hears mom's voice in the hallway. Able to pass blocks back and forth between hands, but then drops them. Verbalizes "mama" "dada", but no other words. Mother states child is read to daily, and likes to turn pages. Anterior fontanel closed. Eyes dull. Unable to assess ears due to child's lack of cooperation. Abdomen soft, flat. Standing in crib.

  1. Notify the health care provider of the child's responses
  2. Provide normal nursing cares
  3. Suggest occupational/physical therapy services while in the hospital
  4. Incorporate frequent reading sessions into the nursing care plan.

5. 1. The child is showing some signs of delayed development. By 14 months, the child should be able to put blocks in a cup. Passing blocks back and forth and saying "dada" and "mama" are typically seen in nine-month-old infants. Not cooperating with an ear exam, dull eyes and crying could be due to an illness. The anterior fontanel closes between 12 and 18 months of age.
CN: Health promotion and maintenance; CNS: None; CL: Analyze

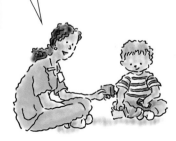

How well should a 14-month-old be able to handle blocks?

CN: Client needs category   CNS: Client needs subcategory   CL: Cognitive level

6. The school nurse overhears a conversation between two eight-year-old boys. Which comment **best** typifies this developmental stage?
1. "Girls are so yucky."
2. "My mommy and I are always together."
3. "I can't decide if I like Amy or Heather better."
4. "I can turn into Batman when I come out of the coat room."

6. 1. During elementary or primary school-age years, the most important social interactions are typically those with peers. Peer-to-peer interactions lead to the formation of intimate friendships between same-sex children. Friendships with children of the opposite-sex are uncommon. At this stage, children socialize more frequently with friends than with parents. Interest in peers of the opposite sex generally doesn't begin until ages 10 to 12. Magical thinking and fantasy play typify the preschool years.
CN: Health promotion and maintenance; CNS: None; CL: Apply

7. The parents of a three-year-old are concerned that the child is not developing normally. Which tasks show a delay in development? Select all that apply.
1. Riding a tricycle
2. Speaking in two-word sentences
3. Requiring help to tie shoelaces
4. Showing early imaginative play
5. Speaking in an incomprehensible manner
6. Requiring assistance with getting dressed.

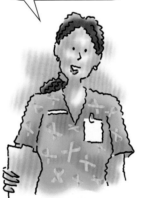

Which statement indicates that the mom understands?

7. 2, 5, 6. At The speech of a three-year-old should be at least 50% intelligible to the nurse, and the child should speak in three-to-four-word sentences. A three-year-old should be able dress themselves with supervision only. The fine motor skills required to tie shoelaces should develop by age five. Gross motor development, and refinement in hand-eye coordination enable a child to ride a tricycle, and cognitively engage in early imaginative behavior by age three.
CN: Health promotion and maintenance; CNS: None; CL: Apply

8. The nurse is providing teaching to the teen mother of a five-month-old infant. The mother understands the teaching on gross motor development when she states:
1. "Since my baby is rolling over, crawling should start next month."
2. "My baby should be able to start sitting alone without help. After that, crawling will start soon."
3. "In the next two months, my baby will start to stand."
4. "My baby still needs to be held for the most part."

8. 2. An infant's gross motor development occurs first by rolling over, then sitting without support, crawling, and finally pulling up to a standing position. Sitting without support occurs in 50 to 90 percent of infants by six months of age. Crawling usually occurs by the eighth month.
CN: Health promotion and maintenance; CNS: None; CL: Analyze

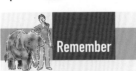

Remember

"'cillins are for killin' bacteria."

They include the following:

Penicillins
- Amoxicillin
- Ampicillin
- Dicloxacillin
- Nafcillin
- Oxacillin
- Penicillin G
- Penicillin VK
- Ticarcillin

9. A nurse is teaching a mom how to administer amoxicillin to her five-year-old son. The child cannot swallow pills. The child weighs 20.6 lb (9.36 kg). The order is for 80 mg/kg/day given in two doses every 12 hours. The medication comes prepared as 250 mg/5 ml. How many teaspoons should the nurse instruct the mom to give with each dose? Record your answer using one decimal place.

_____ tsp

9. 1.5.
Here are the calculations:

$$80\ mg/kg/day \times 9.36\ kg = 748.8\ mg/day$$
$$748.8\ mg/day \div 2\ doses/day = 374.4\ mg/dose$$
Round to 374 mg/dose.

$$250\ mg/5\ ml = 50\ mg/ml$$
$$374\ mg/dose \div 50\ mg/ml = 7.48\ ml/dose$$
Round to 7.5 ml/dose.

$$5\ ml = 1\ tsp$$
$$7.5\ ml/dose \div 5\ ml/tsp = 1.5\ tsp/dose$$

CN: Physiological Integrity; CNS: Pharmacological and Parenteral Therapies; CL: Analyze

CN: Client needs category   CNS: Client needs subcategory   CL: Cognitive level

10. Which behavior is developmentally appropriate for a five-year-old child?
   1. He cries in protest when his mother leaves.
   2. He asks for a bandage after having blood drawn.
   3. He becomes upset about having a scar after surgery.
   4. He wants to know why his friends don't visit.

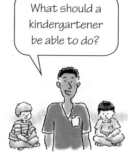

What should a kindergartener be able to do?

10. **2.** A five-year-old typically asks for a bandage after having blood drawn because he has poorly defined body boundaries. He believes he will lose all his blood from the injection site. A toddler cries in protest when a parent leaves. An adolescent might be upset about a surgical scar because he's concerned with body image. A school-age child might ask why his friends don't visit because peers become important at this stage.
CN: Heath promotion and maintenance; CNS: None; CL: Apply

11. A nurse observes parents playing with their 10-month-old infant. Which behavior indicates that this infant will be cruising soon?
   1. The infant is bending her knees and sitting after standing.
   2. The infant bounces up and down while she stands on her father's knees.
   3. The infant is stooping and squatting.
   4. The infant pushes her legs against a hard surface when she's supported under the arms while being held upright.

11. **1.** Bending the knees and learning to sit after standing indicate that a child will soon be cruising. Bouncing up and down helps develop an infant's legs in preparation to roll over, sit and crawl — usually around 6 months of age. Stooping and squatting is a sign that the infant will be walking soon, and usually occurs after the infant starts cruising. Pushing the feet against a hard surface is a newborn reflexive action.
CN: Health promotion and maintenance; CNS: None; CL: Apply

12. A nurse is teaching the parents of a six-month-old infant about age-specific growth and development. Which statements are true regarding infant development? Select all that apply.
   1. A six-month-old infant has trouble holding objects.
   2. A six-month-old infant can usually roll from prone to supine, and supine to prone positions.
   3. A teething ring is appropriate for a six-month-old infant.
   4. Head lag is commonly noted in infants at age six months.
   5. Lack of visual coordination usually resolves by age 6 months.

12. **2, 3, 5.** Gross motor skills of the six-month-old infant include rolling from prone to supine, and supine to prone positions. A teething ring would be appropriate for a six-month old infant. Visual coordination and fine motor skills, including purposeful grasps, usually resolve by six months of age. At this age, a child should have good head control and no longer display head lag when pulled to a sitting position.
CN: Health promotion and maintenance; CNS: None; CL: Apply

13. A nurse is examining an infant. Which anatomical landmark should he use to measure chest circumference?

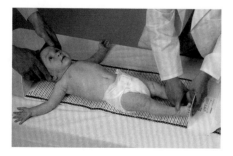

13. Chest circumference is most accurately measured by placing the measuring tape around the infant's chest, with the tape covering the nipples. A false circumference is obtained if measured above or below this landmark.

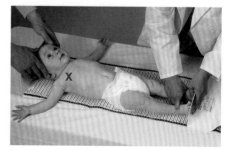

CN: Health promotion and maintenance; CNS: None; CL: Apply

14. The nurse is examining the breasts of an adolescent girl. The nurse classifies this client's sexual maturity as Tanner stage three. Which graphic **best** depicts this stage?

1.

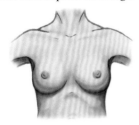

2.

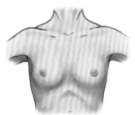

3.

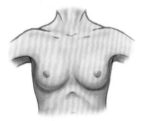

4.

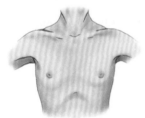

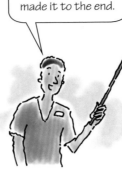

Way to go! You made it to the end.

14. 2. In Tanner stage three, the entire breast enlarges and the nipple does not protrude. In graphic one an adult breast has developed, the nipple protrudes, and the areola no longer appears separate from the breast which illustrates Tanner stage five. Graphic three illustrates Tanner stage four, in which the breast enlarges, nipple and papilla protrude and appear as a secondary mound. Graphic four illustrates Tanner stage two in which breast buds appear, and the areola is slightly widened and appear small mounds.

CN: Physiological integrity; CNS: Reduction of risk potential; CL: Apply

Chapter 27

Cardiovascular Disorders

You've reached our test on cardiovascular disorders in children. Before taking this comprehensive test, why not bolster yourself with a heart-healthy snack of celery and low-fat cream cheese? Yum!

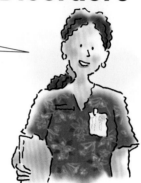

1. The nurse auscultates the first heart sound. When does the first heart sound occur?
1. Late in diastole
2. Early in diastole
3. With the closure of the mitral and tricuspid valves
4. With the closure of the aortic and pulmonic valves

Let's get going! You can do it.

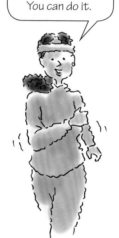

2. The nurse is performing a cardiac assessment on a child and auscultates a grade 1 heart murmur. What is a characteristic of this heart murmur?
1. Equal to the heart sounds
2. Softer than the heart sounds
3. Can be heard with the naked ear
4. Associated with a precordial thrill

3. A graduate nurse has started working in a pediatric intensive care unit and is measuring the client's cardiac output. What factors determine cardiac output? Select all that apply.
1. Contractility
2. Preload
3. Afterload
4. Urine output
5. Heart rate

1. **3.** The S1 occurs during systole with the closure of the mitral and tricuspid valves. The fourth heart sound is heard late in diastole, and may be a normal finding in children. The third heart sound is heard early in diastole. The second heart sound occurs during diastole with closure of the aortic and pulmonic valves.
CN: Health promotion and maintenance; CNS: None; CL: Analyze

2. **2.** A grade 1 heart murmur is commonly difficult to hear, and softer than the heart sounds. A grade 2 murmur is usually equal to the heart sounds. A grade 6 murmur can be heard with the naked ear or with the stethoscope off the chest. A grade 4 murmur is associated with a precordial thrill. A thrill is a palpable manifestation associated with a loud murmur.
CN: Health promotion and maintenance; CNS: None; CL: Analyze

3. **1, 2, 3, 5.** Cardiac output is calculated by taking heart rate times the stroke volume. Stroke volume is the amount of blood ejected by the heart in any one contraction. It's influenced by preload, afterload, and contractility. Cardiac preload is the pressure of the blood on the muscle fibers in the ventricles of the heart at the end of diastole. It, represents the amount of blood volume in the left ventricle of the heart at that particular point in the cardiac cycle (just before the heart contracts, when it is filled with the most blood, which is the end of diastole). Contractility is the ability of the cardiac muscle to act as an efficient pump. Afterload is the resistance the ventricles pump against when ejecting blood. Urine output is used to assess cardiac output, not determine it.
CN: Physiological integrity; CNS: Physiological adaptation; CL: Apply

CN: Client needs category   CNS: Client needs subcategory   CL: Cognitive level

4. A child is diagnosed with cardiogenic shock. What manifestations would the nurse expect to find in this child? Select all that apply.
1. Decreased urine output
2. Bradycardia
3. Tachypnea
4. Bounding peripheral pulses
5. Capillary refill of less than two seconds

5. Which assessment would the nurse consider as a late sign of shock in a six-month-old infant?
1. Heart rate of 172 bpm
2. Blood pressure of 64/36 mmHg in right arm
3. Capillary refill of four seconds
4. Pale, cool, mottled skin

6. A two-year-old child is showing signs of shock. A 10 ml/kg bolus of normal saline solution is ordered. The child weighs 40 lb (18.18 kg). How many milliliters should be administered? Round your answer using a whole number.

_____ ml

7. Which assessment data would lead the nurse to suspect a cardiac defect in a one-month-old infant?
1. Weight gain
2. Mottled skin
3. Poor nutritional intake
4. Pink mucous membranes

8. A nursing student is reviewing electrocardiogram waveforms, of an infant, with the nurse. The student asks the nurse which waveform indicates ventricular depolarization and contraction. What would be the nurse's **best** response?
1. P wave
2. PR interval
3. QRS complex
4. T wave

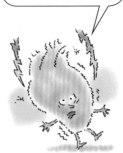

Yikes! Is this what they mean by cardiogenic shock?

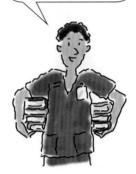

Yes, this is a math question. Stay cool, and you'll do great!

4. 1, 3. Cardiogenic shock occurs when cardiac output is decreased and tissue oxygen needs aren't adequately met. Signs of cardiogenic shock include apprehension, irritability, pallor, decreased urine output, tachycardia, tachypnea, weak pulses, cool extremities, and poor capillary refill.
CN: Physiological integrity; CNS: Physiological adaptation; CL: Analyze

5. 2. Hypotension is considered a late sign of shock in children. This represents a decompensated state and impending cardiopulmonary arrest. Tachycardia, delayed capillary refill, and pale, cool skin are earlier indicators of shock that may show compensation.
CN: Physiological integrity; CNS: Physiological adaptation; CL: Analyze

6. 182.
The correct formula for this calculation is:

$$10\,ml/kg \times 18.18\,kg = 181.8\,ml$$

Round to 182 ml
CN: Physiological integrity; CNS: Pharmacological and parenteral therapies; CL: Analyze

7. 3. Infants and children with heart defects tend to have poor nutritional intake and weight loss, indicating poor cardiac output, heart failure, or hypoxemia. The child appears lethargic or tired because of the heart failure or hypoxia. Mottled skin may be a sign of hypothermia. Pink, moist mucous membranes are normal.
CN: Health promotion and maintenance; CNS: None; CL: Analyze

8. 3. The QRS complex reflects ventricular depolarization and contraction. The P wave represents atrial depolarization and contraction. The PR interval represents the time it takes an impulse to trace from the atrioventricular node to the bundle of His. The T wave represents repolarization of the ventricles.
CN: Physiological integrity; CNS: Reduction of risk potential; CL: Apply

9. Which noninvasive method should the nurse use to evaluate the cardiac status of a child?
1. Transthoracic echocardiogram
2. Cardiac enzyme levels
3. Cardiac catheterization
4. Transesophageal pacing

9. **1.** A transthoracic echocardiogram is a noninvasive procedure to visualize the anatomy of the heart. Blood testing determines cardiac enzyme levels. Cardiac catheterization involves passing a catheter into the chambers of the heart for direct visualization of the heart and great vessels. Transesophageal pacing requires a probe to be placed in the esophagus for high-frequency ultrasound.
CN: Physiological integrity; CNS: Reduction of risk potential; CL: Analyze

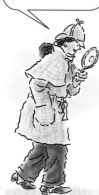

I think I detect the correct statement.

10. An echocardiogram has been ordered for an eight-year-old child. What is the **most** accurate information for the nurse to tell the parents?
1. The child must be sedated in order to get an accurate result.
2. It uses sound waves to measure and evaluate cardiac structures and function.
3. The transthoracic method of echocardiogram is an invasive procedure.
4. It is the most definitive method of evaluating cardiac function.

10. **2.** Echocardiograms use sound waves to measure and evaluate cardiac structures and function. The transthoracic method is not an invasive procedure; however, the transesophageal method is considered invasive. The child does not have to be sedated, but must lay quietly during the procedure. Very young children may need sedation if they are unable to lie still. While an echocardiogram gives the provider a good idea of cardiac function, a cardiac catheterization is the definitive method for a complete and accurate picture.
CN: Physiological integrity; CNS: Reduction of risk potential; CL: Apply

11. The nursing is caring for a school-age child who is scheduled for cardiac catheterization. Prioritize the nurse's steps in preparing this child for this procedure.

| 1. Clean and prep the catheter injection site |
| 2. Give the child a blanket to keep warm |
| 3. Insert an IV |
| 4. Assess vital signs |
| 5. Apply electrocardiograph monitor |
| 6. Ensure the child keeps the leg straight |

11. Ordered Response:

| 4. Assess vital signs |
| 3. Insert an IV |
| 5. Apply electrocardiograph monitor |
| 1. Clean and prep the catheter injection site |
| 2. Give the child a blanket to keep warm |
| 6. Ensure the child keeps the leg straight |

CN: Physiological integrity; CNS: Physiological adaptation; CL: Analyze

12. The nurse is teaching the parents of a child who is scheduled for a cardiac catheterization. Which statement, by the nurse, is **most** accurate regarding the procedure?
1. It is an invasive procedure where the catheter is put directly into the heart muscle.
2. General anesthesia is required for children less than age three.
3. It uses high-frequency sound waves to produce an image of the heart in motion.
4. It provides visualization of the heart and great vessels using radiopaque dye.

12. **4.** Cardiac catheterization provides visualization of the heart and great vessels using radiopaque dye. It's an invasive procedure in which a thin catheter is passed into the chambers of the heart through a peripheral vein or artery, not directly into the heart muscle. Conscious sedation is usually given before cardiac catheterization. General anesthesia may be used for more complex catheterizations, or procedures that place the child at greater risk. High-frequency sound waves describe ultrasound and echocardiography.
CN: Physiological integrity; CNS: Reduction of risk potential; CL: Apply

13. Which nursing intervention would be **most** appropriate for a nurse to implement when caring for a two-year-old child immediately after cardiac catheterization?
1. Allow the child to sit on the parent's lap
2. Allow the parent to lie in bed with the child to keep him flat
3. Assess vital signs every 2 to 4 hours
4. Replace a blood-stained groin dressing with a new dressing

14. The nurse is preparing to discharge a 12-year-old child after cardiac catheterization. What is the **most** important information for the nurse to provide?
1. The child should drink fluids and eat a regular diet.
2. The child may participate in sports once home.
3. The child can routinely bathe after returning home.
4. The child may return to school the next day.

15. A two-year-old child is being monitored after cardiac surgery. Which assessment findings would represent a decrease in cardiac output? Select all that apply.
1. Hypotension
2. Decreased urine output
3. Weak peripheral pulses
4. Capillary refill less than two seconds
5. Warm fingers and toes

16. The nurse is monitoring a three-year-old child who is experiencing distress after having cardiac surgery. Which signs would indicate cardiac tamponade? Select all that apply.
1. Hypertension
2. Muffled heart sounds
3. Widened pulse pressure
4. Decreased chest tube drainage
5. Dyspnea

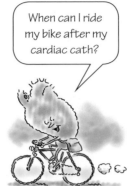

When can I ride my bike after my cardiac cath?

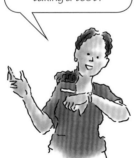

You've already answered 15 questions! See how time flies when you're taking a test?

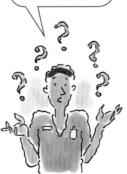

Which signs indicate cardiac tamponade?

13. 2. During recovery, the child should remain flat in bed, keeping the punctured leg straight for the prescribed time. The child should avoid raising the head, sitting, straining the abdomen, or coughing. Vital signs are taken every 15 minutes until the child is awake and stable, then every half hour, and then hourly as ordered. If bleeding occurs at the insertion site, the nurse should mark the margins with a pen and monitor for changes.
CN: Physiological integrity; CNS: Reduction of risk potential; CL: Analyze

14. 1. A regular diet and increased fluids are encouraged after catheterization. Increased fluids help flush the injected dyes out of the system. Normal activities may be resumed, but strenuous physical activities or sports should be avoided for about three days. Prolonged bathing can be resumed in three days. A sponge bath is encouraged until then. The child may return to school three days after discharge.
CN: Physiological integrity; CNS: Physiological adaptation; CL: Analyze

15. 1, 2, 3. Signs of decreased cardiac output include weak peripheral pulses, hypotension, low urine output, delayed capillary refill, and cool extremities.
CN: Physiological integrity; CNS: Physiological adaptation; CL: Analyze

16. 2, 4, 5. Symptoms of cardiac tamponade include muffled heart sounds, hypotension, a narrowing pulse pressure, tachycardia, dyspnea, apprehension, elevated right atrial and left atrial filling pressures, and sudden cessation of chest tube drainage. Cardiac tamponade occurs when a large volume of fluid or clots interferes with ventricular filling and pumping, and then collects in the pericardial sac, decreasing cardiac output.
CN: Physiological integrity; CNS: Physiological adaptation; CL: Analyze

17. A nurse is monitoring fluid and electrolyte balance in a child after cardiac surgery that required cardiopulmonary bypass. Which findings should the nurse expect? Select all that apply.
1. Urine output of 5 ml/kg/hr
2. Glucose level of 153 mg/dl (8.49 mmol/L)
3. Glucose level of 59 mg/dl (3.27 mmol/L)
4. Potassium level of 5.5 mEq/L (5.50 mmol/L)
5. Potassium level of 3.2 mEq/L (3.20 mmol/L)

18. A nurse is teaching wound care to the parents of a child who has undergone cardiac surgery. Which statement, made by the nurse, is **most** appropriate?
1. "It is okay to apply lotions and powders to the incision area when you go home."
2. "Your child may take a tub bath tomorrow."
3. "Your child may report tingling, itching, or numbness at the incision site."
4. "When the adhesive strips over the incision fall off, call the health care provider."

19. Parents ask a nurse about their eight-year-old son's activity level after open cardiac surgery. Which would be the nurse's **best** response?
1. "There are no exercise limitations."
2. "Your child may go back to school in three days."
3. "You should encourage a balance of rest and exercise."
4. "Climbing and contact sports are restricted for one week."

20. The nurse is providing discharge instructions for the parents of an infant who has recently undergone cardiac surgery. The nurse determines that teaching was effective when the parents make which statements? Select all that apply.
1. "I should keep giving my baby all prescribed medicines until the health care provider tells me to stop."
2. "I need to find low-sodium formula to feed to my baby."
3. "I am going to take my baby to church on Sunday so that everyone can see her."
4. "I should wait about six weeks to schedule an appointment for my baby to get her immunizations."
5. "I should place my infant on her stomach when I put her to bed."

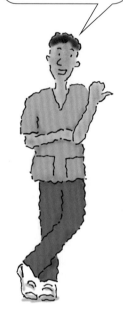

I'm itching to get question 18 correct.

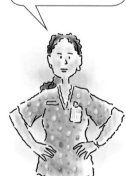

It's important that a child's family understands all discharge instructions.

17. 2, 5. Due to the increased sodium levels, there is a decrease in urine output, which is defined as less than 1 to 2 ml/kg/hr. Hyperglycemia results from the body's decreased release of insulin and stimulation of glycogenolysis. It may also result from the administration of corticosteroids that occurs during the surgery. Hypokalemia is a result of intracellular fluid shifts that occur during bypass.
CN: Physiological integrity; CNS: Physiological adaptation; CL: Analyze

18. 3. As the area heals, tingling, itching, and numbness are normal sensations and will eventually go away. Lotions and powders should be avoided during the first two weeks after surgery. A complete bath should be delayed for the first week, although sponge baths are allowed. Adhesive strips may loosen or fall off on their own. This is a common and normal occurrence.
CN: Physiological integrity; CNS: Physiological adaptation; CL: Analyze

19. 3. Activity should be increased gradually each day, allowing for a sensible balance of rest and exercise. School and large crowds should be avoided for at least two weeks to prevent exposure to people with active infections. Sports and contact activities should be restricted for about six weeks, allowing the sternum adequate time to heal.
CN: Physiological integrity; CNS: Physiological adaptation; CL: Analyze

20. 1, 4. Drugs, such as digoxin and furosemide, shouldn't be stopped abruptly. There are no dietary restrictions. Parents are encouraged to keep their child away from crowds for the first few weeks after surgery in order to prevent exposure to infections such as colds or respiratory syncytial virus bronchiolitis. Immunizations should be delayed for at least six weeks following surgery. Infants should be placed on their backs for sleep; this is the safest position for an infant to sleep.
CN: Physiological integrity; CNS: Reduction of risk potential; CL: Analyze

21. The nurse is caring for a four-year-old client with a chest tube that has been placed on water seal. The nurse assesses the chest tube and determines that it is functioning correctly when:

1. the water level rises with inhalation.
2. bubbling is seen in the suction chamber.
3. bubbling is seen in the water seal chamber.
4. water seal is obtained by clamping the tube.

21. 1. The water seal chamber is functioning appropriately when the water level rises in the chamber with inhalation and falls with expiration. This shows that negative pressure in the lungs is being maintained. Bubbling in the suction chamber should only be seen when suction is being used. Bubbling in the water seal chamber generally indicates the presence of an air leak. The chest tube should never be clamped. A tension pneumothorax may occur. Water seal is activated when the suction is disconnected.
CN: Physiological integrity; CNS: Reduction of risk potential; CL: Apply

22. A child's chest tube becomes dislodged. Prioritize the interventions in the order that they should be performed by the nurse.

1. Place petroleum gauze dressing over the insertion site
2. Call the health care provider
3. Monitor respiratory status and vital signs
4. Prepare for re-insertion of the chest tube
5. Document the incident

22. Ordered Response:

3. Monitor respiratory status and vital signs
1. Place petroleum gauze dressing over the insertion site
4. Prepare for reinsertion of the chest tube
2. Call the health care provide health care provider
5. Document the incident

CN: Physiological integrity; CNS: Reduction of risk potential; CL: Apply

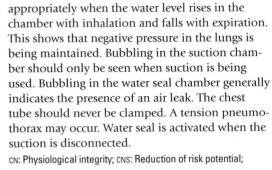

There goes question 23. You're really moving.

23. What are the expected assessment findings of an infant with heart failure? Select all that apply.

1. Heart rate of 100/bpm
2. Respiratory rate of 72 breaths/min
3. Gallop murmur
4. +3 pulses in all extremities
5. Liver palpated at level of umbilicus

23. 2, 3, 5. Tachycardia occurs as a compensatory mechanism to the decrease in cardiac output. This also reflects the body's attempt to increase the force and rate of myocardial contraction and increase oxygen consumption of the heart. The respiratory rate increases in an attempt to increase oxygenation. Pulses are usually weak and thready. When the heart stretches beyond efficiency, an extra heart sound, or S3 gallop murmur, may be audible. This is related to excessive preload and ventricular dilation. Hepatomegaly is due to fluid retention.
CN: Physiological integrity; CNS: Physiological adaptation; CL: Analyze

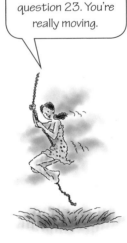

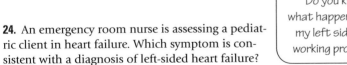

Do you know what happens when my left side isn't working properly?

24. An emergency room nurse is assessing a pediatric client in heart failure. Which symptom is consistent with a diagnosis of left-sided heart failure?

1. Weight gain
2. Peripheral edema
3. Neck vein distention
4. Tachypnea and dyspnea

24. 4. Respiratory symptoms, such as tachypnea and dyspnea, are seen as a result of pulmonary congestion. Peripheral edema, jugular vein distention, and weight gain are seen with systemic venous congestion or right-sided heart failure. Fluid accumulates in the interstitial spaces because of blood pooling in the venous circulation.
CN: Physiological integrity; CNS: Physiological adaptation; CL: Apply

CN: Client needs category   CNS: Client needs subcategory   CL: Cognitive level

25. Which nursing intervention is **most** appropriate when caring for an infant with heart failure?
1. Limit fluid intake
2. Avoid using infant seats
3. Cluster nursing activities
4. Place the infant prone or supine

25. 3. Energy expenditures need to be limited to reduce metabolic and oxygen needs. Nursing care should be clustered, followed by long periods of undisturbed rest. Fluid may be restricted in older children, but infants' nutritional requirements depend on adequate hydration. Infants should be placed in the semi-Fowler's or upright position. Infant seats help maintain an upright position. This facilitates lung expansion, provides less restrictive movement of the diaphragm, relieves pressure from abdominal organs, and decreases pulmonary congestion.
CN: Physiological integrity; CNS: Physiological adaptation; CL: Analyze

26. Which treatment plan is recommended for an infant with heart failure?
1. Restriction of fluids
2. Weigh infant once a week
3. Use of low-sodium formula
4. Use of formula with an increased caloric content

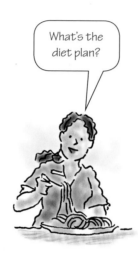

What's the diet plan?

26. 4. Formulas with increased caloric content are given to meet the increased caloric requirements caused by an overworked heart and labored breathing. Fluid restriction and low-sodium formulas aren't recommended. An infant's nutritional needs depend on fluid. Daily weights at the same time of the day, on the same scale, before feedings, are recommended to follow nutritional stability and diuresis trends. Low-sodium formulas may cause hyponatremia and can lead to decreased bone development.
CN: Physiological integrity; CNS: Basic care and comfort; CL: Apply

27. A mother is holding her son, born with patent ductus arteriosus six hours ago. As the nurse enters the room to assess the neonate's vital signs, the mother states, "My doctor says that my baby has a heart murmur. Does that mean he has a bad heart?" What is the nurse's **most** appropriate response?
1. A murmur is caused by an opening in the heart. He'll need more tests to determine his heart condition.
2. Murmurs can mean the blood circulation in the heart is not correct. He'll require oxygen therapy at home for a while.
3. Murmurs in children are usually benign. He'll be fine. Don't worry about him.
4. The murmur is caused by the natural opening for fetal circulation, which can take a day or two to close. It's a normal part of your baby's transition.

27. 4. The most appropriate response would be to explain the neonate's present condition to relieve the mother, and to acknowledge an awareness of the condition. A neonate's vascular system changes following birth. Certain factors help to reverse the flow of blood through the ductus and ultimately induce its closure. This closure typically begins within the first 24 hours following birth, and ends within a few days. Diagnostic tests, especially invasive ones such as a cardiac catheterization, are reserved for a symptomatic infant. Oxygen is contraindicated in infants with this condition as it lowers the pulmonary vascular resistance and will lead to too much blood flow through the lungs.
CN: Health promotion and maintenance; CNS: None; CL: Analyze

28. A teenage client with heart failure is prescribed carvedilol. She asks the nurse, "What is this drug supposed to do?" Which responses by the nurse are correct? Select all that apply.
  1. "Improve the way your heart works"
  2. "Keep you from getting an infection in your heart"
  3. "Increase the amount of blood pumped by your heart"
  4. "Lower your blood pressure"
  5. "Slow your heart rate"

29. Which assessment finding would lead the nurse to suspect a child has a digoxin level greater than 2 mcg/ml?
  1. Weight gain
  2. Tachycardia
  3. Nausea and vomiting
  4. Seizures

30. The nurse will administer a dosage of captopril at 1.5 mg/kg/day, in divided doses, q12h, to an infant who weighs 10 kg. How much would the nurse give per dose? Record your answer using one decimal place.

_____ mg

31. A child with heart failure is taking captopril. What are the desired effects of this medication? Select all that apply.
  1. Increased blood pressure
  2. Decreased blood pressure
  3. Increased preload
  4. Decreased preload
  5. Increased urine output
  6. Decreased urine output

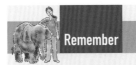

Remember

"Antihypertensives are against (anti) high (hyper) blood pressure (tensives)."

Carvedilol is an antihypertensive, beta-adrenergic blocker that increases left ventricular function and reduces symptoms of heart failure.

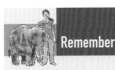

Remember

"ACE inhibitors erase hypertension."

Angiotensin-converting enzymes, such as captopril, reduce blood pressure by interrupting the renin-angiotensin-aldosterone system.

28. 1, 4, 5. Carvedilol is an antihypertensive, beta-adrenergic blocker. It has been shown to increase left ventricular function and reduce the symptoms of heart failure. It reduces cardiac output. Carvedilol will not prevent infection.
CN: Physiological integrity; CNS: Pharmacological and parenteral therapies; CL: Apply

29. 3. Digoxin toxicity in infants and children may present with nausea, vomiting, anorexia, or a slow, irregular apical heart rate. Weight gain, tachycardia, or seizures are not seen in digoxin toxicity.
CN: Physiological integrity; CNS: Pharmacological and parenteral therapies; CL: Analyze

30. 7.5
Here is the calculation:

$$10 \, kg \times 1.5 \, mg/kg/day = 15 \, mg/day.$$

$$15 \, mg/day \div 2 \, doses/day = 7.5 \, mg/dose.$$

CN: Physiological integrity; CNS: Pharmacological and parenteral therapies; CL: Analyze

31. 2, 4, 5. Angiotensin-converting enzyme inhibitors block the conversion of angiotensin I to angiotensin II in the kidneys. This causes vasodilation and decreased secretion of aldosterone. This leads to lowered blood pressure and decreased preload. Renal perfusion is also enhanced, which leads to improved diuresis.
CN: Physiological integrity; CNS: Pharmacological and parenteral therapies; CL: Apply

CN: Client needs category   CNS: Client needs subcategory   CL: Cognitive level

32. The parents of a newborn child have just been told that he has a heart condition known as patent ductus arteriosus. Which statement, made by the parents, indicates an understanding of this condition?
  1. "Heart failure is uncommon in this kind of heart condition."
  2. "The health care provider said if it doesn't close in the next 4 to 6 weeks, our baby might need surgery."
  3. "This kind of opening in the heart can cause a decreased heart and respiratory rate."
  4. "This opening can cause our baby to look blue because of a decreased blood flow to the lungs."

32. 2. At birth, oxygenated blood normally causes the ductus to constrict, and the vessel closes completely by age six weeks. If the open ductus arteriosus fails to close, it can cause an excessive blood flow to the lungs because of the high pressure in the aorta. It typically does not cause cyanosis. Tachypnea and tachycardia may occur as the body tries to compensate. Heart failure is common in premature infants with a patent ductus arteriosus.
CN: Physiological integrity; CNS: Physiological adaptation; CL: Analyze

33. Which intervention is recommended initially, for preterm neonates, to close a patent ductus arteriosus?
  1. Indomethacin
  2. Prostaglandin E1
  3. Surgical ligation
  4. Cardiac catheterization

33. 1. Preterm neonates with good renal function may receive oral indomethacin, a prostaglandin inhibitor, to encourage ductal closure. If this isn't effective, surgery is suggested. Prostaglandin E1 is used in maintaining a patent ductus arteriosus in newborns. This is primarily useful when the threat of premature closure of the ductus arteriosus exists in an infant with ductal-dependent congenital heart disease, including cyanotic lesions. Surgical ligation and a cardiac catheterization procedure may also be performed in infants and children if medication is not effective.
CN: Physiological integrity; CNS: Physiological adaptation; CL: Analyze

34. A nurse is caring for a client with patent ductus arteriosus. What assessment findings would the nurse anticipate with this condition? Select all that apply.
  1. Weak peripheral pulses
  2. Machine-like murmur
  3. Widened pulse pressure
  4. Tachypnea
  5. Cyanosis

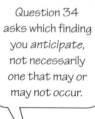

Question 34 asks which finding you *anticipate*, not necessarily one that may or may not occur.

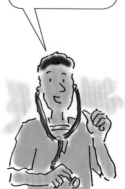

34. 2, 3, 4. The continuous, turbulent flow of blood from the aorta, through the patent ductus arteriosus, to the pulmonary artery, produces a machine-like murmur. The pulse pressure would be widened, and peripheral pulses would be bounding from the runoff of blood from the aorta to the pulmonary artery. Tachypnea is a common finding in all infants and children with heart defects. Cyanosis is not a common finding in children with defects that have increased pulmonary blood flow, such as ductus arteriosus. Cyanosis is common in defects that result in decreased pulmonary blood flow.
CN: Physiological integrity; CNS: Physiological adaptation; CL: Analyze

35. During observation of a child who has undergone cardiac catheterization, the nurse notes significant bleeding from the percutaneous femoral catheterization site. Prioritize the nurse's interventions to treat this finding.

1. Apply direct, continuous pressure
2. Seek the assistance of another nurse
3. Check the pulses in the affected leg
4. Reapply a pressure dressing

35. Ordered Response:

1. Apply direct, continuous pressure
4. Reapply a pressure dressing
2. Seek the assistance of another nurse
3. Check the pulses in the affected leg.

The priority is to stop the bleeding to prevent cardiovascular collapse as a result of blood loss. A pressure dressing will help to maintain a consistent compression and pressure on the area to stop the bleeding. The assistance of another nurse can facilitate calling the health care provider, maintaining pressure on the site, checking pulses, obtaining supplies, and monitoring vital signs.
CN: Physiological integrity; CNS: Reduction of risk potential; CL: Apply

36. What finding would the nurse anticipate while assessing a child with tetralogy of Fallot?
  1. High birth weight
  2. Increased appetite
  3. Delayed growth
  4. Decreased respiratory rate

36. 3. Classic symptoms of tetralogy of Fallot are low birth weight, cyanosis, poor feeding, delayed growth and rapid breathing.
CN: Physiological integrity; CNS: Physiological adaptation; CL: Analyze

37. A nurse is reviewing an infant's progress notes.

Progress notes	
10/15/16 0800	Four-month-old infant admitted last evening. Wt: 4.95 kg. (10%) Ht: 66 cm (95%), Frequent episodes of bradycardia, tachypnea. Breastfeeding every 4 hours for 30 minutes on each side.

What notations would lead the nurse to suspect that this infant has a ventricular septal defect? Select all that apply.
  1. Tachypnea
  2. Plots at 95th percentile for height on growth chart
  3. Plots at the 10th percentile for weight on growth chart
  4. Bradycardia
  5. Increased length of time to finish breastfeeding

37. 1, 3, 5. Children with a ventricular septal defect usually present with symptoms of heart failure, poor growth and development, and failure to thrive. They also have difficulty feeding due to their decreased cardiac output and tachypnea.
CN: Physiological integrity; CNS: Physiological adaptation; CL: Analyze

38. When caring for a child diagnosed with a ventricular septal defect (VSD), which description would the nurse include while teaching the parents about this condition?
1. It is a narrowing of the aortic arch.
2. It is a failure of a septum to develop completely between the atria.
3. It is a narrowing of the valves at the entrance of the pulmonary artery.
4. It is a failure of a septum to develop completely between the ventricles.

38. 4. VSD is a hole in the wall separating the two lower chambers of the heart. In normal development, the wall between the chambers closes before the fetus is born, so that by birth, oxygen-rich blood is kept from mixing with the oxygen-poor blood. In a child with VSD, blood can travel across the hole from the left pumping chamber (left ventricle) to the right pumping chamber (right ventricle) and out into the lung arteries. If the VSD is large, the extra blood being pumped into the lung arteries makes the heart and lungs work harder and the lungs can become congested. The narrowing of the aortic arch describes coarctation of the aorta. Narrowing of the valves at the pulmonary artery describes pulmonic stenosis. When the septum fails to develop between the atria, it's considered an atrial septal defect.
CN: Physiological integrity; CNS: Physiological adaptation; CL: Apply

39. The nurse is caring for a newborn who has been diagnosed with a ventricular septal defect. The newborn is not exhibiting any signs of heart failure. The parents ask the nurse why the health care provider does not want to perform surgery immediately on the newborn. What is the nurse's **most** appropriate response?
1. "Your baby is just too little to have surgery right now."
2. "Waiting will allow you time to bond with your new baby."
3. "The health care provider wants to wait and see if the hole in your baby's heart will close on its own."
4. "Your baby is not sick enough to require surgery at this point in time."

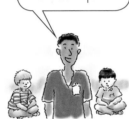

I'm sure you have the answer to this one down pat.

39. 3. Twenty to sixty percent of ventricular septal defects will close spontaneously. While older, bigger infants do have better surgical outcomes, the nurse should avoid saying, "Your baby is too little for surgery." Surgery is not delayed in order to add more bonding time. It is dependent on the infant's symptoms and size. Answer four is correct, but answer three is the most appropriate response.
CN: Physiological integrity; CNS: Physiological adaptation; CL: Analyze

40. A child with a ventricular septal defect repair is receiving dopamine postoperatively. The parents ask the nurse why the child is getting the medication. What is the nurse's **best** response?
1. To decrease heart rate
2. To increase urine output
3. To increase cardiac output
4. To decrease cardiac contractility

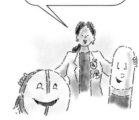

You know more about drugs than you realize!

40. 3. Increased cardiac output is related to the direct inotropic effect of dopamine hydrochloride on the myocardium. Dopamine stimulates β1- and β2- adrenergic receptors. It's a selective cardiac stimulant that will increase cardiac output, heart rate, and cardiac contractility. As a result of improving cardiac output, urine output increases in response to dilation of the blood vessels to the mesentery and kidneys..
CN: Physiological integrity; CNS: Pharmacological and parenteral therapies; CL: Analyze

41. An infant returns to the room after a cardiac catheterization. What **priority** information should the nurse teach the parents about mobility? Select all that apply.
 1. The infant may sit in an infant swing.
 2. The infant may be held as long as the affected extremity is immobilized.
 3. The infant may be maintained on bed rest with the affected extremity immobilized.
 4. The infant may be held upright in arms in order to eat.
 5. The infant may be held as long as both extremities are immobilized.

41. 2, 3. The child should be maintained on bed rest to keep the affected extremity immobilized, and prevent hemorrhage. Allowing the infant to sit in a swing, even with the affected extremity immobilized, places him at risk for hemorrhage. Infants may be held, especially if that keeps the infant calm and the affected extremity remains immobilized. There is no need to keep both extremities immobilized. The infant should not be held upright as that will increase risk of hemorrhage.
CN: Physiological integrity; CNS: Reduction of risk potential; CL: Apply

42. A client with Trisomy 21 comes to the pediatric clinic for a well visit. For which cardiac anomaly would this child be **most** at risk?
 1. Atrial septal defect
 2. Pulmonic stenosis
 3. Coarctation of the Aorta
 4. Atrioventricular canal defect

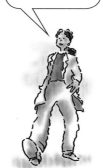

Question 42 already? Wow! You're making great strides!

42. 4. Atrioventricular canal defects are the most common cardiac defect in children with Trisomy 21. Atrial septal defects account for about 10% of all cardiac anomalies. Pulmonic stenosis is responsible for about 8% of all cardiac anomalies. Coarctation of the aorta accounts for 5% to 8% of all congenital heart defects.
CN: Health promotion and maintenance; CNS: None; CL: Apply

43. The nurse is assessing a child one hour after a cardiac catheterization. For which finding would the nurse **immediately** alert the provider?
 1. Weak, thready, unequal dorsalis pedis pulses
 2. Oral temperature of 100° F (37.7° C)
 3. Urine output of 2 ml/kg
 4. Slightly bloody drainage around the catheterization site dressing

43. 1. The pulse below the catheterization site should be strong and equal to the unaffected extremity. A weakened pulse may indicate vessel obstruction or perfusion problems. Slightly elevated temperature and low normal urine output are relatively normal findings after catheterization, and may be the result of decreased oral fluids. A small amount of bloody drainage is normal; however, the site must be assessed frequently for increased bleeding, and the margins of the drainage should be marked on the dressing.
CN: Physiological integrity; CNS: Reduction of risk potential; CL: Apply

44. Which cardiac anomaly produces a left-to-right shunt?
 1. Atrial septal defect
 2. Pulmonic stenosis
 3. Tetralogy of Fallot
 4. Total anomalous pulmonary venous return

44. 1. Atrial septal defects shunt blood from left to right because the pressure is greater on the left side of the heart. Pulmonic stenosis, tetralogy of Fallot, and total anomalous pulmonary venous return will show a right-to-left shunting of blood.
CN: Physiological integrity; CNS: Physiological adaptation; CL: Analyze

CN: Client needs category   CNS: Client needs subcategory   CL: Cognitive level

45. The nurse is assessing a child who has a defect resulting in a left-to-right shunt. Which symptoms would the nurse anticipate in this child? Select all that apply.
1. Weight gain
2. Edema in extremities
3. Tachypnea
4. Retractions
5. Hepatomegaly
6. Decreased activity tolerance

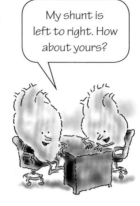

My shunt is left to right. How about yours?

45. 3, 4, 6. Left-to-right shunting leads to increased pulmonary blood flow or blood flow to the lungs. The child's symptoms will mimic respiratory difficulties. Weight gain, extremity edema, and hepatomegaly are more commonly found in children with systemic venous congestion, not pulmonary congestion. Children with left-to-right shunts tend to be small for age because the work of breathing increases metabolic demand, and the child's caloric intake is used for breathing and the work of the heart, leaving few calories left for growth.
CN: Physiological Integrity; CNS: Physiological Adaptation; CL: Analyze

46. A nurse is caring for a child who underwent a ventricular septal defect (VSD) repair.
Based on the note, which sign shows the **most** appropriate outcome for this child?

Progress notes	
10/15/16	Vital signs
1400	Four-year-old male, post-op day one for VSD repair. Pre-surgical weight = 15 kg. Today's weight = 14.7 kg. Oral temp 99.2° F (37.3° C). HR 70, cap refill 4 sec. RR 26. Pain Wong-Baker 5/10. Urine output 26 ml/hr.

1. Capillary refill four seconds
2. Pain score five
3. Urine output 26 ml/hr
4. Heart rate 68 bpm

46. 3. The client should have a urine output of 1 to 2 ml/kg/hr (26 ml/hr ÷ 14.7 kg = 1.77 ml/kg/hr). The capillary refill should be less than three seconds. The nurse should help the client have a lower pain score than five, as pain and can have an impact on the child's recovery. The heart rate should be greater than 70 bpm.
CN: Physiological integrity; CNS: Physiological adaptation; CL: Analyze

47. A six-month-old infant with uncorrected tetralogy of Fallot suddenly becomes increasingly cyanotic and diaphoretic with weak peripheral pulses and an increased respiratory rate. Prioritize the following nursing interventions.

1. Place the infant in a knee-chest position
2. Calm or comfort the infant
3. Administer oxygen per provider order
4. Administer morphine sulfate per provider order

47. Ordered Response:

3. Administer oxygen per provider order
4. Administer morphine sulfate per provider order
1. Place the infant in a knee-chest position
2. Calm or comfort the infant

CN: Safe effective care environment; CNS: Management of care; CL: Apply

48. The nurse is caring for a teen-aged client with a suspected cardiac defect.

Progress notes	
10/15/16	History and physical
1630	Fifteen-year-old male, admitted to unit at
	1415. Reporting headache. Epistaxis just prior
	to admission. Resting quietly. Blood pressure
	120/76 on right arm, 172/98 on left arm,
	84/46 on right leg. Pulses +3 in bilaterally in
	arms and legs.

The nurse suspects coarctation of the aorta when the history and physical reveal which findings? Select all they apply.
1. Warm, flushed skin
2. Blood pressure of 172/98 mmHg in the left arm
3. Blood pressure of 84/46 mmHg in the right leg
4. Reports headache and nosebleed
5. +3 pulses in both arms
6. +3 pulses in both legs

49. What should the nurse assess in a child who has undergone surgical repair of a coarctation of the aorta? Select all that apply.
1. Urine output
2. Neuromuscular function of the lower extremities
3. Neuromuscular function of the upper extremities
4. Heart sounds
5. Lung sounds
6. Bowel sounds

50. The nurse is preparing to assess a child with a possible cardiac anomaly. What is the **priority** assessment for this nurse?
1. Skin turgor
2. Temperature
3. Pupil size and reaction to light
4. Blood pressure in all four extremities

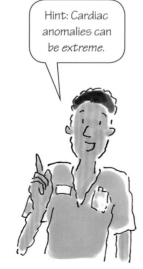

Hint: Cardiac anomalies can be extreme.

48. **2, 3, 4, 5.** Some blood flows to the head and upper extremities as it is pumped from the left ventricle to the aorta, while the rest is impeded by the narrowing of the coarctation and jets through the constricted area. Pressures and pulses are greater in the upper extremities. Decreased or absent pulses are found in the lower extremities. Children who are diagnosed during their adolescent years present with hypertension, headaches, dizziness, fainting, and epistaxis. Cool extremities and muscle cramps are common presentations.
CN: Physiological integrity; CNS: Physiological adaptation; CL: Analyze

49. **1, 2, 4, 5, 6.** Due to the surgical approach in which the surgeon performs a thoracotomy and cross-clamps the aorta while repairing the area of defect, there is lack of blood flow to the lower extremities for a short period of time. The upper extremities are not affected by this. Urine output must be closely monitored as well as reflexes, movement, and sensation of the lower extremities. Cardiovascular status, lung and bowel sounds are important for all postoperative assessments.
CN: Physiological integrity; CNS: Physiological adaptation; CL: Analyze

50. **4.** Measuring blood pressure in all four extremities is necessary to document hypertension and the blood pressure gradient between the upper and lower extremities. Temperature, skin turgor, and pupillary assessment are also important, but are not as specific for cardiac assessment as the blood pressure.
CN: Physiological integrity; CNS: Physiological adaptation; CL: Apply

51. A client has had a surgical repair of coarctation of the aorta. Which intervention would be included in the postoperative care?
1. Administering dopamine
2. Maintaining hypothermia
3. Administering sodium nitroprusside
4. Administering a bolus of IV fluids

51. 3. Blood pressure is tightly managed, and kept low so that there is no excessive pressure on the fresh suture lines, which could lead to rupture and postoperative hemorrhage. Sodium nitroprusside is a potent vasodilator and is used to keep the blood pressure lower than normal. Vasoconstrictors, such as dopamine and epinephrine, would be contraindicated because they would elevate blood pressure. Normothermia is maintained, and diuretics may be given to decrease fluid volume.
CN: Physiological integrity; CNS: Physiological adaptation;
CL: Analyze

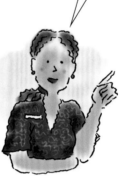

When it comes to assessment, practice makes perfect!

52. What findings should the nurse anticipate while assessing a child with tetralogy of Fallot?
1. Machine-like murmur
2. Eisenmenger's syndrome
3. Cyanosis that increases with crying or activity
4. Higher pressures in the upper extremities than in the lower extremities

52. 3. A child with tetralogy of Fallot will be mildly cyanotic at rest and have increasing cyanosis with crying, activity, or straining. A machine-like murmur is a characteristic of patent ductus arteriosus. Eisenmenger's syndrome is a complication of pulmonary pressure exceeding systemic pressure. Higher pressures in the upper extremities are characteristic of coarctation of the aorta.
CN: Physiological integrity; CNS: Physiological adaptation;
CL: Apply

53. A child with tetralogy of Fallot has clubbing of the fingers and toes. The nurse is aware that the clubbing is **most** likely to be caused by:
1. polycythemia.
2. chronic hypoxia.
3. pansystolic murmur.
4. abnormal growth and development.

53. 2. Chronic hypoxia lasting longer than six months will cause clubbing of the fingers and toes when untreated. Hypoxia varies with the degree of pulmonic stenosis. Polycythemia is an increased number of red blood cells as a result of the chronic hypoxemia. A pansystolic murmur is heard at the middle to lower left sternal border but has no impact on clubbing. Growth and development may appear normal.
CN: Physiological integrity; CNS: Physiological adaptation;
CL: Analyze

54. Which position might a child with tetralogy of Fallot find **most** comfortable following exercise?
1. Prone
2. Semi-Fowler's
3. Side-lying
4. Squatting

54. 4. This child may instinctively squat or assume a knee-chest position to reduce venous blood flow from the lower extremities, and to increase systemic vascular resistance, which diverts more blood flow into the pulmonary artery. Prone, semi-Fowler's, and side-lying positions won't produce this effect.
CN: Physiological integrity; CNS: Physiological adaptation;
CL: Analyze

55. A nurse is describing tetralogy of Fallot to a child's parents. Which statement, by the parents, demonstrates that the teaching has been effective?
1. "The condition is commonly referred to as 'blue tets.'"
2. "A child with this condition experiences hypercyanotic, or 'tet' spells."
3. "A child with this condition experiences frequent respiratory infections."
4. "A child with this condition experiences decreased or absent pulses in the lower extremities."

55. 2. Hypercyanotic, or "tet," spells may occur as a result of increasing obstruction of right ventricular outflow, resulting in decreased pulmonary blood flow and increased right-to-left shunting. Infants with mild obstruction of blood flow have little, or no, right-to-left shunting and appear pink, or "pink tets." Frequent respiratory infections are seen in defects with increased pulmonary blood flow, such as a patent ductus arteriosus. Decreased or absent pulses in the lower extremities are a sign of coarctation of the aorta.
CN: Physiological integrity; CNS: Physiological adaptation; CL: Analyze

56. A child diagnosed with tetralogy of Fallot has been ordered to undergo testing. Which test would **best** indicate the direction and amount of shunting in this child?
1. Chest radiography
2. Echocardiography
3. Electrocardiography (ECG)
4. Cardiac catheterization

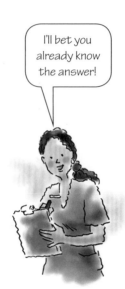

I'll bet you already know the answer!

56. 4. Cardiac catheterization provides specific information about the direction and amount of shunting, coronary anatomy, and each portion of the heart defect. Chest radiographs will show right ventricular hypertrophy pushing the apex of the heart upward, resulting in a boot-shaped silhouette. Echocardiogram scans define such defects as large ventricular septal defects, pulmonic stenosis, and malposition of the aorta. While an echocardiogram can show direction of blood flow, a cardiac catheterization can give more accurate information regarding the flow of blood and the amount of shunting. ECG shows right ventricular hypertrophy with tall R waves, and does not show direction of blood flow.
CN: Physiological integrity; CNS: Reduction of risk potential; CL: Apply

57. A nurse is teaching parents about tricuspid atresia. Which statement indicates that the parents understand this disorder?
1. "There's a narrowing at the aortic outflow tract."
2. "The pulmonary veins don't return to the left atrium."
3. "There's a narrowing at the entrance of the pulmonary artery."
4. "There's no communication between the right atrium and right ventricle."

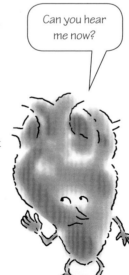

Can you hear me now?

57. 4. Tricuspid atresia is failure of the tricuspid valve to develop, leaving no communication between the right atrium and right ventricle. Narrowing at the aortic outflow tract is aortic stenosis. Total anomalous pulmonary venous return is a defect in which the pulmonary veins don't return to the left atrium but abnormally return to the right side of the heart. The narrowing at the entrance of the pulmonary artery represents pulmonic stenosis.
CN: Physiological integrity; CNS: Physiological adaptation; CL: Analyze

58. Which characteristics would the nurse anticipate in a child diagnosed with tricuspid atresia? Select all that apply.
   1. Cyanosis
   2. Machine-like murmur
   3. Decreased respiratory rate
   4. Capillary refill more than two seconds
   5. Clubbed fingers

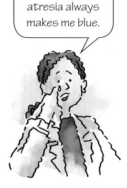

Tricuspid atresia always makes me blue.

58. 1, 4, 5. Cyanosis is the most consistent clinical sign of tricuspid atresia. Tachypnea and dyspnea are commonly present because of the decreased pulmonary blood flow and right-to-left shunting. Tricuspid atresia doesn't have a characteristic murmur. A machine-like murmur is characteristic of a patent ductus arteriosus. Decreased oxygenation would increase capillary refill time. Clubbed fingers in children result from chronic hypoxia, and may be seen in children with this defect.
CN: Physiological integrity; CNS: Physiological adaptation; CL: Analyze

59. The nurse is caring for a child with tricuspid atresia who develops polycythemia. Which statements **most** accurately describe this manifestation? Select all that apply.
   1. The red blood cell count is normal.
   2. There is an increased ability for the oxygen to carry blood.
   3. There is an increased risk of developing a thrombus.
   4. The viscosity of the blood is unchanged.
   5. The condition will cause the child to gain weight.

59. 2, 3. Polycythemia is an increased number of red blood cells, thereby increasing the ability of the blood to carry oxygen to the cells. It is the body's attempt at compensating for the chronic hypoxia associated with this heart defect. Due to this clinical manifestation, the viscosity of the blood increases, which leaves the child at risk for developing a thrombus, particularly when dehydrated. There is also not as much room for clotting factors, which can leave the child at risk for blood clotting disorders. Polycythemia may cause weight loss.
CN: Physiological integrity; CNS: Physiological adaptation; CL: Apply

60. A nurse is teaching the parents of an infant with tricuspid atresia where the defect in the heart is located. In what area on the diagram, would the nurse place an X to identify the site for the parents?

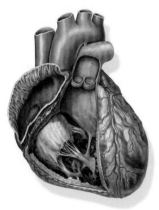

60. Tricuspid atresia entails the complete absence of the tricuspid valve causing an absence of a right atrioventricular connection, leading to a hypoplastic right ventricle. Because of the lack of an A-V connection, an atrial septal defect (ASD) must be present to fill the left ventricle with blood. Also, since there is a lack of a right ventricle, there must be a way to pump blood into the pulmonary arteries. This is accomplished by a ventricular septal defect (VSD).

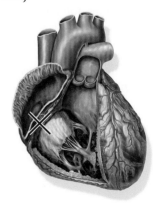

CN: Physiological integrity; CNS: Physiological adaptation; CL: Apply

CN: Client needs category   CNS: Client needs subcategory   CL: Cognitive level

61. The nurse is preparing to administer digoxin to an infant. What is the **most** important intervention by the nurse?
1. Mix the digoxin with the infant's food
2. Double the subsequent dose if a dose is missed
3. Give the digoxin with antacids when possible
4. Withhold the dose if the apical pulse rate is less than 90/bpm

62. A nurse is assessing a child who has undergone complete repair of total anomalous pulmonary venous connection. The nurse should be **most** concerned when the child experiences which sign?
1. Decreased work of breathing
2. Decreased respiratory rate
3. Decreased oxygenation saturation levels
4. Increased urine output

63. The nurse is assessing a child with a total anomalous pulmonary venous return defect. Which finding would the nurse anticipate on assessment?
1. Hypertension
2. Frequent respiratory infections
3. Normal growth and development
4. High activity level

64. The nurse is aware that a client who had a repair of total anomalous pulmonary venous return is at risk for:
1. systemic hypotension.
2. pulmonary hypertension.
3. ventricular arrhythmias.
4. pulmonary vein dilatation.

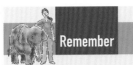

Remember

"Digoxin strengthens contractions of the heart."

Digoxin, a cardiac glycoside, is used to treat heart failure because it strengthens the contraction of the ventricles of the heart.

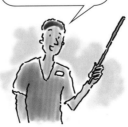

Read this question carefully to make sure you know what's being asked.

61. 4. Digoxin is used to decrease the heart rate; however, the apical pulse must be carefully monitored to detect a severe reduction. Administering digoxin to an infant with a heart rate of less than 90/bpm could further reduce the rate and compromise cardiac output. Mixing digoxin with food may interfere with accurate dosing. Double dosing should never be done. Antacids may decrease drug absorption.
CN: Physiological integrity; CNS: Pharmacological and parenteral therapies; CL: Apply

62. 3. A child who has pulmonary venous obstruction will exhibit signs of increasing respiratory distress, such as increased respiratory rate, dyspnea, and shortness of breath. Oxygen saturation levels will decrease. Urine output will decrease as the heart fails.
CN: Physiological integrity; CNS: Physiological adaptation; CL: Apply

63. 2. Children with total anomalous pulmonary venous return defects are prone to repeated respiratory infections due to increased pulmonary blood flow. Hypertension usually occurs with coarctation of the aorta. Poor feeding and failure to thrive are also signs of this defect. Listlessness may be a sign. Infants often look thin and malnourished.
CN: Physiological integrity; CNS: Physiological adaptation; CL: Apply

64. 2. Pulmonary hypertension, atrial arrhythmias, and pulmonary vein obstruction are complications that may result postoperatively. The left atrium is small and sensitive to fluid volume loading. Increased pressure in the right atrium is required to ensure left atrial filling.
CN: Physiological integrity; CNS: Physiological adaptation; CL: Analyze

65. The parents of an infant recently diagnosed with tricuspid atresia have been told that their child will need a series of surgeries, in three stages, during the first few years of life. Which statements indicate that the parents have an understanding of the procedures? Select all that apply.
1. "My child will have this dusky color for the rest of his life."
2. "These procedures will make my child have a normal heart."
3. "Once fixed, my baby will not have to take any more medicine."
4. "My baby will be just like all of the other children once the surgeries are all done."
5. "My child will have to be closely monitored for signs of a stroke."

65. 1, 5. The child will be dusky, particularly around mucous membranes and nail beds, for the rest of his life as a result of chronic hypoxemia. The resultant polycythemia and increased blood viscosity increase the child's chances of developing a thrombus, leading to a cerebrovascular accident or stroke. The three surgeries do give the child a "normal" heart, as they do not fix the original defect. The child will more than likely be on medications for the rest of his life, and will likely be smaller in stature than other children.
CN: Physiological integrity; CNS: Physiological adaptation; CL: Analyze

66. Which finding would the nurse commonly assess in a child with truncus arteriosus?
1. Weak, thready pulses
2. Narrowed pulse pressure
3. Pink and moist mucous membranes
4. Harsh, systolic regurgitant murmur

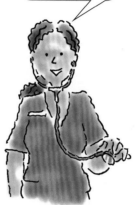

Listen closely and you'll hear the answer to question 66.

66. 4. As a result of the ventricular septal defect, a harsh systolic regurgitant murmur is heard along the left sternal border, and is usually accompanied by a thrill. Increasing pulmonary blood flow causes bounding pulses and a widened pulse pressure. Systemic and pulmonary blood mixing leads to mild or moderate cyanosis, so mucous membranes may appear dull or gray.
CN: Physiological integrity; CNS: Physiological adaptation; CL: Analyze

67. The nurse is preparing to administer digoxin to an infant who weighs 13.7 lb (6.2 kg). The practitioner has ordered 25 mcg/kg divided in three doses with one-half of the total dose for the initial dose, then one-quarter of the total dose for each of two subsequent doses given at eight-hour intervals. The medication comes in an oral solution of 0.05 mg/ml. How many milliliters would the nurse give for the second dose? Record your answer using two decimal places.

_____ ml

67. 0.78.
Here are the calculations:

$$25\,mcg/kg \times 6.2\,kg = 155\,mcg$$

$$0.05\,mg/ml \times 1,000\,mcg/mg = 50\,mcg/ml$$

$$155\,mcg \div 50\,mcg/ml = 3.1\,ml\,(total\,dose)$$

$$3.1\,ml \div 4 = 0.78\,ml\,(one-quarter\,dose)$$

The nurse would give 1.5 ml for the first dose, and then 0.78 ml for the following two doses.
CN: Physiological integrity; CNS: Pharmacological and parenteral therapies; CL: Apply

68. Which change would the nurse anticipate after administering oxygen to a cyanotic infant with uncorrected tetralogy of Fallot?
1. Disappearance of the murmur
2. No evidence of cyanosis
3. Improvement of finger clubbing
4. Less agitation

68. 4. Supplemental oxygen will help the infant breathe more easily and feel less anxious or agitated. Disappearance of the murmur, no evidence of cyanosis, and improvement of finger clubbing would not occur as a result of supplemental oxygen administration. Surgery is the definitive treatment for the cyanotic client with tetralogy of Fallot
CN: Physiological integrity; CNS: Physiological adaptation; CL: Apply

69. A nurse is caring for an infant with transposition of the great vessels. Which illustration shows the defects?

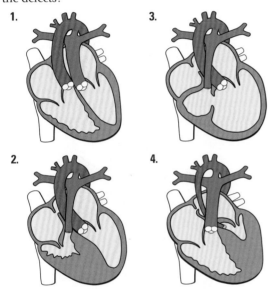

1. 3.

2. 4.

69. 1. The first illustration shows the defect of transposition of the great vessels. Illustration two shows pulmonary atresia. Illustration three shows tricuspid atresia. Illustration four shows hypoplastic left heart syndrome.
CN: Physiological integrity; CNS: Physiological adaptation; CL: Apply

70. A nurse is assessing a child with transposition of the great vessels. A patent foramen ovale is often an associated defect. Identify the location of the patent foramen ovale.

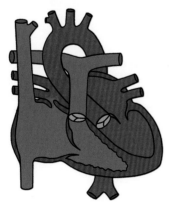

70. A patent foramen ovale, patent ductus arteriosus, and ventricular septal defect are associated defects related to transposition of the great vessels. A patent foramen ovale is the most common and is a hole between the left and right atria (upper chambers) of the heart and allows blood to flow from the right to the left atrium.

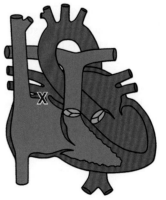

CN: Physiological integrity; CNS: Physiological adaptation; CL: Apply

71. The nurse is caring for a newborn with unre-paired transposition of the great vessels. Which medication should the nurse anticipate giving **first** for treatment of this defect?
  1. Digoxin
  2. Furosemide
  3. Enalapril
  4. Prostaglandin E1

72. A nurse is assessing an infant with unrepaired transposition of the great arteries. Identify the location of the pulmonary artery.

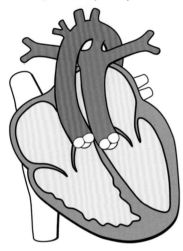

73. Which statement by the nurse **best** describes a characteristic of valvular pulmonic stenosis?
  1. One of the valve cusps is normal; the other two are not.
  2. The pulmonary artery becomes stenotic.
  3. Left ventricular hypertrophy develops.
  4. Divisions between the cusps are fused result-ing in stiffness.

71. 4. Prostaglandin E1 is necessary to maintain patency of the patent ductus arteriosus, and improve systemic arterial flow in children with inadequate intracardiac mixing. Digoxin, furo-semide, and enalapril will treat heart failure when present.
CN: Physiological integrity; CNS: Pharmacological and parenteral therapies; CL: Apply

72. Transposition of the great vessels (TGV) occurs when the pulmonary artery and the aorta are transposed. It is the most common cyanotic heart lesion during the neonatal period. In TGV, the pul-monary artery arises from the left side and carries blood, returning from the lungs, back to the lungs, and eventually to heart failure. The aorta, now arises from the right side and carries de-oxygenated blood back out to the body causing tachypnea. A patent foramen ovale, patent ductus arteriosus, and ventricular septal defect are associated defects related to transposition of the great arteries.

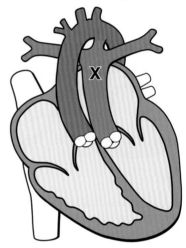

CN: Physiological integrity; CNS: Physiological adaptation; CL: Apply

73. 4. Blood flow through the valve is restricted by fusion of the divisions between the cusps. The valve may be normal or malformed. Right ven-tricular hypertrophy develops due to resistance to blood flow.
CN: Physiological integrity; CNS: Physiological adaptation; CL: Analyze

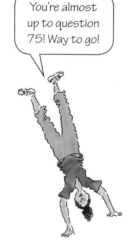

You're almost up to question 75! Way to go!

74. Which findings should the nurse anticipate during the assessment of a child with pulmonic stenosis? Select all that apply.
1. Hyperactivity
2. Normal respiratory rate
3. Systolic ejection murmur
4. Capillary refill more than two seconds
5. Normal pulse oximetry
6. Chest pain

74. 3, 4. A systolic ejection murmur, which may be accompanied by a thrill, can be heard at the upper left sternal border. The decrease in pulmonary blood flow causes fatigue and dyspnea. Systemic cyanosis may result from right ventricular failure that increases the capillary refill time. Lightheadedness, syncope and chest pain are rare even with severe obstruction.

CN: Physiological integrity; CNS: Physiological adaptation; CL: Analyze

75. Which heart defect can potentially causes a cyanotic defect from right-to-left shunting of blood?

1.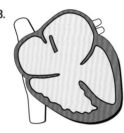
2.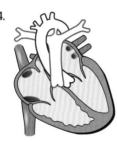
3.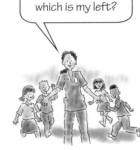
4.

Who can help me remember which is my right and which is my left?

75. 1. Pulmonary valve atresia is a rare abnormality and accounts for only 1% to 3% of cardiac defects. The pulmonary valve is atretic, and there is no exit from the right ventricle. All of the blood flows into the left atrium via the foramen ovale, and the lungs are only perfused via a very wide ductus arteriosus. The other three illustrated defects, ventricular septal defect, atrioventricular septal defect and a patent ductus arteriosus are associated with left-to-right shunting. Left-to-right shunt defects are noted as acyanotic lesions while the right-to-left shunt defects are cyanotic.

CN: Physiological integrity; CNS: Physiological adaptation; CL: Analyze

76. A nurse is caring for a 16-year-old client with aortic stenosis. Which symptoms would this teen experience during physical activity? Select all that apply.
1. Chest pain
2. Dizziness
3. Lack of endurance
4. Dusky lips and fingernail beds
5. Wheezing

76. 1, 2, 3. Children with aortic stenosis may develop chest pain similar to angina when they are active. They may also report dizziness, exercise intolerance or decreased endurance, fatigue, syncope, dyspnea, and palpitations. They do not experience symptoms of wheezing or cyanosis, such as dusky lips or mucous membranes.

CN: Physiological integrity; CNS: Physiological adaptation; CL: Apply

77. A nurse is teaching the parents of a child newly diagnosed with aortic stenosis. Which statements should the nurse include in her teaching of this disorder? Select all that apply.
1. "The aortic valve typically has three leaflets but will commonly have only two in aortic stenosis."
2. "Aortic stenosis can cause an increase in cardiac output."
3. "Your child needs to be encouraged to immediately report any chest pain or nausea and vomiting."
4. "Your child will have blue lips and nail beds as he gets older."

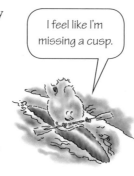

I feel like I'm missing a cusp.

77. 1, 3. Aortic stenosis is often caused by malformed cusps of the valve itself. While the valve is supposed to be tricuspid, it may only be bicuspid. Children with this defect should not participate in strenuous activity, as it can predispose them to myocardial infarction or sudden death. Chest pain or nausea and vomiting are signs of myocardial ischemia, and need to be reported immediately. There is decreased cardiac output as the left ventricle becomes hypertrophied due resistence against the stenotic valve. Children with this defect are not cyanotic, and will have pink mucous membranes.
CN: Physiological integrity; CNS: Physiological adaptation; CL: Analyze

78. What is the **most** important information for the nurse to give the parents of a child with aortic stenosis?
1. Restrict exercise
2. Avoid dental procedure
3. Avoid digoxin
4. Restrict fluid intake

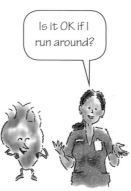

Is it OK if I run around?

78. 1. Exercise should be restricted because of low cardiac output and left ventricular failure. Strenuous activity has been reported to result in sudden death from the development of myocardial ischemia. Dental procedures are not contraindicated, and are advised. The child may need prophylactic antibiotics to prevent bacterial endocarditis. Digoxin may be needed if the child develops heart failure. Fluid restriction is not necessary unless the child develops severe heart failure.
CN: Physiological integrity; CNS: Physiological adaptation; CL: Apply

79. The nurse is planning care for a newly-admitted child with heart failure. Prioritize the nurse's interventions for this child.

| 1. Obtain vital signs, including weight |
| 2. Place child in Semi-Fowler's position |
| 3. Measure abdominal girth |
| 4. Record intake and output |
| 5. Plan play periods |
| 6. Provide skincare |

79. Ordered Response:

| 2. Place child in Semi-Fowler's position |
| 1. Obtain vital signs, including weight |
| 3. Measure abdominal girth |
| 6. Provide skincare |
| 4. Record intake and output |
| 5. Plan play periods |

Placing the child in semi fowlers will help to improve gas exchange. Obtaining vital signs are important to determine baseline status on admission and note changes. Measuring abdominal girth will help to assess fluid retention. Skin care is essential to prevent breakdown that may result from fluid retention or prolonged bedrest. Intake and output will indicate fluid balance or imbalance. Play periods will help as a diversional activity.
CN: Physiological integrity; CNS: Physiological adaptation; CL: Analyze

CN: Client needs category   CNS: Client needs subcategory   CL: Cognitive level

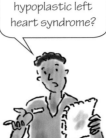

80. A nurse is providing family-centered care for a newborn diagnosed with hypoplastic left heart syndrome. What topic is **most** important to address with these parents?
1. Fears related to death
2. Delayed growth and development
3. Need for continuous oxygen
4. Inability to tolerate activity

80. 1. Without intervention, death usually occurs within the first few days of life as a result of progressive hypoxia, acidosis, and shock as the ductus closes and systemic perfusion diminishes. If the parents choose cardiac transplantation, the child may die waiting for a donor heart. For those who choose surgery, the child may not survive the three stages of the surgery. The other three choices will apply as the infant becomes older and are not the most appropriate at this time.

CN: Physiological integrity; CNS: Physiological adaptation; CL: Analyze

81. The nurse is caring for a child scheduled for a heart transplant. How should the nurse reply when the parents question the prednisone ordered by the provider?
1. It stimulates the appetite.
2. It help prevents organ rejection.
3. It decreases inflammation.
4. It decreases ventilator requirements.

81. 2. The goal of prednisone, for this client, is to suppress the immune system, thereby preventing organ rejection. Prednisone is often used in combination with other immunosuppressant medications to prevent rejection. While corticosteroids do stimulate appetite and decrease inflammation, that is not the desired effect for this child. Prednisone has been shown to decrease ventilator requirements in preterm infants. It would have limited effect on the ventilator requirements of a post-surgical transplant client.

CN: Physiological integrity; CNS: Pharmacological and parenteral therapies; CL: Apply

82. A nurse is caring for a child taking prednisone following a heart transplant. His pre-surgical weight was 25.6 lb (11.6 kg). The practitioner orders the child to receive 2 mg/kg/day divided every six hours. The oral solution comes prepared as 5 mg/5 ml. How many milliliters will the child receive with each dose? Record your answer using one decimal place.

_____ ml

82. 5.8.
Here are the calculations:

$$11.6\,kg \times 2\,mg/kg/day = 23.2\,mg/day$$
$$23.2\,mg/day \div 4\,doses/day = 5.8\,mg/dose$$
$$5\,mg/5\,ml = 1\,mg/ml$$
$$5.8\,mg/dose \times 1\,mg/ml = 5.8\,ml/dose$$

CN: Physiological integrity; CNS: Pharmacological and parenteral therapies; CL: Analyze

83. A child is given 0.5 mg/kg/day of prednisone divided into two doses. The child weighs 22 lb (10 kg). How much is given in each dose?
1. 2.5 mg
2. 5 mg
3. 10 mg
4. 1.5 mg

83. 1. The child should receive 2.5 mg/dose. Here are the calculations:

$$0.5\,mg/kg \times 10\,kg = 5\,kg$$
$$5\,mg/2\,doses = 2.5\,mg/dose$$

CN: Physiological integrity; CNS: Pharmacological and parenteral therapies; CL: Analyze

84. The nurse is caring for three-year-old client who has polycythemia. What is the **most** important intervention for the nurse to include in this child's plan of care?
1. Encouragement of fluid intake
2. Administration of analgesics
3. Sodium-restricted diet
4. Use of a soft toothbrush

84. 1. Dehydration needs to be prevented. The blood of a child with polycythemia is thicker and more viscous, which leaves it prone to thrombus development. Dehydration makes the blood even thicker, leading to increased risk of clot formation. Analgesics are good to include in the plan of care, especially if the child is experiencing pain, but they will not prevent thrombus formation. A soft toothbrush is used when the child is at risk for bleeding and will not be useful in preventing thrombus formation. A sodium-restricted diet will have no effect on clotting, and is not recommended for infants and children.
CN: Physiological integrity; CNS: Reduction of risk potential; CL: Apply

85. How would the nurse **most** accurately describe infective endocarditis?
1. It is most commonly seen in children with a history a rheumatic heart disease.
2. It is an infection of the valves and inner lining of the heart.
3. It is caused by a gram positive organism.
4. It will cause a decrease in the child's systemic oxygen saturation.

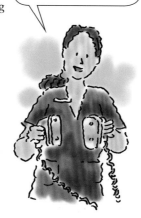

I hope you're finding these questions as stimulating as I am.

85. 2. Infective or bacterial endocarditis is an infection of the valves and inner lining of the heart. It's usually caused by the bacteria *Staphylococcus aureus*, and commonly affects children with acquired or congenital anomalies of the heart or great vessels. Occasionally a gram negative organism will be the cause. Transient bacteremia results in adherence of microbial pathogens to the injured endocardium. Bacteria may grow into adjacent tissues, break off and embolize elsewhere, such as the spleen, kidney, lung, skin, and central nervous system. A decrease in oxygen saturation may occur in children with a cyanotic heart lesion.
CN: Physiological integrity; CNS: Physiological adaptation; CL: Apply

86. A child with suspected infective endocarditis arrives at the emergency department. Which assessment findings would the nurse anticipate in this child? Select all that apply.
1. Weight gain
2. Murmur
3. Low-grade fever
4. Malaise
5. Headache

86. 2, 3, 4, 5. Symptoms may include a low-grade intermittent fever, decrease in hemoglobin level, tachycardia, anorexia, weight loss, malaise, headache, joint and muscle pain, and decreased activity level. Bacteremia leads to these signs of an infection. The murmur is due to damage to the cardiac valves or myocardium.
CN: Physiological integrity; CNS: Physiological adaptation; CL: Apply

87. The nurse is caring for a school-aged child diagnosed with hyperlipidemia. What is the **most** important information the nurse should teach the parents about their child's condition?
1. Increased activity will help decrease the risk of heart disease.
2. A fiber supplement should be used to help decrease lipid levels.
3. A statin will be prescribed to help decrease the risk of heart disease.
4. Increased fish oil will help decrease lipid levels.

87. 1. Lifestyle modification and other non-pharmacologic therapies are the most important intervention in treating high lipid levels. Fiber is thought to bind with cholesterol within bile acids, thus removing it from the enterohepatic circulation; however, fiber supplements are not recommended in children with hyperlipidemia. Omega-3 fatty acids, found in fish, may help decrease cholesterol levels, but lifestyle modification is preferred. Pharmacologic agents such as statins are not recommended until the child at least eight years old.
CN: Physiological integrity; CNS: Physiological adaptation; CL: Apply

CN: Client needs category   CNS: Client needs subcategory   CL: Cognitive level

88. Erythromycin is given to a six-year-old child before dental work to prevent endocarditis. The child weighs 44 lb (20 kg). The order is for 20 mg/kg by mouth two hours before the dental appointment. The bottle comes concentrated as 400 mg/5 ml. How many milliliters should the child receive? Record your answer using a whole number.

_____ ml

89. What adverse reaction might the nurse observe after administering enteric-coated erythromycin to a client?
1. Weight gain
2. Constipation
3. Increased appetite
4. Nausea and vomiting

90. A child is hospitalized with infective endocarditis. Which nursing intervention is **most** appropriate?
1. Increase fluids
2. Provide frequent toileting.
3. Provide diversional activities
4. Give small, frequent meals

91. Which symptoms would the nurse anticipate in a child with Kawasaki disease? Select all that apply.
1. Low-grade fever
2. Strawberry tongue
3. Desquamation of hands and feet
4. Bilateral conjunctival infection with yellow exudates
5. Irritability

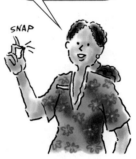

Wow! You finished question 90! The rest should be a snap!

SNAP

88. 5.
Prophylactic antibiotics prior to dental work is reserved for children with the highest risk for infective endocarditis. Here are the calculations: Determine how many milligrams to give:

$$20\,mg/kg \times 20\,kg = 400\,mg$$

Next, determine how many milliliters to give (desired/have × amount on hand = amount to administer):

$$400\,mg \div 400\,mg/5\,ml = 5\,ml$$

CN: Physiological integrity; CNS: Pharmacological and parenteral therapies; CL: Analyze

89. 4. Erythromycin is an antibiotic. Common adverse effects include nausea, vomiting, diarrhea, abdominal pain, and anorexia. It should be given with a full glass of water and after meals, or with food, to lessen gastrointestinal symptoms.

CN: Physiological integrity; CNS: Pharmacological and parenteral therapies; CL: Apply

90. 3. Treatment for infective endocarditis requires long-term hospitalization or home care and IV antibiotics. During this time children may become bored or depressed, and need age-appropriate activities. Excessive fluid volume may be seen with infective endocarditis. Gastrointestinal upset and constipation may be adverse reactions related to the antibiotics. Overeating may occur due to boredom.

CN: Physiological integrity; CNS: Physiological adaptation; CL: Analyze

91. 2, 3, 5. Characteristics of Kawasaki disease include a high fever of five or more days that is unresponsive to antibiotics and antipyretics, dry, red eyes without exudates, inflammation of the pharynx and oral mucosa, strawberry tongue, caused by sloughing of the coating of the tongue, perineal rash, desquamation of the hands and feet, arthritis, cervical lymphadenopathy, and extreme irritability. The cardiac symptoms, such as myocarditis and coronary artery aneurysms, are often subclinical, and are diagnosed with further investigation, such as echocardiogram.

CN: Physiological integrity; CNS: Physiological adaptation; CL: Apply

CN: Client needs category   CNS: Client needs subcategory   CL: Cognitive level

92. A nurse is teaching the parents of a child with Kawasaki disease. Which statement should the nurse include in her teaching?
1. It mostly occurs in the summer and fall.
2. Diagnosis can be made with laboratory testing.
3. It is an acute systemic vasculitis of unknown cause.
4. It manifests in an acute and subacute stage.

92. 3. Kawasaki disease can best be described as an acute systemic vasculitis of unknown cause. Most cases are geographic and seasonal, with most occurring in the late winter and early spring. Diagnosis is based on clinical findings of five of the six diagnostic criteria, and associated laboratory results. There is no specific laboratory test for diagnosis. There are three stages: acute, subacute, and convalescent.
CN: Physiological integrity; CNS: Physiological adaptation; CL: Apply

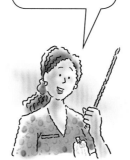

What happens during the subacute phase of this disease?

93. The nurse determines that a child with Kawasaki disease has entered the subacute phase when the assessment includes:
1. polymorphous rash.
2. normal blood values.
3. cervical lymphadenopathy.
4. desquamation of the hands and feet.

93. 4. The subacute phase shows characteristic desquamation of the hands and feet. Blood values return to normal at the end of the convalescent phase. Cervical lymphadenopathy and a polymorphous rash can be seen in the acute phase due to the onset of inflammation and fever.
CN: Physiological integrity; CNS: Physiological adaptation; CL: Analyze

94. A nurse is caring for a child with Kawasaki disease. Which symptom would be **most** concerning to the nurse?
1. Mild diarrhea
2. Pain in the joints
3. Abdominal pain with vomiting
4. Increased erythrocyte sedimentation rate (ESR)

94. 3. The most serious complication of this disease is cardiac involvement. Abdominal pain, vomiting, and restlessness are the main symptoms of an acute myocardial infarction in children. Mild diarrhea can be treated with oral fluids. Pain in the joints is an expected sign of arthritis that usually occurs in the subacute phase. An increased ESR is a reflection of the inflammatory process and may be seen for 2 to 4 weeks after the onset of symptoms.
CN: Physiological integrity; CNS: Physiological adaptation; CL: Analyze

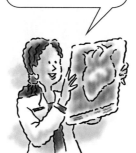

Which tests are best? Remember—select all that apply.

95. A child is undergoing testing to rule out a diagnosis of Kawasaki disease. Which test results would support this diagnosis? Select all that apply.
1. Hematuria
2. Leukocytosis
3. Thrombocytopenia
4. Decreased erythrocyte sedimentation rate
5. Elevated C-reactive protein levels

95. 2, 5. Inflammation of the small vessels, along with pancarditis, leads to an elevated leukocyte count, increased platelet count, increased erythrocyte sedimentation rate, and elevated C-reactive protein levels. Urinalysis would show proteinuria or sterile pyuria.
CN: Physiological integrity; CNS: Physiological adaptation; CL: Analyze

96. Therapy for Kawasaki disease includes a single dose of IV gamma globulin, prescribed at 2 g/kg. The child weighs 32 lb (14.5 kg). How many grams should this child receive? Record your answer using a whole number.

—————— g

96. 29.
Here is the calculation:

$$14.5 \, kg \times 2 \, g/kg = 29 \, g$$

CN: Physiological integrity; CNS: Pharmacological and parenteral therapies; CL: Analyze

97. A child is receiving IV gamma globulin for treatment of Kawasaki disease. The order is for 8 g over 12 hours. The concentration is 8 g in 300 ml of normal saline. How many milliliters per hour will this child receive? Record your answer using a whole number.

_____ ml/hr

98. A child is prescribed high-dose aspirin as part of the therapy for Kawasaki disease. The order is for 80 mg/kg/day PO in four divided doses until the child is afebrile. The child weighs 33.1 lb (15 kg). How many milligrams is given in one dose? Record your answer using a whole number.

_____ mg

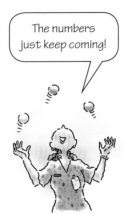

The numbers just keep coming!

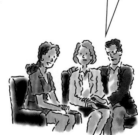

Listen for feedback to find out if your instructions were understood.

99. A nurse is giving discharge instructions to the parents of a child with Kawasaki disease. Which statement, by the parents, shows an understanding of the treatment plan?
  1. "A regular diet can be resumed at home."
  2. "Black, tarry stools are considered normal."
  3. "My child should use a soft-bristled toothbrush."
  4. "My child can return to playing soccer next week."

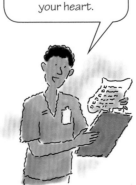

Looks like we'll be seeing you back to take another look at your heart.

100. A nurse is preparing a family for the discharge of a client with Kawasaki disease. What is the **most** appropriate information for the nurse to include?
  1. Stop the aspirin when returning home.
  2. Immunizations can be given in two weeks.
  3. The child may return to school in one week.
  4. Frequent echocardiography will be needed.

97. 25.
Use the following equation:

$$300\,ml/12\,hr = 25\,ml/hr$$

CN: Physiological integrity; CNS: Pharmacological and parenteral therapies; CL: Analyze

98. 300.
Aspirin is used for the treatment of Kawasaki disease due to its anti-inflammatory properties. The benefits of aspirin outweigh the risks in this situation. Use the following equation:
First, determine how many milligrams should be given in one day:

$$80\,mg/kg \times 15\,kg = 1,200\,mg$$

Then, determine how many milligrams should be given in one dose:

$$1,200\,mg/4\,doses = 300\,mg/dose$$

CN: Physiological integrity; CNS: Pharmacological and parenteral therapies; CL: Analyze

99. 3. Because of the anticoagulant effects of aspirin therapy, a soft-bristled toothbrush will prevent bleeding of the gums. A low-cholesterol diet should be followed until coronary artery involvement resolves. Black, tarry stools are abnormal, and are signs of bleeding that should be reported to the provider immediately. Contact sports should be avoided because of the cardiac involvement, and excessive bruising may occur as a result of aspirin therapy.
CN: Physiological integrity; CNS: Physiological adaptation; CL: Analyze

100. 4. Because of the risk of coronary artery involvement and possible aneurysm development, repeat echocardiography and electrocardiography will be required during the first few weeks and at six months. Aspirin therapy may be continued for two weeks after the onset of symptoms. If signs of coronary artery involvement are present, aspirin therapy may be continued indefinitely. Live-virus vaccines should be avoided for 6 to 11 months after gamma globulin therapy because of the increased risk of a cross-sensitivity reaction to the antibodies found in the dose given. Returning to school should be avoided until cleared by the health care provider
CN: Physiological integrity; CNS: Physiological adaptation; CL: Analyze

101. Which rash would the nurse recognize as scarlet fever?

1.

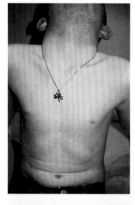

3.

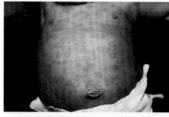

4.

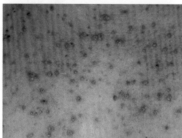

2.

102. Which assessment findings would the nurse anticipate in a child diagnosed with acute rheumatic rever? Select all that apply.
1. Aschoff bodies
2. Arthritis affecting one joint
3. High fever for five or more days
4. Nonpruritic rash
5. Murmur
6. Irregular movements of the extremities

103. What type of isolation precautions would the nurse request for a child diagnosed with group-A beta-hemolytic streptococcus?
1. Universal precautions
2. Droplet precautions
3. Contact precautions
4. Airborne precautions

104. Which manifestations are considered a major Jones criterion for acute rheumatic fever?
1. Carditis
2. Prolonged PR interval
3. Low-grade fever
4. Elevated erythrocyte sedimentation rate (ESR)

101. 1. Scarlet fever is a complication of group-A beta-hemolytic streptococcal infections. The rash of scarlet fever is a diffuse papular erythema with a sandpaper-like texture. Photo three shows erythema multiforme, which is a skin complication of group A beta-hemolytic streptococcal infections. Photo two is the rash typically associated with measles. Photo four is the rash associated with varicella.
CN: Physiological Integrity; CNS: Physiological adaptation; CL: Apply

102. 1, 4, 5, 6. Clinical manifestations associated with Rheumatic Fever include Aschoff bodies, murmur, pericardial rub, polyarthritis that moves to different joints every 1 to 2 days, erythema marginatum, subcutaneous nodules, and chorea. A low-grade fever is a minor manifestation. A high fever of five or more days may represent Kawasaki disease.
CN: Physiological integrity; CNS: Physiological adaptation; CL: Apply

103. 2. Group-A beta-hemolytic streptococcal infections are spread through droplets. Standard and contact precautions would not be sufficient to decrease transmission. Group-A beta-hemolytic streptococcal infections do not require specialized masks.
CN: Physiological integrity; CNS: Physiological adaptation; CL: Apply

I was just trying to "keep up with the Joneses."

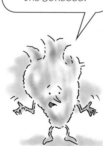

104. 1. Two major, or one major and two minor manifestations from Jones criteria, and the presence of a streptococcal infection justify the diagnosis of rheumatic fever. Carditis is a major diagnostic criteria of acute rheumatic fever. It's the only manifestation that can lead to death or long-term sequelae. Prolonged PR interval, low-grade fever, and elevated ESR are considered minor Jones diagnostic criteria.
CN: Physiological integrity; CNS: Physiological adaptation; CL: Apply

CN: Client needs category   CNS: Client needs subcategory   CL: Cognitive level

105. A nurse is caring for a child with acute rheumatic fever. Which symptom would indicate Sydenham's chorea?
1. Cardiomegaly
2. Regurgitant murmur
3. Pericardial friction rubs
4. Involuntary muscle movements

105. 4. Sydenham's chorea is an involvement of the central nervous system by the rheumatic process. This is seen as muscular incoordination, purposeless, involuntary movements, and emotional lability. A regurgitant murmur, cardiomegaly, and a pericardial friction rub are clinical signs of rheumatic carditis.
CN: Physiological integrity; CNS: Physiological adaptation; CL: Apply

106. What information is **most** important for the nurse to teach an adolescent who is beginning atorvastatin therapy for hyperlipidemia?
1. Pubertal development is not affected by statins.
2. Birth control is important when using a statin.
3. Muscle pain may occur when using a statin.
4. Headaches are a common side effect of statins.

106. 2. Statins decrease the synthesis of cholesterol therefore are contraindicated in pregnancy. Birth control should be utilized in any post-pubertal adolescent female. While the other answers are correct, answer two is the best answer.
CN: Physiological integrity; CNS: Pharmacological and parenteral therapies; CL: Analyze

107. A three-year-old child has a positive culture for a streptococcal organism. What is the **most** important discharge instruction for the nurse to give this child's parents?
1. Administer aspirin as needed for the fever
2. Keep the child home for three days
3. Administer antibiotics for the prescribed amount of time
4. Encourage the child to drink while he is awake

107. 3. Infections caused by Streptococcal organisms are treated with antibiotics. The antibiotics must be administered for the entire course of therapy, and should not be stopped when the symptoms go away. Antipyretics, such as acetaminophen, may be given for fever. Aspirin is not recommended due to the risk of Reye's syndrome. This child should be kept at home for 24 hours after the first dose. Fluid intake is encouraged to prevent dehydration from decreased oral intake due to the sore throat or diarrhea caused by the antibiotics.
CN: Physiological integrity; CNS: Physiological adaptation; CL: Analyze

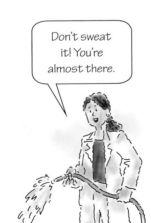

Don't sweat it! You're almost there.

108. The nurse is preparing a child for discharge after being diagnosed with rheumatic fever without carditis. What instructions should the nurse give the parents?
1. Give penicillin for signs of chorea
2. Give penicillin for one month total
3. Give penicillin if exposed to strep throat at school
4. Do not give penicillin before dental work

108. 4. Children who might benefit from prophylactic penicillin include those with unrepaired congenital heart defects, heart defects repaired with synthetic material, or prior infective endocarditis, and some children with heart transplants. Prophylactic antibiotic therapy isn't otherwise recommended.
CN: Physiological integrity; CNS: Pharmacological and parenteral therapies; CL: Apply

109. Which electrocardiogram (ECG) strip would the nurse expect to see from a child with bradycardia?

1.

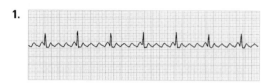

2.

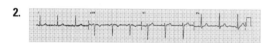

3.

4.

109. 4. Strip four shows sinus bradycardia in an ECG. Strip one shows atrial flutter. Strip two is a normal ECG tracing. Strip three shows heart block.

CN: Health promotion and maintenance; CNS: None; CL: Apply

110. A nurse is teaching the parents of a child who was diagnosed with sinus bradycardia. Which statement about the condition is the **most** correct?
1. It is a heart rate slower than normal for age.
2. It is a heart rate faster than normal for age.
3. It is a variation of the normal cardiac rhythm.
4. It is an increase in sinus node impulse formation.

110. 1. Sinus bradycardia can best be described as a heart rate slower than normal for age. Sinus tachycardia refers to a heart rate faster than normal for age or an increase in sinus node impulse formation. A sinus arrhythmia is a variation of the normal cardiac rhythm.

CN: Physiological integrity; CNS: Physiological adaptation; CL: Apply

111. For which client would sinus bradycardia be a normal finding?
1. A client with hypoxia
2. A client with hypothermia
3. Growth-delayed adolescent
4. Physically-conditioned adolescent

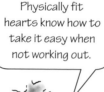

Physically fit hearts know how to take it easy when not working out.

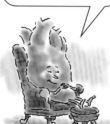

111. 4. A physically-conditioned adolescent might have a lower than normal heart rate. This is of no significance. Hypoxia and hypothermia are pathological states in which a slow heart rate may produce a compromised hemodynamic state. Growth-delayed adolescents won't have bradycardia as a normal finding.

CN: Physiological integrity; CNS: Physiological adaptation; CL: Analyze

112. Treatment for a child with symptomatic bradycardia includes atropine 0.02 mg/kg/dose. If the child weighs 44.1 lb (20 kg), how much should be given per dose?
1. 0.02 mg
2. 0.04 mg
3. 0.2 mg
4. 0.4 mg

112. 4. The child should receive 0.4 mg. Here is the calculation:

$$0.02 \, mg/kg \times 20 \, kg = 0.4 \, mg$$

CN: Physiological integrity; CNS: Pharmacological and parenteral therapies; CL: Analyze

113. Atropine is being administered to a child with sinus bradycardia. Which information is **most** accurate about the administration of this medication?
1. Increases heart rate
2. Raises blood pressure
3. Dilates bronchial tubes
4. Decreases heart rate

114. A nurse has administered atropine to an 11-month-old infant for the treatment of sinus bradycardia. The nurse would be **most** concerned if the infant displayed:
1. lethargy.
2. diarrhea.
3. no tears when crying.
4. increased urine output.

115. A child has an unrepaired heart defect resulting in a right-to-left shunt. As this child grows older, which assessment findings would the nurse anticipate? Select all that apply.
1. Cyanosis of lips and nail beds
2. Auscultation of crackles in lung fields
3. Clubbed fingers
4. Tachypnea
5. Bradycardia

116. The nurse is developing a plan of care for a child with heart failure. How should the nurse plan care for this child? Select all that apply.
1. Cluster all care
2. Weigh the child weekly
3. Maintain the child in a supine position
4. Offer small, frequent feedings
5. Maintain a cool environment

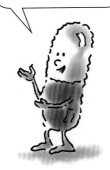

Knowing the classification of a drug can help you remember its actions.

113. 1. Atropine blocks vagal impulses to the myocardium and stimulates the cardioinhibitory center in the medulla, which increases heart rate and cardiac output. Atropine is not given to directly increase blood pressure or dilate the bronchial tubes.
CN: Physiological integrity; CNS: Pharmacological and parenteral therapies; CL: Apply

114. 3. Atropine dries up secretions and reduces the response of ciliary and iris sphincter muscles in the eye, causing mydriasis. It usually causes paradoxical excitement in children. Constipation and urinary retention can be seen due to a decrease in smooth-muscle contractions of the gastrointestinal and genitourinary tracts.
CN: Physiological integrity; CNS: Pharmacological and parenteral therapies; CL: Apply

115. 1, 3, 4. Children who have a heart defect that results in blood shunting from the right side of the heart to the left are cyanotic, and often have pulse oximeter readings in the 70% to 90% range. Clubbing is expected when long-term cyanosis is present. Children become tachypneic in an attempt to improve oxygenation. Tachycardia is the heart's attempt to increase cardiac output. Crackles are usually heard in children with defects that have increased pulmonary blood flow.
CN: Physiological integrity; CNS: Physiological adaptation; CL: Analyze

116. 1, 4. Nursing assessments and interventions should be clustered in order to allow the child opportunities to rest and conserve energy. Small, frequent feedings promote rest while giving the child ample opportunity to consume adequate calories. The child should be weighed daily with the same clothes, and the same scale. The child should be placed at a 30 to 45-degree angle to optimize chest expansion and decrease the work of breathing. Children with heart failure need a normothermic environment to conserve calories otherwise spent on thermoregulation.
CN: Physiological integrity; CNS: Physiological adaptation; CL: Apply

117. How will the Valsalva maneuver decrease cardiac workload for a child with Wolff-Parkinson-White syndrome?
1. Increasing cardiac preload
2. Decreasing cardiac preload
3. Increasing cardiac afterload
4. Decreasing cardiac afterload

118. What is the **most** important information for the nurse to communicate to the parents of a child receiving amiodarone?
1. Amiodarone can be used with antiviral medication.
2. Amiodarone can cause pulmonary toxicity.
3. Amiodarone doses should not exceed 300 mg/day.
4. Amiodarone should be given rapidly by IV means.

119. An unresponsive 41 lb (18.6 kg) child, with supraventricular tachycardia, is prescribed oral amiodarone 5 mg/kg. It comes as a solution of 150 mg/3 ml. How many milliliters should be given? Record your answer using one decimal place.

_____ ml

120. Which finding would the nurse anticipate in a one-year-old child with supraventricular tachycardia?
1. Heart rate of 100 bpm
2. Heart rate of 180 bpm
3. Heart rate of less than 80 bpm
4. Heart rate of more than 240 bpm

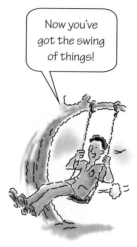

Now you've got the swing of things!

117. 2. A Valsalva maneuver is performed by applying a moderately forceful, attempted exhalation, against a closed airway. The maneuver decreases cardiac preload.
CN: Physiological integrity; CNS: Physiological adaptation; CL: Analyze

118. 2. Amiodarone has a substantial risk of toxicity, and is intended for use in clients with life-threatening arrhythmias. It should not be used with direct-acting antivirals due to the risk of severe bradycardia. Bolus doses should be given ver one hour. The maximum amount of amiodarone to be given is 300 mg/dose.
CN: Physiological integrity; CNS: Pharmacological and parenteral therapies; CL: Apply

119. 1.9.
Here are the calculations:

$$5\,mg/kg \times 18.6\,kg = 93\,mg$$

$$150\,mg \div 3\,ml = 50\,mg/ml$$

$$93\,mg \div 50\,mg/ml = 1.9\,ml$$

CN: Physiological Integrity; CNS: Pharmacological and Parenteral Therapies; CL: Apply

120. 4. Supraventricular tachycardia may be related to increased automaticity of an atrial cell other than the sinoatrial node, or as a reentry mechanism. The rhythm is regular and can occur at rates of 240/bpm or more. A heart rate of 100/bpm is a normal finding for a one-year-old child. In an older child or teenager, sinus tachycardia usually means a heart rate over 100 beats per minute. Babies and younger children have faster resting heart rates, so the criteria for sinus tachycardia is different. For a baby, sinus tachycardia is usually means a heart rate over 160-170 beats per minute. In a school age child, sinus tachycardia is usually considered a heart rate over 120 beats per minute. A heart rate of less than 80/bpm can be characterized as sinus bradycardia.
CN: Physiological integrity; CNS: Physiological adaptation; CL: Analyze

121. An 18-month-old child is experiencing supra-ventricular tachycardia (SVT). What should be the nurse's **first** intervention?
1. Administration of digoxin
2. Administration of adenosine
3. Synchronized cardioversion
4. Placement of a bag of ice over the child's face

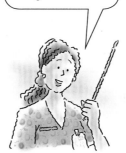

In question 121, the word first is your clue to the right answer.

121. 4. Vagal maneuvers, such as placing a bag of ice over the face for 15 to 30 seconds, or immersing the hands in cold water are commonly the first mechanism used to decrease the heart rate. Other vagal maneuvers include breath-holding, carotid massage, gagging, and placing the head lower than the rest of the body. Synchronized cardioversion may be required if vagal maneuvers and drugs are ineffective. If a child has low cardiac output, cardioversion may be used instead of drugs. Adenosine is the drug of choice for medical conversion of SVT. Verapamil isn't recommended in children under two years of age. Digoxin has a narrow therapeutic margin, has a risk of toxicity, and can delay the attainment of therapeutic levels.
CN: Physiological integrity; CNS: Reduction of risk potential; CL: Apply

122. A two-month-old infant arrives with a heart rate of 180 bpm and a temperature of 103.1° F (39.5° C) rectally. What is the **most** appropriate initial nursing intervention?
1. Give acetaminophen
2. Encourage fluid intake
3. Apply carotid massage
4. Place the infant's hands in cold water

122. 1. Acetaminophen should be given to decrease the temperature. A heart rate of 180/bpm is normal in an infant with a fever. A tepid sponge bath may be given to help decrease the temperature and calm the infant. Carotid massage, and placing the infant's hands in cold water are attempts to decrease the heart rate through vagal maneuvers. This will not work because the source of the increased heart rate is fever. Fluid intake is encouraged after the acetaminophen is given to help replace insensible fluid losses.
CN: Physiological integrity; CNS: Physiological adaptation; CL: Apply

123. A critically ill four-year-old is in the pediatric intensive care unit. Telemetry monitoring reveals junctional tachycardia. Where does this arrhythmia originate?

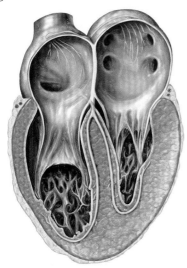

123. In junctional tachycardia, the atrioventricular node rapidly fires.

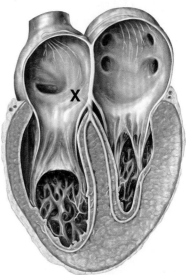

CN: Physiological integrity; CNS: Physiological adaptation; CL: Analyze

124. An infant who weighs 17.6 lb (8 kg) is to receive ampicillin 25 mg/kg IV q6h. How many milligrams should the nurse administer per dose? Record your answer using a whole number.

_____ mg

124. 200.
The nurse should calculate the correct dose using the following equation:

$$25\,mg/kg \times 8\,kg = 200\,mg$$

CN: Physiological integrity; CNS: Pharmacological and parenteral therapies; CL: Apply

125. The nurse is caring for an infant with a heart defect that involves increased pulmonary blood flow. Which illustration shows a congenital heart disorder with increased pulmonary blood flow?

1.

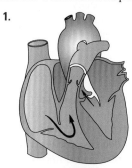

2.

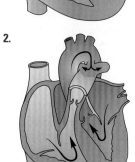

3.

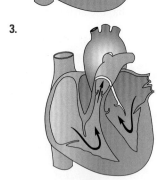

4.

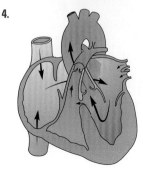

Congratulations! You've finished the test.

125. 2. In patent ductus arteriosus, an accessory fetal structure that connects the pulmonary artery to the aorta fails to close at birth. This allows blood to shunt from the aorta on the left side to the pulmonary artery on the right side. Illustration one depicts aortic stenosis, and illustration three shows pulmonic stenosis. Both disorders obstruct blood flow. Illustration four shows tricuspid atresia, a decreased pulmonary blood flow disorder.
CN: Physiological integrity; CNS: Physiological adaptation; CL: Analyze

CN: Client needs category   CNS: Client needs subcategory   CL: Cognitive level

Chapter 28

Hematologic & Immune Disorders

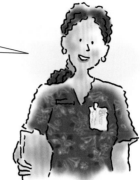

This chapter covers sickle cell disease, varicella, Rocky Mountain spotted fever, leukemia, and many other blood and immune system disorders in kids. It's a whopper of a chapter on a critically important area. If you're ready, let's begin.

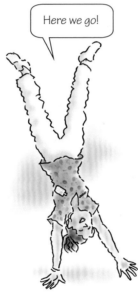

Here we go!

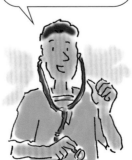

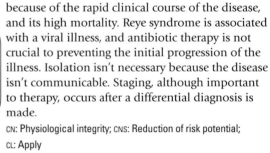

Test-taking tip: Read every question and all the options carefully before selecting your answer.

1. Which laboratory value would indicate inflammation? Select all that apply.
   1. White blood cell count: 14,000/mm³
   2. Red blood cell count: 7.1 million/mm³
   3. C-reactive protein: 5 mg/L
   4. Erythrocyte sedimentation rate: 40 mm/hr
   5. Sodium 132: mEq/L

2. Which is **most** important for successful management of the child with Reye syndrome?
   1. Early diagnosis
   2. Initiation of antibiotics
   3. Isolation of the child
   4. Staging of the illness

1. 1, 3, 4. Inflammation is an indicator of an immune response occurring within the body. There are several laboratory tests that indicate inflammation is present. An elevated white blood cell count could indicate infection or inflammation. An elevated c-reactive protein is a test for inflammation in the body. The elevated erythrocyte sedimentation rate can be used to monitor inflammatory diseases. Red blood cell counts are used to diagnose anemia and other conditions affecting red blood cells, not inflammation. Sodium is an electrolyte required by the body, but an abnormal level does not indicate inflammation.
CN: Physiological integrity; CNS: Physiological adaptation;
CL: Analyze

2. 1. Early diagnosis and therapy are essential because of the rapid clinical course of the disease, and its high mortality. Reye syndrome is associated with a viral illness, and antibiotic therapy is not crucial to preventing the initial progression of the illness. Isolation isn't necessary because the disease isn't communicable. Staging, although important to therapy, occurs after a differential diagnosis is made.
CN: Physiological integrity; CNS: Reduction of risk potential;
CL: Apply

CN: Client needs category   CNS: Client needs subcategory   CL: Cognitive level

3. A child with Reye syndrome is in stage I of the illness. Which intervention should the nurse anticipate to prevent further progression of the illness?
   1. Instituting invasive monitoring
   2. Preparing for endotracheal intubation
   3. Administering hypertonic glucose solution with insulin
   4. Administering pancuronium bromide

3.   3. For children in stage I of Reye syndrome, treatment is primarily supportive and directed toward restoring blood glucose levels and correcting acid-base imbalances. Intravenous administration of dextrose solutions with added insulin will help replace glycogen stores. Noninvasive monitoring is adequate to assess status at this stage. Endotracheal intubation may be necessary later. Pancuronium bromide is used as an adjunct to endotracheal intubation and would not be used in this stage of Reye syndrome.
CN: Physiological integrity; CNS: Reduction of risk potential; CL: Apply

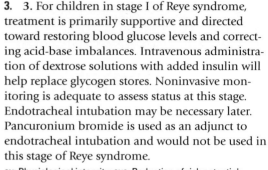

The word *establish* is a big hint.

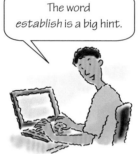

4. The nurse is reviewing lab results of a newly admitted client. Which group of laboratory results and clinical manifestations would establish a diagnosis of Reye syndrome?
   1. Elevated liver enzymes and prolonged prothrombin and partial thromboplastin times
   2. Increased serum glucose and insulin levels
   3. Increased bilirubin and alkaline phosphatase levels
   4. Decreased serum glucose and ammonia levels

4.   1. Reye syndrome causes fatty degeneration of the liver, altering results of liver function studies. Decreased serum glucose levels, with reduced insulin levels, occur secondary to dehydration caused by intractable vomiting. Serum bilirubin and alkaline phosphatase usually are not affected.
CN: Physiological integrity; CNS: Physiological adaptation; CL: Analyze

5. The nurse is caring for a client who is in the latter stages of Reye syndrome. What is the nurse's **most** important intervention to prevent or reduce cerebral edema?
   1. Noninvasive pressure and telemetry monitoring
   2. Paralysis and sedation
   3. Liberal fluid replacement
   4. Non-assisted ventilation

5.   2. Sedation is essential for client comfort when chemical paralytic medications are used. Skeletal muscles are paralyzed with the administration of pancuronium bromide. This prevents activity, especially coughing, that might increase intracranial pressure (ICP). Invasive monitoring is essential to detect increased ICP. Noninvasive pressure monitoring and telemetry may detect global changes but will not prevent edema. Liberal fluid replacement may increase cerebral edema, and should be strictly monitored. Tracheal intubation is performed as soon as possible to prevent hypoventilation and increased carbon dioxide levels.
CN: Physiological integrity; CNS: Reduction of risk potential; CL: Analyze

6. The nurse is assessing a child acutely ill with Reye syndrome. Which assessment change would the nurse be **most** concerned about?
   1. Irritability and quick pupil response
   2. Increased blood pressure and decreased heart rate
   3. Decreased blood pressure and respiratory rate
   4. Sluggish pupil response and decreased blood pressure

6.   2. A marked increase in intracranial pressure (ICP) will trigger this pressure response. Increased ICP produces an elevation in blood pressure with a reflex slowing of the heart rate. The respiratory rate will have increased variability not a decreased rate. Irritability is commonly an early sign, but pupillary response becomes more sluggish in response to increased ICP.
CN: Physiological integrity; CNS: Physiological adaptation; CL: Apply

---

CN: Client needs category   CNS: Client needs subcategory   CL: Cognitive level

7. A client with Reye syndrome is exhibiting increased intracranial pressure (ICP). Which nursing intervention would be the **most** appropriate?
1. Position the child with the head elevated and the neck in a neutral position
2. Maintain the child in the prone position
3. Cluster interventions that may be perceived as noxious
4. Position the child in the supine position, with the child's head turned to the side

8. The goal of nursing care for a client with Reye syndrome is to minimize intracranial pressure (ICP). Which nursing intervention helps to meet this goal?
1. Keeping the head of the bed flat
2. Frequently changing the client's position
3. Positioning to avoid neck flexion
4. Suctioning and chest physiotherapy

9. The nurse is caring for an unconscious child with Reye syndrome. Which nursing interventions are appropriate to prevent skin breakdown? Select all that apply.
1. Keeping the arms and legs flexed
2. Placing the child on a sheepskin
3. Applying lotions on the skin
4. Placing the client in a supine position
5. Frequent change of position

10. A parent asks the nurse if medications can cause Reye syndrome. The nurse's **most** appropriate response is that Reye syndrome has been connected to:
1. acetaminophen.
2. aspirin.
3. ibuprofen.
4. guaifenesin.

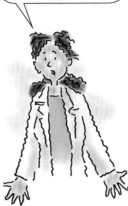

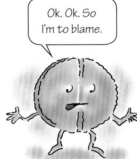

7. **1.** Positioning the child with the head elevated and neck in the neutral position will help decrease ICP. The prone and supine positions will cause increased ICP. Interventions that may be perceived as noxious should be spaced over time because, if clustered, they may have a cumulative effect in increasing ICP. Turning the head to the side may impede venous return from the head and increase ICP.
CN: Physiological integrity; CNS: Physiological adaptation; CL: Apply

8. **3.** Jugular vein compression can increase ICP by interfering with venous return. The head of the bed should be elevated to help promote venous return. Nursing procedures such as frequent repositioning tend to cause overstimulation, and can increase ICP. Suctioning and percussion are poorly tolerated and are contraindicated, unless concurrent respiratory problems are present.
CN: Physiological integrity; CNS: Physiological adaptation; CL: Apply

9. **2, 4.** Placing the child on a sheepskin will help prevent pressure on prominent areas of the body. Keeping extremities in a flexed position can lead to contractures. Rubbing the extremities with lotion stimulates circulation, and will help prevent dry skin. Placing the child supine would be contraindicated because of the risk of aspiration and increasing intracranial pressure (ICP). The supine position puts undue pressure on the sacral and occipital areas. Frequent repositioning causes added stimulation, and could lead to ICP.
CN: Physiological integrity; CNS: Physiological adaptation; CL: Apply

10. **2.** Aspirin administration is associated with the development of Reye syndrome. Acetaminophen, ibuprofen, and guaifenesin have not been associated with the development of Reye syndrome. There has been a decreased incidence of Reye syndrome with the increased use of acetaminophen and ibuprofen for management of fevers in children.
CN: Physiological integrity; CNS: Pharmacological and parenteral therapies; CL: Apply

11. The nurse should tell parents to stop administering aspirin, and notify a provider if their child is exposed to:
1. stress.
2. scabies.
3. influenza.
4. environmental allergies.

12. The nurse is caring for a client with Reye syndrome who is receiving pancuronium bromide. What is the **most** important intervention for the nurse to include in the plan of care?
1. Applying artificial tears as needed
2. Providing regular tactile stimulation
3. Performing active range-of-motion (ROM) exercises
4. Placing the client in a supine position

13. Which goal should be achieved by performing a craniotomy on a client with Reye syndrome?
1. Decreasing carbon dioxide levels
2. Determining the extent of brain injury
3. Reducing pressure from an edematous brain
4. Allowing continuous monitoring of intracranial pressure (ICP)

14. The nurse is aware that the parents of a child with Reye syndrome need a great deal of emotional support. What is the **most** important nursing intervention to support the parent's emotional needs?
1. Not accepting aggressive behavior from the parents
2. Encouraging the parents not to overreact and to hope for the best
3. Letting the parents interpret the child's behaviors and responses
4. Providing education and clarifying or reinforcing the clinical information provided

15. The nurse is planning the administration of vaccinations for a pediatric client. Prioritize the nursing interventions for this client.

1. Wash hands
2. Document the vaccination administered and site on the immunization record
3. Provide vaccine information and handout, to the parent and answer all questions
4. Assess the client for site appropriateness
5. Cleanse the site per protocol

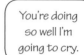

You're doing so well I'm going to cry.

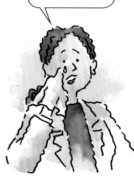

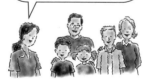

Be sensitive not only to your client's needs but also to the family's needs as well.

11. 3. A strong association exists between influenza and aspirin administration and the development of Reye syndrome. There are no contraindication with the other conditions.
CN: Physiological integrity; CNS: Pharmacological and parenteral therapies; CL: Apply

12. 1. Pancuronium bromide suppresses the corneal reflex, making the eyes prone to irritation. Artificial tears prevent drying. Tactile stimulation isn't appropriate because it may elicit a pressure response. Active ROM exercises may cause an increase in pressure. The head of the bed should be elevated slightly, with the paralyzed client in a side-lying or semi-prone position to prevent aspiration and minimize intracranial pressure.
CN: Physiological integrity; CNS: Pharmacological and parenteral therapies; CL: Apply

13. 3. In severe cases of cerebral edema, a craniotomy is most effective in decreasing ICP. Carbon dioxide levels can be decreased through mechanical ventilation. Most clients with Reye syndrome recover without any resulting brain injury. Continuous monitoring of ICP is implemented through central venous pressure lines.
CN: Physiological integrity; CNS: Reduction of risk potential; CL: Analyze

14. 4. Explaining treatments and therapies will help to alleviate undue stress on the parents. An awareness of the potential for aggressive behaviors provides the nurse with the understanding that allows them to support the parents in their concerns. Being too quick to reassure may block a parent's expression of fears. Parents may need help interpreting their child's behavior to avoid assigning erroneous meanings to the many signs their child exhibits.
CN: Psychosocial integrity; CNS: None; CL: Apply

15. Ordered Response:

3. Provide vaccine information and handout, to the parent and answer all questions.
1. Wash hands
4. Assess the client for site appropriateness
5. Cleanse the site per protocol
2. Document the vaccination administered and site on the immunization record.

CN: Safe and effective care environment; CNS: none; CL: Analyze

CN: Client needs category   CNS: Client needs subcategory   CL: Cognitive level

16. A nurse is administering an immunization to a two-month-old child. Which type of immunity will the child form?
1. Acquired immunity
2. Active immunity
3. Natural immunity
4. Passive immunity

> I'm not immune to the fact that you're doing great!

16. 2. Active immunity occurs when the individual forms immune bodies against certain diseases, either by having the disease, or by the introduction of a vaccine into the individual. Acquired immunity results from exposure to the bacteria, virus, or toxins. Natural immunity is resistance to infection or toxicity. Passive immunity is a temporary immunity caused by transfusion of immune plasma proteins.
CN: Health promotion and maintenance; CNS: None;
CL: Apply

17. A child, diagnosed with thalassemia major will typically suffer complications from the disease and from the treatment. Which potential complications should the nurse be aware of in this child?
1. Hypertrophy of the thyroid
2. Hypertrophy of the thymus
3. Polycythemia vera and thrombosis
4. Chronic hypoxia and iron overload

17. 4. In thalassemia major, increased destruction of red blood cells (RBCs) will cause anemia. RBCs also have a shortened life span. The body responds by increasing its production of RBCs, but it cannot produce enough mature cells to meet the body's demands. This process results in chronic hypoxia. Children with the disorder are given multiple transfusions of packed RBCs. The combination of excessive RBC destruction and multiple transfusions can cause too much iron to be deposited in organs and tissues. This can result in damage to the involved organs. The thymus and thyroid are not involved. Polycythemia vera refers to excessive RBC production, which can result in thrombosis.
CN: Physiological integrity; CNS: Reduction of risk potential;
CL: Analyze

18. Which treatment would the nurse anticipate for the treatment of severe aplastic anemia?
1. Liver transplantation
2. Exchange transfusion
3. Bone marrow transplantation
4. Administration of intravenous immunoglobulins

18. 3. Aplastic anemia refers to either a congenital or an acquired condition in which severe pancytopenia, and/or decrease in cellular components of the blood, occurs. Children with the condition have profound anemia, are susceptible to infections, and risk of bleeding. Transplantation of bone marrow is the treatment of choice when a suitable donor is available. Liver transplantation, exchange transfusion, and the administration of intravenous immunoglobulins are not treatments for aplastic anemia because they will not correct the cause of the anemia.
CN: Physiological integrity; CNS: Physiological adaptation;
CL: Apply

> Looks like you guys are all packed and ready to be transfused.

19. A nurse is caring for a child with sickle cell anemia. Which type of transfusion should the nurse anticipate for this child?
1. Plasma
2. Platelets
3. Whole blood
4. Packed red blood cells (RBCs)

19. 4. Packed RBCs have the plasma removed, yet maintain their oxygen carrying capabilities. These are given to children when their hemoglobin is dangerously low. Severe anemia decreases oxygen perfusion, and leads to increased sickling of cells. If enough whole blood were given to reach the desired hemoglobin level, fluid overload could occur. Platelets are given to children with low platelets, not anemia.
CN: Physiological integrity; CNS: Pharmacological and parenteral therapies; CL: Analyze

CN: Client needs category   CNS: Client needs subcategory   CL: Cognitive level

20. Which information is crucial for the nurse to understand when administering immunizations?
1. Check vaccine was store properly, and follow correct procedure for preparation
2. Monitor clients for adverse reactions for approximately one hour following administration
3. Take the vaccine out of refrigeration one hour before administration
4. Inject multiple vaccines at the same injection site

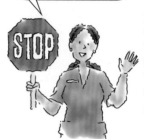
Stop and think: Which direction would be of primary importance?

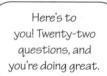

20. 1. Vaccines must be properly stored to ensure their potency. The nurse must be familiar with the manufacturer's directions for storing and reconstituting the vaccine. Faulty refrigeration is a major cause of primary vaccine failure. It is not necessary to monitor the client, but the nurse should teach parents to call the provider to report any adverse effects. If more than one vaccine is to be administered, different injection sites should be used. The nurse should note which vaccine is given, and at what site, in case of a local reaction.
CN: Health promotion and maintenance; CNS: None; CL: Apply

21. A child is admitted to the hospital with a diagnosis of severe combined immunodeficiency disease (SCID). Which symptoms should the nurse monitor during the admission interview and assessment?
1. Bruising
2. Delayed milestones
3. Prolonged bleeding
4. Indicators of current or past infections

21. 4. SCID is characterized by the absence of both humoral and cell-mediated immunity. The most common manifestation is susceptibility to infection early in life, most often by age three months. SCID is characterized by chronic infection, failure to completely recover from an infection, and frequent reinfection. The client's history will reveal no logical source for infection. Delayed milestones is a consequence of persistent illnesses. Prolonged bleeding and bruising indicate abnormalities in the clotting system.
CN: Physiological integrity; CNS: Physiological adaptation; CL: Analyze

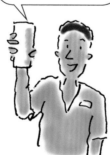
Here's to you! Twenty-two questions, and you're doing great.

22. A child is admitted to the hospital for an asthma exacerbation. The client's history reveals that she was exposed to chickenpox one week ago. The nurse would correctly assign this child to:
1. a semi-private room.
2. an isolated room.
3. an isolated room 10 days after exposure.
4. an isolated room 12 days after exposure.

22. 2. The incubation period for chickenpox is commonly 13 to 21 days. A client is commonly isolated one week after exposure to avoid the risk of an earlier breakout. A person is infectious from one day before the eruption of lesions, to six days after the vesicles have formed crusts.
CN: Safe, effective care environment; CNS: Safety and infection control; CL: Apply

23. On assessment of a child's skin, the nurse notes a papular, pruritic rash with some vesicles. The rash is profuse on the trunk and sparse on the distal limbs. Based on this assessment, which diagnosis should the nurse expect?
1. Measles
2. Mumps
3. Roseola
4. Chickenpox

23. 4. Chickenpox rash is highly pruritic. The rash begins as a macule, rapidly progresses to a papule, and then becomes a vesicle. All three stages are present in varying degrees concurrently. Measles begins as an erythematous maculopapular eruption on the face. The eruption gradually spreads downward. Mumps are not associated with a skin rash. Roseola rash is non-pruritic and is described as discrete rose-pink macules, appearing first on the trunk and then spreading to the neck, face, and extremities.
CN: Health promotion and maintenance; CNS: None; CL: Apply

24. A parent calls the school nurse to ask when her child, who has developed chickenpox, can return to school. What is the nurse's **most** appropriate response?
1. When the child is afebrile.
2. When all vesicles have dried.
3. When vesicles begin to crust over.
4. When lesions and vesicles are gone.

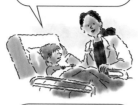

Chickenpox is highly contagious. Teach parents how to assess when it's safe to send kids back to school.

24. 2. Chickenpox is contagious. It is transmitted through direct contact, droplet spread, and contact with contaminated objects. Vesicles can break open and spread the disease until they have dried. It is not necessary to wait until dried lesions have disappeared. Some vesicles may be crusted over, and new ones may have formed. Macules, papules, vesicles, and crusting are present in varying degrees concurrently. A child may be free from fever, but continue to have vesicles. Isolation is usually necessary only for about one week after the onset of the disease.
CN: Health promotion and maintenance; CNS: None; CL: Analyze

25. A parent calls the clinic to ask about the clinical manifestations associated with roseola. What is the nurse's **best** response?
1. Apparent sickness, fever, and rash
2. Fever for 3 to 4 days, followed by rash
3. Rash, without history of fever or illness
4. Rash for 3 to 4 days, followed by a high fever

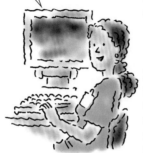

Read each question carefully and don't do anything rash.

25. 2. Roseola is manifested by a persistent high fever for 3 to 4 days in a child who otherwise appears healthy. Fever precedes the rash. When the rash appears, a precipitous drop in fever occurs, and body temperature returns to normal.
CN: Health promotion and maintenance; CNS: None; CL: Analyze

26. The nurse is assessing a child with suspected roseola. Which finding would inform the nurse that this child has a roseola rash?
1. Diffuse pustules
2. Macular and pruritic, with papules and vesicles
3. Rose-pink macules that fade on pressure
4. A red, maculopapular eruption, that begins on the face

26. 3. Roseola rashes are discrete, rose-pink macules or maculopapules that fade on pressure and usually last one to two days. Maculopapular red spots may indicate fifth disease. Chickenpox rash is macular, with papules and vesicles. Roseola is not pruritic. Measles begin as a maculopapular eruption on the face. Pustules are elevated lesions that contain pus, and are not found with roseola.
CN: Health promotion and maintenance; CNS: None; CL: Apply

27. A parent asks the nurse if it is appropriate to allow his child to scratch the chickenpox on her abdomen. The nurse should explain that allowing the child to scratch the chickenpox puts her at risk for:
1. myocarditis.
2. neuritis.
3. obstructive laryngitis.
4. secondary bacterial infection.

27. 4. Secondary bacterial infections can occur as a complication of chickenpox. Irritation of skin lesions can lead to cellulitis or even an abscess. Myocarditis is not considered a complication of chickenpox but has been noted as a complication of mumps. Neuritis has been associated with diphtheria. Obstructive laryngitis occurs as a complication of measles.
CN: Physiological integrity; CNS: Reduction of risk potential; CL: Apply

28. A child with suspected pertussis is admitted to the hospital. The nurse would anticipate a cough associated with pertussis to be:
1. loose and occur throughout the day.
2. loose and nonproductive.
3. frequent throughout the day.
4. harsh with a high-pitched crowing sound.

28. 4. The cough associated with pertussis is a harsh series of short, rapid coughs, followed by a sudden inspiration, and a high-pitched crowing sound. Cheeks become flushed or cyanotic, eyes bulge, and the tongue protrudes. Paroxysm may continue until a thick mucus plug is dislodged. This cough occurs most commonly at night.
CN: Physiological integrity; CNS: Physiological adaptation; CL: Apply

CN: Client needs category   CNS: Client needs subcategory   CL: Cognitive level

29. A preschool teacher has just found out she is pregnant. She asks the school nurse if there are any communicable diseases she could contract from her students that would harm her unborn child. What is the nurse's **most** appropriate response?

1. Pertussis
2. Roseola
3. Rubella
4. Scarlet fever

30. Which medication would the nurse anticipate as the provider's treatment of choice for scarlet fever?

1. Acyclovir
2. Amphotericin B
3. Prednisone
4. Penicillin

31. A school-age child has been diagnosed with scarlet fever. Several parents have called the school and voiced concern over the risk of their children becoming infected. The parents are requesting that the infected child be isolated for one month. It is **most** appropriate for the nurse to tell parents that respiratory isolation of an infected child is necessary until:

1. the associated rash disappears.
2. completion of antibiotic therapy.
3. the client is fever-free for 72 hours.
4. 24 hours after initiation of treatment.

32. Which instruction should the nurse include when teaching parents about the care of a child with chickenpox?

1. Administer penicillin or erythromycin as ordered
2. Administer local or systemic antipruritics as ordered
3. Offer periods of interaction with other children to provide distraction
4. Avoid administering varicella-zoster immune globulin to children receiving long-term salicylate therapy

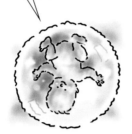

Think before you respond: Can I contract any of these?

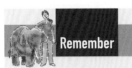

Remember

"Acyclovir assaults herpes simplex virus."

Acyclovir, a synthetic nucleoside antiviral drug, is used to treat severe herpes simplex virus type 2 infections and other herpes-related infections.

29. 3. Rubella (German measles) has a teratogenic effect on the fetus. An infected child must be isolated from pregnant women. Pertussis, roseola, and scarlet fever do not have teratogenic effects on a fetus.
CN: Safe, effective care environment; CNS: Safety and infection control; CL: Apply

30. 4. The causative agent of scarlet fever is Group A beta-hemolytic streptococci, which is susceptible to penicillin. Erythromycin is used for penicillin-sensitive children. Anti-inflammatory drugs, such as prednisone, are not indicated for these clients. Acyclovir is used in the treatment of herpes infections. Amphotericin B is used to treat fungal infections.
CN: Physiological integrity; CNS: Pharmacological and parenteral therapies; CL: Apply

31. 4. A child requires respiratory isolation until 24 hours after initiation of treatment. A rash may persist for three weeks. It is not necessary to wait until the end of treatment. Fever usually breaks 24 hours after therapy has begun. Isolating the child for 72 hours is not necessary.
CN: Safe, effective care environment; CNS: Safety and infection control; CL: Apply

32. 2. Chickenpox is highly pruritic. Preventing the child from scratching is necessary to prevent scarring and secondary infection caused by irritation of the lesions. Penicillin and erythromycin are not usually used in the treatment of chickenpox. Interaction with other children would be contraindicated because of the risk of communication, unless the other children have previously had chickenpox, or have been immunized. Varicella-zoster immune globulin should be administered to exposed children who are on long-term aspirin therapy for its anti-inflammatory or antiplatelet effects, because of the possible risk of developing Reye's syndrome.
CN: Physiological integrity; CNS: Pharmacological and parenteral therapies; CL: Apply

33. A child is admitted with scarlet fever. Which causative agent does the nurse identify as a contributor to this infection?
1. Roseola
2. Staphylococcal parotitis
3. Streptococcal pharyngitis
4. Chickenpox

34. A mother infected with HIV inquires about the possibility of breastfeeding her newborn. What is the nurse's **most** appropriate response?
1. "Breastfeeding is not the best choice in this situation."
2. "Breastfeeding would be best for your baby."
3. "Breastfeeding is only an option if the mother is taking zidovudine."
4. "Breastfeeding is an option if milk is expressed and fed by a bottle."

35. Which assessment finding helps diagnose HIV in children?
1. Excessive weight gain
2. Arrhythmia
3. Intermittent diarrhea
4. Tolerance of feedings

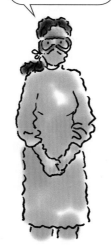

In which body fluids has HIV been isolated?

36. Which approach should be included in the diagnostic workup for a 12-month-old infant suspected of having AIDS?
1. Sputum culture
2. Genetic testing prior to HIV testing
3. Parental counseling prior to testing
4. HIV enzyme-linked immunosorbent assay (ELISA)

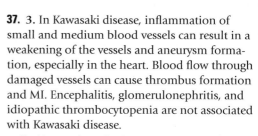

Which approach should the nurse include in the diagnostic workup?

37. The parents of a child with Kawasaki disease should be taught the importance of keeping follow-up appointments to monitor and prevent:
1. encephalitis.
2. glomerulonephritis.
3. myocardial infarction (MI).
4. idiopathic thrombocytopenia.

33. 3. The causative agent of scarlet fever is Group A beta-hemolytic streptococci. Scarlet fever may follow a strep throat infection which is caused by the same bacteria. Roseola, parotitis, and chickenpox are not strep infections and don't contribute to scarlet fever.
CN: Physiological integrity; CNS: Reduction of risk potential; CL: Apply

34. 1. Mothers infected with HIV are unable to breastfeed because HIV has been isolated in breast milk, and could be transmitted to the infant. Taking zidovudine does not prevent transmission. The risk of breastfeeding isn't associated with direct contact with the breast, but with the possibility of the virus contained in the breast milk.
CN: Health promotion and maintenance; CNS: None; CL: Apply

35. 3. A differential diagnosis may be based on the presence of an underlying cellular immunodeficiency-related disease. Symptoms can include intermittent episodes of diarrhea, repeated respiratory infections, and the inability to tolerate feedings. Poor weight gain and failure to thrive are objective assessment findings that result from intolerance of feedings and frequent infections. Arrhythmia is not associated with HIV.
CN: Physiological integrity; CNS: Physiological adaptation; CL: Analyze

36. 3. Before testing, parents should be counseled regarding the disease, the reasons for the tests, confidentiality, and the benefits of early treatment. Sputum culture might help diagnose an upper respiratory infection associated with AIDS but isn't a diagnostic test for AIDS itself. Genetic testing is not indicated. ELISA isn't used diagnostically for children younger than 18 months because of the maternal antibodies in the child's blood.
CN: Psychosocial integrity; CNS: None; CL: Apply

37. 3. In Kawasaki disease, inflammation of small and medium blood vessels can result in a weakening of the vessels and aneurysm formation, especially in the heart. Blood flow through damaged vessels can cause thrombus formation and MI. Encephalitis, glomerulonephritis, and idiopathic thrombocytopenia are not associated with Kawasaki disease.
CN: Health promotion and maintenance; CNS: None; CL: Apply

38. The nurse has just admitted a client with sickle cell crisis. What is the nurse's **priority** intervention?
1. Giving blood transfusions
2. Giving antibiotics and analgesics
3. Increasing fluid intake and giving analgesics
4. Preparing the client for a splenectomy

38. 3. The primary therapy for sickle cell crisis is to increase fluid intake according to age and to give analgesics. Blood transfusions are given conservatively to avoid iron overload. Antibiotics are given to clients with fever. Routine splenectomy is controversial, and not recommended.
CN: Physiological integrity; CNS: Physiological adaptation; CL: Apply

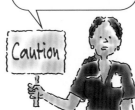

39. The nurse is assessing a client in the emergency department suspected of being in vaso-occlusive crisis. Which assessment findings would indicate that the client is having a vaso-occlusive crisis of an extremity?
1. Hypotension and thready pulse
2. Central pallor and poor capillary refill
3. Anemia, jaundice, and reticulocytosis
4. Acute leg pain and hand-foot syndrome

39. 4. Vaso-occlusive crises are the result of sickled cells obstructing the blood vessels. The major symptoms are fever, acute pain from visceral hypoxia, hand-foot syndrome, and arthralgia. A precipitous drop in blood volume is indicative of a splenic sequestration crisis, and is exhibited by hypotension and a thready pulse. Aplastic crisis exhibits pallor and poor capillary refill and may result in symptoms of shock. Hyperhemolytic crisis is characterized by anemia, jaundice, and reticulocytosis, and may also produce symptoms of shock.
CN: Physiological integrity; CNS: Physiological adaptation; CL: Analyze

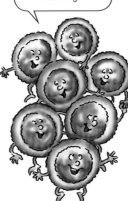

40. A child has tested positive for sickle cell trait. The parent is requesting information on this condition. What is the nurse's **most** appropriate response?
1. "Your child has sickle cell disease."
2. "Your child is a carrier of the disorder but doesn't have sickle cell disease."
3. "Your child is a carrier of the disease and will pass the disease to all offspring."
4. "Your child doesn't currently have the disease, but may show evidence as he gets older."

40. 2. A child with sickle cell trait is only a carrier and may never show any symptoms, except under special hypoxic conditions. A child with sickle cell trait doesn't have the disease and will never test positive for sickle cell anemia. Sickle cell disease would be transmitted to offspring only as the result of a union between two individuals who are positive for the trait. If both parents have sickle cell trait, there is a 25% (1 in 4) chance that any child of theirs will have sickle cell disease. There is the same 25% (1 in 4) chance that the child will not have sickle cell disease or sickle cell trait.
CN: Health promotion and maintenance; CNS: None; CL: Apply

41. The nurse is preparing a treatment plan for a child with sickle cell anemia in vaso-occlusive crisis. What is the **most** important nursing intervention to include?
1. Managing pain
2. Providing a cool environment
3. Immobilizing the affected part
4. Restricting fluids

41. 1. Pain management is an important aspect in the care of a client with sickle cell anemia in vaso-occlusive crisis. The goal is to prevent sickling. This can be accomplished by promoting tissue oxygenation, hydration, and rest, which minimizes energy expenditure and oxygen utilization. A cool environment can cause vasoconstriction, more sickling and pain. Immobilization can promote stasis and increase sickling.
CN: Physiological integrity; CNS: Basic care and comfort; CL: Analyze

42. A nurse is being observed by a group of student nurses while assessing a child in vaso-occlusive crisis. A student asks the nurse why she didn't palpate the child's abdomen. What is the nurse's **most** appropriate response?
1. Risk of splenic rupture
2. Risk of inducing vomiting
3. Increased abdominal pain
4. Risk of blood cell destruction

42. 1. Palpating a child's abdomen in vaso-occlusive crisis should be avoided because sequestered red blood cells may precipitate splenic rupture. Abdominal pain alone would not be a reason to avoid palpation. Vomiting or blood cell destruction would not occur from palpation of the abdomen.

CN: Physiological integrity; CNS: Reduction of risk potential; CL: Apply

43. The nurse is reviewing the interventions listed in the plan of care for a child in vaso-occlusive crisis. Which intervention should the nurse implement **first**?
1. Administering analgesics
2. Monitoring fluid intake
3. Encouraging activity as tolerated
4. Administering antibiotics as prescribed

43. 1. Pain management is a priority intervention when a client is in crisis. Analgesics are used to control pain. Hydration is essential to promote hemodilution and maintain electrolyte balance. Bed rest should be promoted to reduce oxygen utilization. Antibiotics will not be effective in resolving the vaso-occlusive crisis.

CN: Physiological integrity; CNS: Reduction of risk potential; CL: Apply

44. The nurse is providing postoperative care to a client with sickle cell anemia. What is the **most** important intervention for the nurse to include in the plan of care?
1. Increasing fluids
2. Preparing the child psychologically
3. Discouraging coughing
4. Limiting the use of analgesics

44. 1. The main surgical risk of anesthesia is hypoxia. Emotional stress, demands of wound healing, and the potential for infection can each increase the sickling phenomenon. Increased fluids are encouraged because hydration promotes hemodilution, and decreases sickling. Preparing the child psychologically to decrease fear will minimize undue emotional stress, but is not a priority. Deep coughing is encouraged to promote pulmonary hygiene and prevent respiratory tract infection. Analgesics are used to control wound pain and to prevent abdominal splinting and decreased ventilation.

CN: Physiological integrity; CNS: Reduction of risk potential; CL: Apply

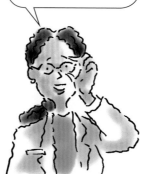

Look carefully at the words *most appropriate*. They will help you find the right answer.

45. The parents of a child with sickle cell anemia ask the nurse what they can do to prevent a sickle cell infection in the future. What is the nurse's **most** appropriate response?
1. Provide adequate nutrition
2. Avoid emotional stress
3. Visit the provider when sick
4. Avoid strenuous physical exertion

45. 1. The nurse should stress adequate nutrition. Avoiding strenuous physical exertion and emotional stress are important aspects to prevent sickling, but adequate nutrition remains a priority. Visiting the provider when sick does not prevent infection.

CN: Health promotion and maintenance; CNS: None; CL: Apply

46. Which assessment finding would indicate vaso-occlusive crisis in a child with sickle cell anemia?
1. Painful urination
2. Pain with ambulation
3. Complaints of throat pain
4. Fever with associated rash

46. 2. Bone pain is one of the major symptoms of vaso-occlusive crisis in clients with sickle cell anemia. Hand-foot syndrome, characterized by edematous painful extremities, is usually exhibited in the refusal of the child to bear weight and ambulate. Painful urination does not occur, but sickle cell anemia can cause kidney abnormalities. Throat pain is not a symptom of vaso-occlusive crisis. Fever commonly accompanies vaso-occlusive crisis but isn't associated with rash.
CN: Physiological integrity; CNS: Physiological adaptation; CL: Analyze

47. The nurse is assessing a child with sickle cell anemia. Which bone-related complication would the nurse be alert for during assessment?
1. Arthritis
2. Osteoporosis
3. Osteogenic sarcoma
4. Spontaneous fractures

47. 2. Sickle cell anemia causes hyperplasia and congestion of the bone marrow, resulting in osteoporosis. Arthritis doesn't occur secondary to sickle cell anemia; however, a crisis can cause localized swelling of joints, resulting in arthralgia. Bones do become weakened, but spontaneous fractures do not occur as a result. Osteogenic sarcoma is bone cancer. Sickle cell anemia isn't a contributing factor to bone cancer.
CN: Physiological integrity; CNS: Physiological adaptation; CL: Apply

48. What role does the nurse play in counseling parents who have a child diagnosed with sickle cell anemia, and who want to have additional children?
1. Encourage selective birth methods or abortion
2. Refer the parents for counseling
3. Encourage the parents to consider a surrogate
4. Reinforcing the idea that transmission is unlikely in subsequent pregnancies

48. 2. The nurse can be instrumental in referring parents for genetic counseling. Genetic counseling should be provided by a medical specialist who has been trained in genetic counseling for hemoglobinopathies. The nurse should not influence alternative birth methods or abortion or surrogacy. These actions are outside the scope of practice. The risk of transmission in subsequent pregnancies remains the same.
CN: Health promotion and maintenance; CNS: None; CL: Apply

49. A child is admitted for sickle cell crisis. Which nursing intervention would be the **priority**?
1. Gathering information about the child's ability to cope with this condition
2. Monitoring the child's temperature, heart rate and blood pressure every two hours
3. Providing adequate oxygenation, hydration, and pain management
4. Making sure the family is involved in every step of the child's care

49. 3. The most critical need of a client in sickle cell crisis is to provide adequate oxygenation, hydration, and pain management until the crisis passes. Obtaining a temperature every two hours would not be the priority intervention. While assessing the client's ability to cope and involving the family in the child's care are important, they are not the priority interventions during a sickle cell crisis.
CN: Safe, effective care environment; CNS: Management of care; CL: Analyze

50. A nurse is administering a blood transfusion to a client with sickle cell anemia. Which assessment findings would indicate that the client is having a transfusion reaction?
1. Diaphoresis and hot flashes
2. Urticaria, flushing, and wheezing
3. Fever, urticaria, and red raised rash
4. Fever, disorientation, and abdominal pain

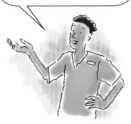

One wrong part of an option makes the entire option wrong.

50. 2. Allergic reactions may occur when the recipient reacts to allergens in the donor's blood. This reaction causes urticaria, flushing, and wheezing. A febrile reaction can occur, causing fever and urticaria, but it isn't accompanied by rash. Diaphoresis, hot flashes, disorientation, and abdominal pain are not symptoms of a transfusion reaction.
CN: Physiological integrity; CNS: Reduction of risk potential; CL: Analyze

51. A mother brings her five-year-old child to the clinic and asks the nurse how often a child should receive the influenza virus vaccine. Which response would be the **most** accurate?
1. Once a year
2. Twice a year
3. It is contraindicated in children
4. Only with the outbreak of illness

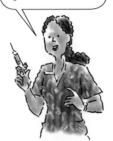

Okay, little fellow. Time for your flu vaccine.

51. 1. The influenza virus vaccine is usually administered once a year. The vaccine isn't contraindicated in children but is targeted at clients with chronic cardiac, pulmonary, hematologic, and neurological problems. The vaccine is given to prevent the onset of illness before an outbreak occurs.
CN: Health promotion and maintenance; CNS: None; CL: Apply

52. The three-year-old sister of a neonate is diagnosed with pertussis. The mother was immunized for pertussis as a child. What information should the nurse provide to the mother about transmitting pertussis to her neonate?
1. The baby will inevitably contract pertussis.
2. Immune globulin is effective in protecting the infant.
3. The risk to the infant depends on the mother's immune status.
4. Erythromycin should be administered prophylactically to the infant.

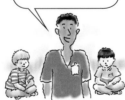

Prevention is commonly the best medicine!

52. 4. In exposed, high-risk individuals, erythromycin may be effective in preventing or lessening the severity of the disease if administered during the preparoxysmal stage. Immune globulin isn't indicated because it's used as an immunization against hepatitis A. Neonates exposed to pertussis are at considerable risk for infections, regardless of the mother's immune status; however, infection is not inevitable.
CN: Health promotion and maintenance; CNS: None; CL: Apply

53. A child has recently been admitted to the pediatric unit with laboratory values indicating an increase in hemoglobin A2. Based on these lab results, the nurse should expect to follow a care plan based on:
1. beta-thalassemia trait.
2. iron deficiency.
3. lead poisoning.
4. sickle cell anemia.

53. 1. The concentration of hemoglobin A2 is increased with beta-thalassemia trait. In severe iron deficiency, hemoglobin A2 may be decreased. The hemoglobin A2 level is normal in lead poisoning and sickle cell anemia.
CN: Physiological integrity; CNS: Reduction of risk potential; CL: Apply

54. A four-year-old child has a petechial rash bilaterally on the lower legs, with no other symptoms. The platelet count is 20,000/ml, the hemoglobin level 13 g/dl and white blood cell count is 8,000/mm³. Which diagnosis is **most** likely?
1. Acute lymphoblastic leukemia (ALL)
2. Disseminated intravascular coagulation (DIC)
3. Idiopathic thrombocytopenic purpura (ITP)
4. Systemic lupus erythematosus (SLE)

54. 3. The onset of ITP typically occurs between ages one and six years. Clients have no symptoms, except for a petechial rash, which typically presents on the lower extremities. ALL occurs when the bone marrow produces a large number of immature lymphoblasts. ALL is associated with a low platelet count, and hemoglobin levels. DIC is secondary to a severe underlying disease. SLE would be rare in a four-year-old child.
CN: Physiological integrity; CNS: Physiological adaptation; CL: Analyze

55. A newborn has been diagnosed with sickle cell anemia. Which instructions should be included in the nurse's discharge teaching for the parents?
1. Importance of iron supplementation
2. Importance of monthly vitamin B$_{12}$ injections
3. Signs of abdominal pain in infants, and demonstration of how to take a temperature
4. Information on immunizations that are contraindicated

55. 3. Acute splenic sequestration is a serious complication of sickle cell anemia. Early detection of splenomegaly by parents is an important aspect of client management. Parents should be able to take the temperature and identify abdominal pain. A temperature of 101.3° F to 102.2° F (38.5° C to 39° C) calls for emergency evaluation, even if the child appears well. Folic acid requirement is increased, and supplementation may be indicated. Vitamin B$_{12}$ supplementation and iron supplementation aren't necessary. Parents should be encouraged to keep immunizations up to date.
CN: Health promotion and maintenance; CNS: None; CL: Apply

56. Which finding would indicate a poor prognosis for a child with leukemia?
1. Presence of a mediastinal mass
2. Increased platelets
3. Normal white blood cell (WBC) count at diagnosis
4. Disease presents between ages 2 and 10 years

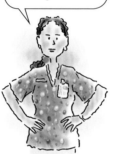

Question 56 asks about a prognosis, not a diagnosis.

56. 1. The presence of a mediastinal mass indicates a poor prognosis for children with leukemia. The prognosis is worse if age at onset is younger than 2 years, or older than 10 years. A WBC count of 100,000/ml or higher also indicate a poor prognosis for a child with leukemia. Platelet levels may be decreased with pancytopenia. An increase would not indicate a poor prognosis.
CN: Physiological integrity; CNS: Physiological adaptation; CL: Analyze

57. A one-year-old boy is in the pediatrician's office for an examination. He is pale, in the 75th percentile for weight, and the 25th percentile for length. His physical examination is normal, but his hematocrit is 24%. Which question should the nurse ask to establish a diagnosis of anemia?
1. "Is the child on any medications?"
2. "What is the child's usual daily diet?"
3. "Did the child receive phototherapy for jaundice?"
4. "What's the pattern and appearance of bowel movements?"

57. 2. Iron-deficient anemia is the most common nutritional deficiency in children between 9 and 15 months. Anemia in a one-year-old child is mostly nutritional in origin, and its cause will be suggested by a detailed nutritional history. None of the other choices would be helpful in diagnosing anemia.
CN: Health promotion and maintenance; CNS: None; CL: Analyze

58. A nurse is providing teaching to the parents of a four-year-old child newly diagnosed with Hodgkin's disease. Which statement should the nurse include in her teaching?
1. Staging laparotomy is mandatory for every client.
2. Excessive weight gain can be a symptom.
3. Hodgkin's disease is rare before five years of age.
4. Incidence of Hodgkin's disease peaks between ages 11 and 15 years.

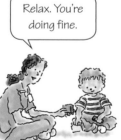

Relax. You're doing fine.

58. 3. Hodgkin's disease is rare before five years of age. Staging laparotomy is not recommended for clients who have obvious intra-abdominal disease. Systemic symptoms of Hodgkin's disease include fever, night sweats, malaise, weight loss, and pruritus. The peak incidence of Hodgkin's disease occurs in late adolescence and young adulthood (ages 15 to 34 years).
CN: Physiological integrity; CNS: Physiological adaptation; CL: Analyze

59. The nurse is caring for a child with perinatally acquired AIDS. The nurse is aware that children usually demonstrate symptoms of AIDS:
   1. within the first month of life.
   2. at 1 to 3 months of age.
   3. at 18 to 24 months of age.
   4. at 3 to 5 years of age.

59. 3. The majority of children with perinatally transmitted AIDS appear normal in early infancy. Symptoms usually develop at 18 to 24 months of age.
CN: Physiological integrity; CNS: Physiological adaptation; CL: Apply

60. Which factors can place adolescent girls at risk for iron deficiency anemia? Select all that apply.
   1. Menses
   2. Vegetarian diet
   3. Weight-loss diets
   4. Participation in sports
   5. Poverty

I can help with iron deficiency anemia.

60. 1, 2, 3, 5. All of the options place adolescent girls, who are still growing, at risk for iron deficiency anemia. That's because these girls lose blood monthly with menstrual periods, and they typically consume inadequate amounts of nutrients because of their eating patterns. Hurried meals, vegetarian diets, and weight-loss diets can also be a contributing factor. Poverty also increases the risk of iron deficiency anemia because of the inability to purchase meats and other iron-rich foods. Participation in sports would not increase the risk of iron deficiency anemia.
CN: Health promotion and maintenance; CNS: None; CL: Analyze

61. Which treatment would be **most** appropriate for a child diagnosed with iron deficiency anemia?
   1. Blood transfusion
   2. Oral ferrous sulfate
   3. An iron-fortified cereal
   4. Intramuscular iron dextran

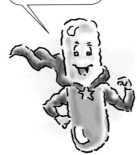

Remember

"Hematinic drugs help hoist hemoglobin levels."

Hematinic drugs, including iron, help the body produce red blood cells by increasing levels of hemoglobin in the blood to treat anemia. Iron preparations include the following:
- Ferrous fumarate
- Ferrous gluconate
- Ferrous sulfate
- Iron dextran
- Iron sucrose
- Leucovorin calcium
- Sodium ferric gluconate complex

61. 2. A prompt rise in hemoglobin level and hematocrit follows the administration of oral ferrous sulfate. Blood transfusion is rarely indicated unless a child becomes symptomatic or is further compromised by a superimposed infection. Dietary modifications are appropriate long-term measures, but they won't make enough iron available to replenish iron stores. Intramuscular dextran is reserved for situations in which compliance can't be otherwise achieved. It is expensive, painful, and no more effective than oral iron.
CN: Physiological integrity; CNS: Physiological adaptation; CL: Apply

62. A child is admitted to the hospital with flu-like symptoms. Diagnostic testing reveals that the IgM antibody parvovirus B19 is present. Which condition would the nurse suspect as a result of this finding?
   1. Roseola
   2. Fifth disease
   3. Varicella
   4. Mumps

62. 2. Fifth disease is known to be caused by human parvovirus B19. Roseola is thought to be caused by the human herpes virus six. Varicella is caused by the varicella-zoster virus. Mumps is caused by the paramyxovirus.
CN: Physiological integrity; CNS: Reduction of risk potential; CL: Apply

63. A six-year-old child has been diagnosed with Rocky Mountain spotted fever. The nurse would be correct when she teaches the parent's that this disease is caused by a bite from a:
1. cat.
2. mosquito.
3. spider.
4. tick.

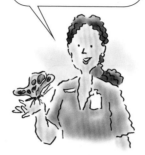

You, my friend, are doing extraordinarily well. Keep up the good work!

63. 4. Rocky Mountain spotted fever is caused by *Rickettsia rickettsii*, which is transmitted by the bite of a tick. Mosquito, spider, and cat bites haven't been known to transmit *R. rickettsii*.
CN: Safe, effective care environment; CNS: Safety and infection control; CL: Apply

64. The parents of an eight-month-old child with iron deficiency anemia have not been compliant with the administration of oral iron supplements. The child must now receive an iron dextran injection. How should the nurse administer this injection?
1. Intradermally
2. Subcutaneously
3. Intravenous
4. Intramuscularly using the z-track method

64. 4. If iron dextran is ordered, it must be injected deep into a large muscle mass, using the z-track method to minimize skin staining and irritation. Neither a subcutaneous nor an intradermal injection would inject the dextran into muscle. The z-track method is preferred over a normal intramuscular injection. Intravenous is not appropriate for this scenario.
CN: Physiological integrity; CNS: Pharmacological and parenteral therapies; CL: Apply

65. The nurse has provided dietary instruction to a client in an attempt to prevent nutritional anemia. The nurse determines teaching has been successful when the client selects:
1. an orange.
2. shrimp.
3. spinach.
4. milk.

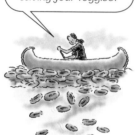

No signs of anemia here. You must have been eating your veggies!

65. 3. Green vegetables are good sources of iron. Citrus foods are not sources of iron, but help with absorption. Fish is not a good source of dietary iron. Milk is deficient in iron, and should be limited in cases of nutritional anemia.
CN: Physiological integrity; CNS: Basic care and comfort; CL: Apply

66. Liquid oral iron supplements have been prescribed for a child. What is the **most** important information for the nurse to provide to this child's parents?
1. Give the supplements with food
2. Stop the medication if vomiting occurs
3. Decrease the dose if constipation occurs
4. Give the medicine via a dropper or through a straw

66. 4. Liquid iron preparations may temporarily stain the teeth. The drug should be given by dropper or through a straw. Iron supplements should be given between meals, when the presence of free hydrochloric acid is greatest. If vomiting occurs, supplementation should not be stopped, but it should be administered with food. Constipation can be decreased by increasing intake of fruits and vegetables.
CN: Physiological integrity; CNS: Pharmacological and parenteral therapies; CL: Apply

67. Which symptom is the **primary** clinical manifestation of hemophilia?
1. Petechiae
2. Prolonged bleeding
3. Decreased clotting time
4. Decreased white blood cell (WBC) count

67. 2. The effect of hemophilia is prolonged bleeding, anywhere from, or within, the body. With severe deficiencies, hemorrhage can occur as a result of minor trauma. Petechiae are uncommon in persons with hemophilia because repair of small hemorrhages depends on platelet function, not on blood clotting mechanisms. Clotting time is increased in a client with hemophilia. A decrease in WBCs is not indicative of hemophilia.
CN: Physiological integrity; CNS: Physiological adaptation; CL: Analyze

CN: Client needs category   CNS: Client needs subcategory   CL: Cognitive level

68. The nurse should be alert to signs and symptoms of internal bleeding in those with hemophilia. From which site does a client with hemophilia **most** commonly bleed?
1. Brain tissue
2. Gastrointestinal tract
3. Joint cavities
4. Spinal cord

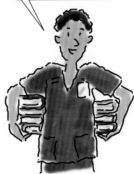

Careful! All of these answers may be accurate, but this question is asking for the *most* common site.

69. The nurse is teaching the parents of a child with hemophilia about the immediate treatment for bleeding. The nurse determines that teaching has been effective when the parents state:
1. "Apply heat to the area."
2. "Withhold factor replacement."
3. "Apply pressure for at least five minutes."
4. "Immobilize and elevate the affected area."

70. Prompt treatment for a two-year-old child with hemophilia, who sustained a joint injury, is essential. Where can this toddler **best** be treated?
1. At home
2. At a clinic
3. In a hospital unit
4. In the emergency department

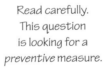

Read carefully. This question is looking for a *preventive* measure.

71. Which nursing measure can prevent the crippling effects of joint degeneration caused by hemophilia?
1. Avoiding the use of analgesics
2. Using aspirin for pain relief
3. Administering replacement factor
4. Using active range-of-motion (ROM) exercises

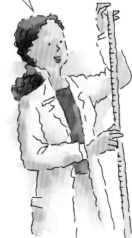

72. The nurse understands that one difference between hemophilia and von Willebrand's disease is where the bleeding tends to occur. From where would the nurse expect a client with von Willebrand's disease to bleed?
1. Brain tissue
2. Gastrointestinal tract
3. Mucous membranes
4. Spinal cord

68. 3. The joint cavities, especially the knees, ankles, and elbows, are the most common site of internal bleeding. This bleeding typically results in bone changes and can cause crippling, disabling deformities. Intracranial hemorrhage is less common because the brain tissue has a high concentration of thromboplastin. Hemorrhage along the gastrointestinal tract and spinal cord can occur but is not common.
CN: Physiological integrity; CNS: Physiological adaptation; CL: Apply

69. 4. Elevating the area above the level of the heart will decrease blood flow. Cold, not heat, should be applied to promote vasoconstriction. Factor replacement should not be delayed. Pressure should be applied to the area for at least 10 to 15 minutes to allow clot formation.
CN: Physiological integrity; CNS: Physiological adaptation; CL: Apply

70. 1. Parents can learn at-home venipuncture techniques to deliver prompt treatment, and prevent joint injury after the child reaches two to three years of age. The child may be transfused on a regular basis to prevent bleeding, and will be given additional doses of the missing factor when an injury occurs. By mid- to late-school age, children can learn to administer their own treatment.
CN: Physiological integrity; CNS: Reduction of risk potential; CL: Apply

71. 3. Prevention of bleeding is the goal, and is achieved by factor replacement therapy. Active ROM exercises are contraindicated after a bleeding episode because the joint capsule can be stretched, causing bleeding. Acetaminophen should be used for pain relief because aspirin has anticoagulant effects. Analgesics should be administered before physical therapy to control pain and provide the maximum benefit.
CN: Physiological integrity; CNS: Physiological adaptation; CL: Apply

72. 3. The most characteristic clinical feature of von Willebrand's disease is an increased tendency to bleed from mucous membranes, which may be seen as frequent nosebleeds or menorrhagia. In hemophilia, the joint cavities are the most common site of internal bleeding. Bleeding into the gastrointestinal tract, spinal cord, and brain tissue can occur, but these are not the most common sites for bleeding.
CN: Physiological integrity; CNS: Physiological adaptation; CL: Apply

CN: Client needs category   CNS: Client needs subcategory   CL: Cognitive level

73. What is the **priority** nursing measure for a client with von Willebrand's disease who is having epistaxis?
1. Lay the client supine
2. Avoid packing the nostrils
3. Avoid pressure to the nose
4. Apply pressure to the nose

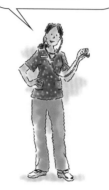

Epistaxis is a term from early in your program. Remember?

73. 4. Applying pressure to the nose may stop the bleeding because most bleeds occur in the anterior part of the nasal septum. Mouth breathing should be encouraged until the bleeding is under control. The child should be instructed to sit up and lean forward to avoid aspiration of blood. Packing with tissue or cotton may be used to help stop bleeding if applying pressure is unsuccessful, but care must be taken while removing packing to avoid dislodging the clot. Pressure should be maintained for at least 10 minutes to allow clotting to occur.
CN: Physiological integrity; CNS: Physiological adaptation; CL: Apply

74. A nurse is providing teaching to the parents of a child with acute lymphoblastic leukemia. The parents ask for information about long-term outcome. The nurse tells the parents that the three most crucial prognostic factors are:
1. histologic type of disease, initial platelet count, and type of treatment.
2. type of treatment, stage at diagnosis, and child's age at diagnosis.
3. the histologic type of disease, initial white blood cell (WBC) count, and client's age at diagnosis.
4. the progression of the illness, WBC count at time of diagnosis, and client's age at diagnosis.

74. 3. Histologic type of leukemia is the factor whose prognostic value is considered to be of greatest significance in determining long-range outcome. Children with a normal or low WBC count appear to have a much better prognosis than those with a high WBC count. Children diagnosed between the ages of 2 and 10 years have consistently demonstrated a better prognosis than those diagnosed before age 2, or after age 10.
CN: Physiological integrity; CNS: Physiological adaptation; CL: Analyze

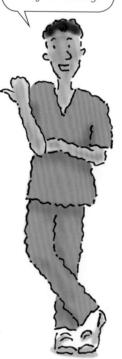

You're already at number 75? Super! You're really something!

75. What are the three main consequences of leukemia?
1. Bone deformities, spherocytosis, and infection
2. Anemia, infection, and bleeding tendencies
3. Lymphocytopoiesis, growth delays, and hirsutism
4. Polycythemia, decreased clotting time, and infection

75. 2. Anemia, caused by decreased erythrocyte production, infection secondary to neutropenia, and bleeding tendencies, from decreased platelet production are the three main consequences of leukemia. Bone deformities don't occur with leukemia, although bones may become painful because of the proliferation of cells in the bone marrow. Spherocytosis refers to erythrocytes taking on a spheroid shape, and is not a feature of leukemia. Lymphocytopoiesis is the production of lymphocytes with leukemia. Mature cells aren't produced in adequate numbers. Hirsutism and growth delay can be a result from large doses of steroids, but aren't common in leukemia. Anemia, not polycythemia, occurs. Clotting times would be prolonged.
CN: Physiological integrity; CNS: Physiological adaptation; CL: Apply

76. A child is seen in the pediatrician's office for reports of bone and joint pain. What other assessment finding by the nurse would indicate that this child may have leukemia?
1. Abdominal pain
2. Increased activity level
3. Increased appetite
4. Petechiae

76. 4. The most common signs and symptoms of leukemia are a result of infiltration of the bone marrow. These include fever, pallor, fatigue, anorexia, and petechiae, along with bone and joint pain. Abdominal pain may be caused by areas of inflammation from normal flora within the GI tract or any number of other causes. Increased appetite can occur, but it usually isn't a presenting symptom.
CN: Physiological integrity; CNS: Physiological adaptation; CL: Apply

77. The nurse is assessing a client with leukemia. What assessment findings may indicate that the cancer has invaded the brain?
1. Headache and vomiting
2. Restlessness and tachycardia
3. Hypervigilant and anxious behavior
4. Increased heart rate and decreased blood pressure

77. 1. The usual effect of leukemic infiltration of the brain is increased intracranial pressure. The proliferation of cells interferes with the flow of cerebrospinal fluid in the subarachnoid space and at the base of the brain. The increased fluid pressure causes dilation of the ventricles, which creates symptoms of severe headache, vomiting, irritability, lethargy, increased blood pressure, decreased heart rate, and, eventually, coma. Children with a variety of illnesses are typically hypervigilant and anxious when hospitalized.
CN: Physiological integrity; CNS: Physiological adaptation; CL: Analyze

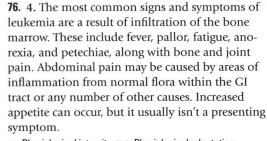

Don't worry. It looks like you're going to be just fine.

78. A student nurse asks the nurse on the hematology unit which type of leukemia has the best prognosis. Which response by the nurse would be the **most** accurate?
1. Acute lymphoblastic leukemia
2. Acute myelogenous leukemia
3. Basophilic leukemia
4. Eosinophilic leukemia

78. 1. Acute lymphoblastic leukemia, which accounts for more than 80% of all childhood cases, carries the best prognosis. Acute myelogenous leukemia, with several subtypes, accounts for most of the other leukemias affecting children. Basophilic and eosinophilic leukemia are named for the specific cells involved. These are much rarer and carry a poorer prognosis.
CN: Physiological integrity; CNS: Physiological adaptation; CL: Apply

79. The nurse is preparing an adolescent client, diagnosed with leukemia, for a lumbar puncture. The nurse determines that the client understands the reason for the procedure when the client states that the procedure is done to:
1. make sure I don't have meningitis today.
2. decrease my intracranial pressure (ICP).
3. find out what kind of leukemia I have.
4. see if the leukemia has spread to my brain.

79. 4. A lumbar puncture is performed to assess for CNS infiltration. It can be done to rule out meningitis, but is not why this test is being done. It would not be done to decrease ICP, nor does it aid in the classification of the leukemia. Lumbar punctures can result in brain stem herniation in cases of increased ICP.
CN: Physiological integrity; CNS: Physiological adaptation; CL: Apply

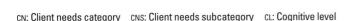

80. The nurse is reviewing the treatment plan for a child recently diagnosed with leukemia. The child is being evaluated for treatment with chemotherapy. Which test does the nurse anticipate before chemotherapy is started?
1. Lumbar puncture
2. Liver function studies
3. Complete blood count (CBC)
4. Peripheral blood smear

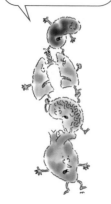

Think back to basic physiology. Which organs metabolize drugs?

80. 2. Liver and kidney function studies are done before initiation of chemotherapy to evaluate the child's ability to metabolize the chemotherapeutic agents. A lumbar puncture is performed to assess for central nervous system infiltration. A CBC is performed to assess for anemia and white blood cell count. A peripheral blood smear is done to assess the maturity and morphology of red blood cells.
CN: Physiological integrity; CNS: Pharmacological and parenteral therapies; CL: Apply

81. A child with pauciarticular juvenile rheumatoid arthritis (JRA) is required to have an eye exam. Which statement, by the nurse, most accurately explains why this exam should take place?
1. Detached retinas are commonly associated with pauciarticular JRA.
2. Painless iritis is commonly seen with pauciarticular JRA.
3. Glaucoma is commonly seen with pauciarticular JRA.
4. Strabismus is commonly seen pauciarticular JRA.

81. 2. Painless iritis may be found in 75% of children with pauciarticular JRA. If it is not detected, and goes untreated, permanent scarring in the anterior chamber of the eye may occur, and vision may be lost. Children should have an annual slit lamp examination by an ophthalmologist. Detached retinas, glaucoma, and strabismus are not commonly associated with the disease.
CN: Health promotion and maintenance; CNS: None; CL: Apply

82. Which medication would the nurse expect the provider to prescribe as prophylaxis against *Pneumocystis carinii* pneumonia for a client with leukemia?
1. Co-trimoxazole
2. Oral nystatin suspension
3. Prednisone
4. Vincristine

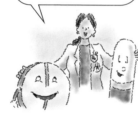

Here's a prescription for the drug of choice. Do you know which one it is?

82. 1. The most common cause of death from leukemia is overwhelming infection. *P. carinii* infection is lethal to a child with leukemia. As prophylaxis against *P. carinii* pneumonia, continuous low dosages of co-trimoxazole are typically prescribed. Oral nystatin suspension would be indicated for the treatment of thrush. Prednisone isn't an antibiotic, and increases susceptibility to infection. Vincristine is an antineoplastic agent.
CN: Physiological integrity; CNS: Pharmacological and parenteral therapies; CL: Apply

83. A four-year-old child is diagnosed as having acute lymphocytic leukemia. The white blood cell (WBC) count, especially the neutrophil count, is low. What is the **most** important intervention the nurse should teach the parents?
1. Protect your child from falls because of his increased risk of bleeding
2. Protect your child from infections because his resistance to infection is decreased
3. Provide rest periods because the oxygen-carrying capacity of your child's blood is diminished
4. Treat constipation, which frequently accompanies a decrease in WBC

83. 2. One of the complications of both acute lymphocytic leukemia and its treatment is a decreased WBC count, especially a decreased absolute neutrophil count. Because neutrophils are the body's first line of defense against infection, the child must be protected from infection. Bleeding is a risk factor if platelets or other coagulation factors are decreased. A decreased hemoglobin level, hematocrit, or both would reduce the oxygen-carrying capacity of the child's blood. Constipation is not related to the WBC count.
CN: Safe, effective care environment; CNS: Safety and infection control; CL: Apply

84. A child with leukemia has been exposed to chickenpox. The child's mother calls the health care provider's office and asks the nurse if her child needs to have anything done. What is the nurse's **most** appropriate response?
1. No treatment is indicated.
2. Acyclovir should be started on exposure.
3. Varicella-zoster immune globulin (VZIG) should be given with evidence of the disease.
4. VZIG should be given within 72 hours of exposure.

85. The client tells the nurse that she frequently experiences nausea and vomiting after receiving radiation and chemotherapy. The nurse adapts the plan of care to include antiemetics. What is the **most** appropriate time for the administration of the medication?
1. Thirty minutes before therapy begins
2. At the same time as therapy
3. Immediately after nausea begins
4. When therapy is completed

86. A child is admitted to the pediatric unit with an unknown mass in her lower left abdomen. Which is the nurse's **priority** action?
1. Obtain the history of the illness
2. Place a "do not palpate abdomen" sign over the child's bed
3. Obtain a complete set of vital signs
4. Schedule a hemoglobin and hematocrit test for early morning

87. Which nursing measure is helpful when mouth ulcers develop as an adverse effect of chemotherapy?
1. Using lemon glycerin swabs
2. Administering milk of magnesia
3. Providing a bland, moist, soft diet
4. Frequently washing the mouth with a hydrogen peroxide solution

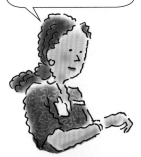

Sometimes, timing is everything!

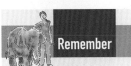
Remember

"Antiemetics arrest nausea and vomiting."

Antiemetic drugs decrease nausea, reducing the urge to vomit. Antiemetic drugs include the following classes and drugs:

Antihistamines
• Cyclizine hydrochloride
• Dimenhydrinate
• Diphenhydramine hydrochloride
• Hydroxyzine
• Meclizine
• Trimethobenzamide

Phenothiazines
• Chlorpromazine
• Perphenazine
• Prochlorperazine
• Promethazine

Serotonin 5-HT₃ Receptor Antagonists
• Dolasetron
• Granisetron
• Ondansetron

84. 4. Varicella is a lethal organism to a child with leukemia. VZIG, given within 72 hours, may favorably alter the course of the disease. Giving the vaccine at the onset of symptoms wouldn't likely decrease the severity of the illness. Acyclovir may be given if the child develops the disease, but not at the time of exposure.
CN: Health promotion and maintenance; CNS: None; CL: Analyze

85. 1. Antiemetics are most beneficial if given before the onset of nausea and vomiting. To calculate the optimum time for administration, the first dose is given 30 minutes to one hour before nausea is expected, and then every two, four, or six hours for approximately 24 hours after chemotherapy. If the antiemetic was given with the medication, or after the medication, it could lose its maximum effectiveness when needed.
CN: Physiological integrity; CNS: Pharmacological and parenteral therapies; CL: Apply

86. 2. The nurse must take measures to prevent palpation of the mass, if possible. If the mass is a malignant tumor, a "do-not-palpate" warning will help prevent trauma and rupture of the suspected tumor capsule. Rupture may cause seeding of cancer cells throughout the abdomen. Obtaining the history, vital signs, and scheduling laboratory work, are important, but not the priority.
CN: Physiological integrity; CNS: Physiological adaptation; CL: Analyze

87. 3. Oral ulcers are red, eroded, and painful. Providing a bland, moist, soft diet will make chewing and swallowing less painful. The use of lemon glycerin swabs and milk of magnesia should be avoided. Glycerin, a trihydric alcohol, absorbs water and dries the membranes. Milk of magnesia also has a drying effect because unabsorbed magnesium salts exert an osmotic pressure on tissue fluids. Frequent mouthwashes without alcohol are indicated. Peroxide should not be used because it is irritating to tissues.
CN: Physiological integrity; CNS: Basic care and comfort; CL: Apply

88. A child undergoing chemotherapy is clinically dehydrated. The provider orders a 200 ml of IV fluid to be administered over 2 hours. The drop factor is 20. At what flow rate should the pump be set? Record your answer as a whole number.

_____ gtts/min

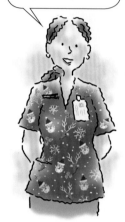

These questions are tough! Hang in there!

88. 33.

$$\frac{Volume\,(ml)}{Time\,(min)} \times Drop\ factor\,(gtts/ml)$$
$$= X\,(Flow\ rate\ in\ gtts/min)$$

$$X = \frac{200\ ml}{120\ min} \times 20\,\frac{gtts}{ml} = 33\,gtts/min$$

CN: Physiological integrity; CNS: Pharmacological and parenteral therapies; CL: Apply

89. The nurse is providing discharge instructions for a client who is receiving chemotherapeutic medications. Which intervention is **most** important to prevent hemorrhagic cystitis?
1. Administering antacids
2. Administering antibiotics
3. Increasing calcium intake
4. Increasing fluid intake

89. 4. Sterile hemorrhagic cystitis is an adverse effect of chemical irritation of the bladder from cyclophosphamide. It can be prevented by liberal fluid intake (at least one-and-a-half times the recommended daily fluid requirement). Antibiotics do not aid in the prevention of sterile hemorrhagic cystitis. Increasing calcium intake does not alter the risk of developing cystitis. Antacids would not be indicated for treatment.

CN: Physiological integrity; CNS: Reduction of risk potential; CL: Apply

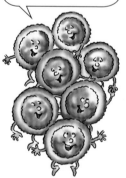

Do you remember what aspirin does to us?

90. The parents of a child diagnosed with leukemia have stated that they'll give aspirin to their child for pain relief. What is the nurse's **most** appropriate response?
1. Aspirin is contraindicated because it decreases red blood cell production.
2. Aspirin is contraindicated because it promotes bleeding tendencies.
3. Aspirin is not a strong enough analgesic.
4. Aspirin decreases the effects of methotrexate.

90. 2. Aspirin would be contraindicated because it promotes bleeding. Aspirin use has also been associated with Reye syndrome in children. For home use, acetaminophen is recommended for mild to moderate pain. Aspirin enhances the effects of methotrexate, and has no effect on red blood cell production. Non-opioid analgesia has been effective for mild to moderate pain in clients with leukemia.

CN: Physiological integrity; CNS: Pharmacological and parenteral therapies; CL: Apply

91. A nine-year-old child has been diagnosed with cancer and is scheduled for chemotherapy. The parents ask the nurse how they should explain the side effect of hair loss to the child. What is the nurse's **best** response?
1. Introduce the idea of a wig after hair loss occurs
2. Explain that hair typically begins to regrow in six to nine months
3. Stress that hair loss during a second treatment with the same medication will be more severe
4. Explain that, as hair thins, keeping it clean and short may camouflage partial baldness

91. 4. The nurse must prepare the parents and child for possible hair loss. Cutting the hair short lessens the impact of seeing large quantities of hair on bed linens and clothing. Sometimes, keeping the hair in a short full style can make a wig unnecessary. Hair usually regrows in six months, depending on the treatment protocol. The child should be encouraged to pick out a wig similar to his own hair color and style before the hair falls out to ease the adjustment to hair loss. Hair loss during a second treatment with the same medication is usually less severe.

CN: Psychosocial integrity; CNS: None; CL: Apply

92. A nurse is discussing childhood cancer with the parents of a child in an oncology unit. Which statement, by the nurse, would be the **most** accurate?
   1. The most common site for children's cancer is the bone marrow.
   2. All childhood cancers have a high mortality rate.
   3. Children with leukemia have a higher survival rate if they're older than 11 years when diagnosed.
   4. The prognosis for children with cancer is not affected by treatment strategies.

92. 1. Childhood cancers occur most commonly in rapidly growing tissue, especially in the bone marrow. Mortality depends on the time of diagnosis, the type of cancer, and the age at which the child was diagnosed. Children who are diagnosed between the ages of two and nine consistently demonstrate a better prognosis. Treatment strategies are tailored to produce the most favorable prognosis.
CN: Physiological integrity; CNS: Physiological adaptation; CL: Apply

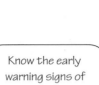
Know the early warning signs of childhood cancer.

93. Which condition, assessed by the nurse, would be an early indicator of childhood cancer?
   1. Difficult swallowing
   2. Nagging cough or hoarseness
   3. Increased appetite
   4. Swellings, lumps, or masses anywhere on the body

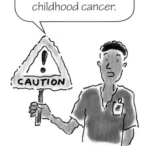

93. 4. By being aware of early signs of childhood cancer, nurses can refer children for further evaluation. Swellings, lumps, or masses anywhere on the body are early warning signals of childhood cancer. Difficulty swallowing, cough, and hoarseness are early signs of cancer in adults. Increased appetite does not occur as an early sign.
CN: Health promotion and maintenance; CNS: None; CL: Apply

94. Which nursing intervention would help to decrease the adverse effects of radiation therapy on the gastrointestinal tract?
   1. Avoiding the use of antispasmodics
   2. Encouraging fluids and a soft diet
   3. Giving antiemetics when vomiting occurs
   4. Avoiding mouthwashes to prevent irritation of mouth ulcers

94. 2. Radiation therapy can cause adverse effects such as nausea and vomiting, anorexia, mucosal ulceration, and diarrhea. Antispasmodics are used to help reduce diarrhea. Encouraging fluids and a soft diet will help with anorexia. Antiemetics should be given before the onset of vomiting. Frequent mouthwashes are indicated to prevent mycosis.
CN: Physiological integrity; CNS: Physiological adaptation; CL: Apply

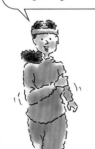
Don't stop now! You're doing a great job!

95. Short-term steroid therapy is used in clients with leukemia to:
   1. increased appetite.
   2. altered body image.
   3. increased platelet production.
   4. decreased susceptibility to infection.

95. 1. Short-term steroid therapy produces no acute toxicities, and results in increased appetite and a sense of well-being. Physical changes caused by steroid use can prompt alterations in body image that can be extremely distressing to children. Prednisone (steroid therapy) has no effect on platelet production, but may increase susceptibility to infection.
CN: Physiological integrity; CNS: Pharmacological and parenteral therapies; CL: Apply

96. Teaching children and parents about the potential adverse effects of treatment for leukemia is important. What is an adverse effect of taking prednisone?
   1. Decreased appetite
   2. Increased blood glucose
   3. Decreased risk of infection
   4. Decreased hair growth

96. 2. Prednisone may cause an increase in blood glucose requiring doses of insulin, especially when other factors are involved. Increased appetite, increased risk of infection, and increased hair growth are also adverse effects of prednisone.
CN: Physiological integrity; CNS: Pharmacological and parenteral therapies; CL: Apply

CN: Client needs category   CNS: Client needs subcategory   CL: Cognitive level

97. Which nursing intervention is a **priority** for a child with hemophilia, who has fallen, and has an acutely bruised leg?
1. Appropriate dose of aspirin and rest
2. Immobilization of the leg and a dose of ibuprofen
3. Heating pad and administration of factor VIII concentrate
4. Pressure on the site and administration of the required clotting factor

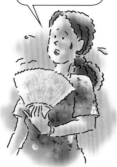

The pressure is really on to prioritize.

97. 4. With any bleeding injury in a client with hemophilia, the first line of treatment is always to replace the clotting factor. Pressure is applied along with cool compresses, and the extremity is immobilized. Aspirin is not used because of its anticoagulant properties and the risk of Reye's syndrome in children. Immobilizing the leg and giving ibuprofen would be done after applying pressure and administering the necessary clotting factor. Heat is not used because it increases bleeding.
CN: Safe, effective care environment; CNS: Management of care; CL: Apply

98. When teaching an adolescent with iron deficiency anemia about diet choices, which menu selection would indicate that more instruction is necessary?
1. Caesar salad and pretzels
2. Cheeseburger with milkshake
3. Red beans and rice with sausage
4. Egg sandwich and snack peanuts

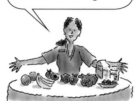

Good diet choices are important for clients of all ages.

98. 1. Caesar salad and pretzels are not high in iron or protein. Meats, including organ meats, eggs, and nuts have high protein and iron.
CN: Physiological integrity; CNS: Basic care and comfort; CL: Analyze

99. The mother of a child diagnosed with leukemia wants to know why her child is susceptible to infection even though he has too many white blood cells (WBCs). Which response, by the nurse, would be **most** accurate?
1. This is an adverse effect of the medication he has to take.
2. He hasn't been able to eat a proper diet since he's been sick.
3. Leukemia is a problem of tumors in the internal organs that decrease his ability to fight infection.
4. Leukemia causes production of too many immature WBCs, which can't fight infection very well.

99. 4. Leukemia is an unrestricted proliferation of immature WBCs, which do not function properly, and are a poor defense against infection. Diet contributes to overall health but does not cause the overproduction of WBCs. There are no solid tumors in the internal organs caused by leukemia. Medications such as chemotherapy can diminish the immune system's effectiveness; however, they don't cause the overproduction of immature WBCs, and the poor resistance to infection, that the mother asked about.
CN: Physiological integrity; CNS: Physiological adaptation; CL: Apply

100. A nurse is developing a teaching plan for the parents of a toddler who was just diagnosed with sickle cell disease. Which statement is important to emphasize in the teaching plan?
1. Other children in the family will also have sickle cell anemia.
2. Knowing how to prevent vaso-occlusive crisis is an important part of the parent's role.
3. The child will have a greater tendency to bleed, and should avoid contact sports.
4. Vaso-occlusive crisis will happen frequently.

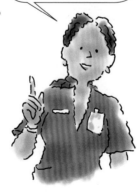

Prevention is the key to avoid pain.

100. 2. It is important to teach the family of a child with sickle cell anemia that prevention is the key. The nurse should emphasize avoidance of dehydration, hypoxia, high altitudes, and cold. These interventions can dramatically reduce the incidence of vaso-occlusive crisis. The disease is autosomal recessive, so each pregnancy has a one-in-four chance of the child having the disease, a one-in-four chance of not having the disease, and a two-in-four chance of carrying the trait. Abnormal bleeding, and the need to avoid contact sports, are associated with hemophilia.
CN: Health promotion and maintenance; CNS: None; CL: Apply

101. A grandmother calls the pediatric clinic to find out whether her three-year-old grandson can get shingles from her. Which response, by the nurse, would be **most** appropriate?
   1. "No, shingles don't occur in small children."
   2. "Yes, the grandson can get shingles from her. Shingles are caused by the herpes zoster virus."
   3. "The grandson could develop shingles if the lesions are on exposed skin areas and are weeping."
   4. "No, but the grandson would be exposed to the varicella-zoster virus, which could lead to the development of chickenpox."

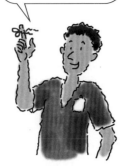

Do you remember that other disease that's caused by the virus that causes shingles?

101. 4. Shingles occur when a dormant varicella-zoster virus in a nerve becomes inflamed. The vesicles of shingles contain the virus and would expose others to it. The grandson could not develop shingles from such exposure. A herpes virus doesn't cause shingles. Shingles can occur in children but only if they have previously had chickenpox. The impetus for the inflammation is internal, not external.
CN: Safe, effective care environment; CNS: Safety and infection control; CL: Analyze

102. A child with idiopathic thrombocytopenic purpura is admitted to the hospital with a platelet count of 20,000/∝l. The nurse is aware that the child should be closely monitored for:
   1. hyperactivity.
   2. proteinuria.
   3. hand-foot syndrome.
   4. a change in level of consciousness (LOC).

102. 4. When the platelet count drops to 20,000/∝l, the child is at risk for spontaneous bleeding, including intracranially. A change in LOC is an important sign of increased intracranial pressure. This child is likely to become somnolent and difficult to arouse, not hyperactive. Proteinuria is more common in glomerulonephritis. With blood in the urine, protein also increases, but this is not the primary concern. Hand-foot syndrome occurs in a child with sickle cell disease.
CN: Physiological integrity; CNS: Reduction of risk potential; CL: Analyze

103. The nurse is caring for a one-month-old infant with signs of increased intracranial pressure (ICP). The nurse is aware that intervention will be necessary if the infant displays:
   1. bulging fontanels, a high-pitched cry, and vomiting.
   2. frequent crying, sunken fontanel, and a pulse rate above 120 bpm.
   3. blood-tinged vomitus, legs flexed to the abdomen, and frequent crying.
   4. somnolence during feeding, a pulse rate above 120 bpm when fussing, and irregular arm and leg movements

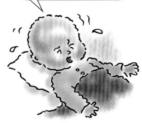

I can't tell you what's wrong, so look for the signs.

103. 1. Because fontanels haven't closed by the age of one month, they bulge with increasing ICP. A high-pitched cry and vomiting also signal increased ICP. Quality of the cry is an important sign in an infant. Vomiting should be distinguished from a small amount of formula regurgitation, which is normal. Frequent crying may result from various stressors, and quality of the cry should be assessed. Blood-tinged vomitus, flexed legs, and crying indicate an abdominal disorder and pain. Infants normally have irregular arm and leg movements. A pulse rate of 120 bpm is normal for a one-month-old infant at rest.
CN: Physiological integrity; CNS: Reduction of risk potential; CL: Analyze

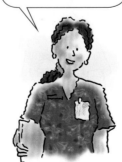

Let's see. Which activity should be restricted?

104. The nurse has just completed discharge teaching for the family of a school-age child with idiopathic thrombocytopenia. The nurse determines that teaching was effective when the family identifies which activity should be restricted?
   1. Swimming
   2. Bicycle riding
   3. Computer games
   4. Exposure to large crowds

104. 2. When routine blood counts reveal the platelet level is 100,000/∝l or less, the child should not engage in contact sports, bicycle riding, climbing, or other activities that could lead to injury. Swimming releases energy, builds muscle, and allows the child to compete without risking injury, as long as she follows normal safety precautions. Computer games do not cause physical injury. There is no need to avoid large crowds because idiopathic thrombocytopenia does not suppress the immune system.
CN: Safe, effective care environment; CNS: Safety and infection control; CL: Apply

CN: Client needs category   CNS: Client needs subcategory   CL: Cognitive level

105. A 17-year-old boy with classic hemophilia (hemophilia A) is admitted to the hospital for surgery. His preoperative preparation should include:
1. bed rest.
2. transfusion of clotting factor VIII.
3. intravenous analgesics given around the clock.
4. hydration at 50% above the normal fluid requirement.

105. 2. In classic hemophilia or hemophilia A, clotting factor VIII is deficient. This factor must be transfused before surgery, and at intervals afterward, to prevent bleeding during and after surgery. Analgesics would be indicated if the child experienced bleeding, especially into the joints. Hydration above the normal requirement is not required. Because the child wasn't admitted for bleeding, bed rest is not necessary.
CN: Physiological integrity; CNS: Reduction of risk potential; CL: Apply

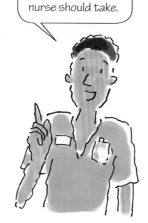

Hint! It's the first action the nurse should take.

106. A child with hemophilia is hospitalized with bleeding into the knee. Which action should the nurse take **first**?
1. Prepare to administer a whole blood transfusion
2. Prepare to administer a plasma transfusion
3. Perform active range-of-motion (ROM) exercise on the affected part
4. Elevate the affected part

106. 4. Bleeding into the joint is the most common type of bleeding episode in the more severe forms of hemophilia. Elevating the affected part and applying pressure and cold are indicated. The nurse should anticipate transfusing the missing clotting factor rather than whole blood or plasma, which won't stop the bleeding promptly, and may pose a risk of fluid overload. Active ROM exercises are contraindicated because they may cause more bleeding, injury, and pain.
CN: Physiological integrity; CNS: Reduction of risk potential; CL: Apply

107. Which intervention is indicated for a child in sickle cell vaso-occlusive crisis?
1. Immobilizing the affected part
2. Applying warm packs to the affected part
3. Applying cool packs to the affected part
4. Performing active range-of-motion (ROM) exercises to the affected part

107. 2. Applying warm packs promotes vasodilation and perfusion, and provides pain relief and comfort. Immobilization leads to stasis, which promotes sickling. Cool packs are contraindicated because they cause vasoconstriction and may precipitate red blood cell sickling. A child in vaso-occlusive crisis experiences acute pain that limits movement of the affected part. After the acute crisis passes, the child should be encouraged to ambulate. Active ROM exercises increase pain in the affected part.
CN: Physiological integrity; CNS: Basic care and comfort; CL: Apply

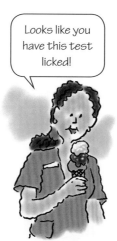

Looks like you have this test licked!

108. A four-year-old child has recently been diagnosed with acute lymphocytic leukemia (ALL). What information about ALL should the nurse provide when educating the child's parents? Select all that apply.
1. Leukemia is a rare form of childhood cancer.
2. ALL affects all blood-forming organs and systems throughout the body.
3. The child shouldn't brush his teeth because of the increased risk of bleeding.
4. Adverse effects of treatment include sleepiness, alopecia, and stomatitis.
5. There's a 95% chance of remission with treatment.
6. The child shouldn't be disciplined during this difficult time.

108. 2, 4, 5. In ALL, abnormal white blood cells proliferate, but they don't mature past the blast stage. These blast cells crowd out the healthy white blood cells, red blood cells, and platelets in the bone marrow, leading to bone marrow depression. The blast cells also infiltrate the liver, spleen, kidneys, and lymph tissue. Common adverse effects of chemotherapy and radiation include nausea, vomiting, diarrhea, sleepiness, alopecia, anemia, stomatitis, mucositis, pain, reddened skin, and increased susceptibility to infection. There's a 95% chance of obtaining remission with treatment. Leukemia is the most common form of childhood cancer. The child still needs appropriate discipline and limits. A lack of consistent parenting may lead to negative behaviors and fear.
CN: Physiological integrity; CNS: Reduction of risk potential; CL: Apply

CN: Client needs category   CNS: Client needs subcategory   CL: Cognitive level

109. A child with sickle cell anemia is being treated for a crisis. The provider orders morphine sulfate 2 mg IV. The concentration of the vial is 10 mg/1 ml of solution. How many milliliters of solution should the nurse administer? Record your answer using one decimal point.

_____ ml

110. A child with sickle cell anemia is being discharged after treatment for a crisis. Which instructions for avoiding future crises should the nurse provide to the client and his family? Select all that apply.
1. Avoid foods high in folic acid
2. Drink plenty of fluids
3. Use cold packs to relieve joint pain
4. Report a sore throat to an adult
5. Restrict activity to quiet board games
6. Wash hands before meals and after playing

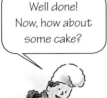

109. 0.2.
The nurse should calculate the volume to be given using this equation:

$$2\ mg/X\ ml = 10\ mg/1\ ml;\ X = (2/10)\ ml = 0.2\ ml$$

CN: Physiological integrity; CNS: Pharmacological and parenteral therapies; CL: Apply

110. 2, 4, 6. Fluids should be encouraged to prevent stasis in the bloodstream, which can lead to sickling. Sore throats, and any other cold symptoms, should be reported because they may indicate the presence of an infection, which can precipitate a crisis. Children with sickle cell anemia should learn appropriate measures to prevent infection, such as proper hand-washing techniques and good nutrition practices. Folic acid intake should be encouraged to help support new cell growth because new cells replace fragile, sickled cells. Warm packs should be applied to provide comfort and relieve pain. Cold packs cause vasoconstriction. The child should maintain an active, normal life. When the child experiences a pain crisis, he should limit his own activity according to his pain level.

CN: Physiological integrity; CNS: Reduction of risk potential; CL: Apply

Chapter 29

Respiratory Disorders

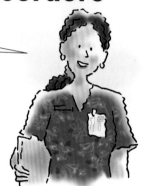

From the simple otitis media to the uncommon and dangerous epiglottiditis, this chapter covers a wide variety of respiratory disorders in children. So, take a deep breath and go for it!

1. An infant has died from sudden infant death syndrome (SIDS). What is the nurse's **best** response to the grieving parents?
1. "You did not cause your infant's death."
2. "An autopsy will confirm the cause of your infant's death."
3. "Don't worry, you'll have more children."
4. "Be sure to place your next infant on his back to sleep."

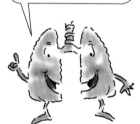

Cool! You made it to Chapter 29. Keep up the good work!

1. 1. The nurse can best support grieving parents by correcting the common falsehood that they could have prevented their infant's death. While an autopsy may need to be performed, it isn't a supportive response to grieving parents. Telling the parents that they will have more children minimizes the death of this infant and belittles the parent's feelings of grief. Instructing the parents to position future infants on their back suggests that the parents could have prevented this child's death.
CN: Psychosocial integrity; CNS: None; CL: Apply

2. Which child has the **highest** risk of sudden infant death syndrome (SIDS)?
1. A neonate born at 32-weeks' gestation weighing 3 lb, 15 oz (1.8 kg)
2. A neonate born at 39-weeks' gestation weighing 7 lb, 14 oz (3.6 kg)
3. A three-month-old infant hospitalized with a temperature of 103.4° F (39.7° C)
4. A first-born child who had a distant half-cousin who died from SIDS

2. 1. Premature infants, especially those with low birth weight, have an increased risk for SIDS. Infants with apnea, central nervous system disorders, or respiratory disorders have a higher risk of SIDS. The peak age for SIDS is two to four months. Hospitalization for fever is insignificant. There's an increased risk of SIDS in subsequent siblings of two or more SIDS victims.
CN: Physiological integrity; CNS: Reduction of risk potential; CL: Apply

3. A six-week-old infant is brought to the emergency department not breathing. A preliminary finding of sudden infant death syndrome (SIDS) is made to the parents. Which **initial** intervention should the nurse take?
1. Call their spiritual advisor
2. Explain the etiology of SIDS
3. Allow them to see their infant
4. Collect the infant's belongings and give them to the parents

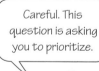

Careful. This question is asking you to prioritize.

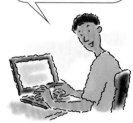

3. 3. The parents need time with their infant to assist with the grieving process. Calling their pastor and collecting the infant's belongings are also important steps in the plan of care, but are not priorities. The parents may be too upset to understand an explanation of SIDS at this time.
CN: Psychosocial integrity; CNS: None; CL: Apply

CN: Client needs category   CNS: Client needs subcategory   CL: Cognitive level

4. The nurse is teaching an infant care course. The parents of a newborn born at 38-weeks' gestational age mention that their niece died of sudden infant death syndrome (SIDS), and that they want to reduce the risk in their own infant. What statement should the nurse make? Select all that apply.

1. Use a pacifier when putting the baby down to sleep
2. Use a cardiac monitor with preterm babies
3. Place the baby on his or her back for 12 months
4. Co-share the room with the baby
5. Reposition the baby onto the back if he or she has rolled over to his or her stomach

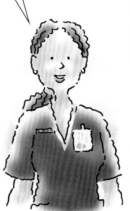

It's important to be sensitive to a family's feelings when they've lost a child to SIDS.

4. 1, 3, 4. Supine positioning is recommended to reduce the risk of SIDS in babies up to one year of age. A protective effect of pacifiers against SIDS has been found. Co-sharing a room, rather than co-sharing a bed, enhances bonding, and ease of breastfeeding at night. It also allows for frequent monitoring, and reduces the risk of smothering from roll over by parents. There is no evidence that repositioning the baby reduces the risk of SIDS.
CN: Physiological integrity; CNS: Reduction of risk potential; CL: Apply

5. An infant is brought to the emergency department (ED) and pronounced dead with the preliminary finding of sudden infant death syndrome (SIDS). Which question should the nurse ask the parents?

1. "Did you hear the infant cry out?"
2. "Was the infant's head buried in a blanket?"
3. "Were any of the siblings jealous of the new baby?"
4. "Was there vomitus in the infant's mouth when you found him?"

5. 4. Only factual questions should be asked during the initial history in the ED. The other questions imply blame, guilt, or neglect.
CN: Psychosocial Integrity; CNS: None; CL: Apply

6. A nurse is teaching parents of an infant with bronchiolitis the proper technique for bulb suctioning. Which statement should be included?

1. Feed the infant 20 minutes prior to suctioning
2. Place the infant in a head down position
3. Suction as often as the infant seems to need it
4. Repeat the suctioning process several times until most of the mucus is removed

6. 4. The parents should repeat the suctioning of each nostril several times until most of the mucus is removed. The infant should be placed on their back. One to two drops of saline may be instilled in each nostril prior to suctioning to help thin the mucus. Bulb suctioning to remove mucus should only be performed two to three times per day to prevent trauma and excess swelling to the nares. It is best to do this before feeding, as the saline and suction process can cause vomiting.
CN: Physiological integrity; CNS: Reduction of risk potential; CL: Apply

7. The nurse in pediatric intensive care is caring for an infant whose respiratory rate is 50 with nasal flaring, grunting and experiencing thick yellow nasal discharge. Vital signs are stable with oxygen saturation of 96% on 0.25 L of oxygen via face mask. Chest physiotherapy has been completed, and the infant is sleeping in the supine position. What should be the nurse's **next** intervention?

1. Call the health care provider
2. Suction the nares
3. Give ordered medications
4. Change the infant's position

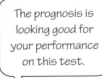

The prognosis is looking good for your performance on this test.

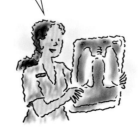

7. 2. The nurse should assess the client for respiratory compromise and clear the airway. Suctioning the nares to remove the thick mucus would be the first intervention. If the infant continues to show labored breathing, the practitioner should be notified and medications given. Repositioning the infant may help but would not be the first intervention.
CN: Physiological integrity; CNS: Reduction of risk potential; CL: Analyze

CN: Client needs category   CNS: Client needs subcategory   CL: Cognitive level

8. The nurse is caring for a seven-month-old infant with bronchiolitis. Which symptoms would the nurse expect to find during his assessment? Select all that apply.
1. Wheezing
2. Respiratory rate of 46
3. Heart rate of 128
4. Respiratory rate of 68
5. Heart rate of 82
6. Poor feeding

8. **1, 3, 4, 6.** Severe bronchiolitis is characterized by increased respiratory effort, including tachypnea, wheezing, nasal flaring and intercostal, subcostal and suprasternal retractions. Lethargy and poor feeding accompany severe cases. The heart rate is typically normal, or slightly increased. A heart rate of 82 is considered bradycardic in this age group and would be a sign of impending cardiac compromise. A respiratory rate of 46 is normal for this age.
CN: Physiological integrity; CNS: Physiological adaptation; CL: Apply

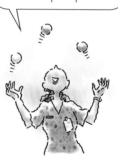

You're juggling these questions like a pro. Keep it up!

9. The nurse is scheduling a home visit to parents who have lost an infant to sudden infant death syndrome (SIDS). How should the nurse plan this visit?
1. One visit in two weeks
2. No visit is necessary
3. As soon after death as possible
4. One visit with parents only, no siblings

9. **3.** When parents return home, a visit is necessary as soon after the death as possible. The nurse should assess what the parents have been told, what they think happened, and how they've explained the death to the other siblings. Not all of these issues will be resolved in one visit. The number of visits and plan for intervention must be flexible. The needs of the siblings must always be considered.
CN: Psychosocial integrity; CNS: None; CL: Apply

10. An infant is brought into the emergency room after an apneic episode. It is later determined to be an apparent life-threatening event (ALTE). What statements are correct regarding an ALTE? Select all that apply.
1. There is a causal relationship between ALTE and sudden infant death syndrome (SIDS).
2. Gagging and color change are often features of ALTE.
3. The infant is usually hypertonic.
4. Stimulation or resuscitation is often required to bring about recovery.
5. Most ALTE episodes occur between 8 am and 8 pm.
6. More males present with ALTE than females.

10. **2, 4, 5.** Studies over the past two decades have not confirmed a causal relationship between pre-existing apnea and SIDS. The features of ALTE can be very frightening to the parents, with limpness and color change often being the initial signs. Most ALTE episodes occur between 8 am and 8 pm, whereas 80% of SIDS deaths occur between midnight and 6 am. Gastroesophageal reflux that causes gagging, or a central nervous system disorder (presenting as seizure), have been diagnosed in 45% to 50% of infants presenting with ALTE. Females present more often with ALTE. Males have a higher incidence of SIDS. Recurrent, severe ALTE events that require cardiopulmonary resuscitation, and that only occur in the presence of a single caretaker, with no reasonable explanation, should alert the nurse to the possibility of medical child abuse through intentional suffocation.
CN: Physiological integrity; CNS: Reduction of risk potential; CL: Apply

CN: Client needs category CNS: Client needs subcategory CL: Cognitive level

11. A nurse is teaching a group of newly-immigrated mothers about basic newborn care. The mothers tell the nurse that they have always been taught to put the infants on their sides to sleep in case the infant vomits. What is the nurse's **best** response?
1. The side-lying position promotes gastric emptying, and should be used for only 30 minutes before putting the baby on his back.
2. Regardless of what was taught in the past, the back is the safest way to position the baby.
3. Placing the infant on the back helps reduce the risk of sudden infant death syndrome (SIDS), and has not been shown to increase the risk of aspiration.
4. The benefits of putting a baby on his side do not outweigh the risk of SIDS.

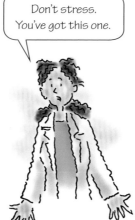

Don't stress.
You've got this one.

12. A nurse is caring for the parents of an infant who died from sudden infant death syndrome (SIDS). Which activity would be **best** for long-term support of these parents?
1. Attending support groups
2. Attending church regularly
3. Attending counseling sessions
4. Discussing feelings with family and friends

13. Which nursing intervention is **best** to help a two-year-old child adapt to hospitalization?
1. Allow the child to have favorite toys
2. Allow the child to play with equipment used on him
3. Explain procedures in simple terms
4. Ask one or both parents to stay with the child

14. A two-year-old child comes to the emergency department with inspiratory stridor and a barking cough. A preliminary diagnosis of croup has been made. What is the nurse's **most** important intervention?
1. Administer IV antibiotics
2. Provide oxygen by face mask
3. Establish and maintain the airway
4. Ask the mother to go to the waiting room

11. 3. Placing the infant on his back for sleeping has been shown to decrease SIDS throughout the world. Side-lying does promote gastric emptying, but the infant would need to be monitored closely while sleeping on his side. While the other responses may be true, the best response is a factual, non-judgmental response.
CN: Health promotion and maintenance; CNS: None; CL: Apply

12. 1. The best support will come from parents who have had the same experience. Attending church and discussing feelings with family and friends can offer support, but they may not understand the experience. Counseling sessions are usually a short-term support.
CN: Psychosocial integrity; CNS: None; CL: Apply

13. 4. The most important factor in helping a child adapt to new and strange surroundings is to allow the parents to be present. This is the hallmark of family-centered care. Placing the child's favorite toys in the room provides distraction, and allows the child to have something of his own with him, but may not alleviate fears. Allowing the child to play with the equipment may pose a safety hazard and isn't appropriate. Explaining procedures in simple terms is important, but a two-year-old has limited understanding.
CN: Physiological integrity; CNS: Physiological adaptation; CL: Apply

14. 3. The initial priority is to establish and maintain the airway. Edema and an accumulation of secretions may contribute to airway obstruction. Antibiotics are not indicated for viral illnesses. Oxygen should be administered as soon as possible to decrease the child's distress. Allowing the child to stay with the mother reduces anxiety and distress.
CN: Physiological integrity; CNS: Physiological adaptation; CL: Apply

15. The parents of a child ask the nurse what the best intervention is if their child is experiencing an episode of midnight croup (acute spasmodic laryngitis). What is the nurse's **best** response?
1. Give warm liquids
2. Raise the heat on the thermostat
3. Provide humidified air with cool mist
4. Take the child into the bathroom with a warm running shower

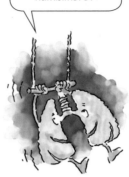

We're on the upswing now. Don't you just love humidifiers?

15. 3. High humidity with cool mist provides the most relief. Raising the heat on the thermostat will result in dry, warm air, which may cause secretions to adhere to the airway wall. A warm, running shower provides a mist that may be helpful to moisten and decrease the viscosity of airway secretions and may also decrease laryngeal spasm, but cool liquids would be best for the child. If unable to take liquid, the child needs to be seen in the emergency department. CN: Physiological integrity; CNS: Physiological adaptation; CL: Apply

16. Which symptom is **most** characteristic of a child with croup?
1. Barking cough
2. Fever
3. High heart rate
4. Respiratory distress

16. 1. A resonant cough described as "barking" is the most characteristic sign of croup. The child may present with a low-grade or high fever depending on whether the etiological agent is viral or bacterial. While the child with croup may have a rapid heart rate, it isn't a characteristic sign of croup. The child may have varying degrees of respiratory distress related to swelling or obstruction. CN: Physiological integrity; CNS: Physiological adaptation; CL: Analyze

17. Which sign should alert a nurse that an 18-month-old child with croup is experiencing increased respiratory distress?
1. A barking cough
2. Intercostal retractions
3. Clubbing of the fingers
4. Increased anterior-posterior chest diameter

17. 2. Intercostal retractions occur as the child's breathing becomes more labored. The use of accessory muscles is necessary to draw air into the lungs. A barking cough occurs in a child with croup, and isn't a sign that the condition is worsening. Clubbing of the fingers and a change in chest diameter occur with chronic respiratory conditions. CN: Physiological integrity; CNS: Physiological adaptation; CL: Analyze

18. What is the **most** important goal for a child with ineffective airway clearance?
1. Reducing the child's anxiety
2. Suctioning the child's secretions
3. Providing adequate oral fluids
4. Administering medications as ordered

I know what's important, but what's the most important?

18. 2. The most important goal is to maintain a patent airway. The child with ineffective airway clearance has secretions which can obstruct the airway. Reducing anxiety and administering medications are necessary after the airway is secure. The child should not be allowed to eat or drink anything to prevent the risk of aspiration. CN: Physiological integrity; CNS: Physiological adaptation; CL: Apply

19. A 19-month-old child with croup is crying as a nurse tries to auscultate breath sounds. What is the nurse's **most** appropriate intervention?
1. Ignore the crying and listen to breath sounds as best as possible
2. Tell the parents that they are upsetting the child and to wait outside the room
3. Tell the child, in a loud and firm voice, that he must sit still and cooperate
4. Hand the stethoscope to the child to examine before auscultating his lungs

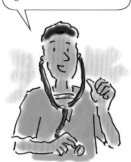

It's important to gain the child's trust.

19. 4. Children at this age are very curious. Encouraging the child to play with the stethoscope will distract him and help gain trust so that the nurse will be able to auscultate the lungs. Ignoring the child's crying may only upset him more, and will not help the nurse gain his trust. The nurse should ask the parents to help quiet and comfort the child. Asking the parents to leave may only upset the child more. The nurse should speak to the child in a soft, comforting tone of voice.
CN: Physiological integrity; CNS: physiological adaptation; CL: Analyze

20. The student nurse asks if any precaution is necessary while caring for children with respiratory infections such as croup in an outpatient setting. What is the **best** information for the nurse to provide?
1. Enforce hand washing
2. Place the child in isolation
3. Teach children to use tissues
4. Constantly run a warm humidifier

20. 1. Hand washing helps prevent the spread of infections. The child's siblings should be placed in separate bedrooms, if possible, but a child with croup does not need to be isolated. Teaching children to properly use tissues is important, but the key is disposal and hand washing after use. The use of cool humidified air is recommended to relax the airways and loosen secretions.
CN: Health promotion and maintenance; CNS: None; CL: Apply

21. A nebulizer treatment has been ordered for a child with croup. What is the **best** time for the nurse to administer this treatment?
1. During naptime
2. During playtime
3. After the child eats
4. After the parents leave

Sometimes a little nebulized air is just what the health care provider ordered.

21. 1. The nurse should administer nebulizer treatments at prescribed intervals. Naptime allows for as little disruption as possible. Administering treatment during playtime will disrupt the child's daily pattern. A child should be given a treatment before eating so the airway will be open, and the work of eating will be decreased. Parents are usually helpful when administering treatments. The child can sit on the parents' lap to help decrease anxiety or fear.
CN: Physiological integrity; CNS: Pharmacological and parenteral therapies; CL: Apply

22. Which intervention should the nurse explain to the parents of a child recovering from croup?
1. Limiting oral fluid intake
2. Recognizing signs of respiratory distress
3. Providing three nutritious meals per day
4. Allowing the child to go to the playground

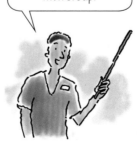

Adequate parent teaching is essential for managing a child with croup.

22. 2. Although most children recover without complications, the parents should be able to recognize signs and symptoms of respiratory distress, and know how to access emergency services. Oral fluids should be encouraged because fluids help to thin secretions. Frequent, small, nutritious snacks are usually more appealing than an entire meal. Children should have optimal rest and engage in quiet play. A comfortable environment free from noxious stimuli lessens respiratory distress.
CN: Physiological integrity; CNS: Physiological adaptation; CL: Apply

CN: Client needs category   CNS: Client needs subcategory   CL: Cognitive level

23. The nurse is planning care for a child admitted to the pediatric unit with neonatal bronchopulmonary dysplasia (chronic lung disease). Which intervention should the nurse perform **first**?
1. Keep fluids at a minimum
2. Provide humidified oxygen
3. Give palivizumab vaccine
4. Keep ambient air temperature cooler than normal

23. 2. Tachypnea, dyspnea, and wheezing are intermittently or chronically present, secondary to airway obstruction and increased airway resistance. Giving humidified oxygen will help keep the airways moist and liquefy secretions. Fluid restriction may be ordered to decrease secondary problems such as heart failure, but it is not in all cases. The palivizumab vaccine is recommended in children with chronic lung disease to prevent respiratory syncytial viral (RSV) infection. It is typically given during RSV season. The ambient air temperature should be kept in a neutral thermal zone to decrease oxygen consumption.

CN: Physiological integrity; CNS: Physiological adaptation; CL: Apply

24. A two-year-old child wakes in the night with a barking cough. Her parents call the pediatric clinic. What instruction should the nurse give these parents?
1. Provide humidified air for the child to breathe
2. Consider calling for an ambulance
3. Place the child in a warm, dry room
4. Give the child a cough suppressant

24. 1. Humidified air reduces laryngeal irritation and spasm, and helps liquefy secretions. The child does not need emergency care at this time; however, if the child develops respiratory distress, the parents should be instructed to call emergency medical services, and not drive the child to the hospital themselves. The child should not be placed in a warm, dry room. Cool, humidified air is used to reduce laryngospasm. Cough suppressants are not recommended for use in children less than 4 to 6 years of age, nor would be helpful, as the cough is due to airway edema and inflammation.

CN: Physiological integrity; CNS: Reduction of risk potential; CL: Apply

25. The nurse is assessing a child recently brought to the emergency department. Based on the notes, which observations would cause the nurse to suspect epiglottitis? Select all that apply.

Progress notes	
4/5/16	History and physical
0215	23-month-old infant brought in by ambulance. Parents noted infant was doing fine when put to bed, but suddenly woke very agitated with breathing difficulties. Mild tactile temperature noted. Child crying excessively. Child tachypneic, drooling. Child refusing to lie down.

1. Excessive crying
2. Drooling
3. Low-grade fever
4. Spontaneous cough
5. Refusal to lie down

25. 2, 5. Drooling of saliva is common due to the pain of swallowing excessive secretions, and a sore throat. The child will usually have a high fever, but no spontaneous cough. The child may place themselves in a tripod position with their mouth open and tongue protruding.

CN: Physiological integrity; CNS: Physiological adaptation; CL: Apply

CN: Client needs category   CNS: Client needs subcategory   CL: Cognitive level

26. Which strategy is the **best** plan of care for a child with acute epiglottitis?
1. Encourage oral fluids for hydration
2. Maintain the client in semi-Fowler's position
3. Administer IV antibiotic therapy
4. Maintain respiratory isolation for 48 hours

27. The nurse walks into the playroom on the hospital unit and finds a toddler unconscious on the floor next to the toy storage chest. Prioritize the nurse's interventions.

| 1. Start mouth-to-mouth resuscitation |
| 2. Begin chest compressions |
| 3. Call for help |
| 4. Open the airway |

28. What pulse should the nurse assess in an infant found in respiratory arrest?

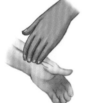

1.

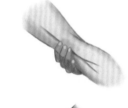

2.

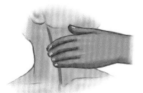

3.

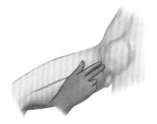

4.

Remember

"Antibiotics are against (anti) life (bio)."

Antibiotics, also known as antibacterials, are medications that either inhibit or kill the living organisms known as bacteria. Classes of antibiotics are listed below.

Antibiotics
- Aminoglycosides
- Penicillins
- Cephalosporins
- Tetracyclines
- Lincomycin derivatives
- Macrolides
- Vancomycin
- Carbapenems
- Monobactams
- Fluoroquinolones
- Sulfonamides
- Nitrofurantoin (nitrofuran)

26. 3. The etiological agent for epiglottitis is usually bacterial. Treatment consists of IV antibiotic therapy. The client should not be allowed anything by mouth during the initial phases of the infection to prevent aspiration. The client should be placed in Fowler's position or any position that provides the most comfort and security. Respiratory isolation is not required.
CN: Physiological integrity; CNS: Physiological adaptation; CL: Apply

27. Ordered Response:

| 3. Call for help |
| 2. Begin chest compressions |
| 4. Open the airway |
| 1. Start mouth-to-mouth resuscitation |

CN: Physiological integrity; CNS: Physiological adaptation; CL: Apply

28. 1. Palpation of the brachial artery is recommended. The radial pulse, shown in graphic two, is not a good indicator of central artery perfusion. The short, chubby neck of an infant, shown in graphic three, makes rapid location of the carotid artery difficult. After age one, the carotid would be used. The femoral pulse, shown in graphic four, is often palpated in a hospital setting, may be difficult to assess because of the infant's position, fat folds, and clothing.
CN: Physiological integrity; CNS: Physiological adaptation; CL: Apply

29. The nurse is teaching the parents of a six-month-old child how to perform CPR prior to discharge. The parents ask why the rescue breaths are so important instead of compressions only. What is the nurse's **best** response?

1. Breathing for the child allows adequate oxygenation to all body systems during CPR.
2. Children, as opposed to adults, often have preceding respiratory failure leading to a decreased oxygen reserve.
3. The child is able to use oxygen from a rescue breath as well as an adult.
4. The standard recommendations for CPR include both compressions and rescue breathing.

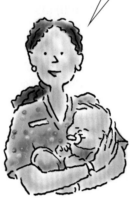

30. The nurse is teaching CPR to parents of a six year old. What is the correct hand position for chest compressions?

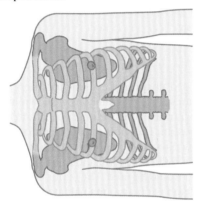

29. 2. Infants and children who develop cardiac arrest often have respiratory failure or shock that reduces the available oxygen supply in the blood prior to the onset of cardiac arrest. As a result, chest compressions alone are not effective in delivering adequate oxygenation to the brain and heart. While the other answers are true, answer two is the best response.

CN: Physiological integrity; CNS: Physiological adaptation; CL: Apply

30. When performing chest compressions on a child, proper hand placement is even more crucial than with adults. Two fingers are placed at the sternum just below the nipple line and then the heel of the other hand is placed directly on top of the fingers. Compressions are done to a depth of 1 to 1½ in (2.5 to 3.5 cm).

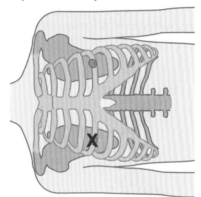

CN: Physiological integrity; CNS: Physiological adaptation; CL: Apply

31. A nurse has noted a sternal depression while examining a child. What is the **most** important information the nurse can teach this child's family about the deformity?

1. "Funnel chest" can be caused by many different defects in structure and growth.
2. The child should be monitored because a severe deformity can cause scoliosis.
3. Some children with this deformity report exercise intolerance and shortness of breath.
4. This deformity may resolve over time; however, it tends to worsen during the rapid growth of adolescence.

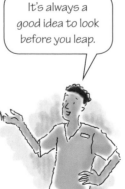

31. 3. Pectus excavatum (PE) is a deformity of the chest wall characterized by a sternal depression beginning over the midportion of the manubrium and progressing inward toward the xiphoid process. It can range in severity from a mild cosmetic concern, to a severe deformity that can affect cardiac and respiratory function. Some children may develop exercise intolerance and shortness of breath which would need further evaluation. While all of the answers are true, the nurse must highlight the risk of respiratory problems due to the deformity.

CN: Physiological integrity; CNS: Physiological adaptation; CL: Apply

CN: Client needs category   CNS: Client needs subcategory   CL: Cognitive level

32. A 10-month-old child is found choking and becomes unconscious. What is the nurse's **priority** intervention after opening the child's airway?
1. Look inside the child's mouth for a foreign object
2. Give five back blows and five chest thrusts
3. Attempt a blind finger sweep
4. Attempt rescue breathing

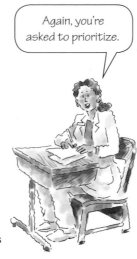

Again, you're asked to prioritize.

32. 1. As soon as the infant is found choking, the nurse should give five back blows and five chest thrusts in an attempt to dislodge the object and open the airway. After the airway is open, the nurse should check for a foreign object and remove it with a finger sweep if it can be seen. After the object is removed, 30 quick compressions should be given before rescue breathing is attempted. Blind finger sweeps should never be performed because this may push the object further into the airway.
CN: Physiological integrity; CNS: Physiological adaptation; CL: Apply

33. The parents of an infant ask the nurse about the risks associated with the DTaP vaccine? What is the nurse's **best** response?
1. "The risk of vaccines are so few, you should not worry."
2. "There is a slight but known risk of seizures."
3. "The risks are few but very substantial."
4. "The benefits of the vaccine outweigh the risks of the vaccine."

33. 4. The benefits of the vaccine, in preventing diphtheria, tetanus and pertussis, outweigh the very small chance of serious complications. The most common problems are a fever, or localized reaction following the vaccination. Seizures and brain damage have been reported; however, these problems have occurred so rarely that the Centers for Disease Control and Prevention do not completely attribute them to the vaccination. Anaphylaxis occurs in fewer than one in a million doses. While all the answer choices are correct, answer four is the best answer.
CN: Physiological integrity; CNS: Pharmocological and parenteral therapies; CL: Apply

34. A three-year-old child is brought to the emergency department not breathing, and is cyanotic. The mother states that her child has likely swallowed a penny. What is the nurse's **first** intervention?
1. Give 100% oxygen
2. Administer five back blows
3. Attempt a blind finger sweep
4. Administer abdominal thrusts

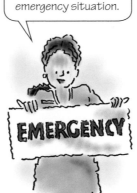

It's important to prioritize in an emergency situation.

34. 4. A child between the ages of one and eight should receive abdominal thrusts to help dislodge the object first. Administering 100% oxygen will not help if the airway is occluded. Infants younger than age one should receive back blows before chest thrusts. Blind finger sweeps should never be performed because this could push the object further back into the airway.
CN: Physiological integrity; CNS: Physiological adaptation; CL: Apply

35. Which statement, made by the parent of a four-year-old boy who just had a tonsillectomy, indicates that a nurse's discharge instructions were understood?
1. "I will keep him flat on his back in bed."
2. "I will sit him in bed at a 45-degree angle."
3. "I will place him on his stomach with his head to the side."
4. "I will place him on his back with his head on a pillow."

35. 3. Laying the child on his stomach with the head turned to the side will allow blood and other secretions to drain from the mouth and pharynx, reducing the risk of aspiration. Placing the child flat on his back, on his back with a pillow, or at a 45-degree angle does not promote drainage, and will increase the likelihood of aspiration.
CN: Physiological integrity; CNS: Reduction of risk potential; CL: Apply

CN: Client needs category   CNS: Client needs subcategory   CL: Cognitive level

36. The nurse receives a prescription for amoxicillin 80 mg/kg/day to be administered in two divided does to an infant who weighs 19 lb 8 oz (9 kg). The medication is supplied as 250 mg/ml. How many milliliters should the nurse administer for one dose? Record your answer using one decimal place.

_____ ml

36. 1.4.
Here are the calculations:

$$80\frac{mg}{kg/day} \times 9\,kg = 720\,mg/day.$$
$$720\,mg/2\,doses = 360\,mg/dose.$$
$$360\,mg/dose \div 250\,mg/ml = 1.4\,ml$$

CN: Physiological integrity; CNS: Pharmacological and parenteral therapies; CL: Apply

37. The parents of a toddler want to know why ear tubes will help prevent otitis media. The nurse should explain that:
1. antibiotics were not working well, and the tubes need to be placed.
2. the middle ear needs to be flushed out to prevent infection.
3. the tubes help relieve the pressure in the ear; thus, prevent infection.
4. the tubes help drain fluid; thus, help to prevent infection.

37. 4. Children with chronic otitis media commonly require a myringotomy and ear tube placement. Antibiotics may, or may not, have helped in the past. Ear tubes allow normal fluid to drain from the middle ear. They provides ventilation, and allows pressure to equalize in the middle ear. A myringotomy does not, necessarily, prevent infection.

CN: Physiological integrity; CNS: Physiological adaptation; CL: Apply

38. A nurse is discharging a 10-month-old client with a prescription for eardrops. The nurse teaches the parents how to correctly administer the drops. Prioritize the steps in correct order of administration.

1. Have the child lie down with the affected ear up
2. Observe the ear for discharge
3. Warm the medication
4. Rub the area anterior to the ear
5. Pull the pinna downward and backward to instill the medication

38. Ordered Response:

3. Warm the medication
1. Have the child lie down with the affected ear up
2. Observe the ear for discharge
5. Pull the pinna downward and backward to instill the medication
4. Rub the area anterior to the ear

CN: Physiological integrity; CNS: Pharmacological and parenteral therapies; CL: Apply

39. A child is diagnosed with right chronic otitis media. After the child returns from his myringotomy and placement of ear tubes, which intervention is appropriate?
1. Apply gauze dressings
2. Position the child on the left side
3. Position the child on the right side
4. Apply warm compresses to both ears

39. 3. The child should be positioned on the right side to facilitate drainage. Gauze dressings are not necessary after surgery. Some health care providers may prefer a loose cotton wick. The left side isn't an area of concern for drainage. Warm compresses may help to facilitate drainage when used on the affected ear.

CN: Physiological integrity; CNS: Physiological adaptation; CL: Apply

40. A parent asks how to reduce the risk of the infant developing otitis media. What critical information should the nurse to provide?

1. Treat all cold symptoms with antibiotics
2. Place the infant in an upright position when feeding from a bottle
3. Avoid washing the ears to keep them dry
4. Swab the outer ear with a cotton-tipped swab

40. 2. Although breast-fed infants have an overall lower incidence of otitis media, the risk can be further reduced by bottle feeding the infant in an upright position. Formula that pools in the nasopharynx is a good medium for bacterial growth. Bacteria can easily move through the shortened, horizontal eustachian tube of an infant. Administering antibiotics with cold symptoms will not reduce the risk of otitis media since colds are most commonly due to viral causes. Washing the ears, or swabbing the outer ear does not contribute to otitis media.
CN: Health promotion and maintenance; CNS: None;
CL: Apply

41. The nurse is using an otoscope to assess a child with otitis media. What assessment finding should the nurse expect?

1.

3.

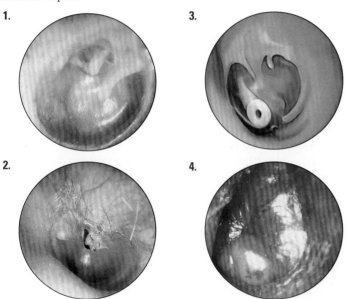

2.

4.

41. 4. With acute otitis media, the tympanic membrane may present as bright red or yellow, bulging or retracted. Photo one shows a normal tympanic membrane. Photo two shows scarring of the membrane. This could be due to a severe past infection or perforation. Photo three shows a tympanic membrane tube often placed to prevent accumulation of fluid in the middle ear; thus, decreasing the likelihood of otitis media.
CN: Physiological integrity; CNS: Physiological adaptation;
CL: Analyze

42. The parents of a one-year-old infant who has otitis media are curious about the factors that predisposed their child to this infection. The nurse knows that teaching has been successful when the parents state:

1. "My child's cartilage needs to develop."
2. "When my child lies down, the fluid drains in the wrong place."
3. "My child has several siblings."
4. "My child's eustachian tubes are short, which increases the risk of infections."

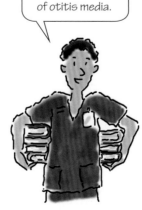

Question 42 is asking about a proximate cause of otitis media.

42. 4. The Eustachian tubes in an infant or child are short, straight, wide, and lie on a horizontal plane. This allows them to be more easily blocked by conditions such as large adenoids and infections. Until the eustachian tubes change in size and angle, children are more susceptible to otitis media. Cartilage lining is underdeveloped, making the tubes more distensible, and more likely to open inappropriately. Many infants favor a supine resting position which allows fluids, such as formula, to pool in the pharyngeal cavity. Immature humoral defense mechanisms increase the risk of infection, as in the case of many siblings, but that does not predispose a child to otitis media.
CN: Physiological integrity; CNS: Physiological adaptation;
CL: Apply

CN: Client needs category   CNS: Client needs subcategory   CL: Cognitive level

43. The nurse is teaching the parents of a child with otitis media steps to decrease the risk of further infection and complications. Which statements should be included in teaching? Select all that apply.
1. Complete all medications as prescribed
2. Clean out the child's ear canals weekly
3. Stop smoking
4. Decrease the amount of time, if possible, at daycare
5. Use a pacifier as much as possible

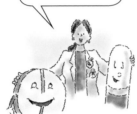

Your body's immune system can collaborate with antibiotics.

43. 1, 3, 4. To prevent complications of otitis media, medications should be used as prescribed. Children who are exposed to smoke, and infants over 12 months of age who use a pacifier have a higher incidence of otitis media. Limiting group contact decreases the amount of exposure to germs. Cleaning the ear canals, whether by using an irrigant, or cotton swabs, increase the chance of infections and can damage to the inner ear.
CN: Physiological integrity; CNS: Physiological adaptation; CL: Apply

44. The parents of a child diagnosed with otitis media ask the nurse why their healthcare provider instructed them to wait 48 hours before filling a prescription for an antibiotic to treat the infection. What is the **best** information for this nurse to give the parents?
1. Ear infections need to fully settle in before antibiotics are effective.
2. Antibiotics may cause drug-resistance later.
3. The child's body may fight the infection on its own without the use of antibiotics.
4. Waiting to fill the prescription will save you money.

44. 3. A child's body may be able to fight the infection on its own without medication. Given the increase in drug-resistant microbes, practitioners are urged to judiciously prescribe antibiotics. Waiting 48 to 72 hours to see if the child is better would reveal if antibiotics are needed. Antibiotics would tend to be effective immediately regardless of whether the infection has "settled in" or not.
CN: Physiological integrity; CNS: Pharmacological and parental therapies; CL: Analyze

45. The nurse is caring for a 12-kg child diagnosed with epiglottitis. Vancomycin 50 mg/kg/day in three divided doses is prescribed. The medication is supplied as 500 mg/100 ml. How many milliliters per dose will the nurse administer? Record your answer using a whole number.

_____ ml

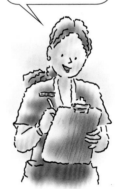

What did I tell you? Here's that formula again.

45. 40.
The child should receive 40 ml per dose. Here are the calculations:

$$50 \ mg/kg/day \times 12 \ kg = 600 \ mg/day$$
$$600 \ mg/day \div 3 \ doses/day = 200 \ mg/dose$$

$$500 \ mg/100 \ ml = 5 \ mg/ml$$

$$200 \ mg/dose \div 5 \ mg/ml = 40 \ ml/dose$$

CN: Physiological integrity; CNS: Pharmacological and parenteral therapies; CL: Apply

46. The nurse notes an erythematous rash on the face of a three-year-old child who is receiving vancomycin for acute epiglottitis. Prioritize the actions this nurse should take in caring for this child.

1. Check the vital signs
2. Call the practitioner
3. Stop the vancomycin
4. Complete a facility incident report

46. Ordered Response:

3. Stop the vancomycin
1. Check the vital signs
2. Call the practitioner
4 Complete a facility incident report

The priority action is to stop the medication as the child may be experiencing a reaction due to the medication. The next priority would be to assess the vital signs to determine hemodynamic stability. After the assessment of vital signs, the practitioner is called to notify of status. The final step would be documentation of the incident.
CN: Physiological integrity; CNS: Pharmacological and parenteral therapies; CL: Analyze

47. A three-year-old child is given a preliminary diagnosis of acute epiglottitis. Which initial nursing intervention is **most** appropriate?
  1. Obtain a throat culture
  2. Place the child in a side-lying position.
  3. Have emergency airway equipment readily available
  4. Obtain blood cultures

47. 3. With acute epiglottitis, the glottal structures become edematous. Emergency airway equipment and humidified oxygen should be readily available. The nurse should not attempt to visualize the epiglottis, use tongue blades or throat culture swabs, which can cause the epiglottis to spasm, and totally occlude the airway. Throat inspection should only be attempted when immediate intubation or tracheostomy can be performed in the event of further or complete obstruction. The child should always remain in a position that provides the most comfort, security and ease of breathing. The child will often assumes a classic tripod posture with the trunk leaning forward, neck hyperextended, and chin thrust forward.
CN: Physiological integrity; CNS: Physiological adaptation; CL: Apply

48. The nurse would withhold a *Haemophilus influenzae* type B (Hib) vaccine for a six-month-old infant if the infant has a:
  1. runny nose and cough.
  2. history of fever of 100.7° F (37.9° C) after the Hib vaccine.
  3. current temperature of 101.8° F (38.7° C).
  4. history of seizures after a previous DTaP administration.

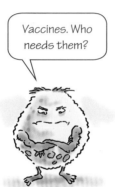

Vaccines. Who needs them?

48. 3. Epiglottitis is caused by *H. influenza* bacteria. The American Academy of Pediatrics recommends that, beginning at age two months, children receive the Hib conjugate vaccine. A decline in the incidence of epiglottitis has been seen as a result of this vaccination regimen. Current symptoms such as a low-grade fever, rhinorrhea or a cough should not preclude the administration of vaccines. A higher fever (over 101° F or 38.3°C) would indicate a need to use precaution before administering the vaccine. Seizures after DTaP vaccination would contraindicate the administration of that vaccine, but not the Hib vaccine.
CN: Physiological Integrity; CNS: Reduction of Risk Potential; CL: Apply

49. A three-year-old child is diagnosed with acute epiglottitis. Which sign would indicate to the nurse that this child's respiratory distress is increasing?
  1. Progressive barking cough
  2. Increasing irritability
  3. Increasing heart rate
  4. Productive cough

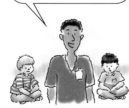

This question is asking about an increase—not just a presence of—symptoms.

49. 3. An increasing heart rate is an early sign of hypoxia. A progressive barking cough is characteristic of spasmodic croup. A child in respiratory distress will be irritable and restless. As distress increases, the child will become lethargic related to the work of breathing, and impending respiratory failure. A productive cough shows that secretions are moving, and the child can effectively clear them.
CN: Physiological integrity; CNS: Physiological adaptation; CL: Apply

50. The nurse is examining a child with acute epiglottitis. What item should the nurse have available?
  1. Cool mist humidifier
  2. Intubation equipment
  3. Tongue blades
  4. Viral culture medium

50. 2. Emergency intubation equipment should be at the bedside to secure the airway if examination reveals further or complete obstruction. Viral culture medium and cool mist humidifiers are recommended for the diagnosis and treatment of croup. Tongue blades are contraindicated, and may cause the epiglottis to spasm.
CN: Physiological integrity; CNS: Physiological adaptation; CL: Apply

CN: Client needs category   CNS: Client needs subcategory   CL: Cognitive level

51. A two-year-old child is brought to the emergency department in respiratory distress. The child is drooling, sitting upright, and leaning forward with chin thrust out, mouth open, and tongue protruding. Which nursing intervention is **most** appropriate?

  1. Check the child's gag reflex with a tongue blade
  2. Allow the child to cry to keep the lungs expanded
  3. Check the airway for a foreign body obstruction
  4. Support the child in an upright position on the parent's lap

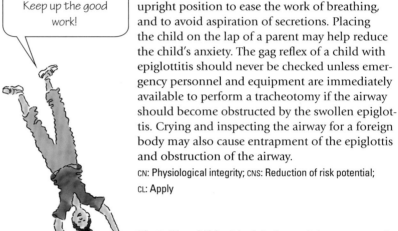

Congratulations! You've finished more than 50 questions! Keep up the good work!

52. How should the nurse position a preschooler with right lower lobe pneumonia?

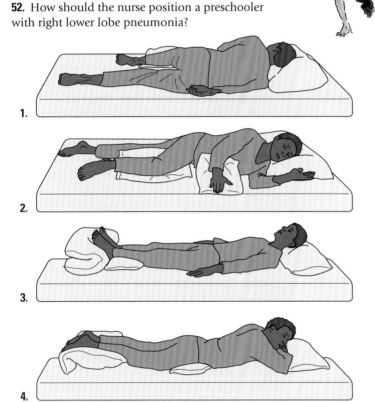

  1.

  2.

  3.

  4.

51. 4. The classic signs of epiglottitis are drooling, sitting upright, leaning forward with chin thrust out, mouth open, and tongue protruding. The child with epiglottitis should be kept in an upright position to ease the work of breathing, and to avoid aspiration of secretions. Placing the child on the lap of a parent may help reduce the child's anxiety. The gag reflex of a child with epiglottitis should never be checked unless emergency personnel and equipment are immediately available to perform a tracheotomy if the airway should become obstructed by the swollen epiglottis. Crying and inspecting the airway for a foreign body may also cause entrapment of the epiglottis and obstruction of the airway.

CN: Physiological integrity; CNS: Reduction of risk potential; CL: Apply

52. 2. The child with right lower lobe pneumonia should be placed on his left side. This places the unaffected left lung in a position so that gravity will promote blood flow to the healthy lung tissue, improving gas exchange. Placing the child on the right side, his back, or his stomach doesn't promote circulation to the unaffected lung.

CN: Physiological integrity; CNS: Physiological adaptation; CL: Apply

53. The arterial blood gas analysis of a child with asthma shows a pH of 7.30, pCO_2 of 56 mmHg, and HCO_3 of 25 mEq/L. Which condition does this child have?
1. Metabolic acidosis
2. Metabolic alkalosis
3. Respiratory acidosis
4. Respiratory alkalosis

54. Which neonate is at highest risk for developing neonatal bronchopulmonary dysplasia?
1. A neonate born at 38-weeks' gestation receiving 1 to 4 L oxygen during feedings
2. A premature neonate born at 34-weeks' gestation receiving supplemental oxygen
3. A premature neonate born at 28-weeks' gestation on a high-pressure ventilator
4. A neonate born at 42-weeks' gestation who requires treatments for respiratory syncytial virus

55. Which nursing intervention is the **priority** for an infant with neonatal bronchopulmonary dysplasia (chronic lung disease)?
1. Weigh the infant on the same scale, at the same time each day
2. Give the infant higher calorie formula as ordered
3. Monitor oxygen status via pulse oximetry
4. Monitor strict input and output

56. A child is newly diagnosed with neonatal bronchopulmonary dysplasia (chronic lung disease). Which intervention should the nurse perform **first** to help the parents?
1. Teach cardiopulmonary resuscitation
2. Refer them to support groups
3. Help parents identify necessary lifestyle changes
4. Evaluate and assess parents' stress and anxiety levels

57. Which nursing action would be **most** appropriate to facilitate gas exchange for an infant with neonatal chronic lung disease (bronchopulmonary dysplasia)?
1. Provide or arrange for chest physiotherapy
2. Provide adequate rest periods
3. Monitor oxygen saturation
4. Promote bonding between parent and child

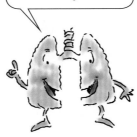

I think I sense an acid–base disturbance coming on.

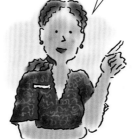

Which management strategy is recommended in question 56?

53. 3. Respiratory acidosis is an acid-base disturbance characterized by excess CO_2 in the blood, indicated by a pCO_2 greater than 45 mmHg. The pH level is usually below the normal range of 7.36 to 7.45. The HCO_3 level is normal in the acute stage, and elevated in the chronic stage.
CN: Physiological integrity; CNS: Physiological adaptation; CL: Analyze

54. 3. Premature neonates with low birth weight on high-pressure ventilators are at highest risk for developing neonatal bronchopulmonary dysplasia (chronic lung disease). Supplemental oxygen, respiratory treatments, and 1 to 4 L oxygen during feedings are not high-risk factors.
CN: Physiological integrity; CNS: Reduction of risk potential; CL: Apply

55. 3. The infant will have impaired gas exchange related to retention of carbon dioxide and borderline oxygenation secondary to fibrosis of the lungs. Although the infant may require increased caloric intake, and may have excess fluid volume, the priority intervention is to maintain effective gas exchange.
CN: Physiological integrity; CNS: Physiological adaptation; CL: Analyze

56. 4. The emotional impact of neonatal bronchopulmonary dysplasia (chronic lung disease) is a crisis situation. The parents are experiencing grief and sorrow over the loss of a healthy child. In addition to evaluating the parent's current stress and anxiety level, it is also helpful to assess their previous coping strategies. The other strategies are more appropriate for long-term intervention.
CN: Psychosocial integrity; CNS: None; CL: Apply

57. 1. All these activities decrease the risk of impaired gas exchange however providing chest physiotherapy actively facilitates gas exchange by mobilizing secretions.
CN: Physiological integrity; CNS: Basic care and comfort; CL: Analyze

CN: Client needs category   CNS: Client needs subcategory   CL: Cognitive level

58. Chlorothiazide is ordered for a one-year-old client with neonatal bronchopulmonary dysplasia (chronic lung disease). The dosage ordered is 30 mg/kg/day. The client weighs 10 kg. How much is given per dose when administered two times per day? Record your answer using a whole number.

_____ mg

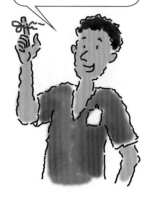

Can you remember the right formula to use here?

58. 150.

Here are the calculations:

$$30 \, mg/kg/day \times 10 \, kg = 300 \, mg/day$$

$$300 \, mg/2 \, doses = 150 \, mg/dose$$

CN: Physiological integrity; CNS: Pharmacological and parenteral therapies; CL: Apply

59. Infants with neonatal bronchopulmonary dysplasia (chronic lung disease) require frequent, prolonged rest periods. Which sign indicates overstimulation?
1. Increased alertness
2. Good eye contact
3. Cyanosis
4. Increased appetite

59. 3. Signs of overstimulation in an infant with chronic lung disease include cyanosis, avoidance of eye contact, vomiting, diaphoresis, or falling asleep. The child may also become irritable and show signs of respiratory distress.
CN: Physiological integrity; CNS: Basic care and comfort; CL: Apply

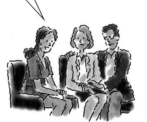

Remember to talk with parents about their care plans, not just their child's.

60. The nurse is preparing a care plan for the parents of a child with neonatal bronchopulmonary dysplasia (chronic lung disease). Which outcome would the nurse anticipate for this child's parents?
1. Report the same levels of stress
2. Make safe decisions with professional assistance
3. Participate in routine caretaking activities
4. Verbalize the causes, risks, therapy options, and nursing care

60. 4. The parents should understand the causes, risks, and care of their infant by the time of discharge. Having the parents verbalize this information is the only way to assess their understanding. The parents should report decreased levels of stress, be capable of making decisions independently, and participate in routine and complex care.
CN: Physiological integrity; CNS: Basic care and comfort; CL: Analyze

61. The nurse is assessing an infant with neonatal bronchopulmonary dysplasia (chronic lung disease). Which symptoms would the nurse expect to find? Select all that apply.
1. Tachypnea
2. Bradypnea
3. Hyperexpansion on chest X-ray
4. Rapid weight gain
5. Wheezing

61. 1, 3, 6. The physical exam of an infant with neonatal chronic lung disease often reveals tachypnea and wheezing. The chest X-ray shows hyperinflation as the disease becomes more severe. Infants often fail to gain weight.
CN: Physiological integrity; CNS: Physiological adaptation; CL: Apply

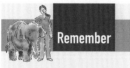

Remember

"Furosemide causes edema to subside."

Loop diuretics, such as furosemide, promote significant urinary excretion by the kidneys and are used to decrease edema, such as pulmonary edema.

62. A nurse is caring for an infant with neonatal bronchopulmonary dysplasia (chronic lung disease) administers furosemide. What is the priority intervention following the administration of this medication?
1. Obtain daily weights
2. Obtain vital signs every two hours
3. Obtain a vision screen
4. Monitor electrolyte status

62. 4. Furosemide is a potent diuretic that, if given in excessive amounts, can lead to a profound diuresis of water, and electrolyte depletion which could lead to life-threatening arrhythmias. Input and output should be monitored along with vital signs. Furosemide can be ototoxic therefore hearing should be evaluated.
CN: Physiological integrity; CNS: Pharmacological and parenteral therapies; CL: Analyze

CN: Client needs category   CNS: Client needs subcategory   CL: Cognitive level

63. A pediatric client is to receive furosemide 4 mg/kg/day in one daily dose. The client weighs 20 kg. The oral solution comes as 8 mg/ml. How many teaspoons should be administered in each dose? Record your answer using a whole number.

_____ tsp

63. 2.
The child should receive 80 mg per dose. Here are the calculations:

$$80 \ mg/dose \div 8 \ mg/ml = 10 \ ml/dose$$

$$5 \ ml = 1 \ teaspoon$$

$$10 \ ml/dose \div 5 \ ml/tsp = 2 \ teaspoons/dose$$

CN: Physiological integrity; CNS: Pharmacological and parenteral therapies; CL: Apply

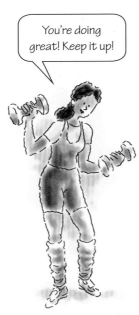

You're doing great! Keep it up!

64. The nurse is educating the parents of a two-year-old child with neonatal bronchopulmonary dysplasia (chronic lung disease) who is placed on furosemide. Which statement by the parents **best** indicates an understanding of this medication?
1. "I need to make sure my child uses the bathroom at least every six hours."
2. "I need to make sure my child gets his blood pressure checked twice a year."
3. "I need to make sure my child wears short sleeves when outside."
4. "I need to make sure my child eats foods rich in potassium."

64. 4. Children should eat foods rich in potassium to replace what is lost through diuresis while taking furosemide. Parents should take their child to the bathroom often if he is toilet trained to prevent accidents. Blood pressure should be checked regularly and sun protection utilized.

CN: Physiological integrity; CNS: Pharmacological and parenteral therapies; CL: Apply

65. An infant with infant with neonatal bronchopulmonary dysplasia has been on a ventilator for eight weeks. The pulmonologist has just informed the parents that the child will require a tracheostomy? What is the **most** likely cause of the tracheostomy?
1. Increased risk of tracheomalacia
2. Inability to wean from the ventilator
3. Need to allow for gastrostomy tube feedings
4. Increased signs of respiratory distress

65. 2. Tracheostomy may be required after a child has been ventilator dependent for six to eight weeks and is unable to wean from the ventilator. This will allow for oral feedings and reduce the risks of tracheomalacia and bronchomalacia.

CN: Physiological integrity; CNS: Physiological adaptation; CL: Analyze

66. A one-year-old infant with neonatal bronchopulmonary dysplasia (chronic lung disease) has just received a tracheostomy. What is the **most** appropriate nursing intervention?
1. Keep extra tracheostomy tubes at the bedside
2. Secure ties at the side of the neck for easy access
3. Change the tracheostomy tube 2 weeks after surgery
4. Secure the tracheostomy ties tightly to prevent dislodgment of the tube

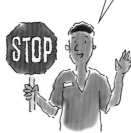

Ask yourself what you would need if the worst occurred.

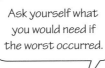

66. 1. Extra tracheostomy tubes should be kept at the bedside in case of an emergency, including one size smaller in case the appropriate size doesn't fit due to edema, or lack of a tract formation. Ties are usually placed at the back of the neck. The ties should be placed securely but should allow the width of a little finger for room to prevent excessive pressure or skin breakdown. The first tracheostomy tube change is usually performed by the health care provider after seven days.

CN: Physiological integrity; CNS: Reduction of risk potential; CL: Apply

---

CN: Client needs category   CNS: Client needs subcategory   CL: Cognitive level

67. An 11-month-old infant with neonatal bronchopulmonary dysplasia (chronic lung disease), and a tracheostomy, experiences a decline in oxygen saturation from 97% to 88%. The infant appears anxious with a heart rate of 180 bpm. Which nursing intervention is **most** appropriate?
  1. Change the tracheostomy tube
  2. Suction the tracheostomy tube
  3. Obtain an arterial blood gas (ABG) level
  4. Increase the oxygen flow rate

67. 2. Tracheostomy tubes, particularly in small children, require frequent suctioning to remove mucus plugs and excessive secretions. The tracheostomy tube can be changed if suctioning is unsuccessful. Obtaining an ABG level may be beneficial if oxygen saturation remains low and the child appears to be in respiratory distress. Increasing the oxygen flow rate will only help if the airway is patent.
CN: Physiological integrity; CNS: Reduction of risk potential; CL: Analyze

68. Which nursing intervention is appropriate when suctioning a tracheostomy tube?
  1. Hyperventilate the child before suctioning
  2. Repeat the suctioning process for two intervals
  3. Insert the catheter 1 to 2 cm below the tracheostomy tube
  4. Inject a small amount of normal saline solution into the tube before suctioning

68. 1. The child should be hyperventilated before and after suctioning to prevent hypoxia. Injecting a small amount of normal saline solution to help loosen secretions for easier aspiration is no longer recommended as it damages bronchial surfactant. It can also flush particles into the lower respiratory tract and increase bacterial colonization. Hydrating the client is the best way to liquefy secretions. The suctioning process should be repeated until the trachea is clear, generally it may clear in 2-3 passes If the catheter is inserted too far, it will irritate the carina and may cause blood-tinged secretions. The catheter should be inserted 0.5 cm beyond the tracheostomy tube.
CN: Physiological integrity; CNS: Reduction of risk potential; CL: Apply

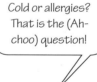

Cold or allergies? That is the (Ah-choo) question!

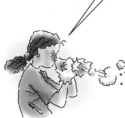

69. A parent asks the nurse which characteristic distinguishes allergies from colds. What is the nurse's **best** response?
  1. Allergies and colds often have the same symptoms.
  2. Colds can be accompanied by high fever.
  3. Allergies can cause itching of the eyes and nose.
  4. Colds can last longer than allergies.

69. 1. The body reacts in the same way to both allergies and colds and they often have the same symptoms. Colds are occasionally accompanied by low grade fever. Fever is rare with allergies. Colds tend to last 7 to 14 days, while allergies may last many months depending on exposure to the allergen.
CN: Health promotion and maintenance; CNS: None; CL: Apply

70. A two-year old with pneumonia is placed on oxygen. Which is the **priority** nursing action?
  1. Humidify the oxygen
  2. Continually monitor oxygen saturation
  3. Avoid the use of equipment or toys that can produce sparks
  4. Keep the face mask as tight fitting as possible

70. 3. While all the interventions are appropriate for caring for a child on oxygen, preventing a fire is the priority. All equipment and toys that may produce a spark should be avoided.
CN: Safe, effective care environment; CNS: Management of care; CL: Analyze

71. A two-year-old child has been diagnosed with asthma. Which are common asthma triggers? Select all that apply.
1. Weather
2. Food allergies
3. Gastrointestinal illness
4. One parent with asthma
5. Cats and dogs

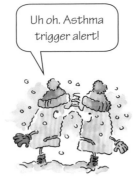

Uh oh. Asthma trigger alert!

71. 1, 3, 5. Triggers are substances, weather conditions, or activities that are harmless to most people, but can lead to coughing, wheezing, and shortness of breath in those with asthma. Excessively cold air, wet or humid changes in weather and seasons, and air pollution are some of the most common asthma triggers. Household pets are also a trigger. Evidence suggests that asthma is partly hereditary in nature but it is not a trigger for attack. Food allergens are rarely responsible for airway reactions in children. Respiratory illness such as colds or influenza can also trigger an exacerbation although other types of illness do not.
CN: Physiological integrity; CNS: Physiological adaptation; CL: Apply

72. The nurse is assessing breath sounds of a child admitted to the unit. Based on the progress notes, which respiratory illness would the nurse suspect?

Progress notes	
10/15/16 2030	Seven-year-old child admitted from ER. Oxygen via mask at 4 L/min. Frequent, tight cough. A/Ox3. Shortness of breath noted while talking to mom. HEENT normal. Lungs with wheezing in bases. Heart RRR, no murmur. Abdomen soft, flat. Active bowel sounds. Moving all extremities well.

1. Pneumonia
2. Croup
3. Pulmonary Edema
4. Asthma

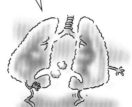

All this wheezing! What's wrong with us?

72. 4. Asthma frequently presents with wheezing and coughing. Airway inflammation and edema increase mucous production. Other signs include dyspnea, tachycardia, and tachypnea. Stridor is heard in croup. Rhonchi and rales are heard with pneumonia and pulmonary edema.
CN: Physiological integrity; CNS: Physiological adaptation; CL: Apply

73. Which circumstance places a child at increased risk for an asthma-related death?
1. One emergency department visit eight months ago
2. One hospital admission for asthma last year
3. Two prior admissions to the general pediatric floor years ago
4. One prior admission to an intensive care unit for asthma

73. 4. Asthma results in varying degrees of respiratory distress. A prior admission to an intensive care unit marks an increased severity and need of immediate therapy. Two or more hospitalizations for asthma, a recent hospitalization or emergency department visit in the past month, or three or more emergency department visits in the past year put a child at high risk for asthma-related death.
CN: Physiological integrity; CNS: Reduction of risk potential; CL: Analyze

74. Which characteristic of status asthmaticus distinguishes it from asthma?
1. Several asthma attacks per month
2. Little or no response to corticosteroids
3. Little response to bronchodilators
4. Constant asthmatic state unrelieved by bronchodilators

75. A two-year-old child with status asthmaticus is admitted to the pediatric unit and begins to receive continuous treatment with albuterol, given by nebulizer. For which clinical manifestation should the nurse watch?
1. Bradycardia
2. Lethargy
3. Tachycardia
4. Tachypnea

76. A 10-year-old child is admitted with asthma. The health care provider orders a methylprednisolone loading dose of 3 mg/kg. The child weighs 30 kg. It comes as a solution of 40 mg/ml. How many milliliters should the child receive? Record your answer using two decimal places.

_____ ml

77. Oral methylprednisolone was recently started for a 10-year-old client with asthma. He begins to vomit and reports that his stomach hurts. Which nursing intervention is appropriate?
1. Check the methylprednisolone level
2. Call the health care provider to decrease the dose
3. Take no action; methylprednisolone can cause nausea
4. Call the health care provider to change the medication form to IV.

78. A nurse is preparing to obtain an arterial blood gas specimen from a child, and plans to perform the Allen's test. Prioritize the nurse's actions to perform this test.

| 1. Apply pressure over the ulnar and radial arteries |
| 2. Ask the child to clench the fist |
| 3. Assess the color of the extremity distal to the pressure point |
| 4. Release pressure from the ulnar artery |
| 5. Explain the procedure to the child and parents |

CN: Client needs category   CNS: Client needs subcategory   CL: Cognitive level

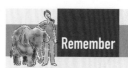

"Bronchodilators open (dilate) the airways (bronchioles)."

Bronchodilators, such as albuterol, are used to dilate the bronchioles and thereby relieve breathing disorders such as asthma.

Bronchodilators
- Albuterol
- Ephedrine
- Formoterol
- Levalbuterol
- Metaproterenol
- Pirbuterol
- Salmeterol
- Terbutaline

74. 4. Status asthmaticus can best be described as constant and unrelieved by bronchodilators. Moderate asthma is characterized by several attacks per month. Little or no response to bronchodilators or corticosteroids would describe severe asthma.
CN: Physiological integrity; CNS: Physiological adaptation; CL: Apply

75. 3. Albuterol is a rapid-acting bronchodilator. Common adverse effects include tachycardia, nervousness, tremors, insomnia, irritability, and headache.
CN: Physiological integrity; CNS: Pharmacological and parenteral therapies; CL: Apply

76. **2.25.**
The child should receive 90 mg per dose. Here are the calculations:

$$3\,mg/kg \times 30\,kg = 90\,mg$$

$$90\,mg/dose \div 40\,mg/ml = 2.25\,ml/dose$$

CN: Physiological integrity; CNS: Pharmacological and parenteral therapies; CL: Apply

77. 4. Nausea and GI upset are adverse effects of methylprednisolone. The treatment of asthma requires treatment of the inflammation that is a hallmark of the disease. If the child cannot tolerate oral corticosteroids, an IV dose is warranted.
CN: Physiological integrity; CNS: Pharmacological and parenteral therapies; CL: Analyze

78. **Ordered Response:**

| 5. Explain the procedure to the child and parents |
| 2. Ask the child to clench the fist |
| 1. Apply pressure over the ulnar and radial arteries |
| 4. Release pressure from the ulnar artery |
| 3. Assess the color of the extremity distal to the pressure point |

CN: Physiological integrity; CNS: Reduction of risk potential; CL: Apply

79. The nurse is caring for a client with atelectasis. What is the nurse's **most** important intervention?
1. Implement chest physiotherapy
2. Give increased IV fluids
3. Administer oxygen
4. Obtain arterial blood gas (ABG) levels

79. 1. Chest physiotherapy and incentive spirometry help to enhance the clearance of mucus and open the alveoli. Intravenous and oral fluids are recommended to help liquefy and thin secretions. Administration of oxygen will not give enough pressure to open the alveoli. Obtaining ABG levels would not assist in resolving the atelectasis.
CN: Physiological integrity; CNS: Physiological adaptation; CL: Apply

80. A 10-year-old child was recently diagnosed with asthma. Her parents ask if she can continue to play sports. What is the nurse's **best** response?
1. "Sports don't cause asthma attacks."
2. "You should limit activities to quiet play."
3. "It's okay to play some sports, but swimming isn't recommended."
4. "Physical activity and sports are encouraged, provided the asthma is under control."

80. 4. Participation in sports is encouraged but should be evaluated on an individual basis if the asthma is under control. Exercise-induced asthma is an example of the airway hyperactivity common to asthmatics. Swimming is well tolerated due to the style of breathing involved, and moisture in the air. Exclusion from sports or activities may hamper peer interaction.
CN: Physiological integrity; CNS: Physiological adaptation; CL: Apply

81. The nurse admits a school-aged child to the emergency department. The child has a respiratory rate of 52 and is in acute respiratory distress. What action will the nurse take **first**?
1. Take a full medical history
2. Give a bronchodilator by nebulizer
3. Apply a cardiac monitor to the child
4. 4 Provide emotional support to the child and family

81. 3. A client in respiratory distress needs to have cardiac monitoring placed immediately followed by oxygen administration. The other interventions follow this initial action.
CN: Physiological integrity; CNS: Physiological adaptation; CL: Apply

82. A nurse is caring for a two-year-old client with asthma. What is the **most** appropriate nursing intervention for this client?
1. Give warm liquids
2. Give cold juice or ice pops
3. Provide three meals and three snacks
4. Give IV fluid boluses

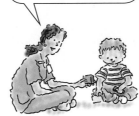

Keep this client's age in mind when answering question 82.

82. 1. Liquids are best tolerated if they are warm. Cold liquids may cause bronchospasm and should be avoided. Dehydration should be corrected slowly. Small, frequent meals should be provided to avoid abdominal distention that may interfere with diaphragm excursion. Over hydration may increase interstitial pulmonary fluid and exacerbate small airway obstruction.
CN: Physiological integrity; CNS: Physiological adaptation; CL: Apply

83. Which intervention, by the parents, is appropriate to "allergy proof" the home?
1. Cover floors with carpeting
2. Designate the basement as the play area
3. Dust and clean the house thoroughly twice a month
4. Use foam rubber pillows and synthetic blankets

83. 4. Bedding should be free from allergens with hypoallergenic covers. Unnecessary rugs should be removed, and floors should be bare, and mopped a few times a week to reduce dust. Basements or cellars should be avoided to decrease the child's exposure to molds and mildew. Dusting and cleaning should occur daily or at least weekly.
CN: Physiological integrity; CNS: Physiological adaptation; CL: Apply

CN: Client needs category   CNS: Client needs subcategory   CL: Cognitive level

84. The nurse is preparing to discharge a client with asthma. Which intervention is **most** important for the nurse to perform prior to discharge?
1. Obtain additional equipment and medication that can be provided at the school
2. Arrange for a thorough, deep cleaning of the home
3. Discuss appropriate sports activities that the child can be involved in
4. Counsel the family in making arrangements to remove the family pet

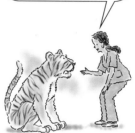

Sorry, Fluffy. Your dander is an asthma trigger. We're going to need to make some changes.

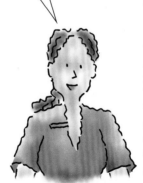

Consider the pathology of bronchiolitis when answering question 86.

84. 1. The child needs to have equipment and medication available at school to treat and prevent asthma attacks. A discussion should be held with the child and family to motivate the child to be involved in as many normal childhood activities as possible. The house should be kept as clean as possible to prevent exacerbations due to dust and pet dander. If the child is allergic to the family pet, the nurse should provide counseling on ways to minimize the risks.
CN: Physiological integrity; CNS: Reduction of risk potential; CL: Apply

85. A nurse is explaining bronchiolitis to the parents of an infant admitted with the condition. What is the **best** information for the nurse to provide?
1. Bronchiolitis is a seasonal viral illness that causes inflammation and obstruction of the small airways.
2. Bronchiolitis causes decreased mucus secretion which causes air trapping and lobular collapse.
3. Bronchiolitis affects premature infants because they lack surfactant.
4. Bronchiolitis is caused by a bacteria that causes epithelial necrosis and damage to the cilia.

85. 1. Bronchiolitis is an infection of the bronchioles, usually caused by a viral infection, most commonly respiratory syncytial virus (RSV). The airways become inflamed, swell and fill with mucus, which can make breathing difficult. It is common in premature infants as a result of their weakened immune systems.
CN: Physiological integrity; CNS: Physiological adaptation; CL: Apply

86. The nurse in the emergency department is caring for a toddler with a preliminary diagnosis of bronchiolitis. Which signs and symptoms should this nurse anticipate during his assessment? Select all that apply.
1. Heart rate of 157
2. Temperature of 101.8° F (38.7° C)
3. Subcostal retractions
4. Poor feeding
5. Diarrhea

86. 3, 4. In bronchiolitis, the bronchioles become narrowed and edematous. This can cause wheezing and retractions. Children will typically have a two- to three-day history of an upper respiratory infection and feeding difficulties with loss of appetite due to nasal congestion and increased trouble breathing. This combination leads to respiratory distress with tachypnea and tachycardia. There is typically a low-grade or no fever with bronchiolitis. Bronchiolitis affects the respiratory tract, not the GI tract.
CN: Physiological integrity; CNS: Physiological adaptation; CL: Apply

87. The nurse is teaching the parents of a seven-month-old child with respiratory syncytial virus (RSV) bronchiolitis. Which statement, by the parents, would **best** indicate understanding of this infection?
1. "RSV bronchiolitis infections usually just cause a bad cold in people."
2. "RSV bronchiolitis infections occur mostly in the fall."
3. "RSV bronchiolitis infections usually only affect preterm infants."
4. "RSV bronchiolitis infections are spread primarily through indirect contact."

87. 1. RSV bronchiolitis infections typically cause cold-like symptoms in people, but can cause severe respiratory illness in infants, especially preterm infants, young children, and the elderly. RSV bronchiolitis is spread through contact with infected droplets and through direct and indirect contact with infected secretions in the environment. The virus is most prevalent in the winter and early spring months.
CN: Physiological integrity; CNS: Physiological adaptation; CL: Apply

88. A student nurse asks the nurse if any precautions are needed when caring for a two-month-old infant with respiratory syncytial virus (RSV) to prevent the spread of infection. What is the nurse's **best** response?
1. Gloves only
2. Gown, gloves, and mask
3. Standard precautions only
4. Proper hand washing between clients

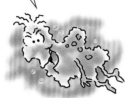

You better take precautions if you want to avoid the likes of me.

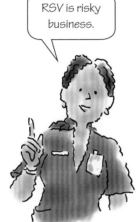

88. 2. RSV is highly contagious, and is spread through direct and indirect contact with infectious secretions via hands, droplets, and fomites. Gowns and gloves should be worn for client care to prevent the spread of infection. Masks should be used, as RSV is easily spread through infected droplets. Proper hand washing, and standard precautions, are essential in all cases to prevent the spread of germs.
CN: Safe, effective care environment; CNS: Safety and infection control; CL: Apply

89. The nurse is preparing a child and family for a nasopharyngeal wash to obtain a specimen. Which statement, by the nurse, would be **most** accurate in explaining this procedure? Select all that apply
1. The child will need to be held still for this procedure.
2. Nasal secretions are aspirated after 3 ml of saline is instilled in each nostril.
3. Nasal secretions are suctioned out of each nostril.
4. The procedure will take only a few minutes.
5. The child will not be able to eat until the gag reflex is assessed.

89. 2. RSV can only be diagnosed with direct aspiration of nasal secretions or nasopharyngeal washings. Positive identification is accomplished using the enzyme-linked immunosorbent assay. The child can be held on the parent's lap or swaddled tightly. Secretions can be obtained using a bulb syringe and should only take a few minutes. Blood, throat, and sputum cultures can't definitively diagnose RSV. The child is not sedated for the test. It is not necessary to test the reflex.
CN: Physiological integrity; CNS: Physiological adaptation; CL: Apply

RSV is risky business.

90. Which child would be at increased risk for a respiratory syncytial virus (RSV) infection?
1. A two-month-old child managed at home
2. A two-month-old child with neonatal bronchopulmonary dysplasia (chronic lung disease)
3. A three-month-old child requiring low-flow oxygen
4. A two-year-old child

90. 2. Infants with cardiac or pulmonary conditions are at highest risk for RSV. Because of their underlying conditions, they usually require mechanical ventilation. Many infants can be managed at home. A three-month-old infant on low-flow oxygen has some risks of progression but is not at a high risk. A two-year-old child has built up the immune system, and can tolerate the infection without major problems.
CN: Physiological integrity; CNS: Reduction of risk potential; CL: Analyze

91. The nurse is preparing discharge plans for the parents of an infant born at 24 weeks' gestation. What **priority** information should the nurse tell these parents regarding vaccinations for their child?
1. Routine vaccines should occur for all babies, regardless of prematurity.
2. Palivizumab should be given to prevent RSV infection in preterm infants.
3. An extra dose of certain vaccines will need to be given to preterm infants.
4. There are some specific contraindications to vaccines for preterm infants.

91. 2. Palivizumab is a monoclonal antibody against the RSV F glycoprotein. It can help to prevent serious lower respiratory tract infections caused by RSV. The first dose is given before RSV season, with monthly doses given throughout the season for protection. This agent is indicated for children with neonatal bronchopulmonary dysplasia (chronic lung disease), who are younger than 24 months of age, who have a history of prematurity (less than 35 weeks), or who have hemodynamically significant congenital heart disease. Routine vaccines are given based on chronological age not corrected age. There are no specific contraindications based on prematurity alone. Certain vaccines such as Hepatitis B may need an extra dose depending on the age or weight of the child at the time of the vaccine. While all the answers are correct, answer two is the priority to include in parent teaching.
CN: Health promotion and maintenance; CNS: Reduction of risk potential; CL: Apply

CN: Client needs category   CNS: Client needs subcategory   CL: Cognitive level

92. What area of the chest would the nurse monitor for suprasternal retractions in an infant diagnosed with bronchiolitis?

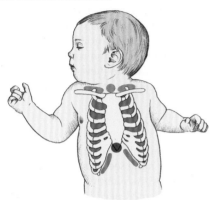

92. Suprasternal retractions can be noted in a child who is experiencing severe respiratory distress, secondary to airway obstruction found with bronchiolitis. The nurse should take measures to prevent worsening distress and possible respiratory failure.

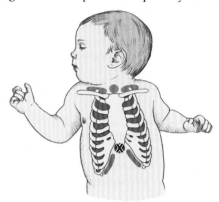

CN: Physiological integrity; CNS: Physiological adaptation
CL: Apply

93. The nurse is planning care for an infant with bronchiolitis who requires monitoring for dehydration. What is the **most** important intervention for the nurse to provide?
1. Daily weight
2. Blood levels every four hours
3. Urinalysis every eight hours
4. Weighing each diaper

93. 1. Weight is a good indicator of hydration in infants. Accurate measurement of intake and output is essential. Weighing diapers is a way of measuring output only. Blood levels may be obtained daily or every other day. A urinalysis every eight hours is not necessary. Urine specific gravities are recommended but can be obtained with diaper changes.
CN: Physiological integrity; CNS: Physiological adaptation;
CL: Apply

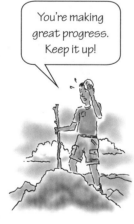

You're making great progress. Keep it up!

94. The nurse is planning care for an infant with bronchiolitis. What is the nurse's **priority** intervention for this child?
1. Position the infant with the head elevated
2. Monitor intake and output
3. Assess respiratory status frequently
4. Incorporate parents into the child's care

94. 3. Infants with bronchiolitis will have impaired gas exchange related to bronchiolar obstruction, atelectasis, and hyperinflation. Changes in respiratory status may occur quickly as energy reserves are depleted; therefore, close monitoring is essential. Positioning the infant, monitoring fluid status and including parents in care plan are necessary, but not the priority.
CN: Physiological integrity; CNS: Physiological adaptation;
CL: Analyze

95. The nurse is teaching home care to the parents of a child with bronchiolitis. What is the **most** important information for the nurse to provide?
1. Place the child in a prone position for comfort
2. Use warm mist to replace insensible fluid loss
3. Recognize the signs of increasing respiratory distress
4. Engage the child in many activities to prevent developmental delay

95. 3. It's essential for parents to be able to recognize signs of increasing respiratory distress and know how to count the respiratory rate. The child should be positioned with the head of the bed elevated for comfort, and to facilitate removal of secretions. The use of a cool mist humidifier may help to replace insensible fluid loss. Quiet play activities are required as the child's energy level permits. An infant with bronchiolitis will show clinical improvement in three to four days; therefore, developmental delay is not an issue.
CN: Physiological integrity; CNS: Physiological adaptation;
CL: Analyze

CN: Client needs category   CNS: Client needs subcategory   CL: Cognitive level

96. The nurse is teaching the parents of a pre-school child with bacterial pneumonia about care at home. Which statement, by the parents, **best** indicates understanding?
1. "I need to give my child smaller amounts of fluid more frequently."
2. "My child should receive the pneumonia vaccine."
3. "Antibiotics are the best treatment for pneumonia."
4. "The cough should go away after 2 or 3 days."

97. The nurse is caring for an infant with bacterial pneumonia. What nursing action is **best** to prevent a fluid volume deficit?
1. Weigh the client daily
2. Assess skin turgor
3. Give small frequent feedings
4. Monitor intake and output

98. The nurse knows that a child with pneumonia is at risk for activity intolerance. What intervention is appropriate for the nurse to minimize this risk?
1. Maintain the child on bed rest
2. Group or cluster care to allow adequate rest periods
3. Allow visitors during daytime hours only
4. Monitor vital signs every two hours

99. The nurse is monitoring a child with a suspected diagnosis of pertussis. The nurse is **most** concerned when the child develops:
1. a barking cough.
2. a whooping cough.
3. a low-grade fever.
4. post-tussive emesis.

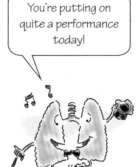

You're putting on quite a performance today!

96. 1. Children with pneumonia should be given plenty of fluids, in smaller amounts, more frequently. Antibiotics are used to treat bacterial pneumonia but are not used with viral pneumonia. The child will usually feel better within 2 to 3 days of antibiotics, however fatigue and cough may last for weeks or even months. Several vaccines may protect against pneumonia. The provider will decide if it is appropriate to give a child a pneumonia vaccination.
CN: Physiological integrity; CNS: Physiological adaptation; CL: Apply

97. 3. Giving small frequent feedings will help ensure that the infant is receiving adequate fluids. The other options will help the nurse maintain fluid balance, but they do not prevent fluid volume deficits.
CN: Physiological integrity; CNS: Physiological adaptation; CL: Apply

98. 2. Nursing care should be grouped or clustered to allow adequate periods of rest. Vital signs may need to be monitored every two hours depending on the severity of the child's illness. The child should be allowed to participate in as many age-appropriate activities as tolerated. Visitors, and especially parents, should be allowed if the child tolerates it.
CN: Physiological integrity; CNS: Physiological adaptation; CL: Apply

99. 2. Pertussis is characterized by consistent short, rapid coughs followed by a sudden inspiration with a high-pitched whooping sound. Post-tussive emesis is common. A barking cough is noted with croup. Pertussis is usually accompanied by a low-grade fever.
CN: Physiological integrity; CNS: Physiological adaptation; CL: Apply

CN: Client needs category   CNS: Client needs subcategory   CL: Cognitive level

100. A nurse is admitting a child to the unit. Based on the history, what illness would the nurse suspect?

Progress notes	
10/15/16	History and physical
1030	Nine-year-old child admitted with frequent
	cough and fever of > 100.5°F (38.1°C) for
	the past month. Child lives with parents and
	with grandparents who recently emigrated
	from SE Asia. Weight = 20 kg. Mom reports
	significant weight loss in child. Child
	reporting fatigue and poor appetite. Denies
	vomiting/diarrhea. Does have some nausea. No
	problems with voiding or stooling. Child does
	well in school.

1. Pneumonia
2. Tuberculosis
3. Asthma
4. HIV

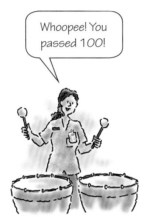

Whoopee! You passed 100!

100. 2. Tuberculosis often presents with a chronic, unremitting cough and fever lasting more than three weeks. Weight loss and fatigue are common symptoms. Risk factors include visiting or living with persons from endemic areas. Pneumonia typically does not produce significant weight loss. Asthma is not usually accompanied by fever. HIV symptoms are varied, non-specific, and seen with specific risk factors such as a mother with HIV at delivery.
CN: Physiological integrity; CNS: Physiological adaptation; CL: Analyze

101. The nurse is educating a teen while preparing to place a tuberculin (TB) skin test. What statement, by the nurse, is the **most** accurate regarding this test?
1. The test is read after a 24 hours.
2. The test is positive if the skin has an induration of 10 or more millimeters.
3. The needle is placed into the fat tissue.
4. A vaccine for TB does not affect the skin test.

101. 2. A reading of 5 to 10 mm, or greater, induration at the site indicates a positive test. The reading is of induration not erythema. It is read between 48 and 72 hours after placement. The medication is placed intradermally. Previous vaccination may sometimes cause a false positive.
CN: Health promotion and maintenance; CNS: None; CL: Apply

102. A two-year-old child has tested positive for tuberculosis (TB), and has been started on rifampin. The child's parents ask the nurse if there is any important information they should know about this medication. What important adverse effect should the nurse inform these parents about?
1. Hyperactivity
2. Orange body secretions
3. Decreased bilirubin levels
4. Decreased levels of liver enzymes

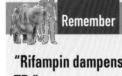

Remember

"Rifampin dampens TB."

Rifampin is an antitubercular drug that can turn urine, feces, sputum, tears, and sweat an orange color.

102. 2. Rifampin and its metabolites will turn urine, feces, sputum, tears, and sweat an orange color. This is not a serious adverse effect. Rifampin may also cause GI upset, headache, drowsiness, dizziness, visual disturbances, and fever. Liver enzyme and bilirubin levels increase because of hepatic metabolism of the drug. Parents should be taught the signs and symptoms of hepatitis and hyperbilirubinemia such as jaundice of the sclera or skin.
CN: Physiological integrity; CNS: Pharmacological and parenteral therapies; CL: Apply

103. The school nurse is providing an in-service program about dietary safety to a group of pre-school teachers and aides who care for children younger than age three. What is the **most** important information for this nurse to provide?
  1. Cut hotdogs in half
  2. Limit popcorn and peanuts
  3. Cut grapes into quarters
  4. Limit hard candy to special occasions

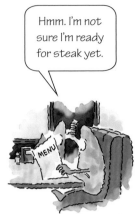

Hmm. I'm not sure I'm ready for steak yet.

104. A child is admitted with a possible occluded trachea. Which assessment findings should the nurse anticipate?
  1. Cough, dyspnea, and drooling
  2. Cough, stridor, and changes in phonation
  3. Expiratory wheeze and inspiratory stridor
  4. Cough, asymmetrical breath sounds, and wheeze

105. Which activity is recommended to prevent foreign body aspiration during meals?
  1. Insist that children are seated
  2. Give children toys to play with
  3. Allow children to watch television
  4. Allow children to eat in a separate room

106. A child is being tested for foreign body aspiration. The nurse explains to the child's parents about the diagnostic tool for this test. Which test should the nurse describe?
  1. Bronchoscopy
  2. Chest X-ray
  3. Fluoroscopy
  4. Lateral neck X-ray

107. A child with cystic fibrosis is having difficulty clearing secretions. Which nursing intervention is **most** appropriate?
  1. Implement chest physiotherapy four times per day
  2. Administer pancreatic enzymes with meals
  3. Provide oxygen by nasal cannula at all times
  4. Provide a high-calorie, high-protein diet at each meal

103. 3. Grapes, hotdogs, and sausage should be cut into many small pieces. Hard candy, raisins, popcorn, and peanuts should be avoided for children age four and younger.
CN: Physiological integrity; CNS: Reduction of risk potential; CL: Apply

104. 3. Expiratory and inspiratory noise indicates that the foreign body is lodged in the trachea. Cough, dyspnea, drooling, and gagging indicate supraglottic obstruction. A cough with stridor and changes in phonation would occur if the foreign body were in the larynx. Asymmetrical breath sounds indicate that the object may be located in the bronchi.
CN: Physiological integrity; CNS: Physiological adaptation; CL: Apply

105. 1. Children should be seated while eating. The risk of aspiration increases if the child is running, jumping, or talking with food in their mouth. Television and toys are a dangerous distraction to toddlers and young children, and should be avoided. Children need constant supervision, and should be monitored while eating snacks and meals.
CN: Safe, effective care environment; CNS: Safety and infection control; CL: Apply

106. 1. A bronchoscopy can definitively detect an obstruction, and is also the best choice for removal of the obstruction with direct visualization. A chest X-ray and lateral neck X-ray may be used, but findings vary. Some films may appear normal or show changes such as inflammation related to the presence of the foreign body. Fluoroscopy is a type of medical imaging that shows a continuous X-ray image on a monitor. Fluoroscopy may be used to guide biopsies or remove fluid from the chest or abdomen.
CN: Physiological integrity; CNS: Physiological adaptation; CL: Apply

107. 1. Chest physiotherapy should be performed to mobilize secretions so they can be more easily cleared. Pancreatic enzymes should be administered with meals to aid in digestion, but do not help clear secretions. Administering oxygen may improve oxygenation but won't help clear secretions. A high-calorie, high-protein diet is important for normal growth and development but will not aid in clearing secretions.
CN: Physiological integrity; CNS: Reduction of risk potential; CL: Apply

CN: Client needs category   CNS: Client needs subcategory   CL: Cognitive level

108. Which statement, made by the parent of a 17-month-old child with cystic fibrosis, should alert a nurse to investigate further?
1. "My child is not walking yet."
2. "My child is saying a few words and short phrases."
3. "My child doesn't interact with other children her age."
4. "My child cries when I leave the room."

108. 1. A toddler should be walking by 15 months. At 10 months, an infant holds on to furniture while walking, walks with support at 11 months, and takes her first steps at 12 months. By 12 months, a child should say a few words, with more words and short phrases being added each month. At 17 months, a child should engage in solitary play and usually has little interaction with other children. Separation anxiety is common in toddlers.
CN: Psychosocial integrity; CNS: None; CL: Analyze

109. A nurse is performing an assessment on a newborn with a delayed passage of meconium. Which condition would the nurse be **most** concerned about?
1. Duodenal atresia
2. Intussusception
3. Pyloric stenosis
4. Cystic fibrosis

109. 4. Meconium ileus is commonly a presenting sign of cystic fibrosis. Infants with duodenal atresia usually pass meconium before presenting with abdominal distention and vomiting. Intussusception is the most common cause of intestinal obstruction in infants between 6 and 36 months of age, and presents with a sudden onset of severe intermittent abdominal pain. Pyloric stenosis is characterized by the classic sign of projectile vomiting in a 3- to 6-week-old infant.
CN: Physiological integrity; CNS: Physiological adaptation; CL: Apply

110. The parents of a child with cystic fibrosis tell the nurse that they are having difficulty coping. Which intervention is **most** appropriate for a nurse to perform?
1. Reassure the parents they will learn to cope
2. Refer the parents to a cystic fibrosis support group
3. Show the parents how to perform chest physiotherapy at home
4. Tell the parents that with good medical care their child can live into adulthood

Are you starting to see the light at the end of the tunnel yet?

110. 2. Support groups can help parents cope with their child's condition, as well as provide them with accurate information on the disorder. Reassuring the family that they will learn to cope is not helpful at this time. Showing the parents how to perform chest physiotherapy is an important intervention but won't help them cope with their child's condition. With good medical care, children with cystic fibrosis can live into adulthood, but telling the parent this does not help their current coping needs.
CN: Psychosocial integrity; CNS: None; CL: Apply

111. Which intervention would the nurse perform to increase airway clearance in a toddler with cystic fibrosis?
1. Monitor oxygen saturation continuously
2. Administer albuterol before chest physiotherapy
3. Administer the influenza vaccine
4. Administer fluids

111. 2. Opening the airways with a bronchodilator prior to chest physiotherapy provides more effective airway clearance. While the other interventions are important, they do not specifically address airway clearance.
CN: Physiological integrity; CNS: Physiological adaptation; CL: Apply

112. The parents of a child with cystic fibrosis ask the nurse which diet is recommended for their child. What is the nurse's **best** response?
1. Fat restricted
2. High calorie
3. Low protein
4. Sodium restricted

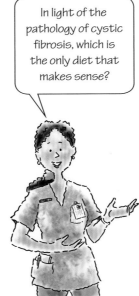

In light of the pathology of cystic fibrosis, which is the only diet that makes sense?

112. **2.** A well-balanced, high-calorie, high-protein diet is recommended for a child with cystic fibrosis due to impaired intestinal absorption. Fat restriction isn't required, because digestion and absorption of fat in the intestine are impaired. The child should usually increase enzyme intake when high-fat foods are eaten. Low-sodium foods can lead to hyponatremia; therefore, high-sodium foods are recommended, especially during hot weather or when the child has a fever.
CN: Physiological integrity; CNS: Basic care and comfort; CL: Apply

113. Which statement concerning pancreatic enzymes, for a cystic fibrosis client, is correct?
1. Capsules may not be opened.
2. Microcapsules can be crushed.
3. The client should be encouraged to eat throughout the day.
4. The client should have enzymes administered at each meal and with snacks.

113. **4.** Enzymes are administered with each feeding, meal, and snack to optimize absorption of the nutrients consumed. Regular capsules may be opened and the contents mixed with a small amount of applesauce or other nonalkaline food. Microcapsules cannot be crushed due to the enteric coating. Eating throughout the day should be discouraged. Three meals, and two or three snacks per day are recommended.
CN: Physiological integrity; CNS: Physiological adaptation; CL: Apply

114. Which information on nutrition should the nurse include in a family's teaching plan for their child with cystic fibrosis?
1. Provide a high-calorie, high-protein diet
2. Place the child on a daily 1,200 ml fluid restriction
3. Restrict daily intake of sodium to 1.5 g/day
4. Provide adequate amounts of fat-soluble vitamins

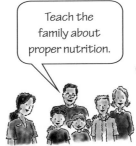

Teach the family about proper nutrition.

114. **1.** To promote growth and development, the child should eat a high-calorie, high-protein diet. The child with cystic fibrosis should also be encouraged to consume higher than usual amounts of fluids and sodium. Malabsorption of fat soluble vitamins is likely in most clients with CF, particularly those who are pancreatic insufficient
CN: Physiological integrity; CNS: Basic care and comfort; CL: Apply

115. A nurse is caring for a client with cystic fibrosis. Ranitidine 4 mg/kg/day q12h is ordered. The child weighs 20 kg. The medication comes as a syrup of 15 mg/ml. How many milliliters are given per dose? Record your answer using one decimal place.

_____ ml

115. 2.7.
The child should receive 40 mg per dose. Here are the calculations:

$$40\,mg/dose \div 15\,mg/ml = 2.7\,ml/dose$$

CN: Physiological integrity; CNS: Pharmacological and parenteral therapies; CL: Apply

116. Which nursing intervention is appropriate for the care of the child with cystic fibrosis?
1. Decrease exercise and limit physical activity
2. Administer cough suppressants and antihistamines
3. Implement chest physiotherapy two to four times per day
4. Administer bronchodilator or nebulizer treatments after chest physiotherapy

116. 3. Chest physiotherapy is recommended two to four times per day to help loosen and move secretions to facilitate expectoration. Exercise and physical activity are recommended to stimulate mucous secretion and to establish a good, habitual breathing pattern. Cough suppressants and antihistamines are contraindicated. The goal is for the child to be able to cough and expectorate mucous secretions. Bronchodilator or nebulizer treatments are given before chest physiotherapy to help open the bronchi for easier expectoration.
CN: Safe, effective care environment; CNS: Management of care; CL: Apply

117. The parents of a child with cystic fibrosis are planning to have a second child. Which statement is appropriate for the nurse to make?
1. Genetic counseling is recommended.
2. There's a 50% chance the child will not have cystic fibrosis.
3. There's a 50% chance the child will have cystic fibrosis.
4. There's a 25% chance the child will only be a carrier.

117. 1. Genetic counseling should be recommended. Cystic fibrosis is an autosomal-recessive disease. Therefore, there is a 25% chance of the child having the disease, a 25% chance the child will have cystic fibrosis, and a 50% chance that the child will carry the disease.
CN: Health promotion and maintenance; CNS: None; CL: Apply

118. Parents ask the nurse about the cause of their child's cystic fibrosis. Which statement **best** describes this autosomal-recessive disorder?
1. The genetic disorder is carried on the X chromosome.
2. Both parents must pass the defective gene or set of genes.
3. Only one defective gene or set of genes is passed by one parent.
4. The disorder is due to an extra chromosome.

118. 2. In recessive disorders such as cystic fibrosis, both parents must pass the defective gene, or set of genes, to the child. Sex-linked genetic disorders are carried on the X chromosome. Dominant disorders are characterized by only one defective gene, or set of genes, passed by one parent. An extra chromosome is called trisomy. Common trisomies include Down's syndrome or Klinefelter's syndrome.
CN: Physiological integrity; CNS: Physiological adaptation; CL: Apply

119. The nurse enters the room of a three-year-old child to administer an antibiotic elixir. The child turns up his nose, refuses the medicine and says, "that medicine is yucky." What is the nurse's **best** response?
1. "Do you want to take the medicine with vanilla ice cream or chocolate ice cream?"
2. "If you don't take the medicine, I will tell your mother."
3. "The health care provider says you must take the medicine."
4. "You need to take this medicine to get better."

119. 1. Offering a choice provides the child with some control. Threatening to tell the child's mother won't help, and erodes any trust between the child and nurse. Telling the child that the health care provider says he must take the medication also is not helpful. At age three, children use concrete thinking. Trying to reason with the child at this age will not be successful..
CN: Psychosocial integrity; CNS: None; CL: Analyze

120. Ceftazidime has been ordered for a client with cystic fibrosis. The order states to give 40 mg/kg q8h. The child is two years old and weighs 38 lb 5 oz (17.5 kg). How many milligrams of the ceftazidime should be given in one dose?
1. 116
2. 233
3. 260
4. 466

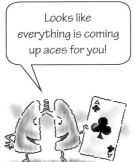

Looks like everything is coming up aces for you!

120. 2. The child should receive 233 mg per dose. Here are the calculations:

$$40\,mg/kg \times 17.5\,kg = 700\,mg$$
$$24\,hr/8\,hr = 3\,doses$$
$$700\,mg/3\,doses = 233\,mg/dose$$

CN: Physiological integrity; CNS: Pharmacological and parenteral therapies; CL: Apply

121. A child with cystic fibrosis is placed on an oral antibiotic to be given in four equally divided doses per day for 14 days. Which time schedule is **most** appropriate?
1. 8 am, 12 pm, 4 pm, 8 pm
2. 8 am, 2 pm, 8 pm, 2 am
3. 9 am, 1 pm, 5 pm, 9 pm
4. 10 am, 2 pm, 6 pm, 10 pm

121. 2. The doses should be given routinely every six hours. This helps maintain a therapeutic blood level of the antibiotic. The other answers have doses only every four hours during the day and no doses for 12 hours at night.

CN: Physiological integrity; CNS: Pharmacological and parenteral therapies; CL: Analyze

122. Which nursing action would the nurse perform to prevent the **most** serious complication of cystic fibrosis?
1. Give enzyme replacements as ordered
2. Implement chest physiotherapy
3. Monitor growth and nutritional status
4. Practice good hand hygiene techniques

122. 2. Pulmonary obstruction related to thickened mucous secretions is the most serious complication, and can lead to a progressive pulmonary disturbance and secondary infections that can lead to death. Rectal prolapse is managed with enzyme replacement therapy. Gastroesophageal reflux can be managed with monitoring, medications and proper reflux precautions. Proper hand hygiene techniques should be used for all clients to minimize the risk of infection.

CN: Physiological integrity; CNS: Physiological adaptation; CL: Analyze

123. Which is the **best** method of evaluation for a six-year-old child with cystic fibrosis who has been placed on an aerosol inhaler?
1. Ask if the parents have any questions
2. Ask if the child can explain the procedure
3. Ask the parents if they understand the usage
4. Ask the client to perform a return demonstration

123. 4. A return demonstration is the best evaluation. The parents should understand how the inhaler should be used, and ask questions, but the child must be able to correctly demonstrate usage first. The child may have difficulty explaining the procedure at age six.

CN: Physiological integrity; CNS: Pharmacological and parenteral therapies; CL: Apply

124. Which intervention is appropriate for a two-year-old client with chest trauma, who has a left lower chest tube in place?
1. Strip or milk the tubing
2. Change the required routine dressings
3. Clamp the chest tube during transport
4. Inspect tubing for kinks or obstructions

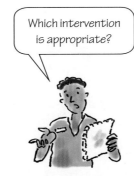

Which intervention is appropriate?

124. 4. Tubing should be inspected for kinks or obstructions so that drainage can flow freely. Manipulation of the tubing should be avoided. The pressure created from stripping the tubing can damage the pleural space or mediastinum. There is no need for routine dressing changes if the dressing isn't soiled, and there's no evidence of infection. The area around the dressing should be routinely inspected. The chest tube should never be clamped because it may lead to a tension pneumothorax. Water seal will protect the client during transit.

CN: Physiological integrity; CNS: Physiological adaptation; CL: Apply

125. A toddler in respiratory distress is admitted to the pediatric intensive care unit. When he refuses to keep his oxygen face mask on, his mother tries to help. Which action by a nurse is **most** appropriate?
1. Give the child his favorite toy to play with
2. Have the mother read the child's favorite book to him
3. Administer a strong sedative so the child will sleep
4. Tell the child that the face mask will help him breathe better

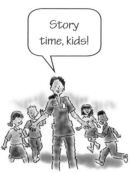

Story time, kids!

125. 2. Having the mother read the child's favorite book will ease his anxiety and provide comfort. Although giving the child a favorite toy is appropriate, the child needs his mother's comfort because the face mask is frightening. Sedation is contraindicated because it can mask signs of respiratory distress. A toddler is too young to understand that something will make him feel better.
CN: Safe, effective care environment; CNS: Management of care; CL: Apply

126. The nurse is performing discharge teaching for a school-aged child who experienced an asthma attack. What is the **most** important information the nurse can provide this client about the prescription for budesonide?
1. Use the medication before using a bronchodilator.
2. This medication is used for acute asthma attacks.
3. There is no need to use a spacer when taking this medication.
4. Rinse the mouth after using this medication.

126. 4. Oral candidiasis or thrush (a fungal infection of the throat) may occur in 1 in 25 persons who use budesonide without a spacer device on the inhaler. The risk is even higher with large doses, but is less in children than in adults. The child should be instructed to rinse the mouth after use and parents should be instructed to monitor the child's mouth for this. The medication should be given after using a bronchodilator to ensure maximum effectiveness.. Corticosteroids should not be used for acute asthma attacks.
CN: Physiological integrity; CNS: Pharmacological and parenteral therapies; CL: Apply

127. A six-year-old with a history of asthma is being evaluated by an allergist. The allergist orders skin testing to be done at the next visit. Which action, by a nurse, will help ensure accurate skin testing results?
1. Making sure the child doesn't have a runny nose
2. Making sure the child hasn't received antihistamines in the past seven days
3. Using the child's posterior legs for testing
4. Limiting testing to environmental allergens

127. 2. Antihistamines may alter results of skin testing and should be withheld for at least one week prior to testing. A runny nose won't alter test results. The forearm and upper back are the best sites for allergy testing. Testing only for environmental allergens precludes a diagnosis of allergies to other substances.
CN: Physiological integrity; CNS: Pharmacological and parenteral therapies; CL: Apply

128. A child received an allergy shot at 4:00 pm. At 5:00 pm the nurse evaluates the child. Which sign should alert the nurse that this child is experiencing a potentially life-threatening complication?
1. Urinary output less than 30 ml/hr
2. Heart rate of 58/bpm
3. Blood pressure of 82/48 mmHg
4. Rash

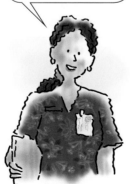

Hint: Start by thinking of life-threatening complications.

128. 3. Anaphylaxis can cause hypotension and tachycardia. Urinary urgency and incontinence, not anuria, may also be reported. A rash may signal an allergic reaction, but not as severe as anaphylaxis.
CN: Physiological integrity; CNS: Physiological adaptation; CL: Analyze

129. The nurse is caring for a 17-year-old female client with cystic fibrosis who has questions about the consequences of the disease. Which statements about the course of cystic fibrosis are true? Select all that apply.
1. Breast development is frequently delayed.
2. The client is at risk for developing diabetes.
3. Pregnancy and childbearing are not affected.
4. Normal sexual relationships can be expected.
5. Only males carry the gene for the disease.
6. By age 20, the client should be able to decrease the frequency of respiratory treatment.

129. **1, 2, 4.** Cystic fibrosis delays growth and the onset of puberty. Children with cystic fibrosis tend to be smaller than average size, and develop secondary sex characteristics later in life. In addition, clients with cystic fibrosis are at risk for developing diabetes mellitus because the pancreatic duct becomes obstructed as pancreatic tissues are destroyed. Clients with cystic fibrosis can expect to have normal sexual relationships, but fertility becomes difficult because thick secretions obstruct the cervix and block sperm entry. Both men and women carry the gene for cystic fibrosis. Pulmonary disease commonly progresses as the client ages, requiring additional respiratory treatment.
CN: Physiological integrity; CNS: Physiological adaptation; CL: Analyze

130. A nurse is preparing to administer the first dose of tobramycin to an adolescent with cystic fibrosis. The order is for 3 mg/kg IV daily in three divided doses. The client weighs 110 lb (50 kg). How many milligrams should the nurse administer per dose? Record your answer using a whole number.

_____ mg

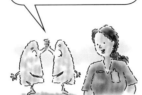

Uh oh. Looks like they squeezed in one last math question here. You can do it!

130. **50.**
To perform this dosage calculation, the nurse should calculate the client's daily dose using this formula:

$$50 \, kg \times 3 mg/kg = 150 \, mg$$

The nurse then should calculate the divided dose:

$$150 mg/3 \, doses = 50 mg/dose$$

CN: Physiological integrity; CNS: Pharmacological and parenteral therapies; CL: Apply

131. A parent is planning to enroll her nine-month-old infant in a day care. She asks the nurse what indicators would ensure that the daycare facility is adhering to good infection control measures. How should the nurse reply? Select all that apply.
1. The facility keeps boxes of gloves in the director's office.
2. Diapers are discarded into covered receptacles.
3. Toys are kept on the floor for the children to share.
4. Disposable papers are used on the diaper-changing surfaces.
5. Facilities for hand hygiene are located in every classroom.
6. Soiled clothing and cloth diapers are sent home in labeled paper bags.

131. **2, 4, 5.** A parent can assess a daycare facility's infection control measures by appraising the steps taken to prevent the spread of potential diseases. Placing diapers in covered receptacles, covering the diaper-changing surfaces with disposable papers, and ensuring that there are hand sanitizers and sinks available for personnel to wash their hands after activities are all good indicators that infection control measures are being followed. Gloves should be readily available to personnel and, should be kept in every room. Typically, toys are shared by numerous children; however, this contributes to the spread of germs and infections. All soiled clothing and cloth diapers should be placed in a sealed plastic bag prior to being sent home.
CN: Safe, effective care environment; CNS: Safety and infection control; CL: Apply

CN: Client needs category   CNS: Client needs subcategory   CL: Cognitive level

132. Which nursing intervention is **most** appropriate when caring for an infant with neonatal bronchopulmonary dysplasia (chronic lung disease)?
1. Provide frequent playful stimuli
2. Decrease oxygen during feedings
3. Place the infant on a set schedule
4. Place the infant in an open crib

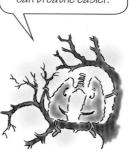

You finished Chapter 29! Now you can breathe easier.

132. 3. Timing care activities with rest periods to avoid fatigue, and decreasing respiratory effort is essential. Early stimulation activities are recommended, but the infant will have limited tolerance for them because of the illness. Oxygen is usually increased during feedings to help decrease respiratory and energy requirements. Thermoregulation is important because both hypothermia and hyperthermia will increase oxygen consumption, and may increase oxygen requirements. These infants are usually maintained on warmer beds or inside isolettes.

CN: Safe, effective care environment; CNS: Management of care; CL: Apply

CN: Client needs category   CNS: Client needs subcategory   CL: Cognitive level

Chapter 30

Neurosensory Disorders

Here are two Web sites you can check for more information about neurosensory disorders in children: **www.add.org** (Attention Deficit Disorder Association) and **www.ndss. org** (National Down Syndrome Society).

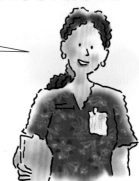

1. A mother of a three-year-old with a myelomeningocele is considering having another baby. She asks the nurse if she should make any changes in her diet. What is the nurse's **best** response?

 1. Increase folic acid to 0.4 mg/day
 2. Increase folic acid to 4 mg/day
 3. Increase vitamin B$_{12}$ to 0.4 mg/day
 4. Increase vitamin B$_{12}$ to 4 mg/day

Remember

"Folic acid axes neural tube defects."

Pregnant women are planning to get pregnant are advised to increase folic acid intake to 4 mg/day 1 month before becoming pregnant and continue this regimen through the first trimester.

1. 2. The American Academy of Pediatrics recommends that a woman, who has had a child with a neural tube defect, increase her intake of folic acid to 4 mg/day one month before becoming pregnant and that she continue this regimen through the first trimester. Health Canada suggests that this supplementation start at least three months before pregnancy. A woman who has no family history of neural tube defects should take 0.4 mg daily. All women of childbearing age should be encouraged to take a folic acid. Vitamin B$_{12}$ is important for neurological development, but the dosages listed are not correct.

CN: Health promotion and maintenance; CNS: None; CL: Apply

2. The nurse is caring for a neonate born 12 hours ago with a myelomeningocele. Which assessment finding should be reported immediately to the primary health care provider?

 1. Axillary temperature 102.2° F (39° C)
 2. Dribbling of urine
 3. No lower limb movement
 4. Talipes equinovarus

Immediately— that's the key phrase for question 2.

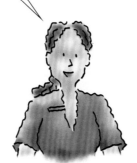

2. 1. During the first 12 hours of life, the most life-threatening event would be an infection. The other findings are consistent with the diagnoses of myelomeningocele.

CN: Physiological integrity; CNS: Reduction of risk potential; CL: Apply

3. A neonate has been brought to the emergency room by his mother. The nurse assesses the child and suspects that he may have hydrocephalus. Which observations, by the nurse, would indicate this condition?

 1. Bulging fontanel, low-pitched cry
 2. Depressed fontanel, low-pitched cry
 3. Bulging fontanel, eyes rotated downward
 4. Depressed fontanel, eyes rotated downward

3. 3. Hydrocephalus is caused from an alteration in the circulation of the cerebrospinal fluid (CSF). The amount of CSF increases, causing the fontanel to bulge. This also causes an increase in intracranial pressure. As the intracranial pressure increases, the neonate's eyes deviate downward, and the neonate's cry becomes high pitched.

CN: Health promotion and maintenance; CNS: None; CL: Analyze

CN: Client needs category   CNS: Client needs subcategory   CL: Cognitive level

4. The nurse is caring for a child following the insertion of a shunt on the right side of the head to relieve hydrocephalus. Which **priority** intervention should the nurse include in the plan of care?
1. Place the child in a supine position
2. Place the child flat in bed on the left side
3. Place the child in a semi-Fowler's position
4. Place the child in an upright position

5. What is an appropriate nursing action for a child experiencing a seizure?
1. Insert a nasogastric tube to prevent emesis
2. Restrain the extremities with a pillow or blanket
3. Insert a tongue blade to prevent injury to the tongue
4. Pad the side rails of the bed to protect the child from injury

6. A mother brings her infant to the emergency department and states that her child has had a seizure. The mother states that she was running out of formula so she stretched the formula by adding three times the normal amount of water. Electrolytes and blood glucose levels are drawn on the infant. Which laboratory value would the nurse anticipate?
1. Blood glucose: 5.5 mmol/L (100 mg/dl)
2. Chloride: 104 mmol/L (1,872 mg/dl)
3. Potassium: 4 mmol/L (72 mg/dl)
4. Sodium: 125 mmol/L (2250 mg/dl)

7. A neonate is admitted to the unit with a diagnosis of bacterial meningitis. On assessment, which symptoms would the nurse anticipate?
1. Hypothermia, irritability, and poor feeding
2. Positive Babinski's reflex, mottling, and pallor
3. Headache, nuchal rigidity, and developmental delays
4. Positive Moro's embrace reflex, hyperthermia, and sunken fontanel

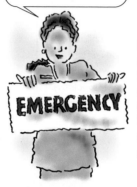

Remember, in emergency situations, your priority is to ensure the client's safety.

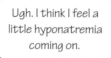

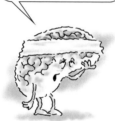

Ugh. I think I feel a little hyponatremia coming on.

4. 2. The child should be placed supine and on the left side in bed to avoid a rapid decompression of cerebrospinal fluid (CSF), and to avoid occlusion of the shunt. Placing the child in a semi-Fowler's or upright position may promote too rapid decompression of CSF.
CN: Physiological integrity; CNS: Reduction of risk potential; CL: Apply

5. 4. A child having a seizure could fall out of bed or injure himself on side rails of the bed. Attempts to insert anything into the child's mouth may cause injury. Attempting to restrain the child won't stop a seizure; in fact, tactile stimulation may increase the seizure activity.
CN: Safe, effective care environment; CNS: Safety and infection control; CL: Apply

6. 4. Diluting formula beyond what's recommended alters the infant's electrolyte levels. Normal serum sodium for an infant is 135 to 145 mmol/L. When formula is diluted, the infant's sodium is also diluted and will decrease. Hyponatremia is one of the causes of seizures in infants. The other values are all within normal limits.
CN: Physiological integrity; CNS: Reduction of risk potential; CL: Analyze

7. 1. The clinical appearance of a neonate with bacterial meningitis is different from that of a child or adult. Neonates may be either hypothermic or hyperthermic. The irritation to the meninges causes the neonate to be irritable and have a decreased appetite. The neonate may be pale or mottled with a bulging, full fontanel. Normal neonates have positive Moro's embrace and Babinski's reflexes. Developmental delays, if present, would appear when the child is older.
CN: Physiological integrity; CNS: Physiological adaptation; CL: Apply

CN: Client needs category   CNS: Client needs subcategory   CL: Cognitive level

8. A school nurse has been asked to assess a six-year-old child. Which behavior may suggest to the nurse that the child may have an attention deficit hyperactivity disorder (ADHD) rather than a learning disability?

1. The child reverses letters and words while reading.
2. The child is easily distracted and reacts impulsively.
3. The child is always getting into fights during recess.
4. The child has a difficult time reading a chapter book.

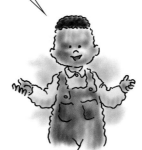

I'm trying to pay attention. Really I am.

8. 2. Two of the most common characteristics of children with ADHD include inattention and impulsiveness. Children who reverse letters and words while reading have dyslexia. Although aggressiveness may be common in children with ADHD, it isn't a characteristic that will help diagnose this disorder. Six-year-old children aren't usually cognitively ready to read a chapter book.
CN: Health promotion and maintenance; CNS: None; CL: Analyze

9. Which statement, by the parent of a child with cerebral palsy, would indicate that a nurse's teaching has been successful?

1. "My child's muscles will get stronger over time."
2. "My child's condition will get progressively worse."
3. "My child will have low intelligence."
4. "My child will need continual therapy to maintain functioning."

9. 4. A child with cerebral palsy will need continual treatment and therapy to maintain or improve functioning. Without therapy, muscles will get progressively weaker and more spastic. Although some children with cerebral palsy have an intellectual disability, many have normal intelligence.
CN: Health promotion and maintenance; CNS: None; CL: Analyze

10. A 12-year-old child, who sustained a spinal cord injury at the level of T1, is showing signs and symptoms consistent with autonomic dysreflexia. What assessment finding is the **most** likely cause?

1. Bladder distention
2. Low blood pressure
3. Large bowel movement
4. Client's head of bed elevated

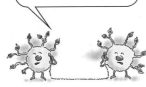

Hey, Stan. Are the reports of unusual electrical activity in your area true?

10. 1. Noxious stimuli that can trigger autonomic dysreflexia are painful or uncomfortable sensations below the level of the SCI. The client is unable to detect these sensations, however, because of the disruption of the nerves in the spinal cord. The first area the nurse should assess is the client's bladder. Bladder distention is a frequent trigger for autonomic dysreflexia and requires intervention. An acute episode of autonomic dysreflexia is characterized by sudden and severe hypertension. The first intervention for autonomic dysreflexia is to raise the head of the client's bed. Impacted bowel is the second most likely cause of autonomic dysreflexia.
CN: Physiological integrity; CNS: Physiological adaptation; CL: Analyze

11. A mother reports that her school-age child has been reprimanded for daydreaming during class. The mother is concerned because her other child has been diagnosed with absence seizures. This behavior is new, and the child's grades are dropping. What is the **most** appropriate action by the nurse?

1. Refer the child to an audiologist for a hearing assessment
2. Refer the child to the special education department to assess for a learning disability
3. Refer the child to the primary care provider to assess for attention deficit hyperactivity disorder (ADHD)
4. Refer the child to the primary health care provider to assess for absence seizures

11. 4. Absence seizures are commonly misinterpreted as daydreaming. The child loses awareness, but no alteration in motor activity is exhibited. A mild hearing problem usually presents as leaning forward, talking loudly, increasing the volume of the TV and radio, and continually asking, "What?" There isn't enough information to indicate a learning disability. ADHD isn't characterized by episodes of daydreaming.
CN: Physiological integrity; CNS: Physiological adaptation; CL: Analyze

12. A two-month-old infant is brought to the well-baby clinic for his first checkup. What is the nurse's **priority** based on nurse's notes?

Nurse's note	
10/15/16	Breast feeding every 2 to 3 hours
1130	during the day and every 3 to 4 hours
	at night; 2 to 4 loose yellowish stools
	and; 8 to 10 wet diapers per 24 hours
	Height/Weight Chart
	Plot height at 50th percentile and
	weight at 75th percentile
	Head Circumference Chart
	Plot head circumference over the
	95th percentile

1. Assess the infant's neurological signs
2. Re-measure the infant's head circumference
3. Collect a stool sample for culture and sensitivity
4. Advise the mother to decrease the frequency of breast feeding

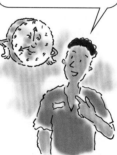

Hmm. Sounds like it's time for a reassessment, to me.

13. The nurse is teaching the mother of a child with cerebral palsy about the condition. Which observation would indicate that the mother needs further instruction?
1. The mother gives the child assistive devices for eating.
2. The mother feeds the child because he is unable to eat without making a mess.
3. The mother provides adequate time for the child to finish eating.
4. The mother provides finger foods.

12. 2. Whenever there is an abnormal finding the nurse should reassess to determine if an error in assessment error occurred. All other information in the chart is normal and would not require follow-up.
CN: Health promotion and maintenance; CNS: None; CL: Analyze

13. 2. Parents should encourage a child with cerebral palsy to be as independent as possible. Assistive devices can help a child with weak or spastic muscles eat independently. A child with cerebral palsy would require more time to bring food to his mouth and chew, and shouldn't be rushed. These parents should provide a calm, stress-free environment for eating. Providing finger foods can help this child eat independently.
CN: Physiological integrity; CNS: Basic care and comfort; CL: Analyze

CN: Client needs category   CNS: Client needs subcategory   CL: Cognitive level

14. A 12-year-old child is admitted to the pediatric unit following a seizure. What is the **priority** nursing action based on these data?

Progress notes	
10/15/16	Vital Signs
1500	T: 104°F (40°C)
	P: 89
	R: 30
	B/P: 80/42
	Nurse's Note
	Difficult to arouse; c/o headache;
	emesis × 2. Exhibiting nuchal rigidity;
	slight petechiae noted on distal
	extremities
	Lumbar Puncture
	Elevated WBCs in CSF
	Decreased glucose in CSF

1. Administer antipyretic therapy
2. Reduce all environmental stimuli
3. Place the child on airborne precautions
4. Position the child in lateral Simm's position

14. 3. The child is exhibiting signs and symptoms of bacterial meningitis. Nurses should take necessary precautions to protect themselves and others from possible infection from the bacterial organism causing the meningitis. The affected child should be placed in respiratory isolation immediately. Although environmental stimuli should be reduced and antipyretics likely administered, this does not take priority over immediate isolation. There is no indication for lateral Simm's position
CN: Safe, effective care environment; CNS: Safety and infection control; CL: Analyze

15. A 12-year-old child is admitted to the pediatric unit with the diagnosis of a possible brain tumor. Which assessment would be the **priority** for the nurse?
1. Bulging fontanel
2. High-pitched cry
3. Behavioral changes
4. Change in vital signs

15. 3. In a school-age child with a closed cranium, a common symptom of a brain tumor is behavior changes due to increased cranial pressure. A bulging fontanel and high-pitched cry are typical signs in an infant. A change in vital signs is a late sign of increased intracranial pressure.
CN: Physiological integrity; CNS: Physiological adaptation; CL: Apply

16. A preschool-age child has just been admitted to the pediatric unit with a diagnosis of bacterial meningitis. What is the nurse's **priority** intervention?
1. Assess LOC every 12 hours
2. Monitor temperature every four hours
3. Decrease environmental stimulation
4. Encourage the parents to hold the child

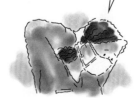

Take the necessary precautions to protect yourself and others from possible infection.

16. 3. A child with the diagnosis of meningitis is more comfortable in an environment with decreased stimuli. Noise and bright lights would stimulate this child and cause the child to cry; in turn, increasing intracranial pressure. Vital signs should be assessed initially every hour and temperature monitored every two hours. Neurosigns should be assessed according to the child's condition, but more frequently that every 12 hours. Children are usually much more comfortable if allowed to lie flat because this position reduces meningeal irritation.
CN: Physiological integrity; CNS: Physiological adaptation; CL: Apply

17. A child has just returned to the pediatric unit following placement of a ventriculoperitoneal shunt for hydrocephalus. The child is placed in a supine position. What is the nurse's **priority** intervention?
1. Assess intake and output
2. Place the child on the side opposite the shunt
3. Offer fluids because the child has a dry mouth
4. Administer oral pain medication as ordered

17. 2. Immediately following shunt placement surgery, the child should be placed supine to prevent to ensure that CSR does not drain too quickly. Upon return to the room, the client can be placed on the side opposite of the surgical site to prevent pressure on the shunt valve. Intake and output should be assessed, but this isn't the priority. Following surgery, the child would likely be NPO until the nasogastric tube is removed and bowel sounds return. Pain medication would initially be administered by IV route postoperatively.
CN: Physiological integrity; CNS: Basic care and comfort; CL: Analyze

18. An otherwise healthy 18-month-old has a history of febrile seizures. The child is visiting the clinic today for a wellness check-up. Which statement, by the child's father, would indicate a need for teaching?
1. "I have ibuprofen available in case it's needed."
2. "My child should outgrow these seizures by age five."
3. " I always keep phenobarbital with me in case of a fever."
4. "The most likely time for a seizure is when the fever is rising."

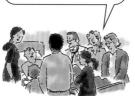

Note that for question 18, you're looking for an incorrect response from the father.

18. 3. Anticonvulsant drugs, such as phenobarbital, are administered to children with prolonged seizures or neurological abnormalities. Ibuprofen, not phenobarbital, is given for fever. Febrile seizures usually occur after age six months, and are unusual after age five years. Treatment would be to decrease fever, because seizures will occur as the temperature rises.
CN: Health promotion and maintenance; CNS: None; CL: Apply

19. The nurse is providing support to the parents of a 15-year-old boy who just underwent successful removal of a brain tumor. Which statements, by the nurse, are appropriate? Select all that apply.
1. "It's difficult, at this point, to accurately determine the residual deficits your son may have."
2. "Your son will have to wear a helmet, until the skull is fully healed, if he participates in physical activities."
3. "The tumor was successfully removed, and there is no chance of recurrence."
4. "Your son can resume his usual activities, within tolerable limits, as soon as possible."
5. "Any residual disabilities will decrease over time, and disappear in adulthood."

19. 1, 2, 4. Long-term survivors of brain tumors may have permanent disabilities in areas such as speech and mobility. A helmet will be necessary until the skull is fully healed. The goal for anyone who undergoes the removal of a brain tumor is for them to return to full activities as soon as possible. It is inappropriate to give false reassurance that the cancer will not return.
CN: Physiological integrity; CNS: Physiological adaptation; CL: Apply

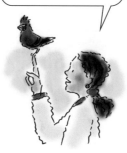

You're through the first 20! Keep going!

20. The nurse is teaching an adolescent, who has just been started on valproic acid for the treatment of seizures, about the medication. What **priority** information should the nurse share with this client?
1. This medication has no adverse effects.
2. A common adverse effect is weight gain.
3. Drowsiness and irritability commonly occur.
4. Early morning dosing is recommended to decrease insomnia.

20. 2. Weight gain is a common adverse effect of valproic acid. Drowsiness and irritability are more commonly associated with phenobarbital. Felbamate commonly causes insomnia.
CN: Physiological integrity; CNS: Pharmacological and parenteral therapies; CL: Apply

CN: Client needs category   CNS: Client needs subcategory   CL: Cognitive level

21. A nurse is teaching the parents of a child recently diagnosed with cerebral palsy (CP) about the diagnosis. Which statements, by the parents, would indicate that teaching was effective? Select all that apply.
1. We will schedule frequent rest periods throughout the day."
2. "Our child will have to spend a lot of time in hospital."
3. "We will have to learn to feed our son through a feeding tube."
4. "Our child will have to learn to read sign language in order to communicate."
5. "We will have to learn exercises and positioning to prevent deformities from occurring."

22. An older child is recovering from a craniotomy performed to remove a brain tumor. Which statement would be appropriate for the nurse to say to this child's parents?
1. "Your child really had a close call."
2. "I'm sure your child will be back to normal soon."
3. "I'm so glad to hear that your child doesn't have cancer."
4. "What has your provider told you about the tumor?"

23. A six-month-old infant is being admitted with a diagnosis of bacterial meningitis. What considerations should be made, by the nurse, regarding the infant's room assignment? Select all that apply.
1. The child will need to be on droplet precautions.
2. The infant's parents will not be allowed in the room.
3. A private room is required.
4. The room should be near the nurses' station.
5. There must be a window in the door to view the child.

24. A nurse is caring for a nine-year-old immediately after a head injury. The nurse notes a blood pressure of 110/60 mmHg, a heart rate of 78 bpm, dilated and nonreactive pupils, minimal response to pain, and a slow verbal response to name. Which symptom would cause the nurse the **most** concern?
1. Vital signs
2. Nonreactive pupils
3. Slow verbal response to name
4. Minimal response to pain

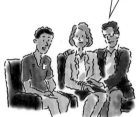

For question 22, keep in mind the difference between the nurse's and health care provider's roles.

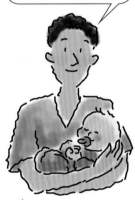

Sick infants are particularly vulnerable. It's a good idea to keep them close.

21. 1, 5. Children with cerebral palsy expend a lot of energy trying to complete the activities of daily living. Physical therapy is necessary to maintain mobility. Cerebral palsy does not require hospitalization unless a complication occurs. Children with CP will require assistance with feeding, but do not need feeding tubes. Cerebral palsy does not cause deafness unless there are repeated ear infections
CN: Physiological integrity; CNS: Physiological adaptation; CL: Apply

22. 4. When comforting parents, it's best to ascertain what information the provider has shared regarding the tumor. Since the outcome of the surgery isn't known, it would be inappropriate to say that the child has had a close call. It will take several weeks or more before the child is back to normal following a craniotomy. The health care provider will inform the parents of final pathology results.
CN: Psychosocial integrity; CNS: None; CL: Apply

23. 1, 3, 4. An infant, diagnosed with bacterial meningitis, should be placed on droplet precautions in a private room until that child has received IV antibiotics for 24 hours. This infant would be contagious. Bacterial meningitis can be quite serious; therefore, the infant's room should be near the nurses' station for close monitoring and easier access. The infant's parents would be permitted to visit as long as they wear the proper PPE. Although a window in the door is ideal, it is not a requirement.
CN: Safe, effective care environment; CNS: Safety and infection control; CL: Apply

24. 2. Dilated and nonreactive pupils indicate that anoxia or ischemia of the brain has occurred. If the pupils are fixed, herniation of the brain stem has occurred. The vital signs are normal. Slow response to pain can be normal following a head injury, and can indicate the child's level of consciousness.
CN: Physiological integrity; CNS: Physiological adaptation; CL: Apply

25. Which assignment, made by a charge nurse, would be **most** appropriate?
1. A registered nurse (RN) assigned to an infant who was newly diagnosed with bacterial meningitis
2. A student nurse assigned to an adolescent with cystic fibrosis who is on many medications
3. A licensed practical nurse (LPN) assigned to a newly-admitted child with acute leukemia who is receiving blood
4. An unlicensed assistive personnel (UAP) assigned to a transfer client with a head injury who has frequent seizures

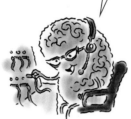

Keep it up! Looks like you're making all the right connections.

25. 1. An RN would be appropriately assigned to care for an infant with meningitis. The RN would make frequent assessments and provide a higher level of care. Student nurses may not be allowed to give medications without supervision, and it may be easier for the RN or LPN to provide care to this client. In many institutions, LPNs aren't allowed to monitor clients receiving blood or blood products. A transfer client with a head injury would need frequent assessments that only an RN or an LPN would be able to provide.
CN: Safe, effective care environment; CNS: Management of care; CL: Apply

26. An infant has returned to the pediatric unit after repair of a myelomeningocele. The nurse notices that the infant has had no urine output in the past two hours. Which nursing intervention would be **most** appropriate?
1. Perform Crede's maneuver on the infant's bladder
2. Catheterize the infant's bladder
3. Ask the mother to breast-feed the infant
4. Increase the IV fluid rate

26. 2. Swelling around the surgical site may cause transient urinary retention, and catheterization would be required to empty the bladder. Credé's maneuver isn't recommended because it can cause renal rupture. Breast-feeding the infant would be inappropriate in this situation. The fluid rate wouldn't be increased because there's no indication that the infant is dehydrated.
CN: Physiological integrity; CNS: Reduction of risk potential; CL: Apply

27. A two-month-old infant, who had an L4-L5 myelomeningocele repair, is brought to the clinic for a well-baby checkup. The mother reports that she catheterizes the infant every two to three hours. Which aspect of care should a nurse discuss with the mother?
1. Changing to a special diet
2. Scheduling immunizations
3. Explaining normal gross motor functions
4. Investigating the possibility of developing a latex allergy

27. 4. Children who are repeatedly exposed to latex products, such as during bladder catheterizations, are at high risk for developing a latex allergy. There's no need for a special diet unless another problem deems it necessary. This infant should receive regularly scheduled immunizations. It is important to discuss what abnormal motor functions the child will display and how to adapt care. Gross motor function will be abnormal in an infant with an L4-L5 repair.
CN: Health promotion and maintenance; CNS: None; CL: Apply

28. The nurse is teaching the parents of a 17-month-old, diagnosed with cerebral palsy, how to prevent the scissoring position. What is the **most** appropriate instruction by the nurse?
1. Keep the child in leg braces 23 hours per day
2. Let the child lay down as much as possible
3. Try to keep the child as quiet as possible
4. Straddle the child on your hip when being carried

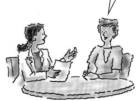

It's important that the parents of pediatric clients have a thorough understanding of their child's care needs.

28. 4. Straddling the child on the hip is an easy way to interrupt the scissoring position. Wearing leg braces 23 hours per day is inappropriate, and doesn't allow the child to move freely. Trying to keep the child quiet and flat are inappropriate. This child needs stimulation and movement to reach the goal of development to the fullest potential.
CN: Physiological integrity; CNS: Basic care and comfort; CL: Apply

CN: Client needs category   CNS: Client needs subcategory   CL: Cognitive level

29. The mother of a child with a ventriculoperi-toneal shunt states that her child has a temperature of 101.2° F (38.4° C), is lethargic and vomited the night before. Other children in the family have had similar symptoms, but are no longer affected. Which nursing intervention is **most** appropriate?
1. Provide symptomatic treatment for the fever
2. Advise the mother that this is a viral infection and it will run its course
3. Tell the mother to isolate the sick child from the other children
4. Have the child assessed by the primary health care provider

29. 4. One of the complications of a ventriculoperitoneal shunt is a shunt infection. Shunt infections can mimic a viral infection. It's best to have this child examined. There is no indication that the other children would need to be isolated from the sick child.
CN: Physiological integrity; CNS: Reduction of risk potential; CL: Apply

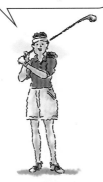

Wow! You've completed 30 questions. You're really in the swing of things.

30. The mother of a 10-year-old child with attention deficit hyperactivity disorder (ADHD) tells the nurse that her husband won't allow their child to take more than 5 mg of methylphenidate each morning. The child's performance in school is suffering. What is the nurse's **best** response?
1. Sneak the medication to the child anyway
2. Put the child in charge of administering the medication
3. Bring the child's father to the clinic to discuss the medication
4. Have the school nurse give the child the rest of the medication

30. 3. Bringing the father to the clinic for a teaching session would help him understand why it's necessary for his child to receive the full dose. A nurse shouldn't advise dishonesty to a client or family. The father should be included in the treatment as much as possible.
CN: Physiological integrity; CNS: Pharmacological and parenteral therapies; CL: Apply

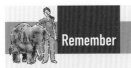

Remember

"Ritalin rocks ADHD."

Methylphenidate (Ritalin) is used to treat attention deficit hyperactivity disorder (ADHD).

31. A hospitalized child is to receive 75 mg/po/q4h of acetaminophen for fever control. How many milliliters per dose should the nurse administer if the available acetaminophen is 40 mg/0.4 ml?
1. 0.37 ml
2. 0.75 ml
3. 1.12 ml
4. 1.5 ml

31. 2. The nurse will administer 0.75 ml. Because 10 mg equals 0.1 ml, then 75 mg equals 0.75 ml.
CN: Physiological integrity; CNS: Pharmacological and parenteral therapies; CL: Apply

32. The nurse is preparing a toddler for a lumbar puncture. In which position should the nurse place this child?
1. Lying prone, with the neck flexed
2. Sitting up, with the back straight
3. Lying on one side, with the back curved
4. Lying prone, with the feet higher than the head

32. 3. A lumbar puncture involves placing a long needle between the lumbar vertebrae into the subarachnoid space. For this procedure, the nurse should position the client laterally, with the back curved. Curving the back maximizes the space between the lumbar vertebrae, facilitating needle insertion. Prone and seated positions don't achieve separation of the vertebrae.
CN: Physiological integrity; CNS: Reduction of risk potential; CL: Apply

33. A nurse makes the following assessment of a school-age child, who has had a brain tumor removed: Pupils equal and reactive to light; motor strength equal; knows name, date, but not location; and reports a headache. Which nursing intervention is **most** appropriate?
  1. Provide medication for the headache
  2. Notify the primary health care provider immediately
  3. Determine the child's baseline level of consciousness (LOC)
  4. Call the child's parents to sit at the child's bedside

34. A child requires IV fluids to infuse at 27 ml/hr. The tubing delivers 60 gtts/ml. How many gtts/min should the nurse count to ensure that the fluid is safely infusing?
  1. 14 gtts/min
  2. 27 gtts/min
  3. 54 gtts/min
  4. 60 gtts/min

35. The parents of a 19-month-old bring their toddler to the clinic for a well-child checkup. What action should the nurse take after assessing that both anterior and posterior fontanels have closed?
  1. Record this finding as normal
  2. Complete a thorough neurological assessment
  3. Refer the child to a primary care provider for further assessment
  4. Ask the parents if they have noted any change in the child's behavior

36. A 10-year-old with a concussion is admitted to the pediatric unit. Which roommate would be **most** appropriate for this child?
  1. A six-year-old child with osteomyelitis
  2. An eight-year-old child with gastroenteritis
  3. A 10-year-old child with rheumatic fever
  4. A 12-year-old child with a fractured femur

37. A nurse notes that a four-year-old child, with cerebral palsy, has a weight at the 30th percentile and a height at the 60th percentile. What is the **most** important information for the nurse to provide this child's family?
  1. The child should eat fewer calories per day.
  2. The child's height and weight are within the normal range.
  3. The child needs to increase his number of calories per day.
  4. The child is small for a four-year-old, and will never be average.

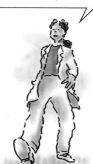

You're making great strides. Keep going.

33. 3. When there's an abnormality in current assessment data, it's vital to determine what the client's previous status was. Determine whether the status has changed or remained the same. Providing medication for the headache would be done after determining the baseline LOC. Contacting the primary health care provider and the child's parents isn't necessary before a final assessment has been made.
CN: Physiological integrity; CNS: Physiological adaptation; CL: Apply

34. 2. The nurse should count 27 gtts/min.

$$27\,ml/h \times 60\,gtts/ml \div 60\,min/h = 27\,gtts/min$$

CN: Physiological integrity; CNS: Pharmacological and parenteral therapies; CL: Apply

35. 1. It is normal, that by age 18 months, the anterior and posterior fontanels have closed. The diamond-shaped anterior fontanel normally closes between ages 9 and 18 months. The triangular-shaped posterior fontanel normally closes between ages 2 to 3 months. There is no need for further assessment or follow-up
CN: Health promotion and maintenance; CNS: None; CL: Apply

36. 4. A child with a concussion should be placed with a roommate who's free from infection and close to the child's age. Osteomyelitis, gastroenteritis, and rheumatic fever involve infection.
CN: Safe, effective care environment; CNS: Management of care; CL: Apply

37. 3. A height and weight between the 25th and 75th percentile would be considered normal for most children. Children with cerebral palsy expend vast amounts of energy performing activities of daily living. The may also have difficulty eating and swallowing due to a lack of motor control of the throat, mouth and tongue. Because of these two factors, this child is at risk of being malnourished. Eating fewer calories per day would result in a greater discrepancy between his height and weight. There is no evidence to suggest that his height and weight will never reach an average range.
CN: Health promotion and maintenance; CNS: None; CL: Apply

CN: Client needs category   CNS: Client needs subcategory   CL: Cognitive level

38. After a pathogen compromises the blood-brain and blood-cerebrospinal fluid (CSF) barriers, infection will spread to the meninges because:
   1. the spinal fluid has a rich erythrocyte content.
   2. glucose content of the spinal fluid is elevated high.
   3. there's a build-up of infectious exudate within the ventricular system.
   4. CSF is devoid of the body's major defense systems.

38. 4. After an organism compromises the natural barriers, the CSF provides an ideal medium for growth. All of the body's major defense systems are essentially absent in normal CSF. A CSF sample from a client with bacterial meningitis has decreased to normal glucose level. Exudate that may be present is the result of the infectious process, but is not the cause.
CN: Physiological integrity; CNS: Physiological adaptation; CL: Apply

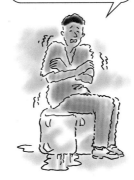

Brain freeze? Take a break and let your mind thaw out.

39. The nurse is caring for a child who has been diagnosed with a brain tumor. Which assessment findings are recognized as **early** signs of increased intracranial pressure? Select all that apply.
   1. Headache
   2. Fixed and dilated pupils
   3. Irritability
   4. Decerebrate posturing
   5. Dizziness

39. 1, 3, 5. Headache, irritability and dizziness are early signs; fixed dilated pupils and decerebrate positioning are late signs.
CN: Physiological Integrity; CNS: Physiological adaptation; CL: Analyze

40. A seven year old has just been admitted to the unit for excessive vomiting. Based on the available chart data, what is the nurse's **most** appropriate action?

Progress notes	
10/15/16	Vital Signs Record
0730	T: 104.9°F (40.5°C)
	P: 98
	RR: 30
	Lab Values
	Serum Potassium: 3.1 mmol/L
	Serum Sodium: 128 mmol/L
	Nurse's Note
	Skin flushed and warm to touch;
	good turgor; petechiae noted over
	entire trunk

   1. Cover the petechiae with dry sterile dressings
   2. Initiate extremity restraints as seizure precautions
   3. Suspect that the child has been abused
   4. Assess the child's neurological status

40. 4. Since fever, seizures, vomiting, and petechiae are signs of meningitis, the nurse should promptly assess the child's neurological status and report the findings to the provider. Petechiae does not require dry sterile dressings, nor are they signs of abuse. Restraints are not used as a seizure precautions, the finding of petechiae wouldn't be a reason to initiate seizure precautions. The lab values are just below normal, and would be expected if the child has been vomiting.
CN: Physiological integrity; CNS: Physiological adaptation; CL: Analyze

41. A nurse is assessing a three-year-old child with suspected nuchal rigidity. Which assessment finding would indicate nuchal rigidity?
  1. Positive Kernig's sign
  2. Negative Brudzinski's sign
  3. Positive Homans' sign
  4. Negative Babinski's sign

41. 1. A positive Kernig's sign indicates nuchal rigidity which is caused by an irritative lesion of the subarachnoid space. A positive Brudzinski's sign indicates meningeal irritation and is often associated with meningitis. Homans' sign would indicate venous inflammation of the lower leg. A negative Babinski reflex is expected after one year of age.
CN: Physiological integrity; CNS: Physiological adaptation; CL: Apply

42. A nurse is caring for a child with spina bifida. The child's mother asks the nurse what she did to cause the birth defect. What is the nurse's **best** response?
  1. Advanced age at conception is one of the major causes of the defect.
  2. It's a common complication of amniocentesis.
  3. It has been linked to maternal alcohol consumption during pregnancy.
  4. Many factors may contribute to it, but the exact cause is unknown.

42. 4. There is no known cause of spina bifida, but scientists believe that it's linked to hereditary and environmental factors. Neural tube defects, including spina bifida, have been strongly linked to low dietary intake of folic acid. Maternal age doesn't have an impact on spina bifida. An amniocentesis is performed to help diagnose spina bifida in utero, but it doesn't cause the disorder. Maternal alcohol intake during pregnancy has been linked to mental retardation, craniofacial defects, and cardiac abnormalities, not spina bifida.
CN: Physiological integrity; CNS: Physiological adaptation; CL: Apply

43. A child diagnosed with meningococcal meningitis has developed signs of sepsis, and has a purpuric rash over both lower extremities. The nurse should notify the primary health care provider immediately because these signs could indicate:
  1. a severe allergic reaction to the antibiotic regimen with impending anaphylaxis.
  2. the onset of the syndrome of inappropriate antidiuretic hormone (SIADH).
  3. fulminant meningococcemia.
  4. adhesive arachnoiditis.

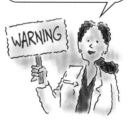

Check these signs carefully. They're critical for answering question 43.

WARNING

43. 3. Meningococcemia is a serious complication usually associated with a meningococcal infection. Anaphylaxis is a severe allergic reaction that occurs rapidly and causes a life-threatening response involving the whole body. This reaction can lead to difficulty breathing and shock ultimately leading to death. SIADH can be an acute complication, but it wouldn't be accompanied by the purpuric rash. Adhesive arachnoiditis occurs in the chronic phase of the disease and leads to obstruction of the flow of cerebrospinal fluid.
CN: Physiological integrity; CNS: Reduction of risk potential; CL: Apply

44. A 14 year old, diagnosed with head trauma following a motor vehicle accident, is prescribed an IV administration of mannitol. Which assessment would help determine the effectiveness of this medication?
  1. BUN
  2. Cardiac rhythm
  3. Urinary output
  4. Serum potassium

44. 3. Mannitol is an osmotic diuretic used to decrease cerebral edema. An increase in urinary output would indicate effectiveness. Cardiac rhythm and serum potassium are important assessments, as diuretics can cause electrolyte losses; however, they do not indicate the effectiveness of these drugs. Kidney function (BUN) would be determined prior to prescribing mannitol.
CN: Physiological integrity; CNS: Physiological adaptation; CL: Apply

45. A child with an elevated temperature and change in behavior is scheduled for a lumbar puncture. Which intervention should the nurse perform to alleviate this child's pain and fear of the lumbar puncture?
1. Sedate the child with fentanyl per order
2. Apply a topical anesthetic to the skin 5 to 10 minutes before the puncture
3. Have a parent hold the child in his or her lap during the tap procedure
4. Have the child inhale small amounts of nitrous oxide gas before the puncture

45. **1.** Sedation with fentanyl or other drugs can alleviate the pain and fear associated with a lumbar puncture. A topical anesthetic can be applied, but it should be done one hour before the procedure to be fully effective. A parent holding a child in his or her lap increases the risk of neurological injury due to the inability to assume and maintain the proper anatomic position required for a safe lumbar puncture. Use of nitrous oxide gas isn't recommended.
CN: Physiological integrity; CNS: Basic care and comfort; CL: Apply

46. The nurse is aware that antimicrobial therapy, to treat meningitis, should be instituted immediately after:
1. admission to the nursing unit.
2. initiation of IV therapy.
3. identification of the causative organism.
4. collection of cerebrospinal fluid (CSF) and blood for culture.

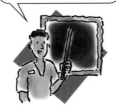

Check out the words *immediately after*, sounds urgent, doesn't it?

46. **4.** Antibiotics are always started immediately after the collection of CSF and blood cultures. Admission and initiation of IV therapy aren't, by themselves, appropriate times to begin antimicrobial therapy. After the specific organism is identified, bacteria-specific antibiotics can be administered if the organism isn't covered by the initial choice of antibiotic therapy.
CN: Physiological integrity; CNS: Pharmacological and parenteral therapies; CL: Analyze

47. A nurse is teaching the parents of a child diagnosed with meningitis about the child's medications. Which statement, by the nurse, is the **most** accurate regarding steroid therapy in conjunction with antimicrobial therapy?
1. It's the treatment of choice in aseptic meningitis.
2. It's used for the prevention of gastrointestinal hemorrhage.
3. It's used for the management of problems related to blood pressure.
4. It's used for the prevention of deafness with *Haemophilus influenzae* meningitis.

47. **4.** Steroids may play a role in the prevention of bilateral deafness in children *with H. influenzae* type B meningitis. Treatment of aseptic meningitis is primarily symptomatic, with acetaminophen for headache and muscle pain, and positioning for comfort. The use of steroids could complicate, rather than prevent, gastrointestinal bleeding and problems related to blood pressure.
CN: Physiological integrity; CNS: Pharmacological and parenteral therapies; CL: Apply

48. A nurse is caring for a client diagnosed with muscular dystrophy. What is the **most** appropriate goal for this client?
1. Acknowledgement of lifelong disabilities
2. Full independence in the activities of daily living
3. Acceptance of the ultimate prognosis of muscular dystrophy
4. Intensive physical therapy to prevent joint contractures

48. **3.** No matter how successful a program is, or how well the client adapts to the physical and emotional problems associated with the diagnosis, there is the constant presence of the ultimate outcome of the disease. The client will have disabilities throughout life that will continually progress and change. It is not realistic for someone with muscular dystrophy to gain full independence. Intensive physical therapy is important to manage joint contractures, but it will not prevent them from occurring.
CN: Psychological integrity; CNS: Physiological adaptation; CL: Apply

49. A child, diagnosed with bacterial meningitis, has been admitted to the unit. What is the **priority** nursing action?
1. Protecting self and others from possible infection
2. Administering intravenous antibiotics
3. Reducing environmental stimuli
4. Avoiding lifting the client's head

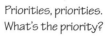
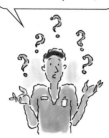

Priorities, priorities. What's the priority?

49. 2. Bacterial meningitis is a medical emergency that requires immediate treatment. If not treated rapidly it may lead to brain damage, deafness, stroke and death. All the other actions are important but only secondary to administering antibiotics.
CN: Physiological integrity; CNS: Basic care and comfort; CL: Apply

50. Which nursing assessment data would be given **priority** for a child with clinical findings related to tubercular meningitis?
1. Onset and character of fever
2. Degree and extent of nuchal rigidity
3. Signs of increased intracranial pressure (ICP)
4. Occurrence of urinary and fecal incontinence

50. 3. Assessment of fever and evaluation of nuchal rigidity are important aspects of care, but assessing for signs of increasing ICP should be the highest priority due to the life-threatening implications. Urinary and fecal incontinence can occur in a child who is ill from nearly any cause. This doesn't pose a great danger to life.
CN: Physiological integrity; CNS: Reduction of risk potential; CL: Analyze

51. The clinical manifestations of acute bacterial meningitis are dependent on which factor?
1. Age of the child
2. Length of the prodromal period
3. Time span from bacterial invasion to onset of symptoms
4. Degree of elevation of cerebrospinal fluid (CSF) glucose compared to serum glucose level

51. 1. Clinical manifestations of acute bacterial meningitis depend largely on the age of the child. These manifestations aren't dependent on the prodromal or initial period of the disease, or the time from invasion of the host to the onset of the symptoms. The glucose level of the CSF is reduced, not elevated. A serum glucose level is drawn one-half hour before the lumbar puncture so that the relationship between the CSF glucose and the serum glucose levels can be compared.
CN: Physiological integrity; CNS: Physiological adaptation; CL: Apply

52. A nurse has just started working in a neurology unit. What statement, by the nurse, would indicate adequate knowledge of seizures?
1. Clonic seizure activity is usually interpreted as falling.
2. It's not unusual to develop seizures after a head injury because of brain trauma.
3. Focal discharge in the brain may lead to absence seizures that can go unnoticed.
4. The epileptogenic focus in the brain needs multiple stimuli because it will discharge and cause a seizure.

52. 2. Stimuli from an earlier injury may eventually elicit seizure activity. Atonic seizures, not clonic, are frequently interpreted as falling. Focal seizures are partial seizures. Absence seizures are generalized seizures. Focal seizures don't lead to absence seizures. The epileptogenic focus consists of a group of hyperexcitable neurons responsible for initiating synchronous, high-frequency discharges leading to a seizure rather than needing multiple stimuli.
CN: Physiological integrity; CNS: Physiological adaptation; CL: Apply

53. A nurse is providing teaching to an adolescent who has been prescribed phenytoin for seizures. What information should the nurse include in this teaching? Select all that apply.
   1. "Brush your teeth using a soft toothbrush."
   2. "You can stop taking this medication when your seizures stop."
   3. "A rash is normal while taking this medication."
   4. "You will need to have bloodwork done frequently."
   5. "You should wear an ID bracelet indicating you are taking this drug."

53. **1, 4, 5.** This drug can cause gingival hyperplasia, so proper dental care is important to prevent infection. This drug has a narrow therapeutic index and many drug interactions. A steady serum level is needed to maintain effectiveness without toxicity, so serum levels should be done frequently. An ID bracelet is necessary because of the numerous drug interactions. This drug should not be stopped abruptly as this may precipitate seizures. A measles like rash may lead to Steven-Johnson syndrome. If this rash occurs, the drug should not be used.
CN: Physiological integrity; CNS: Pharmacological and parenteral therapies; CL: Apply

54. A nurse is providing teaching to the parents of a child diagnosed with muscular dystrophy. Which statements, by the nurse, are correct? Select all that apply.
   1. Braces and mobility aids will be needed to maintain flexibility in the joints.
   2. Continuous exercises will help your child overcome muscle weakness and prevent the progression of the disease.
   3. Monitoring for spinal deformities is very important as they can interfere with respiratory function.
   4. Avoid letting your child stand as this will cause undue stress on the lower extremities.
   5. Eventually your child will have to depend upon a wheelchair for mobility.

Use good judgment when answering question 54. Multiple answers may be right.

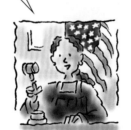

54. **1, 3, 5.** Without braces and mobility aids contractures will readily develop. As spinal deformities such as kyphosis develop, the lungs will not be able to fully expand. There is no treatment to prevent the progression of the disease, and the child will ultimately require a wheelchair. Although exercises will help maintain some mobility, the disease cannot be halted. Standing will help maintain muscle tone rather than putting undue stress on the extremities
CN: Physiological integrity; CNS: Physiological adaptation; CL: Apply

55. A five-year-old child, diagnosed with cerebral palsy, has just been prescribed oral baclofen. Which assessment finding, by the nurse, would indicate effective drug therapy?
   1. The child is exhibiting less spasticity.
   2. The child has less frequent seizures.
   3. The child no longer sleeps during the daytime.
   4. The child is better able to concentrate on mental activities.

55. **1.** Baclofen is a skeletal muscle relaxant that is effective in reducing overall spasticity. It is not an anti-seizure drug. Significant side effects of this drug are drowsiness and confusion, so this child would not be sleeping less, nor demonstrating a better ability to concentrate on mental activities.
CN: Physiological integrity; CNS: Pharmacological and parenteral therapies; CL: Apply

A little bit of me goes a long way.

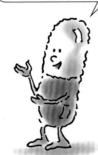

56. The parents of a child with a history of seizures ask the nurse why it's difficult to maintain therapeutic levels of phenytoin. Which statement, by the nurse, would be the **most** accurate?
   1. A drop in the plasma drug level will lead to a toxic state.
   2. The capacity to metabolize the drug becomes overwhelmed in time.
   3. Small increments in dosage lead to sharp increases in plasma drug levels.
   4. Large increases in dosage lead to more rapid stabilizing therapeutic effect.

56. **3.** Phenytoin has a narrow therapeutic range. Small increments in dosage can produce sharp increases in plasma drug levels. The capacity of the liver to metabolize phenytoin is affected by slight changes in the dosage of the drug, not necessarily the length of time the client has been taking the drug. Large increments in dosage will greatly increase plasma levels leading to drug toxicity.
CN: Physiological integrity; CNS: Pharmacological and parenteral therapies; CL: Apply

57. A nurse is caring for a child with a spinal cord lesion at the level of the seventh cervical vertebrae. The child becomes flushed, diaphoretic, hypertensive and reports a headache and blurred vision. What is the **priority** nursing action?
1. Assess the bladder for distension and slowly drain if distended
2. Administer antihypertensive and pain medication
3. Remove external stimulation and tight clothing
4. Administer a stool softener and perform manual anal stimulation

57. 1. This child is exhibiting signs and symptoms of autonomic stimulation. Although it could be caused by fecal impaction, the most common cause is a distended bladder. All other interventions are correct, but the nurse's priority must be to remove the stimulus for the condition.
CN: Physiological integrity; CNS: Physiological adaptation; CL: Analyze

58. The nurse is teaching a 16-year-old client how to self-catheterize following a spinal cord injury. Which statements, by the nurse, are correct? Select all that apply.
1. Always use a latex catheter
2. Drink caffeinated drinks sparingly
3. Use strict sterile technique
4. Self-catheterize according to a schedule
5. Maintain a regular pattern of fluid intake over the day

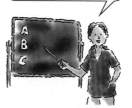

When teaching a client, be sure to stop occasionally and make sure he or she understands what you're saying.

58. 2, 4, 5. Caffeinated drinks should be avoided because their diuretic effect can over distend the bladder. Self-catheterization should be done according to a regular schedule that coincides with a regular pattern of intake. Latex catheters should be avoided because this group is at high risk for latex allergy. Clean technique rather than sterile technique, is used for self-catheterization.
CN: Physiological integrity; CNS: Basic care and comfort; CL: Apply

59. The parents of a 10 year old tell the nurse that they are concerned that their child may have a concussion after being hit in the head by a soccer ball during a game. The child is fully oriented, remembers being hit with the ball, and has vital signs within normal range. What is the nurse's **most** appropriate response?
1. "It is unlikely that your child has a concussion if there was no loss of consciousness."
2. "Your child will need uninterrupted sleep tonight in order for any damage to heal."
3. "Seek medical attention if there is any change in condition in the next 2 to 3 days."
4. "There is no need for concern as children are very resilient at this age."

59. 3. Head trauma can lead to a gradual decline in neurological status 2 to 3 days following the injury. Concussions can occur in the absence of loss of consciousness. It is important that the child is awakened every couple of hours the first night to ensure that there is no decline in neurological status. The child should recognize the caregiver and respond appropriately. Young children are more susceptible to head trauma because of brain immaturity.
CN: Physiological integrity; CNS: Physiological adaptation; CL: Apply

60. The nurse is reviewing assessment data and admission orders of a client. The provider has ordered the IV administration of phenytoin. The nurse determines that further intervention is required when the admission assessment includes which findings? Select all that apply?
1. Episodic nosebleeds
2. History of Stokes-Adams syndrome
3. History of bone marrow depression
4. Attention deficit hyperactivity disorder (ADHD)
5. Increased appetite

60. 1, 2, 3. Intravenous administration of phenytoin can lead to arrhythmia and hypotension, and is contraindicated when a history of sinus bradycardia, sinoatrial block, second or third-degree heart block, or Stokes-Adams syndrome is present. Phenytoin would be administered cautiously in clients with episodic nosebleeds or bone marrow depression due to its adverse effects of leukopenia, anemia, and thrombocytopenia. Phenytoin has no known effect on ADHD but can interfere with cognitive function in excessive doses. There is no increased appetite reported by people who take phenytoin.
CN: Physiological integrity; CNS: Pharmacological and parenteral therapies; CL: Analyze

61. The parents of a child newly diagnosed with a seizure disorder ask the nurse when seizure activity is most likely to occur. Which response, by the nurse, would be the **most** accurate?
1. During the rapid eye movement (REM) stage of sleep
2. During long periods of excitement
3. While falling asleep and on awakening
4. While eating, particularly if the child is hurried

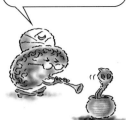
You are beginning to feel verrrry sleepy.

61. 3. Seizure activity is more likely to occur during periods of functional instability in the brain. This instability most often occurs when the child is falling asleep or waking up. Eating quickly, excitement without undue fatigue, and REM sleep haven't been identified as contributing factors.
CN: Physiological integrity; CNS: Physiological adaptation;
CL: Apply

62. The nurse is speaking with the family of a child diagnosed with an epidural hematoma. Which information, regarding this condition, is **most** accurate?
1. Because of the location of the bleed there is no concern for neurologic damage.
2. The best treatment for this type of head injury is rest.
3. Surgery to remove the blood and control the bleeding may be needed.
4. Symptoms should not last longer than 48 hours.

62. 3. Prompt surgical treatment may be needed as brain compression can occur rapidly. There is a high risk for neurological damage as the bleeding is arterial. Unlike a concussion, there is active bleeding with this type of injury, so rest alone is not indicated. The symptom-free period may last longer than 48 hours.
CN: Physiological integrity; CNS: Physiological adaptation;
CL: Apply

63. Which factors can lead to seizure activity in a child with a seizure disorder?
1. Striped wallpaper and ceiling fans
2. Uninterrupted sleep
3. Limiting periods of intense physical play each day
4. Abstaining from soda consumption

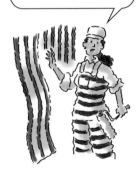
I'm afraid no one will like this pattern … or am I being too sensitive?

63. 1. Striped wallpaper, ceiling fans, and blinking lights on a Christmas tree can all be triggers to seizure activity if the child is photosensitive. Sleep interruption hasn't been identified as a triggering factor. Avoiding fatigue can reduce seizure activity; therefore, intense physical activity for extended periods should be avoided. Restricting caffeine intake by using caffeine-free soda is a dietary modification that may prevent seizures.
CN: Physiological integrity; CNS: Physiological adaptation;
CL: Apply

64. Which nursing intervention would support the goal of avoiding injury, respiratory distress, or aspiration for a child during a seizure?
1. Positioning the child with the head hyperextended
2. Placing a pillow or folded blanket under the child's head for support
3. Using pillows to prop the child into the sitting position
4. Working a padded tongue blade or small plastic airway between the teeth

64. 2. Placing a small cushion or blanket under the child's head will help prevent injury. The child should be positioned with the head in midline, not hyperextended, to promote a patent airway and adequate ventilation. The child should not be propped up into a sitting position, but should be eased to the floor to prevent falling and unnecessary injury. Nothing should be placed in the child's mouth because it could cause infection or obstruct the airway.
CN: Physiological integrity; CNS: Reduction of risk potential;
CL: Apply

65. A child has been admitted to the hospital following a severe concussion. Which nursing interventions are important while caring for this child? Select all that apply.
1. Provide heavy sedation
2. Maintain the child NPO
3. Implement seizure precautions
4. Frequently assess vital and neurological signs
5. Keep the head of the bed slightly elevated

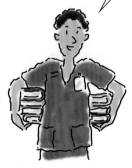

Hang on! You've reached question 65!

65. 3, 4, 5. Seizure precautions are an important safety measure. Frequent assessment of vital and neurological signs are important to detect any deterioration in condition. Bed rest with the head slightly elevated will minimize headache and reduce ICP. Heavy sedation is contraindicated as this may mask signs of deterioration in condition. There is no indication for NPO status.
CN: Physiological integrity; CNS: Physiological adaptation; CL: Apply

66. A nurse is teaching the parents of a child diagnosed with spina bifida. Which description of spina bifida, by the nurse, is **most** accurate?
1. It has little influence on the intellectual and perceptual abilities of the child.
2. It's a simple neurological defect that can be surgically corrected within one to two days after birth.
3. Its presence would indicate that many areas of the central nervous system (CNS) may not develop or function adequately.
4. It's a complex neurological disability that will require the involvement of a collaborative health care team effort for the entire first year of the child's life.

66. 3. When a spinal cord lesion is present at birth, it commonly leads to altered development or function in other areas of the CNS. Spina bifida is a complex neurological defect that heavily impacts the physical, cognitive, and psychosocial development of the child. Collaborative, lifelong management is needed due to the chronicity and multiplicity of the problems involved.
CN: Physiological integrity; CNS: Physiological adaptation; CL: Apply

67. A nurse is counseling a mother who just gave birth to an infant with spina bifida. The mother asks if her child will have leg and foot deformities. What is the nurse's **most** correct response?
1. "Your child will have weakness, and may not be able to walk but there will be no deformities."
2. "Your child will have minor deformities that can be easily corrected by surgery."
3. "Some infants born with spina bifida with have a deformity called club foot."
4. "Your baby's hips and legs will most likely be turned outward."

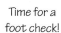
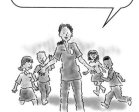

Time for a foot check!

67. 3. A neurogenic form of quinovarus (club foot) may occur in children born with spina bifida and myeleomeningocele. These deformities are not easily corrected by surgery. The hips, if affected, will be internally rotated. It would not be appropriate for the nurse to guarantee that there will be no deformities.
CN: Physiological integrity; CNS: Physiological adaptation; CL: Apply

68. What is the nurse's **priority** when caring for a 10-month-old infant with meningitis?
1. Maintaining an adequate airway
2. Maintaining fluid and electrolyte balance
3. Controlling seizures
4. Controlling hyperthermia

68. 1. Maintaining an adequate airway is always a top priority. Maintaining fluid and electrolyte balance and controlling seizures and hyperthermia are all important, but not as important as an adequate airway.
CN: Physiological integrity; CNS: Reduction of risk potential; CL: Apply

CN: Client needs category   CNS: Client needs subcategory   CL: Cognitive level

69. While caring for an infant with myelomeningocele, the nurse notices a change in the assessment that may indicate a Chiari II malformation. Which change was noted in this assessment?
1. Rapidly progressing scoliosis
2. Changes in urological functioning
3. Back pain below the site of the sac closure
4. Respiratory stridor

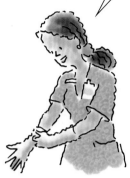

I have to hand it to you. You're doing awesome!

69. 4. Children with a myelomeningocele have a 90% chance of developing a Chiari II malformation. This may lead to respiratory function problems, such as respiratory stridor associated with paralysis of the vocal cords, apneic episodes of unknown cause, difficulty swallowing, and an abnormal gag reflex. Urological function changes and scoliosis occur with myelomeningocele, but these complications aren't specifically related to Chiari II malformation. Lower back pain doesn't occur due to the loss of sensory function related to the cord defect.
CN: Physiological integrity; CNS: Reduction of risk potential; CL: Analyze

70. The nurse is providing support to the parents of an adolescent who has a serious brain injury. The parents have been told that there is damage to the brainstem, and that the prognosis is very poor. Which type of posturing would **most** likely be exhibited by their child?

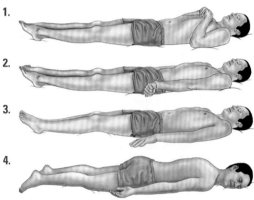

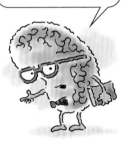

You can tell by a client's posture which part of me is injured.

70. 2. This diagram demonstrates decerebrate posturing which occurs with damage to the brainstem. The client will present with extension and pronation of the arms while the legs are extended. Illustration 1 demonstrates decorticate posturing which occurs with damage to the cerebral cortex. Illustrations 3 and 4 do not demonstrate findings consistent with brain injury.
CN: Physiological integrity; CNS: Physiological adaptation; CL: Apply

71. The parents of a child newly diagnosed with myelomeningocele ask the nurse why surgical repair needs to be done immediately. Which response would be the **most** accurate?
1. It's done to rapidly restore neural pathways to the legs.
2. It's done to decrease the possibility of infection and further cord damage.
3. It's done to expose the spinal cord defect and allow an individualized therapeutic strategy.
4. It's done to remove excess nerve tissue from the vertebral canal, and to decrease pressure on the cord.

71. 2. The myelomeningocele sac presents a dynamic disability and is treated as a life-threatening situation with sac closure taking place within 24 to 48 hours of birth. Early management decreases the possibility of infection and further injury to the exposed neural cord. There's complete loss of nervous function below the level of the spinal cord lesion. The aim of surgery is to replace the nerve tissue into the vertebral canal, cover the spinal defect, and achieve a leak-proof sac closure.
CN: Physiological integrity; CNS: Reduction of risk potential; CL: Apply

72. The nurse is providing preoperative care for an infant with a myelomeningocele. What position is **most** appropriate for this client?
1. Prone position with head turned to the side for feeding
2. Side-lying position with the head at a 30-degree angle to the feet
3. Prone position with a nasogastric (NG) tube inserted for feedings
4. Side-lying position, supported by diaper rolls, both anterior and posterior

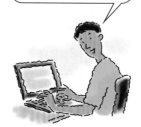

Don't sweat it! Just choose the most appropriate response.

72. **1.** Prone position is used preoperatively because it minimizes tension on the sac and the risk of trauma. The head should be turned to one side for feeding. There's no advantage to positioning the body with a 30-degree head elevation. Although feeding can be a problem in the prone position, it can be accomplished without the need for an NG tube. Side-lying or partial side-lying positions are more appropriate after the repair has been accomplished unless it permits undesirable hip flexion.
CN: Physiological integrity; CNS: Reduction of risk potential; CL: Apply

73. Which nursing intervention is necessary when large body areas of sensory and motor impairment, associated with myelomeningocele, occur in the immediate postoperative period?
1. Gentle range of motion exercises
2. Vigorous stretching of contractures
3. Frequent turning side-to-side and prone-to-supine
4. Keeping skin dry and avoiding the use of emollients and lubricants

73. **1.** Areas of sensory and motor impairment require meticulous care, including gentle range-of-motion exercises to prevent contractures as well as stretching of contractures when indicated. Vigorous exercise should be avoided. Frequent turning is indicated in order to maintain skin integrity, but the supine position shouldn't be used, as it puts pressure on the surgical site. Skin should be kept clean and dry, and lubrication can be used for massage, which increases circulation to the areas involved.
CN: Physiological integrity; CNS: Basic care and comfort; CL: Apply

74. Children with spina bifida are at high risk for developing intraoperative anaphylaxis linked to an allergic response to latex. Which risk factor leads to this allergic response?
1. Weakened immune response
2. Need for lifelong steroid therapy
3. Need for numerous bladder catheterizations
4. Use of large amounts of adhesive tape to attach sac dressings

74. **3.** Children with spina bifida are at high risk for developing a latex allergy because of repeated exposure to latex products during multiple surgeries and from numerous bladder catheterizations related to lack of bladder function. A weakened immune response wouldn't elicit an anaphylactic reaction. Steroid therapy isn't indicated in the management of spina bifida and also wouldn't support an anaphylactic reaction. Sac removal is accomplished as quickly as possible after birth, and the sac usually isn't covered with any type of dressing because it may contribute to trauma to the sac.
CN: Physiological integrity; CNS: Reduction of risk potential; CL: Apply

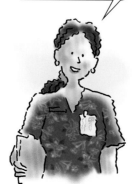

Taking folic acid before conception reduces certain risks in infants.

75. A nurse is counseling the mother of a child born with spina bifida regarding future pregnancies. The mother asks, "How can I avoid giving birth to a second child with spina bifida?" What is the nurse's **best** response?
1. There's no known way to avoid it; adoption is recommended.
2. A previous pregnancy, affected by a neural tube defect, isn't a factor.
3. Pre-pregnancy intake of 4 mg of folic acid daily will reduce the risk of recurrence.
4. Aerobic exercise in the first trimester will decrease the chance of a positive alpha-fetoprotein (AFP).

75. **3.** Studies have shown that the risk for having an infant with a neural tube defect is significantly reduced by taking supplements of folic acid before conception. The chances of having a second affected child are low, but still greater than the chances in the general population. Aerobic exercise won't decrease the chance of a positive AFP.
CN: Health promotion and maintenance; CNS: None; CL: Apply

CN: Client needs category   CNS: Client needs subcategory   CL: Cognitive level

76. A school-age child, with a diagnosis of epilepsy, is admitted to the pediatric unit of a local hospital for evaluation of his anticonvulsant medications. As the nurse enters the child's room, the child begins to have a seizure. What is the **priority** nursing action?
1. Push the call light and ask for help
2. Hold the child down so he doesn't injure himself
3. Loosen any restrictive clothing
4. Force the jaw open to maintain an open airway

76. 3. The primary nursing goal, during a seizure, is to protect the client from physical injury and maintain a patent airway. Loosening clothing will allow free movement and aid in keeping the airway open. After making sure the client is safe from injury, the nurse should push the call light if further assistance is needed. The nurse should never forcibly hold a client down, and shouldn't force the jaw open.

CN: Physiological integrity; CNS: Reduction of risk potential; CL: Apply

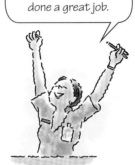

You're almost there, and you've done a great job.

77. A nurse is planning care for a nine-year-old boy with Down's syndrome. What is the **most** appropriate statement regarding nursing interventions?
1. Nursing interventions should be planned at a nine-year-olds developmental level.
2. Nursing interventions should be planned at a seven-year-olds developmental level.
3. The nurse should assess the child's developmental level before planning interventions.
4. The developmental level of the child is not important in planning care.

77. 3. Before developing a care plan, the nurse should assess this child's developmental level and plan care accordingly. The nurse shouldn't plan care geared toward the child's chronological age without first assessing the child. The nurse also shouldn't assume that the child is at a lower developmental level without assessing the child. The child's developmental age is important in planning age-appropriate care and teaching.

CN: Health promotion and maintenance; CNS: None; CL: Apply

78. A six-year-old child is unconscious from a head injury following a bicycle accident. The nurse is assessing the child for increased intracranial pressure (ICP). His baseline vital signs are respirations 20 breaths/min, blood pressure 100/56 mmHg, and pulse 100 bpm. The nurse continues to monitor the child, and is **most** concerned when changing vitals reveal:
1. respirations 12 breaths/min; blood pressure 90/45 mmHg; pulse 80 bpm.
2. respirations 14 breaths/min; blood pressure 130/40 mmHg; pulse 70 bpm.
3. respirations 30 breaths/min; blood pressure 80/45 mmHg; pulse 130 bpm.
4. respirations 14 breaths/min; blood pressure 70/58 mmHg; pulse 102 bpm.

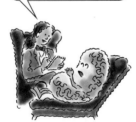

Which vital signs would indicate increased ICP?

78. 2. Classic signs of increased ICP are a decrease in respirations, an increase in blood pressure, and a decrease in pulse rate. Answer one may indicate normal vital signs. Answers three and four may indicate shock.

CN: Physiological integrity; CNS: Physiological adaptation; CL: Analyze

79. When assessing an infant for changes in intracranial pressure (ICP), it's important to palpate the fontanels. Identify the area where a nurse should palpate to assess the anterior fontanel.

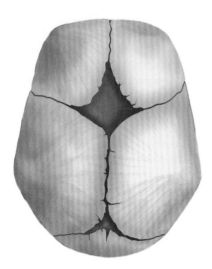

79. The anterior fontanel is formed by the junction of the sagittal, frontal, and coronal sutures. It's shaped like a diamond and normally measures 4 to 5 cm at its widest point. A widened, bulging fontanel is a sign of increased ICP.

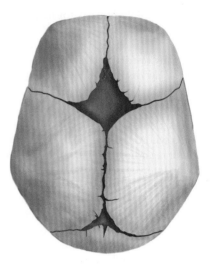

CN: Health promotion and maintenance; CNS: None; CL: Apply

80. A nurse is preparing a dose of amoxicillin for a three year old with acute otitis media. The child weighs 33 lb (15 kg). The dosage prescribed is 50 mg/kg/day in divided doses every 8 hours. The concentration of the drug is 250 mg/5 ml. How many milliliters should the nurse administer? Record your answer using a whole number.

_____ ml

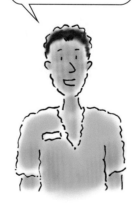

Time for a math question! Put on your number-crunching hat.

80. 5.

To calculate the child's weight in kilograms, the nurse should use the following formula:

$$\frac{1\,kg}{2.2\,lb} = \frac{X\,kg}{33\,lb}$$

$$X = \frac{33}{2.2}\,kg = 15\,kg$$

Next, the nurse should calculate the daily dosage for the child:

$$50\,mg/kg/day \times 15\,kg = 750\,mg/day$$

The medication is divided into three daily doses:

$$750\,mg/day \div 3\,doses/day = 250\,mg$$

The drug's concentration is 250 mg/5 ml, so the nurse should administer 5 ml.

CN: Physiological integrity; CNS: Pharmacological and parenteral therapies; CL: Apply

81. The nurse is providing education for a mother who gave birth to a child with the spinal deformity shown in the illustration. Which statement, by the nurse, is correct?

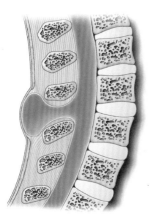

1. The child will require surgery as soon as possible to prevent complications.
2. Surgery is not an option, and unfortunately there is no treatment to prevent complications.
3. This defect can be corrected surgically, and often there are no complications.
4. This defect will not require surgery, and in most cases there are no complications.

81. 4. This illustration depicts spina bifida occulta, which in most cases is benign, asymptomatic and produces no neurologic deficits.

CN: Physiological integrity; CNS: Physiological adaptation; CL: Apply

82. The nurse is assessing the primitive reflexes of a four-month-old. Which reflexes, shown in the photos, should not be present?

1.
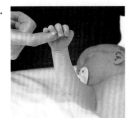

2.
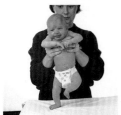

3.
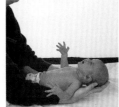

4.
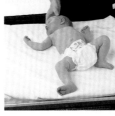

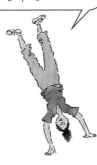

You did it! Now take a break and go play outside.

82. 4. Photo four shows a stepping reflex. Persistence of this reflex beyond two months would suggest asymmetric central nervous system development. Photo one shows the palmer grasp reflex. This reflex disappears around age 3 to 4 months. Photo four shows the tonic neck reflex. This reflex disappears at age 3 to 4 months. Photo three shows the Moro reflex. This reflex disappears around age 3 to 6 months.

CN: Physiological integrity; CNS: Reduction of risk potential; CL: Analyze

Chapter 31

Musculoskeletal Disorders

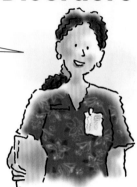

Challenge yourself with these sample questions on musculoskeletal system disorders in children. I'm betting you'll have a blast!

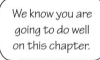

We know you are going to do well on this chapter.

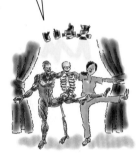

1. A nurse is caring for a 10 year old in Buck's traction for a fractured femur following a bicycle accident. The child reports increasing pain one hour after receiving an IV opioid analgesic. What is the nurse's **most** appropriate action?
  1. Tell the child that he needs to give the analgesic time to work
  2. Perform a neurovascular assessment
  3. Make sure the weights are hanging freely
  4. Administer more analgesics

1. 2. This client's unrelieved pain may be a sign of compartment syndrome if pressure develops within the muscle and its surrounding structures due to the constrictive dressing used in Buck's traction. The nurse should immediately perform a neurovascular assessment to detect signs of impaired circulation and nerve function. The findings should be immediately reported to the provider, and the pressure dressing loosened or removed. Opioid analgesics should provide pain relief within one hour of administration. While the weights in Buck's traction should hang freely, the child should be assessed first. More analgesics may be administered as ordered but only after the neurovascular status is assessed.
CN: Physiological integrity; CNS: Reduction of risk potential; CL: Analyze

2. The nurse is observing an 18-month-old child in Bryant's traction. Which observation would indicate that the traction is properly positioned?
  1. The hips are resting on the bed.
  2. The hips are slightly elevated off the bed.
  3. The hips are elevated above the level of the heart.
  4. The hips are resting on a pillow.

2. 2. In Bryant's traction, the child's hips should be elevated at a 15-degree angle off the bed. The hips shouldn't be resting on the bed or on a pillow, and shouldn't be above the level of the heart.
CN: Physiological integrity; CNS: Basic care and comfort; CL: Apply

3. The mother of a neonate with clubfoot feels guilty because she believes she did something to cause the condition. The nurse should explain that the cause of clubfoot is:
  1. unknown.
  2. always hereditary.
  3. due to unrestricted movement in utero.
  4. caused by the position of the fetus in utero.

3. 1. The definitive cause of clubfoot is unknown. In some families, there's an increased incidence. Some postulate that anomalous embryonic development or restricted fetal movement is the cause. There is no way to predict the occurrence of clubfoot.
CN: Psychosocial integrity; CNS: None; CL: Apply

CN: Client needs category   CNS: Client needs subcategory   CL: Cognitive level

4. Which statement, by the father of an 8-year-old boy with Duchenne's muscular dystrophy, would indicate that he has realistic expectations about the course of this disease?
  1. "My son will gradually lose his ability to walk."
  2. "Corticosteroids will help prevent muscle degeneration."
  3. "Surgery will help my son walk."
  4. "My son will have a normal lifespan."

4. 1. Duchenne's muscular dystrophy is a progressive degenerative disorder in which children lose their ability to walk independently by age 12. Corticosteroids may slow muscle degeneration but won't stop its progression. Surgery may be done to correct contractures, but it doesn't change the course of the disease. Death occurs by early adulthood, usually from respiratory failure.
CN: Physiological integrity; CNS: Physiological adaptation; CL: Apply

5. A nurse is teaching the parents of a three-month-old infant with severe torticollis. The child's head is tilted to the left and the side bent to the right. Which muscle group would the parents identify as being shortened?
  1. Left upper trapezius
  2. Right middle trapezius
  3. Left sternocleidomastoid
  4. Right sternocleidomastoid

5. 4. The right sternocleidomastoid is shortened with the head in this position. The left upper trapezius is not shortened. The middle trapezius is not affected, and the left sternocleidomastoid is in a lengthened position.
CN: Physiological integrity; CNS: Physiological adaptation; CL: Apply

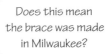

I've heard of muscle strengthening, but what's muscle lengthening?

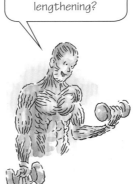

6. A nine-month-old infant's head is rotated to the left and side bending to the right due to torticollis. What is the **most** effective position for the nurse to place this infant in for development of muscle lengthening?
  1. Prone
  2. Supine
  3. Left side-lying
  4. Right side-lying

6. 3. The left side-lying position will help lengthen the muscles because and make it easier to stretch the sternocleidomastoid and upper trapezius. No other positions will assist in increasing muscle length.
CN: Physiological integrity; CNS: Reduction of risk potential; CL: Apply

7. The nurse is teaching a 13-year-old client how to wear a Milwaukee brace for scoliosis. Which statement, by the client, indicates effective teaching?
  1. "I'll have to wear the brace 24 hours a day."
  2. "I should wear soft, non-irritating clothes under my brace."
  3. "I can use powder or lotion if my skin gets dry or itchy."
  4. "This brace will cure my scoliosis."

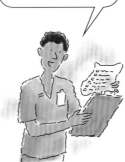

Does this mean the brace was made in Milwaukee?

7. 2. Soft, nonirritating clothing should be worn under the brace to prevent irritation and to absorb moisture. The Milwaukee brace is usually worn from 16 to 23 hours each day per provider's order. The skin should be kept clean and dry, but the client should avoid the use of powders and lotions that can lead to skin breakdown. The Milwaukee brace is not curative, but may slow down the progression of the curvature of the spine, and allow for proper skeletal growth.
CN: Health promotion and maintenance; CNS: None; CL: Apply

8. Which interventions should the nurse include when developing a plan of care for a child who was placed in a hip-spica cast 24 hours ago for hip dysplasia? Select all that apply.
   1. Turn the child at least every two hours
   2. Keep the cast uncovered for six hours
   3. Use a regular fan to help with the drying process
   4. Perform neurovascular checks once a shift
   5. Elevate the lower body and extremities.

8. 1, 3, 5. Turning the child in a plaster cast will allow even drying, and help prevent complications related to immobility. A regular fan will circulate air to facilitate drying. Elevating the lower body and extremities this will promote venous return, decrease edema, and decrease the risk of neurovascular complications. The cast should be kept uncovered for a minimum of 24 to 48 hours to allow for complete evaporation of water. After the cast is applied, a client is at risk for peripheral neurovascular dysfunction due to swelling within the confines of the cast. Neurovascular checks should initially be conducted every 1 to 2 hours to prevent neurovascular complications.
CN: Safe, effective care environment; CNS: Management of care; CL: Analyze

9. What is the **most** important nursing intervention when caring for a child with a newly applied wet hip-spica cast?
   1. Use the abductor bar to help move the child
   2. Cover the cast in plastic to keep it clean
   3. Reposition the child every 1 to 2 hours
   4. Use the fingertips when handling the cast

9. 3. The child in a wet hip-spica cast should be turned every 1 to 2 hours to help dry all sides of the cast and prevent skin breakdown. The abductor bar shouldn't be used for turning the child, even after the cast is dry. A wet cast shouldn't be covered with plastic because this will impede drying, reduce air circulation and allow heat to build up in the cast. A wet cast should be handled using the palms, because fingertips may cause indentations and pressure points.
CN: Physiological integrity; CNS: Basic care and comfort; CL: Apply

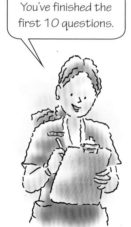

Congratulations! You've finished the first 10 questions.

10. The parents of an infant born with clubfoot express feelings of guilt and anxiety about their child's condition. What is the nurse's **most** appropriate intervention?
   1. Teach them about their child's condition
   2. Introduce them to other parents whose children have the same condition
   3. Ask if they would like to speak with the chaplain
   4. Encourage discussion of their feelings

10. 4. While all the options are appropriate interventions for the nurse to implement, the first step is to encourage the parents to verbalize their concerns and feelings about their child's condition. This will help alleviate anxiety and develop a trusting therapeutic relationship.
CN: Physiological integrity; CNS: None; CL: Analyze

11. The Milwaukee brace is commonly used in the treatment of scoliosis. Which position **best** describes the placement of the pressure rods?
   1. Laterally on the convex portion of the curve
   2. Laterally on the concave portion of the curve
   3. Posteriorly on the convex portion of the curve
   4. Posteriorly along the spinal column at the exact level of the curve

11. 1. Lateral pressure applied to the convex portion of the curve is best at reducing the curvature. Pressure pads applied posteriorly will help maintain erect posture. Pressure applied to the concave portion of the curve will increase the lordosis.
CN: Physiological integrity; CNS: Reduction of risk potential; CL: Apply

CN: Client needs category   CNS: Client needs subcategory   CL: Cognitive level

12. The nurse is working with a client diagnosed with talipes equinovarus. Which muscle group will need to be strengthened?
1. Evertors
2. Invertors
3. Plantar flexors
4. Plantar fascia musculature

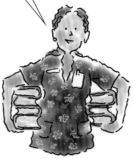

All this studying is strengthening my muscle groups. Oh, goody.

12. 1. Because the foot is held in inversion, it's important to strengthen the evertors to counter the inversion present in the foot. Inversion is incorrect because the foot is already held in this position. Plantar musculature and plantar flexors aren't important because the foot is already in a plantar flexed position.
CN: Physiological integrity; CNS: Reduction of risk potential; CL: Analyze

13. A nurse is caring for a 15-year-old who sustained a fracture of the femur 24 hours ago. Which finding would alert the nurse to an early complication?
1. Pain
2. Local swelling
3. Loss of function
4. Dyspnea

13. 4. After the fracture of a long bone, such as the femur, the client is at risk for fat embolism. Clinical manifestations include dyspnea, hypoxia, tachypnea, tachycardia, and chest pain. Pain, local swelling, and loss of function are all typical findings after a fracture.
CN: Physiological integrity; CNS: Reduction of risk potential; CL: Analyze

14. The nurse determines that an adolescent client with scoliosis understands the treatment plan when the client makes which statement?
1. "I will have to wear a brace for several years."
2. "I can put on the brace after I get home from school."
3. "I should avoid any exercise that will stretch my spine."
4. "I can remove the brace at night."

14. 1. A brace to correct scoliosis must be worn for several years to correct the spinal deformity. The brace should be worn all day, even during school and sleep. Exercises, performed several times per day, are commonly prescribed to stretch and strengthen back muscles. It should only be removed for one hour each day while bathing.
CN: Physiological integrity; CNS: Basic care and comfort; CL: Analyze

15. A child has just returned to his room with a cast on his leg after open reduction of a fractured femur. The nurse notes a 6 cm by 10 cm area of blood on the cast. What is the **most** important action by the nurse?
1. Tape gauze pads over the bloody area
2. Mark the bloody drainage and monitor hourly
3. Assess vital signs
4. Call the provider

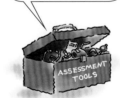

You'll need to pull out your assessment tools for this one.

ASSESSMENT TOOLS

15. 3. The most appropriate action for the nurse to take is to assess the client's vital signs for evidence of hemorrhage, such as tachycardia and hypotension. After the nurse has assessed the client, the provider should be notified with the findings. Gauze pads may be placed over the bloody drainage after the client is assessed and the provider notified. The size of the bloody drainage should be monitored after the client is assessed and the provider notified.
CN: Physiological integrity; CNS: Reduction of risk potential; CL: Analyze

16. Which observation, by a nurse, indicates proper fitting crutches for a nine-year-old boy?
1. The crutches fit snugly under the axilla.
2. The crutches end 2 in (5 cm) below the axilla.
3. The elbow is flexed 60 degrees.
4. The elbow is flexed 90 degrees.

16. 2. The crutches should end 2 in (5 cm) below the axilla, and the elbow should be flexed 20 to 30 degrees. Crutches should not fit snugly under the axilla to avoid potential damage to the neurovascular structures located in the axillary region. Elbow flexion is 15 to 30 degrees, not 60 or 90.
CN: Physiological integrity; CNS: Basic care and comfort; CL: Apply

17. Which technique may assist a three-month-old client diagnosed with torticollis?
1. Lying supine
2. Gentle massage
3. Range-of-motion (ROM) exercises
4. Lying on the side

17. 4. Side-lying, opposite the affected side, may help elongate shortened muscles. Lying supine won't assist with the elongation of muscles. Gentle massage won't assist with the elongation of muscles. ROM exercises won't assist with shortened muscles unless in specific patterns, and with stretching.

CN: Health promotion and maintenance; CNS: None;
CL: Apply

18. A physical therapist has instructed the nursing staff on how to perform range-of-motion (ROM) exercises for an infant with torticollis. The nurse is uncomfortable when the infant cries and grimaces during the exercises. What is the **most** important action for the nurse to take?
1. Check the primary health care provider's orders
2. Call the primary health care provider
3. Call the physical therapist
4. Discontinue the exercises

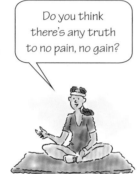

Do you think there's any truth to no pain, no gain?

18. 3. The only cure for the torticollis is exercise or surgery. The physical therapist is the expert in exercise and should be called for assistance in this situation. The primary health care provider should only be called if there is concern over the orders written, or an abnormal development in the child.

CN: Physiological integrity; CNS: Physiological adaptation;
CL: Analyze

19. A client has developed a right torticollis with side bending to the right and rotation to the left. Which exercises may assist in reduction of the torticollis?
1. Rotation exercises to the right
2. Rotation exercises to the left
3. Cervical extension exercises
4. Cervical flexion exercises

19. 1. Performing rotation exercises to the right will help increase the length of the shortened right sternocleidomastoid. Rotation to the left will add to the torticollis because the head is already rotated in that direction. Cervical extension exercises won't lengthen tightened muscles. Cervical flexion will add to shortening of the muscles.

CN: Physiological integrity; CNS: Reduction of risk potential;
CL: Apply

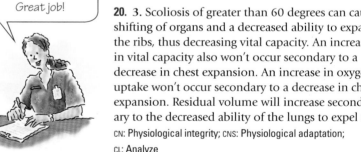

You've done 20 questions already. Great job!

20. The nurse is caring for a client with severe scoliosis. The nurse determines that the client is at risk for:
1. increased vital capacity.
2. increased oxygen uptake.
3. diminished vital capacity.
4. decreased residual volume.

20. 3. Scoliosis of greater than 60 degrees can cause shifting of organs and a decreased ability to expand the ribs, thus decreasing vital capacity. An increase in vital capacity also won't occur secondary to a decrease in chest expansion. An increase in oxygen uptake won't occur secondary to a decrease in chest expansion. Residual volume will increase secondary to the decreased ability of the lungs to expel air.

CN: Physiological integrity; CNS: Physiological adaptation;
CL: Analyze

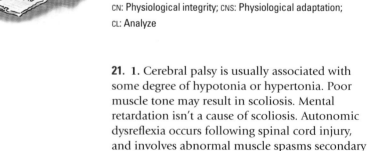

21. The parents of a four-year-old child, diagnosed with cerebral palsy and resultant thoracic scoliosis, ask the nurse what caused the scoliosis. What is the nurse's **best** response?
1. Hypotonia
2. Mental retardation
3. Autonomic dysreflexia
4. Increased thoracic kyphosis

21. 1. Cerebral palsy is usually associated with some degree of hypotonia or hypertonia. Poor muscle tone may result in scoliosis. Mental retardation isn't a cause of scoliosis. Autonomic dysreflexia occurs following spinal cord injury, and involves abnormal muscle spasms secondary to abnormal inhibitory neurons present during stretch reflexes. Increased thoracic kyphosis won't result in scoliosis.

CN: Physiological integrity; CNS: Physiological adaptation;
CL: Apply

22. Which statement, by the parents of a child with crutches, indicates an understanding of how to safely walk down stairs?
  1. First, place the crutches on the lower step
  2. Advance the fractured leg first
  3. Advance the strong leg first
  4. First, place the crutch on the fractured side on the lower step

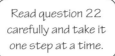

Read question 22 carefully and take it one step at a time.

22. 1. To walk down the stairs with crutches, the crutches are first placed on the lower step. Then the fractured or weaker leg is lowered, followed by the unaffected leg. The arms and unaffected leg share the work of carrying the body weight.
CN: Safe, effective care environment; CNS: Safety and infection control; CL: Apply

23. A school nurse is performing scoliosis screening and notices that an adolescent has a raised iliac crest height. What condition would the nurse suspect?
  1. Forward head posture
  2. Leg length discrepancy
  3. Increased lumbar lordosis
  4. Increased thoracic kyphosis

23. 2. A raised iliac crest may be indicative of a leg length discrepancy, or a curvature in the lumbar spine. It isn't indicative of forward head posture, lumbar lordosis, or thoracic kyphosis.
CN: Health promotion and maintenance; CNS: None; CL: Apply

24. A school nurse is performing a scoliosis screening on a group of students. Which student would **most** commonly develop this condition?
  1. A seven-year-old girl
  2. A seven-year-old boy
  3. A 13-year-old girl
  4. A 13-year-old boy

24. 3. Scoliosis is eight times more prominent in adolescent girls than boys. Peak incidence is between ages eight and 15. Therefore, a 13-year-old girl is at the highest risk. Seven-year-old boys and girls are at lower risk.
CN: Health promotion and maintenance; CNS: None; CL: Analyze

25. The nurse is caring for a child with a Harrington instrumentation rod placement. While assessing the child on the second postoperative day, the nurse is **most** concerned when the assessment data includes:
  1. fever of 99.5° F (37.5° C).
  2. pain along the incision.
  3. decreased urinary output.
  4. hypoactive bowel sounds.

25. 3. Because of extensive blood loss during surgery and possible renal hypoperfusion, decreased urinary output could indicate decreased renal function. A fever of 99.5° F (37.5° C) is of concern, but may be due to decreased chest expansion secondary to anesthesia, surgery, and pain. Pain along the incision site is expected. A paralytic ileus is common after surgery, and the client may have a nasogastric tube for the first 48 hours.
CN: Physiological integrity; CNS: Reduction of risk potential; CL: Analyze

26. What is the **best** landmark for the nurse to observe when performing scoliosis screening on children?
  1. Iliac crests
  2. Spinous processes
  3. Acromion processes
  4. Posterior superior iliac spines

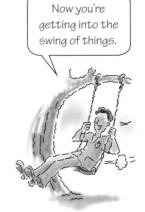

Now you're getting into the swing of things.

26. 2. The spinous processes are the best bony landmarks to identify when attempting to screen for scoliosis, because this will show lateral deviation of the column. Abnormalities in the acromion process, iliac crests, and posterior superior iliac spines may not be indicative of scoliosis.
CN: Health promotion and maintenance; CNS: None; CL: Apply

27. Which intervention may be a possible treatment choice for talipes equinovarus?
1. Traction
2. Serial casting
3. Short leg braces
4. Inversion range-of-motion (ROM) exercises

28. What is the **best** technique for the nurse to use when performing stretches with a child who has scoliosis?
1. Slow and sustained
2. Quick, short movements
3. Quick movements to the end range of pain
4. Slow movements for brief, 3- to 4-second periods

29. Which observation, by a nurse, indicates that the parent of a neonate with developmental dysplasia of the hip understands the discharge teaching?
1. The parent places a folded towel between the infant's legs.
2. The infant is wearing three diapers.
3. The infant is tightly swaddled in a blanket.
4. The infant is placed in a prone position to sleep.

30. A nurse is caring for an infant with suspected developmental dysplasia of the hip (DDH). Which information should the nurse give the parents about diagnostic testing?
1. A diagnosis can't be confirmed until the child begins to walk.
2. Diagnostic testing is performed at six months if the dysplasia hasn't resolved by then.
3. A radiopaque dye will be injected into the subarachnoid space of the spine.
4. An X-ray will confirm the diagnosis.

31. Which hip position should be avoided in an eight-month-old infant who has been diagnosed with developmental dysplasia of the hip?
1. Extension
2. Abduction
3. Internal rotation
4. External rotation

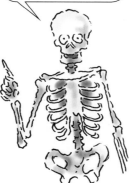

It's all about stability and, in this case, instability.

28. 2. Serial casting is a treatment choice while attempting to change the length of soft tissue. Traction is not an option. Corrective shoes are used instead of short leg braces. Eversion rather than inversion exercises will help.
CN: Physiological integrity; CNS: Reduction of risk potential;
CL: Apply

28. 1. Stretches should be slow and sustained. It's difficult to see changes in muscle length. Stretches shouldn't be performed with quick movements. Stretches should be performed for longer than a few seconds.
CN: Health promotion and maintenance; CNS: None;
CL: Apply

29. 2. Placing several diapers on the infant will keep the hips and knees flexed, and the hips abducted. A towel placed between the legs is not enough to keep the hips abducted. Swaddling the infant tightly straightens the legs and doesn't allow the hips to be abducted. Placing the infant in a prone position will not keep the hips abducted, and isn't recommended due to the increased risk of sudden infant death syndrome.
CN: Physiological integrity; CNS: Basic care and comfort;
CL: Apply

30. 4. X-rays will show the location of the femur head and a shallow acetabulum, confirming the diagnosis DDH. The diagnosis can be made in the neonate and should be made as soon as possible since it becomes more difficult to correct as the child ages. Myelography is an invasive procedure used to evaluate abnormalities of the spinal canal and cord. It isn't used in the diagnosis of congenital hip dysplasia.
CN: Physiological integrity; CNS: Physiological adaptation;
CL: Apply

31. 3. Internal rotation of the hip is an unstable position and should be avoided in infants with hip instability. Hip extension is a relatively stable position. Typically, the child is placed in slight abduction while in a hip-spica cast. External rotation isn't necessarily an unstable position, as long as it isn't externally rotated too far.
CN: Physiological integrity; CNS: Reduction of risk potential;
CL: Apply

CN: Client needs category   CNS: Client needs subcategory   CL: Cognitive level

32. A nurse is planning care for a client who has muscular dystrophy. The nurse would anticipate that this client would initially have difficulty with:
1. breathing.
2. sitting.
3. standing.
4. swallowing.

32. 3. Muscular dystrophy initially affects postural muscles of the hip and shoulder. Sitting may be affected, but a client would have difficulty standing before having difficulty sitting. Swallowing and breathing are usually affected last.
CN: Physiological integrity; CNS: Physiological adaptation;
CL: Apply

33. Which diagnostic test would the nurse anticipate for the diagnosis of suspected developmental dysplasia of the hip (DDH)?
1. X-ray
2. Positive Ortolani's sign
3. Positive Trendelenburg gait
4. Audible clicking with adduction

33. 1. An X-ray will confirm the diagnosis of DDH. All of the options are positive signs of DDH, but only the X-ray will confirm the diagnosis.
CN: Physiological integrity; CNS: Physiological adaptation;
CL: Apply

34. What finding would the nurse anticipate when assessing a neonate with a positive Galeazzi sign?
1. Raised iliac crest
2. Pelvic downward tilt on weight bearing
3. Knees flexed to 90 degrees, with one knee higher
4. Involved leg flexed to 90 degrees, with an audible click during external rotation

34. 3. A positive Galeazzi sign is used to help diagnose hip dislocation. It presents as one knee higher than the other. A raised iliac crest isn't indicative of specific hip pathology. A downward pelvic tilt upon weight bearing is Trendelenburg gait. External rotation of the hip with an audible click is Ortolani-Barlow test.
CN: Health promotion and maintenance; CNS: None;
CL: Apply

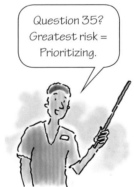

Question 35?
Greatest risk =
Prioritizing.

35. A young child sustains a dislocated hip as well as a subcapital fracture. The nurse is aware that this client is at **greatest** risk for:
1. avascular necrosis.
2. post-surgical infection.
3. hemorrhage during surgery.
4. poor post-surgical ambulation.

35. 1. Avascular necrosis is common with fractures to the subcapital region secondary to possible compromise of blood supply to the femoral head. Post-surgical infection is always a concern, but not a priority. Hemorrhage should not occur. Poor post-surgical ambulation is a concern, but not the priority.
CN: Physiological integrity; CNS: Reduction of risk potential;
CL: Apply

36. How should the femur be positioned in relationship to the acetabulum for a child with developmental dysplasia of the hip (DDH)?
1. Anterior
2. Inferior
3. Posterior
4. Superior

36. 1. The head of the femur should be anterior to the acetabulum in DDH. All other positions are inaccurate.
CN: Physiological integrity; CNS: Physiological adaptation;
CL: Apply

37. The nurse is planning to teach the parents of a child newly diagnosed with muscular dystrophy about the disease. How would the nurse **most** accurately describe this condition?
1. A demyelinating disease
2. Lesions of the brain cortex
3. Upper motor neuron lesions
4. Degeneration of muscle fibers

37. 4. Degeneration of muscle fibers with progressive weakness and wasting best describes muscular dystrophy. Demyelination of myelin sheaths is a description of multiple sclerosis. Lesions within the cortex and in upper motor neurons suggest a neurological, not a muscular, disease.
CN: Physiological integrity; CNS: Physiological adaptation;
CL: Apply

CN: Client needs category   CNS: Client needs subcategory   CL: Cognitive level

38. Which muscles should the nurse anticipate as **first** affected in a child suspected of having muscular dystrophy?
  1. Hip muscles
  2. Foot muscles
  3. Hand muscles
  4. Respiration muscles

39. What information should the nurse provide to the parents of child undergoing testing for a diagnosis of muscular dystrophy?
  1. The genitals will be covered by a lead apron.
  2. A local anesthetic will be used for the test.
  3. Electrode wires will be attached to the scalp.
  4. A fiber-optic endoscope will be inserted into a joint.

40. The nurse is reviewing the laboratory tests of a child diagnosed with muscular dystrophy. Which laboratory test would help verify a diagnosis of this condition?
  1. Bilirubin
  2. Creatinine
  3. Serum potassium
  4. Sodium

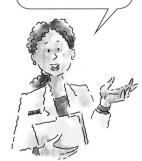

Question 40 asks which lab test helps in diagnosing the condition.

41. The nurse is teaching a student nurse about muscular dystrophy. The student nurse asks, "Which form of muscular dystrophy is most common?" What is the nurse's **most** accurate response?
  1. Duchenne's
  2. Becker's
  3. Limb girdle
  4. Myotonic

38. 1. Positional muscles of the hip and shoulder are affected first. Progression of the disease then advances to muscles of the foot and hand. Involuntary muscles, such as the muscles of respiration, are affected last.
CN: Physiological integrity; CNS: Physiological adaptation; CL: Apply

39. 2. A muscle biopsy, used to confirm the diagnosis of muscular dystrophy, will show the degeneration of muscle fibers and infiltration of fatty tissue. The biopsy is typically performed using local anesthetic. The genitals are covered by a lead apron during an X-ray examination, which is used to detect osseous, not muscular, problems. Electrode wires are attached to the scalp during a EEG to observe brain wave activity, but is not used to diagnose muscular dystrophy. Arthroscopy involves the insertion of a fiber-optic scope into a joint, and isn't used to diagnose muscular dystrophy.
CN: Physiological integrity; CNS: Basic care and comfort; CL: Apply

40. 2. Diagnostic studies for muscular dystrophy include muscle serum enzymes, especially creatine kinase, EMG, muscle fiber biopsy, and ECG abnormalities reflective of cardiomyopathy. Creatinine values will help verify the diagnosis of muscular dystrophy. Creatinine will be elevated in progressive muscular dystrophy, as it is a by-product of muscle metabolism as it hypertrophies. Bilirubin, a pigment derived from the breakdown of hemoglobin, is a by-product of liver function. Potassium and sodium levels can change due to various factors and are not indicators of muscular dystrophy.
CN: Health promotion and maintenance; CNS: None; CL: Apply

41. 1. Duchenne's, also known as pseudohypertrophic, muscular dystrophy accounts for 50% of all cases of muscular dystrophy. It affects the cardiac and respiratory muscles and all voluntary muscles.
CN: Physiological integrity; CNS: Physiological adaptation; CL: Apply

42. Which condition would alert the nurse that a child may have developed muscular dystrophy?
1. Hypertonia of extremities
2. Increased lumbar lordosis
3. Upper extremity spasticity
4. Hyperactive lower extremity reflexes

42. 2. Increased lumbar lordosis is seen in a child affected by muscular dystrophy secondary to paralysis of lower lumbar postural muscles. It also occurs to increase lower extremity support. Hypertonia is not a symptom of muscular dystrophy. Upper extremity spasticity is not a symptom, because this disease isn't caused by upper motor neuron lesions. Hyperactive reflexes are not indications of muscular dystrophy.
CN: Physiological integrity; CNS: Physiological adaptation; CL: Analyze

43. The parents of a child with Duchenne's muscular dystrophy want to know how it is acquired. What is the nurse's **most** accurate response?
1. Virus
2. Hereditary
3. Autoimmune factors
4. Environmental toxins

43. 2. Muscular dystrophy is hereditary, and acquired through a recessive sex-linked trait. It is not viral, autoimmune, or caused by toxins.
CN: Physiological integrity; CNS: Physiological adaptation; CL: Apply

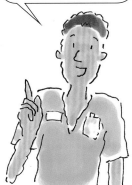

It's all in the jeans ... I mean the genes.

44. A client with muscular dystrophy has lost complete control of his lower extremities. He has some strength bilaterally in the upper extremities, but poor trunk control. Which mechanism would be the **most** important to have on this client's wheelchair?
1. Antitip device
2. Extended breaks
3. Headrest support
4. Wheelchair belt

44. 4. This client has poor trunk control. A belt will prevent him from falling out of his wheelchair. Antitip devices, head rest supports, and extended breaks are all important options, but aren't the most important for this client.
CN: Safe, effective care environment; CNS: Safety and infection control; CL: Apply

Question 44 tests your ability to ensure the client's safety.

45. A two-year-old toddler has muscular dystrophy. His legs are held together, and his knees are touching. Which of this client's muscles are contracted?
1. Hip abductors
2. Hip adductors
3. Hip extensors
4. Hip flexors

45. 2. The hip adductors are in a shortened position. The abductors are in a lengthened position. This position isn't indicative of hip flexor or hip extensor shortening.
CN: Health promotion and maintenance; CNS: None; CL: Apply

46. A 12-year-old child with muscular dystrophy is hospitalized secondary to a fall. This client will require surgery and skeletal traction. For which complication should the nurse be **most** alert?
1. Skin integrity
2. Infection of pin sites
3. Respiratory infection
4. Non-union healing of the fracture

46. 3. Respiratory infection can be fatal for clients with muscular dystrophy due to poor chest expansion and decreased ability to mobilize secretions. Skin integrity, infection of pin sites, and non-union healing are important, but not as important as the prevention of respiratory infection.
CN: Physiological integrity; CNS: Reduction of risk potential; CL: Analyze

47. A nurse is teaching a 12-year-old boy and his parents about his osteogenesis imperfecta. The boy tells the nurse that he likes to swim. What is the nurse's **most** appropriate response?
  1. "You should add a weight-bearing exercises as well."
  2. "Swimming isn't safe for you since you can slip on the wet surfaces around the pool."
  3. "Swimming is the only exercise that you'll need."
  4. "Any form of exercises is not safe for you."

48. The nurse understands that adolescent females with scolioisis are **most** commonly afflicted with:
  1. respiratory distress.
  2. poor self-esteem.
  3. poor appetite.
  4. renal difficulty.

49. A child is having difficulty ambulating, and tends to walk on his toes. This child may require surgical intervention. Which surgical intervention would the nurse anticipate?
  1. Adductor release
  2. Hamstring release
  3. Plantar fascia release
  4. Achilles tendon release

50. The parents of a child with muscular dystrophy ask the nurse what causes this condition. What is the nurse's **best** response?
  1. Gene mutation
  2. Chromosomal aberration
  3. Unknown non-genetic origin
  4. Environmental factors

51. The nurse is assessing a child suspected of having muscular dystrophy for muscle weakness. At which age do the signs usually **first** appear?
  1. 1 year
  2. 2 years
  3. 3 years
  4. 4 years

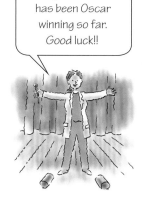

Your performance has been Oscar winning so far. Good luck!!

47. 1. Swimming is a beneficial form of exercise for people with osteogenesis imperfecta, but does little to prevent bone loss. This client should add weight-bearing exercises to his fitness regime. Although wet areas around the pool are a risk for the person with osteogenesis imperfecta, the risk can be minimized by walking carefully and wearing nonskid footwear. Mild forms of exercise are encouraged to improve cardiovascular conditioning, promote bone density and maintain joint mobility.
CN: Health promotion and maintenance; CNS: None;
CL: Apply

48. 2. Poor self-esteem is a major affliction with many adolescents. The use of orthopedic appliances, such as those used to treat scoliosis, can negatively affect body image of many adolescents with scoliosis. Although respiratory distress and poor appetite may be present, they aren't as common as poor self-esteem. Renal problems aren't usually an issue in adolescents with scoliosis.
CN: Health promotion and maintenance; CNS: None;
CL: Apply

49. 4. A shortened Achilles tendon may cause a child to walk on his toes. Surgical release of the tendon may assist this child with proper walking. An adductor release is commonly performed if the legs are held together. A plantar fascia release won't help, and a hamstring release is only done when there's a knee flexion contracture.
CN: Physiological integrity; CNS: Reduction of risk potential;
CL: Apply

50. 1. Muscular dystrophy belongs to a group of genetic diseases that are characterized by the progressive wasting of skeletal muscles, and is a result of a gene mutation. Muscular dystrophy does not come from a chromosomal aberration or environmental factors. It is genetic, and there is a known origin of the disease.
CN: Physiological integrity; CNS: Physiological adaptation;
CL: Apply

51. 3. Studies have shown that children diagnosed with muscular dystrophy usually show some form of weakness around age three.
CN: Health promotion and maintenance; CNS: None;
CL: Apply

CN: Client needs category   CNS: Client needs subcategory   CL: Cognitive level

52. To promote safe transfers for a client with muscular dystrophy a nurse should teach this client exercises to maintain:
1. gastrocnemius muscles.
2. gluteus maximus muscles.
3. hamstring muscles.
4. quadricep muscles.

52. 2. The gluteus maximus is the strongest muscle in the body, and is important for standing as well as for transfers. All muscles are important, but the maintenance of the gluteus maximus will enable maximum function.
CN: Health promotion and maintenance; CNS: None; CL: Apply

53. Which strategy would be the **first** choice in attempting to maximize function in a child with muscular dystrophy?
1. Long-leg braces
2. Motorized wheelchair
3. Manual wheelchair
4. Walker

The words *first choice* can help you focus on the answer to question 53.

53. 1. Long-leg braces are functional assistive devices that provide increased independence and the increased use of upper and lower body strength. Wheelchairs, both motorized and manual, provide less independence and less use of upper and lower body strength. Walkers are functional assistive devices that provide less independence than braces.
CN: Physiological integrity; CNS: Basic care and comfort; CL: Apply

54. A child with muscular dystrophy is having increased difficulty getting out of his chair at school. Which recommendation should the nurse make to assist the child?
1. A seat cushion
2. Long leg braces
3. Powered wheelchair
4. Removable armrests on wheelchair

54. 1. A seat cushion will put the hip extensors at an advantage and make it somewhat easier to get up. Long leg braces wouldn't be the first choice. A powered wheelchair wouldn't be important in assisting with the transfer. Removable armrests have no bearing on assisting the client.
CN: Physiological integrity; CNS: Basic care and comfort; CL: Apply

55. The nurse is palpating the muscles of a child with muscular dystrophy. Which findings should the nurse anticipate?
1. Soft on palpation
2. Firm on palpation
3. Extremely hard on palpation
4. No muscle consistency on palpation

55. 2. Muscles will commonly be firm on palpation secondary to the infiltration of fatty tissue and connective tissue into the muscle. The muscles won't be soft secondary to the infiltration and won't be hard upon palpation. There is some consistency to the muscle, although in advanced stages, atrophy is present.
CN: Physiological integrity; CNS: Physiological adaptation; CL: Analyze

56. A six-year-old client is being discharged following treatment of osteomyelitis caused by *Staphylococcus aureus*. The provider has ordered 300 mg cephalexin bid, for administration at home. The suspension comes in a bottle containing 400 mg/5 ml. How many milliliters should the nurse administer for each dose? Record your answer to the nearest hundredth.

_____ ml

56. 3.75.
The formula to use is:

$$\text{Amount Given} = \frac{\text{Desired}}{\text{Have}} \times \text{Volume}$$

Desired: 300 mg. Have 400 mg. The suspension volume is 5 ml.

$$\text{Amount Given} = \frac{300\,\text{mg}}{400\,\text{mg}} \times 5\,\text{ml}$$

$$X = 3.75\,\text{ml}$$

CN: Physiological integrity; CNS: Pharmacological and parenteral therapies CL: Apply

CN: Client needs category   CNS: Client needs subcategory   CL: Cognitive level

57. How would the nurse **best** describe Gowers' sign to the parents of a child with muscular dystrophy?
1. A clinical sign
2. A waddling-type gait
3. The pelvis position during gait
4. Muscle twitching present during a quick stretch

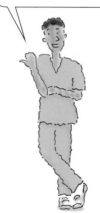

To remember Gowers' sign, think going somewhere— that's a description of what the child is trying to do.

58. A 13-year-old, admitted with a fractured femur, had an open reduction and internal fixation two days ago and is currently in traction. The client asks the nurse, "What would happen to me if a terrorist decided to bomb the hospital." What is the nurse's **best** response?
1. "I wouldn't worry about that. Focus on getting well and going home."
2. "We have plans to call your parents and take care of you if there's a problem."
3. "What do you think might happen if there is a terrorist attack?"
4. "Why are you asking me that question?"

59. A client with bilaterally-fractured femurs is scheduled for a double–hip-spica cast. She says to the nurse, "Only three more months and I can go home." Further conversation reveals that this client and her family believe that she'll be hospitalized until the cast comes off. The nurse should explain that the child:
1. may be hospitalized for 2 to 4 months.
2. will go home 2 to 4 days after casting.
3. will go home 1 week after casting.
4. will go home as soon as she can move.

60. Which observation, by a nurse, indicates that an infant in a hip-spica cast is properly positioned?
1. The infant's upper body and cast are at a 180-degree angle.
2. The infant's hips are higher than the head.
3. The infant's upper body and the cast are at a 45-degree angle.
4. The infant is flat in bed.

57. 1. Gowers' sign is a clinical sign for the manner in which children with well-developed Duchenne's muscular dystrophy rise from a sitting to a standing position by grasping and pulling on body parts from the knees to hips until they are in an erect position. The child turns on the side or abdomen, extends the knees, and pushes on the torso to an upright position by walking his hands up the legs. A waddling-type gait doesn't describe Gowers' sign. The position of the pelvis during gait isn't described by Gowers' sign. Muscle twitching present after a quick stretch is described as clonus.
CN: Physiological integrity; CNS: Physiological adaptation; CL: Analyze

58. 3. Something prompted this question, and the nurse should take this opportunity to explore the teen's concerns and fears. Answer one discounts this teen's feelings, and may increase her anxiety. Answer two doesn't provide reassurance or help build a therapeutic relationship that can promote health and wellness. Answer four is a confrontational response and does not use therapeutic communication technique.
CN: Physiological integrity; CNS: None; CL: Analyze

59. 2. The cast will dry quickly if fiberglass casting material is used. The time spent in the hospital following casting is typically 2 to 4 days. This time will be used to teach the client and her family about home care, and how to evaluate the client's skin integrity and neurovascular status before discharge.
CN: Health promotion and maintenance; CNS: None; CL: Apply

60. 1. Proper positioning will help keep the cast clean and dry during toileting. Keeping your child's head slightly higher than his feet will help drain urine and stool away from the cast. The infant's body and cast should be at a 180-degree angle. While the cast should be kept level with the body, it should be on a slant with the head of the bed elevated so that urine and stool can drain downward and not soil the cast.
CN: Physiological integrity; CNS: Basic care and comfort; CL: Apply

CN: Client needs category   CNS: Client needs subcategory   CL: Cognitive level

61. What is the **most** severe type of muscular dystrophy?

1. Duchenne's
2. Facioscapulohumeral
3. Limb girdle
4. Myotonic

61. 1. Studies have shown that Duchenne's is the most severe form of muscular dystrophy, affecting all voluntary muscles as well as cardiac and respiratory muscles.

CN: Physiological integrity; CNS: Physiological adaptation; CL: Remember

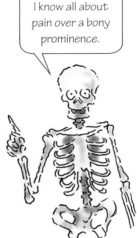

I know all about pain over a bony prominence.

62. The nurse assesses a client with a cast following a fracture of the radius. Which finding would the nurse be **most** concerned about?

1. Discomfort occurring at the site of the fracture
2. Fingers that are pink and warm
3. Swelling that is reduced with cast elevation
4. Pain that occur over a bony prominence

62. 4. Pain over a bony prominence, such as in the wrist or elbow, are signs of an impending pressure ulcer and require prompt attention. Pain or discomfort at the site of a fracture is expected and is relieved by analgesics. Warm, pink fingers are an expected finding. Swelling should be relieved by elevation of the extremity. Swelling that isn't relieved by elevation of the affected limb should be reported to the provider.

CN: Physiological integrity; CNS: Reduction of risk potential; CL: Apply

63. The parents of a child with newly diagnosed developmental dysplasia of the hip (DDH) ask the nurse why their child has this condition. The nurse explains that the majority of cases are caused by:

1. dislocation.
2. subluxation.
3. acetabular dysplasia.
4. dislocation with fracture.

63. 2. Subluxation is a partial or incomplete displacement of the joint surface. Studies show that subluxation accounts for the majority of cases of DDH. Dislocation results in a separation or complete displacement of the articular surfaces of a joint, and often occur with a fracture. The acetabulum connects with the head of the femur to form the hip joint.

CN: Physiological integrity; CNS: Physiological adaptation; CL: Apply

64. Which finding would the nurse anticipate in a client with developmental dysplasia of the hip (DDH)?

1. Ligamentum teres is shortened.
2. Femoral head loses contact with acetabulum and is displaced inferiorly.
3. Femoral head loses contact with the acetabulum and is displaced posteriorly.
4. Femoral head maintains contact with acetabulum, but there's noted capsular rupture.

64. 3. In DDH, the femoral head loses contact with the acetabulum and is displaced posteriorly, not inferiorly, capsular rupture does not occur. Ligamentum teres is lengthened.

CN: Physiological integrity; CNS: Physiological adaptation; CL: Apply

65. A toddler is immobilized with traction to the legs. Which play activity would be appropriate for the nurse to include in the plan of care for this child?

1. Pounding board
2. Tinker toys
3. Pull toys
4. Board games

65. 1. A pounding board is appropriate for an immobilized toddler because it promotes physical development and an acceptable energy outlet. Toys with small parts, such as Tinker toys, aren't suitable because a toddler may swallow the parts. A pull toy is suitable for most toddlers, but not for one who is immobilized. Board games are usually too advanced for the developmental skills of a toddler.

CN: Health promotion and maintenance; CNS: None; CL: Apply

66. An unlicensed assistive personnel (UAP) asks the nurse how to care for a client's hip-spica cast that has been soiled. What is the nurse's **best** response?
1. Clean with damp cloth and dry cleanser
2. Clean with soap and water
3. Don't do anything
4. Change the cast

66. 1. A damp cloth and dry cleanser are best. Water will break the cast down. If nothing is done, the cast will emit a foul odor. Changing the cast is not an option.
CN: Physiological integrity; CNS: Basic care and comfort; CL: Apply

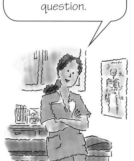

Knowing the shape of a hip-spica cast can help answer this question.

67. A child in a hip-spica cast needs to be toileted. How should the nurse position this child?
1. Supine when using a bedpan
2. Seated in a toilet chair
3. Shoulder lower than buttocks when using a bedpan
4. Head higher than buttocks when using a bedpan

67. 4. Because it's difficult for children to use the bathroom while in a spica cast, a bedpan or urinal is used. To use a bedpan, turn your child to the side and place the bedpan under her buttocks and then turn her back onto the bedpan. Check between her thighs to be sure the bedpan is properly positioned. Always elevate your child's head, so urine flows down and away from the cast. This child isn't able to use a toilet chair.
CN: Physiological integrity; CNS: Basic care and comfort; CL: Apply

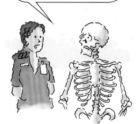

Pulling and pins? This doesn't sound like fun.

68. Which intervention should a nurse perform for a four-year-old child in skeletal traction?
1. Provide daily pin site care
2. Release weights for one hour each day
3. Change the child's position every four hours
4. Unwrap the elastic bandage every shift to assess the skin

68. 1. When a pin is placed into the bone it is called skeletal traction, and requires pin site care. Pin site care involves cleaning the insertion sites to reduce the risk of infection and observing for the signs and symptoms of infection. Weights should hang freely and shouldn't be released. The child's position should be changed every two hours to prevent skin breakdown. Elastic bandages are used in skin, not skeletal, traction.
CN: Physiological integrity; CNS: Basic care and comfort; CL: Apply

69. The nurse observes a client who has a positive Trendelenburg gait. Which characteristic would indicate this gait?
1. Pelvis tilts downward upon weight bearing
2. Pelvis tilts upward upon weight bearing
3. Abnormal height of the iliac crests
4. Leg length discrepancy

69. 1. The pelvis will tilt downward upon weight bearing secondary to a weakness of the abductors on the affected side. The pelvis does not tilt upward with a positive Trendelenburg gait. Leg length and iliac crest height aren't indicative of a positive Trendelenburg gait.
CN: Physiological integrity; CNS: Physiological adaptation; CL: Apply

70. Which complication, involving leg length, should the nurse anticipate in a client with developmental dysplasia of the hip?
1. Increased hip abduction
2. Increased leg length on the affected side
3. Decreased leg length on the affected side
4. No change in muscle length or leg length

70. 3. Internal rotation with subsequent dislocation will cause the leg to be shorter, not longer. There is usually decreased abduction as well as muscle and leg length changes.
CN: Physiological integrity; CNS: Physiological adaptation; CL: Analyze

71. A nurse recognizes that the parent of a child with developmental dysplasia of the hip requires additional teaching when they place their child in a position that encourages:
1. hip abduction.
2. knee extension.
3. external rotation.
4. internal rotation.

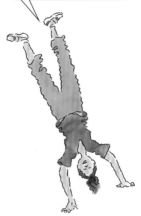

Feeling a little keyed up? Take a break and do a few cartwheels.

71. 4. Internal rotation increases the risk of hip dislocation. Abduction, external rotation, and knee extension will not increase the risk of dislocation.
CN: Health promotion and maintenance; CNS: None; CL: Apply

72. The nurse is caring for a child immediately following a spinal fusion. The nurse understands that **immediate** action is required when the child states:
1. "I'm afraid to move. It's going to hurt."
2. "My feet feel like they are asleep."
3. "I want to sit on the side of the bed."
4. "My feet feel funny and I can't move them."

72. 4. Paresthesia may not subside immediately after surgery; however, the nurse should document any new muscle weakness or paresthesia, and report it to the surgeon immediately. The child should be reassured that there are enough nurses to ease turning and movement. Depending on the healthcare provider's preference, and the type of surgery, the client may be allowed to dangle at the side of the bed, stand, or ambulate the same day as surgery.
CN: Health promotion and maintenance; CNS: None; CL: Apply

73. Which intervention should a nurse implement to prevent a client from developing venous stasis after skeletal traction application?
1. Bed rest only
2. Convoluted foam mattress
3. Vigorous pulmonary care
4. Antiembolism stockings or an intermittent compression device

73. 4. To prevent venous stasis after skeletal traction application, antiembolism stockings or an intermittent compression device should be used on the unaffected leg. Bed rest can cause venous stasis. Convoluted foam mattresses and pulmonary care don't prevent venous stasis.
CN: Health promotion and maintenance; CNS: None; CL: Apply

74. What is the **best** technique for a school nurse to use when assessing a 13-year-old with suspected structural scoliosis?
1. Have the client bend over and touch her toes while the nurse observes from the back
2. Have the client stand sideways while the nurse observes her profile
3. Have the client assume a knee-chest position on the examination table
4. Have the client arch her back while the nurse observes her from the back

74. 1. As the child bends over, the curvature of the spine is more apparent. The scapula on one side becomes more prominent, and the opposite side hollows. The knee-chest position is used for lumbar puncture. Scoliosis cannot be properly assessed from the side or the front.
CN: Health promotion and maintenance; CNS: None; CL: Apply

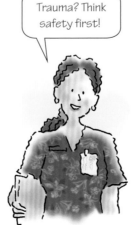

Trauma? Think safety first!

75. Which nursing intervention is appropriate for a child with a suspected fracture due to trauma?
1. Keep the child still
2. Sit the child up to facilitate breathing
3. Immediately move the child to a safe place
4. Immobilize the extremity and then move the child to a safe place

75. 4. The nurse should immobilize the extremity of a child with a suspected fracture and then move him to a safe place. If the child is already in a safe place, don't attempt to move him. Sitting the child up could worsen the fracture.
CN: Safe, effective care environment; CNS: Safety and infection control; CL: Apply

76. A nurse is assessing an 18-month-old infant who is lying on his back in Bryant's traction for a fractured left femur. What is the correct position for this child?
1. Left leg extended 90 degrees off the bed
2. Right leg extended 90 degrees off the bed
3. Both legs extended 90 degrees off the bed
4. Both legs extended at 180 degrees off the bed

77. The nurse is caring for a client in skeletal traction. What is an appropriate nursing intervention for this client?
1. Assessing pin sites every shift and as needed
2. Ensuring that the rope knots catch on the pulley
3. Adding and removing weights per client's request
4. Performing range of motion (ROM) exercise for all joints every shift

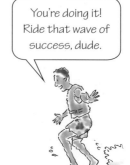

You're doing it! Ride that wave of success, dude.

76. 3. Bryant's traction is for lower extremity fractures in children younger than two years. Both legs are suspended at 90 degrees off the bed. The child's body weight will provide counter traction.
CN: Physiological integrity; CNS: Basic care and comfort; CL: Apply

77. 1. Pin sites should be assessed every shift and as needed. The nurse should also ensure that the knots in the rope don't catch on the pulley. Weights should be added and removed per the primary health care provider's order, and all joints, except those immediately proximal and distal to the fracture, should have ROM exercises each shift.
CN: Physiological integrity; CNS: Basic care and comfort; CL: Apply

78. A nurse is caring for a client immediately following the application of a cast for a fractured femur. Prioritize the nurse's care.

1.	Rest the cast on the bed supported by pillows
2.	Dispose of the plaster water in the sink
3.	Support the cast with palms of hands
4.	Wait until the cast dries before cleaning the surrounding skin

78. Ordered Response:

3.	Support the cast with palms of hands
2.	Dispose of the plaster water in the sink
4.	Wait until the cast dries before cleaning the surrounding skin
1.	Rest the cast on the bed supported by pillows

CN: Physiological integrity; CNS: Reduction of risk potential; CL: Analyze

79. A school-age child tells the nurse that he's experiencing intense itching under his cast. What is the nurse's **most** appropriate response?
1. There's nothing that can be done
2. Place the eraser end of a new pencil under your cast to scratch
3. Elevate the cast above the level of your heart
4. Aim cool air from a hair dryer under the cast

79. 4. Cool air from a hair dryer may soothe the itch. Nothing should be placed under a cast because this can cause skin irritation and breakdown. Elevating the cast above the level of the heart doesn't relieve itching. This position is used to reduce swelling.
CN: Physiological integrity; CNS: Basic care and comfort; CL: Apply

80. A client returns to the unit after the application of a cast. On assessment, the nurse notes that the cast is not dry, and the client reports a sensation of heat from the cast. What is the nurse's **best** intervention?
1. Remove the cast immediately
2. Notify the primary health care provider
3. Assess the client for other signs of infection
4. Explain to the client that this is a normal sensation

80. 4. As the cast dries, the client may report a sensation of heat from the cast. The nurse should reassure the client that this is normal. There is no need to notify the primary health care provider or remove the cast. Heat from the cast isn't a sign of infection.
CN: Physiological integrity; CNS: Reduction of risk potential; CL: Apply

81. How should the nurse prevent foot drop in a casted leg?
1. Encourage bed rest
2. Support the foot with 45 degrees of flexion
3. Support the foot with 90 degrees of flexion
4. Place a stocking on the foot to provide warmth

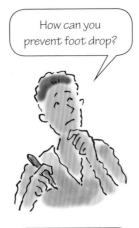

81. 3. To prevent foot drop in a casted leg, the nurse should support the foot with 90 degrees of flexion. Bed rest can cause foot drop. Keeping the extremity warm won't prevent foot drop.
CN: Health promotion and maintenance; CNS: None; CL: Apply

82. The nurse instructs a client with a hip-spica cast to avoid gas-forming foods. The client asks, "What can happen if these foods are consumed?" What is the nurse's **best** response?
1. Flatus
2. Diarrhea
3. Constipation
4. Abdominal distention

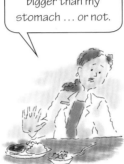

82. 4. A client with a hip-spica cast should avoid gas-forming foods to prevent abdominal distention. Gas-forming foods may cause flatus, but that isn't a reason to avoid them. Gas-forming foods don't generally cause diarrhea or constipation.
CN: Physiological integrity; CNS: Reduction of risk potential; CL: Apply

83. A nurse determines that a client, with a fractured left femur, understands the instructions for touch-down weight bearing when the client states:
1. "I will place full weight on my left leg."
2. "I will place about 30% to 50% of my weight on my left leg."
3. "I will keep my left leg off the floor."
4. "I will allow my left leg to touch the floor without placing weight on it."

83. 4. Touch-down weight bearing allows the client to put no weight on the extremity, but may touch the floor with the affected extremity. Partial-weight bearing allows for only 30% to 50% weight bearing on the affected extremity. Non-weight bearing is no weight on the extremity, and the extremity must remain elevated.
CN: Physiological integrity; CNS: Basic care and comfort; CL: Apply

84. Which strategy should the nurse teach an adolescent to prevent sports-related injuries?
1. Warming up an hour before
2. Pacing activity
3. Building strength
4. Moderating intensity

84. 1. To prevent sports-related injuries, an adolescent client should be instructed to warm up prior to participation in the sport. Pacing activity, building strength, and using moderate intensity are also prevention measures.
CN: Health promotion and maintenance; CNS: None; CL: Apply

85. A child is allowed full activity following the repair of a clubfoot. Which activity would be **most** helpful for this child?
1. Playing catch
2. Standing
3. Swimming
4. Walking

85. 4. Walking will stimulate all of the involved muscles and help strengthen the foot. All of the options are good exercises, but walking is most helpful.
CN: Health promotion and maintenance; CNS: None; CL: Apply

86. The parent of an infant diagnosed with club-foot asks the nurse about the casting treatment regimen. The nurse determines further instruction is not needed when the parent states:
1. "The cast will be changed in eight weeks."
2. "The cast will be changed in two weeks."
3. "The cast will be changed when his child starts to walk."
4. "The cast will be changed when his child starts to crawl".

86. 2. Because an infant grows quickly, a cast change may be needed as often as every two weeks to correct the deformity as the child grows. Eight weeks is too long to leave a cast on the rapidly-growing child. Casting should be complete by the time the child is crawling and walking.
CN: Physiological integrity; CNS: Reduction of risk potential;
CL: Analyze

87. A child fell while playing basketball and sustained a greenstick fracture of the tibia. Which illustration represents a greenstick fracture?

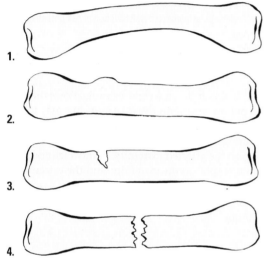

1.

2.

3.

4.

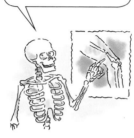

Well looky there. I'd bet my right femur that's one of them greenstick fractures.

87. 3. A greenstick fracture occurs when the bone is bent beyond its limit, causing an incomplete fracture. The first illustration shows a plastic deformation or bend, with a microscopic fracture line where the bone bends. The second illustration shows a buckle fracture, which occurs when porous bone is compressed, causing a raised area or bulge at the fracture site. The fourth illustration shows a complete fracture in which the bone is broken into separate pieces.
CN: Physiological integrity; CNS: Physiological adaptation;
CL: Apply

88. The nurse is preparing a teaching plan for a 10-year-old child who has fractured her radial bone. Which instruction should the nurse include in this teaching plan?
1. Report capillary refill less than three seconds
2. Report warmth under the cast during the first 24 hours after application
3. Report foul odors coming from the cast
4. Report cool fingers that warm within 20 minutes of being covered

88. 3. Foul odors from the cast may be a sign of infection, and should be reported to the provider immediately. Capillary refill less than three seconds is a normal finding. During the first 24 hours, the client may feel warmth under the cast as it dries. After 24 hours, warmth may be a sign of infection and should be reported. Cool fingers that warm up within 20 minutes of being covered is normal. Cool fingers that don't warm up after 20 minutes of being covered may indicate circulatory impairment under the cast and should be reported to the provider.
CN: Physiological integrity; CNS: Reduction of risk potential;
CL: Apply

89. Which factor is the **most** significant for an infant diagnosed with developmental dysplasia of the hip (DDH)?
1. The mother's activity during the third trimester
2. A breech presentation at birth
3. An infant's serum calcium level at birth
4. An Apgar score of 4 at one minute and 6 at five minutes

89. 2. Breech presentation is a factor commonly associated with DDH. The mother's activity during the third trimester, the infant's serum calcium level at birth, and Apgar scores have no bearing on DDH.
CN: Health promotion and maintenance; CNS: None;
CL: Apply

CN: Client needs category   CNS: Client needs subcategory   CL: Cognitive level

90. A 13-year old with structural scoliosis has Harrington rods inserted. Which position would be **best** for this teen during the postoperative period?
1. Supine in bed
2. Side-lying
3. Semi-Fowler's
4. High Fowler's

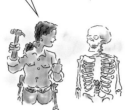

Okay. The rods are inserted. How should we position the client now?

90. 1. After placement of Harrington rods, the client must remain flat in bed. The latch on a manual bed should be taped, and electric beds should be unplugged to prevent the client from raising the head or foot of the bed. Other positions, such as side-lying, semi-Fowler's, or high Fowler's, could prove damaging because the rods may not be able to maintain the spine in a straight position.
CN: Physiological integrity; CNS: Reduction of risk potential; CL: Apply

91. A nurse notes anxiety, dyspnea, tachycardia, tachypnea, hemoptysis and respiratory distress in a client 48 hours after open reduction of a fractured femur. Which complication would the nurse suspect?
1. Fat embolism
2. Deep vein thrombosis
3. Petechiae
4. Acute Osteomyelitis

91. 1. Fat embolism syndrome is a potentially serious complication in which fat globules are released from the yellow bone marrow into the bloodstream. This usually occurs within 12 to 48 hours after a fracture of the long bones. The fat globules clog small blood vessels that supply vital organs, most commonly in the lungs, and impair organ perfusion. Immobility, a fractured femur, and orthopedic surgery all increase the risk of deep vein thrombosis (DVT). Petechiae is a macular rash over the neck, chest and abdomen, and is usually a late sign of fat emboli. Acute osteomyelitis develops rapidly over a period of seven to 10 days. The symptoms for acute and chronic osteomyelitis are very similar and include: Fever, irritability, fever, nausea, tenderness, redness, and warmth in the area of the infection swelling around the affected bon and lost range of motion. Osteomyelitis is an asymptomatic infection in the bone.
CN: Physiological integrity; CNS: Reduction of risk potential; CL: Analyze

92. A six-month-old male with developmental dysplasia of the hip (DDH) has been in treatment for the past six weeks with a Frejka splint. The splint maintains abduction of the hips through padding of the diaper area. During a follow-up visit, the child's mother tells the nurse that she removes the splint and padding when the child gets too fussy to settle him. Which response, by the nurse, would be **most** appropriate?
1. "I can tell you're concerned about his comfort, but he must wear the padded splint except during the three times per day when you perform range-of-motion exercises on his legs."
2. "I'm pleased that you recognize that the padding is too thick, and have adjusted it so he can relax."
3. "Seeing him uncomfortable is difficult for you, but he needs to keep the splint on except when you bathe him or change his diaper."
4. "If he seems uncomfortable while wearing the splint, please call us immediately."

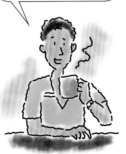

This warming-up activity should keep me awake for the rest of the test.

92. 3. Soft abduction devices, such as the Frejka splint, must be worn continually except for diaper changes and skin care. The abduction position must be maintained to establish a deep hip socket. An appropriate responses during times of discomfort include changing position, holding, cuddling, and providing diversion.
CN: Physiological integrity; CNS: Physiological adaptation; CL: Apply

93. The nurse is caring for an eight-month-old child in Bryant's traction for a congenital abnormality of the hips. Which complications is this child at risk for developing? Select all that apply.
1. Muscle strain
2. Decubitus ulcers
3. Diarrhea
4. Respiratory infection
5. Constipation

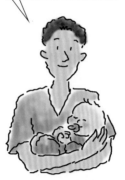

Remember to always be aware of "potential" complications.

Remember

"Docusate softens stuff you ate."

Docusate, an emollient laxative or stool softener, softens the feces, making hard stools easier to pass.

93. **1, 2, 4, 5.** Muscle strain is a potential complication of Bryant's traction, and nurses should use safe handling techniques when working with this child during traction change or rebandage. The weights should be inspected often to make sure they are hanging freely. Skin integrity can be compromised, and the nurse should assess skin integrity for the presence of skin breakdown. Respiratory infections are a potential complication due to immobility. Client care should include coughing and deep breathing exercises. Constipation is a potential complication due to immobility. Client care should include adequate fluid and fiber intake.
CN: Physiological integrity; CNS: Reduction of risk potential; CL: Analyze

94. A 14-year-old client has sustained a femoral fracture and is in a hip-spica cast. The client has been on bed rest and has not had a bowel movement for three days. The provider has ordered docusate sodium 100 mg po bid. The client asks, "Why am I taking this medication?" What is the nurse's **best** response?
1. It causes retention of fluid in the intestinal lumen by osmotic effect.
2. It increases peristalsis by irritating the colon wall and stimulates the enteric nerves.
3. It absorbs water, increasing bulk, which stimulates peristalsis.
4. It lubricates the intestinal tract and softens the feces, making hard stools easier to pass.

94. **4.** A client with a hip-spica cast is at risk for constipation due to decreased physical activity and use of pain medications. If a high-bulk diet is ineffective, the provider may order a stool softener to promote bowel movements. Answer one describes the effect of saline or osmotic solutions. Answer two describes the action of a stimulant. Answer three describes the effect of bulk-forming medications.
CN: Physiological adaptation; CNS: Pharmacology; CL: Apply

95. The nurse is explaining discharge instructions to a client with a fractured right femur who lives alone. Which statements, by the client, lead the nurse to determine that this client understands the instructions? Select all that apply.
1. "I can get the cast wet and allow it to air dry."
2. "I will move the joints above and below the cast regularly."
3. "I can remove the padding at the top of the cast to scratch underneath it if it is bothering me."
4. "I will report any foul odor under the cast to my provider."
5. "I can use a hair dryer on the cool setting for any itching."
6. "I will apply ice directly over the fracture site for 20 minutes each day."

95. **2, 4, 5.** Range-of-motion exercises on the uninvolved joints can be used to offset the effects of prolonged immobility. A foul odor can be a sign of potential infection or complication and should be reported to the provider for further assessment. A hair dryer can be used set on a cool setting with airflow directed under the cast for itching. The cast should be kept dry. A fiberglass cast can be dried by blotting it dry with a towel and then using a hair dryer, on a low setting, until the cast is thoroughly dry. The protective padding should not be removed from the cast in order to scratch. This could predispose the skin to breakdown and infection. Ice, in a plastic bag, should be applied during the first 24 hours postoperatively.
CN: Physiological integrity; CNS: Basic care and comfort; CL: Apply

96. A 15-year-old with structural scoliosis has had surgical placement of Harrington rods. Following routine postoperative care, the nurse monitors the following laboratory values. The nurse notes the lab values three days postoperatively. Which lab values should the nurse report to the health care provider?

1. Hemoglobin (Hgb) 14 g/dl; hematocrit (Hct) 41%
2. Na 135; K+ 4.0 mEq/L
3. White blood cells (WBC) 17,000 × 103/mm³
4. Platelet count 400.00/cu/mm

97. A seven-year-old boy with a fractured right femur has been admitted to the pediatric unit following a car accident. The provider orders morphine 0.02 mg/kg IV for severe pain control. The client weighs 52 lb (23.6 kg) and is experiencing pain of 9 out of 10 on the pain scale. What dosage of morphine should the nurse will administer to this client? Record your answer using two decimal places.

_____ mg

98. The nurse is caring for a 15-year-old female client whose mother and grandmother both have osteoporosis. The client asks the nurse if there are any foods that she could include in her diet to help prevent osteoporosis. What information should the nurse to provide to this client? Select all that apply.

1. American cheese
2. Eight ounces of yogurt
3. Potatoes
4. Sardines
5. Eggs
6. Spinach

99. The nurse is managing the care of a client with osteoarthritis (OA). Which actions are appropriate for a client with OA? Select all that apply.

1. Continuous complete bed rest
2. Administration of muscle relaxants
3. Administration of herbals and nutritional supplements
4. Use of nonsteroidal anti-inflammatory drugs
5. Daily strenuous physical therapy to involved joints
6. Weight reduction

96. 3. A WBC of 17,000 is indicative of an infection and should be reported to the provider. The other laboratory values are within normal range for a 13 to 18 year old.
CN: Physiological integrity; CNS: Reduction of risk potential; CL: Analyze

97. 0.47.
Dosage calculation

$$23.6 \ kg \times 0.02 \ mg/kg = 0.47 \ mg$$

Age: ≥ 1 month but < 12 years: IV/subcutaneous continuous: 0.025 to 0.206 mg/kg/hour (sickle cell or cancer pain) or 0.01 to 0.04 mg/kg/hour (postoperative pain); maximum per 24 hours: 5 mg.
CN: Physiological integrity; CNS: Pharmacological therapies; CL: Apply

98. 1, 2, 4, 6. American cheese, yogurt, sardines, and spinach are all good sources of calcium. Potatoes and eggs are considered poor sources of calcium.
CN: Physiological integrity; CNS: Reduction of risk potential; CL: Analyze

99. 3, 4, 6. Nutritional supplements such as glucosamine and chondroitin sulfate may help some clients improve joint mobility and relieve moderate to severe arthritis pain in the knees. NSAIDs can be used for clients who are not getting adequate pain relief with acetaminophen. If the client is overweight, a plan to reduce the client's weight is an important part of the total treatment plan.
CN: Physiological integrity; CNS: Reduction of risk potential; CL: Analyze

100. A 12-year-old client is two days postoperative from an open reduction, internal fixation procedure for a fractured femur. The client's chart reads:

Progress notes

> Breakfast:
> 1–4 oz cup of hot chocolate (4 oz × 30 ml = 120 ml)
> 1–4 oz carton of milk (4 oz × 30 ml = 120 ml)
> 1 bowl of oatmeal (n/a)
> 1–6 oz glass of orange juice (6 oz × 30 ml = 180ml)
> Additional information for 8-hour shift:
> IV of lactated Ringers is running at 125 ml/hr.
> A 1 g cefazolin injection was administered q8h.
> The pharmacy sent the cefazolin injection 1 g in
> 100 ml 50% dextrose.

Calculate this client's intake for the 7 am to 3 pm shift. Record your answer using a whole number.

_____ ml

100. 1520.
Calculate the breakfast intake in milliliters:
1–4 oz cup of hot chocolate (4 oz × 30 ml = 120 ml)
1–4 oz carton of milk (4 oz × 30 ml = 120 ml)
1 bowl of oatmeal (n/a)
1–6 oz glass of orange juice (6 oz × 30 ml = 180 ml)
Additional information needed: 1,000 (IV 125 ml/hr × 8 hr) plus 100 ml (cefazolin injection, one dose).

$$120 \text{ ml} + 120 \text{ ml} + 180 \text{ ml} + 1{,}000 \text{ ml}$$
$$+ 100 \text{ ml} = 1{,}520 \text{ ml}$$

CN: Physiological integrity; CNS: Pharmacological and parenteral therapies; CL: Apply

101. A 16-year-old male client has fractured his left tibia and fibula in a motorcycle accident. He has been placed in a long-leg cast and reports deep pain unrelieved by analgesics. The nurse suspects this client may be developing:
1. Volkmann's contracture.
2. Dupuytren's contracture.
3. compartment syndrome.
4. peroneal nerve compression.

101. 3. Deep pain unrelieved by analgesics could indicate compartment syndrome. Compartment syndrome occurs when swelling associated with inflammation reduces blood flow to the affected areas. Casting can cause additional constriction of blood flow. Volkmann's contracture is a contraction of the fingers, and sometimes wrist, that occurs after severe injury or improper use of a tourniquet or cast. Dupuytren's contracture is a flexion deformity of the fingers or toes caused by shortening, thickening, and fibrosis of the palmar or plantar fascia. Peroneal nerve compression occurs when the nerve that innervates the calf and foot is compressed.

CN: Physiological integrity; CNS: Physiological adaptation; CL: Analyze

102. A six-year-old boy is admitted to a pediatric unit for treatment of osteomyelitis. The nurse knows that osteomyelitis is **most** commonly caused by:
1. *Staphylococcus epidermidis*
2. *Escherichia coli*
3. *Pneumocystis carinii*
4. *Staphylococcus aureus*

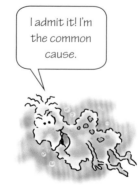

I admit it! I'm the common cause.

102. 4. *Staphylococcus aureus* is the most common causative pathogen of osteomyelitis. The usual source of the infection is an upper respiratory infection. *Staphylococcus epidermidis* is a microorganism found on the skin of healthy individuals. *Escherichia coli*, which is in uncooked meat, can cause a severe case of diarrhea. *Pneumocystis carinii* causes pneumonia in clients with HIV or AIDS, but doesn't normally cause illness in healthy individuals.

CN: Physiological integrity; CNS: Physiological adaptation; CL: Apply

103. A 14-year-old girl was recently fitted with a full back brace for scoliosis. Which response, by the girl, indicates an understanding of when the brace must be worn?
1. "I can leave the brace off for school parties."
2. "I have to wear the brace all the time, except when bathing."
3. "I can take the brace off for a couple of hours if my back starts to hurt."
4. "I only have to wear the brace for a couple of weeks."

103. 2. The brace must be worn at all times except for bathing. It can't be removed for other reasons including parties and discomfort. Most braces must be worn for several months to one year.
CN: Physiological integrity; CNS: Reduction of risk potential; CL: Analyze

104. A 16-year-old client had a full body cast applied three days ago. She's diaphoretic, tachycardic, and tachypneic. The nurse suspects that this client is experiencing:
1. pneumonia.
2. compartment syndrome.
3. anxiety.
4. decreased intestinal motility.

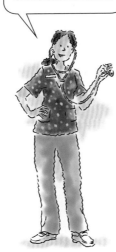

Listening to your client's responses will help you determine if the client understands.

104. 3. This client is exhibiting signs and symptoms of anxiety, most likely caused by the feeling of being claustrophobic. Pneumonia usually presents with fever and coughing. A client with compartment syndrome would exhibit signs of intense pain unrelieved by analgesics. Compression of the mesenteric blood supply can cause constipation, but these symptoms don't suggest that constipation is the most likely condition.
CN: Psychological integrity; CNS: Psychological adaptation; CL: Analyze

105. A nurse is preparing to give an IM injection into the left leg of a two-year-old client. Where should the nurse administer this injection?

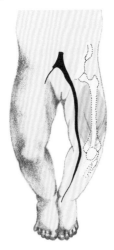

105. The nurse should administer this IM injection in the vastus lateralis, located in the child's thigh. To give the injection, the nurse should first divide the distance between the greater trochanter and the knee joints into quadrants and then inject in the center of the upper quadrant.

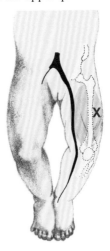

CN: Physiological integrity; CNS: Pharmacological and parenteral therapies; CL: Apply

106. A nurse is caring for a five-year-old client who is in the terminal stages of cancer. Which statements, regarding this child's cancer, are true? Select all that apply.
1. The parents may be at different stages in dealing with their child's impending death.
2. The child is thinking about the future and knows he may not be able to participate.
3. The dying child may become clingy and act like a toddler.
4. Whispering in the child's room will help the child cope.
5. The death of a child may have long-term disruptive effects on the family.
6. The child doesn't fully understand the concept of death.

106. 1, 3, 5, 6. The parents may be at different stages of grief at different times. The child may regress in behavior. The stress of a child's death commonly results in divorce and behavioral problems in siblings. Preschoolers see death as temporary, a type of sleep or separation. They recognize the word "dead" but don't fully understand its meaning. Thinking about the future is typical of an adolescent facing death, not a preschooler. Whispering in front of the child only increases his fear of death.

CN: Psychosocial integrity; CNS: None; CL: Analyze

107. A 13-year-old client admitted with a fractured femur had an open reduction and internal fixation (ORIF) 12 hours ago. The client is reporting pain 8 out of 10 on the numeric pain scale. The provider has ordered ketorolac 20 mg to be administered IV every 6 hours. The pharmacy sends over ketorolac 50 mg/1 ml. How many milliliters will the nurse administer for the correct dosage? Record your answer using one decimal place.

_____ ml

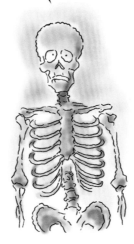

No bones about it. You're doing great!

107. 0.4.
The formula to use is:

$$\text{Amount Given} = \frac{\text{Desired}}{\text{Have}} \times \text{Volume}$$

The amount desired is 20 mg. Divide by 50 mg (sent over by the pharmacy is the amount you have). Then multiply that amount by 1 ml (because the 50 mg is in 1 ml of solution).

$$X = \frac{20\,\text{mg}}{50\,\text{mg}} \times 1\,\text{ml}$$

$$X = 0.4\,\text{ml}$$

CN: Physiological Integrity; CNS: Pharmacological and Parenteral Therapies; CL: Apply

108. A nurse is caring for a two-year-old, who weighs 25 lb (11.3 kg), and has a fractured femur. What is the nurse's **priority** assessment for this client?
1. Length of one leg to the other
2. Affected leg distal to the fracture
3. Affected leg anterior to the fracture
4. Affected leg proximal to the fracture

108. 2. The nurse should focus the assessment on the area distal to the fracture. This area is most at risk for neurovascular compromise. If a fracture severs or obstructs blood vessels or nerves, blood flow is disrupted distal to the site, and may lead to nerve or tissue damage. The unaffected leg should be used for baseline comparison. This client should be assessed for the five "Ps:" pulse, pallor, parathesia, pain and paralysis.

CN: Physiological integrity; CNS: Physiological adaptation; CL: Apply

CN: Client needs category   CNS: Client needs subcategory   CL: Cognitive level

109. What is the nurse's **priority** intervention for a toddler who has just had a hip-spica cast applied?
1. Limit fluids to reduce urine output and risk of getting the cast wet
2. Instruct the parents how to get their child home in the car
3. Assess sensation, circulation, and motion of the child's feet and toes
4. Reduce the risk of constipation by avoiding pain medications

109. 3. Assessing sensation, circulation, and motion is necessary in all children with a cast. Fluids should be encouraged, and careful diapering and padding will keep the child's cast dry. Discharge instructions are not a priority, but should be shared at a later time. Children experiencing pain should receive medication as needed.

CN: Safe, effective care environment; CNS: Management of care; CL: Apply

110. A five-year-old boy was admitted to a pediatric unit four hours ago with reports of pain in his right ankle. Upon assessment, the nurse documents the following findings: VS: 102.8° F (39.3° C), P 112, R 16 BP 96/55, O2 99% on RA, moderate amount of erythema and +2 edema over the lateral aspect of the right ankle, warm to touch, limited range of motion noted. The nurse also reviews the laboratory values. Based on the assessment findings and laboratory data in the chart below, for what is this client at risk?

110. 2. Systemic symptoms such as fever and irritability, and localized symptoms such as edema, swelling and tenderness over the bone are often precursors to osteomyelitis. This child's physical examination should focus on identifying common findings, such as erythema, soft tissue swelling or joint effusion as well as decreased joint range of motion, and tenderness over the bone.

CN: Physiological integrity; CNS: Reduction of risk potential; CL: Analyze

Progress notes

Test Name	Client Results	Units
CBC:		
WBC	17.8	$\times 10^3/\mu l$
RBC	4.8	million/mm^3
Hgb	13.5	gm/dl
HCT	38	%
Bands:	13	PMN%
CRP:	2.8	ng/dl
Blood Culture	Gram positive: Staphylococcus aureus	

1. Aplastic anemia
2. Osteomyelitis
3. Osteogenesis
4. Developmental dysplasia of the hip (DDH)

111. The nurse is evaluating a five-year-old client's response to clindamycin being given IV for osteomyelitis. For which is it important that the nurse monitor this client? Select all that apply.
1. WBC count of 17,000 mm³
2. Creatinine level of 1.2 mg/dl
3. BUN level 1.7
4. Tinnitus and hearing loss
5. Blood sugar level of 80
6. Excessive thirst

111. 1, 2, 4. The length of therapy for osteomyelitis is determined by the duration of the symptoms, the client's response to treatment and the organism's sensitivity. Because of the prolonged duration of high-dose antibiotic therapy, the nurse should monitor for hematologic, renal, hepatic, ototoxic, and other potential side effects. When a client is on aminoglycoside therapy, the nurse should monitor for tinnitus and hearing loss which could indicate ototoxicity. Nephrotoxicity is indicated by rising BUN levels, and increasing creatinine levels. A WBC count of 17,000 mm³ is above the normal range of 5.5 to 15.5. A decrease would indicate the clindamycin is being therapeutic. Normal creatinine ranges from 0.3 to 0.7 mg/dl. Normal BUN ranges from 0.0 to 0.7 mg/dl for children up to 12 years of age.
CN: Physiological integrity; CNS: Reduction of risk potential; CL: Analyze

112. A nurse is instructing a wheelchair-bound client with muscular dystrophy on exercises to prevent skin breakdown. What is the **best** information the nurse should provide?
1. Wheelchair push-ups
2. Leaning side to side
3. Leaning forward
4. Gluteal sets

112. 1. A wheelchair push-up will alleviate the most pressure from the buttocks. Leaning side to side and leaning forward will help, but not as much as wheelchair push-ups. Gluteal sets won't relieve pressure.
CN: Health promotion and maintenance; CNS: None; CL: Apply

113. A client is to receive 100 mg of cefazolin following an open reduction and internal fixation (ORIF) for repair of a fractured femur. The pharmacy has sent 100 mg of cefazolin in 50 ml of dextrose. The medication is to be administered over 30 minutes. Calculate the gtt/min using a 20 gtt/ml set. Record your answer using a whole number.

_____ gtt/min.

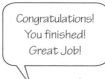

Congratulations! You finished! Great Job!

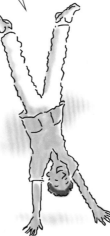

113. 34.
Formula for IV calculations:

$$\frac{\text{Amount}}{\text{Rate}} = \frac{\text{Volume}}{\text{Rate}} \times \text{Set}$$

A medication volume of 50 mL is to be administered in 30 min using a 20 gtt/ml set.

$$X = \frac{50\,\text{ml}}{30\,\text{min}} \times 20\,\frac{\text{gtt}}{\text{min}}$$

X = 33.33. Rounded to : 34 gtt / min.

CN: Physiological integrity; CNS: Pharmacological and parenteral therapies; CL: Apply

Chapter 32

Gastrointestinal Disorders

I'll bet that when you started nursing school, you had no idea kids could be subject to so many GI disorders. This chapter tests you on the most common ones. Good luck!

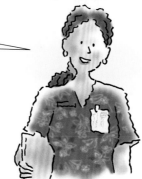

1. The nurse determines that teaching has been effective when the mother of a child with celiac disease states:
  1. "I won't serve wheat, rye, oats, or barley."
  2. "I will provide a diet high in gluten."
  3. "I won't serve potatoes, rice, or corn bread."
  4. "I can safely serve any frozen or packaged food."

In question 2, the word *priority* guides you to the right answer.

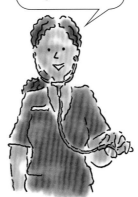

2. The nurse is teaching the parents of a child diagnosed with celiac disease? What is the nurse's **priority** goal?
  1. Promote developmentally appropriate activities for the child
  2. Stress the importance of good health, in preventing infection
  3. Introduce the parents and child to a peer who has celiac disease
  4. Help the parents and child follow the prescribed dietary restrictions

3. The nurse is assessing the stool of a child with celiac disease. Which findings will the nurse expect to record?
  1. Marble-like, hard stool
  2. Clay-colored stool
  3. Red currant jelly stool
  4. Foul-smelling, fatty, frothy stool

1. 1. The child with celiac disease should consume a gluten-free diet, eliminating foods containing wheat, rye, oats, and barley. Foods containing potatoes, rice, and corn flour are permissible. The mother should carefully read all food packaging to ensure the product gluten-free.
CN: Physiological integrity; CNS: Basic care and comfort; CL: Apply

2. 4. It takes a long time to describe the disease process, the specific role of gluten, and the foods that must be restricted. Parents need to carefully read food labels to avoid hidden sources of gluten. Promoting developmentally-appropriate activities for the child, stressing good health, in preventing infection, and meeting a peer who has celiac disease are also important nursing considerations, but are not the priority.
CN: Physiological integrity; CNS: Reduction of risk potential; CL: Analyze

3. 4. Steatorrhea is common because of the body's inability to absorb dietary fat. Profuse and watery diarrhea, not marble-like hard stool, is usually a sign of celiac disease. Clay-colored stools are characteristic of a decrease or absence of conjugated bilirubin. Red currant jelly-type stool is an indication of intussusception.
CN: Physiological integrity; CNS: Physiological adaptation; CL: Apply

CN: Client needs category   CNS: Client needs subcategory   CL: Cognitive level

4. A client with celiac disease is being discharged from the hospital. The nurse determines that discharge instructions are understood when the client makes which statement? Select all that apply.
1. "I will eat oatmeal raisin cookies."
2. "I can eat a bologna sandwich."
3. "I will make pepperoni and cheese pizza with rice flour."
4. "I will have rice cakes for lunch."
5. "I can drink apple juice."

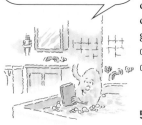

Clients with celiac disease need help learning how to pamper their stomachs.

5. The parents of a child with celiac disease ask the nurse how they can help promote a normal life for their child. What is the nurse's **best** response?
1. "Treat the child in special ways when compared to siblings."
2. "Focus on the restrictions that make him feel different."
3. "Introduce the child to another peer who has celiac disease."
4. "Prevent the child from talking negatively about his gluten-free diet."

6. The nurse is evaluating the effectiveness of nutritional therapy for a child with celiac disease. What is the **most** important assessment?
1. Vital signs
2. Appearance, size, and number of stools
3. Blood urea nitrogen (BUN) and serum creatinine levels
4. Intake and output

7. The nurse is caring for a child with celiac disease. The child was started on a prescribed gluten-free diet two day ago. Which should the nurse expect to find?
1. Diarrhea
2. Foul-smelling stools
3. Improved appetite
4. Weight loss

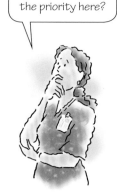

Hmm. What's the priority here?

8. The nurse is planning care for a neonate with a cleft lip and palate. What is the nurse's **priority** action?
1. Inadequate urinary output
2. Operative care
3. Pain management
4. Parental reaction

4. 4, 5. Sources of gluten found in wheat, rye, barley, and oats should be avoided. Rice and corn are suitable substitutes because they don't contain gluten. Pepperoni pizza, luncheon meat, and oatmeal cookies contain gluten and, when broken down, can't be digested by people with celiac disease. Rice cakes and apple juice do not contain gluten.
CN: Physiological integrity; CNS: Basic care and comfort; CL: Apply

5. 3. Introducing the child to peer who has celiac disease will let him know that he is not alone. It will show him how other people live a normal life with similar restrictions. Treat the child no differently than his siblings, and stress appropriate limit setting. Instead of focusing on restrictions that make him feel different, the nurse should encourage the parents to focus on ways that he can be normal. Allow the child with celiac disease to express his feelings about dietary restrictions.
CN: Psychosocial integrity; CNS: None; CL: Apply

6. 2. The fatty, foul-smelling, bulky stools should cease when a child with celiac disease follows a gluten-free diet. Vital signs, BUN and serum creatinine levels, and intake and output aren't affected by a gluten-free diet.
CN: Physiological integrity; CNS: Basic care and comfort; CL: Analyze

7. 3. Within a day or two of starting a gluten-free diet, most children with celiac disease show improved appetite, disappearance of diarrhea, and weight gain. It takes longer than two days for steatorrhea to subside.
CN: Physiological integrity; CNS: Physiological adaptation; CL: Apply

8. 4. Parents typically show a strong negative response to this deformity. They may mourn the loss of a perfect child. Helping the parents cope with their child's condition is a priority. Feeding can be challenging, and can result briefly in reduced fluid intake, but inadequate urinary output is unlikely to occur. Surgical repair is usually delayed until the child is 6 to 12 weeks of age. This deformity is not painful.
CN: Psychosocial integrity; CNS: None; CL: Analyze

CN: Client needs category   CNS: Client needs subcategory   CL: Cognitive level

9. The nurse is assessing an infant who has just returned to the pediatric unit after undergoing a cleft lip repair. Which is the nurse's **best** intervention to prevent trauma to the suture line?
1. Place mittens on the infant's hands
2. Maintain arm restraints on the infant
3. Disallow the parents to touch the infant
4. Remove the lip device from the infant after surgery

9. **2.** Arm restraints are used to prevent the infant from rubbing the sutures. Placing mittens will not prevent the infant from rubbing the suture line. Parental contact will increase the infant's comfort. The lip device should not be removed.

CN: Physiological integrity; CNS: Reduction of risk potential; CL: Apply

10. Which intervention should the nurse use to prevent tissue infection and breakdown after cleft palate or lip repair?
1. Keep the suture line moist at all times
2. Allow the infant to suck on a pacifier
3. Rinse the infant's mouth with water after each feeding
4. Follow orders from the provider to not feed the infant by mouth

10. **3.** To prevent formula buildup around the suture line, the infant's mouth should be rinsed. The sutures should be kept dry at all times. Placing objects in the mouth should be avoided following surgery. Infants are fed by mouth using the syringe technique.

CN: Physiological integrity; CNS: Physiological adaptation; CL: Analyze

11. Which nursing intervention is **priority** for an infant during the first 24 hours following surgery for cleft lip repair?
1. Carefully clean the suture line after feedings to reduce the risk of infection
2. Position the infant in the prone position after feedings to promote drainage
3. Allow the infant to cry to promote lung expansion
4. Encourage the infant to use a pacifier to satisfy the urge to suck

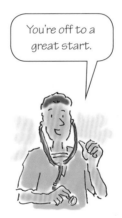

You're off to a great start.

11. **1.** The suture line must be carefully cleaned with a sterile solution after each feeding to reduce the risk of infection, which could adversely affect the healing and cosmetic results. The infant shouldn't be placed in the prone position because this puts pressure on the incision, and may affect healing. Anticipatory care should be provided to reduce the risk of the infant crying, which puts strain on the incision. Pacifiers and other firm objects should not be placed in the infant's mouth because they can disrupt the suture line.

CN: Physiological integrity; CNS: Reduction of risk potential; CL: Apply

12. The nurse is teaching parents how to feed their infant who has a cleft palate. The nurse teaches the parents to apply gentle steady pressure to the base of the bottle. The nurse explains that this will:
1. reduce the risk of choking or coughing.
2. prevent further damage to the affected area.
3. decrease the amount of formula lost while eating.
4. limit the amount of noise the infant makes when eating.

12. **1.** Children with cleft palate or lip have a greater risk of choking while eating, so all measures are used to reduce this risk. Steady pressure creates a seal when the nipple is against the cleft palate or lip, reducing the risk of aspiration. The nurse cannot cause more damage to an infant's cleft lip or palate unless proper precautions aren't followed postoperatively. If the nipple is cut correctly and proper procedures are followed, the infant won't lose a lot of formula during a feeding. Infants with cleft palate or lip usually make more noise while eating.

CN: Physiological integrity; CNS: Reduction of risk potential; CL: Apply

CN: Client needs category   CNS: Client needs subcategory   CL: Cognitive level

13. The pediatric unit has just been notified that they will be admitting an infant with cleft lip and palate. What is the **best** nursing intervention to implement when feeding the infant?
1. Burp the infant often
2. Limit the amount the infant eats
3. Feed the infant at routine unit scheduled times
4. Remove the nipple if the infant makes loud noises

13. 1. Infants with cleft lip and palate have a tendency to swallow excess air, and need to be burped frequently during feedings. The amount of formula they eat at each feeding is the same as an infant without cleft lip or palate. Loud noises are common when these infants eat. It is important to individualize a feeding schedule to meet the infant's needs and metabolic demands. Usually a full term healthy newborn takes about 2 to 3 oz (59 to 89 ml) of breast milk or formula per feeding
CN: Physiological integrity; CNS: Physiological adaptation; CL: Apply

14. Which nursing intervention is **essential** while caring for an infant with cleft lip or palate?
1. Avoid encouraging breastfeeding
2. Cradle the infant horizontally while feeding
3. Involve the parents in feeding as soon as possible
4. Choose a regular nursery nipple for feedings

14. 3. The sooner the parents become involved, the quicker they're able to determine the method of feeding best suited for them and their infant. Breastfeeding, like bottle feeding, may be difficult but can be facilitated if the mother is supported in this decision. If the cleft isn't severe, breastfeeding may be easier than other feeding techniques because the human nipple conforms to the shape of the infant's mouth. Feedings are usually given in the upright position to prevent formula from coming through the nose. Various special nipples have been developed for infants with cleft lip or palate. A regular nursery nipple is not effective.
CN: Physiological integrity; CNS: Physiological adaptation; CL: Apply

15. The parents of an infant born with a cleft lip and palate are seeing the infant for the first time. On which area should the nurse caring for this infant focus?
1. The infant's positive features and attributes
2. Concern for how the infant eats
3. Ambivalence in caring for an infant with this defect
4. Dissatisfaction with the infant's physical appearance

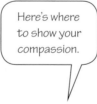
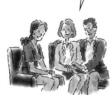

Here's where to show your compassion.

15. 1. To relieve the parents' anxiety, the positive aspects of the infant's physical appearance should be emphasized. Showing optimism toward surgical correction and showing a photograph of possible cosmetic improvements may be helpful. Because this is the parents' first encounter with the infant, helping them appreciate their baby's attributes will support their acceptance of, and bond with, the child. This lays the foundation for coping with challenges the nurse knows lie ahead.
CN: Psychosocial integrity; CNS: None; CL: Apply

16. Following the repair of a cleft lip in a three-month-old infant, the mother asks the nurse what toy would be most appropriate for her infant. What is the nurse's **best** response?
1. A plastic teething ring
2. A stuffed animal
3. A mobile to hang over the crib
4. Children's books

16. 3. Considering the infant's age, a mobile would be the most appropriate toy. The mobile would provide the infant with visual stimulation. A plastic teething ring or a stuffed animal should be avoided because they can disrupt the suture line if the infant sucks on them. The infant would not be able to understand children's stories, but would enjoy the sound of a person's voice.
CN: Physiological integrity; CNS: None; CL: Analyze

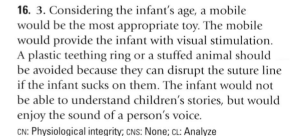

CN: Client needs category   CNS: Client needs subcategory   CL: Cognitive level

17. The mother of a neonate, who was born with a cleft lip and palate, is preparing to feed the baby for the first time. What is the **most** important information for the nurse to give this mother?
   1. Burp the neonate before beginning to feed
   2. Clean the mouth prior to feeding
   3. Hold the neonate in an upright position
   4. Prepare the bottle using a regular nipple

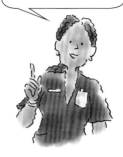

There are many things to teach this mother, so what is most important to teach her first?

17. 3. When neonates are held in an upright position, the formula is less likely to leak out of their nose or mouth. Neonates need to be burped frequently during, but not before, a feeding. There is no need to clean the mouth before eating. After surgical repair, the mouth should be cleaned at the suture site after feeding to prevent infection. The bottle should be prepared using a special nipple or feeding device.
CN: Physiological integrity; CNS: Physiological adaptation; CL: Apply

18. An infant returns from surgery after repair of a cleft palate. What is the **priority** nursing intervention?
   1. Offer a pacifier for comfort
   2. Position the infant on his side
   3. Suction the mouth and nose of all secretions
   4. Remove the arm restraints placed on the infant after surgery

18. 2. The infant should be positioned on his side to allow oral secretions to drain from the mouth. Suctioning should be avoided. Pacifiers should not be used because they can damage the suture line. Arm restraints should be kept on to prevent the infant from disrupting the suture line.
CN: Physiological integrity; CNS: Reduction of risk potential; CL: Analyze

19. A small child has undergone surgical repair of a cleft palate and is ready for discharge. What information is **most** important for the nurse to tell the parents?
   1. Continue a normal diet
   2. Continue using arm restraints at home
   3. Don't allow the child to drink from a cup
   4. Establish good mouth care and proper brushing

19. 2. Continuing to use arm restraints is a priority. They should be used at home to keep the child's hands away from their mouth until the palate is healed. A soft diet is recommended. No foods harder than mashed potatoes should be eaten. Fluids are best taken from a cup. Proper mouth care is encouraged after the palate is healed.
CN: Physiological integrity; CNS: Physiological adaptation; CL: Apply

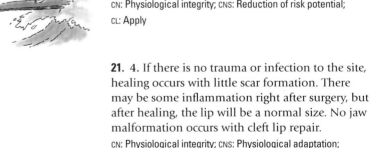

Sweet! You're doing great. Keep it up.

20. Following cleft lip and palate repair, what is the best position for the nurse to place an infant in to allow irrigation of the mouth after feeding?
   1. Supine with the head to the side
   2. Fowler's position with the head to the side
   3. Upright with the head tilted forward
   4. Prone with the head over the side of the bed

20. 3. Following repair of a cleft palate, the nurse should irrigate the infant's mouth with the child in an upright position, and the head tilted forward to prevent aspiration. A supine or Fowler's position, with the head to the side, won't prevent aspiration. The prone position isn't appropriate following cleft lip repair because this may put pressure on the infant's suture line.
CN: Physiological integrity; CNS: Reduction of risk potential; CL: Apply

21. The parents of an infant who had cleft lip repair ask the nurse how the area will appear when it is healed. What is the nurse's **best** response?
   1. A large scar on the lip
   2. An abnormally large upper lip
   3. A distorted jaw
   4. Minimal scarring

21. 4. If there is no trauma or infection to the site, healing occurs with little scar formation. There may be some inflammation right after surgery, but after healing, the lip will be a normal size. No jaw malformation occurs with cleft lip repair.
CN: Physiological integrity; CNS: Physiological adaptation; CL: Apply

CN: Client needs category   CNS: Client needs subcategory   CL: Cognitive level

22. The nurse would advise the parents of a newborn with a cleft lip and palate to schedule an appointment with which specialist?
1. Cardiologist
2. Neurologist
3. Nutritionist
4. Otolaryngologist

22. 4. An otolaryngologist is used because ear infections are common, along with hearing loss in children born with a cleft lip and palate. Cardiac and brain function is usually normal. A nutritionist is not required unless the neonate becomes malnourished.
CN: Safe, effective care environment; CNS: Management of care; CL: Apply

23. The nurse is **most** concerned when a neonate with esophageal atresia and tracheoesophageal fistula presents with:
1. bulging eyeballs.
2. sunken anterior fontanelle.
3. skin that returns briskly when pinched.
4. fluctuating weight gain.

23. 2. A sunken anterior fontanelle is a sign of dehydration in a neonate whose fontanelle has not closed. Bulging eyeballs are sign of over hydration. Fluctuating weight gain is not a sign of dehydration. Skin that returns quickly when pinched is a sign of adequate hydration.
CN: Physiological integrity; CNS: Reduction of risk potential; CL: Apply

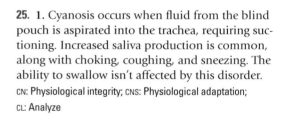

You're making good progress. Keep it up.

24. Feedings are being withheld for a neonate with esophageal atresia and tracheoesophageal fistula until a gastrostomy tube can be placed. What is the **most** appropriate nursing intervention to implement when this neonate is irritable and crying?
1. Offer the neonate a pacifier
2. Encourage the parents to talk to the neonate
3. Encourage the parents to hold the neonate
4. Distract the neonate by placing a mobile over the crib

24. 1. A neonate who is unable to suck to obtain nutrition may be comforted by a pacifier. Encouraging the parents to hold and talk to the neonate, and placing a mobile over the crib are appropriate interventions but won't satisfy a newborn as much as a pacifier.
CN: Physiological integrity; CNS: Basic care and comfort; CL: Analyze

25. Which assessment finding indicates to a nurse that a neonate born with esophageal atresia needs suctioning?
1. Cyanosis
2. Decreased production of saliva
3. Coughing
4. Inadequate swallow

25. 1. Cyanosis occurs when fluid from the blind pouch is aspirated into the trachea, requiring suctioning. Increased saliva production is common, along with choking, coughing, and sneezing. The ability to swallow isn't affected by this disorder.
CN: Physiological integrity; CNS: Physiological adaptation; CL: Analyze

26. A neonate is suspected of having esophageal atresia. Which factor would a definitive diagnostic evaluation include?
1. Decreased breath sounds
2. Absence of bowel sounds
3. How the neonate tolerates eating
4. Ability to pass a catheter down the esophagus

26. 4. A moderately stiff catheter will meet resistance if the esophagus is blocked, and will pass unobstructed if the esophagus is patent. Breath sounds are normal unless aspiration occurs. The intestinal tract isn't affected with this anomaly, so normal bowel sounds will be present. If a neonate does not tolerate eating, it doesn't mean that he has an esophageal atresia.
CN: Physiological integrity; CNS: Physiological adaptation; CL: Analyze

CN: Client needs category   CNS: Client needs subcategory   CL: Cognitive level

27. A neonate has been diagnosed with a tracheo-esophageal fistula. Which will the treatment plan include?
 1. Initiating antibiotic therapy
 2. Keeping the neonate lying flat
 3. Continuing normal feedings
 4. Removing the diagnostic catheter from the esophagus

27. 1. Antibiotic therapy is initiated because aspiration pneumonia is inevitable and soon after diagnosis. The neonate's head is usually kept in an upright position to prevent aspiration. Intravenous fluids are started, and the neonate is not allowed oral intake. The diagnostic catheter is left in the upper esophageal pouch to easily remove fluid that collects there.
CN: Physiological integrity; CNS: Pharmacological and parenteral therapies; CL: Analyze

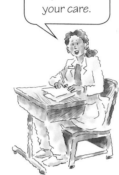

Question 28 asks you to prioritize your care.

28. A nurse suspects an infant may have a tracheo-esophageal fistula or esophageal atresia. What is the **most** important intervention by the nurse?
 1. Give oxygen
 2. Tell the parents
 3. Put the neonate in an isolette or on a radiant warmer
 4. Report the suspicion to the health care provider

28. 4. The provider needs to be told so that immediate diagnostic tests can be done to determine a definitive diagnosis with surgical correction. Oxygen should be given only after notifying the provider, except in an emergency. It is not the nurse's responsibility to inform the parents of the suspected finding. By the time tracheoesophageal fistula or esophageal atresia is suspected, the neonate would have already been placed in an isolette or a radiant warmer.
CN: Physiological integrity; CNS: Physiological adaptation; CL: Analyze

29. The nurse is aware that an infant who had surgical repair of a tracheoesophageal fistula is **most** at risk for:
 1. atelectasis.
 2. choking during feeding attempts.
 3. damaged vocal cords.
 4. infection.

29. 1. Atelectasis is a threat to the neonate's life preoperatively and postoperatively because of the continual risk of aspiration. Choking is more likely to occur preoperatively, although neonates should be carefully monitored postoperatively while eating to be sure they can swallow without choking. Vocal cord damage is not common following this repair. The neonate is generally given antibiotics preoperatively to prevent infection.
CN: Physiological integrity; CNS: Physiological adaptation; CL: Analyze

30. The nurse is caring for an infant suspected of having esophageal atresia and tracheoesophageal fistula. Which sign would the nurse **initially** observe?
 1. Abdominal distention
 2. Decreased oral secretions
 3. Normal respiratory effort
 4. Scaphoid abdomen

I feel so bloated!

30. 1. Crying may force air into the infant's stomach, causing distention. Secretions in a client with this condition may be more visible, although normal in quantity, because of the client's inability to swallow effectively. Respiratory effort is usually more difficult. When no distal fistula is present, the abdomen will appear scaphoid.
CN: Physiological integrity; CNS: Physiological adaptation; CL: Apply

31. The nurse is providing information on dietary management to a child diagnosed with ulcerative colitis. Which diet should this child follow?
 1. High-calorie diet
 2. High-residue diet
 3. Low-protein diet
 4. Low-salt diet

31. 1. A high-calorie diet is given to combat weight loss and restore nitrogen balance. A low-residue, or residue-free diet is encouraged to decrease bowel irritation. The diet should be high-protein not low in protein to promote tissue synthesis Salt reduction is not a factor in this disease.
CN: Physiological integrity; CNS: Basic care and comfort; CL: Analyze

CN: Client needs category   CNS: Client needs subcategory   CL: Cognitive level

32. A neonate returns from the operating room after surgical repair of a tracheoesophageal fistula and esophageal atresia. What is the nurse's **priority** intervention?
1. Maintain a patent airway
2. Start feedings right away
3. Let the parents hold the neonate right away
4. Suction the endotracheal tube, stopping when resistance is met

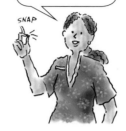

Priority. You know what that means.

SNAP

32. 1. Maintaining a patent airway is essential until sedation wears off. Feedings usually aren't started until 48 hours after surgery. Parents are encouraged to participate in the neonate's care but not immediately following surgery. The catheter should be measured before suctioning so the tube doesn't meet resistance, which could cause damage.
CN: Safe, effective care environment; CNS: Management of care; CL: Apply

33. The nurse is providing discharge instructions to the parents of a neonate who has undergone repair of a tracheoesophageal fistula and esophageal atresia. What is the **most** important information for the nurse to tell these parents?
1. Give antibiotics through the feeding tube
2. Maintain proper care of a chest tube
3. Maintain proper positioning for feedings
4. Utilize tips for preventing crying

33. 3. The neonate should be kept in an upright position after feeding to reduce the risk of refluxed stomach contents and aspiration pneumonia. Although antibiotics are given after surgery, they are discontinued prior to discharge. Because the chest cavity is entered during surgery, the neonate may have a chest tube inserted that will be removed prior to discharge. Because lung expansion is important following chest surgery, vigorous crying helps expand the lungs and should not be discouraged.
CN: Physiological integrity; CNS: Basic care and comfort; CL: Apply

34. Which postoperative nursing intervention should be provided to a neonate after the repair of a tracheoesophageal fistula and esophageal atresia?
1. Withhold mouth care
2. Offer a pacifier frequently
3. Decrease tactile stimulation
4. Use restraints to prevent injury to the repair

34. 2. Satisfying the neonate's oral needs by offering him a pacifier is important because the infant will not be able to drink from a bottle. The nurse should provide mouth care and tactile stimulation to this neonate. Restraints should be avoided when possible.
CN: Physiological integrity; CNS: Physiological adaptation; CL: Apply

35. A baby is admitted with a history of tracheoesophageal fistula and esophageal atresia repair. This history places this client at risk for:
1. oral aversion.
2. gastroesophageal reflux.
3. the inability to tolerate feedings.
4. strictures.

What complication is this client most at risk for?

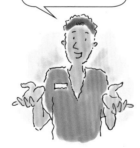

35. 4. Strictures of the anastomosis occur in 40% to 50% of cases. Oral aversion occurs quickly after surgery, and can be a problem. It is common for babies with esophageal atresia and tracheoesophageal fistula to have gastroesophageal reflux. This is due to poor motility, or contractility, of the lower portion of the esophagus. If the neonate is having problems tolerating feedings, it is quickly noted.
CN: Physiological integrity; CNS: Physiological adaptation; CL: Apply

36. The nurse observes a neonate who is having excessive salivation and drooling, accompanied by coughing, choking, and sneezing. Which condition should the nurse suspect?
1. Cleft lip
2. Cleft palate
3. Gastroschisis
4. Tracheoesophageal fistula

36. 4. Because tracheoesophageal fistula causes a slower flow of saliva and secretions through the esophagus, more appear in the mouth and around the lips. Coughing, choking, and sneezing occur for the same reason, and usually follow eating. Cleft lip and palate do not produce excessive salivation. None of these symptoms occurs with gastroschisis.
CN: Physiological integrity; CNS: Physiological adaptation; CL: Apply

CN: Client needs category   CNS: Client needs subcategory   CL: Cognitive level

37. Which nursing action takes **priority** for the first 24 hours following surgical repair of esophageal atresia and tracheoesophageal fistula?
1. Ensuring effective airway clearance
2. Meeting nutritional needs
3. Supporting parenting behaviors
4. Determining effective comfort measures

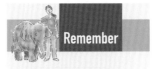

Remember

"Mucolytics mince mucus."

Mucolytics, such as acetylcysteine, break down and loosen mucus in the respiratory system.

37. **1.** The priority nursing action for the first postoperative day is effective airway clearance. The nurse must assess the infant's airway for the buildup of mucus and other secretions. The nurse must also perform a respiratory assessment. Endotracheal suctioning equipment and a laryngoscope should be immediately available. The other nursing actions are all important in the infant in the immediate postoperative period, but assessing and maintaining a patent airway is the highest priority.
CN: Physiological integrity; CNS: Reduction or risk potential; CL: Analyze

38. An infant was born with a portion of an organ protruding through an abnormal opening. The nurse explains to the parents that this structural defect is called:
1. omphalocele.
2. Meckel's diverticulum.
3. gastroschisis.
4. tracheoesophageal fistula.

38. **3.** Gastroschisis is a herniation of the bowel and other abdominal contents through an abnormal opening in the abdominal wall, with no covering membrane. An omphalocele is an abdominal wall defect with herniated viscera with covering membrane. Meckel's diverticulum is a pouch on the wall of the lower intestine. Tracheoesophageal fistula is a malformation of the trachea and esophagus.
CN: Physiological integrity; CNS: Physiological adaptation; CL: Apply

39. When an infant is diagnosed with a diaphragmatic hernia on the left side, which abdominal organ may be found in the thorax?
1. Appendix
2. Descending colon
3. Right kidney
4. Spleen

39. **4.** The spleen has commonly been seen in the thorax of infants with this defect. The appendix and descending colon usually don't protrude into the thorax because of limited space from the other organs. The right kidney wouldn't be seen with a left-sided defect.
CN: Physiological integrity; CNS: Physiological adaptation; CL: Analyze

Hmmm, which way did that mediastinum go?

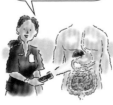

40. The nurse is assessing an infant diagnosed with a diaphragmatic hernia. The nurse would expect the mediastinum to:
1. not shift.
2. shift to the affected side.
3. shift to the unaffected side.
4. partially shift to the affected or unaffected sides.

40. **3.** The increased volume in the chest cavity from the abdominal organs causes the mediastinum to shift to the unaffected side, which causes a partial collapse of that lung. Because of the increased volume on the affected side, the mediastinum cannot shift in that direction.
CN: Physiological integrity; CNS: Physiological adaptation; CL: Analyze

41. What is the **best** way for a nurse to position an infant with a diaphragmatic hernia before surgery?
1. On the affected side
2. On the unaffected side
3. Supine
4. Trendelenburg's position

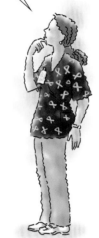

Which position would help the lungs expand?

41. 1. Positioning an infant on the affected side lets the lung on the unaffected side expand, making breathing easier. Positioning the infant on the unaffected side, or in Trendelenburg's position, would further diminish respiration and would increase pressure in the chest cavity. Supine position does not facilitate lung expansion.
CN: Physiological integrity; CNS: Basic care and comfort; CL: Analyze

42. Which nursing intervention should be used for an infant with a diaphragmatic hernia before surgery?
1. Feed the infant clear liquids
2. Provide tactile stimulation
3. Prevent the infant from crying
4. Place the infant on the unaffected side

42. 3. Crying should be avoided to prevent the intestines from being pulled into the infant's chest cavity by the negative pressure. The stomach and intestine may also become distended with swallowed air from crying. The infant usually is not fed until after surgery. Tactile stimulation should be limited because it may disturb the infant's fragile condition. The infant should always be placed on the affected side.
CN: Physiological integrity; CNS: Physiological adaptation; CL: Apply

43. What is the most important intervention for the nurse to implement while caring for a neonate with an omphalocele?
1. Keep the omphalocele dry
2. Cover the omphalocele when parents visit
3. Carefully position and handle the omphalocele
4. Gently palpate the omphalocele to assess for changes

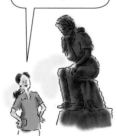

This question calls for a lot of thought.

43. 3. Careful positioning and handling prevents infection and rupture of the omphalocele. The omphalocele should be kept moist until the neonate is taken to the operating room. The parents can see the defect if they so choose. Palpation of the omphalocele increases the risk of rupture and infection.
CN: Physiological integrity; CNS: Physiological adaptation; CL: Apply

44. What is the **most** appropriate toy for a nurse to give to an eight-month-old infant admitted for repair of a diaphragmatic hernia?
1. Large building blocks
2. Crib-attached, multi-activity toy
3. Black-and-white mobile
4. Colorful pull toys

44. 2. By the eighth month, the infant can sit up, change positions, manipulate objects and enjoy different textures, colors and sounds making a multi-activity toy interesting and age-appropriate. Newborns enjoy the visual stimulation of black-and-white mobiles. Large building blocks and pull toys are appropriate for toddlers.
CN: Health promotion and maintenance; CNS: None; CL: Analyze

45. An adolescent who has a nasogastric (NG) tube in place following surgery for a ruptured appendix reports feeling nauseated. What is the nurse's **most** appropriate action?
1. Assess bowel sounds
2. Measure the gastric drainage
3. Assess serum electrolytes
4. Irrigate the tube

You're doing a pear-fect job! Keep it up.

45. 4. When a client with an NG tube reports nausea, the nurse should first determine the position of the tube and then irrigate it to check for patency. A clogged tube allows stomach contents to accumulate, contributing to nausea. Assessing for bowel sounds is something the nurse should do, but not the most appropriate action related to the report of nausea. Measuring gastric drainage is important but will not relieve nausea. Serum electrolytes should be monitored in the client with an NG tube. Although an electrolyte imbalance may cause nausea, the tube should be checked for patency first.
CN: Physiological integrity; CNS: Reduction of risk potential; CL: Apply

CN: Client needs category   CNS: Client needs subcategory   CL: Cognitive level

46. What is the **most** appropriate nursing intervention for an infant with pyloric stenosis who has been vomiting?
1. Place the infant in a supine position to sleep
2. Weigh the infant every eight hours
3. Assess for signs of dehydration
4. Assess vital signs every eight hours

46. 3. Because the infant is vomiting, the nurse should assess for signs and symptoms of dehydration. The infant should be placed on the right side to sleep to prevent aspiration of vomitus. The infant should be weighed daily, not every eight hours. Vital signs should be assessed every four hours until stable.

CN: Physiological integrity; CNS: Reduction of risk potential; CL: Apply

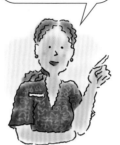

Think! This question is asking about what is abnormal.

47. The nurse is performing an initial assessment on a six-month-old infant being admitted for intestinal obstruction. The nurse is **most** concerned when the assessment reveals:
1. Moro reflex.
2. positive Babinski reflex.
3. eruption of the first tooth.
4. rolling from stomach to back.

47. 1. By six months of age, the Moro reflex should no longer be observed. Positive Babinski reflex, eruption of the first tooth, and rolling from stomach to back are all normal for a six-month-old infant.

CN: Health promotion and maintenance; CNS: None; CL: Analyze

48. The nurse is teaching the parents of an infant with pyloric stenosis. Where does the pyloric canal narrows?
1. Stomach and esophagus
2. Stomach and duodenum
3. Stomach and esophagus as well as the stomach and duodenum
4. Duodenum and jejunum

48. 2. The narrowing of the pyloric canal occurs between the stomach and duodenum, where the pyloric sphincter is located. Hyperplasia and hypertrophy cause narrowing and possible obstruction of the circular muscle of the pylorus.

CN: Physiological integrity; CNS: Physiological adaptation; CL: Apply

49. The nurse is caring for an infant with pyloric stenosis. Which manifestation requires priority attention?
1. Loss of appetite
2. Explosive diarrhea
3. Projectile vomiting
4. Coffee ground emesis

49. 3. The obstruction doesn't allow food to pass through the pyloris to the duodenum. When the stomach becomes full, the infant forcefully vomits for pressure relief. Chronic hunger is commonly seen. There's no diarrhea because food doesn't pass the stomach. Coffee ground emesis is a result of partially digested blood in the stomach, and not an expected finding with pyloric stenosis.

CN: Physiological integrity; CNS: Physiological adaptation; CL: Apply

50. When assessing a neonate, the nurse notes visible peristaltic waves across the epigastrium. Based on this characteristic which disorder would the nurse suspect?
1. Infantile hypertrophic pyloric stenosis
2. Imperforate anus
3. Intussusception
4. Short-gut syndrome

Looks like you're picking all the right answers.

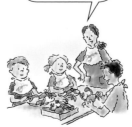

50. 1. Infantile hypertrophic pyloric stenosisis, also known as pyloric stenosis, is a form of gastric outlet obstruction, which means a blockage from the stomach to the intestines. Increased stomach contractions or waves of peristalsis, which move from left to right over the baby's belly, can occur as the stomach tries to empty itself against the thickened pylorus. Imperforate anus, intussusception, and short-gut syndrome are each diagnosed by other characteristics.

CN: Physiological integrity; CNS: Physiological adaptation; CL: Analyze

CN: Client needs category   CNS: Client needs subcategory   CL: Cognitive level

51. How soon after surgical repair of pyloric stenosis, should the nurse resume the infant's normal, full feeding regimen?
  1. Four to six hours after surgery
  2. 24 hours after surgery
  3. 48 hours after surgery
  4. One week after surgery

51. 3. Small, frequent feedings of clear fluids are usually started four to six hours after surgery. If clear fluids are tolerated, the nurse should advance to formula feedings, in gradually increasing amounts, 24 hours after surgery. It usually takes 48 hours to reach a normal, full feeding regimen in this manner. The infant usually goes home on the fourth postoperative day.
CN: Physiological integrity; CNS: Physiological adaptation; CL: Apply

52. A nurse admits an infant diagnosed with pyloric stenosis. What is the nurse's **priority** intervention?
  1. Weigh the infant
  2. Check urine specific gravity
  3. Place an IV catheter
  4. Change the infant and weigh the diaper

52. 1. Weighing the infant would be done first so a baseline weight can be established and weight changes can be evaluated. After a baseline weight is obtained, an IV catheter can be placed because oral feedings generally aren't given. Infants with pyloric stenosis are usually dehydrated, so weighing the diaper or checking the specific gravity, though important, are not a priority.
CN: Physiological integrity; CNS: Physiological adaptation; CL: Analyze

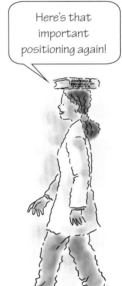

Here's that important positioning again!

53. A nurse is caring for an infant with pyloric stenosis following pyloromyotomy. In which position should the nurse place the baby after feeding?
  1. Prone in Fowler's position
  2. On the back without elevation
  3. On the left side in Fowler's position
  4. Slightly on the right side in high semi-Fowler's position

53. 4. Positioning the infant slightly on the right side, in high semi-Fowler's position, will help facilitate gastric emptying. The other positions won't facilitate gastric emptying, and may cause the infant to vomit.
CN: Physiological integrity; CNS: Physiological adaptation; CL: Apply

54. The nurse is preparing to feed an infant diagnosed with pyloric stenosis prior to surgical repair. What is the nurse's **most** important intervention?
  1. Give feedings quickly
  2. Burp the infant frequently
  3. Encourage parental participation
  4. Don't give more feedings if the infant vomits

54. 2. These infants usually swallow a lot of air from sucking on their hands and fingers because of their intense hunger. Burping frequently will reduce gastric distention, and increase the likelihood that the infant will retain the feeding. Feedings should be given slowly with the infant lying in a semi-upright position. Parental participation should be encouraged to the extent possible, but this will not increase the likelihood that the feeding will be retained. Record the type, amount, and character of the vomit, as well as its relation to the feeding. The amount of feeding volume lost is usually refed to the infant.
CN: Physiological adaptation; CNS: Physiological adaptation; CL: Apply

55. Which finding should the nurse expect up to 48 hours after the surgical repair of pyloric stenosis?
1. Oliguria
2. Oral aversion
3. Scaphoid abdomen
4. Vomiting

55. 4. Most infants will vomit during the first 24 to 48 hours following successful surgery. Oliguria isn't a complication with this surgical procedure. Oral aversion doesn't occur because these infants may be fed up until surgery. Scaphoid abdomen isn't characteristic of this condition. The abdomen may appear distended, but not scaphoid.
CN: Physiological integrity; CNS: Physiological adaptation; CL: Apply

56. Which nursing intervention will help prevent vomiting in an infant diagnosed with pyloric stenosis?
1. Hold the infant for one hour following feeding
2. Handle the infant minimally after feedings
3. Space the feedings out and give them in large amounts
4. Lay the infant prone with the head of the bed elevated

56. 2. Minimal handling, especially after a feeding, will help prevent vomiting. Holding the infant would provide too much stimulation, which might increase the risk of vomiting. Feedings are given frequently, slowly, and in small amounts. An infant should be positioned in a semi-Fowler's position and slightly on the right side after a feeding.
CN: Physiological integrity; CNS: Physiological adaptation; CL: Apply

57. Which nursing intervention would **best** provide support to the parents of an infant diagnosed with pyloric stenosis?
1. Keep the parents informed of their infant's progress
2. Provide all care for the infant during the parent's visit
3. Encourage the parents to minimize handling their infant while awake
4. Ask the provider to keep the parents informed of the infant's progress

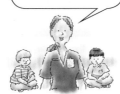

Encourage parents to be involved with their child's care.

57. 1. Keeping the parents well informed will decrease their anxiety. The nurse should encourage the parents to be involved with the infant's care. Telling the parents to minimize handling of the infant isn't appropriate because contact with their child is important. The provider is responsible for updating the parents on the infant's medical condition. The nurse is responsible for updating the parents on the day-to-day progress and activities of the infant.
CN: Psychosocial integrity; CNS: None; CL: Analyze

58. An infant has been diagnosed with pyloric stenosis. For which would the nurse assess the infant?
1. Lack of hunger
2. Bradycardia
3. Dry lips and skin
4. Hypothermia

58. 3. Dry lips and skin are signs of dehydration, which is common in infants with pyloric stenosis. These infants are constantly hungry because of their inability to retain feedings. Bradycardia and hypothermia aren't clinical findings in infants with pyloric stenosis.
CN: Physiological integrity; CNS: Physiological adaptation; CL: Apply

Question 59 asks what's normally found with a disease, not what's normal in a healthy infant.

59. Which assessment finding is considered normal in an infant diagnosed with pyloric stenosis?
1. Diminished bowel sounds
2. Heart murmur
3. Reduced appetite
4. Sleeping for long intervals

59. 1. Bowel sounds decrease because food cannot pass through the pylorus into the intestines. Heart murmurs may be present but aren't directly associated with pyloric stenosis. The infant's desire to eat is increased since feedings are lost when vomiting occurs. Sleeping time is reduced due to hunger.
CN: Physiological integrity; CNS: Physiological adaptation; CL: Analyze

CN: Client needs category   CNS: Client needs subcategory   CL: Cognitive level

60. The nurse is caring for a child who has undergone the first of two planned surgeries to correct Hirschsprung disease. When providing education to the child's parents, including which information is **essential**?
1. Food allergy precautions
2. Colostomy care
3. Central line care
4. Oral administration of iron

60. 2. A temporary colostomy allows the distended bowel to decompress and ready the child for a second procedure to remove the aganglionic portion of the colon. Food allergies do not accompany Hirschsprung disease. A central line would not usually be needed. Iron replacement would not be directly related to this health problem.

CN: Physiologic integrity; CNS: Physiological adaptation; CL: Apply

61. The nurse cares for a child who has been poisoned. Which intervention should the nurse perform **first**?
1. Stabilize the child
2. Notify the parents
3. Identify the source of poison
4. Determine time of poisoning

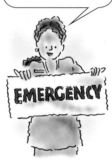

Would you know what to do first in this emergency situation?

EMERGENCY

61. 1. Stabilize the child and begin initial emergency treatment, such as respiratory assistance, circulatory support, or control of seizures. This will prevent the poison from further damaging. If the parents didn't bring the child in, they should be notified as soon as the child is stabilized. Identification of the source of poison is important; however, stabilization is the priority. Determining when the poisoning took place is an important consideration, but emergency stabilization and treatment is the priority.

CN: Physiological integrity; CNS: Physiological adaptation; CL: Analyze

62. A child has ingested a poisonous substance. What is the **priority** intervention?
1. Make the child vomit
2. Contact poison control
3. Give large amounts of water
4. Empty the mouth of any foreign material

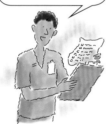

Practice setting priorities because it's part of nursing practice.

62. 4. Emptying the mouth of pills, plant parts, or other material will stop exposure to the poison. Making the child vomit will not remove exposure to the substance, and may be contraindicated with some poisons. Calling poison control for care instruction should occur, but removing any further sources of the poison in the mouth would be the priority. Drinking small amounts of water will confine the poison to the smallest volume. Large amounts of water will allow the poison pass the pylorus and empty into the duodenum. The duodenum will rapidly absorb the poison, increasing potential toxicity.

CN: Physiological integrity; CNS: Physiological adaptation; CL: Analyze

63. The nurse is caring for a child in the recovery phase following an ingestion of drain cleaner. The nurse is aware that the child is at risk for:
1. esophageal strictures.
2. esophageal diverticula.
3. tracheal stenosis.
4. tracheal varices.

63. 1. Scar tissue develops as the burn from the ingestion of drain cleaner heals, leading to esophageal strictures. The formation of esophageal diverticula is rare. Tracheal stenosis may occur, but only if the child vomited and aspirated. Tracheal varices don't commonly occur after drain cleaner ingestion.

CN: Physiological integrity; CNS: Physiological adaptation; CL: Analyze

CN: Client needs category   CNS: Client needs subcategory   CL: Cognitive level

64. A preschooler is brought to the emergency department after ingesting kerosene. The nurse is aware the child is at risk for:
1. pneumonitis.
2. carditis.
3. uremia.
4. hepatitis.

64. 1. Chemical pneumonitis is the most common complication following ingestion of a hydrocarbon, such as kerosene. The pneumonitis is caused by irritation from the hydrocarbon aspirated into the lungs. The other options aren't complications of kerosene ingestion.

CN: Physiological integrity; CNS: Physiological adaptation; CL: Analyze

65. What is the **most** important information for a nurse to tell parents if their child ingests a poison?
1. Administer syrup of ipecac
2. Call the poison control center
3. Transport the child to the emergency department
4. Watch the child for adverse effects

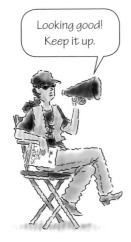

Looking good! Keep it up.

65. 2. The first step parents should take if their child has ingested a poisonous substance is to call the poison control center for instructions. Home administration of syrup of ipecac is no longer recommended by the American Academy of Pediatrics. Parents should contact poison control before transporting their child to the emergency department. Valuable time may be lost if poison control recommends a specific action to remove the poisonous substance from the body. Poison control may recommend watching the child for adverse effects, but parents should not make this decision without consulting poison control.

CN: Physiological integrity; CNS: Reduction of risk potential; CL: Analyze

66. A child has ingested poisonous hydrocarbons. What is the **most** important nursing intervention?
1. Induce vomiting
2. Keep the child calm and relaxed
3. Administer activated charcoal
4. Monitor the parent-child interactions for possible child abuse

66. 2. Keeping the child calm and relaxed will help prevent vomiting. If vomiting is induced, the esophagus will be damaged from regurgitation of the gastric poison. The risk of chemical pneumonitis exists if vomiting occurs. Activated charcoal poorly absorbs hydrocarbons, and it tends to distend the stomach and cause vomiting. The parents should remain with the child to help keep him calm. It is not necessary to monitor parent-child interactions for possible child abuse.

CN: Physiological integrity; CNS: Physiological adaptation; CL: Analyze

67. Shock is a complication of several types of poisoning. Which measure would help reduce the risk of shock?
1. Keep the child on his right side
2. Let the child maintain normal activity as possible
3. Elevate the head and legs to the level of the heart
4. Keep the head flat and raise the legs to the level of the heart

67. 3. Elevating the head and legs to the level of the heart will promote venous drainage and decrease the chance of the child going into shock. The child may safely lie on the side he prefers, and should be encouraged to get plenty of rest.

CN: Physiological integrity; CNS: Physiological adaptation; CL: Apply

68. A seven-year-old child who ingested several leaves of a poisonous plant has arrived in the emergency department. What is the **priority** nursing intervention?
1. Begin teaching accident prevention
2. Provide emotional support to the child
3. Be prepared for immediate intervention
4. Provide emotional support to the parents

68. 3. Time and speed are critical factors in stabilizing the child. The remaining three answers are important nursing functions but don't require the immediate.

CN: Health promotion and maintenance; CNS: None; CL: Analyze

69. A child is being admitted through the emergency department with a diagnosis of suspected accidental poisoning by medication. What is the **most** common cause of accidental poisoning in children?
1. Pain medications
2. Vitamins
3. Laxatives
4. Antibiotics

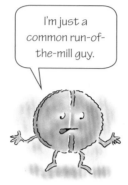

I'm just a common run-of-the-mill guy.

69. 1. The most common accidentally ingested class of drugs is pain medications. The most common pain medications ingested are acetaminophen-containing drugs, nonsteroidal anti-inflammatory drugs, and opioids. The other classes of drugs are less commonly ingested.

CN: Health promotion and maintenance; CNS: None; CL: Apply

70. A client is undergoing tests for a diagnosis of ulcerative colitis. Which symptom would the nurse most likely identify during this **initial** diagnosis?
1. Constipation
2. Diarrhea
3. Vomiting
4. Weight loss

70. 2. Recurrent or persistent diarrhea is a common feature of ulcerative colitis. Constipation doesn't occur because the bowel becomes smooth and inflexible. Vomiting isn't common in this disease. Weight loss will occur after, or during, the episode but not initially.

CN: Physiological integrity; CNS: Physiological adaptation; CL: Analyze

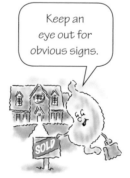

Keep an eye out for obvious signs.

71. A child arrives in the emergency department after ingesting toxic amounts of salicylates. When would the nurse assess this child for obvious signs of toxicity?
1. Immediately
2. Four hours after ingestion
3. Six hours after ingestion
4. 18 hours after ingestion

71. 3. There's usually a delay of six hours before evidence of toxicity is noted. Toxic evidence is rarely immediate. Aspirin will reach peak effect in two to four hours. The effect of aspirin may last as long as 18 hours.

CN: Health promotion and maintenance; CNS: None; CL: Apply

72. The nurse is caring for a client with an extreme case of salicylate poisoning. Which treatments would the nurse anticipate for this client? Select all that apply.
1. Gastric lavage
2. Warming blankets
3. Hemodialysis
4. Vitamin K injection
5. Intravenous diphenhydramine

72. 1, 3, 4. Hemodialysis is usually reserved for life-threatening cases of salicylism. Gastric lavage is used in the immediate treatment for salicylate poisoning, where vomiting will result in the removal of the poison. Cooling blankets may be used to reduce the possibility of seizures. Vitamin K may be used to decrease bleeding tendencies. Diphenhydramine is used for allergic reactions. This is not an allergic response to salicylates.

CN: Physiological integrity; CNS: Physiological adaptation; CL: Analyze

CN: Client needs category   CNS: Client needs subcategory   CL: Cognitive level

73. When a child has been poisoned, it is important for the nurse to identify the ingested poison. Which intervention will appropriately identify the poison?
   1. Call poison control
   2. Ask the child
   3. Ask the parents
   4. Save all evidence of poison

73. 4. Saving all evidence of the toxin (container, vomitus, urine) will help determine the type and quantity ingested. Calling the poison control center may help get information on a specific toxin, but can rarely help determine which one has been ingested. Asking the child may help, but the she may fear punishment, and may not provide an honest answer. The parent may be helpful, but may not have been with the child when the ingestion occurred.
CN: Health promotion and maintenance; CNS: None; CL: Analyze

74. Which nursing responsibility can help prevent salicylate poisoning?
   1. Identify what constitutes a salicylate overdose
   2. Teach children the hazards of ingesting non-food items
   3. Decrease a child's curiosity by having parents keep aspirin and drugs in clear view
   4. Teach parents that salicylate bottles must be kept out of reach of their children

Know your nursing responsibilities.

74. 2. Teaching children the hazards of ingesting non-food items will help prevent the ingestion of poisonous substances. Identifying an overdose won't prevent it from occurring. Aspirin and other drugs should be kept out of a child's sight. Drugs should be securely stored and out of reach for children.
CN: Health promotion and maintenance; CNS: None; CL: Apply

75. The nurse is evaluating the effectiveness of acetylcysteine in a child with acetaminophen poisoning. Which laboratory value should the nurse closely monitor?
   1. Serum alanine aminotransferase
   2. Serum calcium levels
   3. Prothrombin time
   4. Alkaline phosphatase

75. 1. Acetaminophen poisoning damages the liver, leading to elevated serum alanine aminotransferase and aspartate aminotransferase levels. After therapy with acetylcysteine is started, these liver enzymes should begin to fall. Serum calcium levels may fall following chelation therapy in clients with lead poisoning. If the liver enzymes did not begin to decrease, prothrombin time would be measured and followed. These indicate impaired hepatic synthetic function. Alkaline phosphatase levels monitor diseases of the liver or bone, and would not be sensitive enough to indicate response to acetylcysteine therapy.
CN: Physiological integrity; CNS: Reduction of risk potential; CL: Analyze

76. A client is diagnosed with acetaminophen poisoning. Which signs would the nurse expect to assess 12 to 24 hours after ingestion? Select all that apply.
   1. Hyperthermia
   2. Nausea and vomiting
   3. Sweating
   4. Diarrhea
   5. Irritability

Don't sweat it! You know the answer.

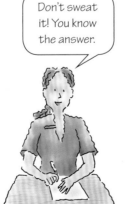

76. 2, 3, 4, 5. The signs and symptoms observed during the first 12 to 24 hours of acetaminophen poisoning are sweating, anorexia, nausea, vomiting, diarrhea, and irritability. Hyperthermia is not a sign.
CN: Physiological integrity; CNS: Physiological adaptation; CL: Analyze

77. A client ingested a large amount of acetaminophen at 1:00 AM. Two hours later, the client comes to the emergency department, and is diagnosed with acetaminophen poisoning. What is the **priority** intervention for this client?
1. Perform gastric lavage
2. Obtain blood work
3. Administer IV fluid
4. Administer N-acetylcysteine

78. The mother of a child admitted for ingesting a caustic cleaning product tells the nurse she feels guilty. What is the nurse's **best** response?
1. "Now you'll know to keep all cleaning products locked up."
2. "Luckily, your child is going to be fine."
3. "You'll need to watch your child more carefully."
4. "Tell me more about your guilty feelings."

79. Which factor **most** influences a child's risk of ingesting lead-containing substances?
1. Age
2. Gender
3. Race
4. Parental eating habits

80. The nurse explains to the mother of a child who has lead poisoning that X-rays can indicate that lead has accumulated in the child's:
1. bones.
2. brain.
3. kidney.
4. liver.

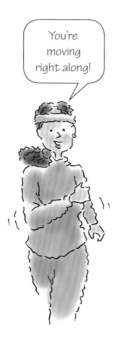

You're moving right along!

77. 4. If the client is seen within one hour of ingestion, activated charcoal can be given to prevent absorption, or gastric lavage can be used. Blood work would be obtained but wouldn't be the first priority. Intravenous fluids would also be administered, but administering N-acetylcysteine, the specific antidote for acetaminophen poisoning, is the priority.
CN: Physiological integrity; CNS: Physiological adaptation; CL: Analyze

78. 4. Encouraging the mother to talk about her feelings shows that the nurse accepts her feelings and is prepared to listen. This also helps establish a trusting nurse–client relationship. Telling the mother she should keep all cleaning products locked up, and that she needs to watch her child more carefully lays fault on the mother, and may block further communication. Telling the mother that her child will be fine dismisses the mother's feelings, and may give false reassurance.
CN: Psychosocial integrity; CNS: None; CL: Analyze

79. 1. The highest risk of lead poisoning occurs in young children who have a tendency to put things in their mouth. Homes built before 1978 often contain lead-based paint. Flaking paint chips may be eaten by the child, or lead dust may cling to toys or hands that are then put into the child's mouth. Poisoning isn't gender-related. African Americans have a higher incidence of lead poisoning, but it can happen in any race. Most parents don't eat lead-based paint or other non-food items intentionally.
CN: Health promotion and maintenance; CNS: None; CL: Apply

80. 1. Ingested lead is initially absorbed by a child's bones. An X-ray will reveal a characteristic lead line at the epiphyseal line. If chronic ingestion occurs, the central nervous, renal, and hematologic systems are affected.
CN: Physiological integrity; CNS: Physiological adaptation; CL: Apply

81. The nurse is evaluating a child for suspected lead poisoning. Which condition is an **initial** sign of lead poisoning?
1. Anemia
2. Constipation
3. Anorexia
4. Paralysis

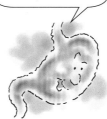

Be aware of the initial signs of lead poisoning.

81. 1. Lead is dangerously toxic to the biosynthesis of heme, and the reduced heme molecule in red blood cells causes anemia. Constipation and anorexia are nonspecific symptoms. Paralysis may occur if toxic damage to the brain occurs.
CN: Physiological integrity; CNS: Physiological adaptation; CL: Analyze

82. The most serious and irreversible adverse effects of lead intoxication affect the:
1. central nervous system (CNS).
2. hematologic system.
3. renal system.
4. respiratory system.

82. 1. Damage that occurs to the CNS is difficult to repair. Damage to the hematologic and renal systems can be reversed if treated early. The respiratory system isn't affected until coma and death occur.
CN: Physiological integrity; CNS: Physiological adaptation; CL: Analyze

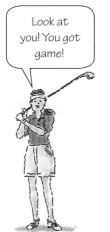

Look at you! You got game!

83. A mother of a recently admitted child asks the nurse about the bluish-black lines along her child's gums. The nurse would respond that the bluish black lines often indicate:
1. acetaminophen poisoning.
2. lead poisoning.
3. plant poisoning.
4. salicylate poisoning.

83. 2. One diagnostic characteristic of lead poisoning is bluish-black lines along the gums. Bluish-black lines don't occur along the gums with acetaminophen, plant, or salicylate poisoning.
CN: Physiological integrity; CNS: Physiological adaptation; CL: Analyze

84. The parents of a child with lead poisoning ask the nurse which procedure is the main treatment for lead poisoning. What is the nurse's **best** response?
1. Exchange transfusion
2. Bone marrow transplant
3. Chelation therapy
4. Dialysis

84. 3. Chelation therapy is the main treatment for lead poisoning, and involves the removal of metal by combining it with another substance. Sometimes, exchange transfusions are used to rid the blood of lead quickly. Bone marrow transplants usually are not needed. Dialysis is not usually part of the treatment.
CN: Physiological integrity; CNS: Physiological adaptation; CL: Apply

85. What is the **most** important nursing intervention for a child with lead poisoning who must undergo chelation therapy with intramuscular edetate calcium disodium? The nurse should prepare the child for:
1. extra bed rest.
2. intravenous fluid therapy.
3. an extended hospital stay.
4. a large number of injections.

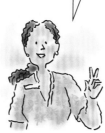

Watch for these two words—most important.

85. 4. Intramuscular chelation therapy for symptomatic children commonly involves a large number of injections in a relatively short period of time. It's traumatic to most children. Edetate calcium disodium can also be given IV. The other components of the treatment plan are important but aren't as likely to cause the same anxiety as multiple injections. Allowing adequate rest to protect painful injection sites is helpful. Physical activity is usually limited. Receiving IV fluid is not as traumatizing as multiple injections.
CN: Physiological integrity; CNS: Physiological adaptation; CL: Analyze

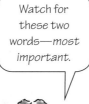

CN: Client needs category   CNS: Client needs subcategory   CL: Cognitive level

86. For which should the nurse monitor in a child receiving chelation therapy with edetate calcium disodium?
1. Hypercalcemia
2. Hypocalcemia
3. Hyperglycemia
4. Hypoglycemia

86. 2. A calcium chelating agent is used for the treatment of lead poisoning, so calcium is removed from the body with the lead. Hypocalcemia can occur. Hyperglycemia and hypoglycemia do not occur as a result of this therapy.
CN: Physiological integrity; CNS: Physiological adaptation; CL: Analyze

87. A nurse is aware that the **best** way to prevent lead poisoning in children is to:
1. educate the child about the dangers of chewing on pencils.
2. educate the public about imported toys containing lead.
3. identify high-risk groups.
4. provide home chelation kits.

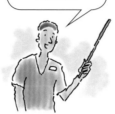

You know the routine; keep on teachin'.

87. 2. Educating others about the risks of lead poisoning risks is important in preventing the poisoning. Identifying high-risk groups including young children will help but won't prevent the poisoning. Pencil lead is graphite, and cannot cause lead poisoning. Home chelation kits are not currently available.
CN: Health promotion and maintenance; CNS: None; CL: Analyze

88. A nurse is planning care for a 14-year-old client following an appendectomy. What is the **most** important intervention?
1. Reduce conflict between the client and his parents
2. Promote the development of an identity and independence
3. Encourage the development of trust
4. Confirm plans for the future

88. 2. Since adolescents are in Erikson's identity versus role confusion stage, planning care should include interventions that promote a sense of identity and independence. During adolescence, conflict is usually intensified, not reduced. Trust is a developmental task of infancy. Plans for the future aren't confirmed at age 14.
CN: Health promotion and maintenance; CNS: None; CL: Apply

89. The nurse tells parents that certain forms of pica are caused by a dietary deficiency. Which nutrients are **most** commonly deficient?
1. Minerals
2. Vitamins
3. Electrolytes
4. Protein

89. 1. Eating clay is related to zinc deficiency. Eating chalk can indicate calcium deficiency, and eating ice, may indicate an iron deficiency. Vitamin, electrolyte, and protein deficiencies are not related to pica.
CN: Health promotion and maintenance; CNS: None; CL: Analyze

90. A child with appendicitis reports a sudden cessation of abdominal pain to the nurse. What is the **most** appropriate nursing intervention?
1. Prepare the child and parents for discharge
2. Begin feeding the child, as tolerated
3. Prepare the child for emergency surgery
4. Begin ambulation, as tolerated

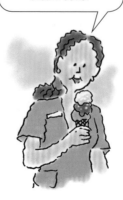

Taking NCLEX practice tests is more fun than eating a triple-decker ice cream cone!

90. 3. The sudden cessation of abdominal pain in the client with appendicitis may indicate perforation or infarction of the appendix, requiring emergency surgery. Therefore, the child should not be prepared for discharge or given oral feedings. The child with a ruptured appendix should be on complete bed rest and be prepared for surgery.
CN: Physiological integrity; CNS: Reduction of risk potential; CL: Apply

91. Which advice should a nurse give over the telephone to the mother of a seven-year-old child who has abdominal pain, a low-grade fever, and is vomiting?
1. "Give prune juice to relieve constipation."
2. "Palpate the abdomen for tenderness several times."
3. "Give fluids in moderate amounts to prevent dehydration."
4. "Seek immediate emergency medical care."

91. 4. The cardinal signs of appendicitis are pain, fever, and vomiting. This mother should seek immediate emergency care to reduce the risk of rupture. Prune juice can increase peristalsis and possible rupture of the appendix. The nurse shouldn't rely on the mother's findings when palpating for tenderness. Palpating repeatedly will increase the child's pain. The child should be given nothing by mouth in case surgery is required.
CN: Physiological integrity; CNS: Reduction of risk potential; CL: Apply

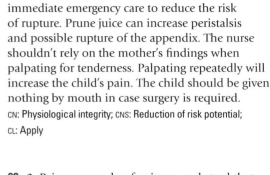

92. The nurse receives a phone call from the mother of a fussy toddler. The mother states that the child has mucus-filled stool that is reddish in color and glistening. The nurse advises the mother to take the child to the nearest urgent-care center. The nurse suspects that the child has:
1. gastroenteritis.
2. hirschsprung disease.
3. intussusception.
4. rotavirus.

92. 3. Pain expressed as fussiness, and stool that is often compared to currant jelly would suggest intussusception. Intussusception can self-resolve or progress to intestinal damage if inadequate circulation to the intestine occurs. The symptoms would require additional assessment. Surgical intervention is sometimes necessary. Constipation is typical of Hirschsprung disease. Gastroenteritis includes diarrhea, fever and often vomiting. Rotavirus presents as gastroenteritis with symptoms including fever and vomiting, followed by three or more days of watery diarrhea. Immunization for rotavirus is given in infancy.
CN: Physiological integrity; CNS: Reduction of risk potential; CL: Analyze

93. The nurse is providing preoperative care for a child diagnosed with appendicitis. What is the **most** appropriate intervention?
1. Give the child's preference of clear fluids
2. Apply heat to the abdomen
3. Maintain complete bed rest
4. Offer an oral antiemetic

93. 3. Bed rest will prevent aggravating the condition. Those with appendicitis should not eat or drink as surgery is likely. Controlling nausea is important, but taking an oral antiemetic will result in fluid ingestion, and may induce vomiting and aspiration while under anesthesia. Cold applications should be placed on the abdomen. Heat increases blood flow to the area and could increase the possibility of spreading infectious disease by promoting perforation of the appendix.
CN: Physiological integrity; CNS: Reduction of risk potential; CL: Analyze

94. Which treatments or interventions should be included in the postoperative care of a child with a ruptured appendix? Select all that apply.
1. Diet as tolerated
2. Ambulation daily
3. Left-side positioning
4. Pain control
5. Parenteral antibiotics

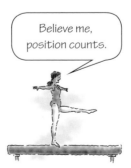

Believe me, position counts.

94. 1, 2, 4, 5. Parenteral antibiotics are used postoperatively to treat and prevent the spread of infection. An adequate diet as tolerated allows for nutritional and fluid intake required for healing. The child is positioned on the right side with his head elevated following surgery to help minimize the spread of infection throughout the abdomen, and development of sub-diaphragmatic abscess. Daily ambulation prevents respiratory and venous complications. Pain control is needed for comfort, promotion of healing and easing ambulation.
CN: Physiological integrity; CNS: Reduction of risk potential; CL: Analyze

95. A one-month-old infant is admitted to the hospital with gastroenteritis. Which intervention should be included on the child's nursing care plan?
1. Blood pressure every four hours
2. Prone positioning
3. Oral glucose feedings
4. Frequent perineal skin care

95. 4. The tender skin of an infant's perineal area will be easily irritated by frequent stooling. Good skin care will promote comfort and desired integrity. Infants are safely positioned when on their backs. Feeding a glucose solution may further diarrhea. The child's blood glucose level is not likely at risk. An oral electrolyte replacement solution would be more appropriate. Checking blood pressure every four hours is not necessary since this infant is not critically ill. Doing so would disrupt sleep and upset the child.
CN: Physiological integrity; CNS: Reduction of risk potential; CL: Analyze

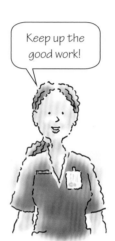

Keep up the good work!

96. A child being treated for pinworms. Which statement by the child's parent would indicate that further teaching is necessary?
1. "I will make my child wash his hands well before meals."
2. "I will tell my child not to share hairbrushes or hats."
3. "I will give my child only one dose of medication."
4. "I will keep my child's nails short."

96. 2. Sharing hairbrushes and hats reduces the spread of lice, not pinworms. Hands should be washed well before food preparation and eating to avoid ingesting eggs that may be under the child's fingernails. Only a single dose of medication, such as mebendazole, is needed to treat pinworms. Keeping the fingernails short is hygienic, and reduces the risk of carrying pinworm eggs under the nails.
CN: Safe, effective care environment; CNS: Safety and infection control; CL: Apply

97. During an initial nursing assessment, a nurse determines that an eight-year-old child has right lower quadrant pain, a low-grade fever, nausea, rebound tenderness, and a positive psoas sign. Which condition would the nurse suspect?
1. Appendicitis
2. Gastroenteritis
3. Pancreatitis
4. Cholecystitis

97. 1. Right lower quadrant pain, a low-grade fever, nausea, rebound tenderness, and a positive psoas sign are all consistent with appendicitis. Gastroenteritis is characterized by generalized abdominal tenderness. Pancreatitis is characterized by pain in the left abdominal quadrant. Cholecystitis is characterized by pain in the right upper abdominal quadrant.
CN: Physiological integrity; CNS: Physiological adaptation; CL: Analyze

98. An order has been written to discontinue an infusion of total parenteral nutrition (TPN) for a child. What is the **priority** nursing action?
1. Gradually reduce the rate of the TPN per health care provider order
2. Prepare to infuse a glucose solution after discontinuing the TPN
3. Notify pharmacy to prevent additional preparation of the expensive fluid
4. Prepare to administer insulin for prevention of hyperglycemia

98. 1. Gradually reducing the rate will avoid a sudden loss of the highly concentrated solution of amino acids, glucose and other nutrients, and allow the child's body to adapt. Infusing a glucose solution after discontinuing TPN is not necessary when if infusion rate has been tapered. A glucose solution may need to be infused if discontinuation was sudden to avoid an abrupt drop in blood glucose. Administering insulin after discontinuing TPN would result in hypoglycemia. The pharmacy should be notified so that additional TPN is not prepared, but that is not a priority nursing action.
CN: Physiologic integrity; CNS: Pharmacological and parenteral therapies; CL: Analyze

CN: Client needs category   CNS: Client needs subcategory   CL: Cognitive level

99. The child's provider orders 720 ml of total parenteral nutrition (TPN) to be infused over the next 24 hours. The nurse will record TPN intake of how many milliliters at the end of the eight hour shift? Record your answer using a whole number.

_____ ml

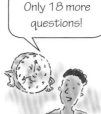

Only 18 more questions!

99. 240.
The nurse may calculate the rate two ways. First method:

$$720 \, ml \; TPN \div 24 \, hours = 30 \frac{ml}{hour}$$

$$30 \frac{ml}{hour} \times 8 \, hours = 240 \, ml$$

Second method:

$$720 \, ml \; TPN \div 3 \; (i.e., \; three \; 8 \; hour \; segments \; in \; 24 \; hours) = 240 \, ml$$

CN: Physiological integrity; CNS: Pharmacological and parenteral therapies; CL: Apply

100. When assessing a client suspected of having pyloric stenosis, which finding should the nurse expect?
   1. An "olive" mass in the right upper quadrant
   2. An "olive" mass in the left upper quadrant
   3. A "sausage" mass in the right upper quadrant
   4. A "sausage" mass in the left upper quadrant

100. 1. Pyloric stenosis involves hypertrophy of the circular muscle fibers of the pylorus. This hypertrophy is palpable in the right upper quadrant of the abdomen. A "sausage" mass is palpable in the right upper quadrant in children with intussusception. A "sausage" mass in the left upper quadrant wouldn't indicate pyloric stenosis.

CN: Physiological integrity; CNS: Physiological adaptation; CL: Apply

101. Which laboratory values should a nurse caring for an infant with pyloric stenosis expect to observe?
   1. pH 7.30; chloride 120 mEq/L
   2. pH 7.38; chloride 110 mEq/L
   3. pH 7.43; chloride 100 mEq/L
   4. pH 7.49; chloride 90 mEq/L

101. 4. Infants with pyloric stenosis vomit hydrochloric digestive acid from their stomach. This causes them to become alkalotic and hypochloremic. Normal serum pH is 7.35 to 7.45. Levels above 7.45 represent alkalosis. The normal serum chloride level is 97 to 107 mEq/L. Levels below 99 mEq/L represent hypochloremia.

CN: Physiological integrity; CNS: Physiological adaptation; CL: Analyze

102. A mother tells the nurse that her toddler had been suffering from diarrhea. The diarrhea has subsided, and the mother asks the nurse what she should feed her child. Which is the nurse's **best** response?
   1. "Give the child clear liquids such as juice, popsicles, and gelatin."
   2. "Offer the child chicken or beef broth and carbonated beverages."
   3. "Give the child cereal, cooked vegetables, soft meats and milk."
   4. "Follow the BRAT diet of bananas, rice, applesauce, toast."

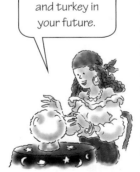

I see a meal of green beans and turkey in your future.

102. 3. This toddler has been rehydrated and can be given a regular diet of easily digested foods including milk. Resuming a regular diet rather than slowly reintroducing foods would have no adverse effects. Clear liquids offer little nutrition, are high in carbohydrates and low in electrolytes. Broth is high in sodium and lacks carbohydrate. Carbonated beverages may contain caffeine which can lead to additional water loss. The BRAT diet provides limited nutrition and is high in carbohydrates and low in electrolytes.

CN: Physiological integrity; CNS: Physiological adaptation; CL: Apply

103. Which findings would the nurse assess in a premature neonate who may have necrotizing enterocolitis?
1. Abdominal distention
2. Metabolic alkalosis
3. Active bowel sounds
4. Guaiac-negative stools

103. 1. Necrotizing enterocolitis is an ischemic disorder of the gut. The cause is unknown, but it's more common in premature neonates who have had a hypoxic episode. The neonate's intestines become dilated and necrotic, and the abdomen becomes very distended. Paralytic ileus develops, causing the neonate to have high gastric residuals. Bowel sounds are diminished. These residual gastric contents, along with any passed stool, will be guaiac-positive. The neonate also develops metabolic acidosis.
CN: Physiological integrity; CNS: Physiological adaptation; CL: Analyze

104. An infant has just been admitted to the hospital's pediatric unit with gastroenteritis. Prioritize the actions that this nurse should take.

| 1. Review arriving laboratory reports |
| 2. Begin ordered rehydration measures |
| 3. Determine comfort interventions |
| 4. Establish intake and output |
| 5. Protect skin from diarrheal stool |

104. Ordered Response:

| 2. Begin ordered rehydration measures |
| 4. Establish intake and output |
| 1. Review arriving laboratory reports |
| 5. Protect skin from diarrheal stool |
| 3. Determine comfort interventions |

CN: Physiological integrity; CNS: Physiological adaptation; CL: Analyze

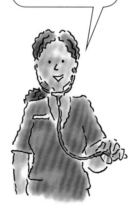

Nursing assessments are so important.

105. A nurse is assessing an infant with gastroenteritis. Toward which potential problem should the nursing assessments be directed?
1. Urinary retention
2. Heart failure
3. Electrolyte imbalance
4. Hyperactive reflexes

105. 3. Diarrhea in infants can rapidly lead to dehydration and electrolyte imbalances, especially hyponatremia and hypokalemia. Urinary retention is not a sign of dehydration, but should be distinguished from kidney failure, which may occur with severe dehydration. Heart failure occurs with fluid volume overload, not fluid volume deficit. Reflexes are typically diminished or absent with hypokalemia.
CN: Physiological integrity; CNS: Reduction of risk potential; CL: Apply

106. A mother calls the health clinic and tells the nurse that she found her toddler with an open and empty bottle of acetaminophen. The mother asks the nurse what she should do. What is the nurse's **priority** intervention?
1. Have the mother give the child syrup of ipecac
2. Tell the mother to get the child to drink a glass of milk
3. Give the mother instructions on how to call poison control
4. Determine whether the mother knows cardiopulmonary resuscitation (CPR)

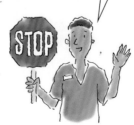

Do you know the priority invention for this toddler?

106. 3. The mother should call poison control and ask what immediate steps she should take to treat this ingestion. Home administration of syrup of ipecac is no longer recommended. Milk is not an antidote for acetaminophen toxicity. Asking about CPR is not appropriate since it would distract from the immediate interventions needed.
CN: Safe, effective care environment; CNS: Safety and infection control; CL: Analyze

CN: Client needs category CNS: Client needs subcategory CL: Cognitive level

107. The nurse is preparing a teaching plan for the parents of a child with celiac disease. What is the **most** important information for the nurse to include in this teaching?
1. "The gluten-free diet alterations must be continued for a lifetime."
2. "The diet needs to be free of lactose because the child is intolerant."
3. "Dietary alterations are necessary when the child reports cramping and bloating."
4. "The diet needs to be low in fat because of the malabsorption problem in the intestines."

107. 1. Celiac disease is the inability to digest gluten. The treatment is a lifelong gluten-free diet. It's important that the gluten-free diet is continued to avoid symptoms and the associated risk of colon cancer. The disease isn't caused by lactose intolerance, or a problem digesting fat.
CN: Health promotion and maintenance; CNS: None;
CL: Apply

108. A pediatrician suspects that a child has pinworms and instructs the nurse to assess the child for their presence. How should the nurse assess for pinworms?
1. A history of itching the anal area, and restlessness sleep
2. A blood culture
3. Eggs retrieved from a piece of cellophane tape placed along the anal edge at night
4. A stool culture

108. 3. Cellophane tape placed near the anal edge will capture the eggs as the female deposits them outside the rectum at night. A history of itching and restlessness isn't enough to definitively diagnosis pinworms. A blood culture or a stool culture would not be helpful.
CN: Physiological integrity; CNS: Reduction of risk potential;
CL: Apply

109. A one-month-old infant is brought to the pediatrician's office. The mother states that the baby is fussy and cries as if in pain. The infant is tolerating normal amounts of formula, gaining weight, and having episodes of paroxysmal abdominal cramping after feedings. Which condition do these sign and symptoms most likely indicate?
1. Intussusception
2. Meconium ileus
3. Colic
4. Pyloric stenosis

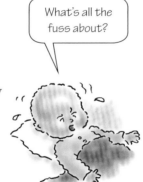

What's all the fuss about?

109. 3. An infant with colic exhibits symptoms of abdominal cramping after feedings, cries as if in pain, and is fussy. An intussusception begins suddenly and leads to bloody stools and vomiting. A meconium ileus is the non-passage of meconium in the first 24 hours. Signs of pyloric stenosis include projectile vomiting and weight loss.
CN: Physiological integrity; CNS: Physiological adaptation;
CL: Analyze

110. A 16-year-old black student visits a school nurse with a report of nausea and fatigue. The nurse assesses for jaundice. Which area of the body should the nurse examine?
1. Sclera of the eye
2. Overall skin color
3. Outer ears and back of the neck
4. Tongue and inside the cheek area

110. 1. The sclera is the best place to check for jaundice in a person of darker skin color. The outer ears and back of the neck, as well as the tongue and inside of the cheek, are not appropriate places to check for jaundice.
CN: Physiological integrity; CNS: Physiological adaptation;
CL: Apply

CN: Client needs category   CNS: Client needs subcategory   CL: Cognitive level

111. A mother brings her four-week-old child to the clinic. She states that the infant hasn't been eating well and is lethargic when she holds him. The infant has lost 7 oz (198.5 g) since birth. The infant is otherwise healthy and has no congenital defects. Which condition would the nurse suspect?
1. Celiac disease
2. Failure to thrive
3. Hirschsprung disease
4. Imperforate anus

112. A 15-year-old client needs a nasogastric tube inserted because of peritonitis caused by a ruptured appendix. The client is afraid that the procedure will hurt. Which statement by the nurse will decrease this client's anxiety?
1. "Breathe deeply through your mouth and relax. It will be over soon."
2. "This is a simple procedure, and it won't hurt."
3. "You'll feel pressure and be uncomfortable for a few minutes, but it shouldn't be painful."
4. "You're old enough now and should be able to handle pain."

113. A mother brings her 18-month-old child to the emergency department and tells a nurse that he has been ill for the past two days. He has a fever of 104.8° F (40.8° C), is irritable, has diarrhea, and hasn't been wetting his diaper much in the past 24 hours. The child is admitted to the pediatric unit for treatment of moderate dehydration and gastro-enteritis. Intravenous therapy and strict intake and output are ordered. As rehydration occurs, the child is started on oral feedings of rehydration fluid. Which action should the nurse take while caring for this child during the later stage of rehydration?
1. Force fluids
2. Allow the client to drink as much as he wants
3. Monitor the client's intake and output
4. Monitor the client's ability to retain fluids

114. A nurse is conducting an infant nutrition class for parents. Which healthy foods should be introduced during the first year of life? Select all that apply.
1. Sliced beef
2. Pureed fruits
3. Fat-free milk
4. Rice cereal
5. Strained vegetables
6. Fruit drinks

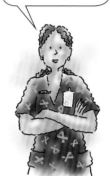

Just a little more to go and you're done with this chapter.

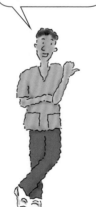

You're being asked for the later stage in question 113.

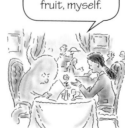

I'm a big fan of the pureed fruit, myself.

111. 2. These signs and symptoms are classic of failure to thrive. Celiac disease presents with steatorrhea, weight loss, and the inability to digest foods containing gluten. Hirschsprung disease and imperforate anus present with abdominal distention and absence of stool. No anal opening is present in imperforate anus.
CN: Physiological integrity; CNS: Physiological adaptation; CL: Apply

112. 3. Discussing the procedure will help the client understand the extent of discomfort. Breathing deeply will help relieve discomfort, but the statement implies that the procedure will be painful. Anticipatory pain will increase the client's anxiety. By saying the procedure is simple, the nurse isn't acknowledging the client's concerns. Telling the client that he is old enough now, and should be able to handle pain is condescending. Any client has the right to express fear, and to have those fears acknowledged.
CN: Psychosocial integrity; CNS: None; CL: Analyze

113. 4. The GI tract may not tolerate a full-liquid diet immediately. Allowing only clear liquids gives the intestine time to heal. Fluids should not be forced, but should be reintroduced slowly to determine the child's ability to tolerate and retain them. Monitoring intake and output is important and was initially ordered. It should continue until discharge.
CN: Physiological integrity; CNS: Basic care and comfort; CL: Analyze

114. 2, 4, 5. The first food provided to a neonate is breast milk or formula. Between ages four and six months, rice cereal can be introduced, followed by pureed or strained fruits and vegetables, and then strained or ground meat. Meats must be chopped or ground prior to feeding them to an infant to prevent choking. When milk is added to the diet it should be whole milk to provide the nutrients needed for development of the myelin sheath. Some fruit drinks provide no nutritional benefit, and may contain only 10% juice.
CN: Health promotion and maintenance; CNS: None; CL: Apply

115. A nurse is teaching an adolescent female with inflammatory bowel disease (IBD) about treatment with corticosteroids. Which adverse effects should concern this client? Select all that apply.
1. Acne
2. Hirsutism
3. Mood swings
4. Osteoporosis
5. Growth spurts
6. Adrenal suppression

116. A mother brings her child to the pediatrician's office for evaluation of chronic stomach pain. The mother states that the pain seems to go away when the child is allowed to stay home from school. The provider diagnoses school phobia. What should the nurse teach the mother to monitor? Select all that apply.
1. Nausea
2. Headaches
3. Weight loss
4. Dizziness
5. Fever

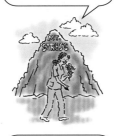

Welcome to the other side of Mt. Stress! Glad you made it.

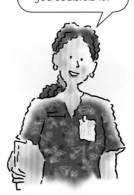

You're done with all those questions? I knew you could do it!

115. 1, 2, 3, 4, 6. The adverse effects of corticosteroids include acne, hirsutism, mood swings, osteoporosis, and adrenal suppression. Steroid use in children and adolescents may cause delayed growth, not growth spurts.
CN: Physiological integrity; CNS: Pharmacological and parenteral therapies; CL: Apply

116. 1, 2, 4. Children with school phobia commonly report vague symptoms, such as stomach aches, nausea, headaches, and dizziness, to avoid going to school. Typically, these symptoms do not occur on weekends. A careful history must be taken to identify a pattern of school avoidance. Such signs as weight loss and fever are more likely to have a physiologic cause, and are uncommon in children with school phobia.
CN: Psychosocial integrity; CNS: None; CL: Analyze

Chapter 33

Endocrine Disorders

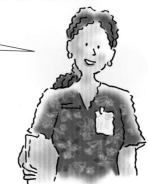

Caring for a child with an endocrine system disorder can be overwhelming. To get started on the right track, check out the Web site of the Juvenile Diabetes Research Foundation at **www.jdrf.org**. Go for it!

1. What information should the nurse share with the parents of an infant, newly-diagnosed, with hypothyroidism?
 1. For some infants, hypothyroidism is temporary, for others it's permanent.
 2. It's likely that there is a family history of this problem on one or both sides.
 3. For many infants, hypothyroidism is linked to a maternal infection during the first trimester.
 4. Prompt use of phototherapy partially relieves the symptoms of hypothyroidism in infants.

1. 1. Congenital hypothyroidism can be permanent or transient and may result from a defective thyroid gland or an enzymatic defect in thyroxine synthesis. There is no known genetic or infectious component to congenital hypothyroidism. Phototherapy is used to treat physiologic jaundice, not hypothyroidism.
CN: Physiological integrity; CNS: Physiological adaptation; CL: Apply

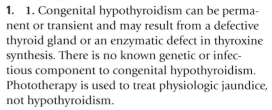

You're off to a good start.

2. An infant with hypothyroidism is receiving oral levothyroxine. Which assessment findings would the nurse be **most** concerned about?
 1. Tachycardia, irritability, and diaphoresis
 2. Bradycardia, excessive sleepiness, and dry scaly skin
 3. Bradycardia, irritability, and cool extremities
 4. Tachycardia, cool extremities, and irritability

2. 1. Clinical manifestations of synthetic thyroid hormone overdose in an infant include tachycardia, irritability, and diaphoresis. Bradycardia, excessive sleepiness, dry scaly skin, and cool extremities are manifestations of hypothyroidism.
CN: Physiological integrity; CNS: Pharmacological and parenteral therapies; CL: Apply

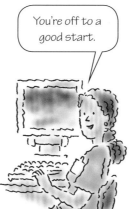

3. A nurse is teaching the parents of a neonate newly diagnosed with hypothyroidism about the condition. What is the **most** important information for the nurse to provide?
 1. A large goiter doesn't present a problem in a neonate.
 2. Preterm neonates usually aren't affected by hypothyroidism.
 3. Usually, the neonate exhibits obvious signs of hypothyroidism.
 4. The severity of the disorder depends on the amount of thyroid tissue present.

3. 4. The severity of the disorder depends on the amount of thyroid tissue present. The more thyroid tissue present, the less severe the disorder. A large goiter in a neonate could possibly occlude the airway and lead to obstruction. Preterm neonates are usually affected by hypothyroidism due to hypothalamic and pituitary immaturity. The neonate doesn't usually exhibit obvious signs of the disorder because of maternal circulation.
CN: Physiological integrity; CNS: Reduction of risk potential; CL: Apply

CN: Client needs category   CNS: Client needs subcategory   CL: Cognitive level

4. A nurse is assessing a neonate with a suspected diagnosis of hypothyroidism. For which sign should the nurse assess in this infant?
  1. Diarrhea
  2. Lethargy
  3. Diaphoresis
  4. Tachycardia

4. 2. Subtle signs of this disorder include lethargy, poor feeding, prolonged jaundice, respiratory difficulty, cyanosis, constipation, and bradycardia. Diarrhea isn't associated with this disorder. The infant would have decreased perspiration rather than diaphoresis. Tachycardia typically occurs in hyperthyroidism, not hypothyroidism.
CN: Physiological integrity; CNS: Physiological adaptation; CL: Apply

5. A nurse is assessing a toddler with hypothyroidism. During the assessment, the nurse is **most** concerned when the toddler presents with:
  1. low hemoglobin and hematocrit.
  2. peripheral cyanosis.
  3. impaired bone and muscle development.
  4. delayed speech and comprehension.

5. 4. The most serious consequence of congenital hypothyroidism is delayed development of the central nervous system, which leads to severe mental retardation. This delay would affect speech and comprehension. The other choices would occur, but aren't the most serious consequences.
CN: Physiological integrity; CNS: Physiological adaptation; CL: Analyze

6. A nurse is counseling the parents of a neonate with congenital hypothyroidism. The parents tell the nurse that they are concerned about the severity of the intellectual deficit. The nurse explains that the deficit is related to:
  1. the duration of the condition prior to treatment.
  2. the degree of hypothermia.
  3. cranial malformations.
  4. the thyroxine (T4) level at diagnosis.

6. 1. The severity of the intellectual deficit is related to the degree of hypothyroidism and the duration of the condition before treatment. Cranial malformations don't affect the severity of the intellectual deficit, nor does the degree of hypothermia as it relates to hypothyroidism. It isn't the specific T4 level at diagnosis that affects the intellect but how long the client has been hospitalized.
CN: Physiological integrity; CNS: Physiological adaptation; CL: Apply

Time to read up about diagnostic tests for neonates.

7. What is the **most** important statement, for the nurse to include, when explaining the screening of neonates for congenital hypothyroidism?
  1. These tests are mandated by law.
  2. An arterial blood sample is most accurate.
  3. The test will usually be done one week to ten days after discharge.
  4. This blood test should be done after the first month of life.

7. 1. A heelstick blood test is mandated by law and is usually performed on neonates between two and six days of age. Specimens are typically taken before the neonate is discharged from the hospital. The test is included with other tests that screen the neonate for errors of metabolism. It is not necessary to obtain an arterial blood sample.
CN: Health promotion and maintenance; CNS: None; CL: Apply

8. The nurse is reviewing the lab results of a neonate who has the possible diagnosis of congenital hypothyroidism. The nurse is **most** concerned by:
  1. high level of thyroxine (T4) and low level of thyroid-stimulating hormone (TSH).
  2. low level of T4 and high level of TSH.
  3. normal TSH and high level of T4.
  4. normal T4 and low level of TSH.

8. 2. Screening results that show a low level of T4 and a high level of TSH indicate congenital hypothyroidism and the need for further tests to determine the cause of the disease.
CN: Health promotion and maintenance; CNS: None; CL: Analyze

CN: Client needs category   CNS: Client needs subcategory   CL: Cognitive level

9. A nurse is teaching the parents of a neonate about the therapeutic management of congenital hypothyroidism. Which response, by a parent, suggests an accurate understanding of their child's diagnosis?

1. "My baby will need regular measurements of his thyroxine (T4) levels."
2. "Treatment involves thyroid hormone replacement therapy whenever his symptoms worsen."
3. "Treatment should begin at 4 to 6 weeks of age."
4. "As my baby grows, his thyroid gland will mature and he won't need medications."

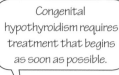

Congenital hypothyroidism requires treatment that begins as soon as possible.

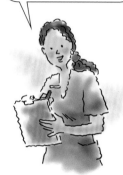

9. 1. Treatment involves lifelong thyroid hormone replacement therapy that begins as soon as possible following diagnosis to abolish all signs of hypothyroidism and to re-establish normal physical and mental development. Regular measurements of T4 levels are important in ensuring optimum treatment.

CN: Physiological integrity; CNS: Reduction of risk potential; CL: Analyze

10. The nurse asks the mother of a neonate how her baby is doing at a two-week office visit. Which statement would prompt the nurse to arrange testing for hypothyroidism?

1. "My baby is unusually quiet and good."
2. "My baby seems to have a stuffy nose a lot of the time."
3. "After feedings, my baby pulls her legs up and cries."
4. "My baby seems to really look at my face during feeding time."

10. 1. Parental remarks about an unusually quiet and good neonate, along with other early physical manifestations, should lead to a suspicion of hypothyroidism which would require additional testing. A stuffy nose is not necessarily suggestive of more serious health problems. If the neonate is pulling her legs up and crying after feedings, she might be showing signs of colic. A neonate likes to look at the human face and should show interest in this at age two weeks.

CN: Physiological integrity; CNS: Reduction of risk potential; CL: Analyze

11. A nurse is caring for preschool-age child. The child's documentation includes the following entry:

Progress notes	
10/15/16 1115	Blood pressure 85/132 mmHg; HR 115/bpm and regular; RR 22 breaths/min. Parent reports child is unusually fatigued for past several weeks; resting hand tremors noted bilaterally; diaphoresis noted.

What is the nurse's **most** appropriate action?

1. Administer levothyroxine as prescribed
2. Arrange testing for syndrome of inappropriate antidiuretic hormone (SIADH)
3. Assess the child for signs and symptoms of infection
4. Facilitate testing of the child's T3 and T4 levels

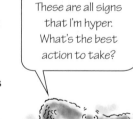

These are all signs that I'm hyper. What's the best action to take?

11. 4. Elevated heart rate and blood pressure, diaphoresis, persistent fatigue and tremors are characteristic of hyperthyroidism. The nurse should arrange the necessary follow up. Infection could yield this change in vital signs, but would not cause long-standing fatigue or tremors. Levothyroxine is used in the treatment of hypothyroidism. SIADH primarily affects fluid balance.

CN: Physiological integrity; CNS: Reduction in risk potential; CL: Apply

CN: Client needs category   CNS: Client needs subcategory   CL: Cognitive level

12. When teaching parents about signs that indicate levothyroxine overdose, which comment from a parent would indicate an accurate understanding?
1. "I should suspect an overdose if my baby's suddenly lethargic."
2. "I'll be concerned if I can feel my baby's heart rate in her arm or wrist."
3. "I should be concerned if my baby loses weight."
4. "I shouldn't worry if my baby does not sleep very much."

12. 3. Parents need to be aware of the signs that indicate overdose; including rapid pulse, dyspnea, irritability, insomnia, fever, sweating, and weight loss. Parents should be given acceptable parameters for heart rate and weight loss or gain. If the heart rate or weight loss is outside the acceptable parameters, the health care provider should be called. A palpable pulse is expected, and does not suggest an overdose of levothyroxine.

CN: Physiological integrity; CNS: Pharmacological and parenteral therapies; CL: Analyze

13. A child's most recent diagnostic testing reveals elevated levels of T3 and T4. When assessing this child for exophthalmos, the nurse should inspect what region?

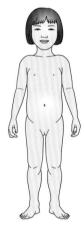

13. Exophthalmos is the abnormal protrusion of the eye globes that occurs when there is an overproduction of thyroid hormone, or hyperthyroidism.

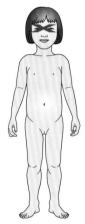

CN: Physiological integrity; CNS: Reduction of risk potential; CL: Apply

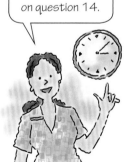

Time is flying! You're already on question 14.

14. A nurse is assessing a child with juvenile hypothyroidism. How can the nurse best address the signs and symptoms of this condition?
1. Promote a high-calorie, high-protein diet
2. Administer antidiarrheal medications as prescribed
3. Teach the parents about the use of skin emollients
4. Teach the parents about the importance of sleep hygiene

14. 3. Children with hypothyroidism will have dry skin, often necessitating skin emollients or other moisturizers. Diarrhea, inadequate nutrition and sleep disturbances are not commonly associated with hypothyroidism.

CN: Physiological integrity ; CNS: Reduction in risk potential; CL: Apply

15. A nurse is observing an infant with thyroid hormone deficiency. Which clinical manifestations would the nurse **most** likely find upon assessment?
1. Tachycardia, profuse perspiration, and diarrhea
2. Lethargy, feeding difficulties, and constipation
3. Hypertonia, small fontanels, and moist skin
4. Dermatitis, dry skin, and round face

15. 2. Hypothyroidism results from thyroid production that inadequately meets an infant's needs. Clinical signs include feeding difficulties, prolonged physiological jaundice, lethargy, and constipation.

CN: Physiological integrity; CNS: Physiological adaptation; CL: Analyze

CN: Client needs category   CNS: Client needs subcategory   CL: Cognitive level

16. What action should the nurse encourage when educating the parents of a neonate with congenital hypothyroidism?
1. Arranging laboratory testing on a scheduled basis
2. Retracing the family tree for others born with this condition
3. Talking to relatives who have gone through a similar experience
4. Seeking alternative therapies for this condition

17. The nurse is providing care for a child diagnosed with hyperthyroidism. The child has been prescribed propylthiouracil to reduce thyroxine production. How can the nurse best address the potential adverse effects of this medication?
1. Encourage small, frequent meals in order to prevent nausea
2. Closely monitor the child's white cell and platelet levels
3. Encourage the use of over-the-counter vitamin D supplements
4. Assess the child's sclerae for signs of jaundice

18. What effect would added physical activity have on a child diagnosed with type 1 diabetes?
1. Increase food intake
2. Decrease food intake
3. Decrease the risk of insulin shock
4. Increase the risk of hyperglycemia

19. A nurse is helping an adolescent deal with diabetes. What important factor should the nurse consider?
1. The adolescent's need for individuality
2. The adolescent's desire to fit in with peers
3. The adolescent's preoccupation with future plans
4. The need to teach peers that this is a serious disease

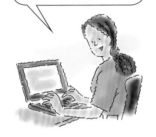

Question 16 is asking for the most appropriate action. In other words, prioritize!

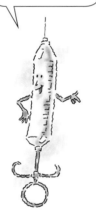

Watch out! I can have adverse effects.

Remember

"-Ide drugs deny thyroid."

Thioamides and iodides are antithyroid drugs, which are used to treat hyperthyroidism.

Thioamides
- Methimazole
- Propylthiouracil

Iodides
- Radioactive iodine (sodium iodide)
- Stable iodine (potassium iodide)

16. 1. Children with hypothyroidism must have their levels of thyroid hormone monitored closely. Retracing the family tree and talking to relatives won't help the parents to become better educated about the disorder. Seeking alternative therapies should be discouraged to prevent possible complications.
CN: Physiological integrity; CNS: Reduction of risk potential; CL: Apply

17. 2. Thrombocytopenia and leukopenia are adverse effects of propylthiouracil therapy. There is no need for vitamin D supplements, and no added risk of jaundice or nausea.
CN: Physiological integrity; CNS: Pharmalogical and parenteral therapies; CL: Apply

18. 1. If a child is more active at one time of the day than another, food or insulin can be altered to meet the activity pattern of the individual. Food should be increased when children are more physically active. The child has an increased risk of insulin shock and a decreased risk of hyperglycemia when he's more physically active.
CN: Physiological integrity; CNS: Reduction of risk potential; CL: Apply

19. 2. Adolescents appear to have the most difficulty adjusting to diabetes. Adolescents feel the need to be "perfect," and have a great desire to fit into a peer group. For many adolescents, having diabetes means being different.
CN: Psychosocial integrity; CNS: None; CL: Apply

CN: Client needs category   CNS: Client needs subcategory   CL: Cognitive level

20. An adolescent with diabetes tells the community nurse that he has recently started drinking alcohol on the weekends. What is the nurse's most appropriate intervention?
1. Recommend a referral to diabetes counseling
2. Create a contract with the adolescent to abstain from alcohol
3. Discuss why the adolescent started drinking
4. Teach the adolescent about the effects of alcohol on diabetes

20. 4. Confusion about the effects of alcohol on blood glucose is common. Teenagers may falsely believe that alcohol increases blood glucose levels. Ingestion of alcohol inhibits the release of glycogen from the liver, resulting in hypoglycemia. Teens who drink alcohol may become hypoglycemic, and some are treated as if they were intoxicated. Behaviors, such as shakiness, combativeness, slurred speech, and loss of consciousness, can cause be mistaken for intoxication. Finding out why the adolescent has started drinking and recommending counseling may be appropriate, but only after education is provided. An adolescent may promise to stop drinking but not follow through.
CN: Health promotion and maintenance; CNS: None; CL: Apply

21. A child has experienced symptoms of hypoglycemia and has eaten sugar cubes. What should the nurse administer to this client **after** ingesting the cubes?
1. Fruit juice
2. Two to three glasses of water
3. Food that are high in protein
4. Complex carbohydrate and protein

21. 4. When a child exhibits signs of hypoglycemia, the majority of cases can be treated with a simple concentrated sugar, such as honey, that can be held in the mouth for a short time. A complex carbohydrate and protein, such as a slice of bread or a cracker spread with peanut butter, should follow the rapid-releasing sugar, or the client may become hypoglycemic again.
CN: Health promotion and maintenance; CNS: None; CL: Apply

22. A nurse is teaching the parents, of a child newly diagnosed with diabetes, to identify the signs and symptoms of hypoglycemia. Which response, by the parents, would indicate that teaching has been effective?
1. "We should watch for symptoms such as irritability, shakiness, hunger, headache, and dizziness."
2. "Drowsiness, lethargy, and decreased urine output need to be reported."
3. "Abdominal pain, nausea and vomiting, and constipation are common findings."
4. "We will report any signs of urinary frequency immediately."

22. 1. Signs of hypoglycemia include irritability, shaky feeling, hunger, headache, and dizziness. Drowsiness, abdominal pain, polyuria, nausea, and vomiting are signs of hyperglycemia.
CN: Physiological integrity; CNS: Physiological adaptation; CL: Apply

23. The nurse is assessing a child, with type 1 diabetes mellitus, who recently came to the emergency department with signs and symptoms consistent with diabetic ketoacidosis. What is the nurse's priority when planning care for this child?
1. Make a referral to the pediatric diabetes nurse
2. Prepare to administer intravenous fluids and insulin per order
3. Teach the family about the prevention of this complication of diabetes
4. Monitor the child closely in the emergency department before transfer to the medical unit

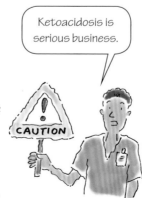

Ketoacidosis is serious business.

23. 2. Diabetic ketoacidosis, the most complete state of insulin deficiency, is a life-threatening condition. The child should be admitted to an intensive care unit for management. Treatment would consist of rapid assessment, adequate insulin to reduce the elevated blood glucose level, fluids to overcome dehydration, and electrolyte replacement. Education would be a priority after the child has stabilized.
CN: Safe and effective care environment; CNS: Management of care; CL: Apply

24. The nurse is teaching an 11-year-old who is newly diagnosed with type 1 diabetes about insulin injections. Which guideline would be **most** appropriate for the nurse to implement?
1. The parents don't need to be involved in education about diabetes management.
2. Self-injection techniques aren't usually taught until the child reaches age 16.
3. The child should be old enough to give most of his own injections.
4. Self-injection techniques should only be taught when the child can reach all injection sites.

24. 3. Parents must be taught to supervise and manage the child's therapeutic program, but the child should assume responsibility for self-management as soon as he's capable. Children can learn to collect their own blood for glucose testing at 4 to 5 years of age, and most are able to check their blood glucose level and administer insulin by age nine.
CN: Physiological integrity; CNS: Pharmacological and parenteral therapies; CL: Apply

25. The nurse suspects that a client has diabetic ketoacidosis. Which laboratory value would be observed with this condition?
1. Blood glucose 39.3 mg/dl (2.2 mmol/L)
2. Potassium 57.6 mg/dl (3.2 mmol/L)
3. Sodium 2,394 mg/dl (133 mmol/L)
4. Blood glucose 419.4 mg/dl (23.3 mmol/L)

25. 4. Diabetic ketoacidosis is determined by the presence of a blood glucose measurement of 298.8 mg/dl (16.6 mmol/L) or higher, accompanied by acetone breath, dehydration, weak and rapid pulse, and a decreased level of consciousness. Alterations in sodium and potassium are not central to the pathophysiology of diabetic ketoacidosis.
CN: Physiological integrity; CNS: Reduction of risk potential; CL: Analyze

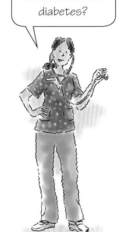

Remember all those "poly's" associated with diabetes?

26. The nurse has just admitted a two-year-old child with a diagnosis of type 1 diabetes mellitus. Which cardinal sign would support this diagnosis?
1. Nausea
2. Seizure
3. Hyperactivity
4. Polyuria

26. 4. Polyphagia, polyuria, polydipsia, and weight loss are cardinal signs of diabetes mellitus. Other signs include irritability, shortened attention span, lowered frustration tolerance, fatigue, dry skin, blurred vision, sores that are slow to heal, and flushed skin.
CN: Health promotion and maintenance; CNS: None; CL: Apply

27. The parent of a child with diabetes asks the nurse why blood glucose monitoring is required. What is the nurse's **best** response?
1. Blood glucose monitoring is an easy method of testing.
2. This is a relatively inexpensive method of testing.
3. Blood glucose monitoring allows children to better manage their diabetes.
4. This gives children a sense of autonomy and helps their development.

27. 3. Blood glucose monitoring improves diabetes management, and is used successfully by children from the onset of their diabetes. By testing their own blood, children are able to change their insulin regimen to maintain a normal glucose level.
CN: Physiological integrity; CNS: Reduction of risk potential; CL: Apply

Teaching clients how to help manage their own conditions is a common subject on the NCLEX.

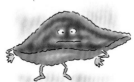

28. What is the nurse's **best** intervention to increase an adolescent's compliance with treatment for type 1 diabetes mellitus?
1. Ask the high school cafeteria to provide a special diet
2. Clarify the adolescent's values to promote involvement in care
3. Identify energy requirements for participation in sports activities
4. Educate the adolescent about long-term consequences of poor metabolic control

28. 2. Adolescent compliance with diabetes management may be hampered by dependence versus independence conflicts and ego development. Attempts to have the adolescent clarify personal values will promote involvement in his care and foster compliance.
CN: Health promotion and maintenance; CNS: None; CL: Apply

CN: Client needs category   CNS: Client needs subcategory   CL: Cognitive level

29. A child, with type 1 diabetes mellitus, reports feeling shaky. The child's skin is pale and sweaty. What is the nurse's **priority** intervention?
1. Give supplemental insulin per order
2. Have the child eat a glucose tablet
3. Administer intravenous dextrose
4. Offer the child a complex carbohydrate snack

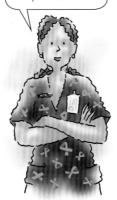

The question is asking you to prioritize.

29. 2. These symptoms are indicative of hypoglycemia. If a client is fully conscious and able to drink and swallow safely, a rapidly-absorbed carbohydrate, such as glucose tablets, glucose gel, table sugar, or fruit juice, should be given by mouth. This will result in a rapid increase in blood glucose. Giving supplemental insulin would lower the blood glucose. Dextrose should only be given if there is a risk of aspiration with oral glucose.
CN: Physiological integrity; CNS: Reduction of risk potential; CL: Apply

30. The parents of a child diagnosed with type 1 diabetes ask the nurse about managing the disease when their child has a minor illness and loss of appetite. What is the nurse's **best** response?
1. "Decrease your child's insulin by half the usual dose during the course of the illness."
2. "Call your health care provider to arrange hospitalization."
3. "Give increased amounts of clear liquids to prevent dehydration."
4. "Substitute beverages sweetened with sugar for uneaten solid food."

30. 4. Drinks containing simple sugars can help maintain normal blood glucose levels as well as decrease the danger of dehydration. The child with diabetes should always take the usual dose of insulin during an illness based on more frequent blood glucose checks. If there is vomiting or a loss of appetite the health care provider should be contacted for any medication adjustments. It is essential to do frequent blood glucose monitoring during the illness.
CN: Safe, effective care environment; CNS: Management of care; CL: Apply

31. The parent of a child asks the nurse about the desired outcome of type 1 diabetes mellitus management. What is the nurse's **best** response?
1. HbA1c level or 7.5 or lower
2. Infrequent occurrences of mild hypoglycemic reaction
3. Hemoglobin A values less than 12%
4. Growth below the 15th percentile

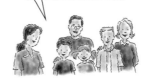

It's important to include a client's family in teaching.

31. 2. Criteria for good metabolic control generally include fewer episodes of hypoglycemia or hyperglycemia, HbA1c values less than 7.0, and normal growth and development.
CN: Physiological integrity; CNS: Reduction of risk potential; CL: Apply

32. A nurse in the neonatal intensive care unit is assessing the infant of a mother with poorly-controlled type 1 diabetes. For which condition should the nurse assess in this neonate?
1. Cataracts
2. Low-set ears
3. Cardiac malformations
4. Cleft lip and palate deformities

32. 3. Cardiac and central nervous system anomalies, neural tube defects and skeletal and gastrointestinal anomalies, are most likely to occur as a result of uncontrolled maternal diabetes.
CN: Physiological integrity; CNS: Physiological adaptation; CL: Apply

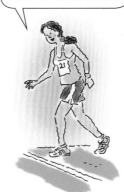

I'm glad I had a snack before I started to race.

33. A client with type 1 diabetes mellitus asks the nurse how to avoid hypoglycemic episodes. What is the nurse's **best** response?
1. "Make sure that you always take enough insulin."
2. "Do all that you can to avoid colds and flu?"
3. "Avoid vigorous exercise without having a carbohydrate snack."
4. "Be very cautious when you go out to eat at a restaurant."

33. 3. Excessive exercise, without having a carbohydrate snack, could cause hypoglycemia. The other options describe situations that cause hyperglycemia.
CN: Health promotion and maintenance; CNS: None; CL: Apply

CN: Client needs category   CNS: Client needs subcategory   CL: Cognitive level

34. The nurse is reviewing the chart of a client with type 2 diabetes prior to a scheduled appointment. The chart states:

Progress notes	
10/15/16	Client states that he has not been following
0245	his prescribed diabetes management program
	for the past 2 to 3 months. Client is aware
	of his blood glucose monitoring regimen and
	diet but has difficulty integrating each into
	his routines. Client denies recent changes in
	urinary function, sensation or vision.

How can the nurse **best** determine this client's glycemic control since the last assessment?
1. Arrange assessment of the client's fasting glucose level
2. Ask the client to complete a 24-hour food recall
3. Review the results of the client's HbA1c
4. Ask the client to describe his recommended diet and glucose monitoring routine

34. 3. An HbA1c provides an overview of a person's blood glucose level over the previous 2 to 3 months. Glycosylated hemoglobin values are reported as a percentage of the total hemoglobin within an erythrocyte. The time frame is based on the fact that the usual life span of an erythrocyte is 2 to 3 months. The client's description of health maintenance will not determine adherence to the prescribed schedule. Fasting glucose gives a point-in-time result. A 24-hour food recall is subjective, and does not help the nurse gauge the client's overall adherence.
CN: Health promotion and maintenance; CNS: None;
CL: Apply

35. A client has received dietary teaching as part of his treatment plan for type 1 diabetes mellitus. Which statement, by the client, would indicate to the nurse that this client requires further teaching?
1. "I'll need a bedtime snack because I take an evening dose of NPH insulin."
2. "I can eat whatever I want as long as I cover the calories with sufficient insulin."
3. "I can have an occasional low-calorie drink as long as I include it in my meal plan."
4. "I should eat meals as scheduled, even if I'm not hungry, to prevent hypoglycemia."

35. 2. The goal of diet therapy in type 1 diabetes mellitus is to attain and maintain ideal body weight. Each client is prescribed a specific caloric intake and insulin regimen to help accomplish this goal.
CN: Physiological integrity; CNS: Basic care and comfort;
CL: Analyze

36. The nurse is caring for a school-age child with diabetes. The child states, "I'm so thirsty this morning, no matter how much I drink." In addition to measuring this child's blood glucose level, what should the nurse do?
1. Assess the client's apical heart rate for one minute
2. Provide a snack containing protein and complex carbohydrates
3. Administer 30 g of simple carbohydrates
4. Assess for signs or symptoms of hyperglycemia

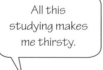

All this studying makes me thirsty.

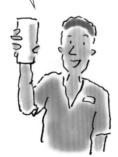

36. 4. Polydipsia is a symptom of hyperglycemia. Snacks containing simple or complex carbohydrates would be contraindicated. A nurse should assess the child's apical heart rate as well as signs and symptoms of hyperglycemia.
CN: Physiological integrity; CNS: Reduction of risk potential;
CL: Apply

37. A client is learning to mix regular insulin and NPH insulin in the same syringe. In what order should the nurse should teach the client to perform these tasks?

| **1.** Inject air into the regular insulin (clear) vial |
| **2.** Inject air into the NPH (cloudy) vial |
| **3.** Draw up regular (clear) insulin |
| **4.** Draw up NPH (cloudy) insulin |
| **5.** Administer the insulins |

37. **Ordered Response:**

| **2.** Inject air into the NPH vial |
| **1.** Inject air into the regular insulin vial |
| **3.** Draw up regular insulin |
| **4.** Draw up NPH insulin |
| **5.** Administer the insulins |

The nurse can memorize this order as "cloudy, clear, clear, cloudy." Inject air into the vial of cloudy (NPH) insulin, then air into the vial of clear (regular) insulin, then draw up the clear (regular) insulin, then draw up the cloudy (NPH) insulin. The final step is to prepare the skin with an alcohol wipe and administer the insulins.
CN: Physiological integrity; CNS: Pharmacological and parenteral therapies; CL: Apply

38. A client is diagnosed with type 1 diabetes mellitus. The nurse administered the prescribed dose of regular insulin at 0745. At what time should the nurse reassess this client's blood glucose for the onset of insulin?
1. 0755
2. 0805
3. 0830
4. 0915

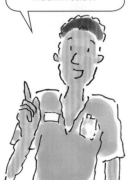

It's important to know how and when different types of insulin react.

38. 3. Regular insulin's onset is 30 minutes to one hour. It peaks at 2 to 4 hours, and lasts for 3 to 6 hours. Lispro insulin has a rapid onset of five minutes. NPH insulin peaks in 4 to 9 hours. Glargine and detemir can last 18 to 26 hours.
CN: Physiological integrity; CNS: Pharmacological and parenteral therapies; CL: Apply

39. Which signs and symptoms of diabetes insipidus should the nurse be aware of when assessing a neonate?
1. Hyponatremia
2. Jaundice
3. Polyuria
4. Hypochloremia

39. 3. The cardinal sign of diabetes insipidus is polyuria, along with polydipsia. Hypernatremia occurs with diabetes insipidus. Jaundice occurs because of abnormal bilirubin metabolism. Hyperchloremia, not hypochloremia, occurs with diabetes insipidus.
CN: Physiological integrity; CNS: Physiological adaptation; CL: Apply

40. The nurse is assessing an infant with diabetes insipidus. What initial symptom or sign should the nurse anticipate?
1. Dehydration
2. Inability to be aroused
3. Extreme hunger relieved by frequent feedings of milk
4. Irritability relieved with feedings of water but not milk

40. 4. An infant with diabetes insipidus will be irritable, with thirst relieved on by water rather than milk. Dehydration and the inability to be aroused are late symptoms.
CN: Physiological integrity; CNS: Physiological adaptation; CL: Apply

41. A nurse is helping parents understand when treatments of their child's growth hormone replacement will stop. What is the **most** important statement for the nurse to include?
  1. The dosage of growth hormone will decrease as the child ages.
  2. The dosage of growth hormone will increase as the time of epiphyseal closure nears.
  3. The dose will be tapered down after one year of treatment.
  4. The dose will be tapered down over several months before it is stopped.

41. 2. To gain the best advantage of the growth hormone it will be increased as the time of epiphyseal closure nears. There is no tapering with growth hormone. It can be abruptly stopped.
CN: Physiological integrity; CNS: Pharmacological and parenteral therapies; CL: Apply

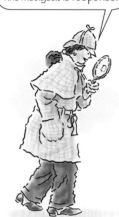

Question 42 asks you to identify a knowledgeable response.

42. A nurse is explaining diabetes insipidus and related diagnostic testing to the parents of an infant suspected of having the disease. Which comment, by the parent, would indicate an understanding of the diagnostic test?
  1. "Fluids will be offered every two hours."
  2. "My infant's fluid intake will be restricted."
  3. "I won't change anything about my infant's intake."
  4. "Formula will be restricted, but glucose water is okay."

42. 2. The simplest test used to diagnose diabetes insipidus is a restriction of oral fluids and observation of consequent changes in urine volume and concentration. A weight loss of 3 to 5% would indicate severe dehydration, and the test should be terminated at this point. This test is performed in the hospital, where the infant is closely observed.
CN: Physiological integrity; CNS: Reduction of risk potential; CL: Apply

43. A nurse has read the chart of a school-age client with a recent diagnosis of hyperthyroidism. Where should the nurse focus his attention when inspecting for the presence of a goiter?

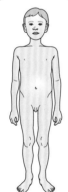

43. Goiter is an abnormal enlargement of your thyroid gland. Your thyroid is a butterfly-shaped gland located at the base of your neck just below your Adam's apple. A goiter can occur in a gland that is producing too much hormone (hyperthyroidism).

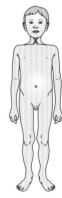

CN: Physiological integrity; CNS: Reduction in Risk Potential; CL: Apply

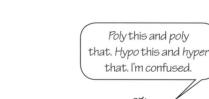

Poly this and poly that. Hypo this and hyper that. I'm confused.

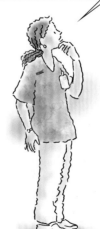

44. An infant has a positive test result for diabetes insipidus. For which medication would the nurse anticipate an order for the treatment of this condition?
  1. Antidiuretic hormone
  2. Biosynthetic growth hormone
  3. Adrenocorticotropic hormone
  4. Aqueous vasopressin

44. 4. If the fluid restriction test is positive, the child should be given a test dose of aqueous vasopressin, which should alleviate the associated polyuria and polydipsia. If the child is unresponsive to exogenous vasopressin, nephrogenic diabetes insipidus is usually suspected. The other choices are used to determine other types of endocrine disorders.
CN: Physiological integrity; CNS: Reduction in risk potential; CL: Apply

CN: Client needs category   CNS: Client needs subcategory   CL: Cognitive level

45. The nurse should teach the parents of an infant diagnosed with diabetes insipidus about the need for:
1. antihypertensives.
2. packed red blood cells.
3. hormone replacement.
4. fluid restrictions.

46. The nurse explains the use of nasal sprays and injections to the parents of a child with diabetes insipidus. What should the nurse teach these parents?
1. Nasal sprays must be instilled 2 to 3 times daily.
2. The infant will require nasal spray throughout the night.
3. Nasal sprays can be given when the child is old enough to self-administer.
4. Injections must be given at the same time every day.

47. A nurse is teaching the parents of an infant with diabetes insipidus about injectable desmopressin. Which statement made by a parent would indicate adequate understanding?
1. "I'll monitor my child's blood glucose levels for the first few weeks of treatment."
2. "I need to be careful that my child eats enough salt while taking this medication."
3. "I need to make sure my child stays out of bright sunlight while taking this medication."
4. "If the injections are too painful, the care team can use nasal spray."

48. The nurse is providing teaching to the parents of an infant newly diagnosed with diabetes insipidus. Which statement, by a parent, would indicate an understanding of this condition?
1. "When my infant stabilizes, I won't have to worry about giving hormone medication."
2. "I don't have to measure my infant's fluid intake."
3. "I realize that treatment for diabetes insipidus is lifelong."
4. "My infant will outgrow this condition."

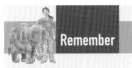

Remember

"-Pressins provide hormone replacement."

Desmopressin acetate and vasopressin are types of antidiuretic hormone and are used for hormone-replacement therapy for clients with diabetes insipidus.

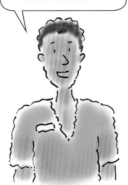

Desmopressin can be delivered by more than one route of administration.

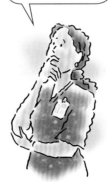

Which of these statements is true?

45. 3. The usual treatment for diabetes insipidus is hormone replacement with vasopressin or desmopressin acetate (DDAVP). Hypertension is not associated with this condition, and fluids should not be restricted. Blood products would not be necessary.
CN: Physiological integrity; CNS: Pharmacological and parenteral therapies; CL: Apply

46. 1. Nasal spray used to treat diabetes insipidus must be instilled every 8 to 12 hours. Injections will last for 48 to 72 hours, and do not need to be given every day. The use of nasal spray must be timed to allow for adequate sleep.
CN: Physiological integrity; CNS: Pharmacological and parenteral therapies; CL: Apply

47. 4. Desmopressin can be given as a nasal spray. There is no particular need to monitor blood glucose or increase sodium intake. Photosensitivity is not associated with therapy.
CN: Physiological integrity; CNS: Pharmacological and parenteral therapies; CL: Apply

48. 3. Diabetes insipidus is a condition that will require lifelong treatment. It is important to record the infant's fluid intake and output to help manage the medication regimen. The infant will not outgrow this condition.
CN: Safe, effective care environment; CNS: Management of care; CL: Apply

49. The nurse has explained the causes of diabetes insipidus to the parents of an infant with the condition. Which statement, made by a parent, indicates a need for further teaching?
1. "This condition could be familial or congenital."
2. "Drinking alcohol during my pregnancy may have caused this condition."
3. "My child might have a tumor that is causing these symptoms."
4. "An infection, such as meningitis, may be the reason my child has diabetes insipidus."

49. 2. Drinking alcohol during pregnancy can lead to a neonate born with fetal alcohol spectrum disorder, but has no known correlation to diabetes insipidus. The other options are possible causes of diabetes insipidus.
CN: Physiological integrity; CNS: Physiological adaptation; CL: Analyze

50. Which assessment finding would advise the nurse of a need to change from the prescribed intranasal route to an injection of desmopressin acetate for a child with diabetes insipidus?
1. Mucous membrane irritation
2. Severe coughing
3. Occasional nosebleeds
4. Pneumonia

50. 1. Mucous membrane irritation, caused by a cold or allergy, can render the intranasal route unreliable. Severe coughing, pneumonia, and nosebleeds shouldn't interfere with the intranasal route.
CN: Physiological integrity; CNS: Pharmacological and parenteral therapies; CL: Apply

51. A nurse is providing in-home management instructions to the parents of a child who is receiving desmopressin acetate (DDAVP). What is the **most** important instruction the nurse to include?
1. Give DDAVP only when urine output begins to decrease
2. Cleanse skin with alcohol before application of the DDAVP dermal patch
3. Increase the DDAVP dose if polyuria occurs just before the next scheduled dose
4. Call the healthcare provider if the child has an upper respiratory infection or allergic rhinitis

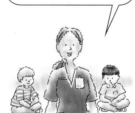

Question 51 asks for a common adverse effect of desmopressin acetate administration.

51. 4. Excessive nasal mucus, associated with upper respiratory infection or allergic rhinitis, may interfere with DDAVP absorption because it is given intranasally. Parents should be instructed to contact the health care provider for advice in altering the hormone dose during times when nasal mucus may be increased. The DDAVP dose should remain unchanged, even if the child is experiencing polyuria just before the next dose to avoid over medicating the child.
CN: Safe and effective care environment; CNS: Management of care; CL: Apply

52. A nurse is assessing a client with suspected hypopituitarism. For which symptom should the nurse observe this child?
1. Sleep disturbance
2. Polyuria
3. Polydipsia
4. Short stature

52. 4. The most common sign, in most instances of hypopituitarism, is short stature. Sleep disturbance may indicate thyrotoxicosis. Polydipsia and polyuria may be indications of diabetes mellitus or diabetes insipidus.
CN: Physiological integrity; CNS: Reduction of risk potential; CL: Apply

53. Which statement, made to a nurse by the parents of a child with idiopathic growth hormone deficiency, would indicate the need for further teaching?
1. "This disorder may be familial."
2. "There is a specific genetic basis for this disorder."
3. "This disorder might be secondary to hypothalamic deficiency."
4. "There may be other disorders related to pituitary hormone deficiencies."

53. 2. The cause of idiopathic growth hormone deficiency is unknown. There's a higher-than-average occurrence of the disorder in some families, which indicates a possible genetic cause. The specifics of the genetic characteristics have not been identified. The condition is commonly associated with other pituitary hormone deficiencies, such as deficiencies of thyroid-stimulating hormone and corticotropin, and may be secondary to hypothalamic deficiency.
CN: Physiological integrity; CNS: Physiological adaptation; CL: Apply

CN: Client needs category   CNS: Client needs subcategory   CL: Cognitive level

54. A nurse is teaching a health class to the parents of school age children. What information is most important for the nurse to include?
   1. There's nothing that a parent can do to influence the child's growth.
   2. Excessive physical activity before the child hits puberty may stunt growth.
   3. All children, who are short in stature, also have parents who are short in stature.
   4. Because this is a time of tremendous growth, there is no need to be concerned about calorie intake.

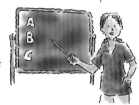

A nurse's responsibility to teach never ends.

54. 2. Intense physical activity that begins before puberty may stunt a child's growth and decrease their height as an adult. Nutrition and environment influence a child's growth. All children who are short in stature don't necessarily have parents who are short in stature. During the school-age years, growth slows, and doesn't accelerate again until adolescence.
CN: Health promotion and maintenance; CNS: None;
CL: Apply

55. While teaching the parents of a child of short stature, the nurse discusses familial short stature. What information is appropriate for the nurse to include in the discussion? Select all that apply.
   1. Short stature occurs in children who are members of a very large family with limited resources.
   2. Short stature occurs in children who have no siblings, and who moved a great deal during their early childhood.
   3. Short stature occurs in children with delayed linear growth and skeletal and sexual maturation.
   4. Short stature occurs in children with ancestors whose adult height is in the lower percentiles, and whose height during childhood is appropriate.
   5. Short stature is unrelated to disease processes or nutritional deficits.

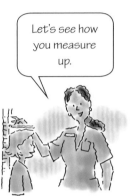

Let's see how you measure up.

55. 4, 5. Familial short stature refers to otherwise healthy children who have ancestors with adult height in the lower percentiles, and whose height during childhood is appropriate for genetic background. This form of short stature is not pathophysiological or related to malnutrition. Children who are members of very large families with limited resources, or who have no siblings, don't fit the description of familial short stature. Children with delayed linear growth and skeletal and sexual maturation are considered to have constitutional growth delay.
CN: Physiological integrity; CNS: Physiological adaptation;
CL: Apply

56. The nurse is assessing a toddler during a routine well-child visit. Which assessment findings cause the nurse to suspect the possibility of growth hormone deficiency?
   1. The child had normal growth during the first year of life, but showed a slowed growth curve below the third percentile for the second year of life.
   2. The child fell below the fifth percentile for growth during the first year of life but, at this check-up, falls below only the 50th percentile.
   3. There has been a steady decline in growth for two years of this toddler's life, but growth has accelerated during the past six months.
   4. Growth was delayed below the fifth percentile for the first and second years of life.

56. 1. Children with growth hormone deficiency generally grow normally during the first year, and then follow a slowed growth curve that's below the third percentile. If growth is consistently below the fifth percentile, it may be an indication of failure to thrive.
CN: Health promotion and maintenance; CNS: None;
CL: Apply

57. A nurse is assessing a child with growth hormone deficiency. What assessment data should the nurse anticipate?
1. Decreased weight with no change in height
2. Decreased weight with increased height
3. Increased weight with decreased height
4. Increased weight with increased height

57. 3. Height may be decreased more than weight. With good nutrition, children with growth hormone deficiency can become overweight or even obese. The well-nourished appearance of these children is an important diagnostic clue to differentiate growth hormone deficiency from other disorders such as failure to thrive.
CN: Health promotion and maintenance; CNS: None; CL: Apply

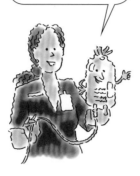

Looks like you're in the flow of things. Keep going!

58. During the assessment of a child with growth hormone deficiency, which physical characteristic should the nurse anticipate?
1. Normal skeletal proportions
2. Edema to the hands, ankles and feet
3. Child appearing older than his age
4. Longer than normal upper extremities

58. 1. Skeletal proportions are normal for age, but these children appear younger than their chronological age. Later in life, premature aging becomes evident in these individuals. Edema is not associated with growth hormone deficiency.
CN: Physiological integrity; CNS: Physiological adaptation; CL: Apply

59. The parents of a child with growth hormone deficiency tell the nurse that their child is interested in playing sports. What is the nurse's **most** appropriate response?
1. "Your child has an increased risk for bone fracture, but should engage in moderate physical activity."
2. "Your child should engage in cardiovascular activity, but weight-bearing exercise should be avoided."
3. "Exercise is beneficial for your child, but activity that could cause skeletal injury should be avoided."
4. "Your child should only engage in sports with children of similar size."

59. 4. Children with growth hormone deficiency can fully engage in size-appropriate sports, such as gymnastics, swimming or wrestling.
CN: Health promotion and maintenance; CNS: None; CL: Apply

60. A nurse is explaining about the social behavior experienced by children with hypopituitarism to the parents of a child affected by the rare disorder. The nurse determines that further teaching is necessary when a parent states:
1. "I understand that my child may have anxiety at school and a low self-esteem."
2. "Because my child is short in stature, some people may expect less of him than his peers."
3. "Because of my child's short stature, he might not be pushed to perform at his chronological age by others."
4. "My child's vocabulary is very well developed, so even though he's short in stature, no one will treat him differently."

60. 4. Height discrepancy has been significantly correlated with emotional adjustment problems and may be a valuable predictor of the extent to which growth hormone-delayed children will have trouble with anxiety, social skills, and positive self-esteem. Also, academic problems aren't uncommon. These children aren't usually pushed to perform at their chronological age but are commonly subjected to juvenilization.
CN: Psychosocial integrity; CNS: None; CL: Apply

CN: Client needs category   CNS: Client needs subcategory   CL: Cognitive level

61. The mother of a child diagnosed with hypopituitarism tells the nurse, "I feel like I should have recognized the signs of this disorder." What is the nurse's **best** response?
1. The exceptional size of children with hypopituitarism is often misattributed to other factors.
2. Children with hypopituitarism are usually small for gestational age at birth.
3. The obstetrician should have recognized the signs of this disorder.
4. The child was a normal size at birth, and there were no other signs at that time.

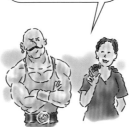

No problem with hypopituitarism here!

61. 4. Children with hypopituitarism are usually normal size for gestational age at birth. Clinical features develop slowly, and vary with the severity of the disorder and deficient hormones.
CN: Psychosocial integrity; CNS: None; CL: Apply

62. The nurse is plotting the height and weight on a four-year-old child's growth chart. What finding should signal, to the nurse, the possibility of a growth hormone deficiency?
1. Upward shift of one percentile or more
2. Upward shift of five percentiles or more
3. Downward shift of two percentiles or more
4. Downward shift of five percentiles or more

62. 3. When the health care provider evaluates the results of a child's growth chart, a downward shift of two percentiles, or more, in children older than three, may indicate a growth abnormality.
CN: Health promotion and maintenance; CNS: None; CL: Analyze

63. The nurse is providing care for a school-age child with hypopituitarism. What is the nurse's **priority** intervention?
1. High-protein, high-calorie diet
2. Vigilant fall precautions and fracture prevention
3. Interventions to enhance the child's self-esteem
4. Education for the child and parents about the importance of weight-bearing exercise

63. 3. Hypopituitarism and reduced stature can have a negative effect on self-esteem and development. Interventions to address these risks are appropriate. There is no need for a high-nutrient diet, and the child is not at high risk for injury. Weight-bearing exercise has no direct effect on the course of the illness.
CN: Psychosocial integrity; CNS: None; CL: Apply

64. The nurse suspects that a child, of small stature, has hypopituitarism. This suspicion would be confirmed if diagnostic testing revealed:
1. hypersecretion of thyroid hormone.
2. pituitary hyperplasia.
3. hyposecretion of antidiuretic hormone (ADH).
4. decreased reserves of growth hormone.

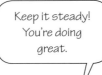

Keep it steady! You're doing great.

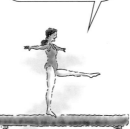

64. 4. Definitive diagnosis is based on absent or subnormal reserves of pituitary growth hormone. Antidiuretic hormone and thyroid hormone levels aren't affected. Pituitary hyperplasia does not lead to a deficiency in growth hormone.
CN: Physiological integrity; CNS: Physiological adaptation; CL: Analyze

65. The nurse is providing teaching to the parents of a child going through testing for hypopituitarism. Which finding would support a diagnosis of hypopituitarism?
1. Growth hormone levels that rise and fall in relation to blood glucose levels
2. Growth hormone levels that are decreased after strenuous exercise
3. Urine growth hormone concentration that increases over night
4. Growth hormone levels that are elevated 45 to 90 minutes following the onset of sleep

65. 4. Growth hormone levels are elevated 45 to 90 minutes following the onset of sleep. Low growth hormone levels following the onset of sleep would indicate the need for further evaluation. Exercise is a natural and benign stimulus for growth hormone release, and elevated levels should be detected after 20 minutes of strenuous exercise in normal children.
CN: Physiological integrity; CNS: Reduction of risk potential; CL: Apply

CN: Client needs category   CNS: Client needs subcategory   CL: Cognitive level

66. A nurse is caring for a school-age client who is in the second percentile of height and weight for age as a result of an endocrine disorder. Which pharmacological intervention should the nurse anticipate?
   1. Treatment with desmopressin acetate (DDAVP)
   2. Replacement of antidiuretic hormone (ADH)
   3. Treatment with testosterone or estrogen
   4. Administration of biosynthetic somatotropin

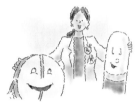

All of these treatments may be used, but only one is *definitive*.

66. 4. The definitive treatment of growth hormone deficiency is the replacement of growth hormone (somatotropin) with biosynthetic somatotropin. This treatment is successful in 80% of affected children. Desmopressin acetate is used to treat diabetes insipidus. A deficiency of antidiuretic hormone causes diabetes insipidus, and isn't related to hypopituitarism. Testosterone or estrogen may be given during adolescence for normal sexual maturation, but neither is the definitive treatment for hypopituitarism.
CN: Physiological integrity; CNS: Pharmacological and parenteral therapies; CL: Apply

67. The nurse is interviewing a child's mother. Which statement, made by the mother, would suggest hypopituitarism in this child?
   1. "I can pass down my child's clothes to his younger brother."
   2. "My child usually wears out his clothes before his size changes."
   3. "I have to buy bigger size clothes for my child about every two months."
   4. "I have to buy larger shirts more frequently than larger pants for my child."

67. 2. Parents of children with hypopituitarism frequently comment that their child will wear out clothing before growing out of the garment, if the clothing fits the child's body, it is frequently too long in the sleeves or legs.
CN: Health promotion and maintenance; CNS: None; CL: Analyze

68. The nurse is teaching the parents of a child with growth hormone deficiency how to administer growth hormone to their child. At what time should the nurse suggest administration of this medication?
   1. At bedtime
   2. After dinner
   3. In the middle of the day
   4. First thing in the morning

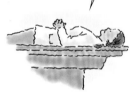

All I can think about is optimum dozing.

68. 1. Optimal therapeutic effect is typically achieved when the prescribed growth hormone is administered at bedtime. Pituitary release of growth hormone occurs during the first 45 to 90 minutes after the onset of sleep, so normal physiological release is mimicked with bedtime dosing.
CN: Physiological integrity; CNS: Pharmacological and parenteral therapies; CL: Apply

69. A nurse is teaching the parents of a child with hypopituitarism about realistic growth expectations. The child is responding well to treatments of growth hormone replacement. What is the **best** information for the nurse to include?
   1. "It is unlikely that your child will reach a normal adult height."
   2. "Your child will attain full adult height, but at an unpredictable rate."
   3. "Your child will attain full adult height at a rate slower than his peers."
   4. "Your child's growth rate will be the same as children without the disorder."

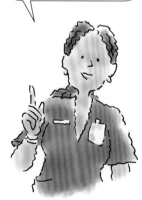

It's important that parents have *realistic expectations* about their child's disorder.

69. 3. These children will attain their full adult height at a slower rate than their peers when hormone replacement is successful. It is important to set realistic expectations regarding improvement.
CN: Psychosocial integrity; CNS: None; CL: Apply

CN: Client needs category   CNS: Client needs subcategory   CL: Cognitive level

70. Which statement, made by a parent of a child with short stature, would indicate to the nurse the need for further teaching?
1. "Blood studies are unlikely to aid in proper diagnosis."
2. "It will not be necessary to discuss a history of my child's growth pattern."
3. "X-rays are not included in my child's diagnostic procedures."
4. "It is not important to share my family history with my child's health care provider."

70. 1. A complete diagnostic evaluation should include family history, a history of the child's growth patterns and previous health status, physical examination, physical evaluation, radiographic survey, and endocrine studies that may involve blood samples.
CN: Physiological integrity; CNS: Reduction of risk potentials; CL: Analyze

71. A child has been diagnosed with type 1 diabetes mellitus. Which signs and symptoms would the nurse manage with this diagnosis? Select all that apply.
1. Polyuria
2. Weakness
3. Abdominal pain
4. Weight loss
5. Postprandial nausea
6. Orthostatic hypertension

71. 1, 2, 4, 5. Polyuria, weakness, weight loss, and postprandial nausea are common symptoms of type 1 diabetes mellitus that would need managed. Abdominal pain is not a symptom of this disease. Orthostatic hypotension, rather than orthostatic hypertension, may occur if extreme fluid loss results.
CN: Safe, effective care environment; CNS: Management of care; CL: Analyze

72. Which metabolic alteration characteristic is often associated with growth hormone deficiency?
1. Galactosemia
2. Homocystinuria
3. Hyperglycemia
4. Hypoglycemia

72. 4. The development of hypoglycemia is often related to growth hormone deficiency. Galactosemia is a rare autosomal recessive disorder with an inborn error of carbohydrate metabolism. Homocystinuria is an indication of amino acid transport or metabolism problems. Hyperglycemia isn't a problem in hypopituitarism.
CN: Physiological integrity; CNS: Physiological adaptation; CL: Apply

73. A nurse is teaching the parents of a child who is receiving growth hormone replacement for hypopituitarism. What action should the nurse include?
1. Explain that growth in height and weight will not begin until puberty
2. Teach the parents how to perform venipuncture for the administration of the growth hormone
3. Stress the importance of interacting with their child according to age rather than size
4. Advise the parents to consider holding their child back in school until linear growth accelerates

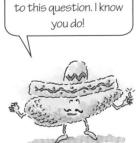

You know the answer to this question. I know you do!

73. 3. To promote the self-esteem and healthy development of a child with growth hormone deficiency, parents should be encouraged to interact with the child according to age, not size. Growth in height and weight will begin soon after treatment begins. Growth hormone administration is subcutaneous, and a child shouldn't be held back in school because of their size.
CN: Psychosocial integrity; CNS: None; CL: Apply

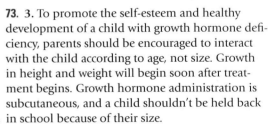

74. The nurse is caring for a neonate diagnosed with diabetes insipidus. Which assessment finding would warrant an **immediate** intervention?
1. Edema
2. Increased head circumference
3. Increased feeding
4. Weight loss

74. 4. Diabetes insipidus has a slow progression. Weight loss can occur when there is a large loss of fluid. Edema isn't evident in the neonate with diabetes insipidus. There should be an increase in head circumference with treatment. A normal neonate should gain weight as he grows. Increased feeding is a positive finding.
CN: Physiological integrity; CNS: Physiological adaptation; CL: Apply

CN: Client needs category   CNS: Client needs subcategory   CL: Cognitive level

75. Which urine characteristics would the nurse anticipate in a client with diabetes insipidus? Select all that apply.
1. Pale
2. Concentrated
3. Specific gravity between 1.000 and 1.015
4. Specific gravity more than 1.03
5. Specific gravity less than 1.006
6. Pink-tinged

75. 1, 5. A client with diabetes insipidus will have excessive urine output that is pale in color, with a specific below 1.01. Pink coloration would suggest the presence of blood, which is atypical.
CN: Physiological integrity; CNS: Reduction of risk potential; CL: Analyze

76. The nurse is obtaining the health history of a child with diabetes insipidus. Which findings would the nurse anticipate? Select all that apply.
1. Rapid onset of nocturia
2. Gradual onset of personality changes
3. Polydipsia
4. Abrupt onset of polyuria
5. Blurred vision

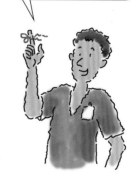

Let's see—what were the symptoms of diabetes insipidus again? Can you remember them all?

76. 1, 3, 4. Diabetes insipidus is characterized by deficient secretion of antidiuretic hormone leading to diuresis. Most children with this disorder experience an abrupt onset of symptoms, including polyuria, nocturia, and polydipsia. The other choices reflect symptoms of pituitary hyperfunction.
CN: Physiological integrity; CNS: Physiological adaptation; CL: Apply

77. The nurse is reviewing the assessment data of a client diagnosed with diabetes insipidus. The client is on fluid restriction for diagnostic testing. The nurse determines further intervention is necessary when the assessment identifies:
1. weight gain of 3 to 5%.
2. weight loss of 3 to 5%.
3. an increase in urine output.
4. generalized edema.

77. 2. A weight loss of 3 to 5% would indicate significant dehydration, and require termination of the fluid restriction. Weight gain would be a good sign. Generalized edema would not occur with fluid restriction, nor would increased urine output.
CN: Physiological integrity; CNS: Physiological adaptation; CL: Analyze

78. A child with diabetes insipidus has a viral illness that includes congestion, nausea, and vomiting. What is the **most** important information for the nurse to tell the parents about administering the child's medications?
1. Monitor the child closely and make no changes in the medication regimen
2. Give medications only once per day until respiratory symptoms resolve
3. Obtain an alternate route for desmopressin acetate (DDAVP) administration
4. Give medication no sooner than one hour after vomiting has occurred

78. 3. Due to nasal congestion, an alternate route for the administration of DDAVP would be required. The other options reflect actions that need to be covered by a health care provider's order.
CN: Physiological integrity; CNS: Pharmacological and parenteral therapies; CL: Apply

79. A child with diabetes insipidus will be receiving injectable vasopressin when discharged from the hospital. What is the **most** important step when teaching injection techniques?
1. Teach injection techniques to the primary caregiver
2. Teach injection techniques to anyone who will provide care for the child
3. Teach injection techniques to anyone who will provide care for the child as well as to the child if he's old enough to understand.
4. Provide information about the nearest home health agency so the parents can arrange for the home health nurse to give the injection

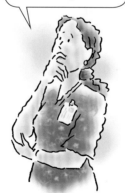

Who needs to know about injection techniques?

79. 3. The most important step is to teach all those who provide care for the child. The child should be included if age-appropriate. It's unrealistic to arrange for a home health nurse to give injections that are required throughout the child's life.
CN: Safe and effective care environment; CNS: Management of care ; CL: Apply

CN: Client needs category   CNS: Client needs subcategory   CL: Cognitive level

80. The nurse is providing care for a school-age client with diabetes insipidus. Which action may be difficult for this child due to delayed growth and development?
   1. Taking desmopressin acetate (DDAVP) when away from home
   2. Taking DDAVP before bedtime
   3. Allowing a parent to administer the vasopressin injection
   4. Self-administration of a vasopressin injection before school starts

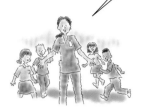

Don't forget to consider how a child's condition affects his or her social life.

80. **1.** Anything that singles a child out, and makes him feel different from his peers may result in noncompliance with the medication regimen. It's important for the nurse to help the client schedule medications around times that he is in school.
CN: Health promotion and maintenance; CNS: None; CL: Apply

81. The parents of a client newly diagnosed with diabetes insipidus ask the nurse about the best method to monitor the condition. What is the nurse's **best** response?
   1. Measure your child's abdominal girths every day
   2. Measure your child's intake, output, and urine specific gravity
   3. Check your child's weight weekly and measure intake carefully
   4. Checking for swelling in your child's lower legs and feet

81. **2.** Measuring intake and output with related specific gravity results and daily weights are the best measurements that will enable close monitoring of the client's condition. All of the other options aren't as accurate for a child with diabetes insipidus.
CN: Physiological integrity; CNS: Reduction of risk potential; CL: Apply

82. A nurse is caring for a neonate with congenital hypothyroidism. Which findings would the nurse anticipate in this client? Select all that apply.
   1. Cool, dry skin
   2. Hyperreflexia
   3. Long forehead
   4. Puffy eyelids
   5. Small tongue
   6. Abdominal distension

82. **1, 4, 6.** Assessment findings would include cool dry skin, puffy eyelids and abdominal distention. Other findings may include a depressed nasal bridge, short forehead, large tongue, thick, dry, mottled skin, coarse, dry, lusterless hair, umbilical hernia, hyporeflexia, bradycardia, hypothermia, hypotension, anemia, and wide cranial sutures.
CN: Physiological integrity; CNS: Physiological adaptation; CL: Apply

83. A child, just been admitted to the emergency department, has the following chart entry:

Progress notes	
10/15/16 1800	Parents describe recent weight loss and lack of energy. Client's ears and cheeks are flushed; acetone-smelling breath noted. Blood glucose 324 mg/dl (18.0 mmol/L), BP: 104/60 mmHg; P: 88/bpm; RR: 16 breaths/min.

What intervention would the nurse should anticipate?
   1. Subcutaneous administration of glucagon
   2. Administration of IV regular insulin by continuous infusion pump
   3. Administration of regular insulin subcutaneously Q4H as needed per sliding scale
   4. Administration of IV fluids in boluses of 20 ml/kg

83. **2.** Weight loss, lack of energy, acetone odor to breath, and a blood glucose level of 324 mg/dl (18.0 mmol/L) would indicate diabetic ketoacidosis. Insulin would be given IV by continuous infusion pump. Glucagon is administered for mild hypoglycemia. Sliding scale insulin isn't as effective as the administration of insulin by continuous infusion pump. Administration of IV fluids in boluses of 20 ml/kg is recommended for the treatment of shock.
CN: Physiological integrity; CNS: Physiological adaptation; CL: Apply

CN: Client needs category   CNS: Client needs subcategory   CL: Cognitive level

84. Which nursing intervention is **most** important when working with neonates who are suspected of having congenital hypothyroidism?
1. Identifying the disorder early
2. Promoting bonding
3. Allowing rooming in
4. Encouraging fluid intake

84. 1. The most important nursing intervention is early identification of the disorder. Nurses caring for neonates must be certain that screening is performed, especially in neonates who are preterm, discharged early, or born at home. Promoting bonding, allowing rooming in, and encouraging fluid intake are all important but are less important than early identification.
CN: Safe and effective care environment; CNS: Management of care; CL: Apply

85. The parents of an infant with hypothyroidism ask the nurse what they should do if the pulse rate is above the provided parameters. What is the nurse's **best** response?
1. Allow the baby to nap and then give the medication
2. Withhold the medication and give a double dose the next day
3. Hold the medication and call the health care provider
4. Give the medication and then consult the health care provider

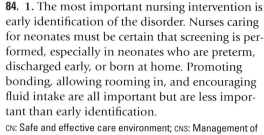

Sweet move! You owned that question.

85. 3. If parents have been taught to count the infant's pulse, they should be instructed to withhold the dose and consult their provider if the pulse rate is above the provided parameter.
CN: Health promotion and maintenance; CNS: None; CL: Apply

86. The care team has determined that an infant, being treated for congenital hypothyroidism, is not responding adequately to treatment. What assessment findings would support this conclusion? Select all that apply.
1. Irritability
2. Fatigue
3. Sleepiness
4. Increased appetite
5. Diarrhea

86. 2, 3. Signs of inadequate treatment are fatigue, sleepiness, decreased appetite, and constipation.
CN: Physiological integrity; CNS: Physiological adaptation; CL: Apply

87. The nurse is assessing a child with Cushing's syndrome. Which findings should the nurse anticipate? Select all that apply.
1. Obesity
2. Moon-shaped face
3. Hypotension
4. Emotional instability
5. Quickened healing
6. Loss of hair

87. 1, 2, 4. Cushing's syndrome occurs as a result of excessive cortisol exposure, through corticosteroid medications or excess production by the adrenal glands. Common findings include obesity, moon-shaped face, and emotional instability. Hypertension, excessive hair growth, and delayed healing are additional findings.
CN: Physiological integrity; CNS: Physiological adaptation; CL: Analyze

CN: Client needs category   CNS: Client needs subcategory   CL: Cognitive level

88. An adolescent with type 1 diabetes mellitus tells the nurse that he will be playing football for his school this year. He asks the nurse what he can do to prevent hypoglycemia. What is the nurse's **best** response?

1. "It's best to limit participation in planned exercise activities that involve competition."
2. "Carry crackers or fruit to eat before or during periods of increased activity."
3. "Increase your insulin dosage before planned or unplanned strenuous exercise."
4. "Check your blood glucose before exercising and eat a protein snack if it's elevated."

88. **2.** Hypoglycemia can usually be prevented if an adolescent with diabetes eats more food before or during exercise. Because exercise with adolescents isn't commonly planned, carrying additional carbohydrate foods is a good preventative measure.

CN: Health promotion and maintenance; CNS: None; CL: Apply

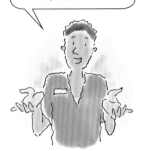

Let's discuss some steps for preventing hypoglycemia.

89. A child with diabetic ketoacidosis is being treated for a blood glucose level of 738 mg/dl (41.0 mmol/L). The nurse should anticipate an order for:

1. normal saline with regular insulin.
2. normal saline with ultralente insulin.
3. 5% dextrose in water with NPH insulin.
4. 5% dextrose in water with PZI insulin.

89. **1.** Short-acting regular insulin is the only insulin used for insulin infusions. Initially, normal saline is used until blood glucose levels are reduced, then a dextrose solution may be used to prevent hypoglycemia. Ultralente, NPH, and PZI insulins have a longer duration of action and shouldn't be used for continuous infusions.

CN: Physiological integrity; CNS: Pharmacological and parenteral therapies; CL: Apply

90. An adolescent client is admitted to the hospital with type 1 diabetes mellitus and unstable blood glucose levels. What is the **most** important question for the nurse to include in the health history?

1. "Do you play any team sports?"
2. "Do you refrigerate your insulin?"
3. "Are you satisfied with your weight?"
4. "Do you smoke tobacco or marijuana?"

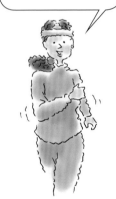

Don't give up now! You're heading down the home stretch.

90. **3.** It's important to ask how the client feels about her body, in particular, her weight. Some female adolescents skip their insulin because they know doing so will result in weight loss. The other issues of sports, drug use, smoking and technique of administering insulin are all relevant, but not as important as knowing what the client is thinking about her own body.

CN: Psychosocial integrity; CNS: None; CL: Apply

91. An adolescent client with type 1 diabetes mellitus plans to join the school basketball team, which practices twice a week with games on Saturdays. The client calls the clinic for advice. What advice should the nurse give this client?

1. "Delay eating a meal until after practice or a game."
2. "Time your insulin to peak at the time of practice and games."
3. "Monitor your blood glucose before, during, and after exercise."
4. "Increase your daily calorie intake by 10% and up your insulin dose by 10%."

91. **3.** An increase in activity would require a snack before the activity and increased insulin. The amount of insulin is the most difficult determination. Monitoring is required for accurate regulation before, during, and after the activity. The client shouldn't delay eating until afterward because the body needs the calories to provide energy to the muscles and tissues. Extreme hypoglycemia may occur if the insulin peaks without extra calories. There's no standard of 10% increase in calories and insulin.

CN: Health promotion and maintenance; CNS: None; CL: Apply

92. A nurse is collecting a health history from the parents of an infant being evaluated for hypopituitarism. What information is **most** important for the nurse to ascertain?
1. If the mother drank alcohol while pregnant
2. If the infant receives multivitamins
3. The infant's growth pattern
4. If the infant was premature

92. 3. Hypopituitarism presents with a slowed growth pattern, appearance that is younger than chronological age, and normal skeletal proportions and intelligence. Serial growth patterns will be crucial to the diagnosis process. It isn't related to maternal alcoholism, use of multivitamins, or prematurity.
CN: Physiological integrity; CNS: Physiological adaptation; CL: Apply

93. A nurse has just finished teaching a family about their child's congenital hypothyroidism. Which actions would indicate that the parents understand their child's diagnosis?
1. Providing a diet including whole grains, fruit, vegetables, and water
2. Anticipating that their child will outgrow hypothyroidism
3. Providing a diet that emphasizes simple and complex carbohydrates
4. Providing a diet high in fat to encourage growth for their child

93. 1. A diet including fruits, vegetables, whole grains, and water will help counteract the trend toward obstinate constipation, resulting from a slowed metabolism and hypotonic bowel. Congenital hypothyroidism isn't outgrown, and thyroid replacement is necessary throughout the life span. A carbohydrate-rich diet involves foods low in fiber, which can lead to constipation. Individuals with hypothyroidism tend to have elevated cholesterol and triglyceride levels. A diet high in fat is contraindicated.
CN: Health promotion and maintenance; CNS: None; CL: Apply

94. A child is being treated for diabetic ketoacidosis. Which finding would the nurse anticipate?
1. Hypercalcemia
2. Hyperphosphatemia
3. Hypokalemia
4. Hypernatremia

94. 3. Hypokalemia occurs as insulin causes potassium and glucose to move into the cells. Insulin doesn't affect calcium or sodium levels. Insulin administration may lead to hypophosphatemia as phosphorus enters the cells with insulin and potassium.
CN: Physiological integrity; CNS: Physiological adaptation; CL: Analyze

95. A nurse is caring for a client with pheochromocytoma. What is the most important intervention by the nurse?
1. Promoting an environment free from emotional distress
2. Avoiding analgesia administration
3. Advising a low-calorie, high-nutrient diet
4. Avoiding parents rooming in because they make the client less dependent on staff

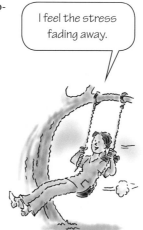

I feel the stress fading away.

95. 1. The child experiencing hyperfunctioning of the adrenal gland, or pheochromocytoma has excessive epinephrine resulting in an accelerated metabolism. Symptoms include hypertension, headaches, hyperglycemia with weight loss, diaphoresis, and hyperventilation. Through provision of a low-stress environment, analgesia as needed, a high-calorie diet, and supportive parents, the child will be able to prepare for surgery to eliminate the tumor causing the hypersecretion of epinephrine.
CN: Safe and effective care environment; CNS: Management of care; CL: Apply

CN: Client needs category   CNS: Client needs subcategory   CL: Cognitive level

96. A nurse is instructing parents about promoting the health of their child with type 1 diabetes. What is the **most** important information for the nurse to include?
  1. Avoid daily bathing so the skin doesn't become too dry
  2. Don't be concerned about cuts and scratches obtained on the playground
  3. Plan for fewer immunizations than other children
  4. Arrange for regular dental and ophthalmo-logic assessments

96. 4. Regular dental care will preserve oral health, and ophthalmologic examinations will ensure visual acuity for reading. Because of their impaired immune system, children with diabetes need to maintain a high level of health to avoid infection. Daily bathing and application of lotion, cleaning minor playground scrapes, applying antibiotic ointments, and keeping immunizations up-to-date are all important.
CN: Health promotion and maintenance; CNS: None; CL: Apply

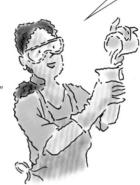

Adjusting insulin reflects that your client understands his disorder.

97. A school-age child monitors and adjusts his own insulin. Which response reflects an understanding of sick day rules?
  1. "I'll withhold my insulin when I'm not eating."
  2. "I'll take my usual dose of NPH insulin and double my dose of regular insulin."
  3. "I'll check my glucose often and keep taking my usual dose of long-acting insulin."
  4. "I'll check my glucose often, and temporarily replace NPH with regular insulin."

97. 3. Because of the stress of illness, serum glucose will likely be elevated. Adjustments may need to be made in insulin doses, but doses of regular insulin are not always doubled. NPH should not be replaced with regular insulin.
CN: Health promotion and maintenance; CNS: None; CL: Analyze

98. The nurse is teaching the parents of a child with hypopituitary dwarfism about the diagnosis. What is the **most** appropriate information for the nurse to provide?
  1. Children with hypopituitary dwarfism are usually low-birth-weight babies.
  2. Symptoms aren't apparent until puberty.
  3. Symptoms include early primary dentition.
  4. Growth is normal until age two, and then lags behind their peers.

98. 4. Generally, hypopituitary children are of average birth weight and grow at a normal pace for the first 2 to 3 years, and then fall behind their peers in height, usually below the third percentile. Dentition of primary teeth is normal. The appearance of permanent teeth is delayed.
CN: Physiological integrity; CNS: Physiological adaptation; CL: Apply

99. A school-age child has been experiencing insatiable thirst and urinating excessively. His serum glucose is 90 mg/dl (5.0 mmol/L). Which condition would the nurse suspect?
  1. Type 2 diabetes mellitus
  2. Type 1 diabetes mellitus
  3. Hyperthyroidism
  4. Diabetes insipidus

99. 4. Polydipsia and polyuria with normal serum glucose may be indicative of diabetes insipidus. Interview and laboratory results can determine whether the origin is neurogenic or nephrogenic. Type 1 or type 2 diabetes mellitus requires an elevation in serum glucose. A child with hyperthyroidism may present as dehydrated from the excessive sweating and rapid respirations that accompany this hypermetabolic state.
CN: Physiological integrity; CNS: Physiological adaptation; CL: Analyze

100. A child with type 1 diabetes is ordered to receive 25 ml/hr of 0.9% IV solution. The nurse is using a pediatric microdrip chamber to administer the medication. What is the correct drip rate for this medication? Record your answer using a whole number.

_____ gtt/min

101. The nurse is preparing to administer IV methylprednisolone sodium succinate to a child who weighs 44 lb (20 kg). The order is for 0.03 mg/kg IV daily. How many milligrams should the nurse prepare? Record your answer using one decimal point.

_____ mg

102. The nurse is providing teaching to the parents of a child admitted with diabetes insipidus. Which statement indicates that the parents understand this condition?
  1. "We know that our child's thyroid is working too much."
  2. "We know that our child's pituitary gland is not working hard enough."
  3. "Our child's pituitary gland is working overtime."
  4. "Our child's parathyroid gland is not doing a good job. It is very lazy."

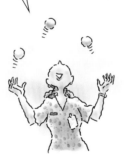

Hooray! Another chapter finished! Good job!

100. 25.
When using a pediatric microdrip chamber, the number of ml/hr equals the number of gtt/min. If 25 ml/hr is ordered, the IV should infuse at 25 gtt/min.
CN: Physiological integrity; CNS: Pharmacological and parenteral therapies; CL: Apply

101. 0.6.
To perform this dosage calculation, the nurse should first convert the child's weight to kilograms:

$$44\,lb \div 2.2\,kg/lb = 20\,kg$$

Then use this formula to determine the dose:

$$20\,kg \times 0.03\,mg/kg = X\,mg$$

$$X = 0.6\,mg$$

CN: Physiological integrity; CNS: Pharmacological and parenteral therapies; CL: Apply

102. 2. The principal disorder of posterior pituitary hypofunction is diabetes insipidus. The disorder results from hyposecretion of antidiuretic hormone, producing a state of uncontrolled diuresis. It is not caused by the thyroid gland or parathyroid gland.
CN: Health promotion and maintenance; CNS: None; CL: Apply

Chapter 34

Genitourinary Disorders

This chapter covers altered patterns of urinary elimination in children and includes glomerulonephritis, hypospadias, and—oh, a whole lot of other conditions. Ready? Let's go!

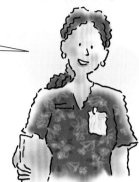

1. The nurse is planning the care of a child who is experiencing impaired urinary elimination, fluid retention and impaired glomerular filtration. What goal is **most** appropriate for this child?
1. Exhibits no evidence of impaired skin integrity
2. Engages in activities appropriate to age and development
3. Demonstrates no periorbital, facial, or body edema
4. Maintains a fluid intake of at least 2,000 ml in 24 hours

If you're having trouble deciding on an answer, begin by eliminating the ones you *know* are incorrect.

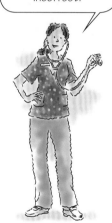

2. The nurse is caring for a child with acute glomerulonephritis. What action is **most** important for the nurse to do?
1. Obtain and monitor daily weight
2. Increase oral fluid intake
3. Provide sodium supplements
4. Monitoring the client for signs of hypokalemia

3. A nurse is taking frequent blood pressure readings on a child diagnosed with acute glomerulonephritis. The parents ask the nurse why this is necessary. Which statement, by the nurse, **most** accurately addresses their concerns?
1. Blood pressure fluctuations are a sign that your child's condition has become chronic.
2. Blood pressure fluctuations are a common adverse effect of the antibiotic therapy your child is on.
3. Hypotension can lead to sudden shock and can develop at any time as part of the disease process.
4. There's a possibility of sudden rises in your child's blood pressure.

1. 3. Interventions such as decreased fluid and salt intake will minimize or prevent fluid retention and edema. The risk of edema is likely higher than that of impaired skin integrity. Activity level is important, but is not directly related to this client's condition. Fluid intake of more than 2,000 ml may be excessive and would exacerbate edema.
CN: Safe and effective care environment; CNS: Management of care; CL: Analyze

2. 1. The child with acute glomerulonephritis should be monitored for fluid imbalance, which is done through daily weights. Increasing oral intake and providing sodium supplements aren't part of the therapeutic management of acute glomerulonephritis. Impaired renal function is associated with increased, not decreased, potassium levels.
CN: Safe and effective care environment; CNS: Management of care; CL: Apply

3. 4. Regular measurement of vital signs, body weight, and intake and output is essential to monitor the progress of the disease, and to detect complications that may appear at any time during the course of the disease. Blood pressure fluctuations don't indicate that the condition has become chronic and aren't common adverse reactions to antibiotic therapy. Hypertension is more likely than hypotension to occur with glomerulonephritis.
CN: Physiological integrity; CNS: Physiological adaptation; CL: Apply

CN: Client needs category   CNS: Client needs subcategory   CL: Cognitive level

4. A nurse is reviewing the urinalysis results of a child diagnosed with acute glomerulonephritis. Based on the results of the routine urinalysis, which finding **best** supports this diagnosis?
1. Specific gravity of 1.036
2. Protein of 10 mg/100 ml
3. Gross hematuria
4. Urine crystals

4. 3. Urinalysis findings consistent with acute glomerulonephritis include low urine specific gravity, mild to moderate proteinuria, gross hematuria, and the presence of RBC casts. The presence of crystals in the urine typically indicates a congenital metabolic problem.
CN: Physiological integrity; CNS: Physiological adaptation;
CL: Analyze

5. Which result would a nurse anticipate when evaluating the urinalysis report of a child with acute glomerulonephritis?
1. Proteinuria and decreased specific gravity
2. Bacteriuria and increased specific gravity
3. Hematuria and proteinuria
4. Bacteriuria and hematuria

5. 3. Urinalysis during the acute phase of this disease characteristically shows hematuria, proteinuria, and increased specific gravity.
CN: Physiological integrity; CNS: Physiological adaptation;
CL: Analyze

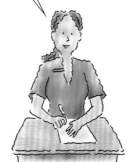

More than one answer may seem correct. It's your job to choose the best answer.

6. What is the nurse's **best** response to a mother who wants to know the first indication that her child's acute glomerulonephritis is improving?
1. "Your child's urine output will increase."
2. "Your child's urine will be free from protein."
3. "Your child's blood pressure will stabilize."
4. "Your child's energy will notably increase."

6. 1. One of the first signs of improvement during the acute phase of glomerulonephritis is an increase in urine output. It will take time for the urine to be free from protein. Increased urine output often precedes the stabilization of blood pressure. Children generally don't have much energy during the acute phase of this disease.
CN: Physiological integrity; CNS: Reduction of risk potential;
CL: Analyze

7. Which statement, by the parents of a child with acute glomerulonephritis, indicates an understanding of the teaching provided by the nurse regarding this diagnosis?
1. This disease occurs after a urinary tract infection.
2. This disease is associated with renal vascular disorders.
3. This disease occurs after a streptococcal infection.
4. This disease is associated with structural anomalies of the genitourinary tract.

7. 3. Acute glomerulonephritis is an immune-complex disease that occurs as a by-product of a streptococcal infection. Certain strains of the infection are usually a beta-hemolytic Streptococcus. The other options are not true of acute glomerulonephritis.
CN: Physiological integrity ; CNS: Physiologic adaptation;
CL: Analyze

8. When obtaining a child's daily weight, the nurse notes a loss of 6 lb (2.7 kg) after three days of hospitalization for acute glomerulonephritis. Which cause is **most** likely?
1. Poor appetite
2. Resolution of edema
3. Decreased salt intake
4. Restriction to bed rest

8. 2. When there's reduction of edema, the client will lose weight. This normally occurs following several days of treatment for acute glomerulonephritis. A poor appetite, decreased salt intake, or a restriction to bed rest would not lead to such a dramatic weight loss.
CN: Physiological integrity; CNS: Basic care and comfort;
CL: Apply

CN: Client needs category   CNS: Client needs subcategory   CL: Cognitive level

9. A nurse is teaching the parents, of a child newly diagnosed with acute glomerulonephritis, about nutrition. The nurse determines that teaching was effective when the parents state the need to:
1. decrease calories being consumed.
2. increase the child's potassium intake.
3. severely limit all sodium intake.
4. moderately restrict sodium intake.

9. 4. Moderate sodium restriction, with a diet that has no added salt after cooking, is usually effective. Calorie consumption doesn't need to decrease and is often increased to compensate for decreased appetite. Potassium consumption shouldn't increase because of the decrease in urinary output. Severe sodium restriction isn't necessary, will make adequate nutrition more difficult, and may result in hyponatremia.
CN: Physiological integrity; CNS: Basic care and comfort; CL: Apply

10. A nurse is evaluating a group of children for the potential development of acute glomerulonephritis. Which client is **most** likely to develop the disease?
1. A client who had pneumonia a month ago
2. A client who was bitten by a brown spider
3. A client who was born with an atrial-septal defect
4. A client who had a streptococcal infection two weeks ago

10. 4. A latent period of 10 to 14 days is common between a streptococcal infection of the throat or skin and the onset of clinical manifestations of acute glomerulonephritis. The peak incidence of disease corresponds to the incidence of streptococcal infections. Pneumonia isn't a precursor to glomerulonephritis, nor is a bite from a brown spider. Cardiac disease does not contribute to acute glomerulonephritis.
CN: Physiological integrity; CNS: Reduction of risk potential ; CL: Analyze

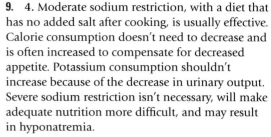

You're making this test look like child's play!

11. The nurse is caring for a 10-year-old child who weighs 82.2 lb (37.3 kg) and is to receive 2.5 ml/kg/hr of 0.45% NaCl solution. How many milliliters per hour should this child receive? Record your answer using a whole number.

_____ ml/hr

11. 93.
To calculate the rate per hour, the nurse should multiply 37.3 kg by 2.5 ml, which equals 93.25 ml/hr; this should be rounded to 93 ml/hr.
CN: Physiological integrity; CNS: Pharmacological and parenteral therapies; CL: Apply

12. The nurse on the pediatric medical unit is admitting a school-age child from the emergency department. The child's chart entry reads:

Progress notes	
10/15/16 1445	Mother reports client has had no urine output for 18 hours. Bladder scan reveals 0 ml residual urine. Pulse 98/bpm and irregular; blood pressure 78/38 mmHg. Client reports abdominal pain described as 'cramps.' Bilateral muscle weakness noted.

What is the nurse's **priority** action?
1. Administer dobutamine as prescribed
2. Administer furosemide as prescribed
3. Administer sodium polystyrene as prescribed
4. Encourage oral fluid intake

12. 3. The client's presentation is consistent with acute kidney injury and accompanying hyperkalemia, which could be addressed with sodium polystyrene. Resolution of this life-threatening complication would be a priority. Inotropic medications like dobutamine are not indicated and oral fluid intake would insufficient. Loop diuretics like furosemide would not resolve hyperkalemia.
CN: Physiological integrity; CNS: Pharmacological and parenteral therapies; CL: Apply

CN: Client needs category   CNS: Client needs subcategory   CL: Cognitive level

13. A nurse is explaining enuresis to a child's parents. What information is **most** appropriate for the nurse to include? Select all that apply.
1. Most children outgrow this distressing problem, but there are treatments available now.
2. Episodes primarily occur when the child is awake and playing vigorously.
3. The child may feel shame, and may withdraw from peers.
4. The condition may respond to tricyclic antidepressants and antidiuretics.
5. The condition may become permanent without appropriate intervention.

14. Which statement, made by a parent, would indicate to the nurse that further teaching about chronic renal failure is necessary?
1. "My child will have to adjust to a diet high in protein and low in fat."
2. "My child's kidneys have lost their ability to make concentrated urine."
3. "It's likely that my child has calcium levels that are lower than normal."
4. "We'll have to watch my child closely for signs of anemia."

15. The nurse is teaching the parents of a three-year-old child how to obtain a clean-catch urine specimen. How should the nurse instruct the parents to proceed?
1. Collect the specimen right after a nap
2. Never use the first voided specimen of the day
3. Collect the specimen at the beginning of urination
4. There is no need to wash the perineal area before collecting the specimen

16. The nurse is providing health education to the parents of a child who was recently diagnosed with chronic renal failure. What meal should the nurse recommend for this child?
1. Baked or grilled chicken breast with vegetables
2. Whole grain breakfast cereal with milk
3. Roasted pork with salad
4. Steamed rice and vegetables

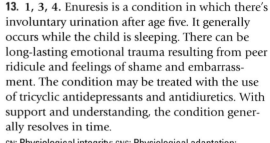

The phrase *further teaching* indicates that question 14 is looking for an inaccurate statement.

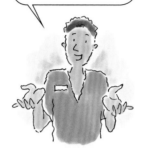

Don't a-void this question. You're doing great!

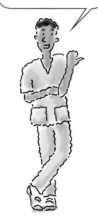

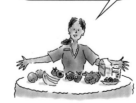

Clients with chronic renal failure should follow a low-protein diet.

13. 1, 3, 4. Enuresis is a condition in which there's involuntary urination after age five. It generally occurs while the child is sleeping. There can be long-lasting emotional trauma resulting from peer ridicule and feelings of shame and embarrassment. The condition may be treated with the use of tricyclic antidepressants and antidiuretics. With support and understanding, the condition generally resolves in time.
CN: Physiological integrity; CNS: Physiological adaptation; CL: Analyze

14. 1. Chronic renal failure causes an inability to produce concentrated urine. Hypocalcemia and anemia are common complications. A high-protein, low-fat diet is not indicated. The child's protein intake should be reduced.
CN: Physiological integrity; CNS: Physiological Adaptation; CL: Apply

15. 2. When collecting a clean-catch urine specimen, the first voided specimen of the day should never be used because of urinary stasis. A specimen should also never been collected following a nap. The specimen should be collected midstream, not at the beginning, or end, of urination. Washing the perineal area before collecting a specimen is very important to make sure there are no contaminants from the skin in the specimen.
CN: Physiological integrity; CNS: Reduction of risk potential; CL: Apply

16. 4. Children with chronic renal failure will benefit from a low-protein diet. Milk and dairy should be limited because of high levels of sodium, potassium, and phosphate. Steamed rice can and vegetables be low in protein and electrolytes.
CN: Physiological integrity; CNS: Basic care and comfort; CL: Apply

17. A nurse is explaining the expected treatment for glomerulonephritis. What is the **most** important information for the nurse to include?
1. Children who have signs of glomerulonephritis are usually hospitalized for 7 to 10 days.
2. Parents should expect children to have a normal energy level during the acute phase.
3. Children who have normal blood pressure and satisfactory urine output can generally be treated at home.
4. Children with gross hematuria and significant oliguria should be brought to the provider's office every two days for monitoring.

18. What is the **most** important nursing intervention for a school-age child with acute kidney injury?
1. Assess blood pressure every four hours
2. Check urine specific gravity every four hours
3. Encourage daily fluid intake of 100 ml/kg/day
4. Provide a 2,500 mg sodium diet

19. A child, with chronic renal failure, is selecting his menu. Which selection would alert the nurse that further teaching is necessary?
1. Turkey sandwich with mayonnaise and celery sticks
2. Hot dog with ketchup and mustard and chips
3. Chocolate cake with white icing and ice cream
4. Apple slices with peanut butter

20. The mother of a child with hypospadias asks the nurse what is wrong with her son's penis. What is the nurse's **most** appropriate response?
1. It is the absence of a urethral opening in the penis.
2. It is a penis that is shorter than usual for the child's age.
3. It is a urethral opening along the dorsal surface of the penis.
4. It is a urethral opening along the ventral surface of the penis.

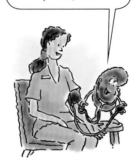

Your blood pressure looks great this time, but we'll keep an eye on it.

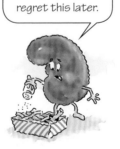

I'll probably regret this later.

17. 3. Children who have normal blood pressure and a satisfactory urine output can generally be treated at home. Parents should expect children to have decreased energy during the acute phase of the disease. Those with gross hematuria and significant oliguria will likely require hospitalization for monitoring. There is no set time frame for hospitalization, and it is not always required.
CN: Health promotion and maintenance; CNS: None; CL: Apply

18. 1. Because hypertension is a complication of acute kidney injury, the nurse should check the child's blood pressure every four hours. Urine specific gravity should also be monitored, but it isn't as high a priority as monitoring the blood pressure. The child may be placed on fluid or sodium restrictions. Fluid intake of 100 ml/kg/day is too much for a healthy child with normal renal function. A sodium intake of 2,500 mg is excessive.
CN: Physiological integrity; CNS: Reduction of risk potential; CL: Apply

19. 2. Foods that are high in sodium, such as hot dogs, should be eliminated from the child's diet. Snacks, such as pretzels and potato chips, should also be discouraged. Any other foods that the child likes should be encouraged.
CN: Physiological integrity; CNS: Basic care and comfort; CL: Apply

20. 4. Hypospadias refers to a condition in which the urethral opening is located below the glans penis, or anywhere along the ventral surface of the penile shaft.
CN: Physiological integrity; CNS: Physiological adaptation; CL: Apply

CN: Client needs category   CNS: Client needs subcategory   CL: Cognitive level

21. Following the acute phase of glomerulonephritis, which discharge instruction should the nurse include?

1. A cystogram will be needed every six months, for follow-up evaluation.
2. Regular visits to the provider may be needed for evaluation.
3. Intermittent urinary catheterization may be necessary to treat urinary retention.
4. Further evaluations are not normally needed for this disease.

22. A newborn has just been diagnosed with chordee. What is the nurse's **most** appropriate action?

1. Prepare the family for the likelihood of surgery
2. Begin educating the parents about urinary catheterization
3. Establish intravenous access, as ordered, to administer a fluid bolus
4. Monitor the neonate for signs of hyperkalemia

23. A toddler weighing 27.6 lb (12.5 kg) is to receive 4 ml/kg/hr of intravenous normal saline solution. The nurse will administer the fluid using microdrip tubing that delivers 60 gtt/ml. How many milliliters per hour should this client receive? Record your answer using a whole number.

_____ ml/hr

24. A nurse is explaining to the parents of a son, born with hypospadias, why surgical repair should be done at such a young age. What is the **best** explanation?

1. To prevent separation anxiety
2. To prevent urinary complications
3. To facilitate hygiene
4. To promote the development of a normal body image

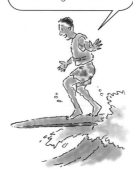

Twenty-one questions done! Looks like you caught the right wave.

21. 2. Weekly or monthly visits to the provider will be needed to evaluate improvement. These visits usually involve the collection of a urine specimen for urinalysis. A cystogram is used to review the anatomic structures of the urinary tract, but isn't helpful in determining the progression of this disease. Catheterization is not normally necessary following recovery from glomerulonephritis.
CN: Safe and effective care environment; CNS: Management of care; CL: Apply

22. 1. Chordee, or ventral curvature of the penis, results from the replacement of normal skin with a fibrous band of tissue, and usually accompanies more severe forms of hypospadias. Surgical correction is normally required. The condition does not usually necessitate catheterization, and it does not create a risk for fluid or electrolyte disturbances.
CN: Safe and effective care environment; CNS: Management of care; CL: Apply

23. 50.
To calculate the rate per hour for the infusion, the nurse should multiply 12.5 kg by 4 ml/kg/hr, which equals 50 ml/hr. The fact that the nurse is using microdrip tubing does not influence the calculation of the rate in milliliters per hour.
CN: Physiological integrity; CNS: Pharmacological and parenteral therapies; CL: Apply

24. 4. Whenever there are defects of the genitourinary tact, surgery should be performed early to promote development of a normal body image. Traumatization is more likely to occur with an older child. A child with normal emotional development will show separation anxiety at 7 to 9 months. Hypospadias doesn't usually put a child at greater risk for urinary complications.
CN: Health promotion and maintenance; CNS: None; CL: Apply

25. The nurse is caring for a neonate who has been diagnosed with a distal hypospadias. At which anatomical position would the nurse anticipate finding the urinary meatus on this child?

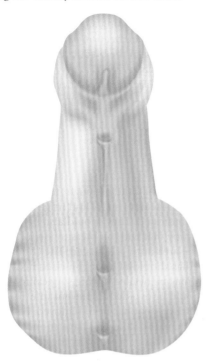

25. In a distal hypospadias, the meatus is on the ventral surface of the glans penis.

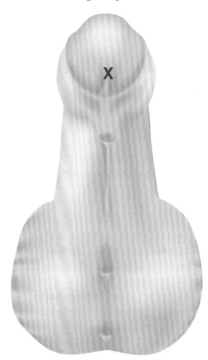

CN: Physiological integrity; CNS: Physiological adaptation; CL: Apply

26. A child is undergoing surgical repair of hypospadias. Which statement, made by this child's parents, implies a need for further teaching?
1. "The surgery will improve the physical appearance of the genitalia for psychological reasons."
2. "The purpose of surgery is to enhance the child's ability to void in the standing position."
3. "The purpose of surgery is to decrease the chance of developing urinary tract infections."
4. "The purpose of surgery is to preserve a sexually adequate organ."

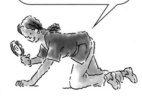

I'm looking for the one inaccurate statement.

26. 3. A child with hypospadias isn't at greater risk for urinary tract infections. The principal objective of surgical correction is to enhance the child's ability to void in the standing position with a straight stream of urine, to improve the physical appearance of the genitalia for psychological reasons, and to preserve a sexually adequate organ.
CN: Physiological integrity; CNS: Reduction in risk potential; CL: Apply

27. What is the **most** important intervention for the nurse to include in the care plan for a male infant following surgical repair of hypospadias?
1. Sterile dressing changes every four hours
2. Frequent assessment of the tip of the penis
3. Removal of the suprapubic catheter on the second postoperative day
4. Urethral catheterization if voiding doesn't occur over an eight-hour period

27. 2. Following hypospadias repair, a pressure dressing is applied to the penis to reduce bleeding and tissue swelling. The tip of the penis should then be assessed frequently for signs of circulatory impairment. The dressing around the penis is initially changed by the surgeon, and shouldn't be changed every four hours thereafter. The provider will determine when the suprapubic catheter will be removed. Urethral catheterization should be avoided after repair of hypospadias to prevent trauma to the repaired urethra.
CN: Physiological integrity; CNS: Reduction in risk potential; CL: Apply

CN: Client needs category   CNS: Client needs subcategory   CL: Cognitive level

28. The nurse is caring for an infant, newly admitted, with a diagnosis of exstrophy of the bladder. Which interventions are **most** appropriate? Select all that apply.
1. Gather supplies in anticipation of Foley catheter insertion
2. Implement a latex-free environment for the infant
3. Maintain the infant in a prone position
4. Cover the defect with a non-adherent dressing
5. Place the infant in a thermo-controlled environment
6. Place a diaper snugly over the genitalia to ensure accurate output monitoring

29. The nurse is providing discharge information to the parents of a child who has had surgical repair of hypospadias. Which instructions would be **most** appropriate? Select all that apply.
1. Care of the circumcision
2. Techniques for providing tub baths
3. Care for the indwelling catheter or stent
4. Encouraging the child to void every two hours
5. Avoiding toys that the child will ride by straddle

30. The nurse is providing discharge instructions to the parents of an older child who has had hypospadias repair. Which activity should be encouraged?
1. Providing a high-potassium diet
2. Soaking the perineum twice daily
3. Increasing fluid intake
4. Providing a high-fiber diet

31. The mother of a neonate, born with hypospadias, is sharing her feelings of guilt about this anomaly with a nurse. What information should the nurse emphasize with this mother?
1. It occurs around the third month of fetal development and was not caused by the mother.
2. It occurs around the sixth month of fetal development and often results from smoking or drinking while pregnant.
3. It's carried by an autosomal recessive gene and may occur with future children.
4. It's hereditary, and can be passed on as an X-linked chromosome from mother to son.

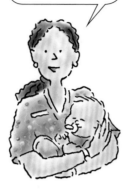

An infant with exstrophy of the bladder needs special protection and care.

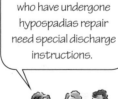

Parents of children who have undergone hypospadias repair need special discharge instructions.

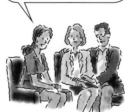

28. 2, 4, 5. Exstrophy of the bladder is a congenital defect in which the bladder is externalized on the abdomen. Treatment requires specialized care, including a latex-free environment, supine positioning, covering the defect with a non-adherent dressing, and maintaining a thermoneutral environment. Catheterization is not performed for these clients, and the bladder defect is never covered with a diaper.
CN: Health promotion and maintenance; CNS: None; CL: Apply

29. 3, 5. Parents should be taught to care for the indwelling catheter or stent, and irrigation techniques, if indicated. They should also be told to avoid any toy that will put pressure on, or irritate, the genital area until it is healed. The child with hypospadias shouldn't be circumcised because the foreskin may be needed during surgical repair. Tub baths should be avoided to prevent infection until the catheter or stent has been removed. Following surgical repair, the child will have an indwelling urinary catheter, so encouraging the child to void isn't appropriate.
CN: Physiological integrity; CNS: Reduction of risk potential; CL: Analyze

30. 3. The family should encourage the child to increase fluid intake. There is no need to increase potassium or fiber intake. Soaking the perineum could inhibit healing.
CN: Health promotion and maintenance; CNS: None; CL: Apply

31. 1. The defect of hypospadias occurs around the end of the third month of fetal development. This defect is not carried by an autosomal-recessive gene. It is also not X-linked or related to smoking or ingestion of alcohol.
CN: Health promotion and maintenance; CNS: None; CL: Apply

32. A mother reports that her six-year-old daughter recently began wetting the bed and running a low-grade fever. A diagnosis of urinary tract infection (UTI) was made following a urinalysis that came back positive for bacteria and protein. Antibiotics have been prescribed for the child. What are appropriate nursing interventions? Select all that apply.
1. Limit fluids for the next few days to decrease the frequency of urination
2. Assess the mother's understanding of UTI and its causes
3. Instruct the mother to administer all the antibiotic as prescribed until the prescription is finished
4. Provide instruction solely to the mother, not the child
5. Discourage the taking of bubble baths
6. Advise wiping from back to the front after voiding and defecation

33. A three-year-old child who had a hypospadias repair yesterday has a suprapubic catheter in place and an IV. The nurse has administered a dose of propantheline bromide. Which assessment finding would indicate that this intervention has been effective?
1. Absence of infection
2. Absence of pain in the meatus and urethra
3. Absence of bladder spasms
4. Increase in urine output

34. The nurse is discussing hypospadias with the parents of a child affected with the condition. Which initial intervention, by the nurse, is **most** appropriate?
1. Refer the parents to a counselor
2. Be there to listen to the parents' concerns
3. Notify the primary care provider of the parents' concerns
4. Suggest a support group of other parents who have gone through this experience

35. The nurse is providing care for a school-age child diagnosed with chronic renal failure. What assessment finding would suggest an exacerbation of the client's condition?
1. Blood pressure 138/89 mmHg
2. Oxygen saturation 91% on room air
3. Reports of bilateral flank pain
4. Apathy toward activities

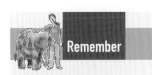

"Propantheline prevents spasms."

Propantheline, a quaternary ammonium drug, is often used to treat spastic or hyperactive conditions of the gastrointestinal tract and urinary tract (including the bladder).

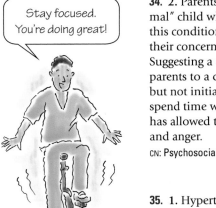

Stay focused. You're doing great!

32. 2, 3, 5. Assessing the mother's understanding of UTIs and their cause will provide a baseline for teaching. The full course of antibiotics must be given to eradicate the organism and prevent recurrence, even if the child's symptoms decrease. Bubble baths can irritate the vulva and urethra, and contribute to the development of a UTI. Fluids should be encouraged to prevent urinary stasis and help flush the organism from the urinary tract. The child should be instructed at her level of understanding to help her understand the treatment and promote compliance. The child should wipe from front to the back to minimize the risk of contamination after elimination.
CN: Health promotion and maintenance; CNS: None; CL: Apply

33. 3. Propantheline bromide is an antispasmodic that works effectively on children. It isn't an antibiotic and will not decrease the chance of infection or the number of organisms in the urine. The drug has no diuretic effect and won't increase urine flow. This medication is not an analgesic and does not decrease pain.
CN: Physiological integrity; CNS: Pharmacological and parenteral therapies; CL: Analyze

34. 2. Parents will grieve the loss of the "normal" child when their neonate is born with this condition. Then nurse should listen to their concerns for their neonate's health first. Suggesting a support group, or referring the parents to a counselor, might be good actions, but not initially. The provider will need to spend time with these parents after the nurse has allowed the parents to express their grief and anger.
CN: Psychosocial integrity; CNS: None; CL: Apply

35. 1. Hypertensive episodes are suggestive of decreasing renal function. Pain, decreased oxygen saturation and apathy are not normally suggestive of decreased renal function.
CN: Physiological integrity; CNS: Physiological adaptation; CL: Analyze

36. A student nurse asks the nurse about the difference between hypospadias and epispadias. What is the nurse's **best** response?
1. Epispadias can only occur in males and may cause sterility.
2. The difference between these conditions is the length of the urethra and size of the urinary meatus.
3. The urinary meatus is on the ventral side of the penis with hypospadias, and on the dorsal side of the penis with epispadias.
4. The urinary meatus is on the dorsal side of the penis with hypospadias, and on the ventral side of the penis with epispadias.

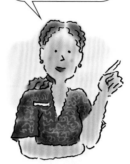

Question 36 is asking you to differentiate between two conditions.

36. 3. Hypospadias results from the incomplete closure of the urethral folds along the ventral surface of the developing penis. Epispadias results when the urinary meatus is on the dorsal surface of the penis. Epispadias can occur in males and females, although it is very rare in females.
CN: Health promotion and maintenance; CNS: None; CL: Apply

37. A school-age child, who weighs 80.5 lb (36.5 kg), has been prescribed a 250 ml bolus of normal saline administered over one hour, followed by a maintenance infusion of 2 ml/kg/hr of the same fluid. The nurse initiated therapy at 1200 and is recording intake and output at 1800. What is the intravenous intake of this child? Record your answer using a whole number.

_____ ml

37. 615.
The nurse should record 250 ml of bolused fluid between 1200 and 1300. To calculate the rate per hour for the infusion, the nurse should multiply 36.5 kg by 2 ml/kg/hr, which equals 73 ml/hr. Five hours at this rate equals 365 ml. Including the bolus, the client's six hour intake is 615 ml.
CN: Physiological integrity; CNS: Pharmacological and parenteral therapies; CL: Apply

38. A nurse is teaching a parent, whose child has had hypospadias repair with a skin graft, about postsurgical care. Which statement, made by the parent, would indicate the need for further teaching?
1. "My child won't be able to take tub baths until healing has occurred."
2. 'I will change the dressing around the penis daily."
3. "I will make sure I change my child's diaper often."
4. "If there's a color change in the penis, I will notify my child's provider."

38. 2. Dressing changes after a hypospadias repair with a skin graft are generally performed by the provider, and are not performed every day because the skin graft needs time to heal and adhere to the penis. Baths aren't given until postoperative healing has taken place. Changing the infant's diapers typically helps keep the penis dry. If the penis color changes, it might be evidence of circulation problems and should be reported.
CN: Health promotion and maintenance; CNS: None; CL: Analyze

39. A nurse is preparing the parents of an infant born with hypospadias for upcoming surgery. The nurse determines further teaching is necessary when the parent states:
1. "Skin grafting may be involved in my infant's repair."
2. "My infant's penis will look perfectly normal following surgery."
3. "Surgical repair may need to be performed in several stages."
4. "My infant will probably be in pain after surgery and may require pain medication."

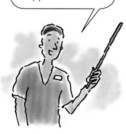

Stay alert for further teaching opportunities.

39. 2. Parents should understand that their infant's penis may not appear normal following surgery. The goals of surgery are to allow the child to void from the tip of his penis, with a straight urine stream, while standing up.
CN: Psychosocial integrity; CNS: None; CL: Apply

40. Which assessment data, collected by the nurse, would inform the provider that a staged, rather than single repair of hypospadias may be required?
1. Chordee is present with the hypospadias.
2. The urinary meatus opens at the scrotum.
3. The urinary meatus is just below the tip of the penis.
4. The infant was circumcised before the defect was discovered.

40. 2. Increased surgical experience and improvements in technique have reduced the number of staged procedures for hypospadias defects. A staged procedure is indicated in severe defects with marked deficits of available skin for mobilization of flaps and inadequate urethral length. Having a chordee present doesn't require a staged hypospadias repair. If an infant has been circumcised, but has a relatively minor hypospadias, the repair can still occur in one stage.
CN: Physiological integrity; CNS: Physiological adaptation; CL: Analyze

41. The nurse is providing health education to an adolescent about the prevention of pelvic inflammatory disease (PID). Which should the nurse address?
1. The relationship between poor hygiene practices and the risk of PID
2. The role of hormonal contraceptives in decreasing the risk of PID
3. The potential long-term complications related to reproductive tract infections
4. The risk of birth defects in infants born to women who have had PID

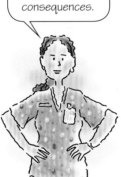

Untreated PID can have long-term and serious consequences.

41. 3. Long-term complications of PID include abscess formation in the fallopian tubes and adhesion formation leading to an increased risk of ectopic pregnancy or infertility. Pelvic inflammatory disease isn't prevented by proper personal hygiene or any form of hormonal contraception. PID does not increase the risk of birth defects in infants born to women who have had PID.
CN: Health promotion and maintenance; CNS: None; CL: Apply

42. The nurse has completed discharge teaching to a teenage client who was treated for a sexually transmitted infection (STI). The nurse determines that teaching was effective when the client states:
1. "I'll be sure to get a penicillin shot at the first sign of infection."
2. "I will inform my sex partners of my infection, and not have unprotected sex from now on."
3. "I will be very careful not to have intercourse with someone who has an STI."
4. "I now know that there are many different kinds of STIs with the same symptoms."

42. 2. Goal achievement is indicated by the client's ability to describe preventive behaviors and health practices. The other options indicate that the client doesn't understand the correct information regarding diagnosis and treatment of STIs.
CN: Health promotion and maintenance; CNS: None; CL: Analyze

43. An adolescent has been referred to a primary care provider with symptoms of a sexually-transmitted infection (STI). Which adolescent should be assessed for a chlamydial infection?
1. Girl with intense pelvic pain and irregular menstrual cycles
2. Boy with a fever and chancre on the shaft of his penis
3. Boy who reports dysuria and urethral itching
4. Girl who has recently developed genital vesicles

43. 3. Clinical manifestations of chlamydia include meatal erythema, tenderness, itching, dysuria, and urethral discharge in the male and mucopurulent cervical exudate with erythema, edema, and congestion in the female. Menstrual cycles are not affected. Vesicles in the genital area are more consistent with herpes simplex virus. Males do not develop chancres as a result of chlamydial infection.
CN: Physiological integrity; CNS: Reduction of risk potential; CL: Analyze

CN: Client needs category   CNS: Client needs subcategory   CL: Cognitive level

44. An adolescent male has presented with several painless chancres on the shaft of his penis. What is the **priority** assessment before treatment for this client?
1. Portal of entry
2. Size and number of the chancres
3. Names of sexual contacts
4. Existence of medication allergies

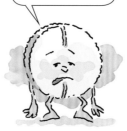

Some people are just hypersensitive—to me, that is.

45. A nurse wants to provide an open environment with adolescents while discussing sex and sexual activities. What is the **best** way for the nurse to obtain this goal?
1. Break the information down into scientific terminology
2. Refer the adolescents to their parents for sexual information
3. Answer only questions that are asked
4. Present sexual information in a straightforward manner using proper terminology

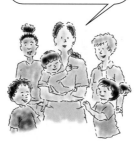

The NCLEX tests your ability to teach clients at different life stages.

46. An adolescent girl is being treated for anogenital warts caused by the human papillomavirus (HPV). What is the nurse's **priority** intervention for this client?
1. Educate the client about the need to adhere to antibiotic therapy
2. Educate the client about the accompanying risk of cervical cancer
3. Assess the client's knowledge of hormonal contraceptives
4. Assess the client for signs and symptoms of systemic infection

47. Which statement, by a nurse, **most** accurately addresses an adolescent female's questions regarding the treatment of gonorrhea?
1. "The disease can be cured by a two week, oral dose of penicillin."
2. "Gonorrhea is easily spread, and I should notify anyone that I've had sex with so they can be treated."
3. "I will need to come into the clinic for several weeks of penicillin injections to treat my gonorrhea."
4. "I may have contracted this disease by not changing my tampons often enough."

44. 4. This client likely has syphilis, and the treatment of choice for syphilis is penicillin. Clients allergic to penicillin must be given another antibiotic. It is not necessary to assess the names of sexual contacts, the portal of entry or the distribution chancres before treatment can begin.
CN: Safe and effective care environment; CNS: Management of care ; CL: Apply

45. 4. Although many adolescents have received sex education from parents and school throughout childhood, they aren't always adequately prepared for the impact of puberty. A large portion of their knowledge is acquired from peers, television, movies, and magazines. Consequently, much of the information they receive incomplete or inaccurate.
CN: Health promotion and maintenance; CNS: None; CL: Apply

46. 2. This client's external lesions should be treated, and she should receive education regarding the relationship between HPV and cervical cancer. Antibiotics are would be ineffective because of the viral etiology of HPV. Hormonal contraceptives are of no benefit, and HPV is not normally the cause of systemic infection.
CN: Safe and effective care environment; CNS: Management of care; CL: Apply

47. 2. Adolescents should be taught that treatment is needed for all sexual partners. Gonorrhea is treated with a single dose of IM ceftriaxone sodium and a single oral dose of azithromycin. Gonorrhea can't be contracted from the use of tampons.
CN: Health promotion and maintenance; CNS: None; CL: Apply

CN: Client needs category   CNS: Client needs subcategory   CL: Cognitive level

48. A nurse is planning education regarding sex and contraceptive use for adolescents. Which factor is **most** important for this nurse to include?
1. Most adolescents will resist dialogue with health care providers regarding the risks of sexuality.
2. Most adolescents are knowledgeable about reproduction.
3. Most adolescents use pregnancy as a way to rebel against their parents.
4. Most adolescents are open to contraception, but are inconsistent with birth control usage.

48. 4. Most teenagers today are open to discussing contraception and sexuality, but may get caught up in the moment and forget about birth control measures. Very few teenagers use pregnancy as a way to rebel against their parents. Most information that adolescents have regarding contraception and sexuality comes from their peers and is often inaccurate.

CN: Health promotion and maintenance; CNS: None; CL: Analyze

49. A sexually active male adolescent is discussing the prevention of sexually-transmitted infections (STIs) with the school nurse. Which statement, by the client, **best** demonstrates an accurate understanding of prevention?
1. "My girlfriend is on the pill, so we aren't worried about contracting diseases from each other."
2. "We practice the rhythm method of birth control, so we don't have sex when we could catch anything."
3. "I prefer using a condom and a spermicide instead of asking my girlfriend to use a sponge."
4. "My friends tell me that if I use the withdrawal method, I am never going to get an STI."

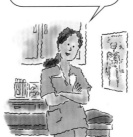

Nice work! You've finished almost 50 questions already!

49. 3. Preventing STIs is the primary concern of health care professionals. Barrier contraceptive methods, such as condoms with the addition of spermicide, offer the best protection against STIs and their complications. Oral contraceptives, the rhythm, or withdrawal method don't prevent the transmission of an STI.

CN: Health promotion and maintenance; CNS: None; CL: Analyze

50. Which developmental rationale **best** explains the risk-taking behavior of adolescents?
1. Adolescents are concrete thinkers and concentrate only on what's happening at the time.
2. Belief in their own invulnerability persuades adolescents that they can take risks safely.
3. The risk of angering and disappointing a parent usually deters an adolescent from engaging in risky behavior.
4. Peer pressure usually doesn't play an important part in an adolescent's decision to become sexually active.

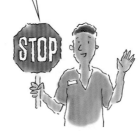

Adolescents may engage in sex as part of risky behavior.

50. 2. Understanding the growth and development of adolescents helps the nurse understand that they often feel invulnerable to risky behavior. Adolescents think about the future, and can become independent and self-governing person *within* relationships. They have gained the ability to make and follow through with their own decisions, live by their own set of principles of right and wrong and have become less emotionally dependent on parents. Peer pressure plays an important role in risk-taking behaviors, more than the fear of angering or disappointing a parent.

CN: Health promotion and maintenance; CNS: None; CL: Analyze

CN: Client needs category   CNS: Client needs subcategory   CL: Cognitive level

51. A nurse is preparing to administer the prescribed dose of erythromycin ointment to a neonate born to an adolescent. Where should the nurse apply this ointment?

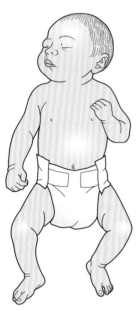

51. To prevent gonococcal ophthalmia neonatorum, a prophylactic agent should be instilled into both eyes of all newborn infants. This procedure is required by law in most jurisdictions. The treatment can be refused by a parent and would require appropriate documentation to be completed.

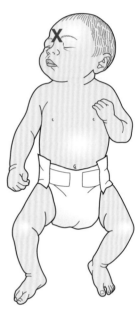

CN: Safe, effective care environment; CNS: Safety and infection control; CL: Apply

52. What information should the nurse include in the discharge teaching for an adolescent client who's taking metronidazole to treat trichomoniasis?
1. Sexual intercourse should be avoided until the medication is completed.
2. Alcohol shouldn't be consumed while taking this medication.
3. Milk products should be avoided since they reduce the effectiveness of the medicine.
4. Exposure to sunlight should be limited to one hour per day.

52. 2. Clients should not consume alcohol for 48 hours following the last dose of metronidazole. The other choices have no effect on the client taking this medication.
CN: Physiological integrity; CNS: Pharmacological and parenteral therapies; CL: Apply

53. The nurse determines that more education about sexually transmitted infections (STIs) is needed when an adolescent states:
1. "The gonorrhea virus is one of the most common STIs in kids my age."
2. "The most common STI in kids my age is chlamydia infection."
3. "Most girls who have chlamydia don't even know it."
4. "Symptoms of gonorrhea can show up a day or a couple of weeks after you're infected."

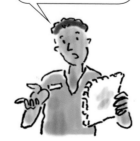

Some sexually transmitted diseases can occur with or without symptoms.

53. 1. Gonorrhea is a bacterial infection, not a viral infection. All of the other statements are accurate.
CN: Health promotion and maintenance; CNS: None; CL: Apply

CN: Client needs category   CNS: Client needs subcategory   CL: Cognitive level

54. A school nurse is developing a new prevention program regarding sexually transmitted infection (STI). Which preventative behaviors should be addressed in this program? Select all that apply.
1. Delaying first sexual intercourse
2. Using the rhythm method safely and effectively
3. Reducing the number of sexual partners
4. Encouraging adolescents to not talk about sex with others
5. Increasing use of condoms

55. A nurse is working with a number of adolescent clients. Which client is at **highest** risk of contracting HIV?
1. A client who lives in crowded housing with poor ventilation
2. A young, sexually active client with multiple partners
3. An adolescent who's homeless and lives in shelters
4. A client who uses marijuana heavily

56. An adolescent female client reports a low-grade fever, lower abdominal pain, and frequent, painful urination. What is the nurse's **priority** action?
1. Assess the client for additional signs and symptoms of pelvic inflammatory disease (PID)
2. Refer the client to be assessed for HIV
3. Educate the client about the prevention of sexually-transmitted infections (STIs)
4. Inspect the client's vulva for the presence of chancres

57. A nurse is preparing to teach an adolescent group about HIV. What is the nurse's **most** appropriate action?
1. Describe the changes in epidemiological trends of HIV that have taken place in recent years
2. Prepare a presentation that accurately describes HIV, using age-appropriate language
3. Reassure participants that anything they disclose will be confidential
4. Emphasize the devastating effects of HIV in an effort to prevent sexual activity

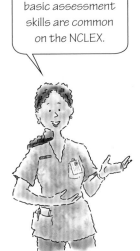

Questions about basic assessment skills are common on the NCLEX.

54. 1, 3, 5. Sexually-transmitted infection prevention programs have had a significant impact on reducing sexual risk behaviors by addressing the importance of condom use, reducing the number of sexual partners, and delaying the initial sexual contact. The rhythm method has no impact on prevention of STIs. Adolescents are less likely to adhere to what is taught if they are not encouraged to discuss sex with other people.
CN: Health promotion and maintenance; CNS: Safety and infection control; CL: Apply

55. 2. The younger the client when sexual activity begins, the higher the incidence of HIV. Also, the more sexual partners he or she has, the higher the incidence of this virus. Neither crowded living environments nor homeless environments, by themselves, lead to an increase in the incidence of HIV. Marijuana use is not an independent risk factor for HIV infection.
CN: Physiological integrity; CNS: Reduction of risk potential; CL: Analyze

56. 1. PID is an infection of the upper female genital tract, most commonly caused by STIs. Chancres are associated with syphilis, which is not a common cause of PID. Similarly, HIV does not normally cause PID. Education is important, but assessment and treatment are short-term priorities.
CN: Safe and effective care environment; CNS: Management of care; CL: Analyze

57. 2. Clear, accurate information using age-appropriate language is most appropriate. The nurse cannot guarantee the confidentiality of information, since some statements must be reported by law. The nurse should not attempt to scare adolescents into changing their behavior. Epidemiological trends are not a priority learning need for adolescents.
CN: Health promotion and maintenance; CNS: None; CL: Apply

CN: Client needs category   CNS: Client needs subcategory   CL: Cognitive level

58. A nurse is planning a program to teach adolescents about HIV. Which action, by the nurse, would enhance this program's success?
1. Survey the community to evaluate the level of education
2. Obtain peer educators to provide information about HIV
3. Set up clinics in community centers and have condoms readily available
4. Have primary health care providers host workshops in community centers

58. 2. Teens are more likely to ask questions of peer educators than of adults. This type of education can change personal teens's attitudes, and their perception of the risk of HIV infection. The other approaches would be helpful, but may not make the outreach program more successful.
CN: Health promotion and maintenance; CNS: None; CL: Apply

59. The nurse has completed teaching an adolescent about syphilis. The nurse determines further teaching is necessary when the adolescent states:
1. "The disease is divided into specific stages."
2. "Affected persons are least infectious during the first year."
3. "Syphilis is easily treated with penicillin or doxycycline."
4. "Syphilis is usually transmitted sexually."

59. 2. Affected persons are most contagious in the first year of the disease. About 95% of syphilis cases are transmitted sexually. There are distinct stages of syphilis, although some people may not experience every stage. The drug of choice for treating syphilis is penicillin or doxycycline.
CN: Health promotion and maintenance; CNS: None; CL: Analyze

Sixty questions down. You deserve a break.

60. A nurse is teaching a group of parents about monitoring for urinary tract infection (UTI) in preschoolers. Which symptom would indicate that a child should be evaluated?
1. The child voids only twice in any six-hour period.
2. The child exhibits incontinence after being toilet trained.
3. The child has difficulty sitting still for more than 30 minutes at a time.
4. The urine has a strong odor of ammonia after standing at room temperature for more than two hours.

60. 2. A child, who exhibits incontinence after being toilet trained, should be evaluated for UTI. Most urine has a strong odor of ammonia after standing for more than two hours, and doesn't necessarily indicate a UTI. The other options aren't a cause for parents to suspect a problem with their child's urinary system.
CN: Physiological integrity; CNS: Reduction of risk potential; CL: Analyze

61. What instruction should the nurse include in a teaching plan for an adolescent client receiving co-trimoxazole for a recurring urinary tract infection caused by *Escherichia coli*?
1. Drink cranberry juice each day to help acidify your urine
2. Take the full course of this medication, even if your symptoms disappear in a few days
3. Return to the clinic in three days for another urine culture
4. Take two pills each day for two days, and save the rest if symptoms reappear within two weeks

Teaching about medications—that's another common NCLEX subject.

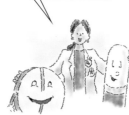

61. 2. Discharge instructions should include taking the full course of the prescribed medication to fully eradicate the causative bacteria. Drinking cranberry juice may help maintain urinary health but won't eliminate and existing infection. Reassessing after three days of treatment will not accurately evaluate the medication's effectiveness. Taking this medication for too brief of a period will not eliminate the infection.
CN: Physiological integrity; CNS: Pharmacological and parenteral therapies; CL: Apply

62. What fact should the nurse include when teaching the parents of a child with recurring urinary tract infections (UTIs)?
1. Antibiotics should be discontinued 48 hours after symptoms subside.
2. Recurrent symptoms should be treated by renewing the antibiotic prescription.
3. Complicated UTIs are related to poor perineal hygiene practice.
4. Follow-up urine cultures are necessary to detect recurring infections and antibiotic effectiveness.

62. 4. A follow-up urine specimen is usually obtained 2 to 3 days after the completion of the antibiotic treatment. The full course of antibiotics should be taken and not stopped if symptoms disappear. If symptoms reappear, a urine culture should be obtained to determine if the infection is resistant to the prescribed antibiotics. Simple UTIs are generally caused by poor perineal hygiene.
CN: Physiological integrity; CNS: Reduction of risk potential; CL: Apply

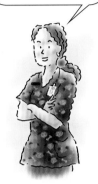

Multiplication is bacteria's favorite function.

63. A nurse is reviewing a child's clean-void urine specimen results. Which result would **best** indicate that the child has a urinary tract infection (UTI)?
1. A specific gravity of 1.020
2. Cloudy appearance without odor
3. A large amount of casts present
4. 100,000 bacterial colonies/ml

63. 4. The diagnosis of a UTI is determined by bacteria in the urine. Infected urine usually contains more than 100,000 colonies/ml, usually of a single organism. Infected urine is often cloudy, odorous, and may have strands of mucus. Casts and increased specific gravity aren't specific to UTI.
CN: Physiological integrity; CNS: Reduction of risk potential; CL: Apply

64. The nurse is providing teaching to the parents of a school-age girl with a urinary tract infection (UTI). Which factor predisposes this child to a UTI?
1. The client was recently treated with antibiotics for a respiratory infection.
2. The client's urethra is comparatively short.
3. The client drinks fruit juices more than water or milk.
4. The client recently received scheduled immunizations.

64. 2. The shorter, female urethra contributes to infection because bacteria have a shorter distance to travel to enter the urinary tract. Recent antibiotic use, recent immunizations and consumption of fruit juices do not predispose this child to UTIs.
CN: Health promotion and maintenance; CNS: None; CL: Apply

65. A nurse is assessing a child with vesicoureteral reflux. For which condition should the nurse be alert to as a potential complication?
1. Glomerulonephritis
2. Hemolytic uremia syndrome
3. Nephrotic syndrome
4. Renal infection

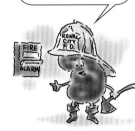

When I get infected, all kinds of alarms go off!

65. 4. The reflux of urine into the ureters, and then back into the bladder after voiding, predisposes this client to a urinary tract infections due to urinary stasis. Reflux can lead to renal damage due to scarring of the parenchyma. Glomerulonephritis is an autoimmune reaction to a beta-hemolytic strep infection. Hemolytic uremia syndrome may be the result of genetic factors. Eighty percent of nephrotic syndrome cases are idiopathic.
CN: Health promotion and maintenance; CNS: None; CL: Analyze

66. The mother of a female child asks the nurse, "How can I prevent my daughter from getting urinary tract infections (UTIs)?" What is the nurse's **best** response?
1. Instruct the mother on the relationship between diet and UTIs
2. Encourage the mother to shower her daughter rather than bathe her
3. Emphasize the correct way for the child to wipe after using the toilet
4. Teach the mother the importance of hand hygiene

66. 3. Girls are higher risk for bacterial invasion of the urinary tract because of basic the female urethra is short and in close proximity to the anus. Wiping toward the anus rather than toward the vagina is important. There is minimal relationship between UTIs and diet. Showering has no notable benefit when compared to bathing. Hand hygiene is a vital aspect of health education, but does not directly relate to UTIs.
CN: Physiological integrity; CNS: Reduction in risk potential; CL: Apply

67. A child has been sent to the school nurse's office after being incontinent of urine three times in the past two days. The nurse should recommend that this child be evaluated for:
1. fluid volume excess.
2. emotional trauma.
3. urinary tract infection (UTI).
4. a structural defect of the urinary tract.

67. 3. Frequent urinary incontinence should be evaluated. The child should be assessed for a UTI. Structural defects may be the cause of a urinary tract infection, but this is not the first consideration. Fluid volume excess will not normally cause incontinence in an otherwise continent child. After infection, structural defect, and diabetes mellitus have been ruled out, emotional trauma should be investigated.
CN: Physiological integrity; CNS: Reduction of risk potential; CL: Apply

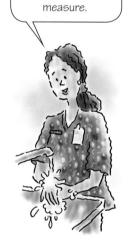

Sometimes, simple hygienic habits offer the best preventative measure.

68. A nurse is teaching a group of parents about recurrent urinary tract infections (UTIs) in their children. What is the **priority** educational goal for this group of parents?
1. Parents will describe laboratory testing related to UTI detection
2. Parents will explain the diagnostic criteria for UTI
3. Parents will identify ways of preventing UTIs
4. Parents will describe the most common treatments for UTI

68. 3. Prevention is the most important goal of teaching about primary and recurrent UTIs. The most preventive measures are simple hygienic practices that should be a routine part of daily care. Treatment, detection, and testing are all important, but are not the priority goal.
CN: Physiological integrity; CNS: Reduction of risk potential; CL: Analyze

69. Which intervention should the nurse recommend to the parents of female children to help prevent urinary tract infections (UTIs)?
1. Limit tub bathing as much as possible
2. Increase fluids and decrease salt intake
3. Have the child wear cotton underpants
4. Have the child clean her perineum from back to front

69. 3. Cotton is a more breathable fabric than synthetic fibers, and allows dampness to be wicked from the perineum. Bathing shouldn't be limited, but bubble baths and whirlpool baths should be infrequent or eliminated if a UTI is present. Increasing fluids is helpful, but there is no need to decrease sodium intake. The perineum should always be cleaned from front to back.
CN: Health promotion and maintenance; CNS: None; CL: Apply

70. Which health education topic is the **priority** when teaching parents ways to prevent urinary tract infections (UTIs) in their children?
1. Teach parents to promote adequate fluid intake
2. Teach parents to limit the frequency of tub baths
3. Encourage parents of male infants to avoid circumcision
4. Educate parents about hand washing, and the use of alcohol-based hand sanitizers

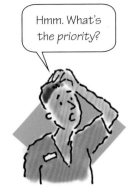

Hmm. What's the priority?

70. 1. Urinary stasis is a major cause of UTIs, and can be partially prevented by increasing fluid intake. Baths and hand hygiene are less significant factors in the development of UTIs. Urinary tract infections are increased in uncircumcised male infants under one year of age, but unaffected thereafter.

CN: Physiological integrity; CNS: Reduction of risk potential; CL: Apply

71. The nurse is assessing an infant for signs of urinary tract infection (UTI). What sign should the nurse anticipate in a child of this age?
1. Abdominal tenderness
2. Feeding problems
3. Frequency
4. Urgency

71. 2. In infants and children less than two years old, the signs of a UTI are characteristically non-specific and can mimic gastrointestinal disorders. A reluctance to take food is often the first indication. Abdominal pain, urinary urgency, and frequency would be observed in the older child with a UTI.

CN: Physiological integrity; CNS: Physiological adaptation; CL: Apply

72. A nurse is caring for a toddler scheduled for a urine culture and sensitivity test. What is the **best** way for the nurse to obtain the sample?
1. Obtain a bagged urine specimen
2. Teach the parent how to obtain a clean-catch urine specimen
3. Monitor the child until a first-voided urine specimen can be obtained
4. Obtain an order for intermittent catheterization

72. 4. The most accurate urine culture tests for bacterial content in children under two years of age are suprapubic aspiration and bladder catheterization. The other methods have a high incidence of contamination not related to infection.

CN: Physiological integrity; CNS: Reduction of Risk Potential; CL: Apply

73. What is the nurse's **most** appropriate action following collection of a urine specimen for a culture and sensitivity test?
1. Arrange for immediate delivery to the laboratory
2. Monitor the client's next voided urine
3. Observe the specimen for cloudiness or sediment
4. Keep the specimen in the refrigerator until it can be taken to the laboratory

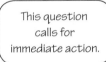

This question calls for immediate action.

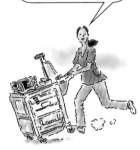

73. 1. Care of urine specimens obtained for culture is an important aspect of nursing related to diagnosis. Specimens should be immediately taken to the laboratory for culture. If the culture is delayed, the specimen can be placed in the refrigerator. Storage can result in a loss of formed elements, such as blood cells and casts. The laboratory will perform an analysis of the sample. There is no need to monitor the client's next void.

CN: Physiological integrity; CNS: Reduction of risk potential; CL: Apply

74. The nurse is teaching the parents of a child with a urinary tract infection (UTI) about fluid intake. Which statement by the parent would indicate the need for further education?
1. "I should encourage my child to drink as much as she possibly can throughout the day."
2. "Clear liquids should be the primary source of hydration for my daughter."
3. "I should offer my child a carbonated or non-carbonated beverages every two hours."
4. "My child should avoid drinking caffeinated beverages."

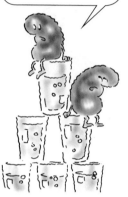

How many glasses of water do you need to drink to keep us healthy?

74. 3. Caffeinated and carbonated beverages should be avoided because of their potentially irritating effect on the bladder mucosa. Children should have between five and eight cups of water each day. Adequate fluid intake is indicated for a client with an acute UTI. The client should primarily drink clear liquids.

CN: Physiological integrity; CNS: Basic care and comfort; CL: Analyze

75. A nurse is planning the care of a child who has a long history of recurrent urinary tract infections (UTIs). The child's care plan would **most** likely include:
1. intermittent catheterization every six hours.
2. administration of prophylactic antibiotics as prescribed.
3. limitation of activities in which there is any risk of genitourinary injury.
4. preparation for a surgical intervention.

75. 2. Children who experience recurrent UTIs may require ongoing antibiotic therapy. A client with a recurring UTI would be investigated for anatomic abnormalities, and a potential surgical intervention. The client would be placed on antibiotics prior to the tests. The child's activities aren't limited, and frequent catheterization predisposes the child to infection.

CN: Physiological integrity; CNS: Pharmacological and parenteral therapies; CL: Apply

76. A nurse is teaching parents about administering medication to their child with a recurring urinary tract infection (UTI). What information should the nurse include?
1. The medication should be given mid-morning.
2. The medication should be given right before bedtime.
3. The medication should be given four times a day.
4. Administration time is unimportant, as long as the proper dose is given.

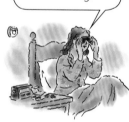

Why do I feel like I'm forgetting something?

76. 2. Medication for a UTI is commonly administered every twelve hours. The benefits of the medication will be greatest if it is given right before bedtime, which is the longest span.

CN: Physiological integrity; CNS: Pharmacological and parenteral therapies; CL: Apply

77. The nurse is providing education to a group of parents about urinary tract infections (UTIs). Which group has the greatest potential for progressive renal injury following a UTI?
1. School-aged children who must get permission to go to the bathroom
2. Adolescent females who have started menstruation
3. Children who compete in competitive sports
4. Young infants or toddlers

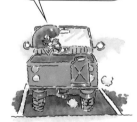

In which type of client am I most likely to be injured following a UTI?

77. 4. The hazard of progressive renal injury is greatest when infection occurs in young children, especially those under two years old. The first two answers might lead to a simple UTI that would require treatment. Competitive sports have no bearing on a UTI.

CN: Safe and effective care environment; CNS: Safety and infection control; CL: Analyze

CN: Client needs category   CNS: Client needs subcategory   CL: Cognitive level

78. A child is in the recovery period following surgery to remove a Wilms' tumor. What is the nurse's **most** appropriate statement, to these parents, regarding this surgery?
1. Children will readily lie in bed and restrict their activities.
2. Recovery is typically fast despite the large abdominal incision.
3. Recovery time is lengthy because of the large incision.
4. Parents should assist their child with activities of daily living (ADLs) for two weeks following surgery.

78. **2.** Children generally recover very quickly from surgery to remove a Wilms' tumor, even though they may have a large abdominal incision. Children are often anxious to return to their routine and play. Though some regression is expected, parents should encourage their child to perform as many ADLs as possible.
CN: Psychosocial integrity; CNS: None; CL: Analyze

79. A nurse is teaching parents about administering co-trimoxazole to their child for the treatment of a urinary tract infection (UTI). What instruction should the nurse include?
1. Give the medication with food
2. Give the medication with a full glass of water
3. Give the medication immediately after a meal
4. Give the medication 60 minutes after a meal

79. **2.** Co-trimoxazole should be administered with a full glass of water on an empty stomach in order to maximize therapeutic benefits and minimize adverse effects.
CN: Physiological integrity; CNS: Pharmacological and parenteral therapies; CL: Apply

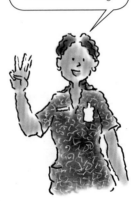

Here's a little hint . . . three of these choices are wrong.

80. A nurse is preparing to assess a child with a history of Wilms' tumor. What information should the nurse consider when planning care for this child?
1. Peak incidence occurs at 10 years of age.
2. It is the least common type of renal cancer.
3. It is the most common type of renal cancer.
4. It has a decreased incidence among siblings.

80. **3.** Wilms' tumor is the most frequent intra-abdominal tumor of childhood, and the most common type of renal cancer. The tumor most commonly appears at three years of age. Siblings and identical twins are also most commonly affected by Wilms' tumor.
CN: Physiological integrity; CNS: Physiological adaptation; CL: Apply

81. A child presents at the emergency room with abdominal pain, blood in the urine, hypertension, and a palpable abdominal mass. What is the nurse's **best** action?
1. Auscultate the child's lungs
2. Prepare the child for an abdominal ultrasound
3. Restrict the child to bed rest pending diagnostic testing
4. Administer a bolus of intravenous normal saline as prescribed

81. **2.** The most common presenting sign of Wilms' tumor is a swelling or mass within the abdomen. The initial diagnostic for Wilms' tumor is typically an abdominal ultrasound. A fluid bolus would be of no benefit. Vigorous activity would be contraindicated, but there is no need for strict bed rest. Chest auscultation would be performed as part of a head to toe assessment, but is not specific to the diagnosis of Wilms' tumor.
CN: Safe and effective care environment; CNS: Management of care; CL: Apply

82. A nurse is explaining a diagnosis of Wilms' tumor to the parents of a child. The nurse determines that further teaching is necessary when the parent states:

1. "Wilms' tumor usually involves both kidneys."
2. "Wilms' tumor occurs slightly more commonly in the left kidney."
3. "Wilms' tumor is staged during surgery for treatment planning."
4. "Wilms' tumor will remain encapsulated for an extended period of time."

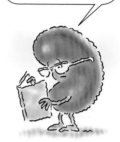

Let me see what I can learn about Wilms' tumor.

82. 1. Wilms' tumor usually involves only one kidney and is usually staged during surgery so that an effective course of treatment can be established. Wilms' tumor has a slightly higher occurrence in the left kidney, and it stays encapsulated for an extended period of time.

CN: Physiological integrity; CNS: Physiological adaptation; CL: Apply

83. The nurse has reviewed the treatment plan of a child with Wilms' tumor on both kidneys. What action would the nurse **most** likely perform?

1. Teach the child and family about peritoneal dialysis
2. Prepare the child for abdominal gavage
3. Describe common side effects of radiation and chemotherapy to the family
4. Administer antibiotics and IV fluid therapy as prescribed

83. 3. If both kidneys are involved, the child may be treated with radiation or chemotherapy preoperatively to shrink the tumor. Peritoneal dialysis would only be needed if the kidneys aren't functioning. Abdominal gavage wouldn't be indicated. Antibiotics aren't needed, because Wilms' tumor isn't an infection.

CN: Safe and effective care environment; CNS: ; CL: Apply

84. A nurse is planning preoperative care for a child diagnosed with Wilms' tumor. What is the nurse's **most** important intervention?

1. Prepare the family for the initiation of chemotherapy and radiation
2. Avoid abdominal palpation or manipulation
3. Insert a nasogastric tube for enteral feedings
4. Begin IV therapy of hyperalimentation and lipids

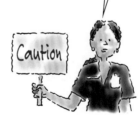

Note the word preoperative in question 84.

Caution

84. 2. After a diagnosis of Wilms' tumor, the abdomen should not be palpated. Palpation of the tumor could lead to rupture, which would spread cancerous cells throughout the abdomen. If surgery is successful, long-term radiation and chemotherapy would not be required. Enteral feedings and total parenteral nutrition are not part of the preoperative treatment of Wilms' tumor. Radiation and chemotherapy are not started preoperatively.

CN: Safe and effective care environment; CNS: Management of care; CL: Apply

85. The nurse is caring for a child in recovery following surgery to remove a Wilms' tumor from one kidney. What nursing action is **most** appropriate?

1. Place the child on protective isolation precautions
2. Tell the family that a kidney transplant will eventually be needed
3. Ensure that the child adheres to a low-protein diet for the next few weeks
4. Prepare the child and family for chemotherapy, and possibly radiotherapy

85. 4. Because radiation and chemotherapy are part of the post-operative treatment for Wilms' tumor, parents should be advised of the expectations, benefits and adverse effects of this treatment. Kidney transplant isn't usually necessary. Standard precautions are sufficient, and there is no need for a low-protein diet.

CN: Safe and effective care environment; CNS: Management of care; CL: Apply

86. The nurse is performing an assessment of a child who has been diagnosed with Wilms' tumor. Which area should not be palpated?

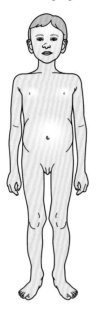

86. To avoid trauma, the nurse should not palpate the abdomen when a Wilms' tumor is suspected or confirmed.

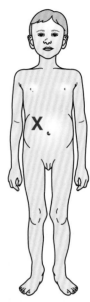

CN: Health promotion and maintenance; CNS: None; CL: Apply

87. The nurse is providing care for a child just diagnosed with Wilms' tumor. The child's family asks the nurse about surgery. What anticipatory guidance should the nurse provide to this family?
1. If chemotherapy and radiation fail, surgery will be performed.
2. Surgery is usually performed within 24 to 48 hours of admission.
3. Targeted therapy has become a first-line treatment for Wilms' tumor.
4. Surgery will be performed within four weeks if the child is in good overall health.

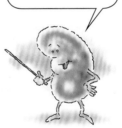

Do you know the preferred treatment for Wilms' tumor?

87. 2. Surgery is the preferred treatment for Wilms' tumor, and is usually scheduled as soon as possible after a renal mass has been confirmed.

CN: Safe and effective care environment; CNS: Management of care; CL: Apply

88. A nurse is caring for a three-year-old child following the removal of a Wilms' tumor. The mother states that her child is in pain, and requests pain medication. What is the nurse's **priority** in regards to this mother's request?
1. Assess the child's pain by asking the child to rate his pain on a 1 to 10 scale
2. Prepare to administer the ordered pain medication
3. Use the Faces Pain Scale to assess the child's degree of pain
4. Document the report of pain, and note the time of the last pain medication

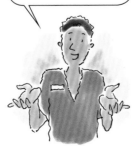

What should you always do before administering a pain medication to a client of this age?

88. 3. The nurse should assess the client's pain level using the age-appropriate Faces Pain Scale. After the pain assessment, the nurse should determine the time previous pain medications were administered and medicate accordingly.

CN: Health promotion and Maintenance; CNS: None; CL: Apply

CN: Client needs category   CNS: Client needs subcategory   CL: Cognitive level

89. The parents of a child, diagnosed with Wilms' tumor refuse to seek treatment because of their religious beliefs. Which statement, by the nurse, indicates a lack of understanding of these parent's decision?

1. "I know you have received a lot of information in a short period of time."
2. "I don't think you have the legal right to make these kinds of decisions."
3. "You don't understand how easily a Wilms' tumor can be treated."
4. "I think you are in shock and don't understand the situation."

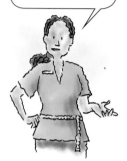

Remember to respect the parents' religious beliefs.

89. 2. Parents have the legal right to make decisions regarding the healthcare of their child. Religion plays an important role in many people's lives, and healthcare decisions are sometimes made that defy scientific reasoning. The parents may be in a state of shock due to the amount of information that has been presented. The decision to treat Wilms' tumor by surgical intervention should be made quickly for optimal results.
CN: Safe, effective care environment; CNS: Management of care; CL: Analyze

90. A child with Wilms' tumor has had a kidney removed, and is now receiving chemotherapy. What **priority** information should the nurse share with this child's family at the time of discharge?

1. Avoid contact sports
2. Limit fluid intake as ordered
3. Decrease sodium intake
4. Avoid contact with other children

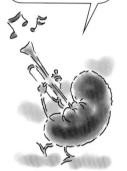

A well-hydrated kidney is a happy kidney.

90. 1. Because the child has only one kidney, certain precautions are recommended to prevent injury to the remaining kidney. Fluid intake is essential for renal function, and should not be decreased. The child's sodium intake shouldn't be reduced. Avoiding other children is unnecessary, may make the child feel self-conscious, and may lead to regressive behavior.
CN: Health promotion and maintenance; CNS: None; CL: Apply

91. Which assessment finding would indicate the need to notify the provider following the removal of a Wilms' tumor?

1. Fever of 101° F (38.3° C)
2. Absence of bowel sounds after 48 hours
3. Slight congestion in the lungs
4. Reports pain when moving

91. 2. This child is at risk for intestinal obstruction. GI abnormalities require notification of the provider. A slight fever following surgery isn't uncommon, nor is slight congestion in the lungs and reports of pain.
CN: Safe and effective care environment; CNS: Management of care; CL: Analyze

92. What should the nurse keep in mind when teaching the family of a child just diagnosed with Wilms' tumor?

1. Because the parents are likely in a state of shock, explanations should be deferred until after surgery.
2. Explanations should be kept simple and should be repeated often.
3. Medical terminology should be supplemented with drawings and models.
4. Because of the quick timeline, education should be delegated to the perioperative nurse.

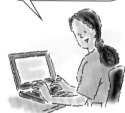

Which finding suggests the need to notify the provider?

92. 2. Decisions are made rapidly after a diagnosis of Wilms' tumor. Parents are typically in shock due to the diagnosis. Explanations should be kept simple, repeated often, and the use of medical terminology should be minimized. It would be inappropriate for the nurse to wholly delegate education.
CN: Health promotion and maintenance; CNS: None; CL: Apply

93. A nurse is providing psychosocial care to a six-year-old child following abdominal surgery for Wilms' tumor. Which activity would be the **most** appropriate?
1. Allow the child to watch a two-hour movie without interruptions
2. Give the child a puzzle with 12 pieces and encourage him to remain in bed
3. Tell the child that you can provide medication that eliminate his pain
4. Provide the child with craft supplies and ask him to draw how he feels

93. **4.** A movie is a good diversion, but giving craft supplies and encouraging the child to draw his feelings is a better outlet. A puzzle with only 12 pieces is too basic for a six-year-old child, and wouldn't hold his interest. The nurse can never guarantee that a client will feel no pain.
CN: Psychosocial integrity; CNS: None; CL: Apply

94. The nurse is teaching the parents of a child with Wilms' tumor about staging. The nurse knows that teaching has been effective when the parents state:
1. "Tumor size has no bearing on my child's stage of cancer or outcome."
2. "Staging is done to help determine how to treat the tumor."
3. "Even if the tumor has spread to other organs, staging is usually the same."
4. "In stage IV, the scar may be larger since the tumor is larger."

94. **2.** Staging of the tumor will help determine the level of treatment because it provides information about the level of involvement. The other choices are inaccurate or irrelevant in staging of the tumor.
CN: Health promotion and maintenance; CNS: None; CL: Analyze

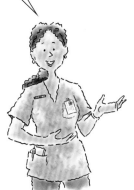

Further teaching is so important that you'll see similar questions more than once.

95. A nurse is educating parents about Wilms' tumor. Which statement, made by a parent, would indicate the need for further teaching?
1. "My child could have inherited this disease."
2. "Wilms' tumor can be associated with other congenital anomalies."
3. "This disease could have been a result of trauma to the baby in utero."
4. "There's no method of identifying gene carriers of Wilms' tumor."

95. **3.** Wilms' tumor isn't a result of trauma to the fetus in utero. Wilms' tumor can be genetically inherited and is often associated with other congenital anomalies. There is no method for identifying gene carriers of Wilms' tumor.
CN: Physiological integrity; CNS: Reduction of risk potential; CL: Analyze

96. Which finding will help differentiate a Wilms' tumor from the liver when performing an abdominal assessment?
1. The liver moves with respiration.
2. The liver is a more encapsulated organ.
3. A Wilms' tumor isn't as deep as the liver.
4. A Wilms' tumor usually isn't well defined.

96. **1.** It's difficult to distinguish a Wilms' tumor from the liver if the tumor is on the right side of the body. The liver will move with respirations and a Wilms' tumor will not. A Wilms' tumor is deep in the abdomen and is usually well defined and encapsulated.
CN: Physiological integrity; CNS: Reduction of risk potential; CL: Apply

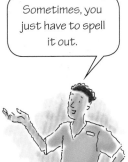

Sometimes, you just have to spell it out.

97. Which action, by a nurse, is **most** appropriate for a child diagnosed with Wilms' tumor?
1. Take blood pressure in the right arm only
2. Offer beverages at room temperature
3. Post a sign over the child's bed that reads, "Do not palpate the abdomen"
4. Encourage the child to participate in group activities in the playroom

97. **3.** To reinforce the need for caution, it may be necessary to post a sign over the bed that reads, "Do not palpate the abdomen." The blood pressure may be taken on any extremity prior to surgery. There are usually no dietary restrictions. Careful bathing and handling are also important to prevent trauma to the tumor site. Group activities should be discouraged.
CN: Safe and effective care environment; CNS: Safety and infection control; CL: Apply

CN: Client needs category   CNS: Client needs subcategory   CL: Cognitive level

98. The parent of a 24-month-old child asks the nurse when to begin toilet training the child. What is the nurse's **most** appropriate response?
1. "It's important that the child is developmentally ready."
2. "Make sure to be consistent in your approach."
3. "Try your best to maintain a positive attitude."
4. "It's best to start at the same age his siblings were trained."

99. The parents of toilet-trained four-year-old child are concerned when the child begins wetting the bed after being hospitalized. Which statement, by the nurse, **best** addresses this concern?
1. Children commonly show regressive behavior following hospitalization.
2. The child is acting out to make the parents feel bad.
3. Sometimes, four-year-olds have accidents.
4. Try decreasing fluids to see if that helps.

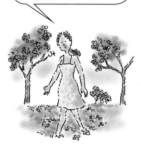

Hey—you're almost done! Finish up, and then go and do something fun.

100. A preschooler is scheduled to have a Wilms' tumor removed. Identify the area where this type of tumor is located.

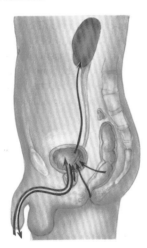

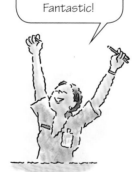

Congratulations! You finished all 101 questions! Fantastic!

101. A three-year-old child weighing 34.2 lb (15.5 kg) is to receive 5 ml/kg/hr of dextrose 5% in normal saline solution. At what rate (in ml/hr) should the nurse set the infusion pump? Record your answer using a whole number.

_____ ml/hr

98. 1. Toilet training should begin when the child is developmentally ready. After training is started, a consistent approach and a positive attitude should be used. Each child's readiness for toilet training is different, and the child shouldn't be compared to his siblings.
CN: Health promotion and maintenance; CNS: None; CL: Apply

99. 1. Young children may exhibit regressive behaviors when under stress. The child may be acting out, but is not likely wetting the bed voluntarily. Four-year-olds should be fully toilet trained. Restricting fluids, as a first step in a hospitalized child isn't appropriate. Other causes of bed-wetting should be considered first.
CN: Psychosocial integrity; CNS: None; CL: Apply

100. Wilms' tumor, also known as nephroblastoma, is a tumor located in the area of the kidney, most commonly on the left side. It is most often found in children ages two to four.

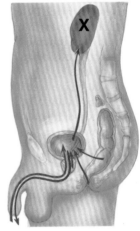

CN: Physiological integrity; CNS: Physiological adaptation; CL: Apply

101. 78.
To calculate the rate per hour for the infusion, the nurse should multiply 15.5 kg by 5 ml, which equals 77.5 ml/hr, which should be rounded to 78 ml/hr.
CN: Physiological integrity; CNS: Pharmacological and parenteral therapies; CL: Apply

Chapter 35

Integumentary Disorders

Skin diseases in children and teens are common and varied. This chapter covers common and uncommon skin disorders among these populations.

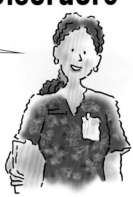

1. The nurse administers 1,500 ml of Lactated Ringers over six hours to a 12-year-old child with partial and full thickness burns over 40% of his body. How many milliters per hour should this child receive? Record your answer using a whole number.

_____ ml/hr

1. 250.

$$\frac{1,500\,ml}{6\,hr} = 250\,ml/hr$$

CN: Physiological integrity; CNS: Pharmacological and parenteral therapies; CL: Apply

2. The nurse is caring for a child with burns. Which statement, by the nurse, **best** describes the nutritional needs of this child?
  1. A child will need 100 cal/kg during the initial hospitalization.
  2. Caloric intake will need to be increased to help with wound healing.
  3. Caloric needs can be lowered by controlling environmental temperature.
  4. Maintaining a hypermetabolic rate will help meet nutritional needs.

2. 2. A burn injury causes a hypermetabolic state leading to protein and lipid catabolism, which affects wound healing. Caloric intake should be one and one half to two times the basal metabolic rate, with a minimum of 1.5 to 2 g/kg of body weight of protein daily. Keeping the temperature within a normal range lets the body function efficiently and use calories for healing and normal physiological processes. If the temperature is too warm or cold, energy must be used for warming or cooling, taking energy away from tissue repair. High metabolic rates increase the need for nutrition and deplete the calories necessary for tissue repair.

CN: Physiological integrity; CNS: Basic care and comfort; CL: Analyze

Measuring burns in children is different than measuring burns in adults.

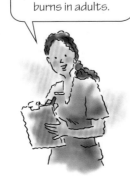

3. What is the **most** accurate way for the nurse to measure the burn size of a two-year-old child who sustained a thermal burn to the anterior surface of the left hand?
  1. The rule of nines
  2. Percentage based on the child's weight
  3. The child's hand equals 1.25% of the child's body surface area
  4. Percentage can't be determined without knowing the type of burn

3. 3. The anterior surface of a child's hand is equal to 1.25% of that child's body surface. The rule of nines is used for children aged 14 years and older. The child's weight is important to calculate fluid replacement for extensive burns, not to estimate total body surface area. The type of burn doesn't determine the percentage of body surface involved.

CN: Physiological integrity; CNS: Physiological adaptation; CL: Apply

CN: Client needs category   CNS: Client needs subcategory   CL: Cognitive level

4. The nurse is caring for an 18-month-old child admitted to the hospital for full-thickness burns to the anterior chest. The mother asks the nurse how the burn will heal. What is the nurse's **best** response?

1. Surgical closure and grafting are usually required.
2. Healing will take 10 to 12 days, and there will be little or no scarring.
3. Pigment in darker-skinned clients will eventually return to the injured area.
4. Healing can take up to six weeks and there will likely be scarring.

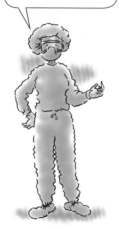

This type of burn requires a major intervention.

4. 1. Full-thickness burns usually require surgical closure and grafting for complete healing. Healing in 10 to 12 days with little, or no, scarring is associated with superficial partial-thickness burns. Pigment is expected to return to the injured area after healing with superficial partial-thickness burns. Deep partial-thickness burns heal in six weeks, with scarring.
CN: Physiological integrity; CNS: Physiological adaptation; CL: Analyze

5. The nurse is assessing a nine-year-old child admitted to the hospital with second degree partial-thickness burns to 25% of his body. What would the nurse expect to assess? Select all that apply.

1. Report of moderate to severe pain
2. Moist blebs, blisters
3. Minimal damage to the epidermis
4. Necrosis through all layers of skin
5. Tissue necrosis through most of the dermis
6. Mottled white, pink to cherry-red color

5. 1, 2, 5, 6. Assessment findings for second degree partial-thickness burns include moist blebs, blisters, mottled white, pink to cherry-red, hypersensitivity to touch or air, moderate to severe pain, blanching with pressure, a client with a second degree partial-thickness burn will have tissue necrosis to the epidermis and dermis layers. The American Burn Association recommends a more precise definition and classifies burns according to depth of skin destruction. Erythema and pain are characteristic of superficial injury. With deep, third and fourth degree burns, the nerve fibers are destroyed and the client won't feel pain in the affected area. Superficial burns are characteristic of slight epidermal damage. Necrosis through all skin layers is seen with full-thickness injuries.
CN: Physiological integrity; CNS: Physiological adaptation; CL: Apply

The word circumferential is a clue, right?

6. The nurse is caring for a four-year-old child admitted to the burn unit with a circumferential burn to the left forearm. Which finding should be reported to the provider?

1. Numbness of fingers
2. +2 radial and ulnar pulses
3. Full range of motion (ROM) and no pain
4. Bilateral capillary refill less than two seconds

6. 1. Circumferential burns can compromise blood flow to an extremity, causing numbness. Normal circulation is indicated by +2 pulses. Absence of pain, and full ROM implies good tissue oxygenation from intact circulation. Capillary refill less than two seconds indicates a normal vascular blood flow.
CN: Physiological integrity; CNS: Physiological adaptation; CL: Apply

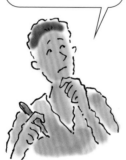

Thorough handwashing can help prevent many infections.

7. What is the **most** important information for the nurse to teach the pregnant mother of a child with Fifth disease?

1. There is a possible reappearance of the rash for up to one week.
2. Isolation of high-risk contacts should be avoided for 4 to 10 days.
3. Pregnant clients are at risk for fetal death if infected with Fifth disease.
4. Children with Fifth disease are contagious only while the rash is present.

7. 3. There's a 3 to 5% risk for fetal death from hydrops fetalis if a pregnant client is exposed during the first trimester. The cutaneous eruption of Fifth disease can reappear for up to four months. The child should be isolated from pregnant women, immunocompromised clients, and clients with chronic anemia for up to two weeks. A child with Fifth disease is contagious during the first stage, when symptoms of headache, body aches, fever, and chills are present, not after the rash.
CN: Safe, effective care environment; CNS: Safety and infection control; CL: Apply

CN: Client needs category   CNS: Client needs subcategory   CL: Cognitive level

8. A mother tells the nurse she is concerned that her child may develop Fifth disease because there was a confirmed case at the daycare center. Which manifestations should the nurse instruct the mother to look for?

1. A fine, erythematous rash with a sandpaper-like texture
2. Intense redness of both cheeks that may spread to the extremities
3. Low-grade fever, followed by vesicular lesions of the trunk, face, and scalp
4. A sustained fever that lasts for two to three days, followed by a diffuse erythematous maculopapular rash

9. A child's parents tell the nurse that their son developed a rash after a tick bite when they were on a recent camping trip. For which finding should the nurse assess?

1. Erythematous rash surrounding a necrotic lesion
2. Erythematous ring with a raised swollen border circling the bite site
3. Onset of a diffuse rash over the entire body two months after exposure
4. A linear rash of papules and vesicles that occur 1 to 3 days after exposure

10. The nurse administered a purified protein derivative (PPD) test to an eight-year-old child. What is the **most** appropriate action by the nurse?

1. Read results within 24 hours
2. Read results 48 to 72 hours later
3. Use the large muscle of the upper leg
4. Massage the site to increase absorption

11. What is the **most** important information for the nurse to teach the parents of a child with Kawasaki disease?

1. It's a highly contagious condition that requires isolation.
2. It's an afebrile condition with cardiac involvement.
3. It usually occurs in children older than five years.
4. There is a prolonged fever, with peeling of the fingers and toes.

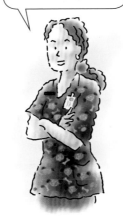

Different symptoms indicate different diagnoses.

8. 2. The classic symptoms of Fifth disease begin with intense redness of both cheeks. It occurs in three stages. During the second stage, the facial rash will begin to fade, and a maculopapular, urticarial, or morbilliform exanthem develops on the extremities and trunk. Pruritus may also be present. An erythematous rash with a sandpaper-like texture is associated with scarlet fever. Children with varicella typically have vesicular lesions of the trunk, face, and scalp after a low-grade fever. An erythematous rash after a fever is characteristic of roseola.
CN: Physiological integrity; CNS: Physiological adaptation;
CL: Apply

9. 2. A bull's-eye rash is a classic symptom of Lyme disease caused by a tick bite. The rash is located primarily at the site of the bite. Necrotic, painful rashes are associated with the bite of a brown recluse spider. A linear, papular, vesicular rash indicates exposure to the leaves of poison ivy.
CN: Physiological integrity; CNS: Physiological adaptation;
CL: Apply

10. 2. The test should be read 48 to 72 hours after placement by measuring the diameter of the induration that develops at the site. The PPD is injected intradermally on the volar surface of the forearm. Massaging the site could cause leakage from the injection site.
CN: Physiological integrity; CNS: Reduction of risk potential;
CL: Apply

11. 4. To be diagnosed with Kawasaki syndrome, the child must have a fever for five days or more, plus four of the following five symptoms: bilateral conjunctivitis, without a thick discharge, changes in the oral mucosa (strawberry tongue), dermatitis of the peripheral extremities, rash, and lymphadenopathy. Desquamation of the fingers and toes often occurs in the second phase of the disease process. Desquamation often occurs in large sheets. The syndrome isn't contagious and doesn't require isolation. Kawasaki syndrome is more likely to occur in children younger than age five years.
CN: Physiological integrity; CNS: Physiological adaptation;
CL: Apply

CN: Client needs category   CNS: Client needs subcategory   CL: Cognitive level

12. A 22 lb (10 kg) child is diagnosed with Kawasaki disease and started on gamma globulin therapy. The provider orders an IV infusion of gamma globulin, 2 g/kg, to run over 12 hours. What is the correct dose? Record your answer using a whole number.

_____ g

13. A mother is concerned because her child was exposed to varicella in daycare. What is the nurse's **best** response?
1. Initially, the rash appears as fluid filled blisters.
2. The treatment of choice is aspirin.
3. Varicella has an incubation period of 5 to 10 days.
4. A child is no longer contagious once the rash has crusted over.

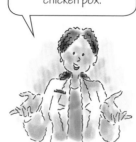

Remember, varicella is the clinical name of chicken pox.

14. The pediatric nurse is assessing a client with varicella zoster. Which findings would be consistent with the varicella rash?
1. Koplik's spots in the oral mucosa
2. The macular papular rash starts on the scalp and hairline and descends
3. The vesicular macular-papular rash appears abruptly on the trunk, face, and scalp
4. The rash appears as yellow ulcers surrounded by red halos on the surface of the hands and feet

15. The nurse is assessing a client who has suspected frostbite. Which assessment findings would be consistent with this diagnosis? Select all that apply.
1. Reddened skin that turns white or pale with tingling, numbness and a burning sensation
2. Mottled or cyanotic skin
3. Raised pink or red papules
4. Blisters that appear in 24 to 36 hours
5. A flat, flesh-colored, or brown scar-like lesion

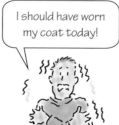

I should have worn my coat today!

12. 20.
Use the child's weight in kilograms.

$$10 \, kg \times 2 \, g/kg = 20 \, g$$

CN: Physiological integrity; CNS: Pharmacological and parenteral therapies; CL: Apply

13. 4. Once every varicella lesion has crusted over, the child is no longer considered contagious. The rash is typically a maculopapular vesicular rash. The rash first appears as pink or red bumps which occur over several days. Following the rash, fluid filled vesicles form over the next 24 hours before breaking and leaking. The use of aspirin has been associated with Reye's syndrome and is contraindicated in varicella. The incubation period for varicella is 10 to 20 days.

CN: Physiological integrity; CNS: Physiological adaptation; CL: Apply

14. 3. Teardrop-shaped vesicles on an erythematous base generally begin on the trunk, face, and scalp, with minimal involvement of the extremities. Koplik's spots are diagnostic of rubeola. A descending macular-papular rash is characteristic of rubeola. Yellow ulcers on the hands and feet are associated with hand-foot-and-mouth disease caused by the coxsackievirus.

CN: Physiological integrity; CNS: Physiological adaptation; CL: Apply

15. 1, 2, 4. Signs and symptoms of frostbite include tingling, numbness, burning sensation, and white skin. When frostbite is in the superficial stage, the skin appears reddened and will turn white or pale. During gradual rewarming, the skin will appear mottled, blue or purple, the client will feel a stinging, burning sensation and edema may be present. After rewarming, fluid-filled blisters may surface in 24 to 36 hours. The raised pink or red papules are associated with varicella zoster. A flat, flesh or brown-colored, scar-like lesion is associated with squamous cell carcinoma.

CN: Physiological integrity; CNS: Physiological adaptation; CL: Apply

16. A child reports pain, redness, and tenderness at the nail bed of her left index finger, and is diagnosed with a paronychia. Which organism **most** likely causes this infection?
1. *Borrelia burgdorferi*
2. *Escherichia coli*
3. *Pseudomonas* species
4. *Staphylococcus* species

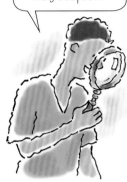

Who is the most likely suspect?

16. 4. A paronychia is a localized infection of the nail bed caused by either staphylococci or streptococci. *Borrelia burgdorferi* is responsible for Lyme disease. *Escherichia coli* is associated with urinary tract infections. Pseudomonas species are associated with ecthyma.
CN: Physiological integrity; CNS: Physiological adaptation; CL: Apply

17. The nurse is instructing the mother of an infant with seborrheic dermatitis of the scalp. Which statement would indicate understanding of the teaching?
1. "Seborrheic dermatitis occurs only on the scalp."
2. "This condition occurs once and will go away on its own."
3. "Seborrheic dermatitis can be treated with baby shampoo and a soft bristled brush."
4. "This condition will require ongoing treatments with medications."

17. 3. Seborrheic dermatitis, also known as cradle cap in infants, can be treated by using non-medicated baby shampoo. The shampoo is applied, and the scales are loosened with a soft-bristled brush before rinsing out the shampoo. Seborrheic dermatitis can occur on other oily areas of the body, such as the face, upper chest and back. Seborrheic dermatitis is also referred to as dandruff, seborrheic eczema and seborrheic psoriasis. For adults, seborrheic dermatitis is usually a long-term condition. Some individuals require repeated treatments and prescription medications before symptoms go away. Others may experience a recurrence of symptoms.
CN: Physiological integrity; CNS: Physiological adaptation; CL: Apply

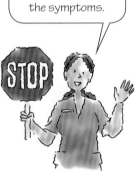

Stop and assess the symptoms.

18. A mother brings her nine-month-old baby to the clinic because she thinks her baby has scabies. Which assessment finding would support the diagnosis?
1. Diffuse pruritic wheals
2. Petechial spotted rash on the bilateral extremities
3. Thrombocytopenic purpura
4. Pruritic papules, pustules, and linear burrows of the finger and toe webs

18. 4. Pruritic papules, vesicles, and linear burrows indicate scabies. Diffuse pruritic wheals are associated with an allergic reaction. Thrombocytopenic purpura is associated with cat scratch, and is caused by *Bartonella henselae*. The petechial-spotted rash associated with Rocky Mountain Spotted Fever may appear two to five days after being bitten by an infected tick.
CN: Physiological integrity; CNS: Physiological adaptation; CL: Apply

19. The home health nurse is reinforcing teaching during a follow-up visit with a mother whose 16-month-old child is being treated for scabies with permethrin 5% cream. The mother is concerned that the cream didn't work because the child is still scratching. Which statement indicates an understanding of the teaching?
1. "I will continue the application daily until the rash disappears."
2. "The itching may be caused by a secondary reaction to the mites, and can last for weeks."
3. "I should stop treatment because the cream is unsafe for children younger than age two."
4. "The itching indicates an allergy to the medicine."

19. 2. Sensitization of the host is the cause of the intense itching, and can last for weeks. One application of the medication usually eliminates the parasites. The home health nurse should instruct the mother that the treatment may need to be repeated after one week, and she should let a provider know if there are any further signs of scabies. Permethrin is the recommended treatment for scabies in infants as young as two months. It can safely be repeated after two weeks.
CN: Physiological integrity; CNS: Pharmacological and parenteral therapies; CL: Apply

20. The mother of a five-month-old infant is planning a trip to the beach. She asks the nurse for advice about sunscreen for her child. What is the **best** information, for the nurse, to give this mother?
1. The sunscreen protection factor (SPF) of the sunscreen should be at least 10.
2. Apply sunscreen to the exposed areas of the skin.
3. Sunscreen shouldn't be applied to infants younger than six months of age.
4. Sunscreen should be heavily applied one-half hour before going out in the sun.

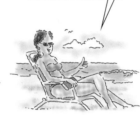

Know the do's and don'ts about sunscreen and its application.

20. 3. Sunscreen isn't recommended for infants younger than six months of age. These children should be dressed in cool light clothes and kept in the shade. The SPF for children should be 15 or greater. Sunscreen should be applied to all areas of the skin. Sunscreen should be applied evenly throughout the day and each time the child is in the water.

CN: Health promotion and maintenance; CNS: None; CL: Apply

21. The nurse at the pediatrician's office is assessing a six-month-old child and notes that the skin in the diaper area is excoriated and red. What is **most** important for the nurse to teach this parent?
1. Expose the diaper area to air between more frequent diaper changes
2. Apply talcum powder with diaper changes
3. Wash the area vigorously with each diaper change
4. Decrease the infant's fluid intake to decrease saturating diapers

21. 1. Simply decreasing the amount of time the skin comes in contact with wet soiled diapers will help heal the irritation. Talc is contraindicated in children because of the risk of inhalation. Gentle cleaning the irritated skin should be encouraged. Infants should have unrestricted fluid intake.

CN: Safe, effective care environment; CNS: Safety and infection control; CL: Apply

22. The nurse is preparing to discharge a nine-year-old child who was hospitalized after experiencing severe urticaria caused by an allergy to nuts. What is the **most** important instruction for the nurse to give this child's parents?
1. Avoid any and all exposure to nuts
2. Apply topical steroids to the lesions as needed
3. Apply over-the-counter products such as diphenhydramine
4. Provide information on how and when to use an epinephrine administration kit

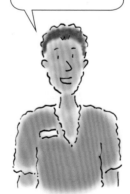

Teaching parents helps keep their children healthy.

22. 4. Children who have urticaria in response to nuts, seafood, or bee stings should be warned about the possibility of anaphylactic reactions to future exposure. Parents and older children should be taught how to use an epinephrine pen. Other treatments, such as diphenhydramine hydrochloride, topical steroids, and emollients, are for the treatment of mild urticaria.

CN: Physiological integrity; CNS: Reduction of risk potential; CL: Apply

23. The nurse is assessing a nursery-school aged child, and finds multiple contusions in various stages of healing over the child's body. Child abuse is suspected. Which assessment data would the nurse document in this child's record?
1. Contusions confined to one body area are typically suspicious.
2. All lesions, including location, shape, and color, should be documented.
3. Natural injuries usually have straight linear lines, while injuries from abuse have multiple curved lines.
4. The depth, location, and amount of initial bleeding is constant, but the noted sequence of skin color change is inconsistent.

23. 2. An accurate examination of all lesions must be properly documented as a legal document. Contusions that result from falls are typically confined to a single body area, and are considered a reasonable finding if the child still learning to walk. Injuries from accidental falls are usually not linear in nature. The bleeding that can result from abuse can cause variations, but the color change is consistent.

CN: Psychosocial integrity; CNS: None; CL: Apply

CN: Client needs category   CNS: Client needs subcategory   CL: Cognitive level

24. The nurse is reinforcing instructions given to the parent of a seven-year-old child recently diagnosed with molluscum contagiosum. Which statement, by the parent, indicates that further teaching is necessary?
1. "This can be spread to other parts of the body by scratching or rubbing the bumps and then touching another part of the body."
2. "Everyone should wash their hands and not share personal items."
3. "I should keep my child home from school until the bumps go away."
4. "Kids can get this from infected children who are coughing and sneezing.'

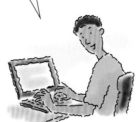

Question 24 already, and you're doing great!

24. 4. Molluscum contagiosum virus (MCV) is a viral infection caused by a member of the poxvirus family, and is spread by direct contact. The appearance of the rash consists of small wart-like bumps and can be pink, white or skin colored. The bumps are usually soft and smooth and may have an indented center. To prevent the spread of the virus, individuals should wash hands frequently, and avoid touching the bumps. Children shouldn't share personal items such as clothing, towels, hair brushes or hats. The bumps should be covered with a water-tight bandage to prevent contact by another person. Because MCV is present only in the top layer of skin, once the lesions are gone, the virus is gone, and it cannot be spread to others. When taking the necessary precautions, there is no reason to keep a child with MCV home from day care or school.
CN: Management of care; CNS: Safe and effective care; CL: Apply

25. The nurse is teaching the mother of a child with lice about treatment options. What is the **most** important information for the nurse to include when discussing the potential side effects of lindane shampoo?
1. It can cause alopecia.
2. It causes hypertension.
3. It has been linked to seizures.
4. It increases liver function test (LFT) results.

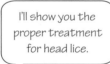

Remember

"Lindane restrains lice and scabies."

Lindane is used as a treatment for lice and scabies.

25. 3. Lindane is associated with seizures after absorption with topical use. Alopecia, increased LFT results, and hypertension aren't associated with the use of lindane.
CN: Physiological integrity; CNS: Pharmacological and parenteral therapies; CL: Apply

26. The nurse is providing instructions to parents about the treatment of head lice. What is the **most** important information for the nurse to provide?
1. The treatment should be repeated in 7 to 12 days.
2. The treatment should be repeated every day for one week.
3. If treated with a shampoo, combing to remove eggs isn't necessary.
4. Anyone in contact with the infested child should be treated.

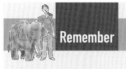

I'll show you the proper treatment for head lice.

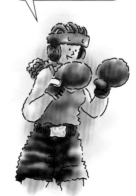

26. 1. Treatment should be repeated in 7 to 12 days to ensure that all eggs are killed. Combing the hair thoroughly is necessary to remove the lice eggs. People exposed to head lice should be examined to assess the presence of infestation before treatment.
CN: Physiological integrity; CNS: Physiological adaptation; CL: Apply

27. During a visit by the home health nurse, the mother reports that her four-year-old child has been scratching at his rectum recently. The nurse notes poor hygiene by the child and numerous other family members. Which infestation, or condition, should the nurse suspect?
1. Anal fissure
2. Lice
3. Pinworms
4. Scabies

27. 3. The clinical indication of pinworms is perianal itching that increases at night. Anal fissures are associated with rectal bleeding and pain with bowel movements. Lice are infestations of the hair. Scabies are associated with a pruritic rash characterized as linear burrows of the webs of the fingers and toes.
CN: Physiological integrity; CNS: Physiological adaptation; CL: Analyze

CN: Client needs category   CNS: Client needs subcategory   CL: Cognitive level

28. The nurse is providing instructions on the diagnoses of pinworms to a parent. The nurse instructs the parent to apply clear cellophane tape to the skin around the anus before the child uses the toilet in the morning. The parent asks how many consecutive days they should use the tape. What is the nurse's **best** response?
1. One
2. Three
3. Five
4. Ten

28. 2. It is recommended that this test be repeated for three consecutive days. The test should be performed in the morning before the child uses the toilet, gets dressed or washes. One test is only 50% accurate. Three tests should detect infestations 90% of the time. Repeating the test 5 to 10 times is not necessary.
CN: Physiological integrity; CNS: Reduction of risk potential; CL: Apply

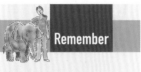

Remember

"Pyrantel pamoate pummels pinworms."

This drug is used for pinworm treatment in humans and a deworming agent in domesticated animals.

29. The nurse is providing teaching to a child's family about the use of pyrantel pamoate. The child has been diagnosed with pinworms. What is the **most** important information for the nurse to give the family?
1. The drug may stain the feces red.
2. The dose may be repeated in two weeks.
3. Fever and rash are common adverse effects.
4. The medicine will kill the eggs in about 48 hours.

29. 2. Pyrantel is effective against the adult worms only, so treatment should be repeated in two weeks to eradicate any emerging parasites. Stained feces is associated with pyrvinium pamoate. Common adverse effects are headache and nausea.
CN: Physiological integrity; CNS: Pharmacological and parenteral therapies; CL: Apply

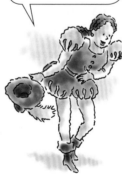

You've completed 30 questions. Take a bow.

30. A nurse in the emergency department is assessing a child who was bitten by a large dog. What type of injury would the nurse expect to assess?
1. Abrasion
2. Crush injury
3. Fracture
4. Contusion

30. 2. Although the bite of a large dog can exert pressure of 150 to 400 psi, the bite causes crush injuries, not fractures. Abrasions are associated with friction injuries. A contusion is injury to tissue usually without laceration or breaking the skin.
CN: Physiological integrity; CNS: Physiological adaptation; CL: Apply

31. What is the nurse's **priority** action when a neighbor frantically rushes over and states, "My child has just been bitten by a dog!"
1. Administer a rabies vaccine
2. Immediately administer antibiotics
3. Clean and irrigate the wounds
4. Nothing; bites from dogs have a low incidence of infection

31. 3. Not every dog bite requires antibiotic therapy, but cleaning the wound is necessary for all injuries involving a break in the skin. Rabies vaccine is used if there is suspicion that the dog has rabies. The infection rate for dog bites has been reported to be as high as 50%.
CN: Physiological integrity; CNS: Reduction of risk potential; CL: Apply

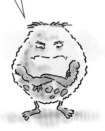

If you think the dog bite was bad, just wait till I get into your system.

32. The nurse is reviewing the wound culture report from a wound caused by a dog bite. Which organism would the nurse suspect as responsible for this infection?
  1. *Escherichia coli*
  2. *Francisella tularensis*
  3. *Pasteurella multocida*
  4. *Bartonella henselae*

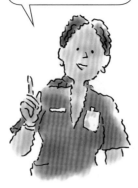

Looks like all the usual suspects. But which one is likely to be present in a dog bite?

32. 3. *Pasteurella multocida* is associated with infection in up to 50% of dog bites. *Escherichia coli* is more likely to cause infections of the urinary tract. *Francisella tularensis* is found in such animals as rabbits, hares, and muskrats. *Bartonella henselae*, a gram-negative rickettsial bacterium, is associated with cat-scratch disease.
CN: Physiological integrity; CNS: Physiological adaptation; CL: Apply

33. A child is brought to a provider's office for multiple scratches and bites from a kitten. Which assessment finding should the nurse anticipate?
  1. Abdominal pain
  2. Adenitis
  3. Diffuse rash and sore throat
  4. Pruritus

33. 2. Adenitis is the primary feature of cat-scratch disease. Although low-grade fever has been associated with cat-scratch disease, it's only present 25% of the time. Pruritus and abdominal pain aren't symptoms of cat-scratch disease.
CN: Physiological integrity; CNS: Physiological adaptation; CL: Analyze

34. The nurse is discussing giardiasis, a parasitic intestinal infection with a group of parents at a community health fair. Several individuals ask the nurse what group is most at risk for developing this infection. What is the nurse's **most** accurate response?
  1. Children riding a school bus
  2. Children playing on a playground
  3. Children attending a sporting event
  4. Children attending group day care or nursery school

34. 4. Giardiasis is most prevalent among children attending group daycare or nursery school. Playgrounds, sporting events, and school buses don't present unusual risk of giardiasis.
CN: Physiological integrity; CNS: Physiological adaptation; CL: Apply

35. A child who has varicella zoster with papules. Which assessment findings would the nurse document?
  1. Palpable elevated masses
  2. Loss of the epidermis layer
  3. Layers of red patches with scales
  4. Non-palpable flat changes in skin color

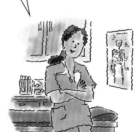

You need to know the correct terms to share information with clients and other health care providers.

35. 1. Papules are elevated up to 0.5 cm. Nodules and tumors are elevated more than 0.5 cm. Erosions are characterized as loss of the epidermis layer. Fluid-filled lesions are vesicles and pustules. Macules and patches are described as non-palpable flat changes in skin color. Layers of reddened patches with silvery scales is symptomatic of psoriasis
CN: Health promotion and maintenance; CNS: None; CL: Apply

36. The nurse is performing an assessment on a child diagnosed with impetigo. How should the nurse document these assessment findings? Select all that apply.
  1. Lesions filled with pus
  2. Reddened patches with sharply marginated, irregular outlines
  3. Pustules with a yellowish-brown crust
  4. Serous-filled lesions greater than 0.5 cm
  5. Reddened patches of skin covered with silvery scales
  6. Reddish macule

36. 1, 2, 3, 6. Pustules are pus-filled lesions, such as acne and impetigo. When the pustules rupture they form a yellowish-brown crust. Impetigo begins as a reddish macule that becomes vesicular. A wheal is a superficial area of localized edema. Vesicles are serous-filled lesions up to 0.5 cm in diameter. Bullae are serous-filled lesions greater than 0.5 cm in diameter. Reddened patches of skin covered with silvery scales are associated with psoriasis.
CN: Physiological integrity; CNS: Physiological adaptation; CL: Apply

CN: Client needs category   CNS: Client needs subcategory   CL: Cognitive level

37. The nurse is assessing a three-month-old infant who is noted to have six café-au-lait-colored lesions greater than 1.5 cm in diameter. How should the nurse interpret this assessment finding?
1. Meningococcemia
2. Neurofibromatosis
3. Tinea versicolor
4. Vitiligo

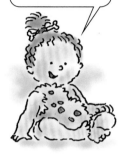

Assessment is an enormously important skill.

37. 2. Six or more uniformly-pigmented patches with irregular borders, known as café-au-lait spots, with diameters greater than 1.5 cm, are associated with neurofibromatosis. Meningococcemia has petechiae, not café-au-lait spots. Tinea versicolor is a superficial fungal infection. Depigmented areas are signs of vitiligo.

CN: Health promotion and maintenance; CNS: None; CL: Analyze

38. The nurse is assessing a child brought to the provider's office for treatment of a rash. Many petechiae are seen over the entire body. What condition would the nurse suspect?
1. Bleeding disorder
2. Scabies
3. Varicella
4. Atopic dermatitis

38. 1. Petechiae are caused by blood outside a vessel, and are associated with low platelet counts and bleeding disorders. Petechiae aren't found with varicella disease or scabies. Petechiae can be associated with vomiting, but would be present on the face, not the entire body.

CN: Physiological integrity; CNS: Physiological adaptation; CL: Analyze

39. The clinic nurse is assessing a child who fell at camp and sustained a bruise to his thigh. Which description would **most** accurately describe this bruise after one week?
1. Resolved
2. Reddish blue
3. Greenish yellow
4. Dark blue to bluish brown

39. 3. After 7 to 10 days, the bruise should become greenish yellow. Resolution can take up to two weeks. Immediately after the fall, there is a reddish-blue discoloration followed by a dark blue to bluish brown color after 1 to 3 days.

CN: Physiological integrity; CNS: Physiological adaptation; CL: Apply

40. The school nurse is assessing a three-year-old child. Which assessment finding would the nurse consider suggestive of child abuse?
1. Multiple contusions of the shins
2. Contusions of the back and buttocks in various stages of healing
3. Contusions at the same stages of healing
4. Large contusion and hematoma of the forehead

40. 2. Contusions of the back and buttocks are highly suggestive of abuse related to punishment. Contusions at various stages of healing are red flags to potential abuse. Contusions of the shins and forehead are usually related to an active toddler falling and bumping into objects.

CN: Psychosocial integrity; CNS: None; CL: Analyze

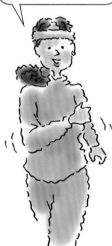

Keep it up. You can go the distance.

41. The nurse is providing discharge instructions to a new mother. Which statement would the nurse include when teaching about telangiectatic nevi?
1. They're benign and may fade in adult life.
2. They're usually associated with syndromes of the neonate.
3. They can cause mild hypertrophy of the muscle associated with the lesion.
4. They're treatable with laser pulse surgery in late adolescence and adulthood.

41. 1. Salmon colored patches occur over the back of the neck in 40% of neonates, are harmless, and require no intervention. Port wine stains are associated with syndromes of the neonate such as Sturge-Weber syndrome. Port wine stains found on the face or extremities may be associated with soft tissue and bone hypertrophy. Laser pulse surgery isn't recommended for salmon patches because they typically fade on their own in adulthood.

CN: Health promotion and maintenance; CNS: None; CL: Apply

42. The nurse is performing an assessment of a neonate. The assessment findings indicate the presence of a blue-black macular lesion over the lower lumbar sacral region. Which term should the nurse use when teaching the parents about this lesion?
1. Café-au-lait spots
2. Mongolian spots
3. Nevus of Ota spot
4. Stork bites

42. 2. Mongolian spots are large blue-black macular lesions generally located over the lumbosacral areas, buttocks, and limbs. Café-au-lait spots occur between ages two and 16 years, not in infancy. Nevus of Ota is found surrounding the eyes. Stork bites, or salmon patches occur at the neck and hairline area.
CN: Health promotion and maintenance; CNS: None; CL: Apply

43. The nurse is admitting a child with severe dehydration. Which integumentary finding should the nurse anticipate?
1. Gray skin and decreased tears
2. Capillary refill less than two seconds
3. Mottling and tenting of the skin
4. Pale skin with dry mucous membranes

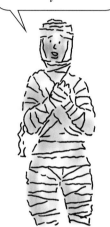

You should have no trouble wrapping up this question.

43. 3. Severe dehydration is associated with mottling and tenting of the skin. Malnutrition is characterized by gray skin and tenting of the skin. Capillary refill less than two seconds is normal. Pale skin with dry mucous membranes is a sign of mild dehydration.
CN: Health promotion and maintenance; CNS: None; CL: Analyze

44. What is the **most** important information for the nurse to include when teaching a 17-year-old female client about the adverse effects of isotretinoin?
1. Diarrhea
2. Gram-negative folliculitis
3. Teratogenicity
4. Vaginal candidiasis

44. 3. The use of even small amounts of isotretinoin has been associated with severe birth defects. Most female clients taking this medication are prescribed hormonal contraceptives. Cleocin T, another medicine used in the treatment of acne, is associated with both diarrhea and gram-negative folliculitis. Tetracycline is associated with yeast infections.
CN: Physiological integrity; CNS: Pharmacological and parenteral therapies; CL: Apply

45. The nurse is developing a teaching plan for adolescents about acne. The nurse understands that many teenagers discontinue treatment because:
1. the medication is applied topically.
2. the medication is a systemic treatment.
3. a parent pushes the teen to use the treatment when the teenager doesn't want to.
4. a parent doesn't push them to continue the treatment.

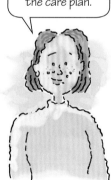

I need to follow the care plan.

45. 3. The active participation of a teenager is needed for the successful treatment of acne. Systemic and topical therapies are needed in most acne treatment.
CN: Health promotion and maintenance; CNS: None; CL: Apply

46. A teenager tells the nurse that he has heard many myths about the cause of acne. He asks the nurse, "What really causes acne?" What is the **most** accurate information the nurse can provide?
1. Diet
2. Gender
3. Poor hygiene
4. Hormonal changes

46. 4. Acne is caused by hormonal changes in sebaceous gland anatomy and the biochemistry of the glands. These changes lead to a blockage of the follicular canal, and cause an inflammatory response. Diet, hygiene, and the client's gender don't cause acne.
CN: Health promotion and maintenance; CNS: None; CL: Apply

47. The nurse reviews information about how to take the prescribed tetracycline. Which statement, by the client, allows the nurse to determine that the client understands the information?
1. "I can take tetracycline with or without meals."
2. "I can take tetracycline with milk and milk products."
3. "I can take tetracycline on an empty stomach with small amounts of water."
4. "I can take tetracycline one hour before or two hours after meals with plenty of water."

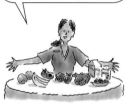

I forget. Does tetracycline pair well with food or is it water?

47. 4. Tetracycline must be taken on an empty stomach to increase absorption, and with ample water to avoid esophageal irritation. Milk products impede absorption.
CN: Physiological integrity; CNS: Pharmacological and parenteral therapies; CL: Apply

48. The nurse is teaching parents how to prevent their children from incurring tap water burn injuries. What is the **most** important instruction for the nurse to include?
1. Set the water heater temperature at 130° F (54.4° C) or less
2. Run the hot water first, then adjust the temperature with cold water
3. Test the water with your hand before putting the infant in the tub
4. Closely supervise the infant while in the bathroom, only leaving him for a few seconds

48. 3. Parents should fill the tub with water first and then test the water with their hand before putting the infant in the tub. Water heaters should be set at 120° F (48.9° C). The cold water should be run first and then adjusted with hot water. Never leave an infant alone in the bathroom.
CN: Health promotion and maintenance; CNS: None; CL: Apply

49. A 2-day-old neonate experiences a color change for approximately two to three minutes while lying on her left side. The nurse interprets this finding as suggestive of:
1. contact dermatitis.
2. environmental conditions.
3. harlequin color change.
4. Tet spells.

49. 3. Harlequin color change is a benign disorder related to the immaturity of hypothalamic centers that control the tone of peripheral blood vessels. A newborn, who has been lying on his side, may appear reddened on the dependent side. The color fades on position change. Contact dermatitis isn't short lived. Changes in environmental conditions can cause diffuse bilateral mottling of the skin. Tet spells are associated with tetralogy of Fallot and cause cyanotic changes.
CN: Health promotion and maintenance; CNS: None; CL: Analyze

50. What is the **most** important treatment information for the nurse to give parents regarding their child's diagnosis of pediculosis?
1. Use lindane
2. Use petroleum jelly
3. Shave the eyebrows
4. No treatment is needed

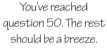

You've reached question 50. The rest should be a breeze.

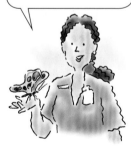

50. 2. Petroleum jelly should be applied twice daily for eight days, followed by manual removal of nits. Lindane is contraindicated because of the risk for seizures. The eyebrows should never be shaved because of an uncertainty of hair return.
CN: Physiological integrity; CNS: Physiological adaptation; CL: Analyze

51. A client is brought to the emergency department after a house fire. What is the **priority** intervention by the nurse?
1. Check the oral mucous membranes
2. Check for any burned areas
3. Obtain a medical history
4. Ensure a patent airway

51. 4. The nurse's priority is to make sure the airway is open and that the client is breathing. Checking the mucous membranes and burned areas is important, but not as vital as insuring a patent airway. Obtaining a medical history can be pursued after ensuring a patent airway.
CN: Physiological integrity; CNS: Physiological adaptation; CL: Apply

52. The nurse is assessing a child suspected of having Kawasaki syndrome. For which should the nurse assess the child's mouth?
1. Koplik's spots
2. Tonsillar exudate
3. Vesicular lesions
4. Strawberry tongue

52. 4. Oral changes associated with Kawasaki disease include reddened pharynx, red, dry fissured lips, and a strawberry tongue. Koplik's spots are consistent with measles. Tonsillar exudate is consistent with pharyngitis caused by group A beta-hemolytic streptococci. Vesicular lesions are associated with coxsackievirus.
CN: Physiological integrity; CNS: Physiological adaptation; CL: Apply

53. The nurse is assessing a three-year-old child and notes palpable purpura on the child's buttocks and lower extremities. Which condition should the nurse suspect with these symptoms?
1. Child abuse
2. Henoch-Schönlein purpura (HSP)
3. Idiopathic thrombocytopenic purpura (ITP)
4. Rocky Mountain spotted fever

53. 2. HSP is a disorder that can cause bleeding and inflammation of the small blood vessels in the skin, joints, kidneys and intestine. The rash associated with HSP is believed to occur in every client, and allows for a definitive diagnosis. It begins as petechiae and progresses to purpuric lesions of the buttocks and lower extremities. The lesions of child abuse are painful and nonraised. Petechiae or purpura associated with ITP are distributed over the entire body. The rash associated with Rocky Mountain spotted fever is a nonraised and macular papular over the body.
CN: Physiological integrity; CNS: Physiological adaptation; CL: Apply

54. A mother asks why she can't use 2.5% hydrocortisone cream prescribed for eczema for longer than one week. What is the nurse's **best** response?
1. The drug loses its efficacy after prolonged use.
2. This reduces adverse effects, such as skin atrophy and fragility.
3. If no improvement is seen, a stronger concentration will be prescribed.
4. If no improvement is seen after one week, an antibiotic will be prescribed.

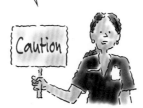

Adverse effects can result from prolonged use of certain medications.

54. 2. Hydrocortisone cream should be used for brief periods to decrease adverse effects such as skin atrophy. The drug doesn't lose efficacy after prolonged use. A stronger concentration may not be prescribed if no improvement is seen, and an antibiotic would be inappropriate.
CN: Physiological integrity; CNS: Pharmacological and parenteral therapies; CL: Apply

55. The A mother brings her nine-year-old child to the ER because she noticed lesions on his tongue. On assessment, the nurse notes painless, slightly depressed, red lesions bordered by white bands. The mother reports that the pattern was different yesterday. Which condition would the nurse suspect?
1. Geographic tongue
2. Koplik's spots
3. Scald burns
4. Stomatitis

55. 1. Geographic tongue is a benign disorder caused by loss of filiform papules. The configuration is known to change from day to day. Koplik's spots and stomatitis lesions don't change patterns. Scald burns are painful lesions caused by hot liquids.
CN: Physiological integrity; CNS: Physiological adaptation; CL: Apply

56. A four-year-old child developed a subungual hemorrhage of the toe after a jar fell on his foot and is scheduled for electrocautery. What is the expected outcome of this procedure?
1. Prevent loss of nail growth
2. Prevent the spread of infection
3. Relieve pain and reduce the risk for infection
4. Prevent permanent discoloration of the nail bed

56. 3. The hematoma is treated with electrocautery to relieve pain and reduce risk for infection. Electrocautery doesn't prevent the loss of the nail. The discoloration seen with subungual hemorrhage is from the collection of blood under the nail bed. It isn't permanent and doesn't affect nail growth.
CN: Physiological integrity; CNS: Physiological adaptation; CL: Apply

57. The nurse is caring for a 12-year-old child diagnosed with eczema. Which nursing intervention is appropriate for the child?
1. Antibiotics as prescribed
2. Antifungals as ordered
3. Tepid baths and application of moisturizers to the skin
4. Hot baths and vigorous drying of the skin

57. 3. Tepid baths and moisturizers are indicated to keep the infected areas clean and minimize itching. Antibiotics are given when superimposed infection is present. Antifungals usually aren't the treatment for eczema. Hot baths can exacerbate the condition and increase itching.
CN: Physiological integrity; CNS: Physiological adaptation; CL: Apply

58. A nine-year-old is brought to the emergency department with extensive burns sustained in a restaurant fire. What is the nurse's **most** important intervention?
1. Administer prescribed antibiotics to prevent superimposed infections
2. Conduct a wound assessment
3. Administer liquids orally to replace lost fluid
4. Administer frequent, small meals to support nutritional requirements

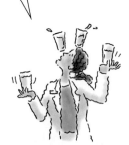

I've heard of maintaining fluid balance, but this is ridiculous!

58. 2. The most important aspect of care for a child with burns is wound management. The goals of wound care are to speed debridement, protect granulation tissue and new grafts, and conserve body heat and fluids. Antibiotics aren't always administered prophylactically. Fluids are administered IV to replace fluid volume according to the child's body weight. Enteral feedings, rather than meals, are initiated within the first 24 hours after the burn to support the child's increased nutritional requirements.
CN: Physiological integrity; CNS: Physiological adaptation; CL: Apply

CN: Client needs category   CNS: Client needs subcategory   CL: Cognitive level

59. The mother of a four-month-old infant asks the nurse about the strawberry hemangioma she noticed on his cheek. What information should the nurse provide to the mother?
1. The lesion will continue to grow for three years and will require surgical removal.
2. If the lesion continues to enlarge, the child should be referred to a pediatric oncologist.
3. Surgery is indicated before age 12 months if the diameter of the lesion is greater than three cm.
4. The lesion will continue to grow until age one year, and will begin to resolve by age two to three years.

59. **4.** These rapidly-growing vascular lesions reach maximum growth by age one year. The growth period is followed by an involution period of 6 to 12 months. Lesions show complete involution by age two or three years. These benign lesions don't require surgical or oncologic referrals.
CN: Health promotion and maintenance; CNS: None;
CL: Apply

60. A three-year-old child is being discharged after receiving sutures for a scalp laceration. What response, by the parent, indicates an understanding of the suture removal?
1. "I will bring the child back in 1 to 3 days."
2. "I will bring the child back in 5 to 7 days."
3. "I will bring the child back in 8 to 10 days."
4. "I will bring the child back in 10 to 14 days."

60. **2.** The recommended healing time for this type of laceration is five to seven days. Sutures require more than one to three days to form an effective bond. Eight to 10 days are needed for sutures of the fingertips and feet, and 10 to 14 days are recommended for extensor surfaces of the knees and elbows.
CN: Physiological integrity; CNS: Physiological adaptation;
CL: Apply

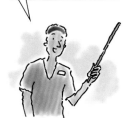

Bolded words in questions are clues to the right answer.

61. Which symptom is an **early** sign of infection of a laceration?
1. Fever
2. Copious drainage
3. Excessive discomfort
4. Local nodal enlargement

61. **3.** The first sign of infection is usually excessive discomfort. Nodal enlargement, fever, and copious drainage are advanced signs of infection.
CN: Health promotion and maintenance; CNS: None; CL: Analyze

62. The nurse is teaching a 17-year-old client how to change a sterile dressing on his right leg. During the teaching session, the nurse notices redness, swelling, and induration at the wound site. How should the nurse interpret these findings?
1. Infection
2. Dehiscence
3. Hemorrhage
4. Evisceration

62. **1.** Infection produces redness, swelling, induration, warmth, and possible drainage. Dehiscence may cause unexplained fever and tachycardia, unusual wound pain, prolonged paralytic ileus, and separation of the surgical incision. Hemorrhage can result in increased pulse and respiratory rate, decreased blood pressure, restlessness, thirst, and cold, clammy skin. Evisceration produces visible protrusion of organs, usually through an incision.
CN: Physiological integrity; CNS: Physiological adaptation;
CL: Analyze

63. The nurse is assessing a six-year-old child diagnosed with herpes zoster of the left anterior chest. Which assessment findings would the nurse document?
1. Bruising and swelling
2. Papulovesicular eruptions with reports of pain and tenderness of the lesion
3. Linear burrows on the fingers and toes
4. Papulovesicular lesions on the chest, trunk, face, and scalp

63. **2.** Herpes zoster is caused by the varicella-zoster virus. It presents with papulovesicular lesions that erupt along a dermatome, usually with hyperesthesia, pain, and tenderness. Contusions are present with bruising and swelling. Scabies appear as linear burrows of the fingers and toes caused by a mite. The papulovesicular lesions of varicella are distributed over the entire trunk, face, and scalp and don't follow a dermatome.
CN: Physiological integrity; CNS: Physiological adaptation;
CL: Analyze

CN: Client needs category   CNS: Client needs subcategory   CL: Cognitive level

64. The nurse notes a flat, dull pink, macular lesion on the forehead of a five-month-old infant. Which condition would the nurse suspect?
1. Cavernous hemangioma
2. Nevus flammeus
3. Salmon patch
4. Strawberry hemangioma

64. 3. Salmon patches are common vascular lesions in infants. They appear as flat, dull pink, macular lesions in various regions of the face and head. When they appear on the nape of the neck, they're commonly called stork bites. These lesions fade by the first year of life. Both strawberry and cavernous hemangiomas are raised lesions. Nevus flammeus, or port wine stains, are reddish-purple lesions that don't fade.

CN: Physiological integrity; CNS: Physiological adaptation; CL: Apply

65. A child's parent asks the nurse for advice on the use of insect repellents that contains DEET. What is the nurse's **best** response?
1. "Spray the child's clothing instead of the skin."
2. "The repellent works better as the temperature increases."
3. "The repellent isn't effective against the ticks responsible for Lyme disease."
4. "Apply insect repellent as you would sunscreen, with frequent applications during the day."

65. 1. DEET spray has been approved for use on children. It should be used sparingly on all skin surfaces. By spraying the clothing and camping equipment, the adverse effects and potential toxic buildup are significantly reduced. Repellent is lost to evaporation, wind, heat, and perspiration. Each 10° F increase in temperature leads to as much as a 50% reduction in protection time. DEET is very effective as a tick repellent.

CN: Physiological integrity; CNS: Reduction of risk potential; CL: Apply

66. A nurse is teaching a parent which DEET-containing insect repellent to use on his child. Which concentration will yield optimal results?
1. 10%
2. 15%
3. 20%
4. 30%

66. 1. For use on children, the highest concentration approved by the Food and Drug Administration and recommended by Health Canada is 10%. Because of thinner skin and greater surface area to mass ratio in children, parents should use DEET products sparingly.

CN: Physiological integrity; CNS: Reduction of risk potential; CL: Apply

67. The nurse is teaching at a community health fair about common skin problems. Which statement, about warts, would the nurse incorporate in this program?
1. Cutting the wart is the preferred treatment for children.
2. There is no specific treatment to kill the wart virus.
3. Warts are caused by a virus affecting the inner layer of skin.
4. Warts are harmless, and usually last three to four years if untreated.

67. 2. The goal of treatment is to kill the skin that contains the wart virus. Cutting the wart is likely to spread the virus. The virus that causes warts affects the outer layer of the skin. Warts are harmless, and last one to two years if untreated.

CN: Health promotion and maintenance; CNS: None; CL: Apply

68. The nurse is assisting with a teaching program for new parents that focuses on oral hygiene. What should the nurse include as a cause of tooth decay and gum disease when allowed to remain on the teeth for prolonged periods?
1. Breast milk
2. Pacifiers
3. Thumb or other fingers
4. Formula

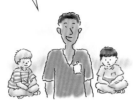

You need to brush those carbs away.

68. 4. Tooth decay and gum disease result when the carbohydrates in formula, cow's milk, and fruit juices are allowed to remain on the teeth for a prolonged period. Studies have shown that breast milk only contributes to dental caries when sugar is already present on the teeth. Breast milk alone promotes enamel growth. Pacifiers and fingers don't cause tooth decay and gum disease, although they may contribute to malocclusion.
CN: Health promotion and maintenance; CNS: None;
CL: Apply

69. The nurse is assessing a child with suspected cellulitis. Which assessment findings, associated with cellulitis, should the nurse document? Select all that apply.
1. Pale skin that is irritated, and cold to touch
2. Vesicular blisters at the site of the injury
3. Edema, tenderness and warmth at the site
4. Swelling, redness, with well-defined borders
5. Blisters and skin dimpling
6. Erythema, and thick patches of plaque

69. 3, 5. Cellulitis is a deep, locally diffuse infection of the skin. It is associated with redness, fever, edema, tenderness, and warmth at the site of the injury. Vesicular blisters suggest impetigo. Cellulitis has no well-defined borders. Thick patches of plaque are associated with psoriasis
CN: Physiological integrity; CNS: Physiological adaptation;
CL: Apply

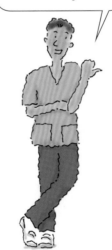

Note that this question asks about the *most likely cause*, not the only one.

70. The nurse is assessing a two-year-old child who was diagnosed with cellulitis of the finger. Which organism or condition is the **most** likely the cause of cellulitis?
1. Parainfluenza virus
2. Respiratory syncytial virus
3. *Escherichia coli*
4. *Streptococcus*

70. 4. *Streptococcus* cause most cases of cellulitis. Parainfluenza and respiratory syncytial virus cause infections of the respiratory tract. *Escherichia coli* is a cause of bladder infections.
CN: Physiological integrity; CNS: Physiological adaptation;
CL: Analyze

71. Which signs and symptoms would indicate that the child is experiencing Stevens-Johnson syndrome?
1. Shedding of the skin
2. Thin, reddened layers of epidermis
3. Thick skin with deep visible burrows
4. Thinning skin that may appear translucent

71. 1. Desquamation is characteristic in diseases such as Stevens-Johnson syndrome. Scaling is thin, reddened layers of epidermis. Thickening of the skin with burrows is defined as lichenification. Thinning skin is best described as atrophy of the skin.
CN: Physiological integrity; CNS: Physiological adaptation;
CL: Apply

72. The nurse is providing information on medication administration to the parents of a child who is to receive nystatin oral solution. Which statement would indicate an understanding of the teaching?
1. "I should give the solution immediately after feedings."
2. "I should give the solution immediately before feedings."
3. "I should mix the solution with small amounts of the feeding."
4. "I should give half the solution before and half the solution after the feeding."

72. 1. Nystatin oral solution should be swabbed onto the mouth after feedings to allow for optimal contact with mucous membranes. Applying the solution before meals and with meals doesn't allow sufficient contact with mucous membranes.
CN: Physiological integrity; CNS: Pharmacological and parenteral therapies; CL: Apply

CN: Client needs category   CNS: Client needs subcategory   CL: Cognitive level

73. The nurse is assessing an infant, and notes the presence of a petechial rash. How would the nurse **most** accurately describe this rash?
1. A purple macular lesion larger than 1 cm in diameter
2. Purple to brown bruises, macular or papular, of various sizes
3. A collection of blood from ruptured blood vessels larger than one cm in diameter
4. A pinpoint, pink to purple, non-blanching macular lesion 1 to 3 mm in diameter

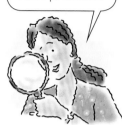

Where are those petechiae?

73. 4. Petechiae are small, 1 to 3 mm macular lesions. Purple macular lesions greater than one cm are defined as purpura. A bruise is defined as ecchymosis. A hematoma is a collection of blood.
CN: Physiological integrity; CNS: Physiological adaptation;
CL: Apply

74. The nurse is inspecting the palms of a child with a rash. With which condition is a rash on the palm unchanging?
1. Coxsackie virus
2. Measles
3. Rocky Mountain spotted fever
4. Syphilis

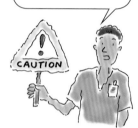

The location of a rash can be critical in identifying its cause.

CAUTION

74. 2. The rash in measles occurs on the face, trunk, and extremities. Rocky Mountain spotted fever, syphilis, and coxsackie virus shows a changing rash on the palms and soles.
CN: Physiological integrity; CNS: Physiological adaptation;
CL: Analyze

75. A mother tells the nurse that her teenager is losing hair in small round areas on the scalp. The nurse interprets this as:
1. Alopecia
2. Scalp psoriasis
3. Atopic dermatitis
4. Seborrhea dermatitis

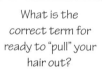

What is the correct term for ready to "pull" your hair out?

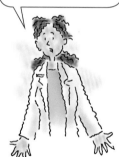

75. 1. Alopecia is the correct term for thinning hair loss. Scalp psoriasis consists of reddened patches of skin that are covered with silvery plaques and a thick crust on the scalp. Atopic dermatitis is eczema and may consist of clusters of small erythematous papules and skin that may appear dry and hyperpigmented. Seborrheic dermatitis is cradle cap and occurs in infants.
CN: Physiological integrity; CNS: Physiological adaptation;
CL: Apply

76. The nurse is teaching the parent of a child diagnosed with eczema how to apply a prescribed topical steroid cream. How should the nurse instruct the parent to apply the cream?
1. Over the entire body
2. Rub a thin layer to the affected area
3. Apply to the infected area without washing the area first
4. Apply a thick layer and allow it to absorb

76. 2. After gently cleansing the affected area, corticosteroid cream should be applied in a thin, not thick, layer and rubbed into the area thoroughly. It shouldn't be applied to the entire body.
CN: Physiological integrity; CNS: Pharmacological and parenteral therapies; CL: Apply

77. The mother of a toddler diagnosed with atopic dermatitis is concerned about how her child acquired the disease. What is the nurse's **best** response?
1. It is a fungal infection.
2. It is a hereditary disorder.
3. It is a sex-linked disorder.
4. It is a viral infection.

77. 2. Atopic dermatitis is a hereditary disorder that isn't sex-linked and is associated with a family history of asthma, allergic rhinitis, or atopic dermatitis. Viral and fungal infections don't cause atopic dermatitis.
CN: Physiological integrity; CNS: Physiological adaptation;
CL: Apply

78. The nurse is providing instruction to the mother of a six-month-old infant with atopic dermatitis. The mother asks the nurse for advice on bathing the child. What is the nurse's **best** response?
  1. "Bathe the infant twice daily."
  2. "Bathe the infant every other day."
  3. "Use coldest water tolerated to decrease itching."
  4. "The frequency of the infant's baths isn't important in atopic dermatitis."

79. A parent asks the nurse why his child with atopic dermatitis needs to keep his fingernails cut short? What is the nurse's **best** response?
  1. To prevent infection of the nail bed
  2. To prevent the spread of the disorder
  3. To prevent the child from causing scarring of the cornea
  4. To prevent breaks in skin from scratching that may lead to secondary bacterial infections

80. The clinic nurse is providing care for a child being treated for common warts. The mother asks the nurse about the cause. What is the nurse's **best** response?
  1. Coxsackievirus
  2. Human herpesvirus
  3. Human immunodeficiency virus
  4. Human papillomavirus

81. The nurse is assessing a six-year-old child with a spiny projection suspended from a narrow stalk of skin on the forehead. Which condition would the nurse suspect?
  1. Filiform wart
  2. Flat wart
  3. Plantar wart
  4. Venereal warts

82. The school nurse is assisting with the annual school physicals. An adolescent tells the nurse that his feet itch, sweat a lot, and have a foul odor. What condition should the nurse suspect?
  1. Candidiasis
  2. Tinea corporis
  3. Tinea pedis
  4. Molluscum contagiosum

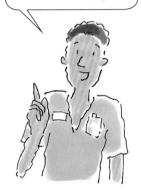

Here's another question pointing out the importance of client teaching.

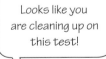

Looks like you are cleaning up on this test!

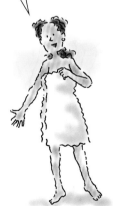

78. 2. Bathing removes lipoprotein complexes that hold water in the stratum corneum and increases water loss. Bathing the child every other day can help prevent the removal of lipoprotein complexes. Soap and bubble bath should be used sparingly while bathing the child.
CN: Physiological integrity; CNS: Basic care and comfort; CL: Apply

79. 4. Keeping fingernails short will prevent breaks in the skin when a child scratches. Cutting fingernails too short, or cutting the skin around the nail can increase the risk of infection. Atopic dermatitis can be found in various areas of the skin, but isn't spread from one area to another. Keeping fingernails short is a good way to reduce corneal abrasions but doesn't apply to atopic dermatitis.
CN: Physiological integrity; CNS: Physiological adaptation; CL: Apply

80. 4. Human papillomavirus is responsible for various forms of warts. Coxsackievirus is associated with hand-foot-and-mouth disease. Human herpesvirus is associated with varicella and herpes zoster. Human immunodeficiency virus infections aren't associated with epithelial tumors known as warts.
CN: Physiological integrity; CNS: Physiological adaptation; CL: Apply

81. 1. Filiform warts are long spiny projections from the skin surface. Flat warts are flat-topped, smooth-surfaced lesions. Plantar warts are rough papules, commonly found on the soles of the feet. Venereal warts appear on the genital mucosa and are confluent papules with rough surfaces.
CN: Physiological integrity; CNS: Physiological adaptation; CL: Apply

82. 3. Tinea pedis is a superficial fungal infection on the feet, commonly called athletes' foot. Candidiasis is a fungal infection of the skin or mucous membranes commonly found in the oral, vaginal, and intestinal mucosal tissue. Tinea corporis, or ringworm, is a flat, scaling papular lesion with raised borders. Molluscum contagiosum is a viral skin infection with lesions that are small red papules.
CN: Physiological integrity; CNS: Physiological adaptation; CL: Analyze

CN: Client needs category   CNS: Client needs subcategory   CL: Cognitive level

83. A nurse is explaining treatments to the parents of a child with hypertrophic scarring. What is the **best** method to control this condition?
1. Compression garments
2. Moisturizing creams
3. Physiotherapy
4. Splints

83. 1. Compression garments are worn for up to one year to control hypertrophic scarring. Moisturizing creams help decrease hyperpigmentation. Physiotherapy and splints help keep joints and limbs supple.
CN: Physiological integrity; CNS: Physiological adaptation;
CL: Apply

84. The nurse is assessing a child and notes nails with pits and ridges. The nails are thick and discolored and have splintered hemorrhages that are easily separated from the nail bed. The nurse would document this condition as:
1. paronychia.
2. psoriasis.
3. scabies.
4. seborrhea.

84. 2. Pitting, brittle nails with changes in color can be caused by systemic diseases, nutritional deficiencies or localized fungal infections. Additionally, pitting of the nail is commonly associated with psoriasis. Paronychia is a bacterial infection of the nail bed. Scabies are mites that burrow under the skin, usually between the webbing of the fingers and toes. Seborrhea is a chronic inflammatory dermatitis often called cradle cap.
CN: Physiological integrity; CNS: Physiological adaptation;
CL: Apply

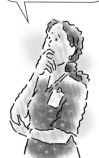

What is the most accurate interpretation?

85. An assessment of a neonate reveals bruising on the scalp, along with diffuse swelling of the soft tissue that crosses over the suture line. The nurse **most** accurately interprets these findings as:
1. caput succedaneum.
2. cephalhematoma.
3. craniotabes.
4. hydrocephalus.

85. 1. Caput succedaneum originates from trauma to the neonate while descending through the birth canal. It's usually a benign injury that spontaneously resolves over time. Cephalhematoma is a collection of blood in the periosteum of the scalp that doesn't cross over the suture line. Craniotabes is the thinning of the bone of the scalp. Hydrocephalus is an increased volume of cerebrospinal fluid (CSF), or the obstruction of the flow of the CSF, and isn't related to soft tissue swelling.
CN: Physiological integrity; CNS: Physiological adaptation;
CL: Analyze

86. The clinic nurse is assessing a child and notes a healed wound from a traumatic injury. The child's mother is concerned because the lesion formed over the wound is pink, thickened, smooth, and rubbery in nature. How would the nurse interpret this finding?
1. Erosion
2. Lichenification
3. Keloids
4. Striae

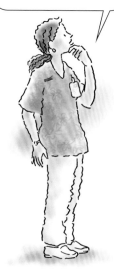

Hmmm, white plaques with an erythematous base. What could that mean?

86. 3. Keloids are an exaggerated connective tissue response to skin injury. An erosion is a depressed vesicular lesion. Lichenification has the appearance of thick, leathery skin and may occur as the result of continuous rubbing and scratching. Striae are linear depressions of the skin.
CN: Physiological integrity; CNS: Physiological adaptation;
CL: Apply

87. A mother reports that her infant has had poor feeding for a few days. A complete physical examination shows white plaques in the mouth with an erythematous base. The plaques stick to the mucous membranes tightly and bleed when scraped. How should the nurse interpret these findings?
1. Aphthous ulcers
2. Herpes lesions
3. Koplik's spots
4. Oral candidiasis

87. 4. Oral candidiasis, or thrush, is a painful inflammation that can affect the tongue, soft and hard palates, and buccal mucosa. Aphthous ulcers are small, shallow lesions that may develop on the soft tissues in the mouth or at the base of the gums. Herpes lesions are usually vesicular ulcerations of the oral mucosa around the lips. Measles that form Koplik's spots can be identified as pinpoint, white, elevated lesions.
CN: Physiological integrity; CNS: Physiological adaptation;
CL: Apply

CN: Client needs category   CNS: Client needs subcategory   CL: Cognitive level

88. The nurse in the emergency department is assessing a child that was found unconscious at home and brought to the emergency department by the fire and rescue unit. Physical examination reveals cherry-red mucous membranes, nail beds, and skin. The nurse suspects the child's condition was the result of:
   1. aspirin ingestion.
   2. carbon monoxide poisoning.
   3. hydrocarbon ingestion.
   4. alcohol ingestion.

89. A 14-year-old client diagnosed with acne vulgaris asks the nurse about the cause. Which factors should the nurse identify for this client? Select all that apply.
   1. Chocolates and sweets
   2. Increased hormone levels
   3. Growth of anaerobic bacteria
   4. Caffeine
   5. Heredity
   6. Fatty foods

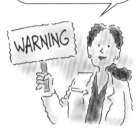

Be careful! There may be more than one correct answer to this question.

WARNING

90. The nurse is assessing a child with a suspected fungal infection on the upper right arm. The assessment reveals a red circular rash with clearer skin in the middle. How should these findings be interpreted?
   1. Tinea capitis
   2. Tinea corporis
   3. Tinea cruris
   4. Tinea pedis

91. The nurse is administering amoxicillin/clavulanate potassium to a child with cellulitis. The provider has ordered 40 mg/kg to be given three times a day over 24 hours. The child weighs 33 lb (15 kg), and the pharmacy has sent amoxicillin/clavulanate 200 mg/5 ml. How many milliliters per dose should the nurse administer? Record your answer using a whole number.

_____ ml/dose

88. 2. Cherry-red skin changes are seen when a child has been exposed to high levels of carbon monoxide. Nausea and vomiting and pale skin are symptoms of aspirin ingestion. A hydrocarbon or petroleum ingestion usually results in respiratory symptoms and tachycardia. A spider bite reaction is usually localized to the area of the bite.
CN: Physiological integrity; CNS: Physiological adaptation; CL: Analyze

89. 2, 3, 5. Acne vulgaris is characterized by the appearance of comedones. Comedones develop for various reasons, including increased hormone levels, heredity, irritation or application of irritating substances, and growth of anaerobic bacteria. A direct relationship between acne vulgaris and consumption of chocolates, caffeine, or fatty foods has not been established.
CN: Physiological integrity; CNS: Physiological adaptation; CL: Apply

90. 2. Tinea corporis describes fungal infections of the body. Tinea capitis describes fungal infections of the scalp. Tinea cruris describes fungal infections of the inner thigh and inguinal creases. Tinea pedis is the term for fungal infections of the foot.
CN: Physiological integrity; CNS: Physiological adaptation; CL: Apply

91. 5.
The dose is calculated by first multiplying the weight times the milligrams. It's then divided by three even doses. The milligrams are then used to determine the milliliters based on the concentration of the medicine.

$$40\,mg/kg \times 15\,kg = 600\,mg$$

$$600\,mg/3\,doses = 200\,mg/dose$$

The concentration is 200 mg in every 5 ml.
CN: Physiological integrity; CNS: Pharmacological and parenteral therapies; CL: Apply

92. The nurse in the emergency department is caring for a five-year-old male who sustained third-degree burns to his right upper extremity after tipping over a frying pan. Which skin structures would the nurse include when explaining a third-degree, full-thickness burn to the child's mother?
1. Epidermis only
2. Epidermis and dermis
3. All skin layers and nerve endings
4. Skin layers, nerve endings, muscles, tendons, and bones

92. 3. A third-degree burn involves all of the skin layers and the nerve endings. First-degree burns involve only the epidermis. Second-degree burns affect the epidermis and dermis. Fourth-degree burns involve all skin layers, nerve endings, muscles, tendons, and bone.
CN: Physiological integrity; CNS: Physiological adaptation; CL: Apply

93. The nurse is caring for a four-year-old child who has a tick embedded in her scalp. How should the nurse remove this tick?
1. Burn the tick at the skin surface
2. Surgically remove the tick
3. Grasp the tick with tweezers and apply slow, outward pressure
4. Grasp the tick with tweezers and quickly pull the tick out

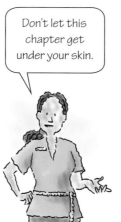

Don't let this chapter get under your skin.

93. 3. Applying gentle outward pressure prevents injury to the skin and the retention of tick parts. Burning the tick and quickly pulling the tick out may cause injury to the skin and should be avoided. Surgical removal is indicated when tick parts have been retained.
CN: Physiological integrity; CNS: Physiological adaptation; CL: Apply

94. A child with hives is prescribed diphenhydramine 5 mg/kg over 24 hours in divided doses every six hours. The child weighs 17.6 lb (8 kg). How many milligrams should be given with each dose? Record your answer using a whole number.

_____ mg

94. 10.
Multiplying 5 mg by the child's weight (8 kg) gives the amount of milligrams for 24 hours (40 mg). Divide this by 4 (doses per day), giving 10 mg/dose.

$$5\,mg/kg \times 8\,kg = 40\,mg$$

$$40\,mg/4\,doses = 10\,mg/dose$$

CN: Physiological integrity; CNS: Pharmacological and parenteral therapies; CL: Apply

95. The nurse is caring for an eight-year-old child who arrived at the emergency department with chemical burns to both legs. What is the **priority** intervention for this child?
1. Diluting the chemicals
2. Applying sterile dressings
3. Applying topical antibiotics
4. Debriding and grafting the burns

95. 1. Diluting the chemical is the priority. It will help remove the chemical and stop the burning process. The remaining treatments are initiated after dilution.
CN: Physiological integrity; CNS: Physiological adaptation; CL: Analyze

96. The nurse in the emergency department is caring for a 12-year-old child with full-thickness, circumferential burns to the chest, and has difficulty breathing. What is the **priority** intervention?
1. Chest tube insertion
2. Escharotomy
3. Intubation
4. Needle thoracocentesis

96. 3. Intubation is performed to maintain a patent airway Escharotomy is a surgical incision used to relieve pressure from edema. It's needed with circumferential burns that prevent chest expansion or cause circulatory compromise. Insertion of a chest tube and needle thoracocentesis are performed to relieve a pneumothorax.
CN: Physiological integrity; CNS: Physiological adaptation; CL: Analyze

CN: Client needs category   CNS: Client needs subcategory   CL: Cognitive level

97. The nurse is providing care for a six-year-old child who is being evaluated after sustaining burns to his left shoulder. The parents are instructed to use moisturizing cream and to protect the burn from sunlight. The parents question the nurse about the purpose of this treatment. The nurse explains that this treatment will decrease:
1. keloids.
2. lichenification.
3. hypopigmentation.
4. hyperpigmentation.

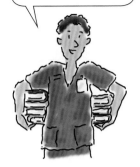

Knowing why something happens allows you to teach more effectively.

97. 4. Healed or grafted burns would require creams and protection from the sun to decrease hyperpigmentation. Scarring, hypopigmentation, and keloids aren't treated with moisturizing creams and avoidance of sunlight.
CN: Physiological integrity; CNS: Physiological adaptation; CL: Analyze

98. A 12-year-old child sustains a moderate burn injury. The mother reports that the child last received a tetanus injection when he was five years old. Which immunization would the nurse anticipate an for this child?
1. 0.5 ml of tetanus toxoid IM
2. 0.5 ml of tetanus toxoid IV
3. 250 units of tetanus immune globulin IM
4. 250 units of tetanus immune globulin IV

98. 1. Tetanus prophylaxis is given to all clients with moderate to severe burn injuries if it has been longer than five years since the last immunization, or if there is no history of immunization. The correct dosage is 0.5 ml IM, one time, if the child was immunized within 10 years. If it has been more than 10 years, or the child hasn't received tetanus immunization, the dosage is 250 units of tetanus immune globulin, one time. There is no IV form of tetanus immune globulin available.
CN: Physiological integrity; CNS: Pharmacological and parenteral therapies; CL: Analyze

99. The nurse is caring for a child who arrives at the emergency department 20 minutes after sustaining a major burn injury to 40% of his body. What is the **priority** action by the nurse?
1. Insert an indwelling catheter
2. Apply silvadene cream to the burn
3. Initiate intravenous access
4. Obtain cultures from the deepest burn area

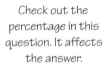
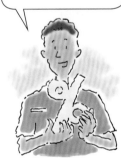

Check out the percentage in this question. It affects the answer.

99. 3. Intravenous fluids must be started immediately on all children who sustain a major burn injury to prevent the child from going into hypovolemic shock. The fluids are titrated based on urine output. To monitor this output exactly, an indwelling urinary catheter must be inserted. The other interventions will be performed but not immediately.
CN: Physiological integrity; CNS: Reduction of risk potential; CL: Apply

100. A nurse in the emergency department is caring for a child who arrives after sustaining a major burn injury. Which conditions should the nurse assess this child for within the first eight hours of admission?
1. Hyponatremia and hypokalemia
2. Hyponatremia and hyperkalemia
3. Hypernatremia and hypokalemia
4. Hypernatremia and hyperkalemia

100. 2. Capillary permeability increases during the first 48 hours postburn, allowing fluids to shift from the plasma to the interstitial spaces. This fluid is high in sodium, causing the client's serum sodium level to decrease. Potassium also leaks from the cells into the plasma, causing hyperkalemia.
CN: Physiological integrity; CNS: Physiological adaptation; CL: Analyze

101. A child weighing 22 lb (10 kg) has a deep, partial-thickness burn to 40% of his body surface area. While titrating this child's IV fluids, the nurse works to maintain which desired hourly urinary output?
  1. 5 ml
  2. 10 ml
  3. 30 ml
  4. 50 ml

102. A team of nurses is preparing a trauma room for the arrival of a child with partial-thickness burns to both lower extremities and portions of the trunk. Which intravenous fluid should the nurse be prepared to administer to this client?
  1. Albumin
  2. Dextrose 5% and half-normal saline
  3. Lactated Ringer's solution
  4. Normal saline with 2 mEq KCl/100 ml

103. A nurse is reinforcing teaching with a mother who states that that hand-foot-and-mouth disease had been diagnosed in a few of her child's pre-school classmates. The nurse should instruct the mother to observe her child for:
  1. a low-grade fever, followed by vesicular lesions on the trunk, face, and scalp.
  2. a mild, self-limiting eruption of vesicles on the buccal mucosa, tongue, soft palate, hands, and feet.
  3. purpuric, maculopapular lesions with GI symptoms and joint pain.
  4. a bright-red rash with a red border that circles a bite mark.

104. The nurse is administering penicillin V potassium to a child with cellulitis. The child weighs 27.5 lb (12.5 kg). The order reads penicillin V potassium 40 mg/kg/day po divided every six hours. How many milligrams of antibiotics should this child receive with each dose? Record your answer using a whole number.

_____ mg

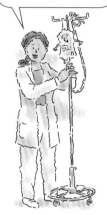

What's the magic urinary output number here?

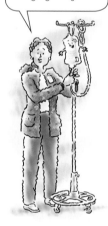

I think I hear something ringing. Do you?

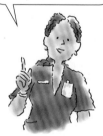

You're being asked about characteristics in question 103.

101. 2. Fluid resuscitation should be started on all clients with burns over more than 20% of their body surface area. In children, an hourly urine output of 1 to 2 ml/kg of body weight shows adequate kidney perfusion and fluid resuscitation. Adults should have an hourly urine output of 30 to 50 ml.
CN: Physiological integrity; CNS: Physiological adaptation; CL: Apply

102. 3. Lactated Ringer's solution is recommended because it replaces the lost sodium and corrects the metabolic acidosis. If albumin is ordered, it's an adjunct therapy and not for primary fluid replacement. The stress from a burn injury affects the glucose metabolism. Dextrose shouldn't be given during the first 24 hours because it can put the client into pseudodiabetes. The client is hyperkalemic from the potassium shift from the intracellular spaces to the plasma, and additional potassium would be detrimental.
CN: Physiological integrity; CNS: Pharmacological and parenteral therapies; CL: Apply

103. 2. Hand-foot-and-mouth disease is caused by coxsackievirus and usually occurs in preschool children. Vesicular lesions accompanied by a low-grade fever are typical signs of varicella. Purpura, GI symptoms, and joint pain are symptoms of Henoch-Schönlein purpura. A bright-red, bull's-eye rash is a classic symptom of Lyme disease.
CN: Physiological integrity; CNS: Physiological adaptation; CL: Apply

104. 125.
40 mg/kg/day equals a total of 500 mg given every six hours or four times in 24 hours. 500 mg divided by four equals 125 mg.
CN: Physiological integrity; CNS: Pharmacological and parenteral therapies; CL: Apply

105. While assessing a two-year-old child brought into the clinic with an upper respiratory infection, the nurse notes bruising on his arms, legs, and trunk. Which findings would prompt the nurse to suspect child abuse? Select all that apply.
1. Superficial scrapes on the lower legs
2. Welts or bruises in various stages of healing on the trunk
3. A deep blue-black patch on the buttocks
4. One large bruise on the thigh
5. Circular, symmetrical burns on the lower legs
6. A parent who is hypercritical of the child and pushes the frightened child away

105. **2, 5, 6.** Injuries in various stages of healing in protected or padded areas can be a sign of inflicted trauma, leading the nurse to suspect abuse. Burns that are bilateral as well as symmetrical are typical of child abuse. The shape of the burn may resemble the item used to create it. Pushing the child away, and being hypercritical are typical behaviors of abusive parents. Superficial scrapes and bruises on the lower legs are normal in a healthy, active child. A deep blue-black macular patch on the buttocks is more consistent with a Mongolian spot rather than a traumatic injury.
CN: Psychosocial integrity; CNS: None; CL: Analyze

106. A 44 lb (20 kg) preschooler is being treated for inflammation. The provider orders 0.2 mg/kg/day of dexamethasone by mouth to be administered every six hours. The elixir comes in a strength of 0.5 mg/5 ml. How many milliliters of dexamethasone should the nurse give this client per dose? Record your answer using a whole number.

_____ ml

106. **1.**
Calculate the total daily dose:
$$20\,kg \times 0.2\,mg/kg/day = 4\,mg/day$$
Next, calculate the amount to be given at each dose:
$$4\,mg/day \div 4\,doses/day = 1\,mg/dose$$
The elixir contains 0.5 mg of drug per 5 ml. To give 1 mg of drug, administer 10 ml to the child at each dose.
CN: Physiological integrity; CNS: Pharmacological and parenteral therapies; CL: Analyze

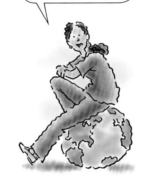

You did it! You should be on top of the world!

107. An infant is being treated with antibiotic therapy for otitis media. During a follow up visit the clinic nurse completes an assessment of a 10-month-old child. Based on the findings, documented by the nurse below, which explanation will **most** likely be given to the mother?

107. **1.** Candidiasis, caused by yeast-like fungi, can occur with the use of antibiotics. The treatment for candidiasis is topical nystatin ointment. Changing the brand of diapers or suggesting that the parent use an over-the-counter remedy would be appropriate for treating diaper rash, not candidiasis. Antibiotic therapy shouldn't be stopped.
CN: Physiological integrity; CNS: Physiological adaptation; CL: Analyze

Progress notes	
10/15/16 0730	A 10-month-old male was brought in for a follow up visit. The infant is currently being treated for otitis media per the mother, and the mother is worried about the rash. There is an erythematous, fine, raised rash in the groin, inguinal folds that extends approximately two inches into the suprapubic area. The rash is sharply demarcated and has several satellite lesions that extend beyond the larger lesion.————— H. Brown, RN

1. The infant has candidiasis
2. Change the brand of diapers
3. Use an over-the-counter diaper remedy
4. Stop the antibiotic therapy immediately

Part VI

Issues in Nursing

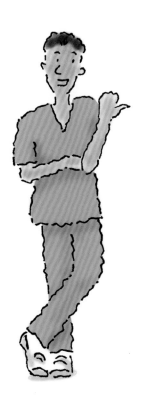

Chapter 36

Management & Leadership

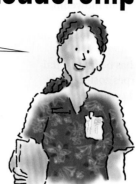

In this chapter, you'll be asked questions about management concepts, methods of coordination, and supervision of care. Take your time here.

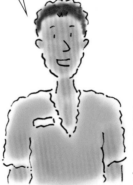

The nurse-manager is accountable 24/7.

1. At the beginning of a shift, the team leader notices that all of the IV antibiotics for a client are still in the medication room. What is the team leader's **first** action?
  1. Ask the client if they received their medications during the previous shift
  2. Return the medications to the pharmacy to reduce hospital expenses
  3. Ask the nurse assigned to this client about the medications
  4. Notify the unit's nurse manager

2. Which is an example of tertiary prevention in disaster planning?
  1. Providing routine tetanus immunizations
  2. Instituting disaster drills
  3. Implementing biohazard precautions
  4. Counseling disaster victims about stress reactions

1. 3. The team leader should attempt to clarify this matter with the assigned staff first. The client would not be an accurate source of information regarding the IV medications. Returning the supplies is secondary to ensuring that the client received the required medications.
CN: Safe, effective care environment; CNS: Safety and infection control; CL: Analyze

2. 4. Tertiary prevention involves reducing the degree and quantity of injury, disability, and damage following a disaster or crisis. Primary prevention focuses on keeping the crisis or disaster from occurring. The goal of secondary prevention is to reduce the duration and intensity of the disaster or crisis. The other choices would take place before a disaster occurs.
CN: Safe, effective care environment; CNS: Management of care; CL: Apply

3. The nurse is triaging clients from a large disaster. Prioritize care for these clients based on the severity of their injuries.

1. A client with a large shard of glass piercing the chest wall with respirations of 32 breaths/min
2. A client with a disfigured forearm with a protruding bone and capillary refill of two seconds
3. A child with one-inch (2.54 cm) laceration on his leg
4. A woman who is two months pregnant with a partial-thickness burn on her forearm

3. Ordered Response:

1. A client with a large shard of glass piercing the chest wall with respirations of 32 breaths/min
2. A client with a disfigured forearm with a protruding bone and capillary refill of two seconds
4. A woman who is two months pregnant with a partial-thickness burn on her forearm
3. A child with 1 in (2.54 cm) laceration on his leg

CN: Safe, effective care environment; CNS: Safety and infection control; CL: Analyze

CN: Client needs category   CNS: Client needs subcategory   CL: Cognitive level

4. There has been a large disaster, and nurses from various units have been assigned to help with the large influx of clients. To whom would it be **most** appropriate to assign an obstetric-postpartum nurse?

1. Male client who is three days post-operative from a hemicolectomy with an indwelling urinary catheter
2. Female in pelvic traction who is three months pregnant without complications
3. Older adult woman who has been hospitalized for two days with herpes zoster
4. Male admitted for hearing command voices to kill himself

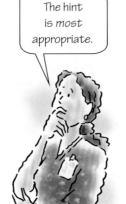

The hint is *most* appropriate.

4. 1. A nurse's current experience should be considered when assignments are made. Caring for a catheterized client who is three days post-operative from a hemicolectomy utilizes skills similar to those required for the care of a client with a cesarean section. Obstetric nurses may have limited experience with traction, and this client has no complications with her pregnancy. This nurse should not care for infectious clients to avoid disease transmission to those on her regular unit. This nurse has no experience with psychiatric clients.
CN: Safe, effective care environment; CNS: Safety and infection control; CL: Analyze

5. Which is an example of the role of an informal leader?

1. Verifying adequate staff coverage for a shift
2. Filling out a discipline form on a nursing assistant
3. Encouraging a peer to join a committee
4. Attending a hospital-wide policy meeting

5. 3. A leader does not always have formal power and authority, but influences the success of a unit by being a role model, and by guiding, encouraging, and facilitating professional growth and development in others. A manager has formal power and authority from the status within the organization. Such power and authority are detailed in the manager's job description.
CN: Safe, effective care environment; CNS: Management of care; CL: Apply

6. A disagreement has arisen over the transfer process of clients between two units of a hospital. What is the **best** way to handle this disagreement?

1. Ask the director of nursing to establish a policy
2. Allow the staff to handle the issue on their own without authoritative interference
3. Arrange managers from involved units to determine a solution
4. Arrange a meeting of staff from the units to identify key issues

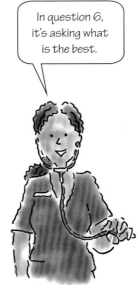

In question 6, it's asking what is the best.

6. 4. In this situation, a democratic approach is best. The staff who handles day-to-day direct client care has the best understanding of the situation, and should have autonomy to resolve this disagreement. Managers, however, should be available to moderate. Asking the director of nursing to resolve the issue reflects an autocratic management style. Without staff input, an autocratic approach won't provide the necessary information to identify the best solution. Allowing staff to determine a solution reflects a laissez-faire style of management. The staff may not have the skills or resources to solve the problem on their own. Limiting decision making to managers can create resentment and frustration among staff. The decision made by the managers may not include necessary input from the staff.
CN: Safe, effective care environment; CNS: Management of care; CL: Analyze

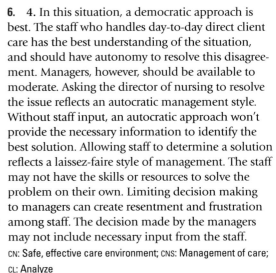

7. A staff nurse receives a phone call, and is told there is a bomb in a client's room. What is the nurse's **priority** action?

1. Put the call on hold and obtain the charge nurse
2. Transfer the call to security
3. Ask the caller for details about the bomb placement
4. Signal to staff to close the client's doors

7. 3. With imminent danger, it is important to determine as much information as possible, as quickly as possible. Transferring the call, or placing the caller on hold could result in a hang-up and loss of information. Clients may need to be evacuated.
CN: Safe, effective care environment; CNS: Safety and infection control; CL: Analyze

CN: Client needs category   CNS: Client needs subcategory   CL: Cognitive level

8. What factors determine which client care delivery system should be used?
1. Staff preference
2. Staff licensure
3. Number of staff
4. Experience of staff

8. **2.** Staff licensure identifies qua[...] staff who are qualified to appropriat[...] ents. Once the qualifications have bee[...] the appropriate nursing care delivery sys[...] be implemented to safely meet the client[...]

CN: Safe, effective care environment; CNS: Management[...]
CL: Apply

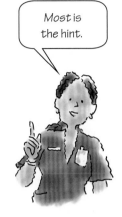

Most is the hint.

9. The nurse-manager is considering a change in the unit's nursing care delivery system from team nursing to primary nursing. Which aspect would make primary nursing **most** appropriate?
1. A common diagnosis among the unit's clients
2. The amount of training available about primary nursing
3. The number of registered nurses
4. The type of documentation system being used

9. **3.** Primary nursing is used for higher-acuity clients, and includes a high registered nurse-to-client ratio. The diagnosis is not directly related to the decision. Training is important, but primary nursing is related to the roles, division of labor, and staffing. Documentation systems are not related to type of nursing delivery system.

CN: Safe, effective care environment; CNS: Management of care;
CL: Analyze

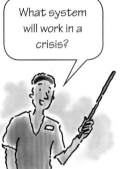

What system will work in a crisis?

10. A winter storm has prevented most of the staff on a busy medical-surgical unit from getting to work. One RN, two LPNs, and three unlicensed assistive personnel (UAP) were able to begin their shift. What nursing care delivery system should be implemented?
1. Team nursing
2. Primary nursing
3. Functional nursing
4. Case management

10. **3.** Functional nursing best uses the skills of limited staff, in a timely manner, during this crisis. This delivery system requires the least staff, and delegates tasks to those who can best perform required functions. Team nursing doesn't allow for the best use of limited staff who must care for a large number of clients. Primary nursing and case management require more registered nurses than are currently available.

CN: Safe, effective care environment; CNS: Management of care;
CL: Analyze

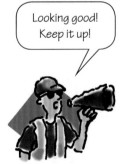

Looking good! Keep it up!

11. A new nurse on orientation asks for an example of a collaborative health care team. Which members would be included on this team? Select all that apply.
1. Case manager
2. Primary care provider
3. Radiology technician
4. Primary nurse
5. Admission manager

11. **1, 2, 4.** The collaborative health care team consists of members that help make decisions regarding the treatment plan, set goals, and solve problems. The radiology technician collects diagnostic images, and plays no role in the treatment plan. The admissions manager ensures that the client's admission paper work is entered into the healthcare record.

CN: Safe, effective care environment; CNS: Management of care;
CL: Analyze

& Leadership

795

ifications of
ely care for cli-
n identified
tem can
needs.
of care.

n calculation
· to admin-
ampicil-
n doses
ient's
ne
, whole

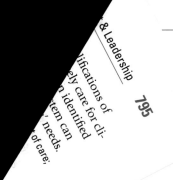

Remember

Ampicillin is for killin' bacterial meningitis."

This penicillin drug is also used in treating the following:

• Respiratory tract infections
• Skin infections
• Gastrointestinal infections
• Urinary tract infections
• Gonorrhea
• Septicemia

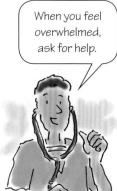

When you feel overwhelmed, ask for help.

12. 2,000.
The nurse should verify that the total dosage will not exceed the maximum dosage of 12 g/day.

$$\frac{150\ mg\,/\,kg}{day} \times 80\ kg = 12{,}000\ \frac{mg}{day} \div 6\,doses$$

$$= 2{,}000\ mg\ per\ dose$$

CN: Safe, effective care environment; CNS: Safety and infection control; CL: Apply

13. A new graduate nurse is completing the scheduled four-week orientation on a medical-surgical unit. Which knowledge deficit should prompt this nurse to request additional orientation?
1. Inability to manage a cardiac arrest independently
2. Unclear how staffing assignments are made
3. Unable to consistently establish a new IV access on the first attempt
4. Unable to simultaneously manage more than two clients

13. 4. Managing the care of multiple clients, and prioritization are skills new graduates commonly need to enhance. Additional time with a helpful preceptor will bolster these skills before a new nurse is independent. New graduates are rarely placed in charge of a client in cardiac arrest. New graduates are not in charge of running the unit. A skill such as IV insertion develops with experience, and is not an essential skill to acquire from orientation.
CN: Safe, effective care environment; CNS: Management of care; CL: Analyze

14. The supervisor is performing a chart review. The nurse can be held legally liable for which documentation?
1. 0800 administered 2 mg hydromorphone IVP per PRN orders of 1 to 2 mg every 4 hours –B Smith, RN
2. 0900 Withheld digoxin dose. Client's apical pulse is 56 beats/min –B Smith, RN
3. 0900 Withheld mononitrate dose. Client's blood pressure is 80/40 mmHg –B Smith, RN
4. 1200 Administered cephalosporin. The client has an allergy to penicillin –B Smith, RN

14. 4. There is a cross-sensitivity between cephalosporin and penicillin, and the drug should not have been given. When a dosage range is ordered, any dose in that range is acceptable. Digoxin is a cardiac glycoside that acts to improve the efficiency of the heart and may slow the heart rate and the drug should not ordinarily be given if the apical pulse is less the 60. Mononitrate is a Nitrate that can cause vasodilation and should not be given when hypotension is present.
CN: Safe, effective care environment; CNS: Management of care; CL: Analyze

15. The nursing team consists of one RN, one LPN, and one unlicensed assistive personnel (UAP). Which assignment should the RN delegate to the LPN?
1. Passing dinner trays
2. Emptying a Foley catheter bag
3. Administering daily am medications
4. Suctioning a client who is one-day postoperative following a tracheostomy

15. 3. LPNs should be assigned higher level skills in stable, predictable situations. Lower level custodial skills should be assigned to UAP. A new tracheostomy may be unstable. The task of suctioning should be retained by the RN.
CN: Safe, effective care environment; CNS: Management of care; CL: Analyze

16. A nurse manager is delegating the revision of the unit's educational policies to staff nurses. What is the **best** instructional guidance the nurse manager can offer?
1. "Let me know if you need anything."
2. "Complete the revision in six weeks."
3. "Give me your suggestions and I'll decide if I like them."
4. "Tell me what you think after looking at everything that has been done."

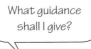

What guidance shall I give?

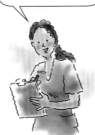

16. 2. Delegation should be done in a clear, precise manner. The nurse manager must first identify the task, and then assign responsibilities to those completing it. The desired outcome should be explained, and the time frame for completion defined. The remaining choices don't clearly define the necessary steps for successful task completion.
CN: Safe, effective care environment; CNS: Management of care; CL: Apply

17. Which task should the RN delegate to the unlicensed assistive personnel (UAP)?
1. Assessing the client's pain level in room 313
2. Advancing the diet for the client in room 212
3. Ambulating the client in room 414
4. Taking a 5 PM tympanic temperature for the client in room 515

17. 4. Taking a tympanic temperature is a specific task that can be delegated. The other options involve nursing judgment, or require evaluation. Ambulation instructions should be more specific.
CN: Safe, effective care environment; CNS: Management of care; CL: Apply

18. The nurse manager is evaluating the performance of a staff nurse who has just completed a six-month probationary period. As part of the evaluation process, the nurse manager should ask the staff nurse to:
1. accept the nurse manager's evaluation by signing in agreement.
2. contribute a self-evaluation with suggestions for future growth.
3. have peers vouch for her performance.
4. give her perception of how the nurse manager is performing.

18. 2. Performance evaluation is a nurse manager's primary managerial function. Professional growth of requires a self-reflective approach, evaluation and goal setting. A staff nurse does not need to fully agree with her performance evaluation. Peer evaluation is used in some settings, but it is done in a systematic way with clear criteria. An evaluation should focus on the staff nurse not the nurse manager's performance.
CN: Safe, effective care environment; CNS: Management of care; CL: Apply

19. A new nurse is improperly changing a client's dressing. What is the nurse manager's **best** approach when addressing this matter?
1. Ask the new nurse how she perceives her performance
2. Tell the new nurse that there are deficiencies in her performance that must be rectified in a timely manner
3. Document the inadequacies in writing, and have the new nurse sign in agreement
4. Ask the nurse educator to schedule a class for the unit on proper dressing change techniques

How do you think you are doing?

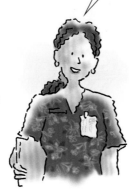

19. 1. Determining how the new nurse perceives her performance, and offering help to correct improper technique is the first step. If the new nurse shows resistance, or fails to improve after initial attempts, a more direct approach should be taken. There is no evidence that the entire unit requires remediation on this topic.
CN: Safe, effective care environment; CNS: Management of care; CL: Apply

CN: Client needs category   CNS: Client needs subcategory   CL: Cognitive level

20. The nurse manager implements new processes to decrease the incidence of central IV line infections. What is the **best** indicator that the measures have been effective?
1. A survey of the unit's nurses indicates a perceived improvement in results.
2. There has been a decrease in the number of central IV line infections on the unit.
3. Retrospective chart audits for infection rates in clients with central IV lines show an improvement.
4. A comparison of the total number of IV antibiotics used between the two time periods shows decreased usage.

20. **3.** A retrospective chart audit is a procedure for evaluating the effectiveness of the care given at a particular institution and for correcting any deficiencies found by reviewing the patient's records after discharge and comparing the data with standards. Opinions from the unit's nurses are useful but do not carry the same validity as evidence-based practice. The absolute number of infections may vary if the number of central IV lines vary. There are many reasons for the use of IV antibiotics other than central line infections.
CN: Safe, effective care environment; CNS: Management of care; CL: Analyze

21. The nurse manager notes an unacceptable number of client falls on the unit. In an attempt to decrease the incidence of falls, the nursing staff is now making hourly rounds. What is the **best** method to determine that hourly rounds have impacted the incidence of falls?
1. Evaluate scores on client satisfaction surveys
2. Survey the staff's perception of the impact
3. Compare the fall rates before and after the rounds were initiated
4. Document that the rounds were completed as scheduled

21. **3.** The best method is to obtain objective evidence that the desired results have been achieved. Objective evidence is more reliable than opinions, or merely determining that an action was completed.
CN: Safe, effective care environment; CNS: Management of care; CL: Apply

22. Which situation **best** exemplifies a nurse manager's autocratic leadership style?
1. Planning vacation time for staff
2. Directing staff activities if a client has a cardiac arrest
3. Evaluating a new medication administration process
4. Identifying the strengths and weaknesses of a client education video

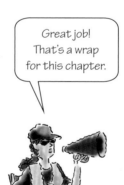

Great job! That's a wrap for this chapter.

22. **2.** In a crisis situation, the nurse manager should take command for the benefit of the client. Planning vacation time, and evaluating procedures and client resources require staff input. Requesting input is a characteristic of a democratic or participative manager.
CN: Safe, effective care environment; CNS: Management of care; CL: Apply

Chapter 37

Ethical & Legal Issues

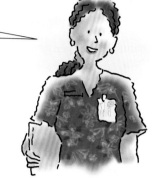

We saved the best, and most challenging, topic for last! Don't stress—you've done an excellent job!

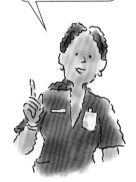

Make sure you choose the most appropriate answer.

1. Following surgery, an older adult client was transferred from post-anesthesia unit to the medical-surgical unit of a hospital. An admission assessment was completed by the nurse, then the client was left unattended with the bed in high position and the side rails down. The client falls from the bed. This nurse's action would be considered:

1. collective liability.
2. willful misconduct.
3. battery.
4. negligence.

2. Which client cannot sign out against medical advice?

1. A pregnant 15-year old with vaginal spotting
2. An adult client with ST elevation on the electrocardiogram
3. A client who drank a bottle of vodka one hour ago
4. A minor who has been emancipated by court order

3. Which circumstance would exempt the nurse from professional negligence following an error in drug administration to a client?

1. Not knowing the drug was contraindicated for this client
2. Lack of harm to the client as a result of the errant drug administration
3. Confirmation by a coworker that the dosage was correct
4. The dosage was inaccurately dispensed by the pharmacy

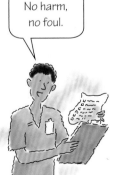

No harm, no foul.

1. 4. Negligence is failure to do what a reasonable, prudent nurse of similar training would do in the same, or similar circumstances. It is a general term that denotes conduct lacking in due care. Carelessness is a deviation from the standard of care that a reasonable person would practice in a particular set of circumstances. Collective liability stems from cooperation by several individuals in a wrongful activity, which by its nature, requires group participation. Willful misconduct is a known violation of an enforced rule or policy. Battery involves harmful or unwarranted contact with the client.

CN: Safe, effective care environment; CNS: Safety and infection control; CL: Analyze

2. 3. A client who is intoxicated is not competent to sign out against medical advice. A pregnant teen is considered an adult. A competent adult client can discharge against medical advice for any reason. A legally emancipated minor is considered an adult.

CN: Safe, effective care environment; CNS: Management of care; CL: Apply

3. 2. The four essential components of a valid lawsuit are duty, breach of duty, injury to the client, and injury to the client as a result of negligence.

CN: Safe, effective care environment; CNS: Management of care; CL: Apply

CN: Client needs category   CNS: Client needs subcategory   CL: Cognitive level

4. The nurse is reviewing orders for a newly-admitted client. Which activity would be **most** appropriate for the nurse to delegate to an unlicensed assistive personnel (UAP)?

1. Infuse 500 ml normal saline (NS) over three hours for dehydration
2. Obtain a portable chest X-ray to rule out pneumonia
3. Collect routine vital signs after the nurse has completed the initial assessment
4. Titrate oxygen per nasal cannula for oxygen (O_2) saturation less than 90%

5. An alert and oriented adult client who is a Jehovah's Witness refuses a life-saving blood transfusion. His wife, who is not a Jehovah's Witness, requests that he receive the blood. Which is the most appropriate action by the nurse?

1. Respect the client's right to refuse the transfusion
2. Honor the wife's request because refusing the transfusion would be suicidal
3. Contact the hospital administrator, and take protective custody of the client
4. See if the client has an advanced directive prior to making the decision

6. A nurse administers incorrect medication to a client. After assessing the client, and completing an incident report, which is the priority action by the nurse?

1. Report the incident to the nursing regulatory agency
2. Complete an adverse drug reaction (ADR) report
3. Anticipate suspension from the facility due to the error
4. Report the incident to risk management

7. At shift change, the departing nurse smells alcohol on the arriving nurse's breath. The departing nurse should:

1. immediately report this finding to the nursing supervisor.
2. observe the night-shift nurse for other signs of intoxication.
3. leave a note for the nurse manager to read in the morning.
4. ask the night-shift nurse if she has been drinking.

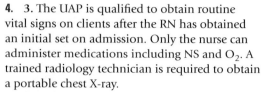
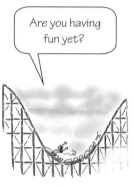

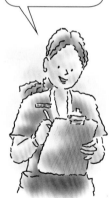

4. 3. The UAP is qualified to obtain routine vital signs on clients after the RN has obtained an initial set on admission. Only the nurse can administer medications including NS and O_2. A trained radiology technician is required to obtain a portable chest X-ray.

CN: Safe, effective care environment; CNS: Management of care; CL: Apply

5. 1. The right to refuse treatment is an ethical principle of respect for the autonomy of a competent individual. This individual must be informed of the risks and complications associated with his decision. A competent adult can refuse treatment even if their spouse does not agree. The right to die involves initiating or withholding treatment for a client who is irreversibly comatose, vegetative, or suffering with end-stage terminal illness. Protective custody is invoked with a minor. A durable power of attorney for health care is utilized when a client is incapacitated and cannot speak for himself.

CN: Safe, effective care environment; CNS: Management of care; CL: Apply

6. 4. The incident should be reported to risk management in order to evaluate care, and determine potential risks, or system problems, that contributed to the error. This type of error will not be reported to the nursing regulatory agency, or result in the nurse's suspension. Some facilities track the number of errors made by a nurse, or that occur on a particular unit, in order to provide appropriate education, and to improve the nursing process. Adverse drug reaction forms are used to report a client's reaction to a medication, not errors.

CN: Safe, effective care environment; CNS: Management of care; CL: Analyze

7. 1. The evening-shift nurse must immediately report any activity that could affect the safety of the client to the nursing supervisor. Observing for other signs of intoxication isn't the evening-shift nurse's responsibility. This situation requires immediate attention. Leaving the nurse manager a note is inappropriate. The evening-shift nurse should not confront the night-shift nurse.

CN: Safe, effective care environment; CNS: Management of care; CL: Analyze

CN: Client needs category   CNS: Client needs subcategory   CL: Cognitive level

8. While administering medication, the client tells the nurse, "I've never seen this pill before." The nurse should:
1. check the medication orders.
2. reassure the client that the health care provider has ordered this medication.
3. teach the client about the effects of the medication.
4. inform the client that pills often look different because of different brands.

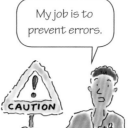

My job is to prevent errors.

CAUTION

8. 1. When a client indicates that something looks different, the nurse should verify the medication before assuming it is a correct.

CN: Safe, effective care environment; CNS: Safety and infection control; CL: Apply

9. What information must be provided to the client before informed consent is given?
1. Facts, consequences, and implications of the scheduled procedure
2. Statistical rate of success for the scheduled procedure
3. The names of health care professionals assisting with the procedure
4. The time of the procedure

9. 1. Informed consent involves providing the client with factual information regarding the treatment, tests or surgery they are about to undergo. It often includes information about the risks versus benefits of a procedure. It does not include statistical data, and the client is given only the name of the main provider, not the names of those assisting with the procedure. The client is often aware of the date and time of the procedure. When the professional nurse is involved in the informed consent process, the nurse is only witnessing the process, and doesn't actually obtain the consent. Obtaining consent is the responsibility of the health care provider.

CN: Safe, effective care environment; CNS: Management of care; CL: Apply

Feeling stressed? Take a deep breath and imagine you're in your favorite place.

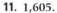

10. The nurse is calculating intake and output for a client. Intake included 1,750 ml of D5W, 500 ml of ceftriaxone, 8 oz of coffee, 4 oz of juice, and 800 ml of water. The client's output included 1,560 ml of urine, and 45 ml of vomitus. What is the total intake for this client? Record your answer using a whole number.

_____ ml

10. 3,410.

$$1,750 \ ml + 500 \ ml + (8 \ oz \times 30 \ ml/oz) + (4 \ oz \times 30 \ ml/oz) + 800 \ ml = 1,750 \ ml + 500 \ ml + 240 \ ml + 120 \ ml + 800 \ ml = 3,410 \ ml$$

CN: Safe, effective care environment; CNS: Management of care; CL: Apply

11. The nurse is calculating intake and output for a client. Intake included 1,750 ml of D5W, 500 ml of ceftriaxone, 8 oz of coffee, 4 oz of juice, and 800 ml of water. The client's output included 1,560 ml of urine, and 45 ml of vomitus. What is the total output for this client? Record your answer using a whole number.

_____ ml

11. 1,605.

$$1,560 \ ml + 45 \ ml = 1,605 \ ouput$$

CN: Safe, effective care environment; CNS: Management of care; CL: Apply

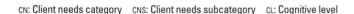

CN: Client needs category   CNS: Client needs subcategory   CL: Cognitive level

12. A client learns that she is pregnant, and asks the nurse for the names of abortion clinics. The nurse does not believe abortion is moral alternative. What is the **most** appropriate response by the nurse?
1. Remind the client that abortion stops a beating heart
2. Tell the client that she will have to ask the health care provider
3. Encourage the client to wait and think about it
4. Give the client the available preprinted list of clinics

12. 4. Nurses should provide nonjudgmental care. A nurse cannot withhold care based on personal religious beliefs. Alternately, the nurse could ask a colleague to provide this client with the information.

CN: Safe, effective care environment; CNS: Management of care; CL: Analyze

13. A client has terminal cancer. Which statement **best** describes the anger stage of grieving according to the Kübler-Ross model?
1. "I've lived a good life and am ready to go."
2. "I need a better doctor so he can cure me!"
3. "I'm not taking any more chemotherapy because the cancer is resistant."
4. "I can't believe God would do this to me!"

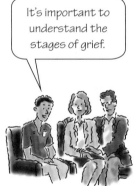

It's important to understand the stages of grief.

13. 4. Anger is the most intense grief reaction. It arises when people realize that death and loss will occur, or has occurred to a family member. Denial is the avoidance of death's inevitability, and is the first step of the grieving process. Bargaining happens when family members attempt to stall or manipulate the outcome or death. Depression is a response to loss that is expressed as profound sadness or deep suffering. Acceptance is the final stage of grieving. It is the ability to overcome grief, and accept what has happened.

CN: Psychosocial integrity; CNS: None; CL: Apply

14. While performing an assessment of a 75-year-old client in the emergency department, a nurse notes several areas of ecchymosis in various stages of healing on the client's body. What is the nurse's **priority** action?
1. Notify the nursing supervisor
2. Notify the health care provider
3. Inquire how these bruises occurred
4. Document the findings

14. 3. The nurse should obtain more information from the client first, in order to complete the initial assessment. The nurse should not assume that the bruises are a result of abuse, and she should not notify the nursing supervisor until additional facts are obtained. The nurse should inform the provider so an examination can be completed. She should follow the facility's policy and procedure for reporting abuse and document the findings.

CN: Psychosocial integrity; CNS: None; CL: Apply

15. An alert and oriented client states that he does not want chemotherapy. His family believes that he should receive it. Which is the nurse's **best** response to the client?
1. "Have you discussed this with your religious advisor?"
2. "How does your family feel about your decision?"
3. "You understand that this decision is ultimately yours to make."
4. "I think that you should carefully consider chemotherapy."

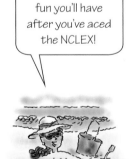

Think of all the fun you'll have after you've aced the NCLEX!

15. 3. A competent client has the right to refuse care. The role of the nurse is to advocate for the client and respect the client's decision. In that role, it is essential for the nurse to make sure that the client is informed regarding the outcome of any choices made. The nurse should not offer advice or attempt to influence the client with personal beliefs or family influence.

CN: Safe, effective care environment; CNS: Management of care; CL: Apply

CN: Client needs category   CNS: Client needs subcategory   CL: Cognitive level

16. What is the nurse's **priority** action in caring for a client who has just had a liver biopsy?
1. Assess the level of pain
2. Monitor vital signs
3. Assess for feelings about body image
4. Instruct the client to avoid alcohol in the future

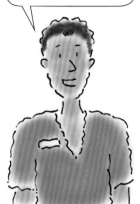

There are legal and ethical issues posed in question 17. Which circumstance can the nurse disclose?

17. A health care provider is legally and ethically required to disclose certain information. Which confidential information should the nurse disclose?
1. A single male client's HIV status to his family members
2. A client's pancreatic cancer diagnosis to the significant other
3. A taxi driver's diagnosis of an uncontrolled seizure disorder to his licensing agency
4. The client is 32 weeks pregnant with twins and is legally separated

18. A competent client in a long-term care facility refuses to take his oral diuretic medication. The nurse informs him that if the medication isn't taken, restraints will be applied, and the medication will be given by injection. Which legal tort **best** describes this nurse's statement?
1. Assault
2. Battery
3. Negligence
4. Autonomy

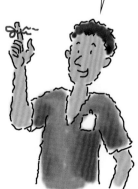

Remember: The neonate's safety and protection is the first priority.

19. A nurse on a maternity unit witnesses a mother slapping the face of her crying neonate. What is the nurse's **priority** action?
1. Take the neonate to the nursery, inform the health care provider of what was witnessed, and notify social services
2. Leave the room without the neonate, and notify the nursing supervisor
3. Ask the mother why she was slapping her child
4. Take the neonate to the nursery, and tell coworkers to observe the mother for further incidents

16. 2. Internal bleeding is a potential complication following a liver biopsy. Elevated pulse and decreased blood pressure are indications that the client may be developing shock, which results in altered circulation. Physiologic needs take priority over psychological needs, Assessing feelings and teaching should be addressed after immediate needs. Pain is considered a psychological reaction unless the client is experiencing an acute episode that is causing physiologic response.
CN: Safe, effective care environment; CNS: Management of care; CL: Apply

17. 3. The health care provider may lawfully disclose confidential information about a client when the welfare of others is at stake. The health care provider is required to inform the Department of Motor Vehicles that the taxi driver has an uncontrolled seizure disorder because it's in the best interest of the public's and client's safety. Confidentiality of HIV testing is required. Disclosing a client's cancer diagnosis to a significant other or pregnancy to a legally separated partner do not affect the welfare of person.
CN: Safe, effective care environment; CNS: Management of care; CL: Apply

18. 1. Assault occurs when one person puts another in fear of harmful or threatening contact. Battery is physical contact with another person. Negligence involves actions that are below the standard of care. Autonomy is an ethical principle of self-determination, and does not constitute a legal issue.
CN: Safe, effective care environment; CNS: Management of care; CL: Apply

19. 1. The neonate's safety and protection are the nurse's first priority. The nurse should immediately take the neonate to the nursery and inform the health care provider of the abuse. As an advocate for the neonate, the nurse provides the health care provider with an opportunity to examine the child for injuries. The nurse should not confront the client. Observing the mother for further incidents may be part of the revised care plan, however this incident requires immediate intervention.
CN: Psychosocial integrity; CNS: None; CL: Analyze

CN: Client needs category   CNS: Client needs subcategory   CL: Cognitive level

20. A mother appears anxious when her neonate cries and says, "I can't handle this." What is the **best** response by the nurse?
1. Discuss anger management therapy with the client
2. Demonstrate proper care of a crying neonate
3. Help the client develop routine bedtime rituals to soothe a crying infant
4. Evaluate the overall coping mechanisms of the client

20. 4. An overall assessment of the mother's strengths, weaknesses, coping mechanisms and support system is imperative, and will provide the basis for ongoing education. It will also help identify stressors. Anger management therapy is unnecessary. Proper care of a crying neonate is important, and would be part of an overall teaching plan.
CN: Psychosocial integrity; CNS: None; CL: Analyze

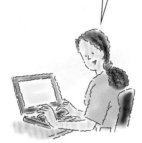

It is important to know who has the power.

21. A male client with a terminal illness is unconscious. His wife wants his status to be full code. His sister, who is the durable power of attorney and healthcare proxy, insists that his status should be do not resuscitate (DNR). Which person has legal precedence?
1. The wife's wishes should be honored as she is closest to the client.
2. The sister's wishes are legally binding.
3. An ethicist should be enlisted to mediate between the two individuals.
4. A chaplain should discuss the implications with both women.

21. 2. The durable power of attorney for health care takes legal precedence. It is often recommended that this role be given to someone objectively distanced from the client.
CN: Safe, effective care environment; CNS: Management of care; CL: Apply

22. A woman arrives at the emergency department with a fractured arm. Her husband is constantly present, and the woman appears anxious. What is the nurse's **priority** action?
1. Privately ask the woman if she is being abused
2. During triage inquire if the woman is in a safe environment
3. Clearly state that all clients are asked about abuse prior to any treatment
4. Provide the woman with a written pamphlet about domestic abuse

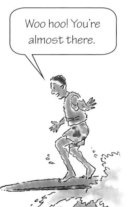

Woo hoo! You're almost there.

22. 1. It is a priority to privately ask the client if she is being abused. Counseling, or printed resources should be given privately. Clarifying that all clients are asked about abuse prior to any treatment allows for the client to understand why these questions are being asked.
CN: Psychosocial integrity; CNS: None; CL: Analyze

23. A client is voluntarily admitted to an inpatient psychiatric facility for the treatment of anxiety. The client is alert, oriented, and denies suicidal ideation. The client states a desire to leave the facility. Which is the **most** appropriate action by the nurse?
1. Inform the client that he is not able to leave against medical advice
2. Contact the attending provider
3. Determine the client's current level of anxiety
4. Provide discharge instructions for the client

23. 2. This client was voluntarily admitted and can leave at will, but his attending provider should be notified first. Determining the client's current level of anxiety and providing discharge instructions are important, but not a priority.
CN: Psychosocial integrity; CNS: None; CL: Apply

CN: Client needs category   CNS: Client needs subcategory   CL: Cognitive level

24. While providing care to a 26-year-old married, female client, the nurse notes multiple areas of ecchymosis on her torso. The bruises were in various stages of healing. When asked how she got these bruises, the client replied, "Oh, I tripped." How should the nurse respond? Select all that apply.

1. Document the client's statement
2. Assess the extremities, and document areas of injury and ecchymosis
3. Ask the client about current antiplatelet medications she may be taking
4. Call the client's husband to discuss the situation
5. Notify local authorities of domestic abuse

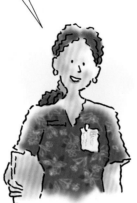

You did it! You finished the final chapter! Now, for more fun, try the comprehensive tests that follow!

24. **1, 2, 3.** The nurse should objectively document her assessment findings. A detailed description of physical abuse is essential in the medical records if legal action is pursued. Potential causes of the ecchymosis should be noted before a determination of abuse is made. Contacting the client's husband without her consent violates confidentiality. Notifying local authorities is not appropriate if domestic abuse is not certain.

CN: Psychosocial integrity; CNS: None; CL: Analyze

CN: Client needs category   CNS: Client needs subcategory   CL: Cognitive level

Appendices

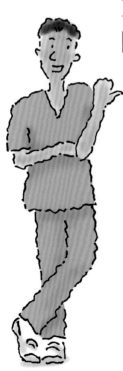

Comprehensive Test 1

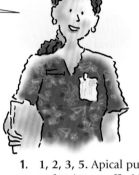

This comprehensive test, the first of three, is just like the shortest NCLEX test: 75 questions. It's a great way to practice!

1. The nurse is assessing a client who sustained blunt chest trauma from a motor vehicle collision. There are no obvious signs of bleeding. The provider diagnoses the client with cardiac tamponade. What assessment data would the nurse anticipate? Select all that apply.
   1. Apical pulse of 156
   2. Blood pressure of 62/48
   3. Muffled heart sounds
   4. Peaked t-waves
   5. Jugular vein distention

1. **1, 2, 3, 5.** Apical pulse of 156, blood pressure of 62/48, muffled heart sounds, and jugular veen distention are associated with a diagnosis of cardiac tamponade. Peaked t-waves are associated with hyperkalemia.
CN: Physiological integrity; CNS: Physiological adaptation; CL: Analyze

2. A nurse asks a nursing assistant to help admit an elderly client diagnosed with pneumonia. Delegation by the nurse is considered appropriate when the nursing assistant is asked to:
   1. obtain the client's height and weight.
   2. obtain a wound culture.
   3. insert a small-bore feeding tube.
   4. assess lung sounds.

2. **1.** Obtaining the client's height and weight are appropriate actions for the nursing assistant. The other options are the responsibility of the registered nurse or other licensed personnel.
CN: Safe effective care environment; CNS: Management of care; CL: Apply

3. A nurse is teaching a client with glaucoma the proper technique for instilling eye drops. The nurse determines that teaching is effective when the client states:
   1. "I should instill the drop directly onto the cornea."
   2. "I should instill the drop in the outer canthus."
   3. "I should instill the drop near the opening of the lacrimal duct."
   4. "I should instill the drop in the lower conjunctival sac."

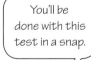
You'll be done with this test in a snap.

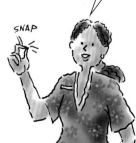
SNAP

3. **4.** Eye drops should be placed in the lower conjunctival sac starting at the inner, not outer, canthus. Placing eye drops on the cornea causes discomfort and should be avoided. Eye drops shouldn't be placed by the opening of the lacrimal ducts to avoid systemic absorption.
CN: Physiological integrity; CNS: Pharmacological and parenteral therapies; CL: Apply

4. A client with HIV is admitted to the hospital with flu-like symptoms, dyspnea, and a cough. A 100% non-rebreather mask and arterial blood gases (ABGs) are ordered. The nurse reviews the results of the ABGs, and is **most** concerned by:
1. PaO_2, 90 mmHg; $PaCO_2$, 40 mmHg
2. PaO_2, 85 mmHg; $PaCO_2$, 45 mmHg
3. PaO_2, 80 mmHg; $PaCO_2$, 45 mmHg
4. PaO_2, 70 mmHg; $PaCO_2$, 55 mmHg

4. 4. An increasing $PaCO_2$ and decreasing PaO_2 indicate poor oxygen perfusion. Normal PaO_2 levels are 80 to 100 mmHg, and normal $PaCO_2$ levels are 35 to 45 mmHg.
CN: Physiological integrity; CNS: Reduction of risk potential; CL: Analyze

5. A client with AIDS has developed a protozoa infection. Which opportunistic infection should the nurse be **most** concerned about?
1. Tuberculosis
2. Histoplasmosis
3. Kaposi's sarcoma
4. *Pneumocystis jiroveci* infection

5. 4. *Pneumocystis jiroveci* infection is caused by protozoa. Tuberculosis is caused by a mycobacterium. Histoplasmosis is a fungal infection. Kaposi's sarcoma is a neoplasm that is associated with HIV.
CN: Physiological integrity; CNS: Physiological adaptation; CL: Apply

6. The nurse is caring for a client who has been intubated. What is the nurse's **priority** intervention?
1. Use lubricant on the lips every eight hours
2. Provide oral care twice a day
3. Suction the oral cavity every four hours
4. Reposition the endotracheal (ET) tube every 24 hours

6. 4. Pressure causes skin breakdown. However, repositioning the ET tube can relieve pressure and decrease this risk. Extreme care must be taken to only move the tube laterally. It must not be pushed in or pulled out. The tape securing the tube must be changed daily. Oral care, suctioning, and lubricant will help keep skin clean, intact and reduce the risk of further infection.
CN: Physiological integrity; CNS: Basic care and comfort; CL: Apply

7. A client with AIDS has developed *Pneumocystis jiroveci* pneumonia and has begun treatment with pentamidine isethionate. When the client develops which side effects should the nurse notify the provider? Select all that apply.
1. Hyperglycemia
2. Tachycardia
3. Tachypnea
4. Hallucinations
5. Leukopenia

7. 2, 4, 5. Tachycardia, hallucinations, and leukopenia are side effects that require provider notification. Side effects such as loss of appetite or an unpleasant taste in the mouth are common, and do not require provider notification. Tachypnea and Hyperglycemia have not side effects with the use of this drug. Other potential side effects include hypoglycemia and wheezing.
CN: Physiological integrity; CNS: Pharmacological and parenteral therapies; CL: Apply

8. A client is receiving pentamidine isethionate. What is the nurse's **priority** assessment?
1. Arterial blood gases (ABGs)
2. Electrolyte levels
3. Blood sugar levels
4. Complete blood count (CBC)

8. 3. Pentamidine isethionate can cause permanent diabetes mellitus. Blood sugar levels should be monitored while taking this medication. The client's electrolyte levels, ABGs, and CBC can be monitored less frequently.
CN: Physiological integrity; CNS: Pharmacological and parenteral therapies; CL: Apply

CN: Client needs category   CNS: Client needs subcategory   CL: Cognitive level

9. A nurse, caring for a client with AIDS, is working with a nursing student. The nurse notes that the student doesn't attempt to suction or assist with the care of this client. What is the **most** appropriate action by the nurse?
1. Talk to the student regarding her feelings about the client
2. Talk to the charge nurse about the student's lack of initiative
3. Address a coworker with the concerns about the student
4. Seek advice from the student's instructor about the student

9. **1.** The nurse should approach the student to determine her feelings and experience in caring for this client. The charge nurse and coworkers aren't familiar with the student's abilities. The instructor should be approached if the nurse cannot communicate with the student.
CN: Safe, effective care environment; CNS: Management of care; CL: Analyze

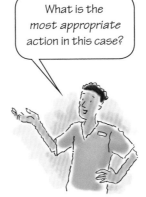

What is the most appropriate action in this case?

10. A client is admitted to the hospital with respiratory failure. He is intubated in the emergency department, placed on 100% FiO_2, and is coughing up copious secretions. What is the nurse's **most** appropriate action?
1. Request a chest X-ray
2. Infuse the ordered antibiotic
3. Suction the client
4. Obtain the ordered arterial blood gas (ABG) analysis

10. **3.** Secretions can cut off the oxygen supply to the client and result in hypoxia. Suctioning the client is the priority. X-rays would be used to check placement of the endotracheal tube. Antibiotics are warranted if sputum reveals bacterial infection. After the client has acclimated to his ventilator settings, ABGs can be drawn.
CN: Physiological integrity; CNS: Reduction of risk potential; CL: Apply

11. The nurse is caring for an intubated client who has copious, brown-tinged secretions. What is the nurse's **most** appropriate action?
1. Use a trap to obtain secretions per protocol
2. Instill saline to break up secretions
3. Call the respiratory therapist
4. Obtain an order for a liquefying agent for the sputum

11. **1.** Suspicious secretions should be sent to the lab for culture and sensitivity using a sterile technique such as a trap. Saline is used to lubricate the catheter, but should not be instilled. A respiratory therapist can choose the correct agent to help break up secretions, but this is not a priority.
CN: Safe, effective care environment; CNS: Safety and infection control; CL: Analyze

12. A nurse is teaching a client's family about tuberculosis and the importance of receiving a Mantoux test to check for tuberculosis (TB). The nurse knows that teaching has been effective when a family member states, "We should all have a Mantoux test to determine:
1. if we have active TB now."
2. if we have have a recently had TB."
3. the extent of TB in our system."
4. if we have had TB at some point."

12. **4.** A positive Mantoux skin test doesn't guarantee that an infection is currently present, but can indicate the presence of tuberculin infection at some point. Individuals may have a false-positive result. If individuals have active TB, it may be viewed on a chest X-ray. Computed tomography or magnetic resonance imaging can evaluate the extent of lung damage.
CN: Safe, effective care environment; CNS: Safety and infection control; CL: Apply

13. A nurse is performing discharge teaching for a client with active tuberculosis (TB). Which intervention should the nurse include in his plan of care?
1. Include daily walking in indoor areas such as malls or health centers
2. Follow a clear liquid diet
3. Take the full course of medications
4. Return to the TB clinic annually for sputum smears

13. **2.** It is important to complete the entire medication regimen. Failure to do so may cause a reinfection to occur. Walking is a benefit, but should take place in areas where others are not present to avoid transmission to others. A clear liquid diet usually does not include all the nutrients needed for healing and nutritional balance. This client needs to return to the TB clinic more frequently for sputum smears.

CN: Physiological integrity; CNS: Pharmacological and parenteral therapies; CL: Apply

14. The family of a client, with a history of Parkinson's disease, explains that the client's condition is getting progressively worse. Which symptom would the nurse anticipate when assessing this client?
1. Impaired speech
2. Muscle flaccidity
3. Confusion
4. Tremors in the fingers that increase with movement

14. **1.** In Parkinson's disease, dysarthria, or impaired speech, is due to a disturbance in muscle control. Muscle rigidity results in resistance to passive muscle stretching. The client may have a mask-like appearance, but is lucid and rational. Tremors should decrease with movement and sleep.

CN: Physiological integrity; CNS: Physiological adaptation; CL: Apply

15. A client is ordered to receive 1,000 ml of 0.45% normal saline with 20 mEq of potassium chloride (KCl) over six hours. The infusion set administers 15 gtt/ml. How many drops per minute should this client receive? Record your answer using a whole number.

_____ gtt/min

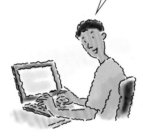

Math alert! Do you remember how to calculate a flow rate?

15. **42.**

The flow rate is determined by the rate of infusion and the number of drops per milliliters of the fluid being administered.

$$\frac{gtt}{ml} \times \frac{amount\ to\ be\ infused}{number\ of\ minutes} = IV\ flow\ rate$$

$$15\,gtt/ml \times 1,000\,ml/360\,min = 42\,gtt/min$$

CN: Physiological integrity; CNS: Pharmacological and parenteral therapy; CL: Apply

16. The nurse is caring for a male client who is 82 years of age. This client has Parkinson's disease and is frequently incontinent of urine. What is the nurse's **most** appropriate intervention?
1. Diaper the client
2. Apply a condom catheter
3. Insert an indwelling urinary catheter
4. Provide skin care every four hours

16. **2.** A condom catheter uses a condom-type device to drain urine away from the client. Diapering the client may keep urine away from the body, but may also be demeaning if the client is alert or the family objects. Because the client with Parkinson's disease is already prone to urinary tract infections, an indwelling urinary catheter should be avoided. Skin care must be provided as soon as the client is incontinent to prevent skin maceration and breakdown.

CN: Physiological integrity; CNS: Basic care and comfort; CL: Analyze

CN: Client needs category   CNS: Client needs subcategory   CL: Cognitive level

17. The nurse is assessing a 30-year-old primigravida client in her second trimester. This client has a history of rheumatic fever. The client tells the nurse that her fingers feel tight and sometimes she feels as though her heart skips a beat. Which assessment finding would be **most** concerning to the nurse?

1. Clear lungs
2. Sinus tachycardia
3. Increased dyspnea on exertion
4. Runs of paroxysmal atrial tachycardia

17. 3. Increasing dyspnea on exertion would alert the nurse to cardiovascular compromise. Cardiac arrhythmias (other than sinus tachycardia or paroxysmal atrial tachycardia), and persistent crackles at the bases are also symptoms of cardiovascular disease.

CN: Health promotion and maintenance; CNS: None; CL: Analyze

18. The nurse is caring for a pregnant client who is suspected of having cardiovascular disease. Which diagnostic test would **best** determine the extent of cardiovascular disease in this pregnant client?

1. Stress test
2. Chest X-ray
3. Echocardiography
4. Cardiac catheterization

18. 3. Echocardiography is less invasive than X-rays and other methods, and provides the information needed to determine the extent of cardiovascular disease, especially valvular disorders. Cardiac catheterization and stress tests may be postponed until after delivery.

CN: Physiological integrity; CNS: Physiological adaptation; CL: Analyze

19. A 25-year-old primigravida client has been in labor for 20 hours with little progress. The health care provider prescribes oxytocin. The order reads 10 units oxytocin in 1,000 ml/NSS to infuse via pump at 1 milliunits/min for 15 minutes; then increase flow rate to 2 milliunits/min. Calculate the flow rate needed to deliver 1 milliunits/minute for 15 minutes? Record your answer using a whole number.

_____ ml/hr

Remember

"Oxytocin is for inducin' labor."

Oxytocin is a hormone that stimulates smooth muscle in the uterus and breast. It is used for inducing labor; treating various pregnancy-related conditions; and stimulating lactation.

19. 6.

First, determine the concentration of the solution with 10 units/1,000 ml as the known factor and X as the unknown factor:

$$\frac{10\ units}{1,000\ ml} = \frac{X}{1\ ml}$$

$$X = 0.01\,units/ml$$

Then, cross-multiply and solve for X. Next, convert to milliunits by multiplying by 1,000.

$$0.01 \times 1,000 = 10\ milliunits/ml$$

Determine flow rate using the following equation:

$$\frac{10\ milliunits}{1\ ml} = \frac{15\ milliunits}{X}$$

$$X = \frac{15\ ml}{10} = 1.5\ ml$$

Convert to an hourly rate by multiplying by 4 (60 min/15 min = 4):

$$\frac{1.5\ ml}{15\ minutes} \times 4 = 6\,ml/hr$$

CN: Physiological integrity; CNS: Pharmacological and parenteral therapies; CL: Apply

CN: Client needs category   CNS: Client needs subcategory   CL: Cognitive level

20. Which statement, by the nurse, **most** accurately reflects subjective data in a nursing assessment?
1. The client's red blood cell count is elevated.
2. The client has a positive Babinski sign.
3. The client's X-ray result showed a fracture present.
4. The client reports that his pain is a 7 on a 1 to 10 scale.

20. 4. Subjective data, also known as symptoms or covert cues, include the client's own verbatim statements about the health problems. Laboratory study results, physical assessment data, and diagnostic procedure reports are observable, perceptible, and measurable and can be verified and validated by others.
CN: Safe, effective care environment; CNS: Management of care; CL: Apply

21. A client arrives at the emergency department in her third trimester with painless vaginal bleeding. The nurse suspects that the client is experiencing:
1. placenta previa.
2. preterm labor.
3. abruptio placentae.
4. a sexually transmitted infection (STI).

21. 1. Placenta previa presents with painless vaginal bleeding. Abruptio placentae usually includes vague abdominal discomfort and tenderness. Preterm labor and STIs usually don't cause bleeding.
CN: Health promotion and maintenance; CNS: None; CL: Analyze

22. The nurse is caring for a client who has been admitted with suspected placenta previa. After assessing vital signs and applying an external monitor, what is the nurse's **most** important action?
1. Insert an indwelling urinary catheter
2. Plan for an immediate cesarean delivery
3. Place the client in Trendelenburg position
4. Obtain blood work and start IV catheters

22. 4. Blood for hemoglobin, hematocrit, type, and crossmatch should be collected and IV catheters inserted. The nurse shouldn't attempt Trendelenburg positioning or urinary catheterization. The client may be placed on her left side. Depending on the degree of bleeding and fetal maturity, a cesarean delivery may be required.
CN: Physiological integrity; CNS: Reduction of risk potential; CL: Apply

23. A pregnant client, who is experiencing vaginal bleeding, has been placed on a fetal monitor. The client asks the nurse how her baby is doing. What is the nurse's **most** appropriate response?
1. "I don't know for sure."
2. "I can't answer that question."
3. "It's too early to tell anything."
4. "Here's what the monitor shows."

23. 4. The client deserves a truthful answer, and the nurse should be objective without giving opinions. Vague answers may be misleading and aren't therapeutic.
CN: Psychosocial integrity; CNS: None; CL: Analyze

24. A neonate requires blood transfusions after delivery. Which cannulation site is **most** appropriate for the nurse to select?
1. Scalp veins
2. Intraosseous
3. Umbilical cord
4. Subclavian cutdown

24. 3. The umbilical cord may be easily cannulated and is the preferred site. Scalp veins may also be used. Intraosseous cannulation is attempted if two attempts at other sites prove inaccessible. A subclavian cutdown takes a prolonged time and is the least desired.
CN: Health promotion and maintenance; CNS: None; CL: Analyze

CN: Client needs category   CNS: Client needs subcategory   CL: Cognitive level

25. A nurse, working in the triage area of an emergency department, sees several pediatric clients arrive simultaneously. Which client should be treated **first**?
1. A crying four-year-old child with a laceration on his scalp
2. A three-year-old child with a barking cough and flushed appearance
3. A three-year-old child with Down syndrome who's pale and asleep
4. A two-year-old child with stridorous breath sounds, sitting up and drooling

26. The nurse is assessing a two-year-old child in the emergency department for epiglottitis. Which assessment finding would the nurse expect to document?
1. Mild fever
2. Clear speech
3. Drooling
4. Gradual onset of symptoms

27. The nurse needs to auscultate a two year old's breath sounds. Which method of approaching the child is **most** appropriate?
1. Tell the child it's time to listen to his lungs now
2. Tell the child to lie down while the nurse listens to his lungs
3. Ask the caregiver to wait outside while the nurse listens to his lungs
4. Ask the child if he would like the nurse to listen to the front or the back of his chest first

28. A mother states that her two-year-old child is up to date with his immunizations. What immunizations should be current for this child?
1. Diphtheria-pertussis-tetanus (DTaP), inactivated polio (IPV), measles-mumps-rubella (MMR)
2. DTaP, IPV, MMR, *Haemophilus influenza* type B (Hib), varicella, pneumococcal, hepatitis B, rotavirus (Rota)
3. DTaP, hepatitis B, IPV
4. MMR, IPV, hepatitis B

29. The nurse is caring for a child with epiglottitis. Which complication is the child at **greatest** risk of developing?
1. Airway obstruction
2. Dehydration
3. Malnutrition
4. Seizures

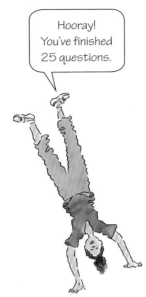

Hooray! You've finished 25 questions.

25. 4. The child with the airway emergency should be treated first because of the risk of epiglottitis. The three-year-old with the barking cough and fever should be suspected of having croup and should be seen promptly, as should the child with the laceration. The nurse would need to gather information about the child with Down syndrome to determine the priority of care.
CN: Safe, effective care environment; CNS: Management of care; CL: Analyze

26. 3. Drooling is a classic sign of epiglottitis. Epiglottitis presents with a sudden onset of inspiratory stridor, high fever, and muffled speech.
CN: Physiological integrity; CNS: Physiological adaptation; CL: Apply

27. 4. The two-year-old child needs to feel in control, and this approach best supports the child's independence. Giving the child no choice may make him uncooperative. The child should be allowed to remain in the tripod position to facilitate breathing. The caregiver should be allowed to remain with the child because fear of separation is common in a two-year-old.
CN: Health promotion and maintenance; CNS: None; CL: Apply

28. 2. By the age of two years, the DTaP, IPV, MMR, Hib, varicella, pneumococcal, hepatitis B, and rotavirus vaccines should have been received. The nurse should clarify this with the mother or caregiver.
CN: Safe, effective care environment; CNS: Safety and infection control; CL: Apply

29. 1. The biggest threat to this child is airway obstruction because of inflammation and swelling of the epiglottis and surrounding tissue. Dehydration can be prevented with IV therapy, and seizures averted by decreasing the fever. Malnutrition is unlikely to occur because epiglottitis is a short-lived condition.
CN: Physiological integrity; CNS: Reduction of risk potential; CL: Apply

CN: Client needs category   CNS: Client needs subcategory   CL: Cognitive level

30. A student nurse and a registered nurse are preparing to assess a child with epiglottitis. The student explains to the child that they need to look at his throat. Which intervention, by the registered nurse, is **most** appropriate?
  1. Hand the student a flashlight and tongue blade
  2. Give the student a sterile tongue blade and culturette swab
  3. Tell the student that the registered nurse will visualize the child's throat
  4. Tell the student that visualization will be done by the anesthesiologist

30. 4. Direct visualization of the epiglottis can trigger a complete airway obstruction and should only be done in a controlled environment by an anesthesiologist or a provider skilled in pediatric intubation.

CN: Safe, effective care environment; CNS: Management of care; CL: Apply

31. The mother of a two-year-old with epiglottitis states that she needs to pick up her older child from school. The two-year-old child begins to cry and appears more stridorous. What is the nurse's **priority** action?
  1. Ask the mother how long she may be gone
  2. Tell the two-year-old child everything will be all right
  3. Tell the two-year-old child the nurse will stay with him
  4. Ask the mother if there's anyone else who can meet the older child

31. 4. Increased anxiety and agitation should be avoided to prevent airway obstruction. A two-year-old child fears separation from parents, and the mother should be encouraged to stay. Other means of picking up the older child should be found. Telling the child that everything will be all right may not decrease agitation. The mother is the primary caregiver and important to the child for emotional and security reasons.

CN: Health promotion and maintenance; CNS: None; CL: Analyze

32. A nurse suspects a client is experiencing alcohol withdrawal syndrome. What is the nurse's **priority** action?
  1. Verify the symptoms with family
  2. Inform social services
  3. Ask the client about his drinking
  4. Tell the client everything will be all right

32. 3. Confirming suspicions directly with the client is the most reliable way to diagnosis and treat withdrawal symptoms. If the client isn't cooperative, verification can be sought from the family. Social services aren't required at this time, but may be helpful in discharge planning. Giving false reassurance isn't therapeutic for the client.

CN: Psychosocial integrity; CNS: None; CL: Apply

33. A client experiencing alcohol withdrawal syndrome says he sees cockroaches on the ceiling. What is the nurse's **most** appropriate response?
  1. Ask the client where he sees them
  2. Ask the client if the cockroaches are still there
  3. Tell the client there are no cockroaches on the ceiling
  4. Turn on the lights and reorient the client

33. 4. Try to reorient the client to reality and minimize distortions. Don't support the client's hallucinations or place the client on the defensive. Present reality gently without agitating the client.

CN: Psychosocial integrity; CNS: None; CL: Apply

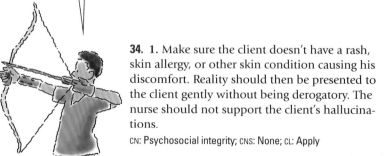

Take aim at success.

34. A client, experiencing alcohol withdrawal syndrome, says that he is itching everywhere from the bugs in his bed. What is the nurse's **most** appropriate action?
  1. Examine the client's skin
  2. Ask what kind of bugs he thinks they are
  3. Tell the client there are no bugs on his bed
  4. Tell the client he's having tactile hallucinations

34. 1. Make sure the client doesn't have a rash, skin allergy, or other skin condition causing his discomfort. Reality should then be presented to the client gently without being derogatory. The nurse should not support the client's hallucinations.

CN: Psychosocial integrity; CNS: None; CL: Apply

CN: Client needs category   CNS: Client needs subcategory   CL: Cognitive level

35. A client, with alcohol withdrawal syndrome, is pulling at his central venous catheter, saying, "I'm swatting the spiders crawling all over me." What is the nurse's **priority** action?
1. Encourage the client to rest
2. Assign a nursing assistant to stay with the client
3. Tell the client there are no spiders
4. Tell the client that he is pulling the IV tubing

35. 2. During periods of alcohol withdrawal syndrome, the client needs to be protected from harm. If the client dislodges the central venous catheter, he may incur an air embolus, which can be life threatening. Although reality should be presented to the client, telling him that there are no spiders and that he's pulling the IV tubing may not make him stop; therefore, his safety is still at risk. The client may need to be restrained if continued observation during this time isn't available. The client should also be encouraged to rest; however, this intervention doesn't take priority over safety.
CN: Psychosocial integrity; CNS: None; CL: Analyze

36. A client, who experienced alcohol withdrawal syndrome, is no longer having hallucinations or tremors. The client states, "I would like to enter a rehabilitation facility to stop drinking." What is the nurse's **most** appropriate intervention?
1. Ask about the client's experience with rehabilitation in the past
2. Tell the client that they should talk with their family
3. Refer this client to Alcoholics Anonymous (AA)
4. Promote participation in a treatment program

36. 4. The client should be encouraged to enter a facility if that's in their best interest. Their past experiences are not relevant to this episode. The client can inform their family, and support should be encouraged. Referral to AA should be considered after rehabilitation takes place.
CN: Psychosocial integrity; CNS: None; CL: Apply

37. A 72-year-old man with cirrhosis is admitted to the hospital in a hepatic coma. What is the nurse's **most** important intervention?
1. Perform a neurological check, cardiovascular check, and gastrointestinal assessment
2. Complete the client admission
3. Orient the client to his environment
4. Check airway, breathing, and circulation

37. 4. Priorities include airway, breathing, and circulation. Once these are ensured, a neurological check is needed to determine status. General orientation and completing the admission may require the help and affirmation of family members. Depending on the client's alertness, orientation to the environment may need to be kept simple.
CN: Physiological integrity; CNS: Reduction of risk potential; CL: Apply

38. The nurse is assessing a client with cirrhosis. Which assessment finding would be **most** indicative of late-stage cirrhosis?
1. Constipation
2. Diarrhea
3. Shortness of breath
4. Vomiting

38. 3. In late-stage cirrhosis, fluid in the lungs and weak chest expansion can lead to hypoxia. Diarrhea, vomiting, and constipation are early signs and symptoms of cirrhosis.
CN: Physiological integrity; CNS: Physiological adaptation; CL: Apply

39. A client with cirrhosis is jaundiced and edematous. She is experiencing severe dry skin and itching. She asks the nurse if anything can be done for her skin. What is the nurse's **best** intervention?
1. Put mittens on his hands
2. Use alcohol-free body lotion
3. Lubricate the skin with baby oil
4. Wash the skin with soap and water

39. 2. Alcohol-free body lotion may be applied to the skin to help relieve dryness, and is absorbed without oiliness. Mittens may help keep the client from scratching his skin. Soap dries out the skin. Baby oil doesn't allow excretions through the skin, and may block pores.
CN: Physiological integrity; CNS: Basic care and comfort; CL: Apply

CN: Client needs category   CNS: Client needs subcategory   CL: Cognitive level

40. The nurse is writing a plan of care for a client who sustained a spinal cord injury and is frequently hospitalized for kidney stones. What is the nurse's **most** appropriate intervention?
  1. Eat yogurt daily
  2. Drink cranberry juice
  3. Eat more fresh fruits and vegetables
  4. Increase the intake of dairy products

40. 2. Acidic urine decreases the risk of kidney stones. The majority of renal calculi forms in alkaline urine. Cranberries, prunes, and plums promote acidic urine. Yogurt helps restore pH balance to secretions in yeast infections. Fruits and vegetables increase fiber in the diet and promote alkaline urine. Dairy products may contribute to the formation of kidney stones.
CN: Physiological integrity; CNS: Reduction of risk potential; CL: Apply

41. The nurse is teaching a client who sustained a spinal cord injury about symptoms that may indicate a urinary tract infection (UTI). The nurse knows that teaching was effective when the client states:
  1. "Pain in my lower back is the initial symptom of a UTI."
  2. "I should not be concerned when I have burning on urination."
  3. "I should be mindful of how frequently I urinate."
  4. "A fever and change in the clarity of my urine are early signs of a UTI."

41. 4. The client with a spinal cord injury should recognize that fever and a change in the clarity of their urine are early signs of a UTI. Lower back pain is a late sign. The client with a spinal cord injury may not have burning or frequency of urination.
CN: Physiological integrity; CNS: Reduction of risk potential; CL: Analyze

42. The nurse is assessing a client with a recent colostomy and finds him tearful. What is the nurse's **most** appropriate intervention?
  1. State that you will come back another time
  2. Ask the client if he's having pain or discomfort
  3. Tell the client you will need to perform an assessment
  4. Sit down with the client and ask if he'd like to talk about anything

42. 4. Asking open-ended questions and taking an interest in what the client has to say will encourage verbalization of feelings. Leaving the client may make him feel unaccepted. Asking closed-ended questions won't encourage verbalization of feelings. Ignoring the client's present state isn't therapeutic for the client.
CN: Psychosocial integrity; CNS: None; CL: Apply

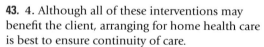

Go on. Give it your best shot.

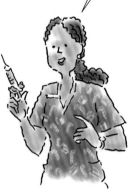

43. After a review of colostomy care, a client tells the nurse that he doesn't know if he will be able to care for himself at home without help. What is the nurse's **most** appropriate intervention?
  1. Review care with the client again
  2. Provide written instructions for the client
  3. Ask the client if there's anyone who can help
  4. Arrange for home health care to visit the client

43. 4. Although all of these interventions may benefit the client, arranging for home health care is best to ensure continuity of care.
CN: Safe, effective care environment; CNS: Management of care; CL: Apply

44. A client is experiencing mild diarrhea through the colostomy. What is the nurse's **most** appropriate instruction for this client?
  1. Eat prunes
  2. Drink apple juice
  3. Increase lettuce intake
  4. Increase intake of bananas

44. 4. Bananas help make formed stool, and aren't irritating to the bowel. Apple juice and prunes can increase the frequency of diarrhea. Lettuce acts as a fiber and can increase the looseness of stools. The BRAT diet (bananas, rice, apple sauce, and toast) used in pediatric clients can be used in any client with diarrhea.
CN: Physiological integrity; CNS: Basic care and comfort; CL: Apply

CN: Client needs category   CNS: Client needs subcategory   CL: Cognitive level

45. A client, recently diagnosed with prediabetes, asks the nurse about the risk factors for developing type 2 diabetes mellitus. Which is this client's **greatest** risk factor?
1. Obesity
2. Japanese descent
3. A great-grandparent with type 2 diabetes mellitus
4. Delivery of a neonate weighing more than 10 lb

45. 1. Obesity is a risk factor associated with type2 diabetes mellitus. Delivery of a neonate weighing more than nine pounds, a family history of type 2 diabetes mellitus (mother, father, or sibling), and those of Native American, Black, Asian, or Hispanic descent are at high risk for developing diabetes mellitus; however, obesity puts this client at greatest risk.
CN: Health promotion and maintenance; CNS: None; CL: Analyze

46. A client with a family history of type 2 diabetes mellitus asks the nurse how to decrease his risk factors. What is the nurse's **best** response?
1. Eat only poultry and fish
2. Omit carbohydrates from your diet
3. Start a moderate exercise program
4. Check blood glucose levels every month

46. 3. Exercise and weight control are the best methods of preventing and treating type 2 diabetes mellitus. Red should be limited because it contributes to cardiovascular disease. Complex carbohydrates account for a large portion of the diabetic diet and shouldn't be omitted. Checking blood glucose levels will help monitor the development of type 2 diabetes mellitus, but won't prevent or decrease the chance of it occurring.
CN: Physiological integrity; CNS: Reduction of risk potential; CL: Apply

47. The nurse is assessing a client's arterial pulses. Which photo illustrates the appropriate site for palpating the dorsalis pedis pulse?

1.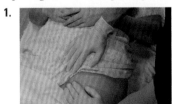
2.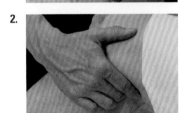
3.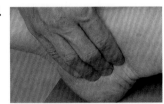
4.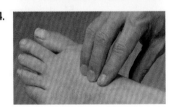

47. 4. To palpate the dorsalis pedis pulse, the nurse places the fingers on the medial dorsum of the foot while the client points his toes down. The first photo illustrates palpation of the femoral, located along the crease, midway between the pubic bone and the anterior iliac crest. The second photo illustrates palpation of the popliteal pulse in the popliteal fossa of the back of the knee. The third photo illustrates palpation of the posterior tibial pulse, slightly below the malleolus of the ankle.
CN: Health promotion and maintenance; CNS: None; CL: Apply

48. A nurse is having lunch in the hospital cafeteria when a visitor, sitting at the next table, begins to choke on his food. According to the American Heart Association (AHA) and the Canadian Red Cross, the nurse should intervene using the actions listed below. Prioritize the actions of this intervention.

| 1. Administer abdominal thrusts until effective or until the client becomes unresponsive |
| 2. Activate the emergency response team |
| 3. Ask the client if he can speak |
| 4. Start cardiopulmonary resuscitation (CPR) |

48. Ordered Response:

| 3. Ask the client if he can speak |
| 1. Administer abdominal thrusts until effective or until the client becomes unresponsive |
| 2. Activate the emergency response team |
| 4. Start cardiopulmonary resuscitation (CPR) |

CN: Physiological integrity; CNS: Physiological adaptation; CL: Apply

CN: Client needs category   CNS: Client needs subcategory   CL: Cognitive level

49. The nurse is performing a cardiac assessment on a client with a suspected murmur. Identify the area where the nurse should place the stethoscope to auscultate the area referred to as Erb's point.

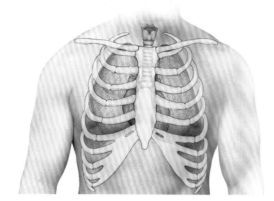

49. Erb's point is located at the third intercostal space, left of, and close to, the sternum. Murmurs of both aortic and pulmonic origin may be heard at Erb's point.

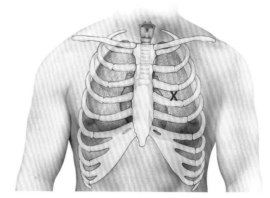

CN: Health promotion and maintenance; CNS: None; CL: Apply

50. A client is undergoing a thoracentesis at the bedside. The nurse assists the client to an upright position with a table and pillow in front of him to support his arms. What is the correct rationale for this intervention?
1. There's easier access to the fluid from this approach.
2. There's less chance to injure lung tissue.
3. It prevents the formation of subcutaneous emphysema.
4. It's less painful for the client in this position.

50. 1. The posterior approach is superior. The posterior gutter is deep, and fluid tends to collect in this dependent area while the client is in an erect position. There's a risk for pneumothorax and subcutaneous emphysema formation regardless of the client's position. This procedure is done using local anesthesia, and is minimally painful.
CN: Physiological integrity; CNS: Physiological adaptation; CL: Analyze

51. Which sport activity would the nurse recommend to parents for a school-age child with hemophilia?
1. Baseball
2. Cross-country running
3. Football
4. Swimming

51. 4. Swimming is a noncontact sport with a low risk for traumatic injury. Baseball, cross-country running, and football all involve a risk for trauma from falling, sliding, or contact.
CN: Physiological integrity; CNS: Physiological adaptation; CL: Apply

52. Which assessment finding would be **most** significant for a child in sickle cell crisis?
1. The child has no bruises.
2. The child has normal skin turgor.
3. The child is ambulatory around the room.
4. The child maintains bladder control.

52. 2. Normal skin turgor indicates that the child isn't severely dehydrated. Dehydration may cause sickle cell crisis or worsen a crisis. Bruising isn't associated with sickle cell crisis. Bed rest is preferable during a sickle cell crisis. Bladder control may be lost when oral or IV fluid intake is increased during a sickle cell crisis, but has no bearing on the primary problem of sickling.
CN: Physiological integrity; CNS: Physiological adaptation; CL: Analyze

CN: Client needs category   CNS: Client needs subcategory   CL: Cognitive level

53. A nurse is giving discharge instructions to the parents of a child who had a tonsillectomy. Which instruction would be **most** important to include?
  1. The child should drink extra milk.
  2. The child should avoid drinking from straws.
  3. Orange juice should be given to provide pain control.
  4. The child's mouth should be rinsed with salt water to provide pain relief.

54. A client with chronic alcohol use is admitted to the hospital for detoxification. Later that day, the client's blood pressure increases and the client is given lorazepam to prevent:
  1. stroke.
  2. seizure.
  3. fainting.
  4. anxiety reaction.

55. An adolescent client ingests a large number of acetaminophen tablets in an attempt to commit suicide. Which laboratory result is **most** consistent with acetaminophen overdose?
  1. Elevated bilirubin levels
  2. Elevated liver enzyme levels
  3. Increased serum creatinine level
  4. Increased white blood cell (WBC) count

56. A client is to take eight ounces of magnesium sulfate solution. The calibrations on the measuring device are in milliliters. How many milliliters should the nurse give?
  1. 8 ml
  2. 80 ml
  3. 240 ml
  4. 480 ml

57. A client with a new colostomy asks a nurse how to avoid leakage from the ostomy bag. What is the nurse's **best** response?
  1. Limit fluid intake
  2. Eat more fruits and vegetables
  3. Empty the bag when it's about half full
  4. Tape the end of the bag to the surrounding skin

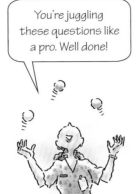

You're juggling these questions like a pro. Well done!

53. **2.** Straws and other sharp objects inserted into the mouth could disrupt the clot at the operative site. Extra milk wouldn't promote healing, and may encourage mucus production. Drinking orange juice and rinsing with salt water will irritate the tissue at the operative site.
CN: Physiological adaptation; CNS: Reduction of risk potential; CL: Apply

54. **2.** During detoxification from alcohol, changes in the client's physiological status, especially an increase in blood pressure, may indicate a possible seizure. Clients are treated with benzodiazepines to prevent this. Stroke, fainting, and anxiety aren't the primary concerns when withdrawing from alcohol.
CN: Physiological integrity; CNS: Pharmacological and parenteral therapies; CL: Apply

55. **2.** Elevated liver enzyme levels, which could indicate liver damage, are associated with acetaminophen overdose. Metabolic acidosis isn't associated with acetaminophen overdose. An increased serum creatinine level may indicate renal damage. An increased WBC count indicates infection
CN: Physiological integrity; CNS: Pharmacological and parenteral therapies; CL: Apply

56. **2.** To determine the amount of milliliters to give, use the following equation: One ounce equals 30 ml.

$$8\,oz \times 30\,ml/oz = 240\,ml$$

CN: Physiological integrity; CNS: Pharmacological and parenteral therapies; CL: Apply

57. **3.** Emptying the bag when partially full will prevent the bag from becoming heavy and detaching from the skin or skin barrier. Limiting fluids may cause constipation but won't prevent leakage. Increasing fruits and vegetables in the diet will help prevent constipation, not leakage. Taping the bag to the skin will secure the bag to the skin but won't prevent leakage.
CN: Physiological integrity; CNS: Basic care and comfort; CL: Apply

CN: Client needs category   CNS: Client needs subcategory   CL: Cognitive level

58. A client reports an inability to sleep while on the medical unit. Which intervention should the nurse perform **first**?
1. Offer a sedative routinely at bedtime
2. Give the client a backrub before bedtime
3. Inquire about the client's sleeping habits
4. Move the client to a bed farthest from the nurses' station

58. 3. Assessing the client's sleeping habits may provide information about the causes of the inability to sleep. Sedatives should be given as a last option. A backrub may promote sleep but may not address this client's problem. Moving the client may not address the client's specific problem.
CN: Physiological integrity; CNS: Basic care and comfort; CL: Apply

59. Three days after discharge, a client who is bottle feeding her neonate, calls the postpartum floor and asks the nurse what she can do for breast engorgement. What is the nurse's **best** response?
1. Use a tight binder around the breasts or wear a snug-fitting bra
2. Take a warm shower and let the water flow over the breasts
3. Stop drinking milk because it contributes to breast engorgement
4. Contact her provider to determine the cause of the engorgement

59. 1. A tight binder or snug bra is recommended for the client bottle feeding her neonate to reduce engorgement. A warm shower will stimulate milk production. It's normal to become engorged during the first few days after delivery. Drinking milk does not cause engorgement.
CN: Physiological integrity; CNS: Basic care and comfort; CL: Apply

60. A pregnant client reports leg cramps that wake her from sleep. What is the nurse's **best** response?
1. Dorsiflex the foot
2. Elevate the legs at night
3. Point the toes until the cramp releases
4. Drink more than one quart of milk a day

60. 1. Dorsiflexion of the foot is the recommended intervention to relieve a leg cramp during pregnancy. Elevating the legs is an uncommon treatment. Drinking more than one quart of milk and pointing the toes can cause leg cramps.
CN: Physiological integrity; CNS: Basic care and comfort; CL: Apply

61. Which behavior is consistent with the diagnosis of conduct disorder in a child?
1. Enuresis
2. Suicidal ideation
3. Cruelty to animals
4. Fear of going to school

61. 3. Cruelty to animals is a symptom of conduct disorder. Enuresis and suicidal ideation aren't usually associated with conduct disorder. Fear of going to school is school phobia.
CN: Psychosocial integrity; CNS: None; CL: Apply

62. Which outcome is **most** appropriate for a client with a diagnosis of depression and attempted suicide?
1. The client will not express suicidal thoughts again.
2. The client will find a group home in which to live for the next year.
3. The client will remain hospitalized for at least six months.
4. The client will verbalize an absence of suicidal ideation, plan or intent.

62. 4. An appropriate outcome is that the client verbalizes a lack of suicidal feelings. It's unrealistic to ask that this client never feels suicidal again. There's no reason for a group home or six months of hospitalization.
CN: Psychosocial integrity; CNS: None; CL: Apply

CN: Client needs category   CNS: Client needs subcategory   CL: Cognitive level

63. Parents of a child with asthma are trying to identify possible allergens in their household. Which inhaled allergen is the **most** common?
1. Perfume
2. Dust mites
3. Passive smoke
4. Dog or cat dander

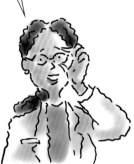

Focus on the words *most common*. They'll help you find the right answer.

63. 2. The household dust mite is the most commonly inhaled allergen that can cause an asthma attack. Animal dander, passive smoke, and perfume are sometimes allergens causing asthma attacks, but aren't as common as dust mites. CN: Safe, effective care environment; CNS: Safety and infection control; CL: Analyze

64. The nurse is devising a meal plan for a child newly diagnosed with celiac disease. What menu choices **best** meets the child's needs?
1. Hamburger on a bun with chips and chocolate milk
2. Cheese pizza with a fruit cup
3. Grilled chicken strips, fries, and a soda
4. Spaghetti with meat sauce and a brownie

64. 3. The intestinal cells of individuals with celiac disease become inflamed when the child eats products such as bagels, bread, crackers, malted breakfast cereals, pasta, and pizza that contain gluten. The child with celiac disease requires normal amounts of fat and protein in their diet for growth and development. Parents should read food labels, and be alert to hidden gluten content. CN: Safe, effective care environment; CNS: Safety and infection control; CL: Apply

65. A man stepped on a sharp piece of glass while walking barefoot. He comes to the emergency department with a deep laceration on the bottom of his foot. What is the **most** important question for the nurse to ask?
1. "Was the glass dirty?"
2. "Are you immune to tetanus?"
3. "When did you have your last tetanus shot?"
4. "How many diphtheria-pertussis-tetanus (DTaP) shots did you receive as a child?"

65. 3. Questioning the client about the date of his last tetanus immunization is important. The client should receive a booster immunization every 10 years in adulthood, or at the time of the injury if the last booster immunization was given more than five years before the injury. All deep lacerations require a tetanus immunization or booster no matter the cleanliness of the inflicting object. It is unlikely that a client would know his tetanus immunity status. DTaP immunizations, given in childhood, don't provide lifelong immunization to tetanus. CN: Safe, effective care environment; CNS: Safety and infection control; CL: Analyze

66. A client, diagnosed with cardiomyopathy, saw a posting on the internet describing research about a new herbal treatment for the disorder. What is the nurse's **best** response regarding this herbal treatment?
1. Herbs are often used to treat cardiomyopathy.
2. Cardiomyopathy can be treated only by heart surgery.
3. The internet is a reliable source of research, so try this treatment.
4. Any research found on the internet should be verified by a provider.

66. 4. Although the internet contains some valid medical research, there's no control over the it's validity. The research should be discussed with the client's provider who has access to the client's history and medical record. This will allow discussion of validity of use, risk, benefits and any contraindications that may exist in the client's history. Herbs are not a standard treatment for cardiomyopathy. Cardiomyopathy is treatable with drugs or surgery. CN: Safe, effective care environment; CNS: Management of care; CL: Apply

67. A registered nurse (RN) is supervising the care of a licensed practical nurse (LPN). The LPN is voicing concerns about a terminal client's end-of-life plan. Which statement, by the LPN, would indicate that further teaching is needed?
1. "Some clients write a living will to indicate their end-of-life preferences."
2. "The law requires that you draft a new living will each time you are admitted to the hospital."
3. "You can designate other people to make end-of-life decisions when you can't make those decisions for yourself."
4. "Some people choose to tell their provider that they don't want to have cardiopulmonary resuscitation."

67. 2. One living will is sufficient for all hospitalizations unless the client wishes to make changes. A living will explains a person's end-of-life preferences. A durable power of attorney for health care can be written to designate who will make health care decisions for the client in the event the client can't make these decisions for himself. The "No-Code" or "Do-Not-Resuscitate" status is discussed with the provider, who then enters the information in the client's chart.
CN: Safe, effective care environment; CNS: Management of care; CL: Analyze

68. A nurse gives the wrong medication to a client. Which communication would the unit's risk manager anticipate as a result of this error?
1. Incident report
2. Oral report from the nurse
3. Copy of the medication record
4. Order change signed by the provider

68. 1. Incident reports are tools used by risk managers when a client may have been harmed. They're used to determine how future problems can be avoided. An oral report won't serve as legal documentation. A copy of the medication record wouldn't be sent with the incident report to the risk manager. A provider will not change an order to cover the nurse's mistake.
CN: Safe, effective care environment; CNS: Management of care; CL: Apply

69. A client in labor is receiving oxytocin to augment her labor. The nurse notes a change in her contraction pattern. The fetal heart monitor indicates that her contractions are lasting two minutes, with a notable rise in the baseline. Based on this finding, what action is the **priority**?
1. Notify the health care provider
2. Give oxygen through a mask
3. Turn oxytocin to the lowest level
4. Turn the client on her left side

69. 3. The first action must be to lower the oxytocin to prevent fetal hypoxia or possible rupture of the uterus. The client would then be placed on her left side and given oxygen to prevent fetal hypoxia. The provider would be notified.
CN: Safe, effective care environment; CNS: Reduction of risk; CL: Analyze

70. After discovering a cleft palate and cleft lip on her newly-delivered neonate, the client has minimal contact with her child. She asks the nurse to provide the neonate's care. The nurse understands that this client is at risk for:
1. depression due to loss of the ideal child.
2. anger due to increased responsibilities.
3. impaired parenting related to birth defect.
4. isolation due to lack of family support.

70. 3. Parents of neonates born with birth defects are at risk for impaired parenting. Parents must work through their issues of not producing the perfect child and the associated guilt. There is no indication that this client feels depressed or is angry about caring for the neonate. Isolation due to lack of family support is not indicated.
CN: Psychosocial integrity; CNS: Management of care; CL: Analyze

CN: Client needs category   CNS: Client needs subcategory   CL: Cognitive level

71. A client with diagnosed substance use is being discharged from a state treatment facility. Which intervention would be included in this client's discharge plans?
1. Referral to Al-Anon
2. Weekly urine testing for drug use
3. Day hospital treatment for six months
4. Participation in a support group like Alcoholics Anonymous (AA)

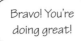

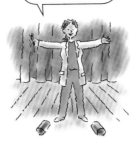

71. 4. Alcoholics Anonymous is a major support group for alcoholics following treatment. Membership in AA is associated with relapse prevention. Al-Anon is a support group for the family of the alcoholic. Weekly urine testing or day hospital treatment is uncommon.
CN: Psychosocial integrity; CNS: Management of care; CL: Apply

72. The registered nurse is caring for a neonate diagnosed with a cardiac anomaly. The pediatrician orders digoxin, 2.5 mg. The nurse questions the order with both the pharmacist and health care provider. The nurse demonstrates an understanding of the:
1. Nurses' Code of Ethics/Code of Ethics for Registered Nurses.
2. Nursing Standards of Practice.
3. National Council of State Boards of Nursing NCLEX Test Plan.
4. Nursing's Social Policy Statement/Canadian Nurses Association Position Statements.

72. 1. Each nurse must practice competent standards based on their state's, territory's, or province's standards of safe practice. The Nurses' Code of Ethics and the Code of Ethics for Registered Nurses articulate the ethical obligations of nurses and do not outline the criteria for safe practice. The National Council of State Boards of Nursing NCLEX Test Plan is used in development of including the nursing licensure examinations. The Social Policy Statement for Nurses and the Canadian Nurses Association Position Statements outline the responsibilities of nurses to the society as a whole, such as the broad issues related to the organization of health care, and do not dictate standards of safe practice.
CN: Safe, effective care environment; CNS: Management of care; CL: Apply

73. During assessment, a client verbally rates the pain as 9 out of 10 on a 0 to 10 pain scale. There is no indication of pain relief, even though the previous nurse signed for an opioid for this client one hour prior. The client denies receiving anything for pain since the previous night. Which action should the nurse take **next**?
1. Notify the provider that an opioid is missing
2. Notify the supervisor that the client didn't receive the prescribed pain medication
3. Notify the pharmacist that the client didn't receive the prescribed pain medication
4. Approach the nurse who signed for the opioid to seek clarification about the missing drug

73. 4. The nurse needs to seek clarification regarding this medication. If the nurse, who signed out the opioid, can't provide a plausible explanation, the nurse who discovered the error must notify the supervisor. The appropriate line of communication is to the hospital supervisor. The provider should be notified if the client didn't receive the prescribed medication. The pharmacist should be notified of discrepancies in the opioid count.
CN: Safe, effective care environment; CNS: Management of care; CL: Apply

CN: Client needs category   CNS: Client needs subcategory   CL: Cognitive level

74. The nurse is assessing a client admitted to the emergency department following a rape. Which are the nurse's client and legal responsibilities? Select all that apply.

1. Place client's clothing in a labeled bag.
2. Have a nurse of the same sex stay with the client.
3. Call for the nurse trained in evaluation of sexual assault victims.
4. Prepare client for complete physical examination including Pap smear.
5. Remind the client to return for follow-up for sexually transmitted disease (STD) testing every 6 weeks for a year.
6. Recognize that assessment charting may be used in legal proceedings.

75. The nursing profession has a responsibility to provide quality cost-effective care. A priority nursing judgment is to recognize that financial reimbursement for care will be lost for certain hospital-acquired conditions if the:

1. client develops a pressure ulcer postoperatively.
2. client admitted with a urinary tract infection (UTI) has a positive urinary culture and sensitivity upon admission.
3. client's peripheral IV infiltrates at the insertion site in the arm after initial 500 milliliter dose of D5 0.9% NaCl with 20 Meq KCL.
4. client feels faint while walking with the nurse and is assisted to the floor.

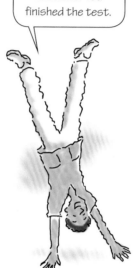

You did it! You finished the test.

74. 1, 2, 3, 4, 6. The nurse should recognize that clothing and physical evidence should be collected and preserved. The nurse should provide supportive care to the client victim of assault. If possible the nurse staying with the client should be the same sex as the client to decrease stress and anxiety. A rape crisis nurse or nurse trained in caring for victims of sexual assault should be called to assess the client and collect and preserve evidence. Accurate charting of physical and emotional findings will be important. The client should be followed for possible STDs within 3 weeks or sooner if any symptoms appear.

CN: Safe, effective care environment; CNS: Management of care; CL: Apply

75. 1. In 2008, Medicare restricted or eliminated reimbursement for certain hospital-acquired events that could have been reasonably prevented. Pressure ulcers are one such condition. The other events are not included in the Centers for Medicare and Medicaid Services guidelines.

CN: Safe, effective care environment; CNS: Management of care; CL: Apply

Comprehensive Test 2

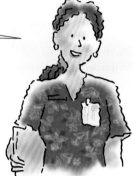

Here's another challenging comprehensive test—this time with 110 questions—just like you may get on the NCLEX. Have a go at it!

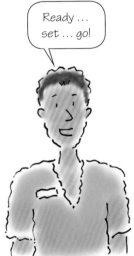

Ready ... set ... go!

1. A nurse suspects that an infant may have transposition of the great vessels (TGV) based on the assessment findings. Which diagnostic test would be performed **first** to detect this defect?
   1. Blood cultures
   2. Cardiac catheterization
   3. Chest X-ray
   4. Echocardiogram

1. 3. Chest X-ray would be done first to visualize congenital heart diseases such as TGV. Blood cultures won't diagnose TGV. Cardiac catheterization and an echocardiogram would be done but would not be the initial diagnostic intervention.
CN: Health promotion and maintenance; CNS: None;
CL: Apply

2. Several four-month-old children have arrived at the clinic for their diphtheria-pertussis-tetanus (DTaP) immunization. Which child can safely receive the immunization at this time?
   1. Temperature of 103° F (39.4° C)
   2. Runny nose
   3. Uncontrolled epilepsy
   4. Difficulty breathing after the last immunization

2. 2. Children with mild acute illness without fever can safely receive DTaP immunization. Children with a temperature of more than 102° F (38.9° C), uncontrolled epilepsy, or serious reactions to previous immunizations shouldn't receive DTaP immunization.
CN: Health promotion and maintenance; CNS: None; CL: Analyze

3. The parents of a two-year-old child, diagnosed with respiratory syncytial virus (RSV), ask the nurse if their eight-year-old child is at risk for RSV. What is the nurse's **best** response?
   1. RSV is not highly communicable in infants and toddlers.
   2. RSV is not communicable to older children and adults.
   3. The two-year-old client must be admitted to the hospital for isolation.
   4. The children should be separated to prevent the spread of the infection.

3. 4. Toddlers easily transmit and contract RSV and should be separated from other children. RSV is transmittable to older children and adults, but may only cause mild symptoms in these individuals. Hospitalization is indicated for children who need oxygen and IV therapy.
CN: Safe, effective care environment; CNS: Safety and infection control; CL: Apply

CN: Client needs category   CNS: Client needs subcategory   CL: Cognitive level

4. A child with asthma uses a peak expiratory flowmeter at school. The results indicate his peak flow is in the yellow zone. Which intervention, by the school nurse, is appropriate?
1. Follow the child's routine asthma treatment plan
2. Monitor the child for signs and symptoms of an acute attack
3. Call 911 and prepare for transport to the nearest emergency department
4. Call the child's mother to take the child to the family health care provider immediately

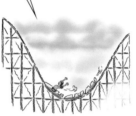

Asthma can be a real rollercoaster ride. Keep an eye on those peak flows.

4. **2.** The child should be monitored to determine if an asthma attack is imminent. The routine treatment plan may be insufficient when the peak flow is in the yellow zone. There's no immediate need to see the health care provider if the child is asymptomatic.
CN: Physiological integrity; CNS: Reduction of risk potential; CL: Apply

5. The nurse suspects that a client is experiencing metabolic alkalosis based on laboratory and physical findings. Which findings **best** indicate this condition?
1. A pH of 7.30; HCO_3 of 20 mEq/L; tachypnea and poor skin turgor
2. A pH of 7.51, HCO_3 of 29 mEq/L; muscle cramps and confusion
3. A pH of 7.32; HCO_3 of 48 mEq/L; shortness of breath and lethargy
4. A pH of 7.46; HCO_3 of 28 mEq/L; dizziness and numbness of hands and feet

5. **2.** A pH greater than 7.45 and a $PaCO_2$ less than 35 mmHg indicate respiratory alkalosis. A pH less than 7.35 and an HCO_3 less than 22 mEq/L indicate metabolic acidosis. A pH greater than 7.45 and an HCO_3 greater than 24 mEq/L indicate metabolic alkalosis. A pH less than 7.35 and a $PaCO_2$ greater than 45 mmHg indicate respiratory acidosis. Physical findings for metabolic alkalosis include muscle spasms, twitching and notable confusion. Rapid breathing and confusion/lethargy are symptoms of metabolic acidosis. Dizziness and numbness of hands and feet are symptoms of respiratory alkalosis. Confusion, lethargy, and shortness of breath are symptoms of respiratory acidosis.
CN: Physiological integrity; CNS: Reduction of risk potential; CL: Analyze

6. A nurse is evaluating the care of a client recently diagnosed with acute pancreatitis. Which statement indicates that a short-term goal of nursing care has been met?
1. The client denies abdominal pain.
2. The client doesn't report thirst.
3. The client denies pain at McBurney's point.
4. The client swallows liquids without coughing.

6. **1.** Pancreatitis is accompanied by acute pain from autodigestion by pancreatic enzymes. When the client denies abdominal pain, the short-term goal of pain control is met. Clients with acute pancreatitis receive IV fluids and may not have a sensation of thirst. Pain at McBurney's point accompanies appendicitis. Clients with acute pancreatitis receive nothing by mouth during initial therapy.
CN: Physiological integrity; CNS: Physiological adaptation; CL: Analyze

7. A client is to take eight ounces of magnesium citrate solution. The calibrations on the measuring device are in milliliters. How many milliliters should the nurse give?
1. 8 milliliters
2. 80 milliliters
3. 240 milliliters
4. 480 milliliters

7. **3.** To determine the amount of milliliters, use the following equation: One ounce equals 30 ml.

$$8\ oz \times 30\ ml/oz = 240\ ml$$

CN: Physiological integrity; CNS: Pharmacological and parenteral therapies; CL: Apply

CN: Client needs category   CNS: Client needs subcategory   CL: Cognitive level

8. A postmenopausal client asks a nurse how to prevent osteoporosis. What is the nurse's **best** response?
1. Take a multivitamin daily
2. After menopause, there's no way to prevent osteoporosis
3. Drink two glasses of milk each day and swim three times a week
4. Do weight-bearing exercises regularly

8. 4. Weight-bearing exercises are recommended for the prevention of osteoporosis. Telling the client that there's no way to prevent osteoporosis would be an incorrect statement. A multivitamin doesn't provide adequate calcium for a post-menopausal woman, and calcium alone won't prevent osteoporosis. Two glasses of milk per day don't provide the daily requirements for adult women, and swimming isn't a weight-bearing exercise.
CN: Health promotion and maintenance; CNS: None; CL: Apply

9. A male client has been diagnosed with pan-hy-popituitarism. Which oral hormone would the nurse anticipate to be given for this condition?
1. Estrogen
2. Levothyroxine
3. Serotonin
4. Testosterone

9. 2. Thyroid hormone release depends on the release of thyroid-stimulating hormone (TSH) by the anterior pituitary. TSH is absent from the pituitary when pan-hypopituitarism exists, so levothyroxine would be given orally. Estrogen isn't indicated for a male client. Serotonin release isn't controlled by the pituitary gland. Testosterone is given by injection or topically by patch.
CN: Physiological integrity; CNS: Pharmacological and parenteral therapies; CL: Analyze

10. Which nursing intervention is appropriate for an adult client with chronic renal failure?
1. Weigh the client daily before breakfast
2. Offer foods high in calcium and phosphorous
3. Serve the client large high-protein/high-fat meals and a bedtime snack
4. Encourage the client to drink large amounts of fluids

> Monitoring of fluid retention is critical in clients with chronic renal failure.

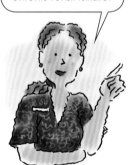

10. 1. Daily weights are obtained to monitor fluid retention. Calcium intake is encouraged, but clients with chronic renal failure have difficulty excreting phosphorous. Therefore, phosphorous must be restricted. To improve food intake, meals and snacks should be given in small portions and fats and protein limited. Fluids should be restricted for the client with chronic renal failure.
CN: Physiological integrity; CNS: Physiological adaptation; CL: Apply

11. A male is diagnosed with a genital chlamydial infection. Which symptom would the nurse antici-pate this client to report?
1. Burning and itching of penis
2. Visible fluid-filled lesions
3. Thick, purulent discharge from the penis
4. Genital warts

11. 1. In men, one of the most common reports with chlamydia is penile itching and burning, especially during urination. There may be a dis-charge, but it is usually clear or white, not yellow or purulent. Genital warts are a sign of human papillomavirus. Fluid-filled blisters are a sign of herpes infection.
CN: Health promotion and maintenance; CNS: None; CL: Analyze

CN: Client needs category   CNS: Client needs subcategory   CL: Cognitive level

12. The nurse is preparing to obtain a urine specimen from an indwelling urinary catheter of a client. What is the nurse's **most** appropriate action?
1. Collect urine from the drainage collection bag
2. Disconnect the catheter from the drainage tubing to collect urine
3. Remove the indwelling catheter and insert a sterile straight catheter to collect urine
4. Insert a sterile needle with syringe through the tubing drainage port after cleaning the port with alcohol to collect the specimen

12. 4. The nurse should wear clean gloves, clean the port with alcohol, and then obtain the specimen with a sterile needle and syringe to ensure that the specimen, and closed drainage system will not be contaminated. The urine specimen must be new urine, and the urine in the drainage collection bag could be several hours old and growing bacteria. The urinary drainage system must be kept closed to prevent microorganisms from entering. It isn't necessary to remove an indwelling catheter to obtain a sterile urine specimen, unless the health care provider requests that the system be changed.
CN: Safe, effective care environment; CNS: Safety and infection control; CL: Apply

13. An older adult client's husband tells a nurse he's concerned because his wife insists on talking about events that happened to her years ago. The nurse assesses the client and finds her alert, oriented, and answering questions appropriately. What is the nurse's **best** response?
1. "Your wife is reviewing her life."
2. "A spiritual advisor should be notified."
3. "You should not encourage conversations about the past."
4. "Your wife is regressing to a more comfortable time in her past."

13. 1. Life review or reminiscing is characteristic of older adults and the dying. A spiritual advisor might comfort the client but isn't necessary for a life review. Discouraging the client from talking would block communication. Regression occurs when a client returns to behaviors typical of another developmental stage.
CN: Health promotion and maintenance; CNS: None; CL: Apply

14. A nurse must obtain the blood pressure of a client in airborne isolation. What is the **best** method to prevent transmission of infection to other clients via shared equipment?
1. Dispose of blood pressure cuff after each use
2. Wear gloves while handling the equipment
3. Use the equipment only with other clients in airborne isolation
4. Leave the equipment in the room for use only with that client

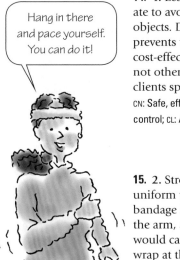

Hang in there and pace yourself. You can do it!

14. 4. Leaving equipment in the room is appropriate to avoid organism transmission by inanimate objects. Disposing of equipment after each use prevents the transmission of organisms but isn't cost-effective. Wearing gloves protects the nurse, not other clients. Sharing equipment with other clients spreads infectious organisms.
CN: Safe, effective care environment; CNS: Safety and infection control; CL: Apply

15. The nurse is applying an elastic wrap to a client's sprained elbow. What is the nurse's **best** action?
1. Wrap the bandage loosely around the arm
2. Apply the bandage while stretching it slightly
3. Apply heavy pressure with each turn of the bandage
4. Start applying the bandage at the upper arm and work toward the lower arm

15. 2. Stretching the bandage slightly will maintain uniform tension on the bandage. Wrapping the bandage loosely wouldn't secure the bandage on the arm, and it will come off. Using heavy pressure would cause circulatory impairment. Starting the wrap at the upper arm would cause an uneven application of the bandage.
CN: Physiological integrity; CNS: Reduction of risk potential; CL: Apply

16. The health care provider's order reads 2 g of cephalexin daily in equally divided doses of 500 mg each. At which frequency should the nurse administer this medication?
1. Three times per day
2. Four times per day
3. Six times per day
4. Eight times per day

16. 2. Two grams is equivalent to 2,000 mg. To give equally divided doses of 500 mg, divide the desired dose of 500 mg into the total daily dose of 2,000 mg. This medication should be given every six hours, four times each day.

CN: Physiological integrity; CNS: Pharmacological and parenteral therapies; CL: Analyze

17. A nurse is assessing the function of a client's optic nerve. What is the **most** important equipment for the nurse to use during this assessment?
1. Finger, to test the cardinal fields
2. Flashlight, to test corneal reflexes
3. Snellen chart, to test visual acuity
4. Piece of cotton, to test corneal sensitivity

17. 3. A Snellen chart is used to test the function of the optic nerve. Testing the cardinal fields assesses the oculomotor, trochlear, and abducens nerves. Corneal light reflex reflects the function of the oculomotor nerve. Corneal sensitivity is controlled by the trigeminal and facial nerves.

CN: Health promotion and maintenance; CNS: None; CL: Apply

18. A nurse is caring for a client following surgery in the post-anesthesia care unit. The nurse observes that the client is gagging on his airway and about to vomit. Which is the **best** position for the nurse to place the client?
1. Prone
2. Trendelenburg
3. Supine
4. Side lying

18. 4. Unless contraindicated, the right or left-side lying position, should be used. This position is commonly called the recovery position because it is used to prevent aspiration of secretions or vomitus during the postoperative phase. The prone position is face down and not appropriate. Trendelenburg position is used for shock, and supine position places the client flat on their back, making aspiration possible.

CN: Physiological integrity; CNS: Reduction of risk potential; CL: Apply

19. Which nursing intervention would **best** help prevent urinary tract infections (UTIs) for a client with an indwelling urinary catheter?
1. Recommend limiting fluid intake
2. Encourage showers rather than tub baths
3. Open the drainage system to obtain a urine specimen
4. Irrigate the catheter twice daily with sterile saline solution

19. 2. A shower would prevent bacteria in the bath water from sustaining contact with the urinary meatus and the catheter. A tub bath should not be given to any client with an indwelling catheter to prevent the transit of bacteria into the urinary tract. Increased fluid intake is recommended for a client with an indwelling urinary catheter because concentrated urine is more likely to become infected. Opening the drainage system would provide a pathway for the entry of bacteria. Catheter irrigation is performed to keep the catheter patent and does not address infection prevention. It should only take place when there is an order from the health care provider.

CN: Physiological integrity; CNS: Reduction of risk potential; CL: Apply

20. Six months after the death of her infant son, a client is suspected of dysfunctional grieving. Which assessment would the nurse expect to find in this client?
1. She goes to the infant's grave weekly.
2. She cries when talking about the loss.
3. She exercises four times a day and ignores her loss.
4. She states the infant will always be part of the family.

20. 3. One of the signs of dysfunctional grieving is over activity without a sense of loss. Including the infant as a part of the family, going to the grave, and crying are all normal responses.

CN: Psychosocial integrity; CNS: None; CL: Apply

CN: Client needs category   CNS: Client needs subcategory   CL: Cognitive level

21. A nurse notices that a hospitalized client has been crying. What is the nurse's **best** response?
1. Respect the client's privacy by saying nothing
2. "It seems like something is bothering you."
3. "Why are you crying and upsetting yourself?"
4. "Being in the hospital is hard, but try to keep your chin up."

21. 2. Therapeutic communication is a primary tool of nursing. The nurse must recognize that this client's nonverbal behavior may indicate a need to talk. Asking "why" is often interpreted as an accusation and should be avoided. Ignoring the client's nonverbal cues, or giving opinions and advice are barriers to communication.
CN: Psychosocial integrity; CNS: None; CL: Apply

22. A nurse gives the wrong medication to a client. Which initial communication will the unit's risk manager anticipate from this nurse?
1. Incident report
2. Oral report from the nurse
3. Copy of the medication record
4. Order change signed by the health care provider

22. 1. Incident reports are tools used by risk managers when a client might be harmed. They're used to determine how future problems can be avoided. An oral report won't serve as legal documentation. A copy of the medication record wouldn't be sent with the incident report to the risk manager. A health care provider won't change an order to cover the nurse's mistake.
CN: Safe, effective care environment; CNS: Management of care; CL: Apply

23. A student nurse witnesses a registered nurse performing a procedure on a client without obtaining informed consent for the procedure. The student nurse recognizes that the registered nurse is guilty of committing:
1. breach of confidentiality.
2. assault and battery.
3. harassment.
4. neglect of duty.

23. 2. Performing a procedure on a client without informed consent can be grounds for charges of assault and battery. Harassment means to annoy or disturb someone, and breach of confidentiality refers to conveying information about the client. Neglect of duty is failure to perform care that a prudent nurse would provide under similar circumstances.
CN: Safe, effective care environment; CNS: Management of care; CL: Apply

24. A surgical client newly diagnosed with cancer tells a nurse that she knows the laboratory made a mistake regarding her diagnosis. Which reaction is this client **most** likely experiencing?
1. Denial
2. Intellectualization
3. Regression
4. Repression

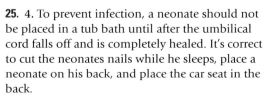

Hey—you've finished 25 questions! Great job!

24. 1. Cancer clients often deny their diagnosis when first made. This response may benefit the client in that it allows energy for surgical healing. Repression describes not remembering being diagnosed, regression describes childlike behavior, and intellectualization describes speaking of the disease as if reading a textbook.
CN: Psychosocial integrity; CNS: None; CL: Apply

25. Which statement, made by a client about her two-day-old newborn, indicates the need for further teaching?
1. "I'll trim the baby's nails when he's sleeping."
2. "I'll remember to place the baby on his back when he sleeps."
3. "Our infant car seat must be placed in the back seat of the car."
4. "The first thing I'm going to do when we get home is give the baby a tub bath."

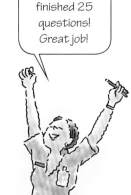

25. 4. To prevent infection, a neonate should not be placed in a tub bath until after the umbilical cord falls off and is completely healed. It's correct to cut the neonates nails while he sleeps, place a neonate on his back, and place the car seat in the back.
CN: Safe, effective care environment; CNS: Safety and infection control; CL: Analyze

26. A client, who just gave birth, is concerned about her neonate's Apgar scores of 7 and 8. She says she's been told scores lower than 9 are associated with learning difficulties later in life. What is the nurse's **best** response?
1. "Why are you worrying? Your infant is perfectly fine."
2. "I understand your concerns. You should ask about placing your infant in a follow-up diagnostic program."
3. "You're right to be concerned, but there are good special education programs available."
4. "Apgar scores are used to indicate a need for resuscitation at birth. Scores of 7 and above indicate that the baby has no problems."

26. 4. Apgar scores don't indicate future learning difficulties. They are used to rapidly assess the need for resuscitation. Asking a client why is confrontational and does not utilize therapeutic communication technique. It's inappropriate to tell a client not to worry. Apgar scores of 7 and 8 are normal, and don't indicate a need for intervention.
CN: Health promotion and maintenance; CNS: None; CL: Apply

27. A prenatal client tells the nurse, "I have tried to become pregnant for the past 10 years, and now I have mixed emotions about the pregnancy. I feel guilt for my conflicting reaction." What is the nurse's **best** response?
1. "You need to talk to your midwife about these unusual feelings."
2. "You're experiencing the normal ambivalence that pregnant mothers feel."
3. "These feelings are expected only in women who have had difficulty becoming pregnant."
4. "Let's make an appointment with a psychologist to help you sort through your feelings."

27. 2. Conflicting, ambivalent feelings regarding pregnancy are normal for all pregnant women. These feelings don't require counseling or other professional interventions.
CN: Psychosocial integrity; CNS: None; CL: Apply

28. A client tells the nurse that her husband is behaving in strange ways since she became pregnant. He's having morning sickness, has put on weight, reports intestinal pains, and acts like he's pregnant. How does the nurse interpret this behavior?
1. Extreme anxiety
2. Normal couvade
3. Signs of reaction formation
4. Abnormal, and in need of counseling

28. 2. The father's adjustment may include behaviors referred to as couvade. Historically, there have been different cultural couvades. Today, the term is associated with a father who develops pregnancy-like symptoms. Because the behavior is normal, and isn't reaction formation or anxiety, there's no need for counseling.
CN: Psychosocial integrity; CNS: None; CL: Analyze

29. A client is being treated for premature labor with ritodrine. After receiving this medication for 12 hours, the client's blood pressure is slightly elevated, her chest is clear, and her pulse is 120 bpm. She reports a little nausea, and the fetal heart rate is 145 bpm. Which intervention is correct?
1. Continue routine monitoring
2. Contact the health care provider immediately.
3. Turn the client on her left side and give oxygen
4. Increase the flow rate of the IV and give oxygen

29. 1. These findings are normal adverse effects to the medication and don't require intervention at this time except continued routine monitoring. Contacting the health care provider, placing the client on her left side, changing the IV flow rate, and giving oxygen are all interventions for abnormal assessment findings.
CN: Physiological integrity; CNS: Pharmacological and parental therapies; CL: Analyze

30. When assessing a client who just delivered a neonate, a nurse notes the following: blood pressure, 110/70 mmHg; pulse, 60 bpm; respirations, 16 breaths/min; lochia, moderate rubra; fundus, above the umbilicus to the right; and negative Homans' sign. What is the **most** appropriate nursing intervention?
1. These findings are all normal
2. Have the client void and recheck the fundus
3. Turn the client on her left side to decrease the blood pressure
4. Rub the fundus to decrease lochia flow and prevent hemorrhage

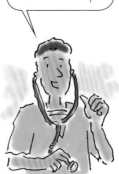

Which of these assessments is abnormal and needs follow-up?

30. 2. A fundus up and to the right indicates a full bladder. The client should empty her bladder and be reassessed. Lochia flow and blood pressure are normal.
CN: Physiological integrity; CNS: Reduction of risk potential; CL: Analyze

31. A client with gestational diabetes delivers an infant weighing 9 lb, 11 oz (4.4 kg) after eight hours of labor and membranes that ruptured three hours ago. Which interventions would be appropriate for this neonate? Select all that apply.
1. Obtain blood cultures for prolonged ruptured membranes
2. Obtain a heel stick for glucose level
3. Maintain a thermo-neutral environment
4. Allow the mother to begin breast feeding the neonate in the delivery room
5. Monitor the neonate for respiratory distress

31. 2, 3, 5. Neonates of mothers with diabetes are at risk for hypoglycemia related to the increased production of insulin by the neonate in utero. Blood glucose must be checked immediately after birth, and interventions implemented if it is low. Maintaining the infant's body temperature will reduce the risk of hypothermia, which can cause increased metabolism and increased burning of glucose. These infants are at increased risk of developing respiratory distress shortly after birth due to decreased surfactant production secondary to increased insulin in the baby's system. Three hours is not a prolonged period for the rupture of membranes. Beginning breast feeding immediately will not prevent hypoglycemic episodes. Providing a standardized glucose source with known glucose amounts is a better solution.
CN: Physiological integrity; CNS: Reduction of risk potential; CL: Apply

32. A 13-year-old, prenatal client asks about getting fat while she's pregnant. The nurse tells her that, due to her age, she needs to gain enough weight to reach the upper portions of her recommended weight to prevent:
1. delivery of a premature neonate.
2. a difficult delivery.
3. delivery of a low-birth-weight neonate.
4. preeclampsia.

32. 3. Adolescent girls, especially those younger than age 15, are at higher risk for delivering low-birth-weight neonates unless they gain adequate weight during pregnancy. Gaining weight isn't associated with an easier delivery, risk for preeclampsia, or risk of delivering a premature neonate.
CN: Physiological integrity; CNS: Reduction of risk potential; CL: Apply

33. The mother of a neonate, receiving phototherapy, asks why her child has developed loose stools. Which response, by the nurse, would be accurate?
1. They're abnormal and may indicate an infection.
2. They're associated with an adverse reaction to formula.
3. They're common when receiving phototherapy treatments.
4. They're abnormal, and phototherapy should be discontinued.

33. 3. While receiving phototherapy, a breakdown of bilirubin often results in loose stools. However, diarrhea is not normal. The neonate must be monitored for diarrhea, skin irritation, and dehydration when under the lights. Loose stools wouldn't be related to infection or formula at this time.
CN: Physiological integrity; CNS: Physiological adaptation; CL: Analyze

CN: Client needs category   CNS: Client needs subcategory   CL: Cognitive level

34. A client, at 36 weeks' gestation, chokes on her food while eating at a restaurant. Which statement is correct regarding the Heimlich maneuver on a pregnant client?
  1. Chest thrusts are used when the client is pregnant.
  2. Only back thrusts are used when the client is pregnant.
  3. The Heimlich maneuver is performed the same as when not pregnant.
  4. The Heimlich maneuver can't be performed on a pregnant client.

34. 1. During pregnancy, chest thrusts are used instead of abdominal thrusts. Abdominal thrusts compress the abdomen, which would harm the fetus. Because of this, the Heimlich is adjusted for the pregnant woman. A fist is made with one hand, placing the thumb side against the center of the breastbone. The fist is grabbed with the other hand and thrust inward. The xiphoid process should be avoided. Back thrusts aren't done because they may result in dislodgment of the obstruction, further obstructing the airway.
CN: Physiological integrity; CNS: Reduction of risk potential; CL: Apply

35. A registered nurse is reviewing the principles of good body mechanics with a student nurse. Which technique is **most** important?
  1. Bending from the waist
  2. Pulling rather than pushing
  3. Stretching to reach an object
  4. Using large muscles in the legs for leverage

35. 4. Keeping the back straight and using the large muscles in the legs will help avoid back injury. The muscles of the back are relatively small compared to the larger muscles of the thighs. Bending from the waist can stress the back muscles, resulting in injury. Pulling may cause muscle strain. If possible, an object should be pushed rather than pulled. Stretching to reach an object increases the risk of injury.
CN: Safe, effective care environment; CNS: Safety and infection control; CL: Apply

36. A community mental health nurse visits a client diagnosed with paranoid schizophrenia in his home. Upon arrival, the client calls the nurse Satan, and shouts, "Get away from me, you evil demon!" What is the nurse's **most** appropriate intervention?
  1. Use the client's phone and call the police
  2. Remain safe by leaving the house
  3. Talk to the client in a calm voice to reduce his agitation
  4. Remind the client who the nurse is and that he has nothing to fear

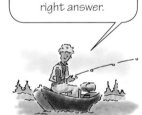

Keep fishing around and you'll hook the right answer.

36. 2. Safety is the first priority during any home visit, so the nurse should leave. Attempting to talk with the client, reminding him who the nurse is, or using the phone, places the nurse at risk for harm. After the nurse has ensured their safety, arrangements should be made to provide help for the client.
CN: Safe, effective care environment; CNS: Safety and infection control; CL: Analyze

37. A client is scheduled to retire in the next month. He phones his nurse therapist and says, "I can't cope with these changes. My whole world is falling apart." The therapist recognizes this reaction as a:
  1. panic reaction.
  2. situational crisis.
  3. separation anxiety.
  4. maturational crisis.

37. 4. A maturational crisis is one that occurs at a predictable milestone such as a birth, marriage, or retirement. A panic reaction would also involve physical symptoms. Situational crisis is caused by events such as an earthquake. Separation anxiety is a childhood disorder.
CN: Health promotion and maintenance; CNS: None; CL: Remember

38. A client, with a phobic condition, is being treated with behavior modification therapy. Which intervention **best** addresses this technique?
1. Suggest she face the phobia head-on
2. Talk to the client and have her identify why she has phobias
3. Recommend gradual and repeated exposure to the source of the phobia
4. Undergo electroconvulsive therapy (ECT) to jump-start the brain

38. 3. Systematic desensitization is a behavior therapy used in the treatment of phobias. Forcing the client to face the phobia head-on, and identifying a phobia do not help eliminate the problem and are not behavior modification methods. ECT is used with depression.
CN: Psychosocial integrity; CNS: None; CL: Apply

39. A nurse is developing a plan of care for a severely depressed client who rarely leaves his chair. What is the **most** important goal for this client?
1. Limit television time
2. Increase calcium intake
3. Rest in bed three times per day
4. Empty the bladder on a schedule

39. 4. To prevent bladder infections associated with stasis of urine, this client should be encouraged to routinely empty his bladder. Calcium intake is not directly related to the psychological effects associated with this condition. Resting in bed is another form of psychomotor retardation. Watching television is merely a distraction and not beneficial to preventing physiological problems.
CN: Health promotion and maintenance; CNS: None; CL: Apply

40. Which intervention is avoided during the termination phase of a therapeutic nurse–client relationship?
1. Referring the client to support groups
2. Addressing new issues with the client
3. Reviewing what has been accomplished during this relationship
4. Having the client express sadness that the relationship is ending

40. 2. During the termination phase, new issues shouldn't be explored. It's appropriate to refer the client to support groups. To review what has been accomplished is a goal of this phase. Sadness is a normal response.
CN: Psychosocial integrity; CNS: None; CL: Apply

In question 42, you are looking for the intervention that should be performed first.

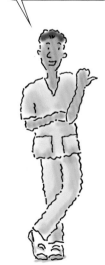

41. The behavior of a client with borderline personality disorder causes a nurse to feel angry toward the client. What is the nurse's **most** appropriate intervention?
1. Ignore the client's irritating behavior
2. Restrict the client to their room until supper
3. Report these feelings to the client's health care provider
4. Tell the client how their behavior makes the nurse feel

41. 4. A nursing intervention used with personality disorders is to help the client recognize how their behavior affects others. Restricting the client to her room, ignoring the client, and reporting feelings to the health care provider aren't appropriate interventions at this time.
CN: Psychosocial integrity; CNS: None; CL: Apply

42. A client with a panic disorder is having difficulty falling asleep. Which nursing intervention should be performed **first**?
1. Call the client's psychotherapist
2. Teach the client progressive relaxation
3. Allow the client to stay up and watch television
4. Obtain an order for a sleeping medication as needed

42. 2. Relaxation techniques work very well with a client showing anxiety. If this doesn't work, then contacting the psychotherapist, diversionary activities, and pharmacological interventions would be in order.
CN: Psychological integrity; CNS: None; CL: Apply

43. The nurse is caring for a client who has just undergone electroconvulsive therapy (ECT). What is the nurse's **most** important intervention?
  1. Assessing the client's vital signs
  2. Leaving the client alone to sleep undisturbed
  3. Allowing the family to visit immediately
  4. Restraining the client until completely awake

43. 1. Vital signs are monitored carefully for approximately one hour after ECT, or until the client is stable. The client shouldn't be restrained or left alone. Visitors should not be allowed until the client is awake and ready.
CN: Physiological integrity; CNS: Reduction of risk potential; CL: Apply

44. A client diagnosed with bipolar disease is receiving a maintenance dosage of lithium carbonate. His wife calls the community mental health nurse and reports that her husband is hyperactive and hyperverbal. What is the **most** appropriate intervention for this client?
  1. Mental status examination
  2. Measurement of lithium blood levels
  3. Evaluation at the local emergency department (ED)
  4. Admission to the hospital for observation

44. 2. Increased activity might indicate a need for an increased dose of lithium, or that the client isn't taking his medication. Blood lithium levels will determine medication levels. The client doesn't need to have a mental status examination, go to the ED, or be admitted to the hospital at this time.
CN: Physiological integrity; CNS: Pharmacological and parenteral therapies; CL: Analyze

45. A nurse is caring for a client with emphysema. Which nursing interventions are appropriate? Select all that apply.
  1. Reduce fluid intake to less than 2,500 ml/day
  2. Teach diaphragmatic, pursed-lip breathing
  3. Administer low-flow oxygen
  4. Keep the client in a supine position as much as possible
  5. Encourage alternating activity with rest periods
  6. Teach the family use of postural drainage and chest physiotherapy

45. 2, 3, 5, 6. Diaphragmatic, pursed-lip breathing strengthens respiratory muscles and enhances oxygenation in clients with emphysema. Low-flow oxygen should be administered because a client with emphysema has chronic hypercapnia and a hypoxic respiratory drive. Alternating activity with rest allows the client to perform activities without excessive distress. If the client has difficulty mobilizing copious secretions the nurse should teach him, and his family how to perform postural drainage and chest physiotherapy. Fluid intake should be increased to 3,000 ml/day, if not contraindicated, to liquefy secretions and facilitate their removal. The client should be placed in high Fowler's position to improve ventilation.
CN: Physiological integrity; CNS: Basic care and comfort; CL: Analyze

46. A nurse is assessing the abdomen of a client who was admitted to the emergency department with suspected appendicitis. Identify the area of the abdomen that the nurse should palpate **last**.

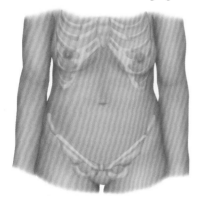

46. An acute attack of appendicitis localizes as pain and tenderness in the lower right quadrant, midway between the umbilicus and the crest of the ilium. This area should be palpated last in order to determine pain present in other areas of the abdomen first.

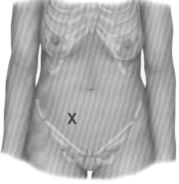

CN: Physiological integrity; CNS: Reduction of risk potential; CL: Apply

47. The nurse is caring for a hospice client who prefers holistic care. The nurse has included complementary and alternative medicine in the plan of care. Which complementary measures are appropriate for this client? Select all that apply.
1. Administering morphine sulfate for breakthrough pain
2. Arranging for music of the client's choice to be played in the room
3. Using aroma therapy
4. Assessing for impaction
5. Providing an air mattress
6. Allowing the family to give oral fluids as needed

47. 2, 3. The use of music, massage, and aroma therapy are considered aspects of complementary medicine. Hospice client care may also include traditional methods of for increased pain relief measures and comfort measures such as air mattresses and family involvement in care. Most beds have an air mattress to decrease pressure on bony prominences. Maintaining the client free from constipation and impaction is not an alternative therapy.
CN: Physiological integrity; CNS: Physiological adaptation; CL: Apply

48. The nurse is caring for a three-year-old with acute lymphocytic leukemia and notes that the child has a decreased appetite. What is the **priority** nursing intervention?
1. Provide oral hygiene after eating
2. Refrain from serving snacks as requested
3. Have the dietician meet with the child and family to provide foods he will eat
4. Encourage the child to eat all his meal to get adequate nutrition

48. 3. The dietician should be involved to help determine foods appropriate for children in different age groups. The child and family should help select preferred foods, identify cultural beliefs and dining habits. Take advantage of a hungry period and serve small snacks. Encourage parents to relax pressures placed on eating by stressing the legitimate nature of loss of appetite. The other responses do not help to stimulate the child's appetite.
CN: Physiological integrity; CNS: Physiological adaptation; CL: Apply

49. The nurse explains the preparation for a bone marrow transplant to a client. Which information is important for the nurse to provide? Select all that apply.
1. An arteriovenous shunt will be established.
2. A course of chemotherapy will be administered.
3. A suitable donor must be identified prior to final preparations for transplant.
4. Total-body radiation will be administered.
5. The donor bone marrow will be injected into the client's bone marrow.
6. The client will be placed in isolation to protect the family.

49. 2, 3, 4. The identified donor's healthy bone marrow is infused intravenously, usually through a peripherally inserted central catheter. An arteriovenous shunt is not established. Chemotherapy and total-body radiation are necessary to prepare the recipient for the healthy bone marrow. Reverse isolation will protect the client from exposure to pathogens from others.
CN: Health promotion and maintenance; CNS: Physiological adaptation; CL: Apply

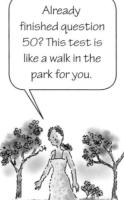

Already finished question 50? This test is like a walk in the park for you.

50. A home care aide notifies the agency that she found a client, newly diagnosed with type 1 diabetes mellitus, lying on the floor. When the home health nurse arrives, she quickly assesses the client, and notes the following: client is semicomatose, apical heart rate is 102 bpm, blood pressure is 84/30 mmHg, and skin is warm and dry. The nurse suspect that the client may be experiencing:
1. hypoglycemia.
2. cardiogenic shock.
3. diabetic ketoacidosis (DKA).
4. hyperosmolar hyperglycemic non-ketotic syndrome (HHNS).

50. 3. DKA develops as a result of severe insulin deficiency. The incidence of DKA generally results from undiagnosed diabetes and inadequacy of prescribed medication and dietary therapies. Signs of DKA include flushed dry skin, restlessness, fruity odor of the breath, and confusion. The client may become unconscious. Hypoglycemia involves episodes of low blood glucose levels caused by erratic or altered absorption of insulin. In cardiogenic shock, the client has pale, cool, and moist skin. HHNS is a deadly complication of diabetes distinguished by severe hyperglycemia, dehydration, and altered mental status.
CN: Physiological integrity; CNS: Physiological adaptation; CL: Analyze

CN: Client needs category CNS: Client needs subcategory CL: Cognitive level

51. A nurse is standing next to a person eating fried shrimp at a parade. Suddenly, the man clutches his throat and is unable to speak, cough, or breathe. The nurse asks the man if he's choking, and he nods yes. What action should the nurse take **next**?

1. Attempt rescue breathing
2. Perform the Heimlich maneuver
3. Deliver external chest compressions
4. Use the head tilt-chin lift maneuver to establish the airway

51. **2.** If a conscious victim acknowledges that he's choking, the best response is to perform the Heimlich maneuver to relieve the airway obstruction. The other options are used for an unresponsive victim with absent heart rate and breathing.
CN: Physiological integrity; CNS: Physiological adaptation; CL: Apply

52. The nurse is preparing a client with sinus tachycardia for cardioversion. What is the nurse's **priority** action?

1. Keep the client awake and alert
2. Keep the side rails up for client safety
3. Set the machine on SYNC and charge at 200 watts
4. Set the machine on DEFIB and charge at 400 watts

52. **3.** If cardioversion is needed, the nurse should set the machine on SYNC and look for a marker on each QRS complex. The nurse should anticipate that the cardioversion will be started at a low energy level and increase as needed. The client will be sedated for this procedure. Lowering the side rails will make it easier to place paddle electrodes.
CN: Physiological integrity; CNS: Physiological adaptation; CL: Apply

53. The healthcare provider orders azithromycin 10 mg/kg PO daily for an 11-year-old child. The client weighs 108 lb (49 kg). How many milligrams should the nurse administer? Record your answer using a whole number.

_____ mg

53. **490.**
Multiply the amount 10 of drug ordered by the child's weight in kilograms to determine the amount per dose per day.

$$10 \text{ mg} / \text{kg} \times 49 \text{ kg} = 490 \text{ mg}$$

CN: Physiological integrity; CNS: Pharmacological and parenteral therapies; CL: Apply

54. A 72-year-old client is being discharged from outpatient surgery after having a cataract removed from his right eye. What is the **most** important information for the nurse to include in this client's discharge instructions?

1. Resume all activities as before
2. Begin eye drops in three days
3. Do not rub or place pressure on the eye
4. Wear eye shields on both eyes at night

54. **3.** Rubbing or placing pressure on the eye increases the risk of accidental injury to ocular structures. An eye shield should be worn on the operative eye at night. Eye drops should be instilled as ordered beginning the day of discharge. Additional teaching includes caution against lifting objects, straining, strenuous exercise, and sexual activity. Such activity can increase intraocular pressure. The client should avoid sleeping on the operative side to reduce the risk of accidental injury to ocular structures. Glasses or shaded lenses should be worn to protect the eye during waking hours after the eye dressing is removed.
CN: Physiological integrity; CNS: Reduction of risk potential; CL: Apply

55. The nurse is preparing to care for a postoperative thyroidectomy client who has just returned to the unit after surgery. What are the **most** important nursing interventions for this client? Select all that apply.
1. Place bed in high Fowler's position
2. Have emergency tracheotomy set on hand
3. Check behind the neck for bleeding
4. Monitor voice quality regularly
5. Observe for sudden increase in temperature, respiratory distress, and tetany.

Congratulations! You're halfway done. Have some cake.

55. 2, 3, 4, 5. Postoperative thyroidectomy clients may need humidified oxygen and should be placed in the semi-Fowler's position. Vital signs will need to be monitored for any changes, and the client should be observed for bleeding behind the neck under the dressing. It is important to observe for signs of respiratory distress and to have tracheotomy equipment on hand. Monitor voice quality for injury to vocal chords. If the client develops postoperative thyroid storm/crisis, the temperature could rise as high as 106° F (41.1° C), and tetany may develop if the parathyroid glands were injured or removed.
CN: Physiological integrity; CNS: Reduction of risk potential
CL: Apply

56. The nurse is planning discharge teaching for a client who will continue taking the prescribed warfarin sodium at home. What is the **priority** teaching?
1. Avoid injury and watch for signs of bleeding
2. Take the medication at 9 am daily
3. Injections may be given in the abdomen
4. Dietary restrictions include tomatoes and cucumbers

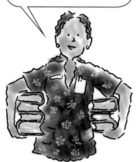

Do you remember what effects warfarin has on a client? Well, then, what teaching would you need to provide?

56. 1. Coumadin is an anticoagulant, so the priority teaching would include watching for signs of hemorrhage and to prevent bleeding. Warfarin is administered orally. The client should have scheduled blood tests for prothrombin time. Consumption of leafy green vegetables should be limited.
CN: Physiological integrity; CNS: Pharmacological and parenteral therapies; CL: Apply

57. The nurse and occupational therapist are planning an outdoor volleyball game and picnic for eight mental health clients. What action should the nurse take for the two clients taking nortriptyline for depression?
1. Be aware that this drug can cause hypotension
2. Recognize that these clients may experience excessive thirst
3. Omit the morning dose on the day of the picnic
4. Provide protective clothing and apply sunscreen before going out

57. 4. A common adverse effect of this drug is sensitivity to the sun. Protective clothing and sunscreen should be worn while the client is exposed to sunlight. Pamelor is a tricyclic antidepressant, often administered at night because it may cause drowsiness. This drug can cause hypertension. Nortripyline takes 2 to 3 weeks to achieve the desired effect.
CN: Physiological integrity; CNS: Pharmacological and parenteral therapies; CL: Analyze

58. The nurse is teaching a client and her family about the total parenteral nutrition (TPN) that the client is receiving. What information should the nurse include in this teaching? Select all that apply.
1. TPN is administered through a large central blood vessel.
2. The solution contains sugar, protein, and fat for increased calories.
3. The client may experience constipation.
4. Tests to monitor blood and urine glucose levels will be done.
5. The client will need insulin to prevent diabetes.

58. 1, 2, 4. There is a possibility of abdominal cramping and diarrhea, not constipation, from TPN. Glucose levels will need to be monitored, and some clients may need insulin to regulate blood glucose levels during TPN, but the client will not develop diabetes from TPN.
CN: Physiological integrity; CNS: Pharmacological and parenteral therapies; CL: Apply

CN: Client needs category   CNS: Client needs subcategory   CL: Cognitive level

59. The nurse is caring for a frail, older adult client who is experiencing pain. At the client care meeting, the family asks if it is safe for the client to receive narcotics. The nurse is aware that the client is receiving hydromorphone hydrochloride for pain. What is the nurse's **most** appropriate response to this family?
1. The narcotic is safe because it does not accumulate in the body.
2. The drug does not cause any problems with breathing.
3. The drug is not as strong as morphine.
4. This drug is similar to methamphetamine.

60. The nurse is instructing a client who will be discharged on anticoagulant therapy. What is the **most** important instruction for this nurse to include?
1. Do not shave with an electric razor
2. Take ibuprofen or aspirin for pain
3. Take the anticoagulant at the same time each day
4. Eat green, leafy vegetables and salad daily

61. A post-operative client has tolerated a full liquid diet for the first meal. Which action, by the nurse, is **best**?
1. Check for bowel sounds
2. Seek an order to advance to full liquids
3. Seek an order to advance to a soft diet
4. Allow the client to select from the menu

62. The home health nurse is instructing the mother of a child diagnosed with juvenile rheumatoid arthritis (JRA) on interventions to reduce the child's pain and stiffness. What is the nurse's **most** appropriate intervention?
1. Hot packs
2. Alternating heat and cold applications
3. Cold compresses
4. A warm bath

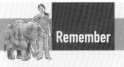

Remember

"Warfarin wars against clots."

Anticoagulant drugs, such as warfarin, decrease the ability of blood to form clots. Anticoagulants include the following:
- Heparin
  - Unfractionated heparin
  - Heparin sodium
  - Dalteparin sodium
  - Enoxaparin sodium
- Warfarin
- Antiplatelet drugs
  - Aspirin
  - Clopidogrel
  - Dipyridamole
  - Ticlopidine
  - Abciximab
  - Eptifibatide
  - Tirofiban
- Thrombin inhibitors
  - Argatroban
  - Bivalirudin
  - Lepirudin
- Factor Xa inhibitor drugs

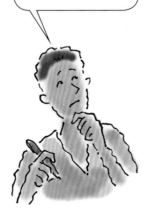

Hmm. What should I tell the family about this client's medication?

59. 1. Hydromorphone is a fast-acting narcotic analgesic drug and is a useful alternative to morphine or meperidine due to its short half-life. Morphine and meperidine can increase the risk of confusion in older adults. Hydromorphone is a synthetic drug similar to morphine with an eight to ten times more potent analgesic effect. Respiratory depression may occur, but is less frequent than with some other narcotics.
CN: Physiological integrity; CNS: Pharmacological and parenteral therapies; CL: Apply

60. 3. It is important to take the anticoagulant at the same time each day to maintain an adequate blood level. An electric razor reduces the risk of cutting the skin. Avoid the use of standard razors. Avoid taking aspirin or ibuprofen because these drugs decrease clotting time. Eating a large amount of green, leafy vegetables that contain vitamin K will increase clotting time, thus requiring more anticoagulants.
CN: Physiological integrity; CNS: Pharmacological and parenteral therapies; CL: Apply

61. 2. Clear liquid diets are nutritionally inadequate but minimally irritating to the stomach. Bowel sounds should be assessed before the client has been given a diet for the first time. Clients should be advanced to a full liquid diet, adding bland and protein foods, followed be a soft diet which omits foods that are hard to chew or digest. A regular or general diet has no limitations. A fluid restriction is ordered in addition to the diet order for clients in renal failure or congestive heart failure.
CN: Physiological integrity; CNS: Basic care and comfort; CL: Apply

62. 4. Heat is beneficial to children with arthritis. Moist heat is best for relieving pain and stiffness. The most efficient and practical method is in the bathtub. Cold, cool, or lukewarm treatments are not beneficial in relieving pain or stiffness in children with JRA. Hot packs and heating pads could burn the child.
CN: Physiological integrity; CNS: Basic care and comfort; CL: Apply

63. The nurse is assessing a client during a home health visit. The client reports a severe burning on urination. What is the **most** important action by the nurse?
1. Have the client drink cranberry juice
2. Have the client take a sitz bath twice daily
3. Obtain a urine specimen from the client
4. Have the client drink 2,500 to 3,000 ml of water per day

63. 3. Though it is suspected that the client has a urinary tract infection (UTI), a urine specimen is needed to determine specific treatment. After obtaining the specimen, comfort measures can be provided pending the results which may take 24 to 72 hours. Drinking large amounts of water will help flush bacteria from the urinary tract, but it is not bacteria specific. Cranberry juice increases the acidity of urine and helps to prevent UTIs; however, it does little to treat a UTI. A sitz bath may provide comfort but does not address the priority need.
CN: Physiological integrity; CNS: Basic care and comfort; CL: Apply

64. The nurse is caring for a client on the rehabilitation unit who has hearing loss. In planning care, the nurse documents ways to minimize the obstacles to successful communication with this client. Select all that may apply.
1. Stand or sit in his line of vision
2. Close the door to the client's room
3. Talk loudly and slowly to the client
4. Minimize the distraction from television and visitors
5. Be certain hearing aids are functioning properly
6. Get the client's attention before communicating

64. 1, 2, 4, 5, 6. It is essential to communicate appropriately with the hearing-impaired client. Face the client and get his attention before speaking to him. Eliminate distractions and background noises. Make sure the client has his hearing aids in, and that the battery is working. Speaking loudly and slowly is not necessary and may interfere with comprehension, as loud sounds may reverberate.
CN: Physiological integrity; CNS: Basic care and comfort; CL: Apply

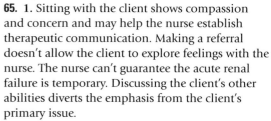

Sometimes what your client needs most from you is just your presence.

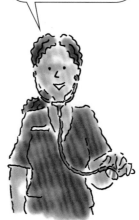

65. A nurse finds a client crying after she was told by the health care provider that she is to start hemodialysis to treat her acute renal failure. What is the nurse's **most** important intervention?
1. Sit quietly with the client
2. Refer the client to the hemodialysis team
3. Remind the client this is a temporary situation
4. Discuss with the client the other abilities she has

65. 1. Sitting with the client shows compassion and concern and may help the nurse establish therapeutic communication. Making a referral doesn't allow the client to explore feelings with the nurse. The nurse can't guarantee the acute renal failure is temporary. Discussing the client's other abilities diverts the emphasis from the client's primary issue.
CN: Psychosocial integrity; CNS: None; CL: Analyze and apply

66. A client is admitted to a mental health unit. While assessing the client, the nurse finds the client exhibiting signs of hyperexcitability, increasing agitation, and distractibility. Based on this assessment, which nursing intervention has **priority**?
1. Involve the client in a group activity
2. Be direct and firm and set rules for the client
3. Use a quiet room for the client away from others
4. Channel the client's energy toward a planned activity

66. 3. Being in a quiet environment away from stimuli will facilitate a sense of control for this client. If the nurse attempts to be firm and set rules, it will most likely heighten the client's agitation. This client is too excited to focus at this time. Group activities or other activities may worsen the client's situation.
CN: Psychosocial integrity; CNS: None; CL: Apply

67. The nurse is reviewing discharge teaching with a client newly diagnosed with type 2 diabetes mellitus. Which statement, made by the client, would indicate the need for further teaching?
1. "I need to check my feet daily for sores."
2. "I need to store my insulin in the refrigerator."
3. "I can eat bread in exchange for rice."
4. "I will see my health care provider for follow-up examinations."

67. 2. Insulin only needs to be stored in the refrigerator if it won't be used within 30 days from time of opening. It should be at room temperature when given to decrease pain and prevent lipodystrophy. The remaining statements show that the client understands his condition and the importance of preventing complications.
CN: Safe, effective care environment; CNS: Safety and infection control; CL: Analyze

68. A client with terminal cancer is receiving large doses of opioids for pain control. He becomes agitated and continues trying to get out of bed but can't stand without the assistance of two people. To reduce the client's risk of falling, which type of restraint should the nurse request for this client?
1. Leg restraints
2. Chemical restraints
3. Mechanical restraints
4. Jacket restraint

68. 2. Antianxiety medication can be used to calm the client. Chemical restraints are effective, especially with highly agitated clients receiving large doses of opioids. Other forms of restraint will increase the client's agitation and hostility, thus increasing the risk of injury.
CN: Safe, effective care environment; CNS: Safety and infection control; CL: Apply

69. A client has returned to his room following a stem cell transplant and is placed in reverse isolation. The nurse understands that implementing this isolation will protect the:
1. client from his own bacteria.
2. hospital staff from the client.
3. other clients on the nursing unit.
4. client from outside infections from others.

69. 4. Immunosuppressed clients need to be protected from infections from others following a stem cell transplant. Infections can occur if strict hand washing techniques aren't observed. Protective isolation is used to protect the hospital staff and other clients from an infected client.
CN: Safe, effective care environment; CNS: Safety and infection control; CL: Remember

70. A health care provider will insert a subclavian central venous catheter into a client to infuse 500 ml of normal saline at 40 ml/hr. Prioritize the nurse's steps in preparing a sterile field for this catheterization.

| 1. Open sterile packs away from self |
| 2. Use correct hand washing technique |
| 3. Put on sterile gloves |
| 4. Place the sterile dressing tray on an over bed table |

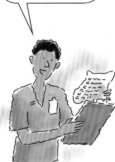
This one is tricky. Put the steps in order.

70. Ordered Response:

| 2. Use correct hand washing technique |
| 4. Place the sterile dressing tray on an over bed table |
| 1. Open sterile packs away from self |
| 3. Put on sterile gloves |

CN: Safe, effective care environment; CNS: Safety and infection control; CL: Apply

71. A public health nurse is visiting a new postpartum client and notes that the client has two other children under age four. One infant is playing in the cabinet under the sink. Which instruction should the public health nurse give to this client?
1. Keep a bottle of ipecac syrup in the house
2. Make sure all liquid cleaners are labeled
3. Tighten all cap tops on the bottles under the sink
4. Remove all cleaners that could be ingested orally

71. 4. All liquid cleaners should be removed to reduce the risk of poisoning. Safety locks should be placed on cabinets to prevent young children from opening the cabinets or the bottles. Infants can't read danger labels. Ipecac is no longer routinely used to induce vomiting in children.
CN: Safe, effective care environment; CNS: Safety and infection control; CL: Apply

CN: Client needs category   CNS: Client needs subcategory   CL: Cognitive level

72. Which nursing action **best** demonstrates the principle of medical asepsis?
1. Return unused linen to the linen supply cart
2. Keep the environment as clean as possible
3. Test for microorganisms in the environment
4. Clean the client's equipment with alcohol as needed

72. 2. Medical asepsis is the process of avoiding contamination from outside sources by keeping the environment clean. A clean environment has a reduced number of microorganisms, but isn't necessarily sterile (the absence of all microorganisms). Testing for microorganisms or culturing isn't indicated in an aseptic environment. Alcohol is not an approved cleansing agent for inanimate objects.
CN: Safe, effective care environment; CNS: Safety and infection control; CL: Apply

73. The nurse has completed an admission assessment on a retired military serviceman who has served two tours in Iraq. The nurse notes that the client continually fidgets, makes no eye contact, and responds to questions with "yes" and "no" answers. What is the **priority** nursing intervention?
1. Determine his plans for civilian life
2. Discuss how his family is adjusting to his return
3. Explore what experiences cause him distress
4. Ask if he is feeling suicidal

73. 3. Explore what causes this client distress and anxiety. Many returning service personnel suffer from posttraumatic stress disorder. Sudden noises and not being able to see who is entering his space could cause further anxiety and flashbacks to wartime experiences. Determining the client's plan for civilian life addresses the future, and is not appropriate at this time. Asking about the family's adjustment does not assess the client at admission. Though suicide is of concern, the priority is to gather more information about the causes of this client's distress.
CN: Psychosocial integrity; CNS: None; CL: Apply

74. The nurse asks the mother of a terminally-ill infant if she would like her child to be baptized. The mother becomes upset and asks to speak to the nurse-manager. What is the nurse-manager's **best** response?
1. Ask the on-duty chaplain to talk to the mother
2. Explain that, since the nurse is catholic, she is only trying to determine the mother's wishes
3. Apologize for the nurse's behavior and assign another nurse to her care
4. Let the mother express her own spiritual beliefs and wishes

74. 4. The best response is to allow the mother to express her own feelings. The chaplain may or may not provide an appropriate response. Explaining and apologizing for another's behavior is not likely to diffuse the situation or help the mother.
CN: Psychosocial integrity; CNS: None; CL: Apply

75. The nurse is preparing to administer 1 unit of whole blood to a client. In which order should the nurse perform these actions?
1. Start an IV of normal saline; assess for a history of blood transfusion reaction; obtain blood from the laboratory; assess vital signs; begin the transfusion
2. Assess for a history of blood transfusion reaction; assess vital signs; start an IV of normal saline; obtain the blood from the laboratory; begin the transfusion
3. Obtain the blood from the laboratory; assess vital signs; start an IV of normal saline; begin the transfusion; assess for a history of blood transfusion reaction
4. Start an IV of normal saline; obtain blood from the laboratory; begin the transfusion; assess for a history of blood transfusion reaction; assess vital signs

75. 2. By obtaining a history and assessing vital signs the nurse can determine any potential problems. Beginning the IV prior to obtaining the blood will provide a patent mode of administration. Blood products should be infused as soon as access is obtained. The transfusion can then be started and the client monitored for any changes.
CN: Physiological integrity; CNS: Pharmacological and parenteral therapies; CL: Analyze

CN: Client needs category   CNS: Client needs subcategory   CL: Cognitive level

76. A new graduate nurse has almost completed orientation on the assigned nursing unit. A skills checklist and performance test are used to identify the new graduate's deficient skills. What is the nurse-manager's **most** appropriate action?
  1. Talk with the supervisor about terminating the new graduate
  2. Discuss the possibility of transferring the new graduate to another unit
  3. Have the graduate's preceptor work with her to meet requirements
  4. Tell the graduate that if performance doesn't improve, employment will be terminated

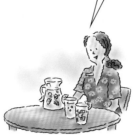

Relax a minute and have some lemonade with me. Everything's going to be okay.

77. The home health nurse is assessing a client and determines that she has an unsteady gait. The client tells the nurse that she has a history of falls. Which nursing action represents an advocacy role for the home health nurse?
  1. Contacting a health care equipment resource to rent a walker for the client to use
  2. Listening to a client express feelings of frustration over increasing limitations
  3. Instructing the client to contact a senior day care service
  4. Reassuring the client that using a walker will prevent falls in the future

78. An elderly client, on bed rest for a week after a bout of pneumonia, has developed a negative nitrogen balance. Which complication has **priority**?
  1. Constipation
  2. Renal calculi
  3. Muscle wasting
  4. Vitamin B_6 deficiency

79. A client has been hospitalized for five days with mononucleosis. Which assessment finding indicates a possibly serious consequence?
  1. Vomiting
  2. Dark brown urine
  3. Temperature of 101° F (38.3° C)
  4. Cervical lymphadenopathy

80. Which condition causes heart failure after a myocardial infarction (MI)?
  1. Increased workload of the heart
  2. Increased oxygen demands of the heart
  3. Inability of the heart chambers to adequately fill
  4. Impairment of contractile function of the damaged myocardium

76. 3. The leader needs to assign a preceptor to work with the new graduate and provide opportunities for the graduate to grow and develop. The other responses wouldn't give the new graduate the opportunity and support needed for improvement.
CN: Safe, effective care environment; CNS: Management of care; CL: Apply

77. 1. Referral to community agencies is an advocacy role for home health nurses. The role of the advocate implies the home care nurse is able to advise clients how to find alternative sources of care. Giving emotional support, giving therapies to clients, and instructing clients about other resources are direct care activities. Reassuring the client is superficial, and using a walker may not prevent falls in the future.
CN: Safe, effective care environment; CNS: Management of care; CL: Apply

78. 3. Negative nitrogen balance leads to muscle wasting. The body breaks down muscle tissue to use as energy. Renal calculi can be a complication of bed rest and demineralization of the bone, but treating a negative nitrogen balance takes priority. Constipation and vitamin B_6 deficiency also need to be corrected but aren't the highest priority.
CN: Physiological integrity; CNS: Physiological adaptation; CL: Analyze

79. 2. Dark brown urine could indicate the presence of bilirubin and implicate liver involvement. The other answers are typical findings for a client with this diagnosis.
CN: Physiological integrity; CNS: Physiological adaptation; CL: Analyze

80. 4. After an MI, the injured myocardium is replaced by scar tissue. This scar tissue causes the ventricle to pump less efficiently. After an MI has resolved, oxygen and workload demands should normalize and the heart's chambers should fill adequately.
CN: Physiological integrity; CNS: Physiological adaptation; CL: Apply

CN: Client needs category   CNS: Client needs subcategory   CL: Cognitive level

81. A client, with a history of myasthenia gravis, is admitted to the emergency department with reports of respiratory distress. The client's condition worsens, and arterial blood gases are drawn. For which condition is this client at risk?
1. Metabolic acidosis
2. Metabolic alkalosis
3. Respiratory acidosis
4. Respiratory alkalosis

81. 3. The client has a restrictive lung problem because of myasthenia gravis. This is aggravated by respiratory distress. Because of the restrictive problem, the client won't be able to exhale efficiently and carbon dioxide will build up, causing respiratory acidosis. Metabolic acidosis is a condition that occurs with either accumulation of acids or excessive loss of bases in the body, such as in diarrhea or renal failure. Metabolic alkalosis occurs due to excessive acid loss or base retention, such as from vomiting. Respiratory alkalosis results from a decreased carbon dioxide level, which could occur if the client were hyperventilating.

CN: Physiological integrity; CNS: Physiological adaptation; CL: Analyze

82. The nurse is teaching another nurse about pulmonary capillary wedge pressure. Which response is the **most** accurate regarding this pressure?
1. It reflects systemic vascular resistance.
2. It reflects right ventricular end pressure.
3. It reflects right atrial presystolic pressure.
4. It reflects left ventricular end-diastolic pressure.

82. 4. The pulmonary capillary wedge pressure is the reflection of the pressure in the left ventricle at rest, which is end diastole. Wedge pressure doesn't reflect pressures in the right side of the heart or systemic vascular resistance.

CN: Physiological integrity; CNS: Physiological adaptation; CL: Apply

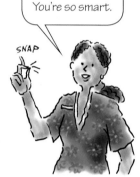

SNAP

You got it! You're so smart.

83. A client is scheduled to have a series of pulmonary function tests (PFTs). For which should the nurse anticipate an order to withhold six hours prior to these tests?
1. Azithromycin
2. Robitussin
3. Albuterol
4. Cefaclor

83. 3. PFTs measure the volume and capacity of air in the lungs. If a bronchodilator is given, it will improve the bronchial airflow and alter the test results. The other drugs have no effect on the bronchial tree with regard to PFT results.

CN: Physiological integrity; CNS: Pharmacological and parenteral therapies; CL: Analyze

84. The nurse receives an order to administer morphine to a client with an acute myocardial infarction. What is the purpose of this medication?
1. To decrease cardiac output
2. To increase preload and afterload
3. To increase myocardial oxygen demand
4. To decrease myocardial oxygen demand

84. 4. Morphine will calm and relax the client and decrease respiratory rate, anxiety, and stress, thus decreasing myocardial oxygen demand. It doesn't have any effect on cardiac output or preload or afterload.

CN: Physiological integrity; CNS: Pharmacological and parenteral therapies; CL: Apply

85. The nurse receives an order to administer 350 mg of amoxicillin to a toddler po/q6h. The pharmacy supplies the amoxicillin with a concentration of 250 mg/5 ml. How many milliliters would the nurse give for each dose? Record the answer using a whole number:

_____ ml

86. A client has just started treatment with rifampin for tuberculosis. Which statement indicates that the client has a good understanding of his medication?
  1. "I won't go to family gatherings for six months."
  2. "My urine will look orange because of the medication."
  3. "Now, I don't need to cover my mouth or nose when I sneeze or cough."
  4. "I told my wife to throw away all the spoons and forks before I come home."

87. During a home health visit, a nurse assesses a client's medication and notes that the client has two prescriptions for fluid retention. One prescription reads, "Lasix, 40 milligrams one tablet daily." The next prescription reads, "Furosemide, 40 milligrams one tablet daily." Which instruction should be given to the client?
  1. Take both medications as ordered
  2. Call the health care provider for verification
  3. Use Lasix one day and furosemide the next day
  4. Throw away one of the drugs to avoid confusing the client

88. A nurse is assessing a client with bipolar disorder. The client tells the nurse his family health care provider prescribed lithium. Which symptom would indicate that the client is developing lithium toxicity?
  1. Lethargy
  2. Hypertension
  3. Hyperexcitability
  4. Low urine output

85. 7.
The nurse would give 7 ml for each dose. Use the following equation:

$$\frac{Dose\ on\ hand}{Quantity\ on\ hand} = \frac{Dose\ desired}{X}$$

In this example, the equation is:

$$\frac{250\ mg}{5\ ml} = \frac{350\ mg}{X}$$

$$X = 7\ ml$$

CN: Physiological integrity; CNS: Pharmacological and parenteral therapies; CL: Analyze

86. 2. Rifampin discolors body fluids, such as urine and tears. The client can go to family functions and eat with normal utensils. The client should cover his mouth and nose when coughing and sneezing until he has been on the medication at least two weeks.

CN: Physiological integrity; CNS: Pharmacological and parenteral therapies; CL: Apply

87. 2. The nurse understands that Lasix and furosemide are the same drug. Calling the health care provider to determine the correct dosage and frequency the nurse's role as a client advocate. Setting up medications in a medication tray, using only one pharmacy to dispense medications, and using all medications until the bottle is emptied will reduce medication errors. However, it is a priority to verify the medication orders first.

CN: Physiological integrity; CNS: Pharmacological and parenteral therapies; CL: Analyze

88. 1. Nausea, vomiting, diarrhea, thirst, polyuria, lethargy, slurred speech, hypotension, muscle weakness, and fine hand tremors are signs of lithium toxicity.

CN: Physiological integrity; CNS: Pharmacological and parenteral therapies; CL: Apply

CN: Client needs category   CNS: Client needs subcategory   CL: Cognitive level

89. A client, with heart failure, is given furosemide 40 mg IV daily. The morning serum potassium level is 2.8 mEq/L. Which nursing action is the **most** appropriate?
1. Question the health care provider about the dosage
2. Give 20 mg of the ordered dose and recheck the laboratory test results
3. Notify the health care provider and obtain additional orders
4. Give the furosemide and get an order for sodium polystyrene sulfonate

89. 3. Furosemide is a loop diuretic. As water is lost, so is potassium. Diuresis is a treatment for heart failure. Notifying the health care provider of the low potassium level and getting an order for potassium chloride are appropriate actions before giving the furosemide. The nurse shouldn't alter the dosage without a provider's order. Giving furosemide and sodium polystyrene sulfonate together would further lower the potassium level.
CN: Physiological integrity; CNS: Pharmacological and parenteral therapies; CL: Apply

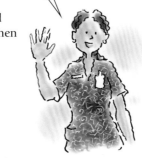

Hey—high-five me! You've finished 90 questions. Way to go!

90. A nurse is assisting a client on a clear liquid diet select his menu. The nurse is concerned when the client selects which choice?
1. Gelatin dessert
2. Milkshake
3. Popsicle or similar frozen dessert
4. Tea

90. 2. Full-liquid diets contain milk, cereal, thin porridge, clear liquids, and plain frozen desserts. The clear liquid diet contains only foods that are clear and liquid at room or body temperature. Gelatin, fat-free broth, bouillon, popsicles or similar frozen desserts, tea, and regular or decaffeinated coffee would be appropriate for this client.
CN: Physiological integrity; CNS: Basic care and comfort; CL: Analyze

91. The assessment of a client on the first day after thoracotomy shows a temperature of 100° F (37.8° C); HR: 96 bpm; BP 136/86 mmHg; and shallow respirations at 24 breaths/min, with rhonchi at the bases. The client reports incisional pain. Which nursing action is **most** important?
1. Medicate the client for pain
2. Help the client get out of bed
3. Give ibuprofen as ordered to reduce the fever
4. Encourage the client to cough and deep-breathe

91. 1. Although all the interventions are incorporated into this client's care plan, the priority is to relieve pain and make the client comfortable. This would give the client the energy and stamina to achieve the other objectives.
CN: Physiological integrity; CNS: Basic care and comfort; CL: Apply

92. A client who had a thoracotomy is using oxygen and having an arterial blood gas (ABG) analysis. What is the **most** appropriate information for the nurse to tell the client?
1. "I will shave the puncture site before the test."
2. "You need to keep the oxygen mask on for the entire test."
3. "You'll be suctioned immediately before the blood is drawn."
4. "You won't be allowed to drink anything for two hours before the blood is drawn."

92. 2. To determine the effectiveness of oxygen therapy, ABGs should be drawn with the oxygen in use. No special preparations for the test, with regard to skin preparation or diet, are needed. Suctioning decreases available oxygen.
CN: Physiological integrity; CNS: Basic care and comfort; CL: Apply

93. A client with chronic obstructive pulmonary disease (COPD) is being discharged from the hospital. The nurse provided teaching on medications, diet, and exercise. Which statement by the client indicates further teaching is necessary?

   1. "I'll eat six small meals a day."
   2. "I'll get a flu shot every winter."
   3. "I'll walk every morning before breakfast."
   4. "I'll call my health care provider if I get cold symptoms."

93. 3. The worst time of the day for a client with COPD is morning. Exercise is important but should be done later in the day. All other choices are appropriate for the client with COPD.

CN: Physiological integrity; CNS: Basic care and comfort; CL: Apply

94. A 42-year-old client who underwent a right modified mastectomy with insertion of a Jackson Pratt drain will be hospitalized overnight because of minor complications. Which goal statement should the nurse include in the plan of care?

   1. Teach proper care of the incision site and drain by third post-operative day
   2. The client will know how to care for the incision site and drain by third post-operative day
   3. The client will demonstrate proper care of the incision site and drain by third post-operative day
   4. The client will care for the incision site and contend with psychological loss by third post-operative day

94. 3. This statement contains a specific, measurable action, clearly identifies the client behavior, and includes a date. Answer one is written as a nursing goal, not a client-centered goal. The client goal of answer two isn't measurable as stated. Answer four includes two goals that need to be addressed separately under the appropriate nursing diagnosis, and it contains non-measurable actions.

CN: Physiological integrity; CNS: Basic care and comfort; CL: Apply

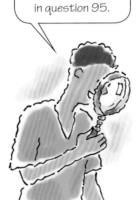

Look carefully for the best approach in question 95.

95. A nurse-manager has identified several interpersonal problems with a staff member. What is the **best** approach for the nurse-manager to take?

   1. Map out a plan of action for each problem and discuss it
   2. Begin to solve the first problem and work through the list
   3. Ask the staff member to select the problem she would like to resolve
   4. Prioritize the problems with the staff member and begin to work on them together

95. 4. It's important for the nurse-manager and staff member to agree on which problem is a priority and work toward its resolution. Mapping out the problem without input from the staff member could result in a lack of commitment from the staff member.

CN: Safe, effective care environment; CNS: Management of care; CL: Apply

96. A team leader notes increasing unrest among staff members. What is the team leader's **best** action?

   1. Discuss the problem with a coworker
   2. Report the problem to the nurse-manager
   3. Bring the group together and discuss the team leader's perception
   4. Ignore the problem and hope the attitude won't interfere with the functioning of the floor

96. 3. The leader should inform the group of the observed behavior. This is a firm approach but one that shows concern. Ignoring problems or discussing them with someone else doesn't confront the issue at hand.

CN: Safe, effective care environment; CNS: Management of care; CL: Apply

97. A health care provider has placed a stat order for a urine specimen for culture and sensitivity stat. What is the **best** way for the nurse to delegate this task to an unlicensed assistive personnel?
1. We need a stat urine culture on the client in room 101.
2. Please get the urine for culture for the client in room 101.
3. A stat urine has been ordered for the client in room 101. Would you get it?
4. We need to collect urine from the client in room 101 for a stat culture. Please tell me when you send it to the lab.

97. 4. This option not only delegates the task but also provides a checkpoint. To effectively delegate, you need to follow up on what someone else is doing. The other options don't provide for feedback, which is essential for communication and delegation.
CN: Safe, effective care environment; CNS: Management of care; CL: Apply

98. Which nursing intervention is **most** important to include in a nursing care plan for a client with atelectasis?
1. Give oxygen continuously at 3 L/min
2. Cough and deep-breathe every four hours
3. Use the incentive spirometer every hour
4. Get the client out of bed to a chair every day

98. 3. Incentive spirometry is used to prevent or treat atelectasis. Done every hour, it will produce deep inhalations that help open the collapsed alveoli. Oxygen use doesn't encourage deep inhalation. Coughing and deep breathing are good interventions but rarely result in as deep an inspiratory effort as using an incentive spirometer, and should be performed more frequently than every four hours. Getting the client out of bed will also help expand the lungs and stimulate deep breathing, but it's done less frequently than incentive spirometry.
CN: Safe, effective care environment; CNS: Management of care; CL: Apply

Howdy, partner. Make sure you have all the right assessment tools before you head out on the range.

99. A client admitted with acute exacerbation of chronic obstructive pulmonary disease (COPD). What assessment data should the nurse expect to observe?
1. Hypothermia, diminished bowel sounds, and urinary frequency
2. Moist mucous membranes, yellow conjunctiva, and bounding radial pulses
3. Dyspnea, hypoxia, and anxiety
4. Reports of dyspepsia, lower left quadrant tenderness, and bradycardia

99. 3. The client with acute exacerbation of COPD will appear anxious, short of breath, and because they are experiencing impaired oxygenation at the cellular level, they will be hypoxic. All other data options have no pulmonary correlations.
CN: Safe, effective care environment; CNS: Management of care; CL: Apply

100. The nurse understands that in order for a client to address all components of health promotion the wellness plan must include all areas associated with:
1. diet, exercise, sleep, and stress.
2. employment, parenting, diet, and exercise.
3. alcohol consumption, over the counter drug ingestion, music appreciation, and stress.
4. bowel habits, eating practices, pain control, and social interactions.

100. 1. Areas of wellness that need to be addressed by each person are diet, exercise, sleep, and stress. Employment, parenting, music appreciation, and pain control are not associated with a wellness plan.
CN: Safe, effective care environment; CNS: Management of care; CL: Apply

CN: Client needs category   CNS: Client needs subcategory   CL: Cognitive level

101. A nurse observes that a client, with a below-the-knee amputation, refuses to look at the stump and changes the subject when the nurse attempts to discuss its care on the third postoperative day. This client's reaction indicates which stage of grief?
1. Anger
2. Depression
3. Denial
4. Acceptance

101. 3. Refusing to look at the stump, or talk about its care are indicative of a state of denial. The question provides no data to support anger, depression, or acceptance.
CN: Safe, effective care environment; CNS: Management of care; CL: Analyze

102. Which client outcome should a nurse identify for a client with disuse syndrome?
1. The client will be free of musculoskeletal complications
2. The client will experience shorter periods of immobility and inactivity
3. The nurse will stress the importance of maintaining adequate fluid intake
4. The nurse will provide holistic care by collaborating with the health care team

102. 2. This is an appropriate outcome for a client with disuse syndrome. Disuse syndrome, a result of prolonged or unavoidable immobility or inactivity, is preventable. Musculoskeletal complications indicate actual disuse or complications of immobility. Stressing the importance of adequate fluid intake, and providing holistic care describe nursing goals, not client outcomes.
CN: Safe, effective care environment; CNS: Management of care; CL: Apply

103. Which goal should a nurse identify for a client who is at risk for an injury related to the lack of awareness of environmental hazards?
1. Encourage the client to discuss safety rules with children
2. Help the client learn safety precautions to take in the home
3. The client will eliminate safety hazards in his surroundings
4. The client will contact community resources for more information

103. 3. This goal is appropriate and measurable as written and focuses on the client. The other options, as written, are nursing interventions.
CN: Safe, effective care environment; CNS: Management of care; CL: Apply

104. After making the bed of a client with dementia, what is the nurse's **priority**?
1. Put the bed in the lowest position
2. Put the call button within the client's reach
3. Put the top side rails in the upright position
4. Put soiled linen in a hamper or biohazard bag

104. 1. To reduce the risk of injury due to falls, the bed should be placed in the lowest position. The call button should be in reach of the client, but the immediate safety of the client comes first. Bed side rails should not be used as a substitute for client protective restraints. Clients who need a protective restraint, such as a vest or wrist/leg device, must be monitored frequently while wearing it. If a protective restraint is used, follow your facility's protocol and the restraint manufacturer's instructions for proper use, in addition to the federal, state, and local regulations regarding the use of protective restraints. Soiled linens should be placed in a hamper or biohazard bag, but client safety is a priority.
CN: Safe, effective care environment; CNS: Management of care; CL: Apply

105. Which situation would warrant the use of a mask and protective eyewear?
1. When strong odors are emitted from an infected wound
2. When the client has an oral temperature greater than 101° F (38.3° C)
3. If needles or other sharp instruments are to be used in the procedure
4. During a procedure where splashing of blood or body fluid is anticipated

105. 4. Eye goggles or face shields should be worn when the possibility of blood or body fluid splashes exist. Odors don't transmit microorganisms. A client with a fever won't transmit microorganisms into the eyes any more frequently than a client without a fever. The use of needles or other sharp instruments doesn't mandate eye protection.
CN: Safe, effective environment; CNS: Management of care; CL: Apply

106. A client returns to a nursing unit after a bronchoscopy, and is expectorating pink-tinged mucus. What is the **most** appropriate nursing action?
1. Notify the health care provider as soon as possible
2. Take the client's vital signs and then call the health care provider
3. Auscultate the client's lung fields for possible pulmonary edema
4. Tell the client this is expected after the procedure but continue to monitor the client

106. 4. Pink-tinged mucus is an expected after a bronchoscopy due to irritation of the bronchial tree. The client should be told that this is common, and it will be monitored. The health care provider shouldn't be called with this finding. This symptom isn't related to pulmonary edema.
CN: Health promotion and maintenance; CNS: None; CL: Apply

107. Two hours after submucous resection, a client's nostrils are packed, and a drip pad is anchored under the nose. Which assessment would alert the nurse that the surgical site is bleeding?
1. Frequent swallowing
2. Dry mucous membranes
3. Decrease in urine output
4. Temperature elevation

107. 1. Frequent swallowing is a sign of hemorrhage following this surgery. Decreased urine output and dry mucous membranes, as well as temperature elevation, are usually signs of dehydration.
CN: Physiological integrity; CNS: Reduction of risk potential; CL: Analyze

108. A nurse is teaching a client about lifestyle changes after a myocardial infarction (MI). Which action is a negative coping mechanism?
1. Reading a book about meal planning
2. Pacing the floor of his room on occasion
3. Sitting quietly in his room for a short time
4. Telling his family he didn't have an MI

108. 4. This action indicates that this client is in denial about his condition. Reading a book on meal planning is a positive intervention. Pacing the floor on occasion is a form of anxiety that's normal for this client to experience. Sitting quietly is a normal behavior. This client needs time to come to terms with his diagnosis.
CN: Psychosocial integrity; CNS: None; CL: Analyze

109. The nurse is assessing a laboring client. The client suddenly screams and exclaims, "My baby is coming." What is the **priority** action by the nurse?
1. Calm the mother
2. Assess for crowning
3. Take the fetal heart tones
4. Administer pain medication

109. 2. The priority nursing action is to assess for crowning of the fetus's head, and prepare for an imminent delivery. The other actions do not respond to the possible spontaneous delivery of the fetus.
CN: Health promotion and maintenance; CNS: Physiological adaptation; CL: Apply

CN: Client needs category CNS: Client needs subcategory CL: Cognitive level

110. The nurse has just received change of shift report. Which client will the nurse see **first**?

1. A client receiving 1 unit of packed red blood cells
2. A client one day post laparoscopic cholecystectomy with an oral temperature of 100.5° F (38° C)
3. A client newly diagnosed with diabetes whose blood glucose is 180 mg/dl
4. A. client scheduled for a bowel resection in two hours who is reporting chills

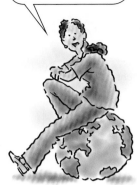

You finished the test! You must feel on top of the world.

110. 4. The client presenting with chills may be experiencing an infection. All other clients are stable or experiencing expected responses.

CN: Safe, effective care environment; CNS: Management of care; CL: Analyze

Comprehensive Test 3

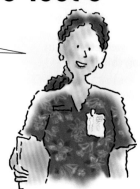

This is the last comprehensive test. It has 265 questions, just like the longest NCLEX test. Good luck! I know you're ready for it.

1. A 67-year-old client asks the nurse, "Do you think it's wrong to masturbate?" What is the nurse's **best** response?
1. "How do you feel about that?"
2. "Do you really want to do that?"
3. "I think you're a little too old for that."
4. "Why don't you ask your health care provider?"

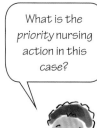

What is the *priority* nursing action in this case?

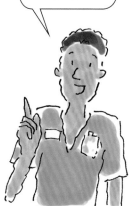

2. An assessment of a client on the first day after a thoracotomy shows a temperature of 100° F (37.8° C); heart rate, 96 bpm; blood pressure, 136/86 mmHg; and shallow respirations at 30 breaths/min, with rhonchi at the bases. The client is diaphoretic, anxious, and reports of incisional pain. Which nursing action is **priority**?
1. Medicate the client for pain as ordered
2. Help the client get out of bed
3. Give ibuprofen as ordered to reduce the fever
4. Encourage the client to cough and deep breathe

3. A bedridden client develops disuse osteoporosis. Which nursing intervention is **most** important for this client?
1. Turn, cough, and deep breathe
2. Increase fluids to 3,000 ml daily
3. Promote venous return by elevating the legs
4. Provide active and passive range-of-motion (ROM) exercises

1. 1. Communication allows the nurse to find out how the client thinks and feels. Telling the client that he's too old, or asking him if he really wants to do that, is biased and puts the client down. The last option tells the client that the nurse isn't interested. The client may be too uncomfortable to discuss this topic with the health care provider.
CN: Psychosocial integrity; CNS: None; CL: Analyze

2. 1. Although all the interventions are incorporated in this client's care plan, the priority is to relieve pain and make the client comfortable. This will relax the client, decrease his respirations, and make deep breathing and coughing more comfortable. In addition, this would give the client the energy and stamina to achieve the other objectives.
CN: Physiological integrity; CNS: Basic care and comfort;
CL: Apply

3. 4. All the interventions listed are good for a bedridden client. However, active and passive ROM exercises provide the mechanical stresses of weight bearing that are absent, and their absence can lead to disuse osteoporosis.
CN: Health promotion and maintenance; CNS: None;
CL: Apply

4. A nurse is assessing a client and notes an increase in the tactile fremitus. Which condition would the nurse suspect with this client?
1. Atelectasis
2. Emphysema
3. Pneumonia
4. Pneumothorax

5. A client, on the orthopedic unit with an arm cast, reports severe pain in the affected extremity. Decreased sensation and motion and swollen fingers are also noted. What is the nurse's **most** important intervention?
1. Elevating the arm
2. Removing the cast
3. Giving an analgesic
4. Calling the health care provider

6. A nurse is teaching a client about lifestyle changes that need to be made following a myocardial infarction (MI). Which action, by the client, suggests they are having difficulty coping with the changes?
1. Reading a book about meal planning
2. Pacing the floor of the room on occasion
3. Sitting quietly in the room for a short time
4. Telling the family he didn't have an MI

7. A client is admitted to the emergency department with severe epistaxis. The health care provider inserts posterior packing. Later, the client is anxious and says they do not feel they are breathing right. Which nursing action is **priority**?
1. Cut the packing strings and remove the packing
2. Reassure the client that what they are experiencing is normal
3. Ask the client to fully explain what they mean by "right"
4. Use a flashlight and inspect the client's posterior oral cavity

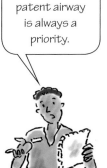

Maintaining a patent airway is always a priority.

8. Which statement, by the nurse, is **most** accurate regarding pulmonary capillary wedge pressure?
1. It reflects systemic vascular resistance.
2. It reflects right ventricular end pressure.
3. It reflects right atrial presystolic pressure.
4. It reflects left ventricular end-diastolic pressure.

4. 3. Pneumonia produces a consolidation of mucus and debris. Mucus causes the lung field to have an increase in tactile fremitus. The other diseases involve air, which would decrease tactile fremitus.
CN: Health promotion and maintenance; CNS: None; CL: Analyze

5. 4. The cast may be too tight and may need to be split or removed by the health care provider. Notify the health care provider when circulation, sensation, or motion is impaired. The arm should already be elevated. Giving analgesics wouldn't be the first step, as it may mask the signs of a serious problem.
CN: Physiological integrity; CNS: Reduction of risk potential; CL: Apply

6. 4. The client is showing the defense mechanism of denial. Reading a book on meal planning is a positive intervention. Pacing the floor on occasion is a form of anxiety that's normal for the client to experience. Sitting quietly is a normal behavior. The client needs time to come to terms with their diagnosis.
CN: Psychosocial integrity; CNS: None; CL: Analyze

7. 4. The nurse must assess the patency of the client's airway. The packing might have become dislodged. The nurse shouldn't remove the packing or give the client false reassurance. The client is too anxious to explain what they mean.
CN: Physiological integrity; CNS: Reduction of risk potential; CL: Analyze

8. 4. The pulmonary capillary wedge pressure is a reflection of the pressure in the left ventricle at rest, which is end diastole. Wedge pressure does not reflect pressures in the right side of the heart or systemic vascular resistance.
CN: Physiological integrity; CNS: Physiological adaptation; CL: Analyze

CN: Client needs category   CNS: Client needs subcategory   CL: Cognitive level

9. Which statement, by the nurse, **best** describes the purpose of diaphragmatic breathing exercises for a client with chronic obstructive pulmonary disease (COPD)?
1. It dilates the bronchioles.
2. It decreases vital capacity.
3. It increases residual volume.
4. It decreases alveolar ventilation.

9. **1.** In COPD, the bronchioles constrict during exhalation due to pressure changes in the lungs. Diaphragmatic breathing exercises keep the bronchioles open during exhalation. These exercises do not impact the other answer choices.
CN: Physiological integrity; CNS: Reduction of risk potential; CL: Apply

10. The nurse is caring for a client showing symptoms of bronchial obstruction. Which assessment finding would the nurse anticipate?
1. Hacking cough
2. Diminished breath sounds
3. Production of rust-colored sputum
4. Decreased use of accessory muscles

10. **2.** Bronchial obstruction means there is no passage of air through the bronchi, so diminished, or no, breath sounds would be heard. A hacking cough is often associated with upper respiratory tract infection and dryness in the upper airways. Rust-colored sputum is a sign of pneumococcal pneumonia. There would be increased use of accessory muscles.
CN: Physiological integrity; CNS: Physiological adaptation; CL: Apply

11. A client has just begun treatment with rifampin for tuberculosis. Which statement indicates that the client has a good understanding of this medication?
1. "I won't go to family gatherings for six months."
2. "My urine will look orange because of the medication."
3. "Now, I don't need to cover my mouth or nose when I sneeze or cough."
4. "I told my wife to throw away all the spoons and forks before I come home."

11. **2.** Rifampin discolors body fluids, such as urine and tears. The client can go to family functions and eat with normal utensils. The client should always cover his mouth and nose when coughing and sneezing, especially until he has been on the medication at least two weeks.
CN: Physiological integrity; CNS: Pharmacological and parenteral therapies; CL: Apply

12. What is the **most** important action for the nurse to implement before feeding a client who has been diagnosed with Parkinson's disease?
1. Sit the client upright
2. Have suction available
3. Acquire an order a clear liquid diet
4. Consult with the health care provider for a swallowing evaluation

12. **4.** A speech therapist should evaluate the client's swallowing and make recommendations before the client is fed. Aspiration due to involuntary movement is common. Sitting the client upright and having suction available are helpful when feeding the client, but evaluation of the client's swallowing ability should come first. Clear liquids may be too difficult for the client. Semisoft foods may be easier to swallow.
CN: Physiological integrity; CNS: Reduction of risk potential; CL: Analyze

13. The nurse is caring for a pregnant client with cardiovascular disease. Which treatment would the nurse anticipate for this client?
1. Scheduled rest periods throughout the day
2. Hospitalization
3. Therapeutic abortion
4. Continuous cardiac monitoring

13. **1.** The goal of antepartum management is to prevent complications and minimize the strain on the client. This is accomplished through rest. Hospitalization may be required in older women or those with previous decompensation. Therapeutic abortion is considered in severe dysfunction, especially in the first trimester. Continuous cardiac monitoring isn't necessary.
CN: Physiological integrity; CNS: Reduction of risk potential; CL: Apply

CN: Client needs category   CNS: Client needs subcategory   CL: Cognitive level

14. Which assessment finding **most** likely indicates a urinary tract infection (UTI) in a five-year-old child?
1. Incontinence
2. Lack of thirst
3. Concentrated urine
4. Subnormal temperature

14. 1. Incontinence in a toilet-trained child is associated with UTI. Lack of thirst wouldn't be expected in a child with UTI. Concentrated urine is a sign of dehydration. Subnormal temperature isn't a sign of UTI.
CN: Health promotion and maintenance; CNS: None;
CL: Apply

15. A school nurse is called to assess a preadolescent newly immigrated from Vietnam and attending a new school. A teacher tells the nurse that the student sits in the back of the class and won't speak when spoken to, although her parents confirmed the student speaks English. Which assessment finding is **most** likely?
1. The student is experiencing cultural shock.
2. The student is developing a peer support system.
3. The student is going through a socialization period.
4. The student is becoming acculturated to the new school.

15. 1. Cultural shock involves feelings of helplessness and discomfort and a state of disorientation when an outsider attempts to comprehend or adapt to a new cultural situation. Peer groups usually develop based on the background, interests, and capabilities of its members. Developing peer cultures is part of the socialization process. Acculturation occurs when there's a blending of cultural or ethnic backgrounds. This process takes time to develop.
CN: Health promotion and maintenance; CNS: None;
CL: Apply

16. A school nurse is screening a group of 11- to 13-year-old students for hearing and vision. What is the **best** technique to effectively communicate with this age group?
1. Give undivided attention to each student
2. Have the parents present during the screening
3. Have several adolescents listen to each other's health histories
4. Use puppets or dolls to show how the screening is going to take place

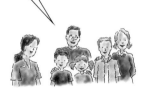

Make good eye contact when communicating with clients of any age.

16. 1. The nurse should give each adolescent undivided attention to communicate effectively, and respect their privacy. The presence of parents, and use of puppets or dolls can be used to effectively communicate with younger children.
CN: Health promotion and maintenance; CNS: None;
CL: Apply

17. A nurse at a rural health clinic is screening an 18-month-old infant for developmental problems. Which developmental screening test is the **most** appropriate?
1. Goodenough-Harris Draw-a-Person Test
2. Denver Developmental Screening Test (DDST)
3. McCarthy Scales of Children's Abilities (MSCA)
4. Preschool readiness screening scales

17. 2. The DDST is applicable for children from birth through age six. The Goodenough-Harris Draw-a-Person Test is used to assess intellectual ability in children ages 3 to 10. The MSCA is a developmental tool for children ages 2.5 to 8.5 years old. Preschool readiness screening scales are used to assess the readiness of five-year-old children for school.
CN: Health promotion and maintenance; CNS: None;
CL: Apply

18. In preparing an educational intervention for college students, a nurse understands that college-age students **most** often drink alcoholic beverages as a relief for:
1. fatigue.
2. anxiety.
3. headache.
4. stomach pain.

18. 2. Students sometimes drink because they think alcohol makes it easier to meet other people, decreases anxiety, relaxes their social inhibitions, and helps them have more fun. These beverages aren't commonly used to relieve fatigue, headache, or stomach pain.
CN: Psychosocial integrity; CNS: None; CL: Apply

CN: Client needs category   CNS: Client needs subcategory   CL: Cognitive level

19. An educational forum about relaxation techniques is being provided to college students who are preparing for their final exams. Which relaxation technique is **most** effective to counteract anxiety?
1. Meditation
2. Music therapy
3. Dance therapy
4. Reality orientation

19. 1. Meditation is a relaxation therapy used to counteract anxiety related to stress-inducing internal and external stimuli. Music therapy, dance therapy, and reality orientation are used as adjuncts to psychiatric care.
CN: Psychosocial integrity; CNS: None; CL: Apply

20. The parents of a nine-year-old child diagnosed with oppositional defiant disorder (ODD) are discussing treatment options with the nurse. What is the **most** appropriate intervention for this child?
1. Administering methylphenidate hydrochloride daily
2. Providing praise to this child for positive behaviors
3. Including this child in group therapy with other children diagnosed with ODD
4. Assigning several household chores to this child to be completed weekly

20. 2. Children with ODD consistently display negativity, defiance to authority, and hostility. Oppositional defiant disorder is best managed with consistent parenting and the establishment of a warm, positive home environment. Medication therapies aren't typically used for children with ODD. Methylphenidate is commonly used to manage attention deficit disorder. The focus of treatment for ODD is on the family unit, not on other children with similar problems. The child should be asked to participate in chores, but the parents need to be aware that overwhelming tasks may cause frustration and more defiance.
CN: Psychosocial integrity; CNS: None; CL: Analyze

21. A 40-year-old female client is admitted to a women's shelter after being raped by her estranged husband. The client describes this traumatic event. What is the nurse's **best** response?
1. Change the subject to prevent the client from crying
2. Listen attentively while the client describes the event
3. Arrange for the client to tell her story in group therapy
4. Medicate the client with a tranquilizer to prevent hysteria

21. 2. Retelling the event is part of the healing process. Giving medication and changing the subject don't allow the client to integrate the experience into her life. Group therapy may be helpful, but the best nursing response is to listen and convey empathy.
CN: Psychosocial integrity; CNS: None; CL: Apply

22. Which nursing intervention is **most** appropriate during the assessment of a pediatric client?
1. Ask the parents to leave the room during health assessment.
2. Position the client on an examination table or bed at all times.
3. Organize the health assessment in the same way for every infant or child.
4. Identify the source (child, parent, caregiver, guardian) and indicate the reliability of the information obtained.

22. 4. Document the source of information obtained for the nursing assessment of a child. Separation from the parent may cause anxiety and increase the child's fear and distrust. Depending on the child's age, parents may help position and hold the child, facilitating assessment. Organization of the assessment is changed to accommodate the individual child's age and development.
CN: Health promotion and maintenance; CNS: None; CL: Apply

23. Which nursing intervention is **most** appropriate during the assessment of an older adult client?
1. Ask the client to change positions quickly
2. Keep the room temperature cool during health assessment
3. Speak loudly and quickly to facilitate understanding of directions
4. Change the height of the examination table or modify the client's position

23. 4. The nurse may need to change the height of the examination table or use a different position when assessing an older adult client. Physiologically, an older client is prone to falls and dizziness due to the decreased ability to respond to sudden movements and position changes. The room temperature should be warm because older clients become hypothermic easily. Speak in a slow, normal tone of voice to facilitate communication.
CN: Health promotion and maintenance; CNS: None;
CL: Apply

24. An intake nurse at a mental health facility is admitting a client with psychosis. Which assessment technique is **most** valuable when planning this client's care?
1. Rorschach test
2. Interview the client
3. Mental Status Examination (MSE)
4. Review the client's previous history

24. 3. The MSE is a basis for planning care with a mental health client who is psychotic. The Rorschach test is used for depression. An interview with a client with psychosis would be unreliable. Reviewing a client's history won't assess the current state on which interventions are planned.
CN: Psychosocial integrity; CNS: None; CL: Apply

25. Which assessment would suggest that a client, with a new diagnosis of breast cancer, is having difficulty coping?
1. The client cries when discussing her diagnosis.
2. The client asks questions about treatment.
3. The client is concerned about missing work during chemotherapy.
4. The client changes the topic when treatment is discussed.

25. 4. By changing the topic when breast cancer treatment is discussed, the client may be denying her condition and having difficulty coping. It is normal to cry, ask questions, and be concerned about missing work when discussing a diagnosis such as breast cancer.
CN: Psychosocial integrity; CNS: None; CL: Apply

26. The nurse is talking with a client who is tearful and having difficulty talking about concerns regarding a recent diagnosis of prostate cancer. What is the **best** nursing action?
1. Ask if he would like to speak with a chaplain
2. Tell the client that you will be back once he has stopped crying
3. Sit and ask him if he would like to talk about his concerns
4. Tell the client that you know how he is feeling

26. 3. By sitting down, the nurse shows the client that he is important. Asking if he would like to talk about his concerns lets the client know that the nurse cares about him and wants to help. Calling a chaplain is appropriate after the nurse has assessed the situation, and the client has verbalized his concerns. Telling the client that you will return after he stops crying does not show concern for his feelings and does not encourage verbalization. Telling the client that you understand how he feels doesn't help him verbalize his feelings.
CN: Psychosocial integrity; CNS: None; CL: Apply

27. A client with heart failure is given furosemide 40 mg IV daily. The morning serum potassium level is 2.8 mEq/L. Which nursing action is the **most** appropriate?
1. Question the health care provider about the dosage
2. Give 20 mg of the ordered dose and recheck the laboratory test results
3. Notify the health care provider and obtain additional orders
4. Give the furosemide and get an order for sodium polystyrene sulfonate

27. 3. Furosemide is a diuretic. Serum potassium is flushed from the body along with excess fluid. Notifying the health care provider of the low potassium level and getting an order for potassium chloride are appropriate actions before giving the furosemide. The nurse should not give half the dose without an order from the provider. Giving furosemide and sodium polystyrene sulfonate together would further lower the potassium level. CN: Physiological integrity; CNS: Pharmacological and parenteral therapies; CL: Apply

28. Which client is at **highest** risk for developing respiratory alkalosis?
1. A client in labor
2. A client with diabetes
3. A client with renal failure
4. An immediate postoperative client

28. 1. A client's respirations, at certain stages of labor, increase in volume and rate, causing the $PaCO_2$ to decrease and the pH to increase. Diabetes often causes a metabolic imbalance, resulting in metabolic acidosis. In renal failure, the inability of the kidneys to eliminate waste increases the risk of developing metabolic acidosis. The respirations of a postoperative client are usually shallow after anesthesia and, because of pain, often cause respiratory acidosis. CN: Physiological integrity; CNS: Physiological adaptation; CL: Analyze

In question 29, you are looking for the answer that indicates contamination.

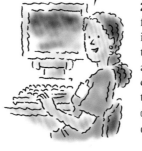

29. Which condition would indicate, to a nurse, that a sterile field has been contaminated?
1. Sterile objects are held above the waist of the nurse.
2. Sterile packages are opened with the first edge away from the nurse.
3. The outer inch of the sterile towel hangs over the side of the table.
4. Wetness on a sterile cloth on top of the non-sterile table has been noted.

29. 4. Moisture outside the sterile package and field contaminates it because fluid can be wicked into the sterile field. Bacteria tend to settle, so there's less contamination above waist level and away from the nurse. The outer inch of the drape is considered contaminated but doesn't indicate that the sterile field itself has been contaminated. CN: Safe, effective care environment; CNS: Safety and infection control; CL: Apply

30. Which intervention should a nurse perform for a client with acute respiratory alkalosis?
1. Have the client breathe into a paper bag
2. Give one ampule of bicarbonate as ordered
3. Give oxygen at three l/min through a nasal cannula
4. Reposition the client in a high Fowler's position

30. 1. By breathing into a paper bag, the client will rebreathe some of his own exhaled carbon dioxide and increase carbon dioxide in his blood. This will correct his respiratory alkalosis. Giving one ampule of bicarbonate will worsen the alkalosis. Giving oxygen won't increase the carbon dioxide to correct the imbalance. Repositioning the client won't help him retain carbon dioxide. CN: Physiological integrity; CNS: Physiological adaptation; CL: Apply

CN: Client needs category   CNS: Client needs subcategory   CL: Cognitive level

31. The nurse is reviewing the laboratory results from a diabetic client admitted to the acute care facility with dehydration. Which laboratory result is consistent with a diagnosis of dehydration?
  1. Serum hematocrit of 42%
  2. Specific gravity of 1.035
  3. Serum creatinine level of 0.8 mg/dl
  4. HbA1c level of 4%

31. **2.** Urine specific gravity reflects the ability of the kidneys to concentrate urine. Normal urine specific gravity is 1.005 to 1.030. A higher urine specific gravity indicates that the urine is more concentrated, and this is consistent with dehydration. The normal hematocrit range is 42% to 52%, so this value is within normal limits. Dehydration would cause an increase in hematocrit. Serum creatinine is used to assess kidney function. The normal range for women is 0.6 to 0.9 mg/dl. HbA1c is used to monitor diabetes treatment and evaluate the average blood glucose over a period of months. The normal range for HbA1c is 4% to 6.7%.
CN: Physiological integrity; CNS: Physiological adaptation; CL: Analyze

32. A client has been admitted with hypoparathyroidism and is being monitored for hypocalcemia. What is the nurse's **priority** assessment?
  1. Battle's sign
  2. Brudzinski's sign
  3. Chvostek's sign
  4. Homans' sign

32. **3.** Hypocalcemia can cause Chvostek's sign, abnormal facial muscle and nerve spasms elicited when the facial nerve is tapped. Battle's sign is bruising over the temporal bone in the presence of a basilar skull fracture. Brudzinski's sign is the flexion of the hips and knees in response to flexion of the head and neck toward the chest, indicating meningeal irritation. A positive Homans' sign indicates deep vein thrombosis.
CN: Physiological integrity; CNS: Reduction of risk potential; CL: Apply

33. A client reports pain one day after a colostomy. The nurse administers 4 mg morphine IV, and reassesses the client 30 minutes later. The following is noted: Respiratory rate at 8 breaths/min. Nasal cannula on floor. Arterial blood gas (ABG) results are: pH, 7.23; PaO_2, 58 mmHg; $PaCO_2$, 61 mmHg; HCO_3 24 mEq/L. Which factors **most** likely contributed to this client's ABG results?
  1. Colostomy, pain, and morphine
  2. Morphine, the nasal cannula on the floor, and the colostomy
  3. Morphine, respiratory rate of 8 breaths/min, and the nasal cannula on the floor
  4. Pain, respiratory rate of 8 breaths/min, and the nasal cannula on the floor

33. **3.** This client has respiratory acidosis. Opioids can suppress respirations, causing retention of carbon dioxide. A PaO_2 of 58 mmHg indicates hypoxemia caused by the removal of the client's supplementary oxygen and decreased respiratory rate. Pain increases the rate of respirations, which causes a decrease in $PaCO_2$. Colostomy drainage doesn't start until 2 to 3 days postoperatively, and this drainage would contribute to metabolic alkalosis.
CN: Physiological integrity; CNS: Physiological adaptation; CL: Analyze

34. Which arterial blood gas (ABG) results should a nurse expect to see in a client with emphysema?
  1. pH, 7.52; $PaCO_2$, 18 mmHg; HCO_3-, 22 mEq/L
  2. pH, 7.50; $PaCO_2$, 38 mmHg; HCO_3-, 38 mEq/L
  3. pH, 7.30; $PaCO_2$, 52 mmHg; HCO_3-, 30 mEq/L
  4. pH, 7.30; $PaCO_2$, 40 mmHg; HCO_3-, 18 mEq/L

34. **3.** Clients with emphysema retain carbon dioxide due to air trapping, causing an elevated $PaCO_2$ and respiratory acidosis. Because emphysema is a chronic disease, the kidneys compensate over time for the increased $PaCO_2$ by retaining HCO_3 in an attempt to normalize the pH. The other ABG results aren't consistent with results found in a client with emphysema.
CN: Physiological integrity; CNS: Physiological adaptation; CL: Analyze

CN: Client needs category   CNS: Client needs subcategory   CL: Cognitive level

35. Which factor does a nurse identify as a major cause of metabolic alkalosis in a client who had a colon resection?
1. Hyperventilation
2. Pain management
3. Nasogastric suction
4. IV therapy

35. 3. Removing acidic gastric secretions from the stomach is a metabolic cause of alkalinization of the blood pH. Hyperventilation decreases carbon dioxide and increases the pH, causing respiratory alkalosis. Pain management may further decrease the respiratory rate. Most IV fluids don't influence pH.

CN: Physiological integrity; CNS: Physiological adaptation; CL: Analyze

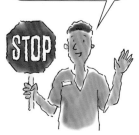
Which of these interventions is best for intracranial pressure?

36. The nurse is developing a plan of care for a comatose client with a closed head injury. What is the nurse's **most** important intervention?
1. Suction the airway every hour to maintain patency
2. Elevate the head of the bed 20 degrees
3. Place in a supine position with the head turned to the side
4. Provide environmental stimulation

36. 2. The head of the bed should be elevated between 15 and 30 degrees to promote venous drainage. Suctioning the airway may increase intracranial pressure (ICP) and should only be performed when needed. Turning the head to the side may cause jugular vein compression and an elevation in ICP. Environmental stimulation should be minimized to reduce any rise in ICP.

CN: Physiological integrity; CNS: Reduction in risk potential; CL: Apply

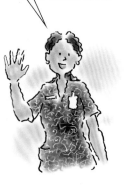
Infection control is completely in your hands.

37. A nurse has emptied urine from the bedpan of a client whose urinary output is being monitored. What should the nurse do **next**?
1. Wash hands thoroughly
2. Apply a clean pair of gloves
3. Report the amount of urine to the nurse in charge right away
4. Document the amount and characteristics of urine in the chart

37. 1. After any procedure is completed, the nurse must wash his hands to prevent transmission of microorganisms. The application of gloves is only necessary if the nurse must attend to another item of personal care before documenting urinary output. Crucial information is reported to the charge nurse, not routine intake and output. Documentation should take place, but hands would be washed first.

CN: Safe, effective care environment; CNS: Safety and infection control; CL: Apply

38. Which client should a nurse place in an orthopneic position?
1. A client with edema of the lower legs and ankles
2. A client with a pressure ulcer on the coccyx and buttocks
3. An immobilized client with calf tenderness due to a thrombus
4. An elderly client with difficulty breathing

38. 4. The orthopneic position is a sitting position with the arms leaning on a bedside table, and is appropriate for a client with breathing difficulty. Sitting with the legs elevated to decrease edema is appropriate for clients with ankle and lower leg edema. A client with a pressure ulcer should be positioned on his side and turned every two hours. Fowler's or semi-Fowler's positions are most appropriate for a client on complete bed rest.

CN: Physiological integrity; CNS: Physiological adaptation; CL: Apply

CN: Client needs category   CNS: Client needs subcategory   CL: Cognitive level

39. A client, preparing to transfer from the bed to a wheelchair, reports feeling light-headed and dizzy as they rise from a supine to a sitting position. Which is an appropriate nursing action?
1. Lift the client quickly into the wheelchair
2. Return the client to the supine position and apply a safety vest
3. Ask the client to dangle their legs at the bedside while leaving the room for a few seconds to get assistance
4. Have the client sit at the side of the bed for a few minutes while supporting their back and shoulders

39. 4. A quick change in position will decrease blood pressure, causing momentary lightheadedness and dizziness. An additional change in position may further reduce this client's blood pressure to a level that may require emergency assistance. The nurse should wait with the seated client until the blood pressure stabilizes. A safety vest isn't necessary. Leaving the room may put the client in danger if the blood pressure drops and the client requires emergency assistance. If the client continues to report dizziness and lightheadedness, the client should be returned to bed.

CN: Physiological integrity; CNS: Reduction of risk potential; CL: Apply

40. What nursing action is **most** effective in controlling and preventing the transmission of infective microorganisms?
1. Change the client's bed linens daily
2. Wash hands before and after client contact
3. Wear sterile gloves when touching a client's skin
4. Wear a mask when in direct contact with infected clients

40. 2. The transmission of microorganisms typically occurs when health care personnel fail to wash their hands before and after touching a client or contaminated objects. A daily linen change isn't the most effective method of controlling infection. Sterile gloves and a mask aren't needed during routine client care.

CN: Safe, effective care environment; CNS: Safety and infection control; CL: Apply

41. The nurse is teaching a student nurse about standard precautions. Which action, by the student nurse, would indicate that teaching has been effective?
1. Wearing eye goggles while giving a complete bed bath
2. Recapping a needle used for an injection before disposal
3. Disposing of blood-contaminated materials in a biohazard container
4. Using alcohol to decontaminate blood-contaminated steel instruments

41. 3. Blood-contaminated materials should be disposed of in a biohazard container. Recapping needles puts the health care provider at risk for a needle stick. Standard precautions are not required during a bed bath because of the low risk for exposure to blood. Blood-contaminated steel instruments are decontaminated in an autoclave.

CN: Safe, effective care environment; CNS: Safety and infection control; CL: Apply

42. A nurse is caring for a client on neutropenic precautions. Where should the nurse remove the barrier protection when leaving the room?
1. Within the client's room, just inside the doorway
2. Out of the client's room, just outside the doorway
3. In the hallway, a significant distance from the client's room
4. At the bedside, immediately after completing work with the client

42. 2. Disposing of gowns and gloves just outside the doorway provides sufficient distance from the client for all but airborne microorganisms. The client is protected from infection by airborne pathogens by keeping the door shut as much as possible to decrease the chance of exposure. Disposal of barriers at the bedside or inside the door negates the effectiveness of wearing barriers in the first place. It's unnecessary to wear the barriers away from the doorway as the door should remain closed.

CN: Safe, effective care environment; CNS: Safety and infection control; CL: Apply

43. What is the **most** appropriate time for teaching a client who is undergoing an open cholecystectomy?
  1. The day of discharge
  2. A day before the surgery
  3. The first 12 hours after surgery
  4. Before discharge and one to two days after the surgery

43. 4. Pain levels should have sufficiently subsided one to two days after the surgical procedure, allowing the client to concentrate on the information. The day of discharge is too late, because it doesn't allow the client sufficient time to ask questions or practice procedures that may be necessary. Also, the individual may be anxious about returning home, which may interfere with learning. A few weeks before surgery is generally too early to retain information, and teaching within the first 12 hours after surgery isn't likely to produce retention of information.
CN: Physiological integrity; CNS: Physiological adaptation; CL: Apply

44. Which technique is **best** for promoting proper breathing in a client experiencing pain or anxiety?
  1. Rapid, light respirations
  2. Rapid, deep respirations
  3. In through the mouth and out through the nose
  4. In through the nose and out through the mouth

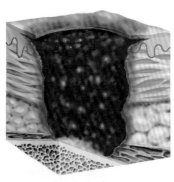

Don't get frightened answering this question.

44. 4. Air inhaled through the nose is warmed, humidified, and filtered for large particles by the nasal hairs, and conditioned for delivery to the lungs. Exhaling through the mouth after inhaling through the nose requires some concentration and provides a welcome distraction to a client experiencing pain and anxiety. This method of breathing is used to control respiratory rates when clients are anxious or in pain and also optimizes air exchange. Rapid, light, or deep respirations reduce the oxygen exchange time while continuing to blow off carbon dioxide. This can lead to hypoxemia and respiratory alkalosis.
CN: Physiological integrity; CNS: Physiological adaptation; CL: Apply

45. The nurse is assessing the skin of a client admitted with a stage II pressure ulcer. Which illustration represents a stage II pressure ulcer?

1.

3.

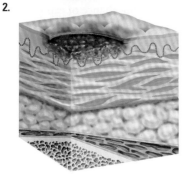

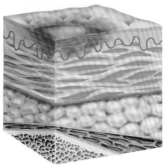

2.

4.

45. 2. Stage II is marked by partial-thickness skin loss that involves the epidermis, dermis, or both, with an abrasion, blister, or shallow crater. The first illustration represents a stage III ulcer, with a full-thickness wound that appears like a deep crater. The third illustration represents a stage IV ulcer, which involves all thicknesses of skin, as well as muscle, bone, and supporting structures. The fourth illustration represents a stage I ulcer, with a reddened area and intact skin. In individuals with dark skin, there may be warmth, edema, discoloration, induration, or hardness.
CN: Physiological integrity; CNS: Physiological adaptation; CL: Analyze

CN: Client needs category   CNS: Client needs subcategory   CL: Cognitive level

46. A 46-year-old single female client is concerned about her 15-year-old son's behavior. He has suddenly decided that his mother should not date or have men in the house. He told his mother that he is the man of the house. What disturbance is occurring in the internal dynamics of this family?
1. Age-appropriate behavior is occurring.
2. The son is powerful in the family system.
3. The son is trying to establish a role reversal.
4. It is culturally acceptable to be the man of the house at age 15.

46. 3. Role reversal occurs when the patterns of expected behavior aren't appropriate to age and ability. Males age 13 to 17 are developing their identities, and separation from parents becomes necessary for individuation to occur. Males have a better understanding of their role in relationships and with families if they're raised around strong male role models. In healthy families, power is shared, appropriate to age until the children are independent.

CN: Psychosocial integrity; CNS: None; CL: Analyze

47. A nurse is reviewing the causes of gastroesoph-ageal reflux disease (GERD) with a client. What area of the gastrointestinal tract causes the reduced pressure associated with GERD?

47. Normally, there is enough pressure around the lower esophageal sphincter (LES) to close it. Reflux occurs when LES pressure is deficient or when pressure in the stomach exceeds LES pressure.

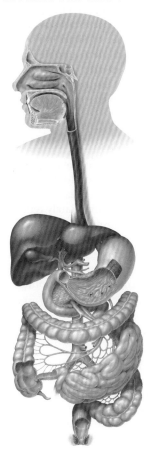

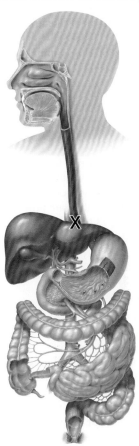

CN: Health promotion and maintenance; CNS: None;
CL: Apply

48. A nurse is preparing a client with a tracheostomy for discharge. The nurses determines that teaching has been successful regarding tracheostomy care when the client states:
1. "I will need to cover the opening when I shower."
2. "I can swim as long as I keep my head above water."
3. "I will need to wash my hands after caring for my tracheostomy."
4. "I will need to take antibiotics to prevent infections."

48. 1. The opening of the tracheostomy will require protection when bathing. Swimming isn't recommended, as drowning can occur even if the client's head isn't submerged. The client should wash his hands before and after caring for the tracheostomy. Prophylactic antibiotics aren't required for the client with a tracheostomy.
CN: Safe, effective care environment; CNS: Safety and infection control; CL: Apply

49. Which assessment data should a nurse report to the health care provider?
1. Blood pressure of 120/72 mmHg in a healthy man
2. Pulse of 110 bpm on awakening in the morning
3. Blood pressure of 110/68 mmHg in a healthy woman
4. Pulse of 120 beats/min immediately after 30 minutes of aerobic exercise

49. 2. The normal range for a pulse is 60 to 100/ bpm, and in the morning, the rate is at its lowest. Blood pressures of 120/72 mmHg for a healthy man and 110/68 mmHg for a healthy woman are normal. Aerobic exercise increases the heart rate over the normal range of 60 to 100 beats/min. The formula for maximum aerobic heart rate is: 210 − age × 80%. A person shouldn't go over the maximum heart rate during aerobic exercise.
CN: Physiological integrity; CNS: Physiological adaptation; CL: Analyze

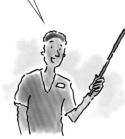

I know you'll get the answer to this one immediately.

50. A client has just returned to the unit following a cardiac catheterization via the femoral artery. Which assessment finding would the nurse **immediately** report to the health care provider?
1. Apical pulse of 98 bpm
2. Dressing with dime-sized red drainage
3. Absence of dorsalis pedis pulse
4. Blood pressure of 105/70 mmHg

50. 3. The dorsalis pedis is the pulse used to determine peripheral circulation to the lower extremities after a cardiac catheterization. Absence of this pulse should be immediately reported to the health care provider. An apical pulse of 98 beats/ min and a blood pressure of 105/70 mmHg are within the normal range. A dressing with dime-sized, red drainage is normal after a catheterization but should continue to be monitored.
CN: Physiological integrity; CNS: Reduction of risk potential; CL: Apply

51. A nurse is preparing to bathe a client who is hospitalized for emphysema. What is the nurse's **most** important intervention?
1. Remove the oxygen and proceed with the bath
2. Increase the flow of oxygen to six l/min via nasal cannula
3. Keep the head of the bed elevated 30 degrees during the procedure
4. Lower the head of the bed and roll the client to their left side to increase oxygenation

51. 3. The best position is one with the head slightly elevated. The elasticity of the lungs is lost for clients with emphysema, and most can't tolerate lying flat because the abdominal organs compress the lungs. The rate of oxygen delivery shouldn't be increased or decreased without an order from the health care provider. Increasing oxygen flow on a client with emphysema may also suppress the hypoxic drive to breathe. Positioning the client on his left side with the head of the bed flat would decrease oxygenation.
CN: Physiological integrity; CNS: Physiological adaptation; CL: Apply

52. The nurse is assessing a 40-year-old client who is scheduled to have elective facial surgery later in the morning and notes a pulse rate of 130 bpm. Which does the nurse suspect as the cause of the increased pulse rate?
1. Age
2. Anxiety
3. Exercise
4. Pain

52. 2. Anxiety tends to increase heart rate, temperature, and respirations. The normal heart rate for a client this age is 60 to 100 bpm. Exercise will temporarily increase the heart rate but most likely won't occur preoperatively. The client shouldn't be in any pain preoperatively.
CN: Physiological integrity; CNS: Physiological adaptation; CL: Apply

53. A thin client who is sitting up in bed, talking on the phone, has a blood pressure of 90/50 mmHg. What is the correct nursing action?
1. Increase fluids
2. Call the health care provider
3. Document the blood pressure
4. Suspect orthostatic hypotension

53. 3. A thin client can have a blood pressure as low as 88/68 mmHg and remain asymptomatic. Calling the health care provider with this information is inappropriate, as is increasing fluids. Orthostatic hypotension is a decrease in blood pressure and increase in heart rate that occurs with a sudden change in position from lying to sitting or standing.
CN: Safety and infection control; CNS: None; CL: Analyze

54. A client has just received morphine IV for postoperative pain. Which assessment finding should alert a nurse to a potential problem?
1. Heart rate 124 bpm
2. Respiratory rate 8 breaths/min
3. Sleeping but easily aroused
4. Blood pressure 90/62 mmHg

54. 2. Since morphine depresses the respiratory center of the brain, the nurse should alert the health care provider of a respiratory rate less than 10 breaths/min. While a heart rate of 124 bpm is considered tachycardia, the nurse should further assess the client before calling the health care provider. Morphine shouldn't be given to a client who is sedated and not easily aroused. Morphine can cause hypotension, but the nurse should further assess the client before calling the health care provider because this may be the client's usual blood pressure.
CN: Physiological integrity; CNS: Pharmacological and parenteral therapies; CL: Analyze

55. A client arrives at the emergency department with profuse, active bleeding from three gunshot wounds to the abdominal area and reports pain and a headache. What would the nurse anticipate? Select all that apply.
1. Rapid infusion of isotonic IV fluids
2. Pulse 44 bpm
3. Elevated oral temperature
4. Blood pressure 96/40 mmHg
5. Biot's respirations

55. 1, 4. Profuse loss of blood would require a rapid replacement of fluids. Isotonic fluids will not alter the fluid balance for this client. A decrease in blood pressure and an increase in pulse would occur as a response to the decreasing loss of blood volume in the body. The remaining options would not be present in this situation. Biot's respiration is an abnormal pattern of breathing characterized by groups of quick, shallow inspirations followed by regular or irregular periods of apnea.
CN: Health promotion and maintenance; CNS: None; CL: Analyze

CN: Client needs category   CNS: Client needs subcategory   CL: Cognitive level

56. A client with type 1 diabetes mellitus is conscious but confused, weak, diaphoretic, and is having heart palpitations. What is the nurse's **priority** action?
1. Administer glucagon intramuscularly (IM) or subcutaneously (subQ)
2. Give an intravenous (IV) bolus of dextrose 50%
3. Provide 15 to 20 g of a fast-acting oral carbohydrate
4. Inject 10 units of fast-acting insulin subcutaneously (subQ)

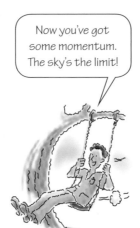

Now you've got some momentum. The sky's the limit!

56. 3. The client is exhibiting signs of hypoglycemia. Since the client is conscious, the first intervention is to give a fast-acting oral carbohydrate, such as orange juice, hard candy, or honey. If the client becomes unconscious, the nurse would administer IM or subQ glucagon or dextrose 50% IV if access is available. Administering insulin wouldn't be appropriate because the client is experiencing hypoglycemia.
CN: Physiological integrity; CNS: Reduction of risk potential; CL: Analyze

57. What is the correct procedure for performing tracheal suctioning for a hospitalized client?
1. Apply suction during insertion of the catheter
2. Limit suctioning to 10 to 15 seconds in duration
3. Re-sterilize the suction catheter in alcohol after use
4. Repeat suctioning intervals every 15 minutes until clear

57. 2. The length of time a client should suctioned is 10 to 15 seconds. Suctioning during insertion can cause trauma to the mucosa, and removes oxygen from the respiratory tract. Suctioning intervals, with supplemental oxygen between suctions, is performed after at least one-minute intervals to allow the client to rest. Suction catheters are disposable and should be cleansed in normal saline solution after each pass and then discarded.
CN: Physiological integrity; CNS: Physiological adaptation; CL: Apply

58. While performing nasopharyngeal suctioning, a nurse notes a client's oxygen saturation reading is 86% by pulse oximeter. What is the nurse's **most** appropriate action?
1. Stop suctioning and give oxygen to the client
2. Withdraw the suction catheter and tell the client to cough several times
3. Continue suctioning for 10 to 15 more seconds and then withdraw the suction catheter
4. Keep the suction catheter inserted and wait a few seconds before restarting suctioning

58. 1. The nurse must stop suctioning and give oxygen to increase the client's oxygen saturation. The normal range for oxygen saturation is 90 to 100%. Suctioning draws air as well as secretions from the lungs, reducing oxygen saturation in the blood. Withdrawing the suction catheter will stop the removal of oxygen, but coughing will delay an increase in saturation. Further suctioning will reduce the oxygen level. The suction catheter occupies space in the airway, making it harder for the client to breathe when it's left in place.
CN: Physiological integrity; CNS: Physiological adaptation; CL: Apply

59. Two hours after starting total enteral nutrition (TEN) through a nasogastric tube, a client starts to have abdominal distention. Which action should the nurse take **first**?
1. Aspirate stomach contents
2. Reposition the nasogastric tube
3. Place client in supine position
4. Stop the feeding

59. 4. Clients receiving TEN are at risk for abdominal distention due to rapid feeding or delayed emptying of the stomach contents. The nurse should stop the feeding to prevent further distention and then continue to assess the cause of the distention. Aspirating the stomach contents and repositioning the tube may be necessary but are not the priority. A client receiving a nasogastric tube feeding should be placed in an upright or Fowler's position to prevent the risk of aspiration.
CN: Physiological integrity; CNS: Basic care and comfort; CL: Analyze

60. What is the nurse's **initial** action when preparing to insert a nasogastric (NG) tube?
1. Wash hands
2. Apply sterile gloves
3. Apply a mask and gown
4. Open all necessary kits and tubing

60. 1. The first intervention before a procedure is hand washing. Clean gloves are used because the mouth and nasopharynx aren't considered sterile. A mask and gown aren't required. Opening all the equipment is the next step before inserting the NG tube.
CN: Safe, effective care environment; CNS: Safety and infection control; CL: Apply

61. As a nurse is inserting a nasogastric tube, the client begins to gag. Which action should the nurse take?
1. Remove the inserted nasogastric tube and notify the health care provider of the client's status
2. Stop the insertion, allow the client to rest, and then continue inserting the tube
3. Encourage the client to take deep breaths through the mouth while the nasogastric tube is being inserted
4. Pause until the gagging stops and then tell the client to take a few sips of water and swallow as the nasogastric tube is inserted

61. 4. Swallowing helps advance the tube by causing the epiglottis to cover the opening of the trachea, thus helping to eliminate gagging and coughing. Removing the tube or stopping the insertion is unnecessary because gagging is an expected response to this procedure. Deep breathing opens the trachea, allowing the tube to possibly advance into the lungs.
CN: Safe, effective care environment; CNS: Safety and infection control; CL: Analyze

62. Which step, if taken by a nurse after the insertion of a nasogastric (NG) tube, could harm the client?
1. Affixing the NG tube to the nose with tape
2. Checking tube placement by aspirating stomach contents using a piston syringe
3. Checking tube placement by instilling 100 ml of water into the tube to check for stomach filling
4. Documenting the insertion method used to check tube placement, and client's response to the procedure

62. 3. If the tube is located in the lungs, instilling water would flood the lungs, precipitating choking, coughing, hypoxemia, and, possibly, pneumonia. Anchoring the tube after placement to the nose with tape or a manufactured device will prevent the tube from becoming dislodged. Withdrawing stomach contents from the NG tube double-checks the correct placement. Documentation is required for any procedure.
CN: Safe, effective care environment; CNS: Reduction of risk; CL: Apply

> Sometimes people just need a little help to overcome their deficiencies.

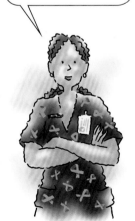

63. A new graduate nurse is assigned to a nursing unit. The nurse-manager notes that the graduate's skills are deficient. Which action is **most** appropriate for the nurse-manager to take?
1. Talk with the nursing supervisor about terminating the new graduate nurse
2. Discuss transferring the new graduate nurse to another unit if necessary
3. Work with the graduate and develop a plan to improve deficient skills
4. Counsel the graduate that, if performance doesn't improve, the graduate will be terminated

63. 3. The leader should work with the new graduate and provide opportunities for the graduate to grow and develop. The other responses wouldn't give the new graduate the opportunity and support needed for improvement.
CN: Safe, effective care environment; CNS: Management of care; CL: Apply

64. The nurse is observing the cardiac monitor of a client whose heart rate is 84 bpm with a normal sinus rhythm. The heart rate suddenly changes to 170 bpm, with frequent premature contractions. What is the nurse's **best** action?
1. Call the client's health care provider immediately
2. Enter the client's room and complete a full assessment
3. Delegate one of the nurses' assistants to take the client's vital signs
4. Notify the supervisor about the change in the client's condition

64. 2. Because a change has occurred in the client's status, the nurse must assess the client first. This shouldn't be delegated to unlicensed personnel. Before the health care provider or supervisor is notified, a full assessment must be made.
CN: Physiological integrity; CNS: Reduction of risk; CL: Analyze

65. An assessment is completed for a client hospitalized with an acute sinus infection. Which finding could indicate a serious complication?
1. Orbital edema
2. Nuchal rigidity
3. Oral temperature 102° F (39° C)
4. Frontal headache

65. 2. Nuchal rigidity indicates neurological involvement, possibly meningitis. The other symptoms are typical of a sinus infection.
CN: Physiological integrity; CNS: Physiological adaptation; CL: Analyze

66. A nurse is providing teaching about postoperative care to a client who had nasal surgery. Which statement would indicate that the client requires additional instruction?
1. "I'll do frequent mouth care."
2. "I'll eat two oranges a day."
3. "I will eat cheese every day."
4. "I'll drink at least eight glasses of water a day."

66. 3. After nasal surgery, the client shouldn't strain or bear down as this will increase the risk for bleeding. Dairy products are one of the causes of constipation which could lead to straining. These include cheese, milk, and yogurt. The other interventions would be appropriate postoperative care for this client.
CN: Physiological integrity; CNS: Reduction of risk potential; CL: Analyze

67. The nurse is collecting a urine specimen from a client's indwelling urinary catheter. Which action should the nurse take?
1. Collect urine from the drainage collection bag
2. Disconnect the catheter from the drainage tubing to collect urine
3. Remove the indwelling catheter and insert a sterile straight catheter to collect urine
4. Insert a sterile needle with syringe through a tubing drainage port cleaned with alcohol to collect the specimen

67. 4. Wearing clean gloves, cleaning the port with alcohol, and then obtaining the specimen with a sterile needle will ensure that the specimen, and the closed urinary drainage system, won't be contaminated. A urine sample must be new urine. The urine in the collection bag could be several hours old and growing bacteria. The urinary drainage system must be kept closed to prevent microorganisms from entering. A straight catheter is used to relieve urinary retention, obtain sterile urine specimens, and measure the amount of postvoid residual urine. It isn't necessary to remove an indwelling catheter to obtain a sterile urine specimen unless the health care provider requests the whole system be changed.
CN: Safe, effective care environment; CNS: Safety and infection control; CL: Apply

CN: Client needs category   CNS: Client needs subcategory   CL: Cognitive level

68. A nurse is teaching a client how to walk with crutches. Which observation would indicate that the client understands these instructions?
  1. The client's axillae rest on the crutches.
  2. The client's hands bear the body weight.
  3. Crutches are 12 inches (30.5 cm) in front of the feet.
  4. The client uses long strides when walking.

68. 2. When using crutches, the client's weight should be on his hands. There should be two inches (5 cm) between the crutch and axilla. The axillae shouldn't rest on the crutches. Crutches should be placed six inches (15 cm) in front of the feet for stability. A short stride provides maximum safety and mobility.
CN: Physiological integrity; CNS: Basic care and comfort; CL: Apply

69. A client, recovering from a knee replacement, has 1,000 ml normal saline solution ordered to run at 125 ml/hr IV. The IV bag was hung at 0800. It's now 1500, and 300 ml have been infused. What is the **most** appropriate action for the evening nurse during the initial assessment at 1500?
  1. Discontinue the IV infusion when the bag is complete
  2. Instruct the client to increase his fluid intake
  3. Speed up the rate of the IV fluids
  4. Assess the IV site

69. 4. At 125 ml/hr over seven hours, 875 ml should have been infused. The infusion is 575 ml behind. The nurse should assess the IV line for possible complications. The health care provider will determine how to adjust the infusion delivery. This order is for IV fluids rather than oral fluids. The route change can only be authorized by a health care provider. The rate of infusion cannot be changed without a provider's order.
CN: Safe, effective care environment; CNS: Management of care; CL: Apply

70. A nurse is removing a client's indwelling urinary catheter. Which action is appropriate?
  1. Don sterile gloves
  2. Cut the lumen of the balloon
  3. Document the time of removal
  4. Position the client on the left side

70. 3. A client should void on their own within eight hours of having an indwelling catheter removed. Documenting the time allows for an accurate measurement of this time lapse. Clean, disposable gloves are required because this isn't a sterile procedure. The catheter Balloon inflation port should be deflated. The client should be in a supine position with privacy provided prior to catheter removal.
CN: Physiological integrity; CNS: Basic care and comfort; CL: Apply

71. The nurse obtains a client's stool sample to test for occult blood. Which diets can cause a false-positive test result?
  1. Red meat, horseradish, and turnips
  2. Dairy products, canned fruit, and pretzels
  3. Cheese, raw fruits, and vegetables
  4. Potatoes, orange juice, and decaffeinated coffee

71. 1. Consumption of red meat has caused false-positive readings. The client should also avoid poultry, fish, turnips, and horseradish. Foods high in iron should be avoided. The other foods don't cause false-positive readings.
CN: Physiological integrity; CNS: Health promotion and maintenance; CL: Apply

72. The nurse is teaching a client about foods that may cause excessive flatulence. Which food is **most** likely to cause this client to be flatulent?
  1. Cauliflower
  2. Rice
  3. Steak
  4. Potatoes

72. 1. Cauliflower is a vegetable of the cruciferous variety (including brussel sprouts, cabbage, and broccoli) that is highly associated with intestinal gas. Besides cruciferous vegetables, foods with these gassy reactions include grains and other starches, onions, artichokes, and pears for their fructose; many fruits for their soluble fiber that creates a gel only broken down in the intestines and dairy. Rice is the only starchy food that does not produce gas
CN: Physiological integrity; CNS: Basic care and comfort; CL: Apply

---

CN: Client needs category   CNS: Client needs subcategory   CL: Cognitive level

73. A nurse is teaching a client postoperative coughing and deep-breathing exercises. What **priority** information should the nurse include?
   1. Splint the incision and cough
   2. Splint the incision, take a deep breath, and then cough
   3. Lie prone, splint the incision, take a deep breath, and then cough
   4. Lie supine, splint the incision, take a deep breath, and then cough

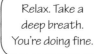
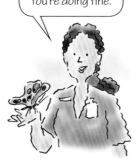

Relax. Take a deep breath. You're doing fine.

73. 2. Splinting with a pillow will protect the incision while the client coughs. Taking a deep breath will help open the alveoli, which promotes oxygen exchange and prevents atelectasis. Coughing and deep-breathing exercises are best accomplished in a seated or semi-upright position. Expectoration of secretions will be facilitated while in a seated position, as will splinting and deep breathing.
CN: Physiological integrity; CNS: Reduction of risk potential; CL: Apply

74. Which care plan goal statement is appropriate for a client?
   1. The nurse will perform the client's bath by 1500
   2. The client will bathe with minimal assistance
   3. The nurse will perform the client's bath
   4. The client will bathe with minimal assistance by discharge

74. 4. All goals should be client focused, with a clear statement of the task to be accomplished and a time frame for that accomplishment. Goals should be realistic and measurable so all staff can evaluate the client's progress. The nurse should be flexible in reassessing needs and approaches to facilitate optimal client recovery. The goal statement should include specific criteria to allow all staff to work from the same data for achieving client goals.
CN: Safe, effective care environment; CNS: Management of care; CL: Apply

75. A cooperative client with AIDS requires assistance with oral care. How should the nurse **best** facilitate this task?
   1. Wear a mask, gown, and gloves
   2. Wear a gown and gloves
   3. Wear a mask with eye shield and gloves
   4. Wear gloves only

75. 4. According to standard precautions, the nurse should wear gloves when coming in contact with a client's blood or body fluids. During oral care with a cooperative client, gloves are sufficient to protect the nurse. A mask is worn when airborne droplets of blood or body fluids are anticipated. A gown and mask with eye shield should be worn when splashing of body fluids is expected.
CN: Safe, effective care environment; CNS: Safety and infection control; CL: Apply

76. A middle-age adult has been identified as being in the stagnation stage of developmental conflict. What evidence would support this assessment? Select all that apply.
   1. Withdrawn from family obligations
   2. Bought a new sports car
   3. Started classes at the community college
   4. Increased nap and sleeping hours
   5. Recently became engaged

76. 1, 4. Clients in the stagnation stage of development will withdraw from activities and relationships. The remaining responses do not express stagnation.
CN: Health promotion and maintenance; CNS: None; CL: Apply

77. A client with pneumonia is having difficulty maintaining airway clearance. What goal would be appropriate for this client?
1. The client will have clear breath sounds by the end of the second day of admission
2. The client will have a respiratory rate of 32 breaths/min by the end of the second day of admission
3. The client will be pain free by discharge
4. The client will have a normal body temperature throughout hospitalization

77. 1. Clear breath sounds in a client with pneumonia would indicate airway clearance. Tachypnea would not indicate clear breath sounds, and may occur because the client has difficulty clearing secretions. Being pain free and having a normal body temperature are appropriate goals for a client with pneumonia but are not an indication that the airway is clear.
CN: Safe, effective care environment; CNS: Management of care; CL: Analyze

78. A client on complete bed rest reports excessive flatulence. What is the **best** position for the nurse to place this client in?
1. Fowler's
2. Knee-chest
3. Semi-Fowler's
4. Trendelenburg's

78. 2. Because gas rises, the knee-chest position will facilitate the passage of flatus. Semi-Fowler's and Fowler's positions inhibit gas passage. In Trendelenburg's position, the client lies flat with his head lower than his feet.
CN: Physiological integrity; CNS: Basic care and comfort; CL: Apply

79. The nurse is assisting with the delivery of a fetus where the mentum is the presenting part. Which illustration shows this fetal presentation?

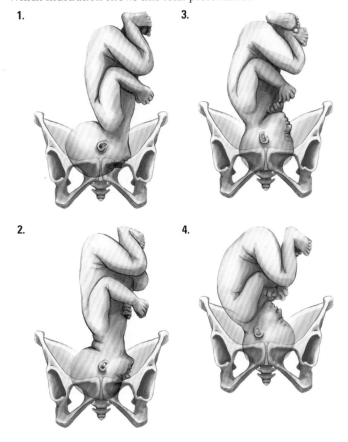

1.   3.

2.   4.

79. 1. In the cephalic, or head-down, presentation, the position of the fetus may be classified by the presenting skull landmark: mentum or chin (illustration one), brow (illustration two), sinciput (illustration three), or vertex (illustration four).
CN: Health promotion and maintenance; CNS: None; CL: Apply

CN: Client needs category   CNS: Client needs subcategory   CL: Cognitive level

80. The nurse is performing percussion and postural drainage on the lower left lobe of a client diagnosed with pneumonia. How should the nurse position the client?
   1. On the right side with the foot of the bed elevated
   2. On the left side with the foot of the bed elevated
   3. On the left side with the head of the bed elevated
   4. Prone with the head of the bed elevated

80. **1.** To mobilize secretions from the left lower lobe, the client should be positioned on the right side. The foot of the bed should be elevated so that gravity can help mobilize secretions. Placing the client on the left side would put the left lobe in a low or dependent position. Elevating the head of the bed wouldn't use gravity to drain the lower lobes.

CN: Physiological integrity; CNS: Basic care and comfort; CL: Apply

81. A client reports moderate pain. Which assessment, by the nurse, would indicate a physiological response to pain?
   1. Restlessness
   2. Decreased pulse rate
   3. Increased blood pressure
   4. Guarding of the painful area

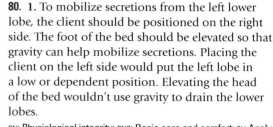

Assessment is always an adventure.

81. **3.** Increased blood pressure is a physiological, or involuntary, response to moderate pain. Restlessness and guarding of the painful area are behavioral responses. Decreased pulse rate occurs when pain is severe and deep.

CN: Physiological integrity; CNS: Physiological adaptation; CL: Analyze

82. A client with long-standing rheumatoid arthritis frequently reports joint pain. The nurse's plan of treatment should be based on an understanding that chronic pain is **most** effectively relieved when analgesics are administered:
   1. conservatively.
   2. intramuscular (IM) alternating with intravenous (IV).
   3. on an as-needed basis.
   4. at regularly scheduled intervals.

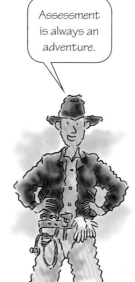

82. **4.** To control chronic pain and prevent cycled pain, regularly scheduled administration is most effective. Conservative and as-needed administration aren't effective means to manage chronic pain because the pain isn't relieved regularly. Intramuscular administration isn't practical on a long-term basis.

CN: Physiological integrity; CNS: Pharmacological and parenteral therapies; CL: Apply

83. A nurse notes crackles in the lung bases and pedal edema during a client assessment. Which factor is a common cause of fluid volume excess?
   1. Prolonged fever
   2. Hyperventilation
   3. Excessive IV infusion
   4. Fluid volume shifts secondary to vomiting

83. **3.** Fluid volume excess can result from excess IV fluids, especially in a compromised client. Vomiting, fever, and hyperventilation will result in a loss of body fluids, leading to a fluid volume deficit.

CN: Physiological integrity; CNS: Basic care and comfort; CL: Apply

84. A client is to receive IV therapy. Prioritize these nursing actions to ensure client safety.

1. Check the order
2. Set the rate as ordered
3. Label the site with the date
4. Connect IV tubing to the insertion site
5. Select a viable site distal to proximal

84. Ordered Response:

1. Check the order
5. Select a viable site distal to proximal
4. Connect IV tubing to the insertion site
2. Set the rate as ordered
3. Label the site with the date

CN: Physiological integrity; CNS: Pharmacological and parenteral therapy; CL: Apply

85. A nurse is teaching a client how to follow a low-sodium diet. Which statement would indicate that the client understands this teaching?
1. "Meat, fish, and chicken are high in sodium."
2. "I'll miss eating fruits."
3. "I'll enjoy eating at restaurants more often now."
4. "I'll avoid dairy products, potato chips, and carrots."

85. 4. Dairy products, potato chips, carrots, and restaurant food are all high in sodium. Meat, fish, chicken, and fruits are better alternatives.
CN: Physiological integrity; CNS: Basic care and comfort;
CL: Apply

86. To reduce the risk of aspiration in a client with impaired swallowing, the nurse should:
1. provide a straw for drinking liquids.
2. remove dentures before eating.
3. position the client in High Fowlers.
4. place food on the paralyzed side of the mouth.

86. 3. When feeding a client with impaired swallowing, the nurse should position the client in High Fowlers to reduce the risk of aspiration. Straws shouldn't be used because they increase the risk of aspiration by sending liquids directly to the back of the mouth. Dentures should be well-fitting and in place for eating. If one side of the mouth is paralyzed, food should be placed on the unaffected side.
CN: Physiological integrity; CNS: Basic care and comfort;
CL: Apply

87. A client must choose a meal that follows a high-calorie, high-protein, low-sodium, and low-potassium diet. Which choice would indicate that the client understands these dietary guidelines?
1. Halibut, salad, rice, and instant coffee
2. Crab, beets, spinach, and baked potato
3. Salmon, rice, green beans, sourdough bread, coffee, and ice cream
4. Sirloin steak, salad, baked potato with butter, and chocolate ice cream

87. 3. The best choice of these meals is salmon with rice and green beans, which are high in protein, and the sourdough bread and ice cream add calories. Halibut, instant coffee, and potatoes are high in potassium, and beets are high in sodium.
CN: Health promotion and maintenance; CNS: None; CL: Analyze

88. A client with terminal cancer tells the nurse, "I've given up. I have no hope left. I'm ready to die." What is the nurse's **most** appropriate response?
1. "It sounds like you've given up hope."
2. "You should talk about dying to a social worker."
3. "You should talk to your health care provider about your fears of dying."
4. "New cures for cancer are found every day."

88. 1. The use of reflection invites the client to talk more about his concerns. Deferring the conversation to a social worker or health care provider closes the conversation. Telling the client the cure for cancer is right around the corner gives false hope.
CN: Psychosocial integrity; CNS: None; CL: Analyze

89. A nurse is preparing a teaching plan for a client with a platelet count of $25,000/mm^3$, and a petechial rash on the legs, arms, and neck. What instruction should be included in this plan?
1. Take an iron supplement daily
2. Take acetaminophen rather than aspirin for headache
3. Stay away from crowds during the flu season
4. Avoid fresh salads

89. 2. A client with thrombocytopenia has a low platelet count and should avoid products containing aspirin due to the risk of increased bleeding. Iron supplements would be helpful for a client with anemia. Staying away from crowds and avoiding fresh salads to reduce the risk of infection would be important for the client with leukopenia.
CN: Physiological integrity; CNS: Reduction of risk potential;
CL: Analyze

CN: Client needs category   CNS: Client needs subcategory   CL: Cognitive level

90. A client is newly diagnosed with type 2 diabetes mellitus. Which laboratory value should the nurse report to the health care provider?
1. pH, 7.45
2. Sodium, 118 mEq/L
3. Glucose, 120 mg/dl
4. Potassium, 3.9 mEq/L

90. 2. The normal range for sodium is 135 to 145 mEq/L. The rest of the results are within normal limits.
CN: Physiological integrity; CNS: Reduction of risk potential; CL: Analyze

91. A client is two days postoperative from a femoral popliteal bypass. During assessment, the nurse finds the client's left leg is cold and pale. What is the nurse's **initial** action?
1. Check distal pulses
2. Notify the health care provider
3. Elevate the foot of the bed
4. Wrap the leg in a warm blanket

91. 1. The nurse must assess the client for post-surgical complications. Before the health care provider is notified, the nurse must assess circulation by checking for distal pulses which could be altered by a clot. Elevating the foot of the bed would promote venous return but decrease arterial blood flow and should be avoided. The leg should be lightly covered after circulation is assessed.
CN: Physiological integrity; CNS: Physiological adaptation; CL: Analyze

92. Which mediation can the nurse administer through a nasogastric (NG) tube?
1. Enteric-coated aspirin
2. Acetaminophen
3. Regular insulin
4. Sublingual nitroglycerin

92. 2. Most oral medications can be given through an NG tube because they're intended for passage into the stomach. Some oral drugs have special coatings intended to keep the pill intact until it passes into the small intestine. These enteric-coated pills shouldn't be crushed and put through an NG tube. Some parenteral medications, such as insulin, may be destroyed by gastric juices. Sublingual medications must be given under the tongue.
CN: Physiological integrity; CNS: Pharmacological and parenteral therapies; CL: Apply

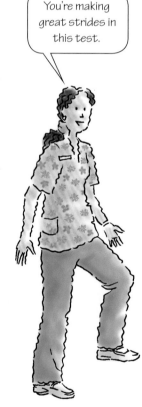

You're making great strides in this test.

93. What is the **most** effective way for a client to receive oxygen delivery at a FiO$_2$ of 92%?
1. Face tent
2. Venturi mask
3. Nasal cannula
4. Mask with reservoir bag

93. 4. A mask with a reservoir bag administers 70 to 100% oxygen at flow rates of 8 to 10 l/min. Maximum delivery using a face tent is 22 to 34%. The maximum rate using a Venturi mask is 24 to 55%, and the maximum rate using a nasal cannula is 44% at six l/min.
CN: Physiological integrity; CNS: Pharmacological and parenteral therapies; CL: Analyze

94. A client returns from surgery with acute pain. What is the **most** effective method of pain relief for this client?
1. Morphine sulfate 10 mg intramuscularly
2. Morphine sulfate 0.2 mg/ml via client-controlled analgesia
3. Dilaudid 2 mg IV every 2 hours
4. Percocet five mg orally every 4 to 6 hours

94. 2. Clients who have ready access to an analgesic are more likely to medicate themselves before the pain becomes severe, and may require reduced amounts of pain medication. Having control over drug administration reduces anxiety, which helps to relieve pain.
CN: Physiological integrity; CNS: Pharmacological and parenteral therapies; CL: Apply

95. A client with dyspnea has a respiratory rate of 34 breaths/min and is becoming anxious. He's refusing all medications, claiming they're making him worse. What is the nurse's **best** action?
1. Notify the health care provider of the status of this client
2. Withhold the medication until the next scheduled dose
3. Encourage the client to take some of his medications.
4. Put the medicine in applesauce to give it without the client's knowledge

95. 1. Notifying the health care provider of the client's condition and his refusal to take his medications will allow the health care provider to decide what alternatives should be instituted. The health care provider should be notified if a medication is withheld, or if a client takes only a portion of the medication. The nurse should explore why the client believes the medications are making him worse. The client has the right to refuse medication and should not be forced or tricked into taking them.
CN: Physiological integrity; CNS: Pharmacological and parenteral therapies; CL: Analyze

96. Which statement is an example of a measurable outcome for a client's plan of care?
1. Advance diet to regular as tolerated
2. Ambulate 30 feet (9 m) with walker by discharge
3. Give furosemide 40 mg IV now
4. Discontinue IV fluids when tolerating oral fluids

96. 2. Ambulating 30 feet with a walker by discharge is a realistic, measurable outcome or goal, a key element of a nursing care plan. Other key elements include a nursing diagnoses and interventions. The other options are health care provider's orders, and not key components of a care plan.
CN: Safe, effective care environment; CNS: Management of care; CL: Apply

97. A client, who was recently hospitalized, has constipation related to her medical regimen. Which medication may contribute to this problem?
1. Folic acid
2. Iron
3. Potassium
4. Vitamin E

97. 2. Iron may cause constipation when supplements are taken at 100% of the recommended daily allowance. Folic acid, potassium, and vitamin E don't increase the likelihood of constipation.
CN: Physiological integrity; CNS: Pharmacological and parenteral therapies; CL: Apply

98. A healthy, young client had an appendectomy 24 hours ago. Which nursing goal is appropriate for this client?
1. The client will be able to walk in the hallway on the first post-operative day.
2. The client will be able to attend physical therapy on the third post-operative day.
3. The client will be able to accomplish all activities of daily living by discharge.
4. The client will be able to state the rationale for all postoperative medications by discharge.

98. 1. A 24-hour postoperative client is expected to be able to walk in the hallway. A client who just had an appendectomy shouldn't need physical therapy unless deconditioning was evident. A client should begin to assume responsibility for activities of daily living but shouldn't necessarily be responsible for all activities at 24 hours. It's too early to expect a client to state the rationale for all postoperative medications, especially if the client is elderly.
CN: Physiological integrity; CNS: Basic care and comfort; CL: Apply

99. A client is being discharged with a full leg cast. Which instruction is **most** important for the nurse to give this client?
1. Observe activity restrictions
2. Maintain proper nutrition
3. Limit weight bearing on affected leg
4. Report signs of impaired circulation

99. 4. The nurse should include all these instructions in the teaching plan; however, the highest priority is report the signs of impaired circulation in order to prevent permanent neurovascular damage, including loss of the leg.
CN: Physiological integrity; CNS: Reduction of risk potential; CL: Analyze

CN: Client needs category   CNS: Client needs subcategory   CL: Cognitive level

100. The nurse is performing an admission assessment. What question would yield the **most** information regarding the reason for this client's admission?
1. "Does your abdomen have sharp pains?"
2. "Are you noticing more flatulence with this condition?"
3. "How have things been going for you?"
4. "May I question you further about your pain?"

100. 3. This is an open-ended question that will encourage the client to talk and express concerns. Answers one and two are close-ended questions that can be answered with a one-word answer. This will not yield the information necessary for an admission assessment. Answer four is not asking for any information and can be answered with one word.

CN: Psychosocial integrity; CNS: None; CL: Apply

101. A registered nurse (RN) is supervising an unlicensed assistive personnel (UAP). Which principle would the nurse follow when delegating tasks?
1. The RN must directly supervise all delegated tasks
2. After a task is delegated, it's no longer the RN's responsibility
3. The RN delegates a task based on the UAP's skill set
4. Follow-up with a delegated task is only necessary if the UAP is untrustworthy

101. 3. The RN must delegate tasks that are within the scope of practice of the unlicensed personnel. The RN need not directly supervise all delegated tasks, as this would negate the benefits of delegation. When a task is delegated, the RN retains responsibility for the successful completion of the task. The RN must always follow up with the UAP to ensure the task was completed appropriately.

CN: Safe, effective care environment; CNS: Management of care; CL: Apply

102. An elderly client had recent hip surgery and is now on bed rest. Which nursing intervention is **most** important to include in the care plan for this client?
1. Daily assessment of the wound site
2. Foot and ankle range-of-motion (ROM) exercises
3. Wound cleaning with hydrogen peroxide
4. Coughing and deep breathing in the prone position

102. 2. Foot and ankle ROM exercises are standard protocol for clients who remain in bed for an extended period of time. ROM exercises promote blood flow to the area, prevent atrophy, and lessen the potential for edema. The wound site should be assessed every shift. Wound cleaning with hydrogen peroxide isn't generally recommended. Coughing and deep breathing aren't generally recommended in the prone position.

CN: Physiological integrity; CNS: Reduction of risk potential; CL: Apply

103. A client receiving phenothiazine has become restless and fidgety, and is anxiously pacing the hallway. What adverse effect of phenothiazine would the nurse suspect, based on this behavior?
1. Dystonia
2. Akathisia
3. Parkinsonian effects
4. Tardive dyskinesia

103. 2. Akathisia is an adverse effect of phenothiazines. Dystonia appears as excessive salivation, difficulty speaking, and involuntary movements of the face, neck, arms, and legs. Parkinsonian effects include a shuffling gait, hand tremors, drooling, rigidity, and loose arm movements. Tardive dyskinesia is characterized by odd facial and tongue movements.

CN: Physiological integrity; CNS: Pharmacological and Parental Therapies; CL: Apply

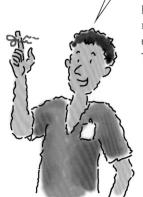

Don't forget to look over all of the answer options first and to eliminate as many wrong ones as you can before making your choice.

CN: Client needs category   CNS: Client needs subcategory   CL: Cognitive level

104. A client who had an open cholecystectomy two days ago reports pain in his right calf. Which is the nurse's **priority** intervention?
1. Assess the leg for swelling and redness
2. Instruct the client to flex his knee and hip
3. Apply a warm compress and call the health care provider
4. Gently massage the calf and notify the health care provider

104. 1. The nurse must further assess the pain in the calf to determine if this symptom is caused by a possible deep vein thrombosis. Assessing the client for redness and swelling would be the next intervention. Making the client flex his knee and hip will not help assess for the presence of a clot. Warm compresses may be ordered after a diagnosis of deep vein thrombosis is made. Never massage the calf muscle because the clot could be dislodged.
CN: Physiological integrity; CNS: Reduction of risk potential; CL: Analyze

105. Which nursing goal is the **priority** for a client with a new tracheostomy?
1. Developing an effective means of communication
2. Maintaining a patent airway
3. Preventing infection
4. Gaining independence in self-care

105. 2. Maintaining a patent airway is the highest priority in a client with a new tracheostomy since drainage and edema can obstruct the airway. The other goals are important, but only after airway patency has been assured.
CN: Physiological integrity; CNS: Reduction of risk potential; CL: Analyze

106. A nurse is providing teaching to a client with chronic arterial disease. Which statement would indicate that the client requires additional teaching?
1. "I'm going to stop smoking."
2. "I'm going to have the podiatrist check my feet."
3. "I'm going to keep the heat in my house at 80° F (26.6° C)."
4. "I'm going to walk short distances every morning."

106. 3. Clients with peripheral vascular disease need to be at a comfortable temperature because of impaired circulation. Having the heat at 80° F is too warm. The other choices are all appropriate interventions for a client with peripheral vascular disease.
CN: Physiological integrity; CNS: Reduction of risk potential; CL: Analyze

107. The nursing team consists of one RN, one LPN, and a UAP. Which activities should the RN perform?
1. Consoling a grieving visitor
2. Assessing a newly admitted client
3. Tabulating the hourly intake and output
4. Administering a tap water enema to a preoperative client

107. 2. Assessment of a new admission can't be delegated to an LPN or a UAP. Consoling a visitor and giving a tap water enema are within the scope of practice of an LPN or UAP. Tabulation of hourly intake and output amounts are within the scope of practice of an LPN and a UAP.
CN: Safe, effective care environment; CNS: Management of care; CL: Apply

108. A six-year-old client requires diabetes teaching. What factor should the nurse consider when planning this teaching?
1. Another child with diabetes can teach the client.
2. The child can teach his parents after the nurse teaches him.
3. The child and parents should both receive this teaching.
4. Teaching should be directed to the parents, who can then teach the child.

108. 3. The parents and child should both participate in the nurse's teaching to ensure accuracy of teaching. A school-aged child shouldn't be the sole provider of teaching to the parents. Another school-aged child couldn't be entrusted to teach this child, although their input would be valuable. Parents should be included in the teaching plan but shouldn't be responsible for the teaching.
CN: Health promotion and maintenance; CNS: None; CL: Apply

CN: Client needs category   CNS: Client needs subcategory   CL: Cognitive level

109. The parents of a toddler are having problems putting their child to bed at night. What is the nurse's **most** appropriate recommendation?
1. Discontinue afternoon naps
2. Allow the toddler to have a tantrum for 30 minutes
3. Encourage the parents to develop nighttime rituals
4. Allow the toddler to have some control over the time he goes to bed

109. 3. Rituals are extremely important for toddlers to feel secure and relaxed. Allowing a toddler to make small decisions, such as choosing the order of the ritual and color of pajamas, will give him the feeling of some control. However, control over the bedtime is outside the decision process of a toddler. Discontinuing naps may be helpful, depending on the toddler's needs. The toddler must clearly understand that tantrums won't get him what he wants.
CN: Health promotion and maintenance; CNS: None; CL: Apply

110. A client is displaying maladaptive coping behavior in response to body changes related to abdominal surgery for an ileostomy. Which nursing intervention is **best**?
1. Let the client express his feelings
2. Explain that a psychological referral would be beneficial
3. Instruct the client on how to use positive coping strategies
4. Encourage the client to participate in diversionary activities

110. 1. Allowing the client to verbalize feelings is the most therapeutic nursing intervention. Making a referral may help, but initially, this client should be allowed to express feelings. Giving advice may halt therapeutic communication. Providing diversionary activities doesn't foster effective coping.
CN: Psychosocial integrity; CNS: None; CL: Analyze

111. A new graduate nurse has started at a medical center and is assigned to a preceptor. The preceptor and other staff report that the new graduate nurse is uncooperative and unwilling to take direction. Which action, by the preceptor, is appropriate?
1. Explain the behavior won't be tolerated
2. Ask the new graduate nurse why he wants to work here
3. Reestablish goals with the new graduate nurse
4. Begin the disciplinary process with this new graduate nurse

111. 3. The preceptor should help this new graduate nurse learn the responsibilities, routines and goals of the unit. If the behavior continues, the new nurse may need career counseling. The new graduate isn't experienced and therefore shouldn't be reprimanded. Asking the new nurse why he wants to work there is inappropriate. Disciplining a new graduate nurse is not an initial action.
CN: Safe, effective care environment; CNS: Management of care; CL: Apply

112. A client with a history of bipolar disorder rushes into the mental health clinic waiting room scantily dressed and makes loud, obscene remarks to other clients. What is the nurse's **most** appropriate intervention?
1. Encourage the other clients to ignore the behavior
2. Confront the behavior and make the client take a seat
3. Tell the client to sit down and stop upsetting the others
4. Quietly escort the client to a private area and help put on a gown

112. 4. The client with bipolar disorder is highly excitable. The nurse needs to be firm yet distracting in a private area that preserves the client's dignity. Having the others ignore the client won't alter the problem. Confronting the behavior isn't recommended, as this client lacks judgment and insight. Telling the client to sit down may cause more resistance and even heighten the behavior.
CN: Psychosocial integrity; CNS: None; CL: Analyze

113. A nurse is reviewing the treatment for hyper-cyanotic spells (tet spells) with the parents of a four-month-old client being discharged from the hospital. What **priority** information should the nurse share with these parents?
1. "Calm your baby down by holding her and placing her knees up to her chest."
2. "Call 911 immediately and begin cardiopulmonary resuscitation (CPR) on your baby."
3. "You'll need to administer four back blows to the baby if she begins having a tet spell."
4. "You don't need to worry about these spells yet because the baby is too young. You'll need to watch for them when she becomes more mobile."

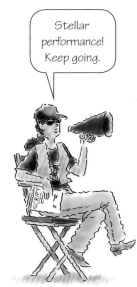

Stellar performance! Keep going.

113. 1. Tet spells are acute episodes of cyanosis and hypoxia that occur when the infant's oxygen demand exceeds the available supply. They may occur when the infant is crying or eating. Tet spells are emergency situations that require immediate intervention. Begin by calming the infant down and placing the infant in the knee-chest position, which increases systemic vascular resistance by limiting venous return. This decreases the right to left shunting and improves oxygenation. CPR won't calm the infant down or improve oxygenation. Back blows are given to infants who have something lodged in their trachea.
CN: Physiological integrity; CNS: Health promotion and maintenance; CL: Apply

114. A nurse is caring for a client with gout. Which nursing intervention should the nurse include in the plan of care?
1. Administer antibiotics
2. Restrict fluid intake
3. Encourage a low-purine diet
4. Administer opioids

114. 3. A low-purine diet decreases uric acid formation and should be encouraged. Antibiotics aren't used to treat gout. Fluid intake should be encouraged to flush out the uric acid. Anti-inflammatory medications are used during acute phases, but because this is a long-term condition, opioids aren't generally given.
CN: Physiological integrity; CNS: Reduction of risk potential; CL: Apply

115. The nurse is evaluating a client who is two days post-crush injury to his right leg. The nurse is **most** concerned when the assessment includes:
1. sudden decrease in pain.
2. swelling in toes or fingers.
3. inability to move fingers or toes.
4. diminished distal pulses.

115. 4. Compartment syndrome is a complication of a cast that places pressure on the blood vessels and nerves to the extremity. Symptoms include pain not relieved by analgesics and swelling of the extremity. A late symptom is a change in skin color with diminished distal pulses. After a fracture, some swelling and pain result, but pulses need to be monitored as well as color, sensation, and movement.
CN: Physiological integrity; CNS: Reduction of risk potential; CL: Apply

116. A client with an arm cast reports severe pain in the affected extremity, and decreased sensation and motion. Swelling in the fingers is also increased. What is the **priority** nursing intervention?
1. Elevate the arm
2. Remove the cast
3. Give an analgesic
4. Call the health care provider

116. 4. The cast may be too tight and may need to be split or removed by the health care provider. The arm should already be elevated. Notify the health care provider if circulation, sensation, or motion are impaired. Giving analgesics wouldn't be the first step as they may mask the signs of a serious problem.
CN: Physiological integrity; CNS: Reduction of risk potential; CL: Apply

CN: Client needs category   CNS: Client needs subcategory   CL: Cognitive level

117. The nurse is planning teaching for a four-year-old child scheduled for cardiac catheterization. How should the nurse approach this child's pre-operative teaching plan?
1. Keep the information basic and share it close to the time of the procedure
2. Share the information several days before the procedure so the child will have time to prepare
3. Provide detailed information so the child will know exactly what to expect
4. Direct the information at the child's parents because the child is too young to understand the procedure

117. 1. Four-year-old children are in Piaget's cognitive stage of preoperational thought. Their thinking is concrete and tangible, and they're unable to make deductions or generalizations and are egocentric. They don't have a concept of the future so explanations need to be done close to the time of the procedure. They need simple explanations of procedures in relationship to how the procedure will affect them. A four-year-old child is old enough to understand basic teaching close to the implementation of the procedure.
CN: Health promotion and maintenance; CNS: None; CL: Apply

118. A registered nurse is directing an unlicensed assistive personnel (UAP) to draw the morning blood work for a four-year-old child in the hospital. The nurse emphasizes that the procedure is to be done in the treatment room. Which rationale is correct?
1. The procedure will be faster.
2. It establishes the child's bed as a safe zone void of pain.
3. The child can only be restrained on the examination table.
4. The parents won't observe the procedure and upset the child.

118. 2. This implementation is based on the concept of atraumatic care, and growth and development principles. Small children need to consider their bed as a safe zone where they can relax and rest. The treatment room should be used instead. It will not be faster to draw blood in the treatment room. The child could be restrained in his room, but it isn't appropriate. Parental support is important and needs to be encouraged during stressful and painful procedures.
CN: Psychosocial integrity; CNS: None; CL: Apply

119. A client tells the nurse, "My medical illness is the result of something bad I did to someone in the past." Which response, by the nurse, is the **most** appropriate?
1. "What did you do wrong?"
2. "Let's talk about your concerns."
3. "That's a silly comment."
4. "You're suffering from a psychiatric delusion."

119. 2. Asking the client to talk about his concerns allows an opportunity for the nurse to clarify issues. Saying a comment is silly, or asking the client what he did wrong would likely escalate the client's concerns. Telling the client that this is a delusion is inappropriate.
CN: Psychosocial integrity; CNS: None; CL: Apply

120. A client on a psychiatric unit asks the nurse about the medications another client takes. What is the nurse's **best** response?
1. "How close are the two of you?"
2. "I respect her privacy and can't share that information."
3. "Let me ask her if it's okay for me to tell you about her condition and medications."
4. "The client is taking insulin for her diabetes and digoxin for her heart condition."

120. 2. Revealing one client's medication to another client is violating procedures of client confidentiality. Asking the nature of his relationship to the other client won't explain the purpose of protecting confidentiality. Seeking the client's permission to release confidential information is an inappropriate action. Assuring the client that the hospital has an obligation to protect the confidentiality of all clients will provide a sense of reassurance and comfort.
CN: Safe, effective care environment; CNS: Management of care; CL: Apply

---

CN: Client needs category   CNS: Client needs subcategory   CL: Cognitive level

121. A client's goal is to verbally interact, at least once, in each group therapy session by a certain date. For a goal to be completely met, the client must show the subjective and objective data. The client attended the group session, maintained eye contact with the group members, followed the conversation non-verbally as indicated by head nodding, and responded once to the group leader with a one-word answer. How should the nurse interpret this client's goal attainment?
   1. The goal was partially met.
   2. The goal was completely met.
   3. The goal was completely unmet.
   4. New problems have developed.

122. A client is prescribed heparin subQ 6,000 units/q12h for deep vein thrombosis prophylaxis. The pharmacy dispenses a vial containing 10,000 units/ml. How many milliliters of heparin should a nurse administer? Record your answer using one decimal place.

_____ ml

123. A client is prescribed lisinopril for the treatment of hypertension. What are the potential adverse effects of this medication? Select all that apply.
   1. Constipation
   2. Dizziness
   3. Headache
   4. Hyperglycemia
   5. Hypotension
   6. Impotence

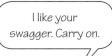

I like your swagger. Carry on.

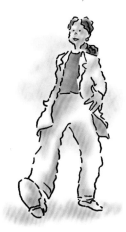

121. 1. This goal was partially met because the client verbally participated in a group therapy session. For a goal to be completely met, the client must show the subjective and objective data indicating the goal has been clearly attained. A completely unmet goal indicates the client's complete lack of behavior change and absence of subjective and objective data to indicate the achievement of the goal. In this case, no new problems or new nursing diagnoses were evident.
CN: Psychosocial integrity; CNS: None; CL: Analyze

122. 0.6.
The following formula is used to calculate drug dosages:

$$\frac{Dose\ on\ hand}{Quantity\ on\ hand} = \frac{Dose\ desired}{X}$$

The nurse should use the following equations:

$$\frac{10,000\ units}{1\ ml} = \frac{6,000\ units}{X}$$

$$X = \frac{6,000\ units \times 1\ ml}{10,000\ units} = 0.6\ ml$$

CN: Physiological integrity; CNS: Pharmacological and parenteral therapies; CL: Analyze

123. 2, 3, 5, 6. Dizziness, headache, and hypotension are all common adverse effects of lisinopril and other ACE inhibitors. Lisinopril may cause diarrhea, not constipation. Adverse effects are possible with lisinopril. Sexual side effects, while rare, include a decreased sex drive and erectile dysfunction or impotence. Lisinopril isn't known to cause hyperglycemia.
CN: Physiological integrity; CNS: Pharmacological and parenteral therapies; CL: Apply

CN: Client needs category   CNS: Client needs subcategory   CL: Cognitive level

124. The nurse is teaching a client about hypertension and associated risk factors. Which client response identifies a non-modifiable risk factor associated with hypertension?
1. High sodium intake
2. Sedentary lifestyle
3. Tobacco use
4. Family history

124. 4. Family history is a risk factor for hypertension that can't be modified. Risk factors that can be modified include high sodium intake, sedentary lifestyle, and tobacco use.
CN: Health promotion and maintenance; CNS: None; CL: Apply

125. A client has experienced an acute inferior myocardial infarction at a community hospital. After thrombolytic therapy fails, the health care provider wants to transfer the client to another hospital for emergency cardiac catheterization. Which member of the health care team must accompany this client?
1. Health care provider
2. Paramedic
3. Registered nurse (RN)
4. Licensed practical nurse (LPN)

125. 3. During transfer, the client must receive the same level of care that he received in the hospital; therefore, an RN must accompany him. It isn't necessary for a health care provider to accompany the client. A paramedic, although not required, will most likely accompany the nurse. An LPN's scope of practice is below the standard of care in this situation.
CN: Safe, effective care environment; CNS: Management of care; CL: Apply

126. A client with heart failure is allergic to sulfa-based medications. Which diuretic would the nurse anticipate ordered as an alternate?
1. Osmotic diuretics
2. Thiazide and thiazide-like diuretics
3. Potassium-sparing diuretics
4. Carbonic anhydrase inhibitors

126. 2. Thiazide and thiazide-like diuretics are sulfonamide derivatives, so they can be used, but used cautiously in clients allergic to sulfa-based medications. Osmotic, potassium-sparing, and carbonic anhydrase inhibitor diuretics can be safely administered to these clients.
CN: Physiological integrity; CNS: Pharmacological and parenteral therapies; CL: Apply

127. A client, with heart failure, tells the nurse that he props himself up with two pillows at night because he has difficulty breathing when lying flat. How would the nurse document this condition?
1. Bradypnea
2. Dyspnea on exertion
3. Paroxysmal nocturnal dyspnea
4. Orthopnea

127. 4. A client with orthopnea has shortness of breath when lying flat, and prefers sleeping with his upper body elevated. Bradypnea is decreased but regular breathing. Dyspnea on exertion occurs when the client has difficulty breathing with activity. Paroxysmal nocturnal dyspnea occurs when the client awakens at night and feels short of breath.
CN: Health promotion and maintenance; CNS: None; CL: Apply

128. During the initial assessment of a neonate, the nurse notes a respiratory rate of 52 breaths/min. What is the **most** appropriate nursing intervention?
1. Notify the health care provider immediately
2. This is a normal respiratory rate for a neonate
3. Position the isolette so the neonate's head is elevated
4. Prepare for emergency endotracheal (ET) intubation

128. 2. A normal respiratory rate for a neonate is 30 to 60 breaths/min, so notifying the health care provider or elevating the neonate's head isn't necessary. The nurse should prepare for ET intubation if the neonate shows signs of imminent respiratory distress such as an expiratory grunt.
CN: Health promotion and maintenance; CNS: None; CL: Analyze

CN: Client needs category   CNS: Client needs subcategory   CL: Cognitive level

129. During a neonate's one-month checkup, the pediatrician flexes the neonate's legs to right angles at the hips and knees, and abducts both hips until the knees touch the table. Which statement **best** describes the purpose of this test?
  1. To check the neonate's flexibility
  2. To assess leg strength
  3. To check for developmental dysplasia of the hip
  4. To examine the neonate for a hydrocele

129. 3. This test assesses for the developmental dysplasia of the hip. If dysplasia is present, the health care provider can see, feel, and, sometimes, hear a click. Although a neonate's flexibility and leg strength may be assessed at one month, the examination techniques differ from those described here. To identify a hydrocele, the health care provider palpates the neonate's testes.
CN: Physiological integrity; CNS: Physiological adaptation; CL: Analyze

130. At what age should a nurse initially screen a child for idiopathic juvenile scoliosis?
  1. 7 years
  2. 10 years
  3. 13 years
  4. 16 years

130. 2. Children should have initial screening at age 10, before the adolescent growth spurt, when promontory signs of scoliosis may become apparent. By age 13, a child may have significantly developed scoliosis that requires surgery.
CN: Health promotion and maintenance; CNS: None; CL: Apply

131. The nurse is screening a 10-year-old client for scoliosis. How should the nurse position the client?
  1. Facing away from the examiner, standing upright with arms held out straight in front of the body
  2. Facing away from the examiner, bending forward in flexion with arms and head dangling
  3. Facing the examiner, standing upright with arms held straight at his sides
  4. Sitting in a chair with feet flat on the floor and back at a 90-degree angle

131. 2. Assessing a client's back for asymmetry, or a hump, is best done with the client bending at the waist in 50% flexion with the arms and head dangling. This assessment can also be done with the arms hanging dependently at the sides so the examiner can check for asymmetry at the shoulders, waist folds, and space between the arms and waist.
CN: Health promotion and maintenance; CNS: None; CL: Apply

132. Parents have brought their infant to the clinic for a checkup after hospitalization for a new onset of type 1 diabetes mellitus. Which statement, to the nurse, indicates an understanding of this child's current condition?
  1. "The health care provider was wrong about the diagnosis because all of my child's fingersticks have been normal."
  2. "My child has experienced a honeymoon period and hasn't required any insulin injections."
  3. "Nobody in our family has diabetes, so we do not understand how our child can be a diabetic."
  4. "If our child lives a careful, sedentary lifestyle, she won't need as much insulin."

132. 2. A honeymoon phase, in which injected insulin seems to wake up the islet cells and cause them to secrete insulin, is common with type 1 diabetes mellitus. This phase has given many parents false hope that their child has been cured. Type 1 diabetes mellitus isn't a genetic trait. A sedentary lifestyle will increase the secondary effects of diabetes.
CN: Physiological integrity; CNS: Physiological adaptation; CL: Analyze

133. The nurse is preparing to administer an injection subcutaneously. Which illustration shows the appropriate needle selection for this type of injection?

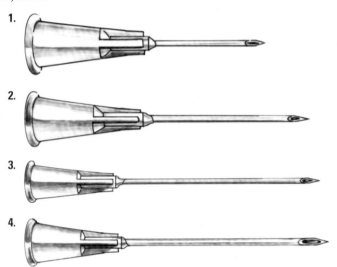

1.

2.

3.

4.

133. 2. When choosing a needle, consider its purpose as well as its gauge, bevel, and length. Illustration two shows a subcutaneous needle with a length of 1/2 to 5/8 in (1.27 to 1.59 cm) and a medium bevel. The first illustration shows an intradermal needle, with a length of 3/8 to 5/8 in (0.95 to 1.59 cm) and a short bevel. The third illustration shows an intramuscular needle, which is 1 to 3 in (2.54 to 7.62 cm) in length and a medium bevel. The fourth illustration shows an intravenous needle, which is 1 to 3 in (2.54 to 7.62 cm) in length with a long bevel.

CN: Physiological integrity; CNS: Pharmacological and parenteral therapies; CL: Apply

134. A two-year-old child has been admitted with a diagnosis of Wilms' tumor. Which intervention should the nurse include in this child's plan of care?
1. Prepare the family and child for surgery to begin within 24 to 48 hours
2. Palpate the abdomen to monitor tumor size
3. Massage the abdomen to relieve pain
4. Place a tight binder around the abdomen for support

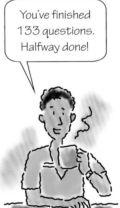

You've finished 133 questions. Halfway done!

134. 1. The nurse should tell the parents that their child will be scheduled for a nephrectomy within 24 to 48 hours. Metastasis occurs quickly with Wilms' tumor. To reduce the risk of disseminating cancer cells, abdominal palpation should be avoided. A tight binder would put pressure on the tumor, increasing the risk of cancer cell dissemination.

CN: Safe, effective care environment; CNS: Management of care; CL: Apply

135. A charge nurse is developing the client care assignments for the shift. Which client is **most** appropriately assigned to a licensed practical nurse (LPN)?
1. A client who experienced a cerebral vascular accident and has a do-not-resuscitate (DNR) status
2. A client who underwent cerebral arteriography one hour ago
3. A client who underwent carotid endarterectomy four hours ago
4. A client who underwent craniotomy three days ago and has just been transferred from the intensive care unit (ICU)

135. 1. The most appropriate client to assign to the LPN is the newly-admitted client with DNR status. Typically, a newly admitted client is assigned to a registered nurse (RN) because the client requires frequent assessments. The client who recently underwent cerebral arteriography, and the client who recently underwent carotid endarterectomy will require frequent assessments by an RN. The client just transferred from the ICU has the potential for becoming unstable, and should be assigned to an RN.

CN: Safe, effective care environment; CNS: Management of care; CL: Analyze

136. A health care provider prescribes carbamazepine 1,200 mg/po/q12h for a client with trigeminal neuralgia. Which action should the nurse take **first**?
1. Administer the medication with meals or with a bedtime snack
2. Encourage the client to promptly report unusual bleeding
3. Question the dose; it exceeds the recommended daily dose
4. Store the drug in a cool, dry place away from sunlight

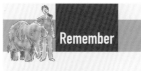

Remember

"Iminostilbenes impede seizures."

Iminostilbenes, such as carbamazepine, are anticonvulsant drugs, which are used to treat seizures.

136. 3. The nurse should verify the dose with the provider as it exceeds the standard prescribed dosage. Clients with trigeminal neuralgia should receive no more than 1,200 mg/po/daily. After the nurse confirms the order, he should encourage the client to take the drug at the same time each day with food to avoid gastrointestinal distress. The nurse should also encourage the client to promptly report unusual bleeding. The drug should be stored in a cool, dry place.
CN: Physiological integrity; CNS: Pharmacological and parenteral therapies; CL: Analyze

137. Emergency medical system personnel have used the Cincinnati Prehospital Stroke Scale to assess a client, and have alerted the hospital that they're transporting a client with a possible stroke. The goal of the emergency department (ED) nurse should be to administer the ordered fibrinolytics within:
1. 4 hours of the onset of symptoms.
2. 60 minutes of arrival in the ED.
3. 2 hours of arrival in the ED.
4. 25 minutes of arrival in the ED.

137. 2. The goal for initiating fibrinolytic therapy is within 60 minutes of arrival in the ED. Fibrinolytics must be administered within three hours of the onset of symptoms.
CN: Physiological integrity; CNS: Pharmacological and parenteral therapies; CL: Apply

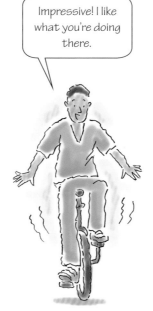

Impressive! I like what you're doing there.

138. A client with an above-the-knee amputation (AKA) visits the orthopedic surgeon for a follow-up. Which statement, by the client, would indicate proper knowledge of stump and prosthetic leg care?
1. "I inspect my stump weekly to look for signs of redness, blistering, or abrasions."
2. "I put my prosthesis on before I get out of bed."
3. "I wash the stump every day with an antiseptic soap."
4. "I wipe out the socket of my prosthesis with a damp, soapy cloth weekly."

138. 2. The prosthesis should be applied upon rising in the morning. The stump and prosthesis should be inspected, cleaned and washed with a mild soap daily. The prosthesis should be kept clean to prevent irritation or pressure caused by dirt or bacteria.
CN: Health promotion and maintenance; CNS: None; CL: Analyze

139. A nurse is caring for a client using a continuous passive motion (CPM) machine after a total knee replacement. Which action is one of the nurse's responsibilities?
1. Check the cycle and range-of-motion settings every morning
2. Increase the degrees of flexion daily, guided by the client's level of tolerance
3. Decrease the degree of extension daily
4. Turn the machine off when the client is eating a meal

139. 4. The CPM machine can be turned off during meals to improve client comfort. The cycle and degrees of flexion should be checked every shift, and either the health care provider or physical therapist determines how and when the degrees of flexion can be increased. Usually, extension, as well as flexion, are increased on a regular basis.
CN: Physiological integrity; CNS: Basic care and comfort; CL: Apply

CN: Client needs category   CNS: Client needs subcategory   CL: Cognitive level

140. Which action should alert the nurse that a client, diagnosed with multiple myeloma, may be having difficulty coping with his prognosis?
1. The client becomes tearful when discussing this condition.
2. The client asks questions about the prognosis.
3. The client shows concerns about their family.
4. The client avoids any conversation concerning their health.

140. 4. A client who avoids conversation about their health may be denying their condition and not coping well with the prognosis. Crying is a normal response to this disease. Asking questions about the prognosis and showing concern for family are normal coping responses.
CN: Psychological integrity; CNS: None; CL: Analyze

141. Which client is **most** likely to develop ankylosing spondylitis?
1. White female, age 16, with knee pain
2. Black male, age 50, with hip pain
3. Asian female, age 70, with chest pain
4. White male, age 23, with back pain

141. 4. Ankylosing spondylitis usually begins between ages 15 and 30 years, and the prevalence is highest in white males. Back pain is the characteristic feature.
CN: Health promotion and maintenance; CNS: None; CL: Analyze

142. After undergoing a gastrectomy, a client develops pernicious anemia. Which route should the nurse use to administer cyanocobalamin (vitamin B_{12})?
1. Buccal route
2. Transdermal route
3. Oral route
4. Parenteral route

142. 4. A client who has undergone gastrectomy is no longer able to produce the intrinsic factor necessary for vitamin B_{12} absorption through the gastrointestinal tract; therefore, supplementation via parenteral route is required. This medication isn't available for buccal or transdermal routes.
CN: Physiological integrity; CNS: Pharmacological and parenteral therapies; CL: Apply

143. The nurse has just completed teaching a client with diverticular disease about dietary changes. The nurse determines further teaching is needed when the client's lunch selection includes which food choices?
1. Tossed salad with tomatoes, sunflower seeds, and tuna
2. Egg salad on whole-wheat bread and an apple
3. Cottage cheese with apple, pear, and plum slices
4. Ham salad served with whole-wheat crackers and a banana

143. 1. Clients with diverticular disease should avoid high-roughage foods, such as nuts, seeds, popcorn, and raw celery. They should consume high-fiber foods, such as fresh fruit with skins on, bananas, dried fruits, whole-wheat bread and crackers, and raw vegetables.
CN: Physiological integrity; CNS: Basic care and comfort; CL: Apply

144. A nurse is teaching a community group about maintaining a healthy liver. Which measure should the nurse include in the teaching?
1. Take over-the-counter medication as needed
2. Take prescribed medications according to instructions
3. Add a nutritional supplement to the diet to ensure adequate nutrition
4. Consume a low-protein diet that contains moderate carbohydrate and fat

144. 2. Prescribed medications should be taken as directed. Over the counter medications that could damage the liver should be avoided. A balanced diet that's moderate to high in protein, moderate in carbohydrate and fat, and adequate in vitamins should be consumed. A nutritional supplement should only be taken if advised to do so by a health care provider.
CN: Health promotion and maintenance; CNS: None; CL: Apply

CN: Client needs category   CNS: Client needs subcategory   CL: Cognitive level

145. Admission assessment data for a client on the telemetry unit includes the following:

Assessment data	
10/15/16	Reports of racing heart and nervousness
1415	that have occurred several times before.
	Telemetry monitor: sinus tachycardia
	Heart rate: 130 bpm
	Skin: warm and dry
	Eyes: appear bulging

What is the most important initial nursing action?

1. Inserting a urinary catheter and assessing appearance of urine
2. Observing the client's gait and speech
3. Palpating the client's neck
4. Standing behind the client and gently palpating the cricothyroid area

146. A client has not taken her prescribed levothyroxine for some time. She states, "I've been getting sicker by the day." Which symptom is **most** likely related to not taking this medication?
1. Diarrhea and vomiting
2. Rapid heart rate
3. Warm, dry, flushed skin
4. Tympanic temperature of 94° F (34.4° C)

147. A child with chronic renal failure is scheduled for hemodialysis with an external shunt three times per week. What is the **most** important information for the nurse to give this family at discharge?
1. Inspect the site daily for symptoms of redness
2. Wash the serum at the shunt site with normal saline
3. Assess the child's blood pressure on the same side as the shunt
4. Keep a clean dressing in place over the shunt site

148. A 17-year-old client tells the nurse that she has vulvar itching and a thick, whitish, vaginal discharge. The nurse anticipates treating this client with:
1. metronidazole.
2. erythromycin.
3. miconazole.
4. amoxicillin.

145. 4. This client shows signs of hyperthyroidism. Standing behind him and palpating the cricothyroid area is the correct way to assess for an enlarged thyroid gland. Inserting a catheter isn't necessary. Assessing the client's urine, which would be concentrated because of dehydration, can be done after he voids. Observing the client's gait isn't necessary at this time.
CN: Physiological integrity; CNS: Physiological adaptation; CL: Analyze

146. 4. Hypothyroidism leads to a hypodynamic state, so a low body temperature is expected after the levothyroxine has been metabolized. Each of the other symptoms is indicative of a hypermetabolic state, and, although the client may exhibit these problems, they're probably related to infection and dehydration.
CN: Physiological integrity; CNS: Physiological adaptation; CL: Apply

147. 1. The child and parents should assess the shunt site for redness daily because a color change may indicate infection. Serum at the shunt site should be washed away with half-strength hydrogen peroxide, and then an antibiotic ointment and sterile dressing should be applied. Blood pressure shouldn't be taken in the arm with the shunt.
CN: Safe, effective care environment; CNS: Safety and infection control; CL: Apply

148. 3. The client most likely has candidiasis, which produces a thick, whitish vaginal discharge, and is treated with miconazole or nystatin. Metronidazole is used to treat Trichomonas vaginalis. Erythromycin, amoxicillin, or other antibiotic therapy can contribute to candidiasis, and isn't used to treat this fungal infection.
CN: Physiological integrity; CNS: Pharmacological and parenteral therapies; CL: Apply

CN: Client needs category   CNS: Client needs subcategory   CL: Cognitive level

149. Which finding would prompt a nurse to notify the healthcare provider when assessing a five-hour-old neonate born via vaginal delivery?
1. Color is dusky, axillary temperature is 96.8° F (37° C), and the baby is spitting up mucus
2. Hands and feet are cyanotic, abdomen is rounded, and the infant hasn't voided or passed meconium
3. Anterior fontanel is 3/4-in (2 cm) wide, head is molded, and sutures are overriding
4. Irregular abdominal respirations and intermittent tremors in the extremities are present

149. 1. The neonate's skin color should be pink tinged or ruddy, and saliva should be scant. The normal axillary temperature should range from 97.7° to 98.6° F (36.5° to 37° C). Acrocyanosis may be present for 2 to 6 hours. The neonate should pass meconium within 24 hours. Overriding sutures and molding may persist for a few days. Neonatal tremors are normal; however, they must be evaluated to rule out seizures.
CN: Safe, effective care environment; CNS: Management of care; CL: Analyze

150. A mother calls the pediatrician because there's an outbreak of scabies at her child's school. The nurse would teach the mother to check for:
1. pain, erythema, and edema at the site of the bite.
2. oval white dots that adhere to hair shafts.
3. diffuse pruritic wheals.
4. raised skin areas and lines on the finger and toe webs.

150. 4. The mother should check her child for pruritic papules, vesicles, and linear burrows on the finger and toe webs. Oval white dots that adhere to the hair shaft can indicate head lice.
CN: Safe, effective care environment; CNS: Safety and infection control; CL: Apply

151. The school nurse assesses a young child with a raised rash that has circumscribed areas filled with fluid. The nurse documents this finding as a:
1. vesicular rash.
2. papular rash.
3. macular rash.
4. petechial rash.

151. 1. A vesicular rash contains small, raised, circumscribed lesions filled with clear fluid. A papular rash contains raised solid lesions with color changes in circumscribed areas. A macular rash is flat with color changes in circumscribed areas. Petechiae are pinpoint purple or red spots on the skin caused by multiple hemorrhages.
CN: Safe, effective care environment; CNS: Safety and infection control; CL: Apply

152. A 20-month-old toddler has been treated with permethrin for scabies. The toddler's mother asks, "Is this medication working? My child is still itching." Which response, by a nurse, is **most** appropriate?
1. Stop treatment because the drug isn't safe for children under age two.
2. Pruritus can be present for weeks after treatment.
3. Apply the drug every day until the rash and itching disappear.
4. Pruritus is common in children under age five treated with permethrin.

152. 2. Pruritus may be present for weeks following treatment with permethrin. The drug is safe for use in infants as young as age two months. Treatment with permethrin can be safely repeated in two weeks. Pruritus is caused by secondary reactions of the mites.
CN: Physiological integrity; CNS: Pharmacological and parenteral therapies; CL: Apply

153. An eight-year-old child was sent home after the school reported the presence of head lice. Which information is **most** helpful to the parents?
1. The child should remain isolated for one week following treatment.
2. Lindane is the treatment of choice for head lice.
3. Treatment with a pediculicide followed by removing the nits with a fine-tooth comb.
4. The only way to get rid of head lice is to cut the hair.

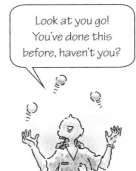

Look at you go! You've done this before, haven't you?

153. 3. Treatment with a pediculicide, followed by removing the nits with a fine-tooth comb will usually kill all lice and remove the nits. Retreatment in 7 to 10 days may be necessary to kill newly-hatched lice. After the infestation has been appropriately treated, there's no reason to isolate the child. Lindane isn't the drug of choice because of its potential for neurotoxicity. The hair should be cut in severe cases only.
CN: Safe, effective care environment; CNS: Safety and infection control; CL: Apply

154. Which should the nurse assess prior to administering disulfiram to a client with a history of alcohol abuse?
1. The client's commitment to attend Alcoholics Anonymous (AA) meetings
2. Whether the client admits to a problem with alcohol
3. When the client's last alcoholic beverage was consumed
4. The client's nutritional status

154. 3. The client must be alcohol free for 12 hours before starting therapy with disulfiram. Assessing the client's commitment to attend AA meetings, the client's perception of his problem, and nutritional status are all important interventions, but they aren't necessary prior to starting disulfiram.
CN: Physiological integrity; CNS: Pharmacological and parenteral therapies; CL: Apply

155. The nurse is assessing a schizophrenic client who exhibits negativism, rigidity, excitement, stupor, and posturing. Which type of schizophrenia would the nurse suspect?
1. Catatonic
2. Undifferentiated
3. Disorganized
4. Paranoid

155. 1. Catatonic schizophrenia is a state of psychologically-induced immobilization, which can be interrupted by episodes of extreme agitation, such as negativism, rigidity, excitement, stupor, or posturing. Undifferentiated schizophrenia occurs when no single clinical presentation dominates. Disorganized schizophrenia is characterized by disorganized speech, disorganized behavior, and inappropriate affect. The dominant theme in paranoid schizophrenia is one of delusions and hallucinations.
CN: Psychosocial integrity; CNS: None; CL: Apply

156. Which statement is an example of a **key** element in a nursing care plan?
1. Advance diet to regular as tolerated
2. Ambulate 30 feet (9.1 m) with walker by discharge
3. Administer furosemide 40 milligrams IV now
4. Discontinue IV fluids when tolerating oral fluids

156. 2. A key element of a nursing care plan is a measurable expected outcome or goal. Other key elements include a nursing diagnoses and planned interventions. The other options are the health care provider's orders, not key elements of nursing care plans.
CN: Safe, effective care environment; CNS: Management of care; CL: Apply

157. A client reports chronic lower back pain and fatigue, and has been seen by multiple care providers without relief of symptoms. The client insists that something is terribly wrong. Which action should the nurse take **first**?
1. Refer the client for a psychiatric evaluation
2. Initiate group therapy for behavior modification
3. Obtain a thorough health assessment to rule out physical illnesses
4. Refer the client to physical therapy

157. 3. The first action by the nurse should be to take a thorough health assessment including laboratory studies to rule out physical illnesses. The other actions aren't appropriate until a diagnosis is made.
CN: Safe, effective care environment; CNS: Management of care; CL: Analyze

CN: Client needs category   CNS: Client needs subcategory   CL: Cognitive level

158. Which physical assessment data would alert the nurse to a possible mild toxic reaction in a client receiving lithium?
  1. Vomiting and diarrhea
  2. Hypertension
  3. Seizures
  4. Increased appetite

158. **1.** Vomiting and diarrhea are signs of mild to moderate lithium toxicity. Hypotension and seizures occur with moderate to severe toxic reactions. Anorexia occurs with mild toxic reactions.
CN: Physiological integrity; CNS: Pharmacological and parenteral therapies; CL: Apply

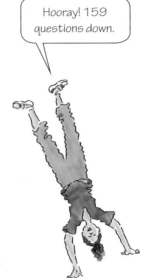

Hooray! 159 questions down.

159. A client with bipolar disorder is taking lithium and tells the nurse, "I can stop taking the medicine when I feel better." What is the nurse's **best** response?
  1. "That's correct. When you feel better, you can stop taking the medication."
  2. "Take the medication for one week after you feel better to be sure there's enough medication in your system."
  3. "You must take the medication as prescribed to prevent relapses."
  4. "This medication is given as needed. That means that you can take it when you feel that you need it."

159. **3.** Lithium, which helps clients with bipolar disorder stabilize their mood swings, is a long-term treatment. Blood measurements are taken regularly to monitor lithium levels in the client's body. The client shouldn't stop taking lithium when he feels better because the therapeutic blood level will decrease. Stopping the medication one week after the client feels better, or taking it as needed, will also decrease the therapeutic level of lithium.
CN: Physiological integrity; CNS: Pharmacological and parenteral therapies; CL: Analyze

160. A client's condition is stabilizing after an episode of substance-induced delirium. For which psychosocial health problem should the nurse assess during the **initial** recovery period?
  1. Flashbacks
  2. Depression
  3. Nightmares
  4. Dissociation

160. **2.** Depression and anxiety are common mental health problems seen immediately after substance withdrawal. Flashbacks and nightmares are commonly observed in clients with posttraumatic stress disorder. Dissociation occurs when a client undergoes prolonged physical and sexual abuse.
CN: Psychosocial integrity; CNS: None; CL: Analyze

161. A client with a history of depression demonstrates inconsistent symptoms of cognitive impairment that looks like dementia. The client is diagnosed with pseudodementia. What outcome would the nurse anticipate from the treatment of this depression?
  1. Delusional thinking ceases
  2. Recognition of objects improves
  3. Memory problems resolve
  4. Suicidal ideation is no longer a problem

161. **3.** Pseudodementia is a situation where a person who has depression also has cognitive impairment that looks like dementia. In this condition, a client treated for depression will have a dramatic improvement in memory. Delusional thinking and object recognition aren't characteristic of pseudodementia. The nurse must assess all clients with depression for suicidal ideation because they're at some degree of risk for suicide.
CN: Psychosocial integrity; CNS: None; CL: Analyze

162. A client with borderline personality disorder has extreme views of himself and his situation. Which behavior would indicate that the client is a candidate for medication?
  1. Disorientation
  2. Hyperactivity
  3. Regression
  4. Mood swings

162. **4.** Medications aren't typically given to clients with personality disorders. However, clients with mood swings, hallucinations, or psychotic behaviors are appropriate candidates for medications. Disorientation, hyperactivity, and regression aren't necessarily seen in clients with borderline personality disorders.
CN: Psychosocial integrity; CNS: None; CL: Apply

CN: Client needs category   CNS: Client needs subcategory   CL: Cognitive level

163. A client has traits of an avoidant personality disorder. Which intervention, for the client's family, should the nurse give **priority**?
1. Explain that they should teach the client social skills
2. Recommend that they recognize the client's high sensitivity to criticism
3. Explore ways to help the client express true feelings
4. Ask them to keep a daily log of the client's adjustment difficulties

163. **2.** A client with traits of an avoidant personality disorder is very sensitive to criticism and disapproval, but doesn't typically have problems with learning or social skills. Such a client may have difficulty expressing feelings, and may have few friends or only family members for interaction. Having the family keep a log of the client's adjustment difficulties isn't an appropriate intervention. The log may be interpreted as a statement of rejection.
CN: Safe, effective care environment; CNS: Management of care; CL: Analyze

164. A client with a substance use disorder reports that the problem doesn't really exist. What is the nurse's **priority** intervention?
1. Educating about the principles of mental health
2. Examining the use of defense mechanisms
3. Recognizing and discussing feelings of resentment
4. Discussing the need for a caretaker while in recovery

164. **2.** Defense mechanisms contribute to the client's denial. Education won't be well received unless the client recognizes the problem and determines that the nurse's teaching would be useful. The client can't recognize and discuss feelings of resentment when denying that a problem exists. The client needs to become responsible for his own behavior and take care of himself.
CN: Psychosocial integrity; CNS: None; CL: Apply

165. A nurse is evaluating the effectiveness of drug therapy for a client undergoing alcohol detoxification. Which finding would indicate that this client's drug therapy needs to be adjusted?
1. There are signs of toxicity from the drug.
2. There are signs that the drug has prevented the occurrence of further problems.
3. The client has tolerated dosage increase during treatment.
4. The medication has allowed the client to have appropriate interactions with staff.

165. **1.** If signs of toxicity exist during the detoxification period, drug therapy needs to be adjusted. Drug therapy is effective if it prevents further problems. Medication dosage may require adjustment to obtain the maximum benefit. If the drug enables the client to have therapeutic interactions with the staff, the client is benefiting from the therapy.
CN: Physiological integrity; CNS: Pharmacological and parenteral therapies; CL: Apply

166. A nurse explains the unit's rules to a client with bulimia nervosa. Which action, by the client, indicates an understanding of the rules?
1. The client asks to be accompanied to the bathroom after lunch.
2. The client writes down every food item eaten in the past 24 hours.
3. The client decides to help the dietitian plan the unit's meals.
4. The client discusses current problems with the nurse before mealtime.

166. **1.** When the client asks to be accompanied to the bathroom after a meal, the client is following the unit's protocol for restoring healthy eating, and indicates the client's commitment to not purging after a meal. Recording the food eaten in a 24-hour period would be appropriate for a client with anorexia nervosa, not a client with bulimia nervosa. It's inappropriate for a client to plan meals for the unit's clients. The client can discuss problems any time, not just before mealtimes.
CN: Psychosocial integrity; CNS: None; CL: Analyze

167. A nurse is teaching a client with an eating disorder about cues that trigger unhealthy eating behaviors. The nurse includes which example of a social cue?
1. Diet advertisements
2. Troublesome memories
3. Interpersonal conflict
4. Frustration fatigue

167. **3.** Social cues that trigger maladaptive behavior include feelings of isolation and conflict with family or friends. Diet advertisements are considered situational cues. Troublesome memories are psychological cues. Frustration fatigue is an example of a physiological cue.
CN: Psychosocial integrity; CNS: None; CL: Apply

CN: Client needs category   CNS: Client needs subcategory   CL: Cognitive level

168. A schizophrenic client states, "The voices keep talking to me. They're telling me that I have to leave here, and that I shouldn't talk to you. Don't you hear what they're saying?" Which is the nurse's **best** response?
1. "Did you take your medicine this morning?"
2. "The voices you hear aren't real, and are a part of your illness."
3. "Are you hearing voices again?"
4. "I don't hear the voices, but can I see that you are upset."

168. 4. The nurse should tell the client that she doesn't hear the voices while acknowledging the client's feelings. Asking if the client took his medication, or explaining that this symptom is part of his illness minimizes the client's feelings. The client explained that he is hearing voices, and should not be asked something that he's already explained.
CN: Psychosocial integrity; CNS: None; CL: Apply

169. The nurse is teaching caregivers which signs and symptoms of schizophrenia should be reported to a mental health professional. Which signs and symptoms should be reported?
1. Changes in appetite resulting in weight loss or gain
2. Loss of interest in sexual activities
3. Increased socialization
4. Difficulty sleeping

169. 4. Signs and symptoms of schizophrenia relapse include difficulty concentrating and sleeping, a feeling of tension, an increase in bizarre thinking and withdrawal. People with schizophrenia can have delusions that are quite bizarre, such as believing that neighbors can control their behavior with magnetic waves, people on television are directing special messages to them, or radio stations are broadcasting their thoughts aloud to others. They may also have delusions of grandeur and think they are famous historical figures. The other choices aren't signs and symptoms of schizophrenia.
CN: Psychosocial integrity; CNS: None; CL: Analyze

170. A client with schizophrenia has been prescribed risperidone. The client's symptoms include hallucinations, delusions, and withdrawal. The nurse should explain that this medication will help improve which symptoms?
1. Negative symptoms only
2. Positive symptoms only
3. Negative and positive symptoms
4. Paranoid symptoms

170. 3. Risperidone targets both negative and positive symptoms. Positive symptoms include delusions, hallucinations, and bizarre behaviors. Negative symptoms indicate a loss or lack of normal functioning such as lack of motivation and social withdrawal.
CN: Physiological integrity; CNS: Pharmacological and parenteral therapies; CL: Apply

171. A new graduate nurse is caring for a client recently diagnosed with dissociative identity disorder. The new graduate nurse asks the preceptor how to discuss the client's traumatic childhood with the client. Which advice, from the preceptor, is **best**?
1. Ask pointed questions and demand specific answers
2. Listen and be supportive of the client's explanation
3. Tell the client that you suspect much of his memory regarding childhood is exaggerated
4. Tell the client that traumatic childhood issues should only be discussed with a health care provider

171. 2. The client will discuss this painful subject when he feels comfortable and ready. Forcing the client to talk about the subject will cause severe anxiety and distrust. The other choices don't facilitate a trusting relationship between the nurse and the client.
CN: Safe, effective care environment; CNS: Management of care; CL: Apply

172. A client with dissociative identity disorder frequently switches from one personality to another. How can the nurse **best** identify a switch in personalities?
1. Episodes of orthostatic hypotension
2. Blinking eyes frequently
3. Dystonic reactions
4. Episodes of tachycardia

172. 2. Switching from one personality to another is evident in a number of ways including blinking, facial movements, and changes in voice. Changes in blood pressure or pulse or dystonic reactions aren't indicative of switching from one personality to another.
CN: Psychosocial integrity; CNS: None; CL: Apply

173. A 38-year-old female client, who is scheduled to have a hysterectomy, is concerned about no longer being a "whole" woman. What is the nurse's **best** intervention?
1. Advise the client to explain the new physiological changes in her body with her husband
2. Refer the client to group therapy
3. Encourage the client to discuss her concerns and feelings about the surgery
4. Provide printed information for the client to read regarding her surgery

173. 3. The nurse should encourage this client to express her feelings. Telling her to talk to her husband will cause increased concern and anxiety. Referring her to group therapy isn't an appropriate intervention at this time. Giving her information, then leaving the room doesn't allow for questions or dialog between the client and the nurse.
CN: Psychosocial integrity; CNS: None; CL: Analyze

174. A 23-year-old female client is seen in the emergency department for sexual assault. The woman appears emotionally unaffected by the event and very calm. Which assessment, of this client's behavior, is **most** appropriate?
1. The client is telling a falsehood, and is trying to frame the perpetrator.
2. The client was a willing participant in the sexual act.
3. The client's calm demeanor is masking her distress, denial and emotional shock.
4. The client is trying to claim an existing pregnancy is the result of this assault.

174. 3. One of the immediate reactions to sexual assault is deceptive calmness. This behavior usually masks emotional shock, denial, or distress. The other responses are judgmental opinions. Nurses should remain nonjudgmental in providing care.
CN: Psychosocial integrity; CNS: None; CL: Analyze

175. A full-term neonate was just admitted to the transitional nursery. The newborn has a large meningomyelocele covered by an intact sac. The nurse immediately places the neonate in a prone position with her hips slightly elevated. Which statement **best** describes the rationale for this position?
1. To prevent the sac covering the defect from rupturing
2. To preserve urine and bowel control
3. To assess neurological functioning more easily
4. To prevent further neurological damage

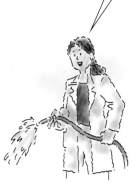

Don't get hosed by this question. Take your time and read it carefully.

175. 1. The damage to the neurological system happened in utero, and the nurse should prevent further damage by placing the infant in a side-lying or prone position until after surgery to prevent sac rupture The sac covering the defect is the only barrier preventing bacteria from directly entering the neonate's central nervous system and causing meningitis and encephalitis. A large defect will result in loss of urine and bowel control.
CN: Physiological integrity; CNS: Reduction of risk potential; CL: Analyze

CN: Client needs category   CNS: Client needs subcategory   CL: Cognitive level

176. The nurse is teaching the mother of a neonate born with a cleft palate how to feed her child. Which instruction should the nurse give this mother?
  1. Feed the neonate in a semi-reclining position with his head resting on the curve of the mother's elbow
  2. Feed the neonate in an upright position
  3. Feed the neonate lying on his stomach with his head turned toward the mother
  4. Feed the neonate in any position in which the mother and child are comfortable

176. 2. The neonate with a cleft palate should be fed in an upright position. Incorrect feeding can allow formula to slip through the palate opening, and enter the upper respiratory tract and lungs, causing aspiration pneumonia. Any of the other positions place the neonate at risk for aspiration pneumonia.
CN: Physiological integrity; CNS: Reduction of risk potential; CL: Analyze

177. A nurse is observing a group of school-age children playing. Which toy is **most** appropriate for this age group?
  1. Barbie dolls
  2. Game of Operation
  3. Game of solitaire
  4. Hot Wheels cars

177. 2. School-age children will engage in competitive play with established rules and goals. The game of Operation® is an example of play that uses simple rules with an established goal. Playing with Barbie® dolls exemplifies associative play. Solitary play of card games is preferred by adolescents. Playing with Hot Wheels® cars is more exemplary of toddlers' parallel play.
CN: Health promotion and maintenance; CNS: None; CL: Apply

178. A nurse is assessing an infant's growth and development. Which action, by the nurse, would promote appropriate growth and development for a four month old?
  1. Eliciting a social smile
  2. Allowing the infant to hold his own bottle
  3. Playing peekaboo with the infant
  4. Letting the infant sit without support

178. 1. A social smile should be seen in a four-month old. An infant cannot hold his own bottle until age 6 to 7 months. The child should engage in peekaboo activities at age 10 to 12 months, and sit without support at eight months of age.
CN: Health promotion and maintenance; CNS: None; CL: Apply

179. The nurse is caring for an 11-year-old client, with cerebral palsy, who has a pressure ulcer on the sacrum. When teaching the client's mother about dietary intake, which foods should the nurse plan to emphasize?
  1. Legumes and cheese
  2. Whole-grain products
  3. Fruits and vegetables
  4. Lean meats and low-fat milk

179. 4. Although this client should eat a balanced diet with foods from all food groups, the diet should emphasize complete protein, such as lean meats and low-fat milk. Protein helps repair body tissue, and promotes healing. Legumes provide incomplete protein. Cheese contains complete protein but also fat, which should be limited to 30% or less of total caloric intake. Whole-grain products supply incomplete proteins and carbohydrates. Fruits and vegetables mainly provide carbohydrates.
CN: Physiological integrity; CNS: Basic care and comfort; CL: Apply

180. A client has just been diagnosed with pneumonia. What is the nurse's **priority** action?
1. Reverse fluid volume excess
2. Maintain airway clearance
3. Incrementally increase activity tolerance
4. Provide information about how to avoid a recurrence

180. **2.** Pneumonia refers to inflammation of the lungs and can produce copious amounts of tracheobronchial secretions. These secretions interfere with airway patency and gas exchange. Airway clearance is a priority. The client may experience decreased fluid volume, not an excess, due to increased temperature and respiratory rate. The client may also experience activity intolerance and deficient knowledge, but neither is the priority diagnosis.

CN: Safe, effective care environment; CNS: Management of care; CL: Analyze

181. A nurse is caring for a client in active labor. Which observation would cause the nurse to suspect fetal distress?
1. Fetal heart rate of 144 bpm
2. Accelerations of the fetal heart rate with contractions
3. Fetal scalp pH of 7.14
4. Presence of long-term variability

181. **3.** A scalp pH below 7.25 indicates acidosis and fetal hypoxia. A fetal heart rate of 144 bpm, acceleration of the fetal heartbeat with contractions, and the presence of long-term variability with contractions are normal responses of a healthy fetus to labor.

CN: Health promotion and maintenance; CNS: None; CL: Apply

182. During a routine examination, the mother of a three-month-old child asks the nurse, "When will she get her first tooth?" Which response, by the nurse, is **most** accurate?
1. Four months
2. Five months
3. Six months
4. Seven month

182. **3.** The first tooth typically erupts at age six months, although some infants do get their first tooth when a little younger or older.

CN: Health promotion and maintenance; CNS: None; CL: Apply

183. A nurse assesses an 18-month-old toddler. Which activity would indicate, to the nurse, that the child is exhibiting normal growth and development patterns?
1. Running and jumping in place
2. Jumping down from a chair
3. Naming a specific color
4. Saying his full name

183. **1.** An 18-month-old child should be able to run and jump in place. Typically, a child of 30 months is able to jump down from a chair, can name one color, and knows his full name.

CN: Health promotion and maintenance; CNS: None; CL: Apply

184. A mother was diagnosed with polyhydramnios during her pregnancy, and just delivered a preterm male neonate. How should the nurse assess a neonate for tracheoesophageal atresia?
1. Observe the neonate during the first formula feeding for difficulties in swallowing
2. Determine if cyanosis of the extremities and mouth are present at birth
3. Attempt to insert a catheter from the mouth through the esophagus to the stomach
4. Assess lung sounds to determine if possible pneumonia is present

184. **3.** Esophageal atresia is present if a catheter can't be passed through the neonate's mouth to the stomach. A barium swallow or a bronchial endoscopy examination will reveal the blind-end esophagus. The condition should be diagnosed before the infant is fed; otherwise, the infant will be unable to retain the feeding. If a tracheoesophageal fistula is present, the infant may choke, or gag, and become cyanotic during feeding. Immediately after birth, pneumonia should not be present if the infant has an esophageal atresia with a tracheoesophageal fistula. Emergency surgery will be essential to create a patent gastrointestinal tract.

CN: Health promotion and maintenance; CNS: None; CL: Analyze

CN: Client needs category   CNS: Client needs subcategory   CL: Cognitive level

185. Which instruction should the nurse include in the care plan for a client following total hip replacement?
1. Keeping the legs adducted
2. Avoid bending at the hip more than 90 degrees
3. Keeping the hips lower than the knees when seated
4. Teaching how to bend forward to put on socks and shoes

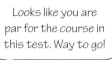

Looks like you are par for the course in this test. Way to go!

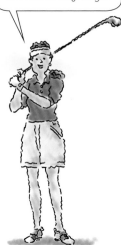

185. 2. Following total hip replacement, the client should be instructed to avoid bending more than 90 degrees at the hip. The legs should be kept abducted to prevent dislocation of the prosthesis. The hips should be kept higher than the knees when seated to minimize hip flexion. The client should be instructed not to bend forward at the hip to put on shoes and socks. Assistive devices can be used to help the client safely dress below the waist.
CN: Physiological integrity; CNS: Reduction of risk potential; CL: Apply

186. The nurse reviews the arterial blood gas results of a client with asthma. The nurse is aware that the client's partial pressure of arterial oxygen (PaO$_2$) result will provide information about:
1. respiratory status.
2. the degree of dyspnea.
3. efficiency of gas exchange.
4. effectiveness of ventilation.

186. 3. The PaO$_2$ reflects the gas exchange ventilation and perfusion. It doesn't measure the respiratory status, degree of dyspnea, or effectiveness of ventilation.
CN: Physiological integrity; CNS: Reduction of risk potential; CL: Apply

187. What is the **most** common cause of myocarditis?
1. Bacteria
2. Parasite
3. Fungus
4. Virus

187. 4. Myocarditis is usually caused by a virus. Coxsackie viruses and echoviruses are the most common agents. Bacteria, parasites, and fungi may cause myocarditis, but aren't the most common causes.
CN: Physiological integrity; CNS: Physiological adaptation; CL: Remember

188. A nurse is caring for a seven-year-old client receiving cyclophosphamide. In addition to administering mesna, which action should the nurse take?
1. Transfuse platelets before administering the drug
2. Give the child cranberry juice to drink
3. Encourage the child to void frequently
4. Limit the child's fluid intake

188. 3. Hemorrhagic cystitis can result when the by-products of cyclophosphamide metabolism remain in the bladder; therefore, emptying the bladder at least every two hours, when the child is awake, can help prevent this painful condition. The child should be encouraged to void as soon as the urge is felt. Bacteria or low platelets do not cause the condition, so transfusing platelets and giving cranberry juice aren't correct. Fluids should not be limited. The child should be given liberal amounts of fluid, usually by IV infusion.
CN: Physiological integrity; CNS: Pharmacological and parenteral therapies; CL: Analyze

189. Protective isolation is not required for a child receiving chemotherapy. Which activity should the nurse plan for this child during treatment?
1. Bed rest
2. Activity as tolerated
3. Walk to bathroom only
4. Out of bed only to shower

189. 2. Children receiving chemotherapy should be able to engage in activities of interest and maintain as much independence and autonomy as possible. They should limit their activity when feeling tired or ill. Limiting activities to bed rest, walking to bathroom only, or only out of bed for brief periods isn't necessary, and restricts activity unnecessarily. Children should be included in care planning whenever possible. These children should avoid adults and other children with infections.
CN: Health promotion and maintenance; CNS: None; CL: Apply

190. A child is intubated and placed on a ventilator after a near drowning. The health care provider's order is to suction every three to four hours. The child's parents ask the nurse why the suctioning is necessary. Which response, by the nurse, is the **most** accurate?
1. To keep the client free of infection
2. To keep the client from experiencing cardiac arrhythmias
3. To keep the client's airway patent
4. To maintain fluid and electrolyte balance

191. A child with cystic fibrosis has been prescribed a bronchodilator, steroids by metered-dose inhaler, and chest physiotherapy. Prioritize the administration of these medications and treatments.

| 1. Perform chest physiotherapy |
| 2. Administer the bronchodilator |
| 3. Administer the steroid |
| 4. Let the client eat lunch |

192. A nurse is teaching a student nurse about a ketogenic diet. The nurse knows that a ketogenic diet is sometimes used to treat:
1. Anorexia nervosa
2. Nephrotic syndrome
3. Epilepsy
4. Ulcerative colitis

193. A child is unable to walk without assistance because of decreased oxygen at birth. Which disorder is characterized by a malfunction of the brain's motor center caused by hypoxia?
1. Down syndrome
2. Cerebral palsy
3. Sickle cell anemia
4. Osteogenesis imperfect

194. A 17-year-old client, who injured his right knee during a basketball game, is scheduled for an arthroscopy. The nurse is teaching the client about this procedure. Which response, about arthroscopy, would be accurate?
1. Taking an X-ray with a contrast medium
2. Visualizing of the joint with a small instrument
3. Inserting a needle and withdrawing fluid for biopsy
4. Aspirating synovial fluid from the bursa

190. 3. Because of the increased secretions from drowning, the airway is more prone to obstruction, and suctioning is essential to maintain patency. Suctioning won't prevent infection and may increase the risk. Suctioning can cause bradycardia; therefore, pre-oxygenation is essential to prevent arrhythmias. Suctioning doesn't affect fluid and electrolyte balance.
CN: Physiological integrity; CNS: Reduction of risk potential; CL: Apply

191. Ordered Response:

| 2. Administer the bronchodilator first |
| 3. Administer the steroid first |
| 1. Perform chest physiotherapy first |
| 4. Let the client eat lunch |

CN: Physiological integrity; CNS: Pharmacological and parental therapies; CL: Apply

192. 3. A ketogenic diet is typically suggested as a method of treatment for epilepsy. Anorexia nervosa is treated with counseling and by slowly reintroducing food to the diet. Children with nephrotic syndrome are usually on a low-sodium diet. Ulcerative colitis is treated with a low-residue diet.
CN: Physiological integrity; CNS: Reduction of risk potential; CL: Apply

193. 2. Cerebral palsy affects the motor center of the brain and is usually caused by brain trauma. Down syndrome is a chromosomal abnormality. Sickle cell anemia is a genetic disorder of red blood cells. Osteogenesis imperfecta is a congenital anomaly involving decreased calcium in the bones and leads to multiple fractures at birth.
CN: Physiological integrity; CNS: Physiological adaptation; CL: Apply

194. 2. After a small incision is made in the knee, a small tube-shaped instrument is inserted for viewing the knee and surrounding cartilage, tendon, and ligaments. Contrast media are typically used for X-rays of joints. Biopsies are taken if cancer is a concern. Synovial fluid is collected for culture if an infection or inflammation is a concern.
CN: Physiological integrity; CNS: Physiological adaptation; CL: Apply

CN: Client needs category   CNS: Client needs subcategory   CL: Cognitive level

195. A nurse is assessing a 13-year-old boy with a compound fracture of the right arm 12 hours after surgical repair. Which assessment finding requires **immediate** attention?
1. Bruising of the fingers
2. Capillary refill of three seconds
3. Pallor of the nail beds
4. Edema of the extremity

195. 3. Pallor suggests a decrease in circulation to the extremity, and the surgeon should be notified. Bruising is expected with a compound fracture. The fingers should be observed for further discoloration indicating decreased circulation. Capillary refill of three seconds is normal. Edema is expected but should be monitored.
CN: Physiological integrity; CNS: Reduction of risk potential; CL: Apply

196. A three-year-old child has diarrhea, and the pediatrician has recommended the BRAT diet for the next 24 hours. The nurse teaches the parents about the diet. Which response, by the parents, indicates that teaching has been effective?
1. "The diet consists of bran, crispy-rice cereal, apple juice, and tomato juice."
2. "The diet consists of beans, red meat, apples, and tomatoes."
3. "The diet consists of bananas, rice, apple-sauce, and toast."
4. "The diet consists of broccoli, red ice pops, apple butter, and tacos."

196. 3. BRAT is an acronym for bananas, rice, applesauce, and toast. This diet is commonly used for children with diarrhea because these foods add form to the stool without further irritating the bowel. The other diet choices can cause gas, irritation, and inflammation in the already inflamed bowel.
CN: Physiological integrity; CNS: Basic care and comfort; CL: Apply

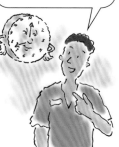

Time for some math. Do you remember how to calculate a drip rate?

197. After undergoing small-bowel resection, a client is prescribed metronidazole 500 mg IV The mixed IV solution contains 100 ml. A nurse is to run the drug over 30 minutes. The drip factor of the available IV tubing is 15 gtt/ml. What is the drip rate? Record your answer using a whole number.

_____ gtt/min

197. 50.
Use the following equation:

$$\frac{100\ ml \times 15\ gtt/ml}{30\ min} = 50\ gtt/min$$

CN: Physiological integrity; CNS: Pharmacological and parenteral therapies; CL: Apply

198. A nurse is caring for a client whose cultural background is different from her own. Which actions are appropriate? Select all that apply.
1. Consider that nonverbal cues, such as eye contact, may have different meanings in different cultures
2. Respect the client's cultural beliefs
3. Ask the client if he has cultural or religious requirements that should be considered in his care
4. Explain your beliefs so that the client will understand the differences
5. Understand that all cultures experience pain in the same way

198. 1, 2, 3. Nonverbal cues may have different meanings in different cultures. In one culture, eye contact is a sign of disrespect. In another culture, eye contact shows respect and attentiveness. The nurse should always respect the client's cultural beliefs, and ask if he has cultural or religious requirements. This may include food choices or restrictions, body coverings, or time for prayer. The nurse should attempt to understand the client's culture. It isn't the client's responsibility to understand the nurse's culture. Culture influences a client's experience of pain.
CN: Psychosocial integrity; CNS: None; CL: Analyze

199. A young adult client received her first chemotherapy treatment for breast cancer. Which statement, if made by the client, requires further assessment by the nurse?
1. "I think I will postpone my dance club practices for now."
2. "I don't think I'm going to work tomorrow."
3. "I don't care about the side effects of the drugs."
4. "I want to return to school for a college degree."

199. 3. Adverse effects of chemotherapy may occur after treatment, and should be discussed with the client because some can be treated, controlled, or prevented. The nurse should explore what the client means by this statement. Joining social clubs is typical behavior for a young adult. The client may feel poorly after chemotherapy and may want to take time off from work until feeling better. Returning to school is also typical of a young adult.
CN: Health promotion and maintenance; CNS: None; CL: Analyze

200. Which assessment finding, by the nurse, would indicate an increased risk for skin cancer in a client?
1. A deep sunburn
2. A small café-au-lait spot on the client's back
3. An irregular scar on the client's abdomen
4. Irregular white patches on the client's arm

200. 1. A deep sunburn is a risk factor for skin cancer. An irregular scar is a benign finding, and café-au-lait spots are suggestive of neurofibromatosis, not cancer. Irregular white patches are abnormal, but aren't a risk factor for skin cancer.
CN: Health promotion and maintenance; CNS: None; CL: Apply

201. An elderly client's husband tells the nurse that he's concerned because his wife insists on talking about events that happened to her in the past. The nurse assesses the client and finds that she's alert, oriented, and answering questions appropriately. What is the nurse's **best** response?
1. "Your wife is reviewing her life."
2. "A spiritual advisor should be notified."
3. "You should not encourage conversations about the past."
4. "Your wife is regressing to a more comfortable time in the past."

201. 1. Life review or reminiscing is characteristic of elderly people and the dying. A spiritual advisor might comfort the client, but isn't necessary for a life review. Discouraging the client from talking would block communication. Regression occurs when a client returns to behaviors typical of another developmental stage.
CN: Health promotion and maintenance; CNS: None; CL: Apply

202. A breastfeeding client asks how she can do breast self-examination (BSE) while nursing. Which response would be the **most** accurate?
1. "You should do BSE after the infant has emptied the breast."
2. "You don't have to do BSE until after you stop breastfeeding."
3. "You should continue to do BSE the way you did before becoming pregnant."
4. "Your health care provider will examine your breasts until after you stop breastfeeding."

202. 1. This client should perform the examination after the neonate has emptied the breast. Women must continue to examine their breasts, even if they're lactating. Breast self-examination should be done on the same day of the month until the menstrual cycle returns. Breast examination shouldn't be done solely by the health care provider.
CN: Health promotion and maintenance; CNS: None; CL: Apply

203. The nurse assesses a client's intake and output at end of the 7 am to 3 pm shift. The recorded intake is as follows: milk, 180 ml; orange juice, 60 ml; 1 serving scrambled eggs; 1 slice toast; 1 can nutritional supplement, 240 ml; IV dextrose 5% in water at 100 ml/hr; 50 ml water after twice daily medications. Medications are given at 9 am and 9 pm. The nurse totals the intake at the end of shift as:

1. 1,000 ml
2. 1,250 ml
3. 1,330 ml
4. 1,305 ml

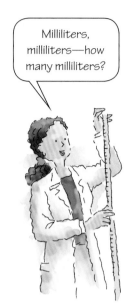

Milliliters, milliliters—how many milliliters?

203. **3.** The client's total intake is 1,330 ml. Use the following equation:

$$180 + 60 + 240 + 800 + 50 = 1,330$$

Eggs and toast do not count towards intake. Only one dose of medication was administered during the shift; 100 ml/hr times the eight hour shift equals 800 ml.

CN: Physiological integrity; CNS: Basic care and comfort; CL: Apply

204. A client is admitted to a mental health unit. While assessing the client, the nurse finds the client exhibiting signs of hyperexcitability, increasing agitation, and distractibility. Based on this assessment, what is the nurse's **priority** intervention?

1. Involve the client in a group activity
2. Be direct and firm and set rules for the client
3. Use a quiet room, away from others, for this client
4. Channel the client's energy toward a planned activity

204. **3.** Being in a quiet environment away from stimuli will help the client regain a sense of control. If the nurse attempts to be firm and set rules for this client, it will most likely heighten the agitation. The client is too excited to focus on group activities or other activities at this time, and it may worsen the client's symptoms.

CN: Psychosocial integrity; CNS: None; CL: Apply

205. A public health nurse, visiting a new postpartum client, notices that the client has two children under age four. The nurse notices that one infant is playing in the cabinet under the sink. Which instruction should the public health nurse give this client?

1. Keep a bottle of ipecac syrup in the house
2. Make sure all liquid cleaners are labeled
3. Tighten all cap tops on the bottles under the sink
4. Safety locks should be placed on cabinets to

205. **4.** Safety locks should be placed on cabinets to prevent young children from opening the cabinets or the bottles. All liquid cleaners must be removed to reduce the risk for poisoning. Infants can't read danger labels. Ipecac is no longer routinely used to induce vomiting in children.

CN: Safe, effective care environment; CNS: Safety and infection control; CL: Apply

206. A school nurse has provided vision and hearing screenings for elementary school children at the beginning of the school year. Later in the year, the nurse offers an immunization clinic during the evening hours. What type of preventions strategy is an immunization clinic?

1. Primary
2. Secondary
3. Tertiary
4. None of the above

206. **1.** Primary prevention strategies are aimed at preventing a disease by avoiding or modifying risk factors. Screening is a secondary prevention strategy aimed at the early detection and treatment of illness. Tertiary prevention strategies focus on rehabilitation and prevention of complications arising from advanced disease.

CN: Health promotion and maintenance; CNS: None; CL: Apply

CN: Client needs category   CNS: Client needs subcategory   CL: Cognitive level

207. A local community health nurse is asked to speak to a group of adolescent girls on the topic of pregnancy prevention. Which statement would indicate that the adolescents need more information on this topic?
  1. "I can get pregnant even on the first time we have sex."
  2. "I can get pregnant even though I don't have sex regularly."
  3. "I can get pregnant only when my menstrual cycle becomes regular."
  4. "I can get pregnant even if my boyfriend withdraws before he ejaculates."

208. A nurse, working in a public health clinic, is planning tuberculosis (TB) screening. Which group is **most** susceptible to TB?
  1. All clients coming into the clinic
  2. People living in a homeless shelter
  3. Clients who haven't received the TB vaccine
  4. Clients suspected of having HIV

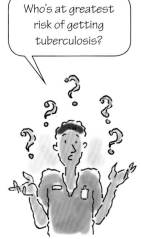

Who's at greatest risk of getting tuberculosis?

209. A public health nurse has obtained a sputum culture from a client. The sputum culture tests positive for tuberculosis (TB). The nurse must report these positive results to the health department within:
  1. 12 hours.
  2. 48 hours.
  3. 1 week.
  4. 10 to 14 days.

210. During an assessment, a home health nurse notices that a client as an unsteady gait. The client tells the nurse that she recently fell. Which action represents an advocacy role for the home health nurse?
  1. Contacting the local church to borrow a walker for the client
  2. Listening to the client express her feelings of frustration over increasing limitations
  3. Instructing the client to contact the senior day care
  4. Reassuring the client that using a walker will prevent falls in the future

207. 3. Many adolescents have misunderstandings related to risk periods and timing, including periods of susceptibility during the menstrual cycle, age-related susceptibility, and timing of male ejaculation.
CN: Health promotion and maintenance; CNS: None; CL: Analyze

208. 4. Clients with HIV infection, or who are suspected of having HIV, are at greater risk for developing TB. A screening test should be done and, if positive, treatment with isoniazid given. Clients coming to the clinic don't need to be tested unless they're at high risk, such as those living with someone infected with TB, IV drug users, or those with chronic health conditions, such as diabetes mellitus and end-stage renal disease. Clients living in a homeless shelter aren't necessarily at greater risk unless other residents in the shelter have TB.
CN: Health promotion and maintenance; CNS: None; CL: Apply

209. 2. The results of this test must be reported to the health department within 24 to 48 hours. The smear or culture may not have grown an organism in 12 hours. One week or 10 to 14 days is too long, and would allow the contagious individual to further spread the disease.
CN: Safe, effective care environment; CNS: Safety and infection control; CL: Analyze

210. 1. A referral to a community agency is an advocacy role for the home health nurse. The role of an advocate includes advising clients on how to find alternate sources of care. Giving emotional support, providing therapies, and instructing clients about other resources are direct care activities. Reassuring a client is superficial, and using a walker does not necessarily prevent falls.
CN: Safe, effective care environment; CNS: Management of care; CL: Apply

211. A nurse at a prenatal clinic is assessing a young pregnant client who exhibits behaviors related to drug and alcohol abuse. Which statement would indicate that this client's child is at high risk of fetal alcohol spectrum disorder?
1. "I just snort once or twice a day."
2. "I was afraid to have one sip of wine with dinner last week."
3. "I drink a six pack of beer daily to settle my nerves."
4. "I smoke marijuana with my boyfriend and his friends."

211. 3. Ingestion of alcohol on a daily basis increases the risk of fetal alcohol spectrum disorder. Other forms of addictive behavior, such as the ingestion of cocaine and smoking marijuana, increase the risk of fetal abuse, not fetal alcohol syndrome.

CN: Health promotion and maintenance; CNS: None; CL: Analyze and apply

212. For which client would a nurse in the public health clinic provide preventive therapy for tuberculosis (TB)?
1. A clients with HIV
2. A client who has had tuberculin skin tests and is at low risk
3. Persons who have had no contact with infectious TB clients
4. A client with an abnormal chest X-ray

212. 1. Preventive therapy should be initiated for clients infected with HIV because latent TB can become active if the immune system is weakened. Clients with low risk and negative skin tests are unlikely to be infected with TB, .Clients who have had no contact with those infected with TB are not at high risk for developing the disease. Although clients with active TB may have abnormal chest X-rays, many other conditions can cause these abnormalities.

CN: Health promotion and maintenance; CNS: None; CL: Apply

213. A nurse is assessing an older adult client in the emergency room and notices that the client is fearful and non-communicative. The nurse suspects that this client is intimidated by the presence of her family members. What is the **most** appropriate nursing intervention?
1. Continue the assessment
2. Be supportive and non-threatening
3. Ask the supervisor to talk to the family
4. Call for the social worker to do a family assessment

213. 2. It is most important to provide emotional support in a non-threatening manner when interacting with a client who may have experienced family violence. It is also important to provide a private, secure environment to establish trust and a therapeutic relationship with this client. Approaches that may be interpreted as threatening, aggressive, or punitive can increase the anxiety for the perpetrator, and increase the risk of violence for the client.

CN: Psychosocial integrity; CNS: None; CL: Apply

214. The mother of a middle school boy tells the school nurse she is concerned because her 13-year-old son is depressed. Which behavior would the nurse anticipate in this boy?
1. Becomes angry at peers easily
2. Seeks out support from peers
3. Eats several small meals daily
4. Feels he can control everything in his life

214. 1. Adolescents experiencing depression may experience and express anger at peers. Adolescents feel a lack of control over their current situation, so they isolate themselves from peers. These adolescents will often have an intake of nutrients insufficient to meet metabolic needs.

CN: Psychosocial integrity; CNS: None; CL: Analyze and apply

215. The home health nurse is visiting a 72-year-old client with severe osteoarthritis. During the visit, the client tells the nurse that his wife died one year ago. Which statement, by the client, requires further intervention?
1. "My children live close but are very busy."
2. "I really don't have anything to live for."
3. "My health isn't very good, and I don't like to have pain."
4. "I relied on my wife to remember where I placed things."

215. 2. Wishing for death is a sign of depression and should alert the nurse to a potential risk for suicide. Most individuals accept the death of their loved ones and begin restoring their lives within a year. Expressing how he is adapting to his health and family situation may be a sign of accepting his new life experiences after the loss of his wife. Memory loss can be a sign of dementia or depression.
CN: Psychosocial integrity; CNS: None; CL: Analyze and apply

216. The nurse is admitting a 35-year-old client, diagnosed with alcohol dependence, to a substance use unit. Which comment, by the client, would the nurse interpret as supportive of this diagnosis?
1. "I don't drink more than two beers when I'm out."
2. "I always remember what happens the next day."
3. "I always ask a friend to drive me home when I'm drinking."
4. "I had four tickets for driving while intoxicated last month."

216. 4. Driving while intoxicated can be seen as a symptom of alcohol dependence. Designating drivers and limiting alcohol consumption don't address the underlying problem. An alcoholic will experience periods of amnesia while intoxicated. A client with alcohol dependence will rationalize their behavior by being responsible, and asking someone to drive them home when their intoxicated.
CN: Psychosocial integrity; CNS: None; CL: Analyze and apply

217. A nurse, on an acute care mental health unit, is caring for a client diagnosed with alcoholism. The client has been referred to Alcoholics Anonymous (AA). Which statement **best** indicates that the client is ready to begin the AA program?
1. "I know I need help since I can't control my drinking."
2. "I think joining AA will be interesting and helpful."
3. "I'd like to sponsor another alcoholic with the same problem."
4. "My family is very supportive and will attend meetings with me."

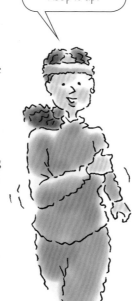

You're covering a lot of ground. Keep it up!

217. 1. In step one of AA, a person admits that he is powerless over alcohol, and ready to accept help. This should occur before he begins AA. A supportive family, and a desire to help others with the same problem are good for the client, but they don't necessarily indicate readiness to participate in the program.
CN: Psychosocial integrity; CNS: None; CL: Apply

218. The psychiatric home health nurse is planning care for a client, recently discharged from a mental health facility, with paranoid schizophrenia. Which nursing action should be included in the plan of care?
1. Confront the client about her hallucinations
2. Ask the minister to provide spiritual direction
3. Instruct family members to discourage delusions
4. Affirm this client's perceptions and thinking when they are in touch with reality

218. 4. The nursing plan of care focuses on reinforcing perceptions and thinking that are in touch with reality. Confronting a client about her hallucinations and delusions isn't effective or therapeutic. Spiritual direction is important, but a client with paranoid schizophrenia may have issues surrounding her religious or spiritual orientation. Asking a minister to provide spiritual direction may not be effective or therapeutic. Using family members could create distrust between the client and the family.
CN: Psychosocial integrity; CNS: None; CL: Apply

CN: Client needs category   CNS: Client needs subcategory   CL: Cognitive level

219. The psychiatric home health nurse is visiting a client with bipolar disorder. The client is swinging rapidly on the porch swing. She is wearing a red polka dot dress, large yellow hat, and heavy makeup with large gold jewelry. The nurse interprets this client's behavior as evidence of:

1. delusions.
2. depression.
3. mania.
4. paranoia.

219. 3. An extremely labile mood is a characteristic of the manic phase of bipolar disorder. Hyperactivity, verbosity, and attention seeking through unusual dress are also typical of the manic phase. Delusions and suspicion may be seen in bipolar disorder, but are more common in schizophrenia. In the depressive phase, clients withdraw, cry, and may not eat. Visual or auditory hallucinations, delusional thoughts, and extreme suspiciousness are behaviors seen in clients with paranoid schizophrenia.
CN: Psychosocial integrity; CNS: None; CL: Apply

220. A pediatric nurse is caring for a four-week-old neonate with severe colic. Which assessment finding would the nurse interpret as a sign of acute pain?

1. Whimpering
2. Eyes opened wide
3. Limp body posture
4. Inability to retain feedings

220. 1. Crying, whimpering, and groaning are vocal expressions of acute pain in the neonate. Eyes tightly closed, changes in feeding behavior, and fist clenching with rigidity also are signs of acute pain in the neonate.
CN: Health promotion and maintenance; CNS: None; CL: Apply

221. A 52-year-old female arrived at the emergency room in cardiac arrest. Which interventions should the nurse implement? Select all that apply.

1. Establish oxygen via nasal cannula
2. Apply electrodes for the cardiac monitor
3. Draw venous blood to evaluate blood gases
4. Establish an IV line
5. Insert a Foley catheter
6. Administer IV medications

221. 2, 4, 5, 6. In the emergency room, these activities could be employed during cardiac resuscitation. An endotracheal tube would be inserted for oxygenation, and arterial blood gases would not be evaluated for this client.
CN: Physiological integrity; CNS: Reduction of risk potential; CL: Apply

222. The nurse is caring for a client who had a pacemaker inserted more than 20 years ago. The client was admitted to the cardiac care unit with possible bacterial endocarditis. Which test would the nurse anticipate as confirmation of this diagnosis?

1. Electrolytes
2. Blood cultures
3. Prothrombin time (PT)
4. Venereal Disease Research Laboratory (VDRL)

222. 2. Blood cultures are crucial in diagnosing bacterial endocarditis. Electrolyte levels would indicate abnormalities that occur with drug therapy, as well as with complications associated with heart failure. Prothrombin time values are useful in monitoring anticoagulant therapy. A positive VDRL may be evidence of syphilitic heart disease.
CN: Physiological integrity; CNS: Reduction of risk potential; CL: Apply

223. The nurse is preparing a client for cardiac catheterization. What is the **priority** nursing communication?

1. "Do you have allergies to shellfish or contrast dye?"
2. "Have you had this procedure before?"
3. "You will need to fast for 24 hours before the procedure."
4. "You'll be given medication to help you sleep during the procedure."

223. 1. The nurse must assess this client for allergies to shellfish or iodine before the procedure because the dye used during catheterization contains iodine. Knowing the client's history and prior experience with this procedure would be helpful, but knowing the client's allergies is the priority. The client will be instructed to fast for six hours before the procedure, and asked to empty his bladder before the procedure. The client needs to stay awake during the procedure to follow directions, such as taking a deep breath and holding it during injection of the dye, and to report chest, neck, or jaw discomfort.
CN: Physiological integrity; CNS: Reduction of risk potential; CL: Apply

CN: Client needs category   CNS: Client needs subcategory   CL: Cognitive level

224. The nurse is caring for a client suspected of having coronary artery disease. The health care provider has ordered a noninvasive diagnostic test to evaluate cardiac changes. The nurse prepares the client for:
  1. a cardiac biopsy.
  2. cardiac catheterization.
  3. magnetic resonance imaging (MRI).
  4. pericardiocentesis.

224. **3.** An MRI is a noninvasive procedure that aids in the diagnosis and detection of thoracic aortic aneurysm, and the evaluation of coronary artery disease, pericardial disease, and cardiac masses. Cardiac biopsy, cardiac catheterization, and pericardiocentesis are invasive techniques used to evaluate cardiac changes.

CN: Health promotion and maintenance; CNS: None; CL: Apply

225. A nurse, working in the telemetry unit, notices a premature ventricular contraction (PVC) on the client's monitor. While assessing the client, the client states that he felt something "flip flop" in the chest. There are no other PVCs noted in the following hour. Which documentation, by the nurse, would be **most** appropriate?
  1. One PVC occurred today between 1 and 2 pm. There was no preceding P wave, and the QRS complex was wide and inverted.
  2. One PVC was observed on monitor between 1 and 2 pm. today. The client stated that they felt a "flip flop" in their chest. No changes in vital signs. No chest pain or shortness of breath was reported.
  3. Client had one PVC today, observed closely, no other PVCs noted.
  4. Only one PVC was observed on monitor between 1 and 2 today.

225. **2.** It is important to chart about the client and their condition, and to note frequency and any abnormal symptoms with premature ventricular contractions (PVCs). Answer one describes the PVC but not the client. Answers three and four are brief and incomplete. PVCs are caused by an ectopic cardiac pacemaker located in the ventricle. PVCs are characterized by premature and bizarre-ly-shaped QRS complexes usually wider than 120 millisecond on the width of the electrocardiogram. These complexes are not preceded by a P wave, and the T wave is usually large, and its direction is opposite the major deflection of the QRS. The clinical significance of PVCs depends on their frequency, complexity, and hemodynamic response.

CN: Physiological integrity; CNS: Reduction of risk potential; CL: Apply

226. A nurse is recording an electrocardiogram (ECG) for a client with a pacemaker in the cardiac clinic. The client has had the fixed-rate pacemaker for many years, and states that at times she feels funny and gets nauseated. Which ECG pattern would the nurse interpret as possible pacemaker malfunction?
  1. Short T waves
  2. Absent P waves
  3. Pacing spikes that appear at different times during a cardiac cycle
  4. Pacing spike that are followed by a wide QRS complex

226. **3.** When pacing spikes appear at different times during a cardiac cycle, it indicates a failure to capture. Failure to capture may result in inappropriate pacing. The ECG would show a pacing spike delivered on time but not followed by a wide QRS complex. Tall T waves or an irregular heart rate would indicate a failure-to-sense malfunction. P waves are not expected. The pacemaker takes over for the sinoatrial node. A pacing spike followed by a QRS indicates a paced beat.

CN: Physiological integrity; CNS: Reduction of risk potential; CL: Apply

Here's one of those "select all that apply" questions. Look out for multiple correct answers.

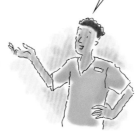

227. The nurse is reviewing discharge teaching for an older adult client who was treated for arterial insufficiency and has undergone an endarterectomy. What important information should the nurse provide? Select all that apply.
  1. "You may leave your feet open to the air."
  2. "Sit and rest for several hours a day."
  3. "Avoid crossing your legs at the knees or ankles."
  4. "The physical therapist will come three times a week for two weeks."
  5. "Avoid constrictive clothing, such as tight elastic on socks."

227. **3, 4, 5.** Leg crossing should be avoided because it compresses the vessels in the legs. Feet and extremities must be protected to reduce the risk of trauma. Clients usually go home on physical therapy to improve mobility and circulation. Sitting for several hours isn't recommended. Constrictive clothing, such as tight elastic on socks, should be avoided to prevent compression of vessels in the legs.

CN: Physiological integrity; CNS: Reduction of risk potential; CL: Apply

CN: Client needs category   CNS: Client needs subcategory   CL: Cognitive level

228. The nurse on the rehabilitation unit has admitted a visually-impaired, older adult client for cardiac rehabilitation therapy. What plan should the nurse include to reduce sensory deprivation for a visually-impaired client?
1. Keep the lights dimmed
2. Close the curtains or window blinds to reduce glare
3. Open the hospital door so bright light can shine in the room
4. Open the curtains during the day so the sun can shine brightly

228. 2. Closing curtains or window blinds can reduce glare and improve vision for the older client. Controlled lighting can help the older client see better in the hospital. Adequate background lighting helps the older client decrease visual accommodation when moving from brightly lit to dimly lit rooms and hallways.
CN: Physiological integrity; CNS: Reduction of risk potential; CL: Apply

229. The nurse is caring for a hearing-impaired client on the coronary care unit. To reduce sensory overload for this client, it is **most** important for the nurse to:
1. reduce the overhead light to dim.
2. keep the client's door open at all times
3. do not allow family members to stay with the client.
4. limit bedside conversation to that directed to the client.

229. 4. Sensory overload occurs when one or more of the body's senses experiences over-stimulation from the environment. It is most important to limit bedside conversation to that directed to the client to create fewer disturbances, and reduce sensory overload. Conversations at the bedside that do not include the client may increase anxiety and heighten the senses as the client tries to understand. Denying family visitation may cause stress and stimulate anxiety. Keeping the door open at all times may contribute to increased stimulation from observed activity.
CN: Physiological integrity; CNS: Reduction of risk potential; CL: Apply

230. The nurse is assessing a prenatal client who is at 37 weeks' gestation. The nurse performs Leopold's maneuvers to assess the position of the fetus. After performing the maneuvers, the nurse anticipates that the health care provider will attempt external version because the head of the fetus is at the:
1. symphysis pubis.
2. top of the uterus.
3. on the mother's left side.
4. vertex position.

230. 3. If the fetal head is palpated at the top of the uterus, the fetus is in the breech position. The health care provider may consider external version to convert the fetus to a vertex lie, or head-down position. This is accomplished by applying pressure on the maternal abdomen to turn the infant over, in somersault fashion.
CN: Physiological integrity; CNS: Reduction of risk potential; CL: Apply

231. The pediatric nurse is caring for a 10-month-old infant. The health care provider orders an IV infusion of dextrose 5% in 0.45% NaCl solution to be infused at 7 mg/kg/hr. The infant weighs 22 lb (10 kg). How many ml/hr of the ordered solution should the nurse infuse? Record your answer using a whole number.

_____ ml/hr

231. 70.
To perform this dosage calculation, the nurse should first convert the infant's weight to kilograms:

$$\frac{1\,kg}{2.2\,lb} \times 22\,lb = 10\,kg$$

Next, the nurse should multiply the infant's weight by the ordered rate:

$$10\,kg \times ml/kg/hr = 70\,ml/hr$$

CN: Physiological integrity; CNS: Pharmacological and parenteral therapies; CL: Apply

232. The health clinic nurse returns from lunch and finds telephone messages from four clients. Which call should the nurse return **first**?
1. A 47-year-old client newly diagnosed with type 2 diabetes mellitus, who has questions about diet selection
2. A 20-year-old female experiencing intermittent abdominal pain
3. The mother of a seven-year-old who states that her son has a harsh, high-pitched wheeze on inspiration
4. A 67-year-old diagnosed with chronic obstructive pulmonary disease (COPD) reports increased respiratory secretions

232. 3. This mother's description indicates inspiratory stridor and a narrowing airway. The mother should be instructed to take the child to the nearest emergency department for assessment and treatment. The increased secretions of a COPD client may indicate an airway issue as well, but not as significant as the abnormal inspiratory sounds. The client with abdominal pain and diet questions are not the priority.

CN: Safe and effective care environment; CNS: Management of care; CL: Analyze

233. The nursing team for the next shift consists of one RN, one LPN, and one unlicensed assistive personnel (UAP). What is the nurse's **priority** action after receiving shift report?
1. Call the nursing supervisor to determine if any new admissions are anticipated
2. Schedule lunch time and break time for each of the team's members
3. Pass all the medications that are currently due
4. Assess an elderly client who has been combative during the previous shift

233. 4. A combative client is a safety concern for the client and others. Though it is proactive to determine if, and how many new admissions can be anticipated, it does not take precedence over the safety concern. The nurse should pass all medications that are due; however, it does not take priority over a safety issue. Scheduling of team member's break times is the least important action.

CN: Safe and effective care environment; CNS; Management of care; CL: Analyze

234. The nurse makes initial rounds for his clients. Five medication are scheduled for administration at the same time to five different clients. Which medication should the nurse administer **first** after initial rounds?
1. A maintenance dose of digoxin to the client with congestive heart failure
2. Morphine sulfate to a client with a myocardial infarction reporting chest pain
3. Naproxen to the client with rheumatoid arthritis
4. Ondansetron to a diabetic client reporting nausea

234. 2. Morphine sulfate relieves pain which immediately decreases myocardial oxygen demand and decreases preload and afterload pressure. The digoxin is a maintenance dose and does not elicit an immediate reaction. Though administration of naproxen and ondansetron are next in the order urgency, they are not the priority.

CN: Physiologic integrity; CNS: Reduction of risk; CL: Analyze

235. A registered nurse from the pediatric unit is reassigned to the oncology unit for one shift. Which assignment is **most** appropriate for the reassigned nurse?
1. A 70-year-old female one day post colectomy for colon cancer
2. A 60-year-old male receiving methotrexate IV
3. A 45-year-old female in the terminal stages of breast cancer
4. A 20-year-old male newly diagnosed with acute leukemia

235. 1. The client who is one day post colectomy is a stable surgical client with predictable outcomes. The client receiving methotrexate should be cared for by a nurse experienced in oncology medications and their possible side effects. The client in the terminal stages of cancer needs a nurse experienced in end stage cancer care. The client with a new cancer diagnosis needs a nurse who can answer questions, and is experienced with this type of client.

CN: Safe and effective care environment; CNS: Management of care; CL: Analyze

CN: Client needs category   CNS: Client needs subcategory   CL: Cognitive level

236. A nurse is caring for clients on a medical/surgical unit. Which client should the nurse see **first**?
1. A 65-year-old female two days postoperative for a coronary artery bypass graft (CABG) with a temperature of 100.2° F (37.89° C)
2. A 35-year-old female scheduled for a laparoscopic cholecystectomy with chills
3. A 50-year-old male admitted for dizziness and hypertension with a blood pressure of 160/90
4. A 60-year-old male admitted with second degree burns covering the arms, chest, neck, and face

236. 4. The client with burns to the face, neck, and chest is at risk for developing airway edema and subsequent breathing difficulty. The nurse should assess this client for airway and respiratory status first. The other three clients need to be seen soon, but do not take priority over a possible airway obstruction.

CN: Physiological integrity; CNS: Physiological adaptation;
CL: Analyze

237. The nurse needs to insert a preoperative indwelling urinary catheter for a client undergoing a scheduled caesarean section. Prioritize the steps for catheter insertion.

1. Inflate the balloon with the syringe of sterile water

2. Cleanse the labia and urinary meatus with a single swipe going anterior to posterior

3. Secure the catheter with tape to the thigh

4. Position the client in a supine position with knees and hips flexed

5. Separate the labia with one hand and expose the urinary meatus

6. Insert the lubricated catheter into the urinary meatus

7. Explain the procedure to the client

8. Collect equipment and perform hand hygiene

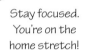

Stay focused. You're on the home stretch!

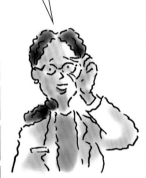

237. Ordered Response:

7. Explain the procedure to the client

8. Collect equipment and perform hand hygiene

4. Position the client in a supine position with knees and hips flexed

5. Separate the labia with one hand and expose the urinary meatus

2. Cleanse the labia and urinary meatus with a single swipe going anterior to posterior

6. Insert the lubricated catheter into the urinary meatus

1. Inflate the balloon with the syringe of sterile water

3. Secure the catheter with tape to the thigh

CN: Health promotion and maintenance; CNS: none; CL: Apply

238. The health care provider orders documentation of a client's intake and output. Using the following information, calculate this client's intake in milliliters. Record your answer using one decimal place.
8 oz (250 ml) decaffeinated coffee 4 oz (125 ml) green jello
2 oz (62.5 ml) apple juice 4 oz (125 ml) lemon-lime soda
8 oz (250 ml) beef broth 300 ml of urine output

_____ ml

238. 812.5.

$$250 \text{ ml coffee} + 62.5 \text{ ml apple juice}$$
$$+ 250 \text{ ml beef broth} + 125 \text{ ml jello}$$
$$+ 125 \text{ soda} = 812.5 \text{ ml}$$

The 300 milliliters of urine output does not calculate into the client's input.

CN: Health promotion and maintenance; CNS: none; CL: Apply

239. The postpartum nurse is about to perform the initial assessment of the four clients. Which client should the nurse see **first**?
1. 35-year-old multipara who is three hours postpartum after delivery of a 36-week infant weighing five pounds six ounces
2. A 29-year-old multipara who is four hours postpartum after delivery of a 39-week infant weighing 10 pound two ounces
3. A 20-year-old primipara who is six hours postpartum after delivery of a 40-week infant weighing seven pound five ounces
4. A 15-year-old primipara who is three hours postpartum after delivery of a 38-week infant weighing six pound two ounces

240. The nurse is caring for a client in the process of having peritoneal dialysis, and is in the out flowing phase. The nurse notes that there is no longer any fluid flowing out from the peritoneum. Of the 2,000 ml instilled only 1,500 ml have returned. What is the nurse's **most** appropriate action?
1. Push the drainage catheters in two ml to access the hidden fluid
2. Irrigate the drainage catheters with 10 ml of sterile water to dislodge any obstructions
3. Reposition the client every 30 minutes to facilitate drainage
4. Call the health care provider for further orders

241. A nurse is providing discharge instructions for a client diagnosed with cataracts. The client has just undergone extra-capsular extraction with lens implantation. What **priority** information should be included in this client's discharge?
1. Restrict fluids to 1,500 ml/day beginning the first post-operative day
2. Instill prescribed eye drops in affected eye beginning on the second post-operative day
3. Avoid straining and heavy lifting until cleared by the health care provider
4. Try to sleep on affected side for the first two post-operative weeks

242. A nurse walks into the room of a client diagnosed with congestive heart failure (CHF). The client is lying supine and is diaphoretic, anxious, and dyspneic. What is the nurse's **priority** action?
1. Administer oxygen at 4 L/min
2. Administer 0.5 mg of lorazepam
3. Raise the head of the bed to 45°
4. Draw arterial blood gases

239. 2. The 29-year-old multiparous mother who recently delivered a large infant is at risk for postpartum hemorrhage. The other multiparous mother has less of a risk for postpartum hemorrhage since her infant was small. The two primiparous mothers are not at risk for postpartum hemorrhage.
CN: Health promotion and maintenance; CNS: none; CL: Analyze

240. 3. Turning and placing the client in different positions will encourage drainage of fluid dwelling into different areas of the peritoneum. A nurse should never irrigate or push drainage catheters further into the abdomen, as this increases the risk of introducing bacteria. A nurse should not call a health care provider before all interventions have been implemented.
CN: Physiological integrity; CNS: Reduction of risk; CL: Apply

241. 3. Straining and heavy lifting increases interocular pressure which can dislodge the new lens. Restriction of fluids may lead to constipation and increase the risk of straining. Eye drop instillation should begin within 24 hours post-operatively. Sleeping on the affected side can increase pain and swelling.
CN: Physiological integrity; CNS: Reduction of risk potential; CL: Apply

242. 3. Raising the head of the bed will help the client's lungs expand and allow for deeper breaths. The nurse would need a provider's order for oxygen, and it may not be most beneficial if the head of the bed is not elevated. Lorazepam may decrease the client's anxiety, but it may also diminish respirations and increase dyspnea. Arterial blood gases are not a priority.
CN: Physiological integrity; CNS: Physiological adaptation; CL: Apply

243. The nurse discusses appropriate dietary needs with a client with iron-deficiency anemia. Which meal selection is **most** appropriate for this client?
1. Chicken noodle soup, saltine crackers, and a toasted cheese sandwich on multigrain bread
2. Oatmeal, 2% milk, dried cranberries, and whole wheat toast
3. Lasagna with eggplant in tomato sauce and garlic bread
4. Ribeye steak, green beans, baked potato, and sliced tomatoes

243. 4. Absorption of iron found in the steak is facilitated by the 20 to 30 mg of vitamin C found in the potato and tomatoes. The chicken and cheese are good sources of protein; however, there is no vitamin C to enhance iron absorption. Oatmeal and lasagna with eggplant in tomato sauce contain no appreciable amounts of iron.
CN: Physiological integrity; CNS: Physiological adaptation; CL: Apply

244. A nurse smells smoke in the hallway of the hospital and, on investigation, realizes the source of the smoke is a fire in a client's room. What is the nurse's **priority** action?
1. Remove the client from the room
2. Extinguish the fire
3. Activate the fire alarm
4. Shut the doors to all other client rooms

244. 1. Client safety is always the top priority. Though the nurse should activate the fire alarm, attempt to extinguish the fire, and prevent the fire from spreading to other areas by shutting the doors of other client's rooms.
CN: Safe and effective care environment; CNS: Management of care; CL: Apply

245. One day after a client's thyroidectomy, the nurse notes that the client has developed tremors. What is the appropriate nursing action?
1. Check the client's serum glucose level
2. Check the client's serum calcium level
3. Check the client's hemoglobin and hematocrit
4. Check the client's serum potassium level

245. 2. Thyroidectomies may cause injury to the parathyroid resulting in decreased calcium levels. Hypoglycemia causes sweating, trembling, and weakness. Hypokalemia causes fatigue, muscle weakness, and dysrhythmias. Low hemoglobin and hematocrit levels cause pallor, fatigue, and tachycardia.
CN: Physiological integrity; CNS: Physiological adaptation; CL: Analyze

246. A local chemical plant has had an environmental leak requiring the mass evacuation of its employees and neighbors in the surrounding area. The emergency room nurse is in the triage area when the first client is brought to the hospital. What should the nurse do **first**?
1. Cut off the client's clothing and dispose of them in hazardous waste containers
2. Place the fully clothed client in a shower for decontamination
3. Determine what decontamination measures took place in the field before approaching the client
4. Discharge or admit all current clients in the emergency department

246. 3. During a disaster the nurse's priority is personal safety. Determining what decontamination measures have already taken place will inform the nurse of necessary precautions. The nurse should not cut off the clothing or place the client in the shower until an assessment of the hazardous material has been completed. Containing the exposed clients in one area, free from other clients, is important, but the safety of the healthcare workers is the priority.
CN: Safe and effective care environment; CNS: Management of care; CL: Apply

247. A client diagnosed with systemic lupus erythematosus (SLE) has been admitted to the hospital. Her lab values indicate: Hgb 10.4 g/dl; Hct 34%; WBC 4,000/mm³; platelets 90,000/mm³. What is the **most** appropriate room assignment for this client?
1. With a client who has toxic hepatitis
2. With a client who has a venous stasis ulcer
3. With a client who has an upper respiratory infection (URI)
4. With a client one day post-operative following an ileostomy

247. 1. A client with SLE will require placement in a "clean" room because they frequently receive immunosuppressive medications. Since toxic hepatitis is a noninfectious inflammation of the liver that is usually drug-induced, this room can be considered "clean." The rooms with an venous ulcer, URI, and a new ileostomy cannot be considered "clean."

CN: Physiological integrity; CNS: Reduction of risk potential; CL: Analyze

248. A new nurse is about to initiate an IV of 0.9% NaCl. The peripheral IV must be initiated first. Prioritize the steps for the initiation of a peripheral IV.

1. Secure the catheter and IV tubing
2. Prime the IV tubing with 0.9% NaCl
3. Place a tourniquet approximately two inches above the insertion site
4. Cleanse the insertion sight per hospital protocol
5. Palpate the location for a possible insertion site
6. Pierce the skin at a 15 to 20° angle with the intravenous needle
7. Attach the IV tubing after establishing intravenous access

248. Ordered Response:

2. Prime the IV tubing with 0.9% NaCl
5. Palpate the location for a possible insertion site
3. Place a tourniquet approximately two inches above the insertion site.
4. Cleanse the insertion sight per hospital protocol
6. Pierce the skin at a 15 to 20° angle with the intravenous needle
7. Attach the IV tubing after establishing intravenous access
1. Secure the catheter and IV tubing

CN: Health promotion and maintenance; CNS: none; CL: Apply

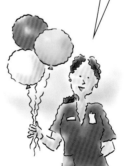

Wow! You've finished 249 questions. Great job!

249. A client's medication orders reads: Administer amoxicillin trihydrate 20 mg/kg PO q8h. The client weighs 75 lb (34 kg). How many milligrams of amoxicillin should the nurse administer for each dose? Record your answer using a whole number.

_____ mg

249. 680.

$$20 \, mg/kg \times 34 \, kg = 680 \, mg$$

CN: Health promotion and maintenance; CNS: none; CL: Apply

250. A 10-hour-old newborn female presents to the nursery with the following: axillary temperature 97.1° F (36.2° C); apical pulse 132; respirations irregular at 40/min; blood glucose 58 mg/dl; wet diaper with a pink-tinged discoloration. What is the **priority** nursing action?
1. Call the health care provider immediately about the pink-tinged discharge
2. Feed the infant 15 ml of glucose water
3. Place the infant under an oxygen hood with 30% oxygen
4. Double wrap the infant and apply a cap to the head

250. 4. The infant's axillary temperature indicates hypothermia and measures to increase the infant's temperature should be taken. There is no need to call the health care provider since pink or rust tinged discharge is normal in female infants. There is no need to feed the infant or place the infant under an oxygen hood because the blood glucose level and the respiratory rate are within normal limits.
CN: Health promotion and maintenance; CNS: none; CL: Apply

251. The nurse is reviewing a client's medication list and providing instruction on how to take each medication. Which medication should not be taken with grapefruit juice? Select all that apply.
1. Digoxin
2. Simvastin
3. Fexofenadine
4. Buspirone
5. Erythromycin
6. Levothyroxine

251. 2, 3, 4, 5. Digoxin is a cardiac glycoside and simvastin is a thyroid preparation. Neither drug interacts with grapefruit.
CN: Health promotion and maintenance; CNS: none; CL: Apply

252. A client taking sulfisoxazole for a bladder infection calls the nurse to explain that she woke up this morning with a fine, itchy macular rash on her torso. What is the nurse's **best** response?
1. "What have you eaten that is different?"
2. "Have you been exposed to poison ivy within the past 24 hours?"
3. "Have you changed clothing detergent?"
4. "Discontinue the medication."

252. 4. The fine, itchy macular rash may indicate hypersensitivity to the medication. The client should discontinue the medication, and seethe health care provider. It is important to first rule out drug hypersensitivity before investigating other possible sources of the rash.
CN: Physiological integrity; CNS: Reduction of risk potential; CL: Apply

253. An infant is admitted to the newborn nursery. During the initial assessment, the nurse finds a 2.5 in (6.35 cm) dark blue, discolored area over the infant's sacral area. What is the nurse's **most** appropriate action?
1. Call the health care provider immediately for orders
2. Document the findings in the medical record
3. Obtain an order for an X-ray of the affected region
4. Question the mother about any injuries within the past week

253. 2. The nurse understands that this is a typical Mongolian spot seen in non-Caucasian ethnicities. There is no need to call the health care provider, question the mother, or X-ray the affected area.
CN: Health promotion and maintenance; CNS: none; CL: Analyze

CN: Client needs category   CNS: Client needs subcategory   CL: Cognitive level

254. A 40-week-gestation newborn presents with a heart rate of 60 bpm; flaccid muscle tone, pink body with blue extremities, a weak cry, and slow, irregular respirations at 20 breaths/min. What is the infant's APGAR score?
1. 7
2. 6
3. 4
4. 9

254. 3. The infant's score is derived from: 1 for a heart rate under 100; + 0 for flaccid muscle tone; + 1 for a pink body with blue extremities; + 1 for a weak cry; + 1 for slow, irregular respirations at 20 breaths per minute. Therefore the total is 4.
CN: Health promotion and maintenance; CNS: none; CL: Apply

255. A client reveals that he is a lacto-ovo vegetarian. Which meal should the nurse order to accommodate this client's dietary preferences?
1. Scrambled eggs, veggie sausage patty, whole wheat toast, skim milk, and orange juice
2. Chicken salad sandwich with lettuce and tomato, carrot and celery sticks, ranch dressing, and lemonade
3. Fruit salad, melba toast, and iced tea
4. Lasagna with meat sauce, garlic toast, and a soft drink

255. 1. A lacto-ovo vegetarian diet includes all foods on a vegan diet, along with milk, cheese, yogurt, other milk products, and eggs, as the only sources of animal protein. Answer three is a vegan diet. Answers two and four include meat as a significant part of the meal.
CN: Health promotion and maintenance; CNS: none; CL: Apply

256. A client has recently been placed on a low sodium diet. He asks the nurse about appropriate drinks for his diet. What is the **best** choice for this client?
1. Two-percent skim milk
2. Fresh lemonade
3. Sports drink
4. Diet soda

256. 2. Fresh lemonade is low in sodium. Milk, sports drinks and soda are all high sodium beverages.
CN: Health promotion and maintenance; CNS: none; CL: Apply

257. The nurse is teaching the normal physical and developmental changes that occur in a preschool child to the mother of a three-year-old. The nurse knows that teaching has been effective when the mother delivers states:
1. "For a safe, healthy snack, I will serve my son slices of cooked turkey hotdog."
2. "For a safe, healthy snack, I will serve my son the large marshmallows."
3. "For a safe, healthy snack, I will serve my son O-shaped dry cereal."
4. "For a safe, healthy snack, I will serve my son chicken nuggets."

257. 3. O-shaped dry cereal are smaller than a three year old's esophagus and trachea, making it a good choice for reduced risk of choking and aspiration. Hotdogs are too large and, if not chewed properly, can be a choking hazard. Large marshmallows are sticky and may create a choking hazard as well. Unless chicken nuggets are chewed completely they can be a choking hazard.
CN: Health promotion and maintenance; CNS: none; CL: Analyze

258. A sixteen-year-old male student asks the school nurse to dress a minor thermal burn from a Bunsen burner. While dressing the burn, the nurse discusses safety issues with the student. Which question should the nurse ask to provide anticipatory guidance?
1. "Do you currently have a girlfriend?"
2. "How well are you doing in your school work?"
3. "Do you wear your seat belt every time you ride in an automobile?"
4. "What extracurricular activities are you involved in?"

258. 3. The number one cause of death for adolescent males is automobile accidents; therefore, inquiring about seatbelt use is the priority. Though the other questions could elicit additional information about possible safety issues, none take priority over automobile safety.
CN: Psychosocial integrity; CNS: none; CL: Analyze

259. An 18-month-old is diagnosed with otitis media, and his mother asks what she can do to help ease his pain. Which medication would the nurse anticipate for pain relief?
1. Children's liquid acetaminophen 5 ml q4h
2. Children's chewable acetylsalicylic acid one 80 mg q4h
3. Amoxicillin trihydrate 20 mg/kg p0 q8h
4. Cetirizine 1.3 ml q4h

259. 1. Children's acetaminophen is an anti-inflammatory and will decrease inflammation and pain. Children's acetylsalicylic acid is contradicted in all children due to the risk of Reye's syndrome. Amoxicillin is an antibiotic used to treat bacterial infections of the middle ear and cetirizine is an antihistamine used to dry up secretions. Neither of these relieve pain.
CN: Physiological integrity; CNS: Physiological adaptation; CL: Analyze

260. A low-fat diet has been ordered for a client. Which meal choices is **best** for this client?
1. Baked tilapia, steamed broccoli, white rice, and watermelon slices
2. Hamburger on a bun, French fries, and a piece of chocolate cake
3. Scrambled eggs, bacon, and buttered wheat toast
4. Hotdog with meat sauce, deep-fried onion rings, chocolate pudding

260. 1. Baked tilapia, broccoli, and white rice have limited fat content. Hamburger, bacon, and hotdogs are high in cholesterol and fat.
CN: Health promotion and maintenance; CNS: none; CL: Analyze

261. A client with mitral valve prolapse is three days post-operative from a mechanical mitral valve replacement. The nurse is reviewing discharge teaching with the client and realizes that teaching has not been effective when the client states:
1. "I will no longer need to take penicillin prophylactically prior to dental work."
2. "I will need to have my INR checked regularly."
3. "I should not take ibuprofen for pain."
4. "I should try to take my warfarin at the same time each day."

261. 1. The client with a mechanical valve replacement must take penicillin prophylactically prior to dental work to prevent oral bacteria from entering the blood system. The client will need to have regular INR measurements. Ibuprofen can potentiate the effects of warfarin and should be avoided. Warfarin should be taken at the same time each day to maintain titer levels.
CN: Physiological integrity; CNS: Reduction of risk potential; CL: Apply

262. In order for pravastatin to have maximum effect, the nurse should administer this medication:
1. early in the morning prior to breakfast.
2. two hours after the afternoon meal.
3. at bedtime.
4. with breakfast.

262. 3. Cholesterol is manufactured in the liver just after midnight each day; therefore, statin medications are best taken just before bedtime.
CN: Safe and effective care environment; CNS: Management of care; CL: Apply

CN: Client needs category   CNS: Client needs subcategory   CL: Cognitive level

263. Which clients does the nurse identify as at risk for the development of metabolic acidosis? Select all that apply.
1. A client with type 1 diabetes mellitus
2. A client with continuous nasogastric drainage
3. A client who is on thiazide diuretic therapy
4. A client with acute renal failure
5. A client experiencing an acute panic attack
6. A client with severe diarrhea

263. **1, 4, 6.** The client with diabetes is at risk for ketoacidosis. In renal failure the kidneys are unable to excrete acids or retain bicarbonate. The client experiencing acute diarrhea is losing bicarbonate. Continuous nasogastric suction, diuretic therapy, and acute panic attacks place the client at risk for the development of alkalosis.
CN: Physiological integrity; CNS: Reduction of risk potential; CL: Apply

264. A client receives a lactated Ringers IV infusion at 100 ml/hr. Ninety minutes later, the nurse notes the client has crackles in both lungs that do not clear with coughing. The client reports shortness of breath. What action is **most** important for the nurse to take?
1. Continue to monitor the client to for changes
2. Place the patient in high Fowler's position
3. Discontinue the IV
4. Administer 20 mg oral metolazone

264. **2.** Priority action is to improve the client's respiratory status. This is an immediate action. The client is experiencing an acute episode which requires action. It is important to have IV access for administration of medications. The onset of oral medication would not give an immediate effect.
CN: Physiological integrity; CNS: Physiological adaptation; CL: Apply

265. The nurse is preparing to instruct a postoperative client about the use of an incentive spirometer. Place the nurse's actions in correct order.

| 1. Explain procedure to the client |
| 2. Have the client cough and deep breathe |
| 3. Place the client in high Fowler's position |
| 4. Instruct the client to inhale and hold the breath for 3 seconds |
| 5. Have the client firmly seal the lips around mouthpiece |
| 6. Instruct the client to exhale air |

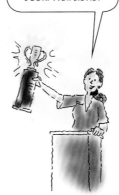

Congratulations! You finished the final test in the book. Well done!

265. Ordered Response:

| 1. Explain procedure to the client |
| 3. Place the client in high Fowler's position |
| 5. Have the client firmly seal the lips around mouthpiece |
| 4. Instruct the client to inhale and hold the breath for 3 seconds |
| 6. Instruct the client to exhale air |
| 2. Have the client cough and deep breathe |

CN: Health promotion and maintenance; CNS: None; CL: Apply

Commonly Used Abbreviations

kg = kilogram	mm = millimeter
g = gram	mm Hg = millimeters of mercury
mg = milligram	mmol = millimole
mcg = microgram	fl = fluid liter
mEq = milliequivalent	fmol = fluid mole
l = liter	pg = picogram
dl (deciliter) = 100 milliliters	kPa = kilopascal
ml = milliliter	

Commonly Used English to Metric Conversion Equations

1 inch (in) = 2.5 centimeters (cm)	1 ounce (oz) = 28 grams (g)
$d_{(in)} = d_{(cm)} / 2.54$	$m_{(oz)} = m_{(g)} / 28.34952$
$d_{(cm)} = d_{(in)} \times 2.54$	$m_{(g)} = m_{(oz)} \times 28.34952$

1 pound (lb) = 0.45 kilogram (kg)	Temperature (Fahrenheit, Celsius)
$m_{(lb)} = m_{(kg)} / 0.45359237$	$T_{(°C)} = (T_{(°F)} - 32) \times 5/9$
$m_{(kg)} = m_{(lb)} \times 0.45359237$	$T_{(°F)} = T_{(°C)} \times 9/5 + 32$

Normal Adult Laboratory Values*

Determination	Conventional Unit	Reference Range, SI
Hematologic Values (Complete Blood Count)		
Hematocrit	Male: 42%–50% Female: 40%–48%	Male: 0.42–0.52 Female: 0.37–0.48
Hemoglobin	Male: 13–18 g/dL Female: 12–16 g/dL	Male: 8.1–11.2 mmol/l Female: 7.4–9.9 mmol/l
Leukocyte count	5,000–10,000/mm^3	4.3–10.8 × 10^9/l
Erythrocyte count	4.2 million–5.9 million/mm^3	4.2–5.9 × 10^{12}/l
Mean corpuscular volume (MCV)	80–94 mcm^3	80–94 fl
Mean corpuscular hemoglobin (MCH)	27–32 pg	1.7–2.0 fmol
Mean corpuscular hemoglobin concentration (MCHC)	33%–38%	19–22.8 mmol/l
Erythrocyte sedimentation rate (Zeta Centrifuge)	41%–54%	Male: 1–13 mm/h Female: 1–20 mm/h
Hematologic Values (Hemoglobin Studies)		
Platelet count	100,000–400,000/mm^3	150–350 × 10^9/l
Blood, Plasma, or Serum Values		
Carbon dioxide content	24 mEq–32 mEq/l	24–30 mmol/l
Chloride	95–105 mEq/l	100–106 mmol/l
Cholesterol	<200 mg/dl	
Creatinine	0.7–1.4 mg/100 ml	60–130 mcmol/l
Glucose	Fasting: 60–100 mg/dl	3.9–5.6 mmol/l
Glycated hemoglobin (HbA1c)	4.0%–5.6%	None
Lipids, total	400–1,000 mg/dl	3.10–5.69 mmol/l
Magnesium	0.33–2.4 mEq/l	0.8–1.3 mmol/l
Oxygen saturation (arterial)	95%–100%	0.96–1.00 l
PCO$_2$	35–45 mm Hg	4.7–6.0 kPg
pH	7.35–7.45	Same
PO$_2$	95–100 mm Hg (dependent on age while breathing room air) >500 mm Hg while on 100% O$_2$	10.0–13.3 kPa
Phosphorus (inorganic)	3.0–4.5 mg/100 ml	1.0–1.5 mmol/l
Potassium	3.8–5.0 mEq/l	3.5–5.0 mmol/l
Albumin	3.5–5.0 g/100 ml	33–50 g/l
Sodium	135–145 mEq/l	135–145 mmol/l
Urea nitrogen (BUN)	10–20 mg/100 ml	2.9–8.9 mmol/l
Urine Values		
Calcium	150 mg/day or less	3.8 mmol/day or less
Creatine	0–200 mg/24 hr	<0.75 mmol/day

*Laboratory values may vary according to techniques used in different laboratories.

Adapted from: Taylor, C., Lillis, C., Lynn, P., LeMone, P. (2015). *Fundamentals of nursing: the art and science of person-centered nursing care* (8th ed.). Philadelphia, PA: Wolters Kluwer.

Normal Pediatric Laboratory Values*

Vital Sign	Infant 0 to 12 months	Child 1 to 11 years	Pre-Adolescent/Adolescent 12 and Older
Heart Rate	95–170 bpm	70–150 bpm	Female: 55–110 bpm Male: 50–105
Respiration (breaths)	30–45 bpm	14–45 bpm	12–20 bpm
Blood Pressure (systolic/diastolic)	65–100/45–65 mm Hg	90–110/55–75 mm Hg	110–135/65–85 mm Hg
Temperature	96–99.9°F 35.6–37.7°C	95.9–99°F 35.5–37.2°C	96.4–99.6°F 35.8–37.6°C

*Laboratory values may vary according to techniques used in different laboratories.

Erikson's Stages of Psychosocial Development

Approximate Age	Virtues	Psychosocial Crisis
0–2 years	Hope	Basic trust vs. mistrust
2–4 years	Will	Autonomy vs. shame and doubt
4–5 years	Purpose	Initiative vs. guilt
5–12 years	Competence	Industry vs. inferiority
13–19 years	Fidelity	Identity vs. role confusion
20–39 years	Love	Intimacy vs. isolation
40–64 years	Care	Generativity vs. stagnation
65-death	Wisdom	Ego integrity vs. despair

From: Erikson, E. H. (1959). *Identity and the life cycle.* New York: International Universities Press.

Heart Sounds

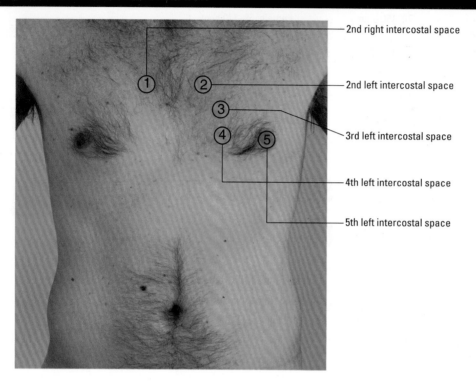

- 2nd right intercostal space
- 2nd left intercostal space
- 3rd left intercostal space
- 4th left intercostal space
- 5th left intercostal space

Breath Sounds

Sites and Sequence for Posterior Auscultation

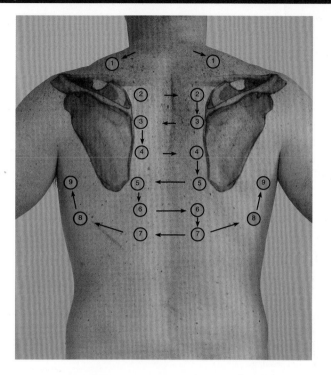

Sites for Anterior Chest Palpation, Percussion, and Auscultation

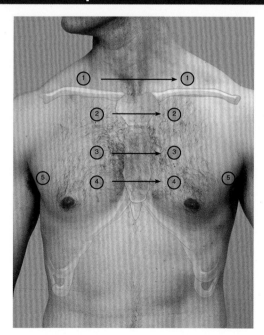

From: Jensen, S. (2015). *Nursing health assessment: a best practice approach* (2nd ed.). Philadelphia, PA: Wolters Kluwer.